VOLUME
7

FOWLER'S
Zoo and Wild
Animal Medicine
CURRENT THERAPY

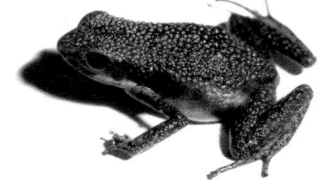

VOLUME
7

FOWLER'S
Zoo and Wild
Animal Medicine
CURRENT THERAPY

R. Eric Miller, DVM, DACZM
Senior Vice President for Zoological Operations
Director, WildCare Institute
Saint Louis Zoo
Forest Park
St. Louis, Missouri;
Adjunct Associate Professor of Veterinary Medicine and Surgery
College of Veterinary Medicine
University of Missouri
Columbia, Missouri

Murray Fowler, DVM, DACZM, DACVIM, DABVT
Professor Emeritus, Zoological Medicine
School of Veterinary Medicine
University of California
Davis, California

with 280 illustrations

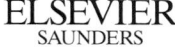
ELSEVIER
SAUNDERS

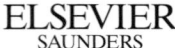

ELSEVIER
SAUNDERS

3251 Riverport Lane
St. Louis, Missouri 63043

Vice President and Publisher: Linda Duncan
Editor: Penny Rudolph
Associate Developmental Editor: Brandi Graham
Publishing Services Manager: Catherine Jackson
Senior Project Manager: Rachel E. McMullen
Design Direction: Karen Pauls
Back Cover Photography: Thane G. Johnson

Printed in China

Last digit is the print number: 9 8 7 6 5 4 3 2 1

Contributors

Michael J. Adkesson, DVM
Associate Veterinarian
Chicago Zoological Society
Brookfield Zoo
Brookfield, Illinois;
Adjunct Clinical Assistant
    Professor
Department of Veterinary Clinical
    Medicine
College of Veterinary Medicine
University of Illinois
Urbana, Illinois
**Degenerative Skeletal Diseases of
    Primates**

Amy Alexander, DVM
Associate Veterinarian
Florida Veterinary Specialists
**Digital Radiography of the
    Elephant Foot**

Jill Allread, APR
Owner
Public Communications Inc.
Chicago, Illinois
**Culture and Media Shifts:
    Challenges and Opportunities
    for Veterinarians**

Cheryl Asa, BA, MS, PhD
Adjunct Professor
Department of Biology
Saint Louis University;
Director of Research AZA Wildlife
    Contraception Center
Research Department
Saint Louis Zoo
St. Louis, Missouri
Contraception

Anne E. Ballmann, DVM, PhD
Wildlife Disease Specialist
U.S. Geological Survey
National Wildlife Health Center
Madison, Wisconsin
**White-Nose Syndrome in Cave
    Bats of North America**

Ursula Bechert, DVM, PhD
Director of Off-Campus Programs
College of Science
Oregon State University
Corvallis, Oregon
**Noninvasive Techniques to
    Assess Health and Ecology of
    Wildlife Populations**

Roy G. Bengis, BVSc, MSc, PhD
Chief State Veterinarian
Department of Agriculture,
    Forestry and Fisheries
Kruger National Park
South Africa
**Anthrax in Free-Ranging Wildlife
Cyanobacterial Biointoxication
    in Free-Ranging Wildlife**

Rui I. Bernardino, DVM
Invited Assistant Professor
Department of Surgery
Faculty of Veterinary Medicine,
    Universidade Lusófona de
    Humanidades e Tecnologias;
Staff Veterinarian
Lisbon Zoo
Lisbon, Portugal
**Fundamentals of Zoo Animal
    Surgery**

Sally Boutelle, MS
Program Coordinator
AZA Wildlife Contraception
    Center
Saint Louis Zoo
St. Louis, Missouri
Contraception

Elizabeth L. Buckles, DVM, PhD,
    DACVP
Assistant Professor
Department of Biomedical
    Sciences
College of Veterinary Medicine
Cornell University
Ithaca, New York
**White-Nose Syndrome in Cave
    Bats of North America**

Mitchell Bush, DVM, ACZM
Senior Veterinarian Emeritus
Smithsonian Conservation Biology
    Institute
National Zoological Park
Front Royal, Virginia
**The Use of Butorphanol in
    Anesthesia Protocols for Zoo
    and Wild Mammals**

Peter E. Buss BVSc, MMedVet
Veterinary Wildlife Services
Kruger National Park Veterinary
    Unit
South African National Parks
Mpumalanga, South Africa
**Cyanobacterial Biointoxication
    in Free-Ranging Wildlife**

Kenneth N. Cameron, DVM
Field Veterinarian
Global Health Program
Wildlife Conservation Society
Bronx, New York
Ebola Hemorrhagic Fever

Norin Chai, DVM, MSc, PhD
Veterinary Department Head
Senior Veterinarian of the
    Research Facilities
Ménagerie du Jardin des Plantes
Muséum National d'Histoire
    Naturelle
Paris, France
Mycobacteriosis in Amphibians

Scott B. Citino, DVM, DACZM
Veterinarian
White Oak Conservation Center
Yulee, Florida
The Use of Butorphanol in Anesthesia Protocols for Zoo and Wild Mammals

Robert A. Cook, VMD, MPA
General Director Living
    Institutions & Executive Vice
    President
Wildlife Conservation Society
Bronx, New York
Emerging Diseases at the Interface of People, Domestic Animals, and Wildlife

Graham Crawshaw, BVM, MS,
    MRCVS, DACZM
Head of Veterinary Services
Animal Health Centre
Toronto Zoo
Scarborough, Ontario, Canada
Amphibian Viral Diseases

Carolyn Cray, PhD
Professor of Clinical Pathology
Department of Pathology
Division of Comparative
    Pathology
Miller School of Medicine
University of Miami
Miami, Florida
Diagnosis of Aspergillosis in Avian Species

Mark W. Cunningham, DVM, MS
Wildlife Veterinarian
Fish and Wildlife Research
    Institute
Florida Fish and Wildlife
    Commission
Gainesville, Florida
Primer on Tick-Borne Diseases in Exotic Carnivores

Sharon L. Deem, DVM, PhD,
    DACZM
Adjunct Associate Professor
Department of Biology
College of Veterinary Medicine
University of Missouri;
Veterinary Epidemiologist
Saint Louis Zoo
St. Louis, Missouri
Disease Risk Analysis in Wildlife Health Field Studies

Ann Duncan, DVM
Senior Veterinarian
Detroit Zoological Society
Royal Oak, Michigan
Reptile and Amphibian Analgesia

Gregory J. Fleming, DVM, DACZM
Department of Animal Health
Disney's Animal Programs and
    Environmental Initiatives
Bay Lake, Florida
Behavioral Training of Reptiles for Medical Procedures

Deidre K. Fontenot, DVM
Veterinarian
Department of Animal Health
Disney's Animal Programs and
    Environmental Initiatives
Bay Lake, Florida
Alternatives for Gastrointestinal Parasite Control in Exotic Ruminants

Jeanette Fuller, RVT
San Diego Zoo's Wild Animal
    Park
San Diego, California
Practical Aspects of Ruminant Intensive Care

Laurie J. Gage, DVM, DACZM
Lecturer
Department of Medicine and
    Epidemiology
College of Veterinary Medicine
University of California
Davis, California;
Carnivore and Marine Mammal
    Field Specialist
APHIS Animal Care
USDA
Fort Collins, California
Ocular Disease and Suspected Causes in Captive Pinnipeds

Kathryn C. Gamble DVM, MS,
    DACZM
Director of Veterinary Services
Lincoln Park Zoo
Chicago, Illinois
Squamous cell carcinoma in _Buceros_ hornbills

Brett Gartrell, DVM, PhD
Senior Lecturer
Department of Animal and
    Biomedical Sciences
Massey University
New Zealand
Veterinary Care of Kakapo

Martin Gilbert, MRCVS, BVMS
Associate Director–Asia
Global Health Program
Wildlife Conservation Society
Bronx, New York
Avian Influenza H5N1 Virus: Epidemiology in Wild Birds, Zoo Outbreaks and Zoo Vaccination Policy

Gwendolyn Griffith, DVM, MS
Program Director
Cumberland River Compact
Nashville, Tennessee
Sustainable Practices for Zoological Veterinary Medicine

Catherine Hadfield, MA, VetMB,
 MRCVS
Associate Veterinarian
Animal Health Department
National Aquarium
Baltimore, Maryland
**Quarantine of Fish and Aquatic
 Invertebrates in Public Display
 Aquaria**

Elizabeth E. Hammond, DVM
Staff Veterinarian Maned Wolf SSP
 Veterinary Advisor
Lion Country Safari
Loxahatchee, Florida
**Medical Management of Maned
 Wolves**

Jean-Michel Hatt, DACZM,
 DECZM, Prof Dr Med Vet, MSc
Professor
Department of Small Animals
University of Zurich
Zurich, Switzerland
**Depth of Anesthesia Monitoring
 by Bispectral Analysis in
 Zoo Animals**

Michelle G. Hawkins, VMD, DABVP
Associate Professor
Department of Medicine and
 Epidemiology
School of Veterinary Medicine
University of California
Davis, California
Avian Analgesia

Gary S. Hayward, PhD
Professor
Department of Oncology
The Johns Hopkins University
 School of Medicine
Baltimore, Maryland
Elephant Herpesviruses

Dean A. Hendrickson, DVM, MS,
 DACVS
Professor
Department of Veterinary Clinical
 Sciences
James L. Voss Veterinary Teaching
 Hospital
Colorado State University
Fort Collins, Colorado
**Laparoscopic Surgery in
 Elephants and Rhinoceros**

Robert Hermes, Dr Med Vet, MRCVS
Reproduction Management
Leibniz Institute for Zoo and
 Wildlife Research
Berlin, Germany
Rhinoceros Theriogenology

Sonia M. Hernandez, DVM, PhD,
 DACZM
Assistant Professor of Wildlife
 Disease
Daniel B. Warnell School of
 Forestry and Natural Resources
Southeastern Cooperative of
 Wildlife Disease Study
College of Veterinary Medicine
University of Georgia
Athens, Georgia
**Wildlife Disease Ecology: What
 Can Zoo and Wildlife
 Veterinarians Learn from this
 Discipline?**

Thomas Bernd Hildebrandt, DVM
Research Society Leibniz
Association of Governmental
 Research Institutes
Head of Reproduction
 Management
Leibniz Institute for Zoo and
 Wildlife Research
Berlin, Germany
**Female Elephant Reproduction
Rhinoceros Theriogenology**

Robert Hilsenroth, DVM
Executive Director
American Association of Zoo
 Veterinarians
Yulee, Florida
**Culture and Media Shifts:
 Challenges and Opportunities
 for Veterinarians**

Peter H. Holz, BVSc, DVSc, DACZM
Senior Veterinarian
Werribee Open Range Zoo
Werribee, Victoria, Australia;
Veterinarian
Australian Wildlife Health Centre
Healesville Sanctuary
Healesville, Victoria, Australia
**Tasmanian Devil Facial Tumor
 Disease**

Lauren L. Howard, DVM, DACZM
Associate Veterinarian
Department of Veterinary Services
Houston Zoo
Houston, Texas
**Treatment of Elephant
 Endotheliotropic Herpesvirus
 (EEHV)**

Ramiro Isaza, DVM, MS
Associate Professor
Department of Small Animal
 Clinical Sciences
College of Veterinary Medicine
University of Florida
Gainesville, Florida
**Digital Radiography of the
 Elephant Foot
Treatment of Elephant
 Endotheliotropic Herpesvirus
 (EEHV)**

Richard Jakob-Hoff, BVMS, ACVSc
Senior Veterinarian
Conservation and Research
New Zealand Centre for
 Conservation Medicine
Auckland Zoological Park
Auckland, New Zealand
**Conservation Medicine for Zoo
 Veterinarians
Veterinary Care of Kakapo**

Stephanie B. James, DVM, DACZM
Director of Animal Health
Pittsburgh Zoo and PPG
 Aquarium
Pittsburgh, Pennsylvania
Children's Zoo Medicine

Donald L. Janssen, DVM
Corporate Director of Animal
 Health
San Diego Zoo
Escondido, California
**Guidelines for the Management
 of Zoonotic Diseases**

Christine K. Johnson, VMD,
   MPVM, PhD
Assistant Professor
Wildlife Health Center
College of Veterinary Medicine
University of California
Davis, California
**Approaching Health Problems at
   the Wildlife–Domestic Animal
   Interface**

Randall E. Junge, MS, DVM, DACZM
Adjunct Assistant Professor
Department of Veterinary
   Medicine and Surgery
College of Veterinary Medicine
University of Missouri
Columbia, Missouri;
Director of Animal Health
Saint Louis Zoo
St. Louis, Missouri
Hellbender Medicine

Olga Martin Jurado, Dr Med Vet
Clinic of Zoo Animals
Exotic Pets and Wildlife
Vetsuisse Faculty
University of Zurich
Zurich, Switzerland
**Depth of Anesthesia Monitoring
   By Bispectral Analysis in Zoo
   Animals**

Jacques Kaandorp, Dr Med Vet
Zoo Animal Manager
Safaripark Beekse Bergen and
   Dierenrijk Europa
Hilvarenbeek, Netherlands
**Veterinary Challenges of Mixed
   Species Exhibits**

Petra Kaczensky, Dr Med Vet
Zoo and Wildlife Biologist
Zoo Salzburg
Anif, Austria
**Asian Wild Horse Reintroduction
   Program**

William B. Karesh, DVM
Executive Vice President for
   Health and Policy
Ecohealth Alliance
New York, New York
**Emerging Diseases at the
   Interface of People, Domestic
   Animals, and Wildlife**

Gretchen E. Kaufman, DVM
Director of Tufts Center for
   Conservation Medicine
Assistant Professor
Department of Environmental and
   Population Health
Tufts Cummings School of
   Veterinary Medicine
North Grafton, Massachusetts;
Education Director
Tufts Institute of the Environment
Tufts University
Medford, Massachusetts
**Sustainable Practices for
   Zoological Veterinary
   Medicine**

David E. Kenny, VMD
Conservation Veterinary
   Coordinator
Conservation Biology Department
Denver Zoological Foundation
Denver, Colorado
**Thiafentanil Oxalate (A3080) In
   Nondomestic Ungulate
   Species**

Pia Krawinkel, DVM, PhD
Zoo and Wildlife Veterinarian
   (FTA)
Zoom Erlebniswelt Gelsenkirchen
Germany
**Feather Follicle Extirpation:
   Operative Techniques to
   Prevent Zoo Birds from Flying**

Andreas Kurth, DVM
Centre for Biological Safety
German Consultant Lab for
   Poxviruses
Robert Koch Institute
Berlin, Germany
Cowpox in Zoo Animals

Nadine Lamberski, DVM, DACZM
Veterinary Clinical Operations
   Manager
San Diego Zoo's Wild Animal Park
Escondido, California
**Updated Vaccination
   Recommendations for
   Carnivores
Practical Aspects of Ruminant
   Intensive Care**

William R. Lance DVM, MS, PhD
Chief Executive Officer
Wildlife Pharmaceuticals Inc
Fort Collins, Colorado
**The Use of Butorphanol in
   Anesthesia Protocols for Zoo
   and Wild Mammals
Thiafentanil Oxalate (A3080) In
   Nondomestic Ungulate
   Species**

Jennifer N. Langan, DVM, DACZM
Clinical Assistant Professor
Department of Veterinary Clinical
   Medicine
University of Illinois
Urbana, Illinois;
Associate Veterinarian
Chicago Zoological Society's
   Brookfield Zoo
Brookfield, Illinois
Integrated Pest Management

Iris I. Levin, PhD
Department of Biology
University of Missouri
St. Louis, Missouri
**Haemosporidian Parasites:
   Impacts on Avian Hosts**

Mark Lynn Lloyd, DVM
Medical Director
Disaster and Emergency Services
Humane Society of the
   United States
Gaithersburg, Maryland;
Independent Contractor and
   Strategic Disaster Planning
   Consultant
Wildlife Conservation,
   Management and Medicine
Athens, Georgia
**Disaster Preparation for Captive
   Wildlife Veterinarians**

Lesa Longley, MA, BVM&S,
   DZooMed (Mammalian), MSC,
   MRCVS
RCVS Recognised Specialist in Zoo
   & Wildlife Medicine
Head of Veterinary Services
Twycross Zoo
Atherstone, Warwickshire,
   United Kingdom
Aging in Large Felids

Linda Lowenstein, DVM, PhD
Professor
Department of Pathology,
 Microbiology and Immunology
College of Veterinary Medicine
University of California
Davis, California
**Cardiovascular Disease in Great
 Apes**

Imke Lueders, DVM
Department of Reproduction
 Management
Institute of Zoo and Wildlife
 Research
Berlin, Germany
Female Elephant Reproduction

Elizabeth J.B. Manning, MPH,
 MBA, DVM
Senior Scientist
Department of Pathobiological
 Sciences
School of Veterinary Medicine
University of Wisconsin
Madison, Wisconsin
**Johne's Disease and Free-
 Ranging Wildlife**

Jonna A.K. Mazet, DVM, PhD
Director
Wildlife Health Center
University of California
Davis, California
**Approaching Health Problems at
 the Wildlife–Domestic Animal
 Interface**

James F. McBain, DVM
Vice President
Corporate Director of Veterinary
 Service
Sea World Inc.
Orlando, Florida
**Longitudinal Monitoring of
 Immune System Parameters of
 Cetaceans and Application to
 Their Health Management**

Stephanie McCain, DVM
Associate Veterinarian
Birmingham Zoo
Birmingham, Alabama
Pyometra in Large Felids

Rita McManamon, DVM
Clinical Instructor
Department of Small Animal
 Medicine & Surgery
Anatomic Pathology Resident
Department of Pathology
College of Veterinary Medicine
University of Georgia
Athens, Georgia
**Cardiovascular Disease in Great
 Apes**

Thomas P. Meehan, DVM
Adjunct Assistant Professor
Department of Veterinary Clinical
 Medicine
College of Veterinary Medicine
University of Illinois
Urbana, Illinois;
Vice President of Veterinary
 Services
Chicago Zoological Society
Brookfield, Illinois
**AAZV Guidelines for Zoo and
 Aquarium Veterinary Medical
 Programs and Veterinary
 Hospitals**

Carol Uphoff Meteyer, DVM,
 DACVP
Biological Resources Division
USGS National Wildlife Health
 Center
Madison, Wisconsin
**Nonsteroidal Anti-inflammatory
 Drugs in Raptors**

James E. Miller, DVM, MPVM,
 PhD
Professor
Department of Pathobiological
 Sciences
College of Veterinary Medicine
Louisiana State University
Baton Rouge, Louisiana
**Alternatives for Gastrointestinal
 Parasite Control in Exotic
 Ruminants**

Michele A. Miller, DVM, MS, PhD
Chief Veterinary Officer and
 Director of Conservation
 Medicine
Melvin J and Claire Levine Animal
 Care Complex
Palm Beach Zoo
West Palm Beach, Florida
**Elephant Neonatal and Pediatric
 Medicine**

Hayley Weston Murphy, DVM
Director of Veterinary Services
Zoo Atlanta
Atlanta, Georgia
**Dangerous Animal Crisis
 Management**

Natalie D. Mylniczenko, MS,
 DVM, DACZM
Veterinarian
Department of Animal Health
Disney's Animal Programs and
 Environmental Initiatives
Lake Buena Vista, Florida
Medical Management of Rays

Nicole M. Nemeth, DVM, PhD
Research Scientist
Department of Biomedical
 Sciences
College of Veterinary Medicine
Colorado State University
Fort Collins, Colorado;
Resident
Department of Pathology
Southeastern Cooperative Wildlife
 Disease Study
College of Veterinary Medicine
University of Georgia
Athens, Georgia
West Nile Virus in Raptors

Andreas Nitsche, DVM
Centre for Biological Safety
German Consultant Lab for
 Poxviruses
Robert Koch Institute
Berlin, Germany
Cowpox in Zoo Animals

Terry M. Norton, DVM, DACZM
Director and Veterinarian
Georgia Sea Turtle Center
Jekyll Island, Georgia;
Wildlife Veterinarian
St. Catherines Island Foundation
Midway, Georgia
Sea Turtle Rehabilitation

J. Lindsay Oaks, DVM, PhD,
   DACVM
Associate Professor
Department of Veterinary
   Microbiology and Pathology
College of Veterinary Medicine
Washington State University
Pullman, Washington
**Nonsteroidal Anti-inflammatory
   Drugs in Raptors**

Justine O'Brien, BVSc, PhD
Research Fellow
Faculty of Veterinary Science
University of Sydney
Sydney, Australia
**Importation of Nondomestic
   Ruminant Semen for
   Management of Zoological
   Populations Using Artificial
   Insemination**

Patricia G. Parker, BS, PhD
Des Lee Professor of Zoological
   Studies
University of Missouri
Columbia, Missouri;
Senior Scientist
Saint Louis Zoo
St. Louis, Missouri
**Haemosporidian Parasites:
   Impacts on Avian Hosts**

Joanne Paul-Murphy, DVM,
   DACZM
Clinical Associate Professor
Department of Surgical Sciences
School of Veterinary Medicine
University of Wisconsin
Madison, Wisconsin
Avian Analgesia

Linda M. Penfold, PhD
Research Coordinator
White Oak Conservation Center
Yulee, Florida
**Importation of Nondomestic
   Ruminant Semen for
   Management of Zoological
   Populations Using Artificial
   Insemination**

Allan P. Pessier, DVM, DACVP
Associate Pathologist and Scientist
Wildlife Disease Laboratories
San Diego Zoo's Institute for
   Conservation Research
San Diego, California
**Diagnosis and Control of
   Amphibian Chytridiomycosis**

Johann "Joost" Philippa, DVM,
   PhD
Wildlife Veterinarian
Global Health Program
Wildlife Conservation Society
Bogor, Java Barat, Indonesia
**Avian Influenza H5N1 Virus:
   Epidemiology in Wild Birds,
   Zoo Outbreaks and Zoo
   Vaccination Policy**

Shane R. Raidal, BVSc, PhD,
   FACVSc
Associate Professor
Veterinary Diagnostic Laboratory
Charles Sturt University
Wagga Wagga, New South Wales,
   Australia
**Avian Circovirus and
   Polyomavirus Diseases**

Edward C. Ramsay, DVM, DACZM
Professor
Department of Small Animal
   Clinical Sciences
College of Veterinary Medicine
University of Tennessee
Knoxville, Tennessee
Pyometra in Large Felids
**Management of Crytosporidiosis
   in a Hoofstock Contact Area**

Leslie Anne Reddacliff, BVSc, PhD
Senior Research Scientist
Elizabeth Macarthur Agricultural
   Institute
NSW Department of Primary
   Industries
Camden, New South Wales,
   Australia
**Viral Chorioretinitis of
   Kangaroos**

Patricia E. Reed, DVM
Global Health Program
Wildlife Conservation Society
Bronx, New York
Ebola Hemorrhagic Fever

Laura K. Richman, DVM, PhD,
   DACVP
Smithsonian Research Fellow
Department of Pathology
Smithsonian National Zoological
   Park
Washington, DC
Elephant Herpesviruses

Gary Riggs, DVM, DABVP
Veterinarian
North Coast Bird & Exotic
   Specialties
Akron, Ohio;
President
Wild4Ever: Wildlife Conservation
   Foundation
Norton, Ohio
Avian Mycobacterial Disease

Nadia Robert, Dr Med Vet, DACVP
Assistant Professor
Institute of Animal Pathology
Vetsuisse Faculty
University of Bern
Bern, Switzerland
Stargazing in Lions

David A. Rubin, MD
Professor of Radiology
Mallinckrodt Institute of
    Radiology
Washington University School of
    Medicine;
Chief, Musculoskeletal Radiology
    Section
Barnes-Jewish Hospital;
Consulting Radiologist
Saint Louis Zoo
St. Louis, Missouri
**Degenerative Skeletal Diseases of
    Primates**

Charles E. Rupprecht, VMD, MS,
    PhD
Chief, Rabies Program
Division of Viral & Rickettsial
    Diseases
Centers for Disease Control &
    Prevention
Atlanta, Georgia
**Rabies Management in Wild
    Carnivores**

Stephanie Sanderson, MA, VMB,
    MSc, MRCVS
Head of Conservation Medicine
Chester Zoo
Chester, United Kingdom
**Bluetongue: Lessons from the
    European Outbreak 2006-2009**

Michael Schlegel, DVM, PhD
Animal Nutritionist
San Diego Zoo's Wild Animal
    Park
Escondido, California
Advances in Giraffe Nutrition

Kent J. Semmen, BS
Chemist Manager
The Seas with Nemo & Friends
    Pavilion at Epcot
Orlando, Florida
**Basic Water Quality Evaluation
    for Zoo Veterinarians**
**The Mechanics of Aquarium
    Water Conditioning**
**Advanced Water Quality
    Evaluation For Zoo
    Veterinarians**

Jessica L. Siegal-Willott, DVM,
    DACZM
Associate Veterinarian
Department of Animal Health
National Zoological Park,
    Smithsonian Institution
Washington, DC
**Digital Radiography of the
    Elephant Foot**

Dennis Slate, MS, PhD
National Rabies Management
    Coordinator
US Department of Agriculture
Animal Plant Health Inspection
    Service
Wildlife Services
Concord, New Hampshire
**Rabies Management in Wild
    Carnivores**

Jonathan Mark Sleeman, MA,
    VetMB, DACZM, DECZM,
    MRCVS
Center Director
US Geological Survey
National Wildlife Health Center
Madison, Wisconsin
**Johne's Disease and Free-
    Ranging Wildlife**

Andrea Brenes Soto, BSc, Lic
Professor and Researcher
Pet, Zoo and Wildlife Nutrition
    and Management Program
Animal Science Department
University of Costa Rica
San Jose, Costa Rica
**Feeding and Nutrition of
    Anteaters**

M. Andrew Stamper, DVM,
    DACZM
Clinical Veterinarian
Research Biologist
The Seas with Nemo & Friends
    Pavilion at Epcot
Lake Buena Vista, Florida
**Basic Water Quality Evaluation
    for Zoo Veterinarians**
**The Mechanics of Aquarium
    Water Conditioning**
**Advanced Water Quality
    Evaluation for Zoo
    Veterinarians**

Hanspeter W. Steinmetz, Dr Med
    Vet, M Sc
Assistant Professor
Clinic for Zoo Animals, Exotic
    Pets and Wildlife
University of Zurich
Zurich, Switzerland
Zurich Zoo
Zurich, Switzerland
**Computed Tomography for the
    Diagnosis of Sinusitis and Air
    Sacculitis in Orangutans**

Mark Stetter, DVM, DACZM
Director
Department of Animal Health
Disney's Animal Programs
Lake Buena Vista, Florida
**Laparoscopic Surgery in
    Elephants and Rhinoceros**

Jeffrey L. Stott, MS, PhD
Professor of Immunology and
    Director of the Laboratory for
    Marine Mammal Immunology
Department of Pathology,
    Microbiology & Immunology
School of Veterinary Medicine
University of California
Davis, California
**Longitudinal Monitoring of
    Immune System Parameters of
    Cetaceans and Application to
    Their Health Management**

Cynthia Stringfield, DVM, BS
Professor
Department of Animal Science
Staff Veterinarian
America's Teaching Zoo
Moorpark College
Moorpark, California
**The California Condor
    (*Gymnogyps californianus*)
    Veterinary Program: 1997-2010**

Meg Sutherland-Smith, DVM,
   DACZM
Veterinary Clinical Operations
   Manager
Veterinary Services
San Diego Zoo
San Diego, California
**Prehatch Protocols to Improve
   Hatchability**

Susan J. Tornquist, DVM, MS,
   PhD, DACVP
Associate Dean of Academic
   Affairs
Department of Veterinary
   Medicine
College of Veterinary Medicine
Oregon State University
Corvallis, Oregon
***Mycoplasma haemolamae* in New
   World Camelids**

Eduardo V. Valdes, PhD
Nutritionist
Disney's Wild Animal Kingdom
Buena Vista, Florida
**Feeding and Nutrition of
   Anteaters**
Advances in Giraffe Nutrition

Michael T. Walsh, DVM
Associate Professor
Associate Director of Aquatic
   Animal Health Program
Department of Large Animal
   Clinical Sciences
College of Veterinary Medicine
University of Florida
Gainesville, Florida
Sea Turtle Rehabilitation

Christian Walzer, DVM
University Professor
Chair Conservation Medicine
Research Institute of Wildlife
   Ecology
University of Veterinary Medicine
Vienna, Austria;
Director Science and Research
International Takhi Group
Takhiin Tal, Mongolia
**Asian Wild Horse Reintroduction
   Program**

Kristen S. Warren, BSc, BVMS,
   PhD
Senior Lecturer
Program Chair
Postgraduate Studies in
   Conservation Medicine
School of Veterinary and
   Biomedical Sciences
Murdoch University
Murdoch, WA, Australia
**Conservation Medicine for Zoo
   Veterinarians**

Martha A. Weber, DVM
Veterinarian
Saint Louis Zoo
St. Louis, Missouri
**Elephant Neonatal and Pediatric
   Medicine**

Jim Wellehan, DVM, MS,
   DAACZM, DACVM
Alumni Fellow
Zoological Medicine Service
College of Veterinary Medicine
University of Florida
Gainesville, Florida
**Virology of Nonavian Reptiles:
   An Update**

Christian J. Wenker, Dr Med Vet
Zoo Veterinarian
Basel Zoo
Basel, Switzerland
Stargazing in Lions

Ellen Wiedner, VMD, DACVIM
Director if Veterinary Care
Ringling Brothers and Barnum &
   Bailey Center for Elephant
   Conservation
Polk City, Florida
**Treatment of Elephant
   Endotheliotropic Herpesvirus
   (EEHV)**

Pat Witman
Animal Care Manager
San Diego Zoo
San Diego, California
**Prehatch Protocols to Improve
   Hatchability**

Michael J. Yabsley, MS, PhD
Assistant Professor
Warnell School of Forestry and
   Natural Resources
University of Georgia
Athens, Georgia
**Wildlife Disease Ecology: What
   Can Zoo and Wildlife
   Veterinarians Learn from This
   Discipline?**
**Primer on Tick-Borne Diseases
   in Exotic Carnivores**

Nina Zimmermann, Med Vet
University of Zürich
Clinic for Zoo Animals, Exotic
   Pets and Wildlife
Zürich, Switzerland
**Computed Tomography for the
   Diagnosis of Sinusitis and Air
   Sacculitis in Orangutans**

Jeffery R. Zuba, DVM
Associate Professor
Wildlife Health Center
University of California
Davis, California
Senior Veterinarian
Department of Veterinary Services
San Diego Zoo's Wild Animal
   Park
Escondido, California
**Hoof Disorders in Nondomestic
   Artiodactyls**

Preface

This is the Seventh Volume of *Fowler's Zoo and Wild Animal Medicine* and it is again in the Current Veterinary Therapy format. The Editors, with the assistance of six Consulting Editors, selected topics to represent current issues, as well as an overview of the practice of zoo and wildlife medicine, particularly as these two fields evolve and share more and more in common.

A particular emphasis has been placed on the challenges of conserving so many threatened and endangered species. As that is truly an international effort, the 102 authors represent 12 countries (Austria, Australia, Canada, France, Germany, New Zealand, Portugal, South Africa, Switzerland, The Netherlands, the United Kingdom, and the United States of America).

Many of the topics address "cutting edge" issues such as white-nose disease in bats and updates on Ebola virus in wild great apes and chytrid fungus in amphibians. Others address the broader field that recognizes the interface between wildlife, livestock, human, and ecosystem health and are based on a growing body of literature regarding the "One Medicine" concept. In summary, zoo and wildlife veterinarians are well positioned to fulfill not only the technical aspects of veterinary medicine, but also to be integral members of the overall biologic team needed to rescue many threatened and endangered species from extinction. The Editors hope that the readers will find the diversity of topics in this edition of *Fowler's Zoo and Wild Animal Medicine* useful in that mission.

Acknowledgments

The Editors offer a sincere thank you to the 102 authors who contributed 83 chapters to the Seventh Volume of *Fowler's Zoo and Wild Animal Medicine*. This contribution is especially significant since all of the royalties from this and past editions of this book go to support research on the health of wild animals, with none going to the authors or editors. We also thank the many researchers whose research and scientific data on the biology and medicine of wild animals allowed these chapters to be written.

The Editors also extend a special thank you to the six Consulting Editors who contributed suggestions for topics for this volume: Paul Calle, Scott Citino, Richard Jakob-Hoff, Don Janssen, Jacques Kaandorp, and Michele Miller.

Once again, we thank our wives, Mary Jean and Audrey, for moral support while we took the time way from family activities to complete the task of editing and bring this volume to completion.

A final and personal acknowledgment from one of the Editors (REM) is to Murray Fowler. Dr. Fowler initiated the first edition of *Zoo and Wild Animal Medicine* in 1978 when few texts existed in this field. In the subsequent 32 years, he has shown an unwavering dedication to the dissemination of this information with six subsequent volumes of this text (not to mention many other related texts authored by him). He has been, and continues to be, a mentor and an inspiration to many in our field, myself included.

General

CHAPTER 1

Disease Risk Analysis in Wildlife Health Field Studies

Sharon L. Deem

Although risk may be defined many ways, it always denotes the possibility of loss or injury. In mathematical terms, a risk is calculated as the probability of an outcome multiplied by the impact if the outcome occurs. We calculate risks in all aspects of our lives. There are risks in walking across a highway (e.g., risk of being hit by a car) or putting money in the stock market (e.g., risk of losing money). With each of these actions, there is an uncertain possibility of injury or loss because the outcome cannot be known beforehand. Rather, we may have a subjective impression (qualitative) or use a calculated probability (quantitative) as an indicator of the risks associated with the action.

As zoological and wildlife veterinarians, we perform risk analyses daily. With each of our decisions, whether working with captive or free-living animals, we weigh the benefits versus risks (a form of risk analysis) for every diagnostic and therapeutic option. We do this knowing that no medical action is risk-free. For example, there are risks when we anesthetize an animal to perform diagnostics. However, there are also risks if we do not anesthetize the animal because we may not be able to collect the biomaterials necessary for making a sound diagnosis leading to proper treatment. Veterinarians are aware of these risks and must often defend their medical decisions to curators, park managers, and politicians based on the risks associated with each of their informed medical actions.

To calculate and manage risks better, the use of disease risk analysis has become an important tool in many areas of the veterinary sciences.[21] Disease issues are often complex and predictive models, using a disease risk analysis format, may be highly effective in dealing with these disease-related challenges. Within wildlife veterinary medicine, risk analysis has also become a highly valued tool.[1,2,20] Many wildlife health field studies are now directed at understanding the following:

(1) diseases in wildlife populations; (2) links among wildlife, domestic animal, and human health; and (3) links between the health of captive and free-living wildlife species. Illustrative examples for each of these three areas of study include an understanding of the following: (1) the conservation implications of *Batracho-chytrium dendrobatidis* in amphibian species; (2) tuberculosis in African wildlife and people; and (3) herpesviruses in captive and free-living elephants. Additionally, we often must make medical management decisions based on findings from wildlife health studies. For example, is vaccination a viable medical decision, or does one let nature take its course during a disease epidemic in a wild canid population? These risk management decisions may best be answered using disease risk analysis.

The growth in awareness, interests, and efforts directed at wildlife health field studies may be viewed as positive for biodiversity conservation; however, this growth is most likely the result of a significant increase in disease-related conservation challenges.[8] These field studies provide a scientific process that may better direct wildlife conservation initiatives. With the current extinction crisis, limited funds for wildlife health and conservation field projects, and the zoonotic connection of diseases found in many species of conservation concern, disease risk analyses should be used to direct and perform wildlife health field studies more effectively.

DISEASE RISK ANALYSIS

Risk analysis is a formal procedure for estimating the likelihood and consequences of adverse effects occurring in a specific population, taking into consideration exposure to potential hazards and the nature of their effects.[23] Disciplines as diverse as economics, engineering, business, environmental science, and health all commonly apply this technique. In the health sciences,

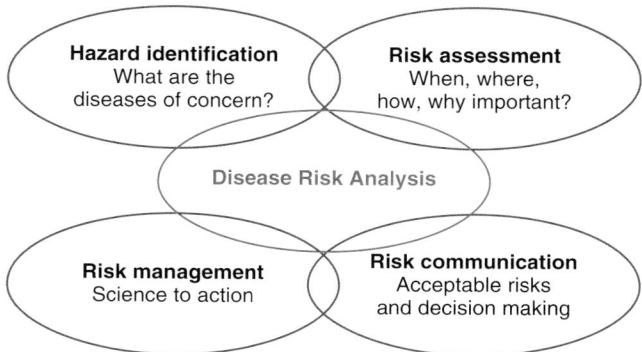

Figure 1-1

Disease risk analysis consists of four interconnected phases that include hazard identification, risk assessment, risk management, and risk communication.

a disease risk analysis is defined as a multidisciplinary process used to evaluate existing knowledge to prioritize risks associated with the spread or occurrence of diseases.

A risk analysis consists of four interconnected phases: (1) hazard identification; (2) risk assessment; (3) risk management; and (4) risk communication (Fig. 1-1). All the phases are interactive with the others—the process should not simply flow from phase 1 to phase 4 in chronologic order. A disease risk analysis is structured similar to that for other risk analyses.

Hazard identification is the identification of what may go wrong. We must identify what diseases have potential effects harmful enough to warrant inclusion in the risk analysis. Some criteria used for ranking infectious disease hazards include prevalence and incidence data, infectivity, pathogenicity (e.g., morbidity, mortality, fitness costs, reproductive costs), transmissibility (e.g., routes, rates, competent vectors), susceptibility (e.g., species, humans), and economic impacts associated with wildlife species, domestic animals, humans, and the ecosystem. Ranking of noninfectious diseases may include species susceptibility to injuries, physiologic stress, and genetic defects.

Risk assessment is the range of calculations required to estimate release, exposure, and consequence parameters for infectious diseases of concern. The process of assessing the risk will help understand the when, where, how, and why of a potential disease risk. With noninfectious diseases, it may involve calculations of the likelihood and consequences of the disease occurring (e.g., capture myopathy, toxicity) in a certain population or community. A subsequent estimate of the total risk may

then be calculated based on the parameters for each of the identified hazards.

Risk management focuses on responses that may decrease the likelihood of an adverse outcome and reduce the consequences if such an outcome occurs. This element of risk analysis may best be viewed as the reason for performing the analysis so that science may move into action. Risk management may be the single most important component because it translates the identification of diseases and assessment of associated risks into management actions that may mitigate these risks.

Risk communication is a continuous process, necessitating respectful communication among the multiple stakeholders throughout the risk analysis.[21] Risk communication should occur among field staff (those on the ground collecting data), modelers (those using data for a quantitative risk analysis), managers, laypersons, politicians, and all potentially affected parties to ensure that management policies and efforts are equitably based on the risk assessment outcome. To be of value, this requires a real-time communications network. All stakeholders must know about and understand the risks and options, with a clear statement of acceptable risk. Additionally, it must be clear as to who makes the risk management decisions. Different stakeholders often hold very different views on which risks are acceptable and who is in charge.

Hazard identification and risk assessment are sometimes grouped together because they are clearly interrelated. The criteria used to identify diseases of concern may also be used to assess the level of their associated risks. In many risk analyses, hazard identification and risk assessment are performed based solely on expert opinion or literature review. One of the most valuable products of disease risk analysis is the identification of missing data points that if obtained, would enhance a broader understanding of disease risks for a population or project. For a disease risk analysis to provide the highest quality outputs, hazard identification and risk assessments should be based on scientific data collected from the field and pertinent to the analysis in question. Providing these necessary data points for disease risk analysis are best performed by implementing standardized disease surveillance and monitoring systems.[6,15,22]

Performing a disease risk analysis may involve data input from literature reviews, expert opinion, direct knowledge of the species, ecosystem, or project of interest, and extrapolation from other similar studies. It is often best to start with a specific question or hypothesis and to know the assumptions (e.g., data from the literature, expert opinion versus real data) used in the risk analysis. For example, prior to a pronghorn *(Antilocapra americana)* relocation project, the risks associated with the project should be analyzed. If the expert opinion (assumption) provided during the analysis is that pronghorns are not susceptible to capture myopathy, then the value of the risk analysis may be flawed from the start. It is also crucial to assess the reliability of the data to be used in the risk analysis. In the pronghorn example, do we have data on the capture technique, mode of transport, and personnel that will be used in the relocation effort? Each of these variables will influence the outcome of the project and need to be factored into the risk analysis to help determine whether to conduct the relocation. There are other factors that must be weighed into this decision—for example, why the pronghorns are being relocated and the health risks if the group is not moved.

Outputs of a disease risk analysis may include the following: (1) a visual representation (e.g., flow charts, tables, graphs) of the analysis; (2) identification of relationships that may not have been immediately obvious; (3) identification of missing data points necessary to better understand disease risks (e.g., need for further studies); and (4) identification of critical control points to facilitate the development of cost-effective management strategies. Critical control points are any location, practice, procedure, or process at which control may be implemented over one or more factors and, if controlled, may minimize or prevent a hazard.[23] Therefore, critical control points are important in the context of planning strategies that may minimize the risks of disease by identifying those actions that should be taken (e.g., risk management).

Disease risk analyses may be qualitative or quantitative. Qualitative analyses indicate the likelihood of an outcome expressed in terms such as high, medium, low, or negligible. Quantitative analyses indicate an outcome expressed numerically (e.g., there is a 10% chance that 5% of the pronghorns will develop capture myopathy). A quantitative disease risk analysis may be time-consuming and require large amounts of resources and possibly advanced training in modeling and epidemiology. Fortunately, there are a number of quantitative risk analysis software programs that go beyond deterministic models, providing stochastic capabilities (Table 1-1). In quantitative analyses, numeric values are attached to various stages of release, exposure, and consequence pathways to generate a numeric estimate of total risk.

If it is not possible or desired to perform a quantitative analysis, a qualitative disease risk analysis is often adequate. A qualitative analysis may simply demand paper and pen and some time for analytic thought. Every good quantitative analysis begins with a qualitative visual representation. In many cases, just the process of specifying the model provides insights that might have been previously missed. It provides a visual summary of what we believe the relationships to be in a complex situation and may stimulate discussion, among all the stakeholders, about the problem being modeled.

Semiquantitative disease risk analyses, in which scores are assigned based on expert opinion, are also available and have the advantage of quantitative analyses but, like qualitative analyses, are easier to perform.[19] However, the limitations of semiquantitative approaches, because of a possible lack of transparency if numbers are assigned and because the method of combination is arbitrary, should be minimized when performing semiquantitative analyses.

Finally, it is important to know how the findings from a qualitative, quantitative, or semiquantitative disease risk analysis will be used. There is both art and science to the proper application of results from the hazard identification and risk assessment phases to direct effective risk management and risk communication. For example, if a risk is determined with a large potential loss and a low probability of occurring (e.g., there is a 2% chance that all 50 pronghorns will develop capture myopathy during translocation), it is often treated differently from a risk determined with a low potential loss and a high likelihood of occurring (e.g., 75% chance of two pronghorns developing capture myopathy during translocation). A risk matrix shows the probability of a risk occurring in relationship to the severity (impact) of its consequences and helps in deciding how findings should direct risk management actions.[23]

EXAMPLES OF DISEASE RISK ANALYSIS IN WILDLIFE HEALTH FIELD STUDIES

The following examples demonstrate the application of disease risk analysis in wildlife health field studies. The overall objective of each of these examples is to understand disease risks for wildlife species, domestic animals, humans and/or ecosystems better and to ensure proper disease management.

TABLE 1-1	Software for Performing Quantitative Disease Risk Analyses			
Package	Cost ($)	Software Developer	URL	Description
Outbreak	None	Conservation Breeding Specialist Group	http://www.vortex9.org/outbreakinstall.zip	Made specifically for the wildlife health community; may stand alone or work within Vortex
Stella	2000	High Performance Systems	http://www.hps_inc.com/edu/stella/stella.htm http://www.iseesystems.com/softwares/Education/StellaSoftware.aspx	Highlights critical data points; predicts consequences; evaluates effectiveness of interventions
Vensim	0-2000	Ventana Systems	http://www.vensim.com	Highlights critical data points; predicts consequences; evaluates effectiveness of interventions
@Risk	2000	Palisade Corporation	http://www.palisade.com/risk	Monte Carlos simulation modeling
Precision Tree	2000	Palisade Corporation	http://www.palisade.com/precisiontree/	Add-in to Microsoft Excel; relatively easy to use
Risk Matrix	Free	MITRE Corporation	http://www.mitre.org/work/sepo/toolkits/risk/ToolsTechniques/RiskMatrix.html	Construction of risk matrices to identify, prioritize, and manage key risks

Conservation Breeding Specialist Group Workbooks

The Conservation Breeding Specialist Group (CBSG) workbook on animal movements and associated disease risks provides a thorough overview of how to perform a disease risk analysis, introduction to quantitative software programs, and real case study examples (e.g., mountain gorilla and tracker health; wildlife disease issues on islands). This workbook may be downloaded[1] or a hard copy may be ordered from CBSG. A separate CBSG workbook on disease risks associated with biomaterial transportation may also be downloaded.[17] This workbook provides an overview of the disease risk analysis method and examples related to biomaterial transportation, such as the international transport of semen. As noted by Miller,[20] the tools provided by the CBSG were designed to enable professionals to incorporate not only published, statistically valid data, but also to make reasonable decisions under conditions of uncertainty and to capture valuable information from more basic field or clinical experiences.

Carnivore Conservation

Diseases challenging the conservation of wild ungulate and carnivore populations have been identified as a primary threat to a number of these species; possibly due to the close genetic relationship between these taxa and their domestic relatives.[4] The critically endangered Ethiopian wolf *(Canis simensis)* is one canid species in which diseases (e.g., canine distemper and rabies viruses) have been shown to have significant conservation implications.[14] A population viability assessment (PVA) Vortex-based model performed in the 1990s only included disease as a single mortality factor.[18] Improving on this model, diseases were incorporated directly into a PVA that provided a much more reliable estimate of viability because diseases are known to be a key factor affecting the viability of this species.[11]

Human Activities and Health

A number of qualitative and semiquantitative disease risk analyses have been performed to understand the implications of human activities as related to the health of domestic animals, wildlife, and humans.[3,5,19] Using relatively simple analyses, each of these examples demonstrates how we may direct risk management better to minimize or mitigate disease threats challenging wildlife conservation, agricultural production, and public health.

Galapagos Avifauna

In the Galapagos Islands, a primary threat to endemic bird conservation is the introduction of novel pathogens.[24] Disease risk analyses provide a means to understand these disease-related threats. A qualitative disease risk assessment, based on literature review and expert opinion, was performed as a first step to inform decision makers and direct risk management.[7] This basic qualitative analysis allowed ranking of pathogens based on potential harm and determination of missing data to direct future studies better, especially for those diseases of high conservation concern (e.g., *Philornis downsi*, avian pox virus; *Plasmodium* sp.).

A quantitative analysis was performed to explore the most likely routes of introduction of West Nile virus into the Galapagos Islands.[13] The findings from this study, which demonstrated air transport as the most likely route, were instrumental in improving risk management, including the requirement of disinsection of all planes entering Galapagos.

Great Ape Conservation

A number of disease risk analyses for free-living primate populations are available in the literature. One example is an analysis using retrospective health data from the long-running Gombe chimpanzee study.[16] This study provides an excellent example of how retrospective data may be used within a disease risk analysis framework. The analysis enumerates various factors, including a better understanding of disease threats to an endangered species, a guide to improve health data collection, and proper risk communication to advance high-quality health care standards.

A second example is a study derived from a workshop on Southeast Asian Macaque Risk Analysis. Field and laboratory data and expert opinion were combined to develop a model to predict transmission of simian foamy virus between temple macaques and humans accurately.[9] This study provides an example of integrating real data with expert opinion for a better understanding of zoonotic pathogens at the interface of semiwild primates and humans.

Translocation Projects

A number of translocation and reintroduction studies have used disease risk analysis.[10,12] These studies demonstrate the application of disease risk analysis, prior to animal movements, that may help minimize the inherent risks and disease-related causes of past translocation failures.[25]

CONCLUSIONS

Health professionals conducting wildlife field studies are constantly confronted with uncertainty related to the complexity of disease issues and the ecology of study populations. The use of disease risk analysis provides a tool for directing these studies better and for understanding these complex disease issues. Disease risk analysis offers a theory to field and field to theory connection. Whether the disease risk analysis output is descriptive or analytic, the underlying objective should be to ensure management actions that are based on scientific evidence.

To be most effective, a disease risk analysis should be performed based on epidemiologic standards, including monitoring, surveillance, and real data. However, expert opinion and literature review may be the only source for some analyses; these often provide the stimulus for additional field studies to gather the missing, but important, real data.

The science in disease risk analysis is only one factor, because management and communication skills are equally important. The need for clear communication and agreement among all stakeholders about the level of risk that is acceptable and identification of the decision maker(s) must be discussed from the start, and possibly continually revised throughout the project.

In this day of increasingly complex conservation challenges that are often associated with disease threats, limited conservation funds, and the zoonotic link of many wildlife diseases, the use of disease risk analyses may direct our efforts more effectively. Whether we perform a qualitative risk analysis with pencil, paper, and a few minutes of thought, or a quantitative analysis using one of the available software packages, risk analysis offers a visual representation, with determination of critical control points that could translate science into conservation action.

REFERENCES

1. Armstrong D, Jakob-Hoff R, Seal US, editors: Animal movements and disease risk: A workbook, ed 5, 2003 (http://www.cbsg.org/cbsg/content/files/Disease_Risk/disease.risk_manual.pdf).
2. Ballou JD: Assessing the risks of infectious diseases in captive breeding and reintroduction programs. J Zoo Wildl Med 24:327–335, 1993.
3. Bridges VE, Akkina J, Grannis J, et al: A qualitative assessment tool for the potential of infectious disease emergence and spread. Prev Vet Med 81:80–91, 2007.
4. Cleaveland S, Laurenson MK, Taylor LH: Diseases of humans and their domestic mammals: pathogen characteristics, host range and the risk of emergence. Philos Trans R Soc Lond B Biol Sci 356:991–999, 2001.
5. Coburn HL, Snary EL, Kelly LA, et al: Qualitative risk assessment of the hazards and risks from wild game. Vet Rec 157:321–322, 2005.
6. Deem SL, Karesh WB, Weisman W: Putting theory into practice: wildlife health in conservation. Cons Biol 15:1224–1233, 2001.
7. Deem SL, Cruz M, Jiménez-Uzcátegui G, et al: Pathogens and parasites: an increasing threat to the conservation of Galapagos avifauna. In Informe Galapagos 2007–2008. Ingala, Puerto Ayora, Galapagos, 2008, Ecuador, pp 125–130.
8. Deem SL, Ezenwa VO, Ward JR, et al: Research frontiers in ecological systems: evaluating the impacts of infectious disease on ecosystems. In Ostfeld RS, Eviner VT, Keesing F, editors: Infectious disease ecology: effects of ecosystems on disease and of disease on ecosystems, Princeton, NJ, 2008, Princeton University Press, pp 304–318.
9. Engel G, Hungerford LL, Jones-Engel L, et al: Risk assessment: A model for predicting cross-species transmission of simian foamy virus from macaques (*M. fascicularis*) to humans at a monkey temple in Bali, Indonesia. Am J Primatol 68:934–948, 2006.
10. Fernández N, Kramer-Schadt S, Thulke H-H: Viability and risk assessment in species restoration: planning reintroductions for the wild boar, a potential disease reservoir (http://www.ecologyandsociety.org/vol11/iss1/art6/, 2006).
11. Haydon DT, Laurenson MK, Sillero-Zubiri C: Integrating epidemiology into population viability analysis: managing the risk posed by rabies and canine distemper to the Ethiopian wolf. Cons Biol 16:1372–1385, 2002.
12. Jakob-Hoff R: Disease risk assessment for translocation of kaki (black stilt), *Himantopus novaezelandiae*, from captivity to the wild. Department of Conservation (Science Internal Series 16), Wellington, New Zealand, 2001.
13. Kilpatrick AM, Daszak P, Goodman SJ, et al: Predicting pathogen introduction: West Nile virus spread to Galapagos. Cons Biol 20:1224–1231, 2006.
14. Laurenson MK, Sillero-Zubiri C, Thompson H, et al: Disease threats to endangered species: Ethiopian wolves, domestic dogs, and canine pathogens. Anim Cons 1:273–280, 1998.
15. Leendertz FH, Pauli G, Maetz-Rensing K, et al: Pathogens as drivers of population declines: the importance of systematic monitoring in great apes and other threatened mammals. Biol Cons 131:325–337, 2006.
16. Lonsdorf EV, Travis D, Pusey AE, et al: Using retrospective health data from the Gombe chimpanzee study to inform future monitoring efforts. Am J Primatol 68:897–908, 2006.
17. Loskutoff NM, Holt WV, Bartels P, editors: Biomaterial transport and disease risk: workbook development, 2003 (http://www.omahazoo.com/iets/biomaterialsanddiseaseriskworkbook.pdf).
18. Mace G, Sillero-Zubiri C: A preliminary population viability analysis for the Ethiopian wolf. In Sillero-Zubiri C, Macdonald DW, editors: The Ethiopian wolf: status survey and conservation action plan, Gland, Switzerland, 1997, World Conservation Union, pp 51–60.
19. McKenzie J, Simpson H, Langstaff I: Development of methodology to prioritise wildlife pathogens for surveillance. Prev Vet Med 81:194–210, 2007.
20. Miller PS: Tools and techniques for disease risk assessment in threatened wildlife conservation programmes. Int Zoo Yb 41:38–51, 2007.
21. Office of International Epizootics: Import risk analysis. In Terrestrial animal health code, ed 13, Paris, 2004, Office of International Epizootics.
22. Spalding MG, Forrester DJ: Disease monitoring of free-ranging and released wildlife. J Zoo Wildl Med 24:271–290, 1993.
23. Thrusfield M: Risk analysis. In Veterinary epidemiology, ed 3, Oxford, England, 2007, Blackwell, pp 482–502.
24. Wikelski M, Fousopoulos J, Vargas H, et al: Galapagos birds and diseases: invasive pathogens as threats to island species (http://www.ecologyandsociety.org/vol9/iss1/art5, 2004).
25. Woodford MH: International disease implications for wildlife translocation. J Zoo Wildl Med 24:265–270, 1993.

CHAPTER 2

Contraception

Cheryl Asa and Sally Boutelle

Contraception has become integral to the reproductive management of mammals. Contraception recommendations are incorporated into animal care manuals and master plans, and almost all zoos and aquariums use contraception to control reproduction. We use the term *contraception* to refer to methods that are designed to be reversible, so that animals may return to reproduction at a later date if recommended to breed. In contrast, we use the term *sterilization* for methods that are considered permanent. For more extensive discussions of the issues surrounding contraceptive use and available methods, as well as complete citations, see *Wildlife Contraception: Issues, Methods and Application*[1] and *Wild Mammals in Captivity.*[2]

FEMALE CONTRACEPTION

Permanent Methods

Permanent sterilization may be the best choice for those not likely to receive breeding recommendations in the future or that may have clinical conditions that make reproduction inadvisable. Ovariectomy removes the source of gametes as well as reproductive hormones, eliminating estrous behavior and secondary sex characteristics, such as perineal swelling. Although removal of the uterus in addition to the ovaries is common for domestic dogs and cats in the United States, a comparative study of the two procedures in dogs has found no differences in prevalence of any of the anticipated side effects.[17] Information on potential side effects of ovariectomy is available primarily for dogs, cats, and humans. No data, however, are available on the potential for decreased bone density following removal of the ovaries in long-lived animals such as great apes, but it may be assumed equivalent to the results for humans.

Tubal ligation or blocking the oviducts by other means may be an option for species in which gonadal hormones are not associated with pathology, such as primates. However, it should not be used in female carnivores, because the repeated cycles of elevated estrogen and progesterone levels increase the risk of mammary tumors and uterine infection and tumors.

Reversible Contraception

Steroid Hormones

Progestins

Synthetic progestins (Table 2-1) have proven effective in all mammalian species that have been treated. Progestins may prevent ovulation by negative feedback on luteinizing hormone (LH), but they also thicken cervical mucus so that sperm passage is impeded, interrupt sperm and ovum transport, and interfere with implantation.[12] Because higher doses are needed to block ovulation than to affect the other endpoints, ovulation may occur in animals that are adequately contracepted.[7] Progestins cannot completely suppress follicle development and the resulting estradiol secretion may stimulate physical and behavioral signs of estrus, so those indications cannot be used to judge efficacy.

The progestin most commonly used by zoos has been the melengestrol acetate (MGA) implant introduced by Seal in the mid-1970s and now available from Wildlife Pharmaceuticals (Fort Collins, Colo). MGA is also available incorporated into a commercial hoofstock diet (Mazuri, Purina Mills, St. Louis) and as a liquid to be added to food (Wildlife Pharmaceuticals). A disadvantage of this approach is confirming that the animal consumes the dose needed each day. In a herd setting, it is important that the more subordinate animals eat an adequate dosage, which may result in dominant animals consuming more than the recommended

TABLE 2-1 Currently Available Synthetic Progestin Products Used as Contraceptives

Synthetic Progestin	Product Name	Manufacturer or Supplier
Melengestrol acetate	MGA implants	Wildlife Pharmaceuticals
	MGA feed (Mazuri)	Purina Mills Inc.
	MGA 200 or 500 Pre-mix	Pharmacia and Upjohn
	MGA liquid	Wildlife Pharmaceuticals
Megestrol acetate	Megace	Par Pharmaceuticals
Altrenogest	Regu-mate oral solution	Merck Intervet
Medroxyprogesterone acetate	Depo-Provera injections	Pharmacia and Upjohn
Proligestone	Delvosteron injections (Europe)	Intervet
Levonorgestrel	Jadelle implants (Europe)	Wyeth-Ayerst
Etonorgestrel	Implanon implants (Europe, Australia, Indonesia)	Organon

dosage. However, data from studies of domestic cows have shown no deleterious effects at as much as three times the minimal effective dose.

Equids are the exception to the species successfully treated with MGA. However, altrenogest (Regu-Mate, Intervet, Boxmeer, The Netherlands), the only synthetic progestin effective in domestic horses for synchronizing estrus, should also be effective as a contraceptive, but at a higher dose. However, cost and the necessity for daily delivery have limited its use.

Depo-Provera (medroxyprogesterone acetate, Pharmacia & Upjohn, Bridgewater, NJ), the second most commonly used progestin in zoos, is often chosen because it is injectable and thus may be delivered by dart. In particular, it has been used for some seasonally breeding species (e.g., prosimians), species in which anesthesia for implant insertion is problematic (e.g., giraffes, hippos), and as an immediately available interim contraceptive. Another synthetic progestin, megestrol acetate, is an option for those that may be administered a daily pill.

The various synthetic progestins differ in degree of binding to receptors of other hormones such as glucocorticoids and androgens, and there are likely also species differences. One concern is possible side effects, such as symptoms of diabetes, as compared with gestational diabetes when endogenous progesterone is elevated. U.S. Seal chose MGA rather than medroxyprogesterone acetate (MPA, the synthetic progestin in Depo-Provera) to use in implants because MPA altered cortisol levels in that study.

A further problem with MPA is androgenic activity, equated in some tests with dihydrotestosterone, a natural androgen with potent morphologic effects, especially during development. For example, Depo-Provera treatment of female black lemurs resulted in male-like pelage darkening.[3] Another progestin with androgen effects, levonorgestrel, has the highest binding affinity to androgen receptors of current progestins and is considered a potential health risk because of its effect on lipids and the cardiovascular system.[24] Although Norplant implants are no longer available in the United States, some progestin-only birth control pills contain levonorgestrel, its active ingredient.

The major side effect reported for progestins is weight gain, and one product (megestrol acetate, Megace, Par Pharmaceuticals, Woodcliff Lake, NJ) is marketed specifically to increase appetite. Progestin supplementation may help maintain pregnancy in some species, whereas in others, especially early in gestation, they have been associated with embryonic resorption.[4] Progestins may interfere with parturition via suppression of uterine smooth muscle contractility, as documented in white-tailed deer,[20] but primates treated with progestins have given birth without incident.[1] This species difference may be related to the patterns of progesterone near term. In general, species other than primates experience a decline in progesterone before the onset of parturition, which may be necessary to release the myometrium from suppression. In contrast, progestins appear to be safe for lactating females and nursing young. They do not interfere with milk production, and no negative effects on the growth or development of nursing infants have been found.

Although MGA implants have been used since the mid-1970s, proper analyses of reversibility by species have been difficult because of the variables that must be considered. First, there must be a sufficient number of attempts to breed, but other factors include matching contracepted and noncontracepted groups on age and parity prior to MGA use. In addition, although MGA implants are recommended to be replaced every 2 years, this is a conservative estimate and in many cases is effective considerably longer. Thus, reversal may only be reasonably expected if the implant is removed. Such analyses have been performed only on golden lion tamarins and tigers. Wood and colleagues[25] have found that 75% of the tamarins conceive within 2 years, a rate comparable to nontreated females, but treated females have higher rates of miscarriage and stillbirths. Chuei and associates[9] have found that only 62% of tigers give birth 5 years after implant removal compared with 85% of nontreated females after 2.7 years. Possible reasons for poorer recovery in tigers were not tested directly but may be related to the high risk of uterine pathology in felids, which might interfere with pregnancy maintenance.

Estrogens

Estrogens may prevent ovulation by suppressing follicle growth, but at contraceptive doses they have been associated in many species with serious side effects. The estrogens diethylstilbestrol (DES), mestranol, estradiol benzoate, and estradiol cypionate may block implantation following mismating in dogs. However, their tendency to stimulate uterine disease, bone marrow suppression, aplastic anemia, and ovarian tumors makes them inappropriate contraceptive compounds.

Estrogen-Progestin Combinations

Some of the deleterious effects associated with estrogen treatment (e.g., overstimulation of the uterine endometrium in primates) may be mitigated by adding a progestin. However, progestins are synergistic, not inhibitory, to estrogen effects in carnivores, making the combination even more likely to result in uterine and mammary disease. Because this synergy occurs in canids when progestin-only methods are initiated during proestrus, when natural estrogen levels are elevated, treatment should be initiated well in advance of the breeding season if progestins must be used. When treatment is begun during deep anestrus, the side effects of synthetic progestins are minimized, even when continued for several years, a regimen that has been used for domestic dogs in Europe for several decades.

There are numerous orally active contraceptive products containing various combinations of an estrogen and a progestin at various doses that are approved for human use in the United States. Ethinyl estradiol is the most common form of estrogen, although a few products use mestranol. Norethindrone is the most common progestin ingredient; others include levonorgestrel, desogestrel, norgestrel, norgestimate, and ethynodiol

diacetate. Oral contraceptive regimes designed for humans were originally intended to simulate the 28-day menstrual cycle, with 21 days of treatment followed by 7 days when either a placebo or no pill is taken, resulting in withdrawal bleeding that resembles menstruation. However, more recently, products have been introduced that only include 1 week of placebo (Seasonale, Duramed Pharmaceuticals, Pomona, NY) every 3 months.

Androgens

Both testosterone and the synthetic androgen mibolerone (Cheque Drops, Pharmacia & Upjohn) are effective contraceptives (gray wolf, *Canis lupus*; leopard, *Panthera pardus*; jaguar, *P. onca*; and lion, *P. leo*), but masculinizing effects have included clitoral hypertrophy, vulval discharge, mane growth (female lion), mounting, and increased aggression. Mibolerone is approved for use in dogs but not cats, and is contraindicated for females that have impaired liver function or are lactating or pregnant, because female fetuses may be virilized. Mibolerone use in wildlife is inadvisable, especially because of the potential for increased aggression.

Gonadotropin-Releasing Hormone Analogues

Synthetic analogues of gonadotropin-releasing hormone (GnRH) may be antagonists that block the action, or agonists, that have the same effects as the natural hormone on target tissue. Although antagonists would be the more logical selection for contraception, they are considerably more expensive and shorter acting, which limits their application. In contrast to antagonists, GnRH agonist administration is followed first by an acute stimulatory phase, when pituitary LH and follicle-stimulating hormone (FSH) levels are elevated, which may result in estrus and ovulation. Continued treatment using long-acting preparations, such as implants or microspheres, causes failure of stimulation of FSH and pulsatile LH secretion because of downregulation of GnRH receptors on pituitary gonadotrophs.[14] The observed effects in the animal are similar to those following ovariectomy, but are reversed after the hormone content of the implant or microspheres is depleted.

The stimulatory phase may be prevented by treatment with the synthetic oral progestin megestrol acetate given for 1 week before and 1 week following implant insertion. This method has successfully prevented proestrus and estrus[26] when tested in domestic dogs and has been successful in many carnivores in zoos.[1]

TABLE 2-2	Number of Males and Females Treated with Deslorelin (Suprelorin) by Taxonomic Group	
Taxon	No. of Males Treated	No. of Females Treated
Bears	6	17
Canids	22	72
Felids	12	127
Small carnivores	63	137
Prosimians	2	27
Old World primates	20	68
New World primates	14	92
Apes	0	7
Artiodactyls	0	58
Pinnipeds	6	3
Cetaceans	7	12
Rodents	8	13
Bats	5	7
Totals by gender	165	640
Total for all individuals	805	

Numerous GnRH agonist products are available, but most are expensive because they were approved for treatment of prostate cancer in humans. Leuprolide acetate, as Lupron Depot injection (TAP Pharmaceuticals, Deerfield, Ill), has been used in zoos and aquariums for a variety of species, but results are not available except for some marine mammals.[8] Deslorelin implants (Suprelorin, Peptech Animal Health, Macquarie Park, Australia), available in the United States by arrangement with the AZA Wildlife Contraception Center (St. Louis), have been effective in many mammalian species[5,6] (Table 2-2). They have been used primarily in carnivores as an alternative to progestins that were associated with uterine and mammary pathology in that taxon. The major problem has been determining an effective dose across species and individuals. Some species were not suppressed at doses that were effective for other species of similar weight. For example, Mexican wolves required four implants for complete suppression, whereas domestic dogs of a similar size would only require one or at most two implants.[1]

Although contraceptives are used primarily in mammals, there has been increasing interest in Suprelorin for use in birds, especially psittacines, ducks, and

ostriches. Results have not been encouraging. No effects were reported for most ducks, but suppression of egg laying, feather plucking, aggression, or molting has been reported for runner ducks as well as psittacines, but the effects were not sustained with subsequent treatment, suggesting habituation or desensitization. Similarly, testosterone levels declined in male ostriches following first treatment, but returned to untreated levels after placement of the second implant.

The length of efficacy of Suprelorin implants is affected by several factors. First, they are produced in two formulations, one intended to last a minimum of 6 months and the other for 12 months. However, these are minimal, and individuals vary considerably in the actual duration of suppression. Whether this variability is caused by individual differences in absorption or drug metabolism or to varying release rates by the implant is unknown. It also appears that higher doses may be effective for longer periods of time.[1]

There have been few attempts to reverse Suprelorin treatment. Most of the eleven females and nine males were carnivores and primates, with only two ungulates,[1] but the ratios are representative of the numbers treated in those taxa. Difficulty in removing Suprelorin implants further complicates timing or judging reversal. The 6- and 12-month designations of the two types of implants indicate only the observed minimum durations of efficacy, with considerable variability observed on an individual basis.

Immunocontraception
Zona Pellucida Vaccines
Immunization with zona pellucida (ZP) proteins results in antibodies that reversibly interfere with binding of sperm to the ZP, the glycoprotein coating of the mammalian oocyte, or egg. Initial treatment requires at least two injections, approximately 1 month apart, with subsequent boosters needed annually for seasonal breeders but perhaps more frequently for continuous breeders. Porcine ZP (PZP) has been effective in a wide variety of ungulates and some carnivores, is safe when administered during pregnancy or lactation, and is reversible after short-term use. However, long-term studies with white-tailed deer (*Odocoileus virginianus*) and feral horses (*Equus caballus*) reveal that treatment for 5 years or longer is increasingly associated with ovarian failure.[15] Ovarian damage may occur with even short-term treatment in dogs, so PZP vaccines are not recommended for carnivores. However, those early studies did not use a very specific antibody.[16] Studies are planned for rhesus macaques and select carnivore

species with a more specific formulation. However, the possibility of permanent ovarian changes makes this method unsuitable for animals that are genetically very valuable, but is a good choice in particular for ungulates not needing long-term treatment.

When the effect is restricted to preventing sperm entry so that ovarian activity is not disrupted, ovulatory cycles with estrous behavior continue. In some species, failure to conceive results in a longer than usual breeding season, with continued estrous cycles accompanied by courtship and mating. Continued breeding activity may be desirable in some situations in which it is seen as more natural than suppression, but it can also result in increased aggression and social disruption.

Gonadotropin-Releasing Hormone Vaccines

Immunization against GnRH can interrupt reproductive processes in much the same way as GnRH analogues, but efficacy rates are variable because of individual differences in immune response. No GnRH vaccine is approved for use in U.S. zoos at this time.

Mechanical Devices

Intrauterine Devices

Intrauterine devices (IUDs) prevent pregnancy primarily by local mechanical effects on the uterus that impede implantation. Most designs include an electrolytic copper coating, with increased efficacy because the copper ions are spermicidal. Although some IUD designs were associated with pelvic inflammatory disease in humans, attention to aseptic technique during insertion, with or without prophylactic antibiotics, is critical to preventing infection.[22] IUDs can be ideal for lactating females. The IUDs marketed for humans may be appropriate for species with a uterine size and shape comparable to that of humans, such as great apes. An IUD developed for domestic dogs (Biotumer, Buenos Aires) was found to be safe and effective in limited trials.

Effects on Behavior

Few studies of contraceptive use have focused on behavior. The most obvious effect of ovariectomy and GnRH agonists is elimination of sexual activity, which also occurs when using continual combination birth control pills, although estrous behavior may occur during the placebo week. Progestins also may suppress estrus, but typically only at higher doses. IUDs and PZP vaccine should not affect estrous cycles or behavior.

Research with humans has linked progestin use, especially MPA, with mood changes, depression, and lethargy. In addition, feral domestic cats treated with

megestrol acetate, a progestin similar to MGA, were described as more docile. However, studies of social groups of hamadryas baboons, *Papio hamadryas*,[21] Rodrigues fruit bats, *Pteropus rodricensis*,[13] golden lion tamarins, *Leontopithecus rosalia*,[4] golden-headed lion tamarins, *Leontopithecus chrysomelas*,[11] and lions[18] have found no significant effects on behavior or interactions of group members when some or all females were treated with MGA implants.

MALE CONTRACEPTION
Permanent Methods

Male castration is a simple procedure, except in species with undescended or partially descended testes (e.g., pinnipeds, cetaceans, elephants). The effect of the subsequent decline in testosterone on secondary sex characteristics will cause the loss (e.g., lion's mane) or disruption of the seasonal cycle (e.g., deer antlers).

Vasectomy may be an option for males when secondary sex characteristics and male-type behavior are desirable. Although potentially reversible, the technique requires highly skilled microsurgery, but high pregnancy rates have been achieved postreversal.[10,23] Success rates may be improved if the vasectomy is done with reversal in mind, because one of the primary reasons for permanent damage is the pressure increase in the epididymis and testis following vas obstruction. Hence, leaving the testis end of the vas open lessens the chance of pressure-related damage and increases the likelihood of successful reversal.

Sperm passage also may be permanently obstructed by injecting a sclerosing agent into the cauda epididymis or vas deferens. Treatment of the epididymis may be more successful, because the tubule lumen may be crossed multiple times during the injection. Treatment of a discrete area of the vas might be amenable to reversal by excision and reanastomosis, but might not be as effective as ensuring sperm blockage.

Vasectomy is not recommended for species in which females have induced ovulation (e.g., carnivores such as felids and bears). Vasectomy permits copulation to continue, which for these species means repeated periods of elevated progesterone levels associated with the induced pseudopregnancies in their female partners, progesterone that increases the risk of uterine or mammary gland pathology. In canids as well, the obligate pseudopregnancy with elevated progesterone levels following spontaneous ovulation increases the risk of uterine pathology.

	Some Areas of Zoo Veterinary
BOX 3-1	Involvement in Conservation
	Medicine Programs

- Health assessment and monitoring of wildlife and/or domestic animal populations
- Research on zoonotic and interspecies disease transmission
- Creation of health screening and quarantine protocols for wildlife translocations
- Disease risk analyses of wildlife translocation projects
- Technical advice on welfare and production aspects of wildlife utilization projects
- Training and capacity building, particularly in developing countries
- Interdisciplinary collaboration in conservation research and captive breeding programs
- Diagnostic and other scientific data collection, management, and interpretation
- Development of diagnostic capabilities to improve identification of disease agents in wildlife species
- Passive (e.g., through rehabilitation programs) and active (targeted) wildlife disease surveillance
- In situ and ex situ reproductive and health management of threatened species
- Planning of import and export protocols for wildlife species
- Policy development at local, national, and international levels

Data from references 8, 10-12, 22, 29, and 30.

freshwater fish. By definition, a hotspot region must contain at least 1500 endemic plant species and have lost 70% of its original habitat.[23] Although New Zealand and southwest Australia are included as hotspot regions, most biodiversity hotspots are located in developing countries. Many conservationists argue that global biodiversity conservation outcomes may be maximized by concentrating conservation efforts and limited resources in these biodiversity hotspot regions.[23,24]

Zoo veterinarians in developing countries, therefore, have a particularly important role to play in biodiversity and endangered species conservation programs. In developing countries, in particular, effective long-term environmental conservation may usually only be achieved by working with local communities to conserve endangered species, protect habitats, and promote sustainable development. Increasingly, human-wildlife conflicts in these countries are intensifying, associated with the proximity of rural farming communities to wildlife populations living in diminishing remnant habitats. Innovative wildlife conservation policies and practices are needed to address these conflicts if there is to be any possibility of ensuring environmentally sustainable development for rural communities along with biodiversity conservation. Zoo veterinarians in developing countries are in the best position to apply their knowledge and skills to specific wildlife conservation dilemmas faced by their countries. Zoo veterinarians elsewhere may build collaborative links with their colleagues in developing countries and assist with capacity building and resource support (see later). In doing so, it is important that they channel resources into projects that address local conservation priorities rather than projects based on personal interest or institutional bias.[25] Kock and Kock[19] have discussed conservation initiatives in developing countries and outlined the need for adaptive action that encourages home-grown solutions to problems. They warn against transfer of technology and practices from developed countries that may be inappropriate, impractical, and unsustainable within the context of the country's resources and capabilities.

CONSERVATION MEDICINE IN PRACTICE

Some examples of how zoo veterinarians are practicing the collaborative, ecosystem-based approach of conservation medicine on behalf of biodiversity conservation are presented here. These are drawn from a combination of our personal experiences in Australasia and augmented by the work of our colleagues elsewhere. These represent a small selection of the many projects and programs now taking place around the globe.

Establishing a Conservation Medicine Infrastructure in New Zealand

Objective
The objective is to promote the collaborative methodology of Conservation Medicine in New Zealand in an effort to minimize disease risks to threatened native wildlife species.

Collaborators
In partnership with the New Zealand Department of Conservation (DOC), Auckland Zoo's veterinarians have led this ongoing project for 20 years. To date, over 60 individuals and 30 local, national, and international agencies have been involved. These have brought together expertise in veterinary medicine, disease ecology, conservation biology, epidemiology, wildlife

management, pathology, clinical pathology, database development, and indigenous Maori protocols.

Activities

In 1990, the Auckland Zoo embarked on a mission to develop close collaborative relationships with key stakeholders involved in native species conservation. A significant contributor has been research and training by its veterinarians to conduct disease surveillance and establish baseline health profiles for threatened native species (Fig. 3-3).[15] Training of DOC staff, university researchers, and others in diagnostic sample collection and field necropsy methodology has been a key strategy. In 1999, zoo veterinarians, commissioned by the DOC, developed a disease risk assessment tool for wildlife translocations.[16] This was further refined in collaboration with the International Union for Conservation of Nature (IUCN) Conservation Breeding Specialist Group (CBSG)[1,21] and is now standard operating procedure for all wildlife translocations within New Zealand.[4] To raise awareness of conservation medicine, Auckland Zoo and Unitec New Zealand hosted a national symposium in 2005, drawing participants from human, animal, and environmental sectors in Australasia.[14] At the same time, a public fundraising campaign culminated in the establishment of the zoo's clinical, research, and teaching facility, the New Zealand Centre for Conservation Medicine (NZCCM), opened by the Prime Minister in August 2007. A key objective

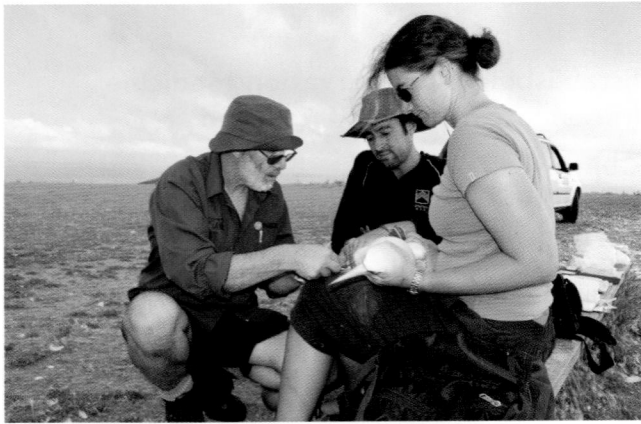

Figure 3-3

Collecting baseline health data. The gathering of baseline health and disease surveillance data has become a significant vehicle for cross-sectoral collaboration in New Zealand. (*Courtesy the Auckland Zoo, Auckland, New Zealand.*)

of this center is to provide a hub to facilitate collaborative networks in support of wildlife health teaching and research for biodiversity conservation. In 2009, a national wildlife health database to collate and disseminate wildlife health and surveillance data was launched by DOC and is managed, on contract, by the Auckland Zoo. Further information may be found at http://www.conservationmedicine.co.nz.

Development of Wildlife Disease Investigation Capability in Southwest Western Australia

Objective

The objective is to combine ecologic health investigations and interventions in support of critically endangered wildlife endemic to southwest Western Australia.

Collaborators

These include Perth Zoo, Western Australian Department of Environment and Conservation (DEC), and Murdoch University.

Activities

As noted, the southwest of Western Australia is one of 34 global biodiversity hotspot regions.[23] The collaborators are involved in several conservation medicine projects promoting recovery of endangered fauna, including a small macropod, the woylie, or brush-tailed bettong (*Bettongia penicillata ogilbyi*). From an estimated population of 40,000 in 1996, the woylie suffered a precipitous decline of more than 80% over the following decade.[31] In response, Perth Zoo veterinarians conducted field examinations and collected biologic samples to enable comparison of disease prevalence and health parameters among populations at different geographic sites and at different stages of decline. Veterinary staff also developed disease investigation protocols and strategic plans for field work and sample collection. Although research findings indicated that the primary cause of the woylie decline is predation, critical analysis and interpretation of the health data has proved invaluable in identifying health factors that may be predisposing woylies to predation. Equally important, the positive collaboration of Perth Zoo veterinary staff with DEC and Murdoch University has resulted in a new appreciation of the role of veterinarians in the woylie conservation effort. This has culminated in the recent appointment of a veterinarian to the position of disease investigator to collate the epidemiologic data collected over several years. Further information may be found at http://www.perthzoo.wa.gov.au/Conservation-Research/Projects-in-the-Wild/Woylie-Conservation-Research-Project.

Capacity Building for Wildlife Disease Diagnostics in Southern Africa

Objective
The objective is to develop the skills and resources of veterinarians and veterinary pathologists working in the Great Limpopo Transfrontier Conservation Area (GLTFCA) and facilitate retrospective and prospective research on wildlife diseases.

Collaborators
These include the National Zoological Gardens of South Africa, Faculty of Veterinary Science-University of Pretoria, Wildlife Conservation Society, U.S. Fish and Wildlife Service, Agricultural Research Institute (Maputo), and Wildlife Unit (Harare).

Activities
The Animal and Human Health for the Environment and Development (AHEAD) initiative in the GLTFCA provides a forum to address disease transmission risks among humans, domestic animals, and wildlife, as well as how the development needs of southern Africa can be met without compromising its environmental heritage. The wildlife disease diagnostics project, led by Pretoria Zoo pathologist Dr. Emily Lane, provides theoretical and practical training, training resources, and necropsy field kits for wildlife disease investigation in South Africa, Mozambique, and Zimbabwe. Further information may be found at http://www.wcs-ahead.org.

Health Surveillance of Common Dormice in England

Objective
The objectives are to reduce the probability that reintroduced dormice *(Muscardinus avellanarius)* harbor alien parasites that could harm the recipient population, ensure that dormice are healthy on release, and monitor the effects of translocation on their health and welfare.

Collaborators
These include the Zoological Society of London (ZSL) in partnership with North of England Zoological Society (Chester Zoo), Paignton Zoo, People's Trust for Endangered Species, and the Common Dormouse Captive Breeders Group.

Activities
Translocation of animals presents serious disease risks and requires careful evaluation before, during, and after the translocation process. For the common dormouse reintroduction, a disease risk analysis was performed to highlight diseases of concern, with concomitant screening of the captive population and postmortem examination of wild dormice found dead. Subsequently, a health monitoring protocol was formulated to address particular parasites of concern; this was modified as more information was gained. Over the past 10 years, selected captive-bred dormice have entered quarantine at London and Paignton Zoos for health monitoring and screening, with detailed clinical examinations performed under anaesthesia. Dormice with abnormalities that could affect postrelease welfare have been held in captivity. One potential alien cestode parasite has been eliminated from dormice prior to release. The levels of a nematode parasite are closely monitored to ensure that dormice are as fit as possible at release and do not introduce potentially alien pathogens, which could affect population viability and conservation status of wild conspecifics and other native rodents. Further information may be found at http://www.zsl.org/conservation/regions/uk-europe/native-habitat-conservation/species-recovery-programme.

Indonesian Veterinary Training Program

Objective
The objectives of the Indonesian Veterinary Training Program (IVPT) are the professional development and support of Indonesian veterinarians.

Collaborators
These include the Woodland Park Zoo, Indonesian Veterinary Medical Association/PDHI, individuals and organizations involved in disaster preparedness, government organizations, universities, agriculture, zoos, wildlife rehabilitation centers, and public health facilities.

Activities
Species biodiversity and habitat conservation initiatives are central to the IVPT, a joint collaboration between the Indonesian Veterinary Medical Association and the U.S.-based, Woodland Park Zoo. Established in 1999,

this partnership was an outcome linked to professional development for Indonesian veterinarians to diversify their professional capabilities and strengthen their economic output. IVTP and grantees work to involve veterinary professionals in the design and evaluation of projects, ensure that the work meets their needs, and addresses the realities that they face in their practice settings. IVTP builds the professional network knowledge base through workshops and international exchanges and connects animal health professionals through ongoing and new initiatives, such as microfinance and digital distance learning, to achieve long-term, sustainable results for the economy and the environment. Further information may be found at http://www.zoo.org/Page.aspx?pid=968.

Cat Ba Langur Conservation Project

Objective
The objectives of the Cat Ba Langur Conservation Project (CBLCP) are to conserve the critically endangered Cat Ba langur (*Trachypithecus poliocephalus poliocephalus*) and contribute to the conservation of the overall biodiversity at the Cat Ba Archipelago.

Collaborators
These include the Muenster Zoo (Germany), Zoological Society for the Conservation of Species and Populations (Germany), and community groups such as the Langur Guardians and commune forest protection groups supported by local Vietnamese authorities.

Activities
The Cat Ba Langur is an endemic primate on Cat Ba Island, North Vietnam. Because of poaching, habitat fragmentation, and disturbance through an increasing number of immigrants and tourists, the population of the Cat Ba langur has been classified as critically endangered by the IUCN. Only 60 to 70 individuals remain in the wild. Since the CBLCP started in 2000, the number of individuals has increased continuously. In addition to the establishment of a strictly protected area, a community-based protection network was initiated. Almost 200 local people are involved in the protection of this langur species and its habitat. In addition to the protection of Cat Ba's forest, the CBLCP focuses on in situ population management of the Cat Ba langur, environmental education to raise awareness about the plight of this primate species, and combating the illegal wildlife trade. Further information may be found at http://www.catbalangur.org.

Disease Surveillance for Tuberculosis Infection in Captive Indian Elephants in Nepal

Objective
The objective is to evaluate serologic techniques as screening tools to identify tuberculosis infection in Indian elephants (*Elephas maximus indicus*) accurately and quickly.

Collaborators
These include Elephant Care International, Disney's Wild Animal Kingdom (Orlando, Florida), Busch Gardens (Tampa, Florida), Institute of Agriculture and Animal Science (Nepal), Department of National Parks and Conservation (Nepal), and Tufts Center for Conservation Medicine (North Grafton, Mass), and others.

Activities
This research team conducted the first comprehensive range country elephant tuberculosis survey in 2006. Biologic samples were collected from 120 elephants, 49 owned by the Nepalese government and 71 owned by 13 private organizations. All elephants were given physical examinations, photographed, and had trunk washes for culture and blood samples collected. Samples were tested in Nepal and imported to the United States for comparative work. The research study compared the results of Elephant TB Stat-Pak (Chembio Diagnostic Systems, Medford, NY), multiantigen print immunoassay (MAPIA), and immunoblot serologic tests with culture results from laboratories in Nepal and the United States. Additional samples were collected to develop RNA-based immunologic assays. This project is ongoing under the supervision of Dr. Susan Mikota, Elephant Care International, who is developing a national elephant tuberculosis program in Nepal based on these preliminary studies. Further information may be found at http://www.elephantcare.org.

BUILDING AND NURTURING RELATIONSHIPS

Just as conservation medicine concerns itself with interconnections in nature, so the successful practice of this discipline is dependent on the development and nurturing of relationships among its practitioners. To describe this challenge, we could do no better than to quote Cook and coworkers in summing up the Manhattan Principles:

It is clear that no one discipline or sector of society has enough knowledge and resources to prevent the emergence or resurgence of diseases in today's globalized world. No one nation may reverse the patterns of habitat loss and extinction that may and do undermine the health of people and animals. Only by breaking down the barriers among agencies, individuals, specialties and sectors may we unleash the innovation and expertise needed to meet the many serious challenges to the health of people, domestic animals and wildlife and to the integrity of ecosystems. Solving today's threats and tomorrow's problems cannot be accomplished with yesterday's approaches. We are in an era of "One World, One Health" and we must devise adaptive, forward-looking and multidisciplinary solutions to the challenges that undoubtedly lie ahead.[3]

This is a formidable challenge, particularly for those of us brought up in cultures that emphasize individual advancement, self-enrichment, and competition over joint responsibility, shared resources, and collaboration, organizational silos that embed an artificially fragmented view of the world, and an economic philosophy that fails to count the environmental, animal welfare, or human social costs of our choices.

Zoo veterinarians who involve themselves in transdisciplinary conservation medicine projects will, in addition to their technical skills, continually need to develop their communication, interpersonal, diplomacy, and negotiation skills to reconcile differing and often polarized views for the achievement of longer term conservation objectives.[8] Scientific reports of conservation medicine projects rarely, if ever, provide readers with an appreciation of the hardship and personal sacrifice that is so often involved when undertaking work on these types of projects. There are often many institutional obstacles that need to be overcome. These include those imposed by competitive research funding, need for personal recognition, and rules about intellectual property, all of which may influence our willingness and ability to share data and work collaboratively in cross-organizational teams. Other potential challenges may include a lack of effective management of staff workload, predisposing individuals to burn out, and failure of conservation institutions to appreciate the value of veterinary involvement in wildlife conservation projects at all levels of project planning and implementation.

Despite this, as illustrated in the World Association of Zoos and Aquariums (WAZA) Conservation Strategy,[34] many zoos and aquaria have a strong and growing culture of information exchange and resource sharing, and zoo veterinarians should take every opportunity to promote and support this trend in their own organizations. Veterinarians are trained problem solvers and this training, when combined with a willingness to consider new approaches, value diversity of opinion, embrace continuous learning, and work collaboratively in a team, can, in our experience, achieve greater conservation outcomes and higher levels of personal satisfaction than any individual endeavor.

CONSERVATION MEDICINE TRAINING RESOURCES

To foster and grow the next generation of conservation medicine practitioners, a number of institutions are leading the way. In this section we provide a brief synopsis of some key training resources for those who wish to pursue this topic further.

The Center for Conservation Medicine at Tufts University (Tufts CCM; http://www.tufts.edu/vet/ccm) offers an interdisciplinary approach to ecosystem health at undergraduate level. Founded in 1997, the CCM has been a signature program that has been incorporated into the Cumming's School undergraduate DVM degree program. Based at its North Grafton campus (North Grafton, Mass), the Tufts CCM course has been structured so that all undergraduate veterinary students are taught conservation medicine, and students committed to pursuing a career in this field are able to select further elective study units in the discipline.[17] Tufts CCM is developing a Master of Science program in Conservation Medicine that will be available for study in 2011.[18]

Murdoch University's School of Veterinary and Biomedical Sciences (VBS; Perth, Western Australia; http://www.vetbiomed.murdoch.edu.au) offers training in conservation medicine at both undergraduate and postgraduate level.[33] Conservation medicine field trips to New Zealand and South Africa are held on an annual basis for undergraduate veterinary students. These field trips were collaboratively established between Murdoch University's School of VBS, the New Zealand Centre for Conservation Medicine, Wildlifevets (http://wildlifevets.com), and the University of Pretoria, respectively, to provide undergraduate veterinary students with insights into innovative conservation medicine initiatives being undertaken in these countries. The University also offers Master's and postgraduate certificate level training in conservation medicine for Australian and overseas veterinarians via distance education or on-campus study. Perth Zoo veterinary staff are involved collaboratively in the development and delivery of some units offered in the postgraduate degrees in Conservation Medicine.

The NZCCM (http://www.conservationmedicine. co.nz), based at the Auckland Zoo, hosts a 3-year postgraduate Residency in Conservation Medicine program in collaboration with New Zealand and Australian universities. The program offers a combination of research on a conservation medicine project and hands-on training in zoological medicine. The center also offers field placements and externships for postgraduate and undergraduate students.

The Institute of Zoology of the Zoological Society of London and Royal Veterinary College (http:// www.zsl.org/science/postgraduate-study/msc-courses) offer a Master of Science (MSc) degree in Wild Animal Health and MSc in Wild Animal Biology, which have been designed for veterinarians and nonveterinarians, respectively.

The University of Liverpool (http://www.liv.ac.uk/ vets/study/vcm1.htm), offers a veterinary conservation medicine program as an intercalated honors Bachelor of Science (BSc) course for undergraduate veterinary students. A 3-year postgraduate program in conservation medicine is also provided in collaboration with Chester Zoo.

The Envirovet Summer Institute (http://www.cvm. uiuc.edu/envirovet) provides 7 weeks of intensive lecture, laboratory, and field experiences to veterinarians, veterinary students, and wildlife biologists in terrestrial and aquatic ecosystem health in developed and developing country contexts. The 2010 program highlights the transdisciplinary cooperative nature of work required for effective wildlife and ecosystem research, management, and long-term problem solving.

Acknowledgments

We thank all those who have made contributions to the development of conservation medicine to date. For contributions to this chapter, we are indebted to the following: Dr. Simone Vitali, Dr. Emily Lane, Dr. Steve Osofsky, Dr. Michelle Miller, Dr. Gretchen Kaufman, Dr. Rebecca Vaughan, Dr. Ivan Rubiano, Dr. Danielle Schrudde, and Dr. Darin Collins. We also thank our institutions and colleagues for support during the preparation of this manuscript.

REFERENCES

1. Armstrong D, Jakob-Hoff R, Seal US, editors: Animal movements and disease risk: a workbook, Apple Valley, Minn, 2001, Conservation Breeding Specialist Group.
2. Cook RA, Karesh WB: Emerging diseases at the interface of people, domestic animals and wildlife. In Fowler ME, Miller RE, editors: Zoo and wild animal medicine: current therapy, vol 6. St. Louis, 2008, Saunders Elsevier, pp 55–65.
3. Cook RA, Karesh WB, Osofsky SA: Conference summary: one world, one health: building interdisciplinary bridges to health in a globalized world. 2004 (http://www. oneworldonehealth.org/2004).
4. Cromarty P, McInnes K: Standard operating procedure for the health management of terrestrial vertebrate species protected under the wildlife health act (wildlife health SOP). Wellington, New Zealand, 2004, Department of Conservation.
5. Daszak P, Cunningham AA: Extinction by infection. Trends Ecol E 14:279, 1999.
6. Daszak P, Cunningham AA, Hyatt AD: Emerging infectious disease of wildlife—threats to biodiversity and human health. Science 287:443–449, 2000
7. Daszak P, Tabor GM, Kilpatrick AM, et al: Conservation medicine and a new agenda for emerging diseases. Ann N Y Acad Sci 1026:1–11, 2004.
8. Deem SL: Role of the zoo veterinarian in the conservation of captive and free-ranging wildlife. Int Zoo Yb 41:3–11, 2007.
9. Deem SL, Kilbourne AM, Wolfe ND, et al: Conservation medicine. Ann N Y Acad Sci 916:370–377, 2000.
10. Deem SL, Karesh WB, Weiseman W: Putting theory into practice: wildlife health in conservation. Cons Biol 15:224–1233, 2001.
11. English AW: The role of the veterinarian in the preservation of biodiversity. In editors: Proceedings of the annual conference of the Australian association of veterinary conservation biologists. Queensland, Australia, 1994, School of Animal Studies, University of Queensland, pp 5–10.
12. Franzmann AW: Veterinary contributions to international wildlife management. In Fowler ME, editor: Zoo and wild animal medicine: current therapy, vol 3. Philadelphia, 1993, WB Saunders, pp 42–44.
13. Friend M: Disease Emergence and resurgence: the wildlife-human connection. Reston, Va, U.S. Geological Survey, Circular 1285, 2006.
14. Jakob-Hoff R: First New Zealand symposium on conservation medicine. EcoHealth 2:372, 2005.
15. Jakob-Hoff R: Establishing a health profile for the North Island brown kiwi, *Apteryx australis mantelli*. Proceedings of veterinary conservation biology: wildlife health and management in Australasia, Taronga Zoo. Sydney, Australia, 2001, pp 135–139.
16. Jakob-Hoff R, Goold M, Reed C: Translocation of brown teal from captivity to the wild: the application of a new process for developing quarantine and health screening protocols. Proceedings of veterinary conservation biology: wildlife health and management in Australasia, Taronga Zoo. Sydney, Australia, 2001, pp 231–235.
17. Kaufman GE, Else J, Bowen K, et al: Bringing conservation medicine into the veterinary curriculum: the Tufts example. Ecohealth 1(Suppl 1):43–49, 2004.
18. Kaufman GE, Epstein JH, Paul-Murphy J, Modrall JD: Designing graduate training programs in conservation medicine—producing the right professionals with the right tools. EcoHealth 5:519–527, 2008.
19. Kock MD, Kock RA: Softly, softly: veterinarians and conservation practitioners working in the developed world. J Zoo Wildl Med 4:1–2, 2003.
20. Meffe GK: Conservation medicine. Cons Biol 13:53–954, 1999.
21. Miller PS: Tools and techniques for disease risk assessment in threatened wildlife conservation programmes. Int Zoo Yb 41:38–51, 2007.

22. Miller RE: Zoo veterinarians—doctors on the ark? JAVMA 200:542–547, 1992.
23. Mittermeier RA, Gil PR, Hoffman M, et al: Hotspots revisited: earth's biologically richest and most threatened terrestrial ecoregions. Chicago, 2005, Chicago University Press.
24. Myers N, Mittermeier RA, Mittermeier CG, et al: Biodiversity hotspots for conservation priorities. Nature 403:853–858, 2000.
25. Osofsky SA: Think link: critically evaluating linkages between conservation and development. J Zoo Wildl Med 28:141–143, 1997.
26. Osofsky SA, Karesh WB, Deem SL: Conservation medicine: a veterinary perspective. Cons Biol 14:336–337, 2000.
27. Ostfeld RS, Meffe GK, Pearl MC: Conservation medicine: the birth of another crisis discipline. In Aguirre AA, Tabor GM, Pearl MC, et al, editors: Conservation medicine: ecological health in practice, New York, 2002, Oxford University Press, pp 17–25.
28. Rabinowitz PM, Conti LA: Human-animal medicine—clinical approaches to zoonoses, toxicants, and other shared health risks. 2010, Saunders Elsevier.
29. Seebeck JH, Booth R: Eastern barred Bandicoot recovery: the role of the veterinarian in endangered species management. Proceedings of the annual conference of the Australian association of veterinary conservation biologists. Queensland, Australia, 1994, School of Animal Studies, University of Queensland, pp 50–51.
30. Sleeman JM: Use of wildlife rehabilitation centres as monitors of ecosystem health. In Fowler ME, Miller RE, editors: Zoo and wild animal medicine: current therapy, vol 6. St. Louis, 2008, Saunders Elsevier, pp 97–104.
31. Smith A, Clark P, Averis S, et al: Trypanosomes in a declining species of threatened Australian marsupial, the brush-tailed bettong *Bettongia penicillata* (Marsupialia: Potoroidae). Parasitology 135:1329–1335, 2008
32. Tabor GM: Defining conservation medicine. In Aguirre AA, Tabor GM, Pearl MC, et al, editors: Conservation medicine: ecological health in practice, New York, 2002, Oxford University Press, pp 8–14.
33. Warren K: Postgraduate veterinary training in conservation medicine: an interdisciplinary program at Murdoch University, Australia. EcoHealth 3:57–65, 2005.
34. World Association of Zoos and Aquariums: Building a Future for Wildlife—The World Zoo and Aquarium Conservation Strategy, 2005 (http://www.waza.org/files/webcontent/documents/cug/docs/WAZA%20CS.pdf).

CHAPTER 4

Veterinary Challenges of Mixed Species Exhibits

Jacques Kaandorp

Modern zoos like to show larger groups of animals, preferably in natural habitat–like mixed species exhibits, but it is not always easy to combine different species in one exhibit. The size of an exhibit is essential when mixing animals, especially when mixing larger mammals. Aviaries and aquaria are examples with a long-standing experience of combining various species, but in mammals this experience is often poor. Most often, zoos still show single species exhibits because of lack of space or simply to prevent problems associated with mixing different species. Safari parks in Europe were very popular in the 1960s, showing more natural displays of animals. However, because of the difficulties of handling animals in mixed exhibits, many of these parks later closed their gates. The parks that remained and still exist gained experience regarding which species may be kept together with others and which species shouldn't be mixed. The main advantage of mixed species enclosures is behavioral enrichment (Fig. 4-1) and the obvious educational value. There are even mixed species exhibits of carnivores. For example, Dierenrijk in Nuenen, The Netherlands, combines European grey wolves (*Canis lupus*) with European brown bears (*Ursus arctos*; Fig. 4-2) and Gelsenkirchen Zoo, Germany, combines arctic foxes (*Vulpes lagopus*) with Kodiak bears (*Ursus arctos middendorffi*; Fig. 4-3).

In this chapter, an incomplete listing of diseases and problems is presented to make the reader aware of the broad variety of veterinary challenges of mixed species exhibits. It is meant to encourage ideas and suggest further reading in veterinary literature about specific diseases and problems when mixing different species of animals. Veterinary problems arising because of keeping different species together may be categorized as trauma, nutrition-related problems, infectious diseases, and parasitic diseases.

TRAUMA

In mixed species exhibits, trauma is the most frequent and serious cause of health problems (Fig. 4-4).[6] Competition for nesting sites in birds, establishment of territories, and competition for food and watering stations in all taxa may provoke fighting and trauma in mixed exhibits such as aviaries and large exhibits of mammals. For example, young antelopes born outside will be chased in the beginning of their lives by curious zebras, leading to death or a fatal myopathy, as has also been seen in young or newborn giraffes[1] and antelopes. Play of young animals may not be understood by other species (Fig. 4-5). Pinioned birds fly in unrecognizable ways in the eyes of other animals and may become victims of other birds or mammals. Another factor is that when animals are frightened because of thunder or other events, or when animals are chased by other animals because of unexpected or differing circumstances, fleeing against fences or walls may cause fatal trauma.

Seasonal aggression, especially in deer (rut), may lead to interspecies conflicts, but different males of the Artiodactylae family will fight intraspecifically over their territory or interspecifically with other animals to protect their herd (Fig. 4-6). Antlers and horns are weapons capable of causing stab wounds, fractures, or even immediate death. Capping horns and cutting of antlers may limit the severity of trauma.[6]

After traumatic injuries, pathologic studies should always be carried out. For example, when birds kill one another, pathology often reveals underlying disease and explains the noticed aggression.[6]

To prevent trauma, next to appropriate size of the exhibit, pole gates (creeps), where small animals can flee from larger animals, creation of large obstacles in

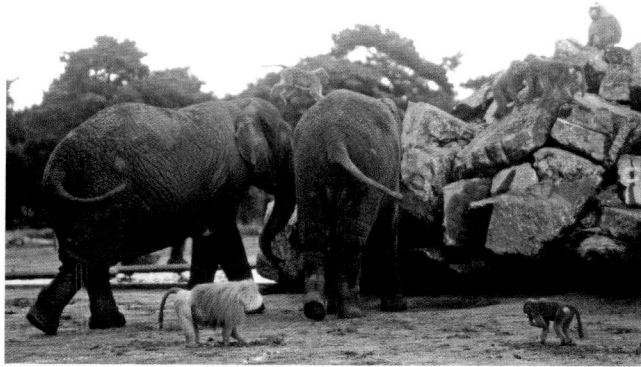

Figure 4-1

Hamadryas baboons *(Papio hamadryas)* enriched by living together with African elephants *(Loxodonta africana)* at Safaripark Beekse Bergen, Hilvarenbeek, The Netherlands.

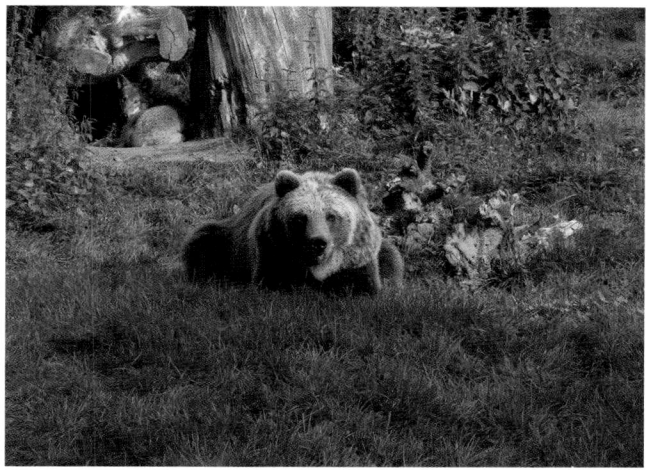

Figure 4-2

European grey wolves *(Canis lupus)* in "discussion" with European brown bears *(Ursus arctos)* at Dierenrijk, Nuenen, The Netherlands.

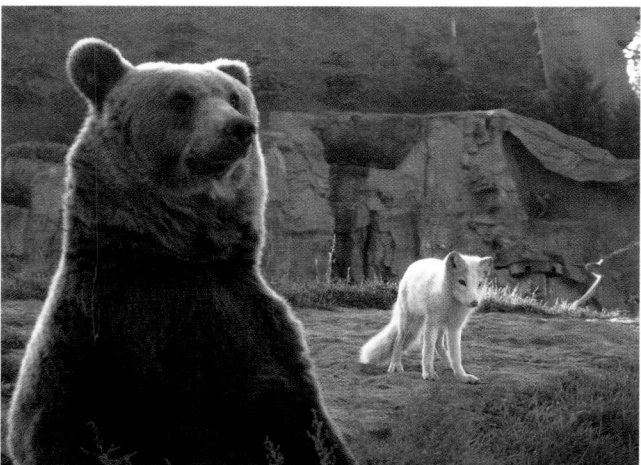

Figure 4-3

Arctic foxes *(Alopex lagopus)* peacefully living together with Kodiak bears *(Ursus arctos middendorffi)*, Gelsenkirchen, Germany.

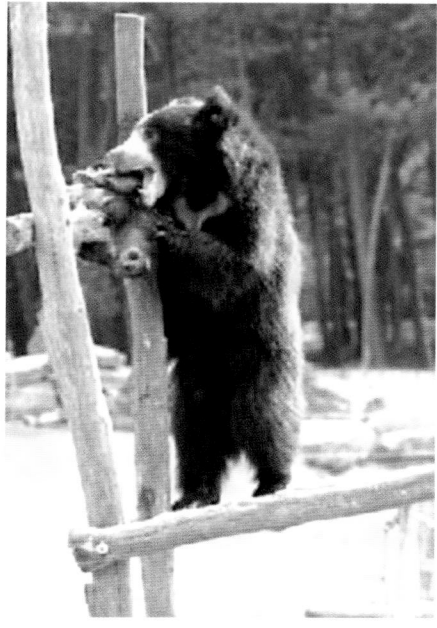

Figure 4-4

Sloth bear *(Ursus ursinus)* catching and eating a stump-tailed macaque *(Macaca arctoides)* at Safaripark Beekse Bergen, Hilvarenbeek, The Netherlands.

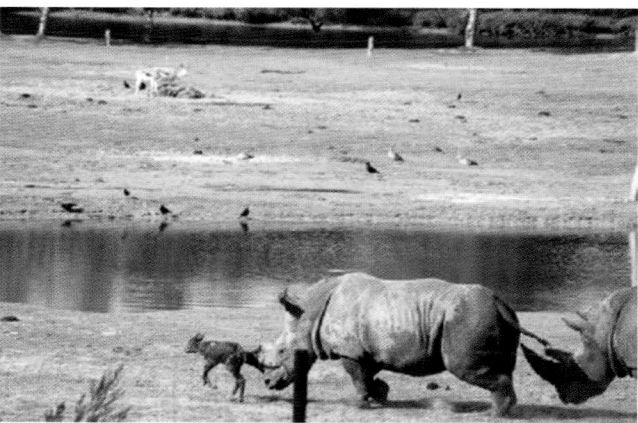

Figure 4-5

White rhinoceros *(Ceratotherium simum)* throwing a newborn African Ankole-Watusi calf *(Bovis Taurus[Watusi])* playfully around, but this caused no injury, at Safaripark Beekse Bergen, Hilvarenbeek, The Netherlands.

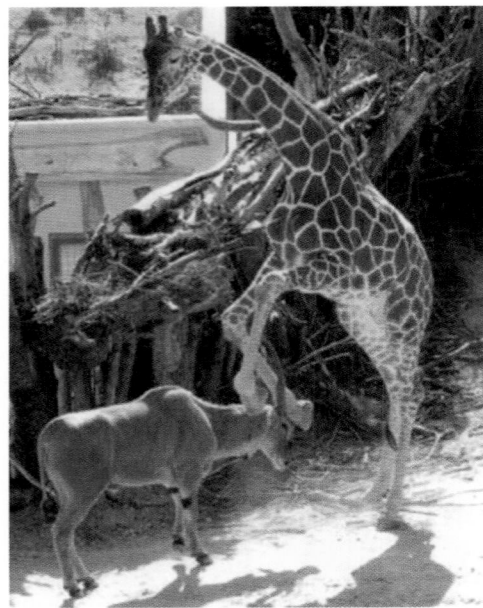

Figure 4-6

Giraffe *(Giraffa camelopardalis)* kicking an eland antelope *(Taurotragus oryx)* with the front legs.

exhibits so animals may circle around these when chased, hiding places, and provision of multiple feeding and watering sources are workable preventive measures when planning mixed exhibits.[6] There is no definition of an appropriate size, but for animal welfare reasons and to avoid trauma, exhibits should be as large as possible.

NUTRITION-RELATED PROBLEMS

Adequate nutrition is vital for every living being. In mixed exhibits, a sufficient number of feeding stations is essential to ensure that all animals may eat and at the same time prevent that some don't overeat.[6] Also, to prevent interspecies aggression, a sufficient number of feeding stations is necessary. Spreading food over larger areas in aviaries or among hoofstock prevents aggressiveness, and is even more effective when food is provided several times a day.

Free-flying wild birds may be a nuisance when feeding, such as kangaroos and birds (e.g., storks and cranes). A special configuration of feeding places may be helpful to prevent this. Precautions should be taken to prevent animals from not being able to eat enough and losing too much weight.

Requirements of trace minerals and other nutrients such as vitamins differ among species. Deficiencies such as copper deficiency in blesbok *(Damaliscus pygargus*

phillipsi) and sable antelope *(Hypotrachus niger)*, or toxicities such as vitamin E toxicity in pelicans or iron storage disease in birds and some primate species, should be avoided when developing feeding protocols for mixed species exhibits.[6] These should incorporate the specific needs and required feeding supplementations of the various species in a mixed exhibit.

INFECTIOUS DISEASES

Various herpesviruses are known to be responsible for disease outbreaks in mixed species exhibits. Other viruses such as rabies or bacteria (e.g., *Mycobacterium tuberculosis* complex) or a variety of endoparasite, ectoparasite, or fungal infections (e.g., aspergillosis) may each be detrimental in mixed exhibits, because not only one species will be infected, as in single-species exhibits. Measures to control these diseases may have an enormous impact on a collection and demands for an effective preventative veterinary protocol. Decisions about which species are to be housed together should be made based on this information.

Mammals

Malignant catarrhal fever (MCF) is probably the first infectious disease that a zoo veterinarian thinks of when asked about the risks of mixed exhibits. The gammaherpesvirus hosted by wildebeest *(Connochaetes* spp.), topi *(Damaliscus* spp.), hartebeest *(Alcelaphalus* spp.); (Alcelaphine herpesvirus 1 [AIHV-1]), sheep (subfamily Ovinae; ovine herpesvirus 2 [OvHV-2]) and goats (subfamily Caprinae; caprine herpesvirus 2 [CpHV-2]) is shed (mostly) around parturition and may infect other species. Giraffes *(Giraffa camelopardis)*, muskox *(Ovibos moschatus)*, European and American bison *(Bison bonasus* and *Bison bison)*, muntjac *(Muntiacus* species), Pere David's deer *(Elaphurus davidianus)*, moose *(Alces alces)*, kudu *(Tragelaphus* spp.) and other deer *(Cervidae* spp.), gaur *(Bos gaurus)*, and banteng *(Bos javanicus)* are especially susceptible to these diseases.[4,5] In white-tailed deer *(Odocoileus virginianus)*, a new MCF virus has been recognized that causes classic MCF. Do not mix wildebeest with giraffes and preferably get rid of all sheep and goats in a zoo collection. Carrier species should at least not be in breeding situations in direct contact or close to susceptible species. There are examples of zookeepers owning sheep at home that transmitted the virus to giraffes, resulting in high mortality.[7] It is questionable whether zookeepers should be allowed to take care of household sheep and goats at home.

Equine herpesvirus 1 has led to problems with Bactrian camel *(Camelus bactrianus)*, llama *(Lama glama)*, and a Thompson's gazelle *(Gazella thomsoni)*.[6] The virus is shed by infected horses *(Equus caballus)*, zebra *(E. grevyi, E. zebra, E. quagga)*, and onager *(E. hemionus)* during respiratory infection, parturition, and abortion. Vaccination is no guarantee for preventing an outbreak. When introducing equids into mixed exhibits, it is advisable to use only seronegative equids.

Mixed exhibits with ruminants should be monitored serologically for diseases such as leptospirosis, brucellosis, infectious bovine rhinotracheitis (IBR; bovine herpesvirus 1 [BHV-1]), bovine virus diarrhea (BVD), tuberculosis *(Mycobacterium tuberculosis, M. bovis)*, paratuberculosis *(M. avium* subsp. *paratuberculosis)*, leucosis (enzootic bovine leucosis, bovine leukemia virus), neosporosis *(Neospora caninum)*, bovine respiratory syncytial virus (BRSV; e.g., ovine lentivirus, Maedi–Visna)—because most of these diseases spread between different ruminant species. Brucellosis, leptospirosis, and tuberculosis will also affect numerous other mammalian species.[4]

The following are other mammalian diseases[4]:

- CWD (chronic wasting disease) or TSE (transmissible spongiform encephalopathy) is a prion-caused disease capable of spreading in mixed deer exhibits possibly by the fecal-oral route. This has occurred and is still occurring in the U.S. deer population.
- EMC *(Encephalomyocarditis virus)* causes mortality in Suidae, Proboscidea, Pongidae, Cercopithecidae, Antelopidae, Camelidae, Tapiridae, Lemuridae, Cebidae, Rodentia, and Marsupialia. Rodents are thought to be the vector of the disease. Vector control is essential, especially in mixed exhibits.
- Cowpox (cowpox virus) spreads in many species from squirrels *(Sciuridae)* to okapi *(Okapia)*, (Asian) elephants (Elephantidae), rhinoceroses *(Rhinocerotidae)*, and many cats *(Felidae* spp.).
- Parapoxvirus is seen in Ovidae, Capridae, and muskox *(Ovibos moschatus)*, spreads among these animals, and causes ulcerative dermatosis and contagious ecthyma (orf).
- Monkeypox (monkeypox virus) may infect humans, nonhuman primates, rodents, lagomorphs, and even anteaters *(Vermilingua* spp.). African rodents appear to be natural hosts. Prairie dogs were well-known victims in the 2003 U.S. outbreak.

Rotaviruses (neonatal calf diarrhea syndrome) and coronaviruses are found in many different mammalian species. There are many carriers of these viruses. Coronaviruses are also known to cause winter dysentery in adult ruminants.[6]

Primates

Spider monkeys (subfamily Ateles) and squirrel monkeys *(Saimiri sciureus)* should not be placed in mixed exhibits with other primates. Squirrel monkeys are hosts of two herpesviruses *(Herpesvirus tamarinus, H. saimiri)* and spider monkeys may transfer *H. ateles* to callitrichids, aotids, marmosets, and tamarins, causing fatal disease in these species.[6]

Rhesus macaques *(Macaca mulatta)* and other macaques may host *H. simiae* (HVB or, most recently, cercopithecine HV-1) and is transmitted by biting and scratching and by dried secretions—for example, to Colobus monkeys *(Colobus guereza)*.[6] Do not mix African and Asian monkeys. At least, macaques should be seronegative for HVs when housed in mixed exhibits. Another herpesvirus, the simian varicella group (SVV), is hosted by macaques; it produces mild, self-limiting signs in the host species but may be fatal in patas monkeys *(Erythrocebus patas)* and other African cercopithecines. Simian hemorrhagic fever (SHF) and simian immunodeficiency virus (SIV) are other reasons not to mix African and Asian monkeys, because they will spread among these primates.

In mixed primate exhibits, salmonellosis, campylobacteriasis, bordetellosis, and shigellosis should be monitored as preventive measures.[4]

Marine Mammals

In marine mammals (cetaceans, pinnipedia), *Morbillivirus, Orthopoxvirus,* and *Parapoxvirus* infections may occur when water systems are connected between basins.[6] The *Morbillivirus* outbreak in the north of the Netherlands, Germany, and Denmark has shown that vaccination using canine distemper virus (CDV–ISCOM) (immune-stimulating complex) vaccine is effective in protecting harbor seals *(Phoca vitulina)* from phocid distemper in 1988. This vaccine from Erasmus University, Rotterdam, The Netherlands, halted the spread of the disease. Using inactivated canine distemper virus will do the same, but is not allowed for use in the European Union (EU).

Birds

Avian herpesviruses such as the Pacheco disease virus may be carried by conures and should be taken into account when mixing birds; they may cross to different species and cause devastating outbreaks in other species of psittacine birds.[6] Avipoxvirus infections are seen in mixed aviaries because a variety of birds are susceptible to the virus.[4]

Amphibians and Reptiles

Tortoises are also known for herpesviruses that will spread among different species. Some species act as reservoirs, whereas other species show high mortality.[6] Another herpesvirus causing fibropapillomatosis is seen in various marine turtles.[4] Gray patch disease in marine turtles is probably also caused by a herpesvirus. It requires the same strict regimen of hygienic measures and quarantine as the other herpesviruses when mixing these animals.

Ophidian paramyxovirus may be transmitted between snakes. Viperids show a variety of susceptibility to this virus and may infect other groups of snakes, such as boids, elaphids and colubrids.[4] Mixed exhibits of amphibian species may have an extra chance of outbreaks of chytridiomycosis caused by *Batrachochytrium dentrobatidis*. Frogs, toads, salamanders, and others are susceptible. In amphibians, the spread of adenovirus infections among lizards, snakes, and crocodiles may only be prevented by in-house biosecurity measures.

Broad Interspecies Infectious Diseases

West Nile virus (WNV) is a vector-borne disease noted in almost 300 species of birds and a variety of domestic and exotic mammals. Using the U.S. data acquired after the WNV outbreak in recent years, vaccination protocols and vector control should be proactively discussed before WNV becomes endemic in Europe.[4]

Salmonella spp. (especially *S. typhimurium* and *S. enteridius*) in mixed bird exhibits and in reptile departments in zoos are difficult to control. Also, among mammals, different *Salmonella* spp. may result in high morbidity and mortality.[4]

Yersinia pseudotuberculosis and *Y. enterocolitica* are responsible for mortality in various species of birds, rodents, and primates (e.g., squirrel monkeys, *Saimirinae*). Often, transmission occurs through uninvited vector species (e.g., rats, mice, wild birds) who share a mixed exhibit with collection species.[4]

Chlamydophila psittaci affects psittacines, passerines, and columbiformes. This well-known zoonosis may also cause significant infections in other nonavian species.[4]

Fungal diseases are seen in all taxa. *Trichophyton* spp., *Microsporum* spp., aspergillosis, candidiasis, *Malassezia*,

cryptococcosis, and histoplasmosis are examples of pathogens and diseases that may cause severe problems in mixed species exhibits.[4]

Mycobacteriosis in the form of paratuberculosis or the mycobacteriaceae responsible for the tuberculosis complex are not easy to control in mixed species exhibits.

Bacterial infections such as leptospirosis, erysipelas, listeriosis, pseudomoniasis, and infections caused by enterobacteria and *Clostridia* are found in many species. They are responsible for an enormous variety of disease problems, especially in mixed species exhibits.[4]

Almost all notifiable diseases as listed in Table 4-1 are enemies of mixed species exhibits. Famous examples are foot-and-mouth disease, African horse sickness, avian influenza, vesicular stomatitis, rabies, anthrax, and Newcastle disease.[2]

PARASITIC DISEASES

Many parasites have a broad host range and are a threat in mixed species exhibits. One animal imported into a collection may be hazardous not only to its own species, but also other species in mixed species exhibits.

Protozoal parasites easily contaminate exhibit substrates. Preventive protocols should be taken to avoid serious problems. In mixed primate exhibits, various protozoal infections may be seen and may cause problems such as gastric amoebiasis, giardiosis, hexamitiasis, trichomoniasis, and cryptosporidiosis. It is popular to mix gorillas in exhibits with other African species such as Colobus monkeys *(C. guereza)* and mangabeys (Fig. 4-7). However, be careful when mixing them, because cercopithecine monkeys are often carriers of *Balantidium coli*. All great apes, especially gorillas, may become very ill from these infections.[4,6]

Toxoplasmosis may be found in all vertebrates and may be spread by all felid species. In mixed aviaries, *Trichomonas* spp. are common in columbiforms but may spread to passeriforms or psittacines, who may become seriously ill.[6] Puffins and penguins are very susceptible to *Plasmodium* infections causing avian malaria. The infection is endemic in many continental birds in Europe and North America and, from these carrier birds, the disease is spread to the susceptible penguins and puffins by mosquito vectors. Antimalarial drugs as a preventive measure are widely used in these birds. Another protozoal parasite, *Neospora caninum*, causes abortions in some herbivores.

Endoparasites such as nematodes, trematodes, and cestodes should also be monitored in mixed species

TABLE 4-1	Notifiable Diseases (in Europe)*
Disease	**Affected Animals**
African horse sickness	Equidae
African swine fever	Suidae and Tayassuidae
American foul brood	*Apis* spp.
Anthrax	Bovidae, Camelidae, Cervidae, Elephantidae, Equidae, and Hippopotamidae
Avian influenza	Aves
Blue tongue	Antilocapridae, Bovidae, Cervidae, Giraffidae, and Rhinocerotidae
Brucella abortus	Antilocapridae, Bovidae, Camelidae, Cervidae, Giraffidae, Hippopotamidae, and Tragulidae
Brucella melitensis infection	Antilocapridae, Bovidae, Camelidae, Cervidae, Giraffidae, Hippopotamidae, and Tragulidae
Brucella ovis infection	Camelidae, Tragulidae, Cervidae, Giraffidae, Bovidae, and Antilocapridae
Brucella suis infection	Cervidae, Leporidae, *Ovibos moschatus*, Suidae, and Tayassuidae
Classic swine fever	Suidae and Tayassuidae
Contagious bovine pleuropneumonia	Bovidae (including zebu, buffalo, bison, and yak)
Foot-and-mouth disease	Artiodactyla and Asian elephants
Infectious hematopoeitic necrosis	Salmonidae
Lumpy skin disease	Bovidae and Giraffidae
Monkeypox	Rodentia and nonhuman primates
Mycobacterium bovis infection	Mammalia—in particular Antilocapridae, Bovidae, Camelidae, Cervidae, Giraffidae, and Tragulidae
Newcastle disease	Aves
Peste des petits ruminants	Bovidae and Suidae
Porcine enterovirus encephalomyelitis	Suidae
Psittacosis	Psittaciformes
Rabies	Carnivora and Chiroptera
Rift Valley fever	Bovidae, Camelus spp., and Rhinocerotidae
Rinderpest	Artiodactyla
Sheep and goat pox	Bovidae
Swine vesicular disease	Suidae and Tayassuidae
TSE	Bovidae, Cervidae, Felidae, and Mustelidae
Vesicular stomatitis	Artiodactyla and Equidae

*In the context of Council Directive 92/65 EC, July 1992 (http://eur-lex.europa.eu/LexUriServ/LexUriServ.do?uri=CONSLEG:1992L0065:20040703: EN:PDF).[2,5]

exhibits because many of them cross species lines. Every large animal practitioner knows not to keep horses and donkeys together—donkeys are carriers of lungworms, without clinical problems, but horses are vulnerable to these parasites. Mixing a variety of artiodactylids will lead to a burden of possible parasitical infections, especially enteric nematode infections.[6] In mixed aviaries, helminths are potentially lethal among birds (especially *Capillaria* spp. and *Syngamus trachea*) and preventive measures are a necessity.

Ectoparasites such as *Sarcoptes* and *Chorioptes* spp. are capable of affecting different, often related species and are not always easy to control in larger mixed species exhibits.

TOOLS FOR VETERINARIANS IN MIXED SPECIES EXHIBITS

Veterinary population management of mixed species exhibits pose a challenge for zoo veterinarians. Preventive measures and monitoring on an annual basis are necessary to prevent infectious disease outbreaks and parasitologic overload. Some tools that may be used are the following:

1. Observation, common sense, knowledge gained by experience, and the use of as many academic information sources as possible are important tools for a zoo veterinarian. To observe and understand gathered knowledge is to learn to

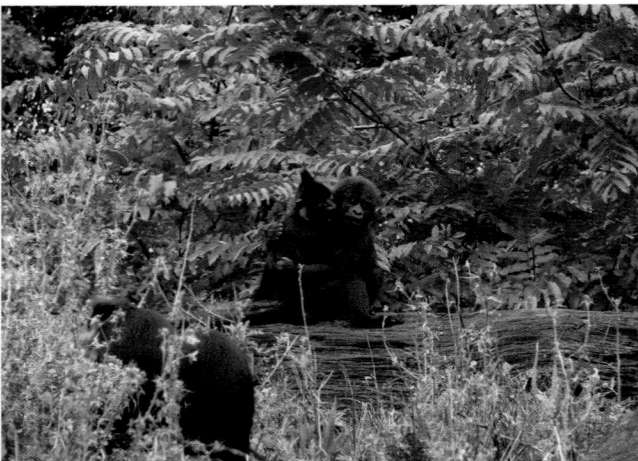

Figure 4-7

Black-crested mangabey *(Lophocebus aterrimus)* in heat presenting to a silverback Western lowland gorilla *(Gorilla gorilla gorilla)* at GaiaPark, Kerkrade, The Netherlands.

adjust and apply protocols to avoid problems. The European Association of Zoo and Wildlife Veterinarians (EAZWV)—Infectious Diseases Working Group (IDWG) *Transmissible Diseases Handbook*[2] is available at http://www.eaza.net and http://www.eazwv.org. It includes chapters on cleaning and disinfection, vaccination, postmortem procedures, blue tongue, tuberculosis, and European legislation. Various links to important associations and the OIE (Office International des Epizooties [World Animal Health Organisation]) may be found, along with a list of national and OIE laboratories. Fact sheets on diseases lists experts to contact when disease outbreaks occur.

2. Laboratory studies using feces, saliva, hair, soil, water, vectors, environment, plants, and postmortem samples and more invasive sampling for bacteriology, skin scraping, blood work, serology, and biopsy are diagnostic tools that provide information about whether diseases may affect other species in an exhibit.
3. In a preventive regimen, vaccination may be used against a variety of infections such as pseudotuberculosis caused by *Yersinia pseudotuberculosis*, blue tongue virus (various serotypes), Q fever, avian influenza (H5N2), avipox, cowpox (e.g., in elephants), tetanus, other Clostridiae (cocktails), pasteurellosis,

bordetellosis, canine distemper, parvovirosis, leptospirosis, rabies, feline panleucopenia, feline HV and calicivirus (feline rhinotracheitis), feline leukemia (FeLV), chlamydophila (cats), and dermatophytosis (ringworm). Many of these vaccines prevent diseases that may occur in different species, spread by animals directly or by humans by carrying them into exhibits. Vector control is an important tool to prevent diseases such as pseudotuberculosis, tularemia, pox in elephants, malaria, blue tongue virus, rabies, and lymphocytic choriomeningitis in callitrichids. In general, vectors capable of bringing pathogens into exhibits are numerous. Insects, rodents, free-flying birds, feral cats and dogs, foxes, and raccoons are known vectors; in addition, humans may transport pathogens into exhibits.[6] Many great ape diseases are directly related to human-animal contacts and pathogens may be transported by humans from elsewhere in the zoo and/or imported from outside the zoo, as noted earlier. Of known infectious diseases, 70% are zoonotic.

4. Quarantine and pretransport measures such as deworming and pretransport diagnostics (e.g., serology, bacteriology, parasitology) are essential tools to prevent potential hazards when introductions are planned into mixed exhibits. Preshipment protocols are especially important for megavertebrates when quarantine is not easily performed.
5. Parasite control, pathology, and necropsy programs are essential preventive tools. The adequate administration of results may lead to proper and timely adjustments of preventive measures.[6]
6. Foot baths and other hygienic measurements as part of a well-controlled biosecurity protocol are tools that may be used not only when disease outbreaks occur.[4,6]

Zoo veterinarians need to be supported by zoo directors, curators, zookeepers, and architects when designing and developing mixed species exhibits to avoid wrong choices and establish a preventive regimen beforehand.[3]

Acknowledgment

I would like to thank Christine Kaandorp-Huber for her patience, support, positive criticism, and technical assistance.

REFERENCES

1. Kaandorp-Huber CM: Personal communication, 2008.
2. Kaandorp J: Transmissible diseases handbook: European association of zoo and wildlife veterinarians, ed 2, Houten, The Netherlands, 2004, Van Setten Kwadraat, pp 74–75.
3. Kaandorp J: GVP (good veterinary practice) regarding (emerging) infectious diseases—a political issue? Presented at the 7th Scientific Meeting of the European Association of Zoo and Wildlife Veterinarians, Leipzig, Germany, Apil-May 2008.
4. Kaandorp J: Transmissible diseases handbook, ed 4, Hilvarenbeek, The Netherlands, 2010, European Association of Zoo and Wildlife Veterinarians–Infectious Diseases Working Group.
5. Kik MJL, Kaandorp S, Melissen A: Malignant catarrhal fever in two closely related zoos in The Netherlands. Presented at the 42nd Scientific Meeting of the Institute for Zoo and Wildlife Research, Prague, 2005.
6. Lowenstine LJ: Health problems in mixed-species exhibits. In Fowler ME, Miller RE editors: Zoo and wild animal medicine: current therapy, vol 4. Philadelphia, 1999, WB Saunders, pp 26–29.
7. Schaftenaar W: Personal communication, 1995.

CHAPTER 5

Cowpox in Zoo Animals

Andreas Kurth and Andreas Nitsche

CAUSE

Cowpox virus (CPXV) belongs to the genus *Orthopoxvirus* (OPV) of the family Poxviridae. Virions are enveloped with a high tenacity, appear brick-shaped, have a size of approximately 200 nm in diameter and 350 nm in length, and carry their genomes of approximately 230 kbp in single, linear, double-stranded segments of DNA.[10] Other members of the OPV are important pathogens in veterinary and human medicine, including monkeypox, vaccinia, and camelpox virus and, with lesser importance, raccoon pox, skunk pox, and vole pox virus. The different species of OPV are serologically indistinguishable from each other. Although taxonomically classified as cowpox virus, the terms *elephantpox*, *catpox*, and *ratpox virus* are used synonymously in the scientific community, depending on the animal species from which the respective virus was isolated.

HISTORY

Attention was first drawn to poxviruses infecting exotic zoo animals in 1960, still in the era of smallpox vaccination, when two captive Asian elephants died at the Zoological Garden in Leipzig, Germany.[22] At that time, the causative agent was believed to be vaccinia virus (VACV) that had most probably been transmitted to the elephants by recently vaccinated children. However, this hypothesis was never verified. The fact that mandatory smallpox vaccination was abolished in Europe in 1980, with poxvirus outbreaks still occurring in continental European and British zoos and circuses, argues against VACV as the causative agent. To date, more than 30 such outbreaks have been reported, affecting various species (Table 5-1). Virus isolates obtained from these animals have been retrospectively characterized as CPXV. Several often fatal infections in zoo and circus elephants have been reported mainly from Germany (see Table 5-1).

EPIDEMIOLOGY

CPXV are endemic in Europe and western parts of Russia[10] and naturally infect a broad range of host species, including domestic animals (cats and pet rats) and zoo animals, as well as humans. Interestingly, cowpox is not enzootic in cattle. Instead, cattle, like humans, are merely incidental hosts of CPXV. Almost 50 years after CPXV was first detected in a species other than cattle, new CPXV hosts are still being discovered and reported, and serologic studies have determined more wild and exotic animals that are potentially susceptible to CPXV. Elephants are the most frequently infected exotic animals. Over 60 cases of elephantpox virus infections have been reported from Germany. Therefore, today, most elephants are regularly vaccinated with vaccinia virus, which provides reliable protection against OPV infections. Hence, only sporadic cases still occur in unvaccinated elephants. The second most frequently infected group are exotic felids, with CPXV outbreaks being reported from the United Kingdom, continental Europe, and Russia. In general, exotic zoo animals that are housed in close proximity to other zoo animals and come into direct contact with wild rodents and animal keepers are likely to have a higher risk of acquiring a CPXV infection. Such circumstances were key factors for larger outbreaks involving animals of different species in Moscow in 1973-1974, Berlin in 1997, Almere, The Netherlands, in 2003, and Krefeld, Germany, in 2008.[11,15,17,18] An intraspecies transmission could be observed repeatedly, with varying clinical symptoms, indicating different virus susceptibilities among vertebrates that possibly depend on the specific CPXV strain. Nevertheless, despite the wide host range of CPXV, only few infections of different animal species have been reported to be caused by the same CPXV strain. Similarly, conclusive evidence for the cocirculation of different CPXV strains

TABLE 5-1 Cowpoxvirus-Infected Exotic Animals (Except Muroidae)

Study (Year)	Order/Family	Species	Geographic Origin (No. of Outbreaks)	No. of Animals With Clinical Signs/Fatal Cases
Schüppel et al (1994)[24]	Artiodactyla/Camelidae	Llama (Lama glama pacos)	Germany	7/5
Basse et al (1963)[1]	Artiodactyla/Giraffidae	Okapi (Okapia johnstoni)	Denmark	2/1
Zwart et al (1968)[27]	Artiodactyla/Giraffidae	Okapi (Okapia johnstoni)	The Netherlands	5/1
Hentschke et al (1997)[11]	Carnivora/Ailuridae	Red panda (Ailurus fulgens)	Germany	2/2
Marennikova et al (1973)[17]	Carnivora/Felidae	Lion (Panthera leo)	Russia	3/3
Marennikova et al (1973)[17]	Carnivora/Felidae	Black panther (Panthera padus)	Russia	1/1
Marennikova et al (1973)[17]	Carnivora/Felidae	Cheetah (Acinonyx jubatus)	Russia	2/2
Baxby et al (1977)[2]	Carnivora/Felidae	Cheetah (Acinonyx jubatus)	England	3/2
Baxby et al (1978)[2]	Carnivora/Felidae	Cheetah (Acinonyx jubatus)	England	3/2
Marennikova et al (1973-1974)[17]	Carnivora/Felidae	Puma (Felis concolor)	Russia	5/3
Marennikova et al (1973)[17]	Carnivora/Felidae	Jaguar (Felis onca)	Russia	2/0
Marennikova et al (1973)[17]	Carnivora/Felidae	Ocelot (Felis pardalis)	Russia	2/1
Marennikova et al (1974)[17]	Carnivora/Felidae	Far eastern cat (Felis bengalis)	Russia	nk/ euthanized
Kurth et al (2008)[15]	Carnivora/Felidae	Jaguarundi (Herpailurus yagouaroundi)	Germany	2/1
Kurth et al (2008)[15]	Carnivora/Herpestidae	Banded mongoose (Mungos mungo)	Germany	13/13
Eulenberger et al, Pilaski and Jacoby (1977, 2004)[9,21]	Perissodactyla/ Rhinocerotidae	Black rhinoceros (Diceros bicornis)	Germany	2/1
Pilaski and Jacoby (1977)[21]	Perissodactyla/ Rhinocerotidae	White rhinoceros (Ceratotherium s. simum)	Germany	2/0
Marennikova et al (1973)[17]	Pilosa/ Myrmecophagidae	Anteater (Myrmecophaga tridactyla)	Russia	2/2
Martina et al (2003)[18]	Primate/ Cercopithecidae	Macaques (Macaca spec.)	The Netherlands	3/3
Matz-Rensing et al (2002)[19]	Primate/Callitrichidae	New world monkeys	Germany	nk/30
Kurth et al, Pilaski and Jacoby, Wisser et al (1960-2007)[15,21,25]	Proboscidea/ Elephantidae	Asian elephant (Elephas maximus)	Germany	>45/>8
Kubin et al (1974)[13]	Proboscidea/ Elephantidae	Asian elephant (Elephas maximus)	Austria	1/0
Essbauer (nk)*	Proboscidea/ Elephantidae	Asian elephant (Elephas maximus)	France	nk/nk
Pilaski and Jacoby (1973)[21]	Proboscidea/ Elephantidae	Asian elephant (Elephas maximus)	The Netherlands	nk/nk
Pilaski and Jacoby (1977)[21]	Proboscidea/ Elephantidae	Asian elephant (Elephas maximus)	Poland	nk/nk
Pilaski and Jacoby (1972)[21]	Proboscidea/ Elephantidae	Asian elephant (Elephas maximus)	Czech Republic	nk/nk
Pilaski and Jacoby (1960-1990)[21]	Proboscidea/ Elephantidae	African elephant (Loxodonta africana)	Germany (7)	>15/2
Hentschke et al (1997)[11]	Rodentia/Castoridae	Beaver (Castor fibor canadensis)	Germany	10/10
Kik et al (2006)[12]	Rodentia/Caviidae	Patagonian cavy (Dolichotis patagonum)	The Netherlands	5/5
Nitsche (2007)*	Rodentia/Caviidae	Patagonian cavy (Dolichotis patagonum)	Germany	6/6

nk, Not known.
*Unpublished.

within the same geographic region has only rarely been provided.[4]

A definite source of infection has only occasionally been identified. Although serologic surveys have demonstrated a high proportion of seropositive bank voles *(Clethrionomys glareolus)*, field voles *(Microtus agrestis)*, and wood mice *(Apodemus sylvaticus)*,[3,5,7,15,20,23] no CPXV isolate has been obtained from these species so far. Because mice have never been found to be CPXV-positive, both wild rats[16,18] and white rats bred as food for carnivores[15,17] have to be considered the most likely source in transmitting a CPXV infection to exotic animals. In this respect, the role of rats remains to be elucidated. Rats could be either a primary reservoir or an amplifying host. However, in most reports, it is only speculated that the source of infection are wild rodents, particularly mice, as they are believed to be the main reservoir for CPXV.

PATHOGENESIS

The clinical picture of CPXV infection in different animals is rather similar, regardless of the infected species, and mostly results in localized or multiple lesions on the skin (Fig. 5-1) and mucous membranes (Fig. 5-2). Less often, animals suffer from pulmonary symptoms without skin lesions or from a generalized rash (Fig. 5-3). CPXV infections are epitheliotropic, often starting as vesicular lesions and then developing

into a pustule with an indented center and a raised erythematous border. This may be followed by a secondary bacterial infection. On the cellular level, CPXV infections result in the production of strongly eosinophilic A–type inclusion bodies in the cytoplasm of infected cells. The mortality among exotic animals and felids is high, although in most reports exact data are lacking.

DIAGNOSIS

Swab or biopsy samples can be used to confirm a cowpox virus infection. Direct poxvirus detection methods include histopathologic examination of biopsy tissues for typical inclusion bodies, electron microscopy for the detection of typical poxvirus particles, or polymerase chain reaction (PCR) assay (real-time PCR) for the detection of OPV DNA (summarized by Kurth and Nitsche[14]). Several real-time PCR-based assays have been published that identify and type OPV in less than 2 hours after the specimen's arrival in the laboratory, either by specific amplification or detection of the virus species or by fluorescence melting curve analysis following the PCR reaction. Recently, pyrosequencing-based techniques have found their way into rapid viral typing. However, the best PCR-based approach established to identify OPV species is by sequencing the open reading frame of the hemagglutinin gene and comparing the sequences obtained to the 193 sequences that have been published in GenBank, the National Institutes of Health

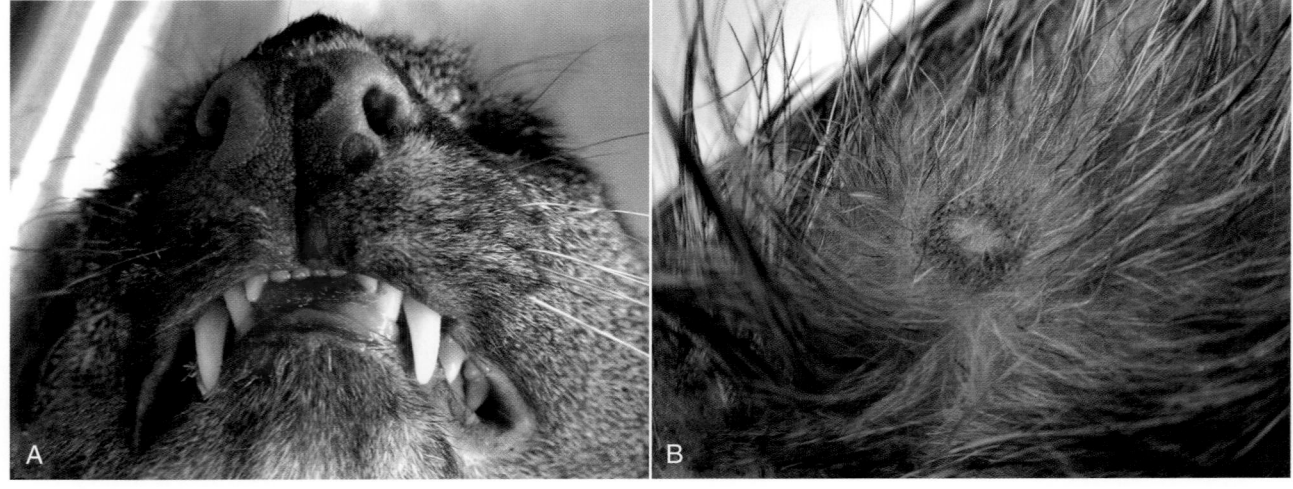

Figure 5-1

Typical cowpoxvirus lesions in zoo animals. **A,** Multiple cutaneous lesions. Note the round punched-out erosions at the mucosal surface of nose and lips of this jaguarundi. **B,** Localized subacute to chronic epidermal lesion with scarring on the body of a mongoose. *(Courtesy Dr. A. Kuczka.)*

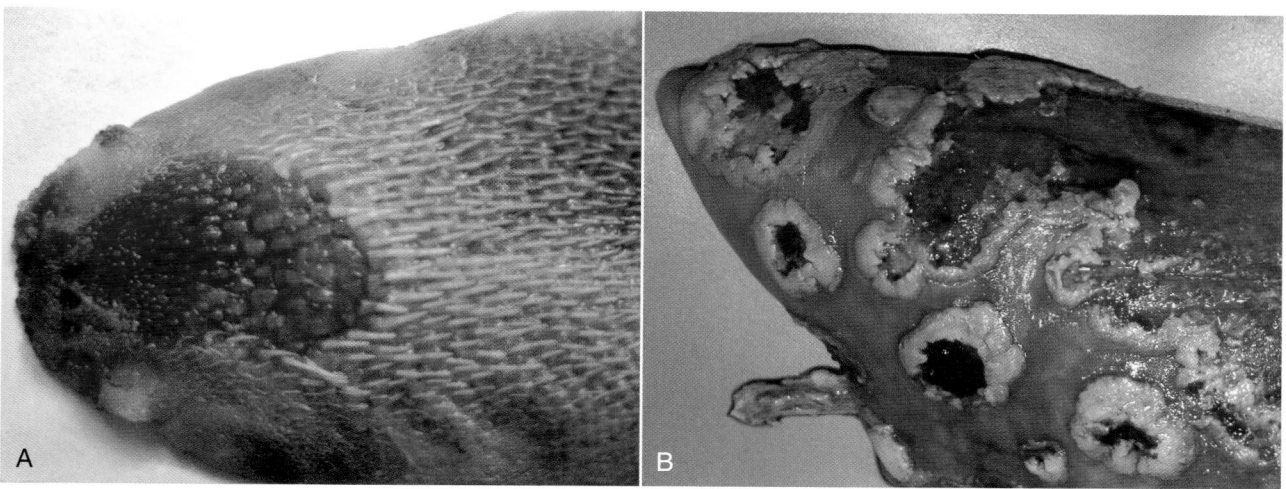

Figure 5-2

Cowpoxvirus lesions on mucous membranes. **A,** Typical lesions at the dorsal aspect of the tongue of a jaguarondi. **B,** Pathognomonic poxvirus lesions with extensive ulceration of the mucosal membrane of the tongue in an Asian elephant. *(A Courtesy Dr. A. Kuczka; B courtesy Dr. G. Wibbelt.)*

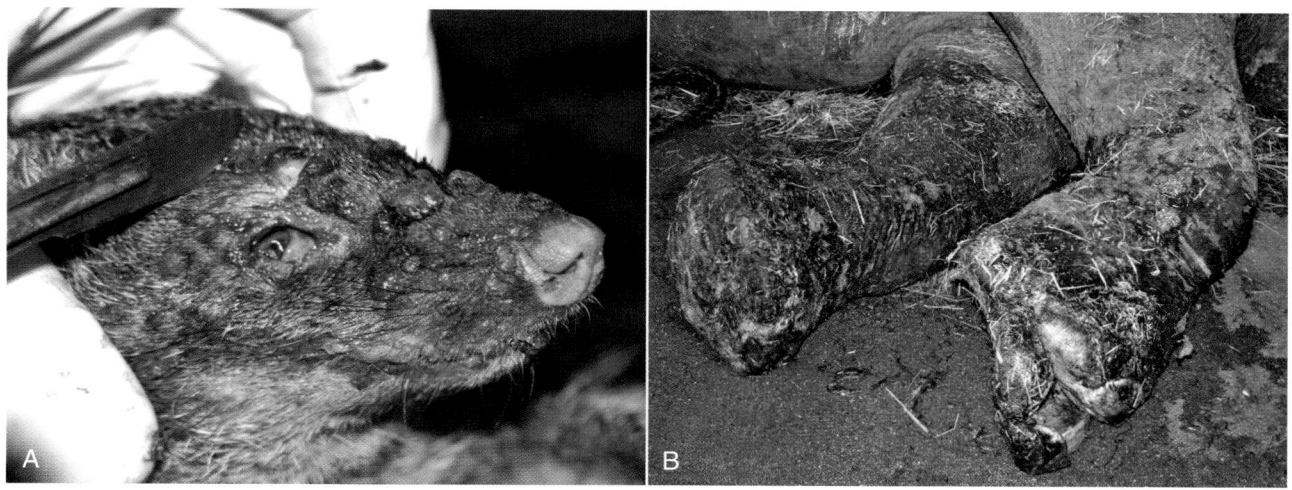

Figure 5-3

Generalized cowpoxvirus infection. **A,** Acute lesions on the head of a mongoose. **B,** Severe skin ulcerations and laminitis with sloughing (left leg) or loss (right leg) of hoof shoes in an Asian elephant. *(A Courtesy Dr. A. Kuczka; B courtesy Dr. G. Wibbelt.)*

genetic sequence database, to date (March 2010). Comprehensive virologic and serologic poxvirus testing is currently only available on a case by case basis in specialized laboratories. After the onset of clinical symptoms in an animal, poxvirus-specific antibodies in sera can be determined by immunofluorescence assay, plaque reduction test, or enzyme-linked immunosorbent assay (ELISA). Detected antibodies are not cowpox virus–specific but can indicate an OPV infection and are therefore useful tools in retrospective studies.

TREATMENT AND VACCINATION

Because no effective and approved treatment for animals in case of CPXV infection is available (e.g., previous trials with gammaglobulin were not successful[2] and the new therapeutic compound ST-246 is not yet approved[26]), only prophylactic vaccination might protect susceptible zoo animals. Elephants have been routinely vaccinated with the attenuated modified vaccinia virus Ankara (MVA) strain of vaccinia virus,[8,15,25] resulting in a prolonged immune response that protects the immunized animals from a symptomatic CPXV infection—there have been no reports of vaccinated elephants becoming infected by CPXV. For other exotic zoo animals, very little is known about successful vaccination and immune response to a cowpox infection. As recognized in a jaguarundi during a CPXV outbreak,[15] the early establishment of a significant OPV-specific antibody titer during a CPXV infection seems crucial for survival. This case highlights the need for further extended vaccination studies leading to increased efforts toward the general vaccination of potentially susceptible and rare exotic animals. In a study without CPXV challenge,[15] a significant increase of the antibody titer was achieved in all vaccinated felids (including cheetah, jaguar, tiger, snow leopard, and serval) but also in red pandas, which had previously been reported as being susceptible to CPXV in two fatal cases.[11] Secondary bacterial infections can be medicated with broad-spectrum antibacterial therapy. Importantly, glucocorticoid treatment should be avoided. Glucocorticoids are among the most widely used drugs that are applied to suppress autoimmune and inflammatory responses and therefore result in a significantly higher viremia and mortality.

As a first countermeasure, animals known to be or suspected to be susceptible to CPXV that reveal typical signs of an infection should immediately be separated from other animals by applying strict quarantine measures. They should be treated with antibiotics against secondary bacterial infections and observed closely for at least 3 weeks. Nevertheless, prompt segregation of potentially infected animals may not be possible because of the lack of separate pens available at the crucial time point. Furthermore, it is impossible to segregate zoo animals permanently from wild rodents that can move freely around the zoo enclosures, transmitting CPXV to other species. A continuous control of food animals might be hard or impossible to accomplish, especially when purchased from different wholesale dealers or animal husbandries.

ZOONOTIC POTENTIAL

Since the first scientific reports of human cowpox in the first half of the 20th century,[10] infections of humans have become more numerous during the last decade, perhaps because of the absent or inadequate immune status of the population after abrogating the cross-protective smallpox vaccination in the 1980s. In humans, CPXV infections usually remain localized and are self-limiting but can become fatal in immunosuppressed patients.[6] General universal precautions should be followed to protect staff from possible CPXV infection.

REFERENCES

1. Basse A, Freundt EA, Hansen JF: [Ein Ausbruch von Pockenkrankheit bei Okapis im Kopenhagener Zoo.] Verh ber Erkrg Zootiere 6:55–62, 1964.
2. Baxby D, Ashton DG, Jones DM, et al: An outbreak of cowpox in captive cheetahs: virological and epidemiological studies. J Hyg (Lond) 89:365–372, 1982.
3. Baxby D, Bennett M: Cowpox: A re-evaluation of the risks of human cowpox based on new epidemiological information. Arch Virol Suppl 13:1–12, 1997.
4. Becker C, Kurth A, Hessler F, et al: Cowpox virus infection in pet rat owners: not always immediately recognized. Dtsch Arztebl Int 106:329–334, 2009.
5. Coras B, Essbauer S, Pfeffer M, et al: Cowpox and a cat. Lancet 365:446, 2005.
6. Eis-Hubinger AM, Gerritzen A, Schneweis KE, et al: Fatal cowpox-like virus infection transmitted by cat. Lancet 336:880, 1990.
7. Essbauer S, Hartnack S, Misztela K, et al: Patterns of orthopox virus wild rodent hosts in South Germany. Vector Borne Zoonotic Dis 9:301–311, 2009.
8. Essbauer S, Meyer H: Genus orthopoxvirus: cowpox virus. In Mercer AA, Schmidt A, Weber O, editors: Poxviruses, Basel, 2007, Birkhäuser, pp 75–88.
9. Eulenberger K, Bernhard A, Nieper H, et al: An outbrack of cowpox virus infection in a black rhino (Diceros bicornis) at Leipzig Zoo. Verh ber Erkrg Zootiere 42:77–85, 2005.
10. Fenner F, Wittek R, Dumbell KR: The orthopoxviruses, San Diego, 1989, Academic Press.
11. Hentschke J, Meyer H, Wittstatt U, et al: [Kuhpocken bei kanadischen Bibern (Castor fiver canadensis) und Katzenbären (Ailurus fulgens).] Tierärztl Umschau 54:311–317, 1999.
12. Kik MJ, Liu PL, van Asten JA: Cowpoxvirus infection in the Patagonian cavy (Dolichotis patagonum): emerging disease in an educational animal park—the first reported case. Vet Q 28:42–44, 2006.
13. Kubin G, Koelbl O, Gerstl F: [Charakterisierung eines vom Elefanten isolierten Pockenvirusstammes.] Wien Tieraerztl Mschr 62:271–276, 1975.
14. Kurth A, Nitsche A: Fast and reliable diagnostic methods for the detection of human poxvirus infections. Future Virology 2:467–479, 2007.
15. Kurth A, Straube M, Kuczka A, et al: Cowpox virus outbreak in banded mongooses (Mungos mungo) and jaguarundis (Herpailurus yagouaroundi) with a time-delayed infection to humans. PLoS ONE 4:e6883, 2009.
16. Kurth A, Wibbelt G, Gerber HP, et al: Rat-to-elephant-to-human transmission of cowpox virus. Emerg Infect Dis 14:670–671, 2008.
17. Marennikova SS, Maltseva NN, Korneeva VI, et al: Outbreak of pox disease among carnivora (felidae) and edentata. J Infect Dis 135:358–366, 1977.
18. Martina BE, van Doornum G, Dorrestein GM, et al: Cowpox virus transmission from rats to monkeys, the Netherlands. Emerg Infect Dis 12:1005–1007, 2006.
19. Matz-Rensing K, Ellerbrok H, Ehlers B, et al: Fatal poxvirus outbreak in a colony of New World monkeys. Vet Pathol 43:212–218, 2006.
20. Pelkonen PM, Tarvainen K, Hynninen A, et al: Cowpox with severe generalized eruption, Finland. Emerg Infect Dis 9:1458–1461, 2003.
21. Pilaski J, Jacoby F: [Die Kuhpocken-Erkrankungen der Zootiere.] Verh ber Erkrg Zootiere 35:39–50, 1993.

22. Potel K, Voigt A, Hiepe T, et al: Eine bösartige Haut- und Schleim-hauterkrankung bei Elefanten. Der Zoologische Garten 27:1–103, 1963.

23. Sandvik T, Tryland M, Hansen H, et al: Naturally occurring ortho-poxviruses: potential for recombination with vaccine vectors. J Clin Microbiol 36:2542–2547, 1998.

24. Schüppel KF, Menger S, Eulenberger K, et al: [Kuhpockeninfektion bei Alpakas (Lama glama pacos).] Verh ber Erkrg Zootiere 38:259–264, 1997.

25. Wisser J, Pilaski J, Strauss G, et al: Cowpox virus infection causing stillbirth in an Asian elephant (Elphas maximus). Vet Rec 149:244–246, 2001.

26. Yang G, Pevear DC, Davies MH, et al: An orally bioavailable anti-poxvirus compound (ST-246) inhibits extracellular virus forma-tion and protects mice from lethal orthopoxvirus challenge. J Virol 79:13139–13149, 2005.

27. Zwart P, Gispen R, Peters JC: Cowpox in okapis (Okapia john-stoni) at Rotterdam. Zoo Br Vet J 127:20–23, 1971.

CHAPTER 6

Disaster Preparation for Captive Wildlife Veterinarians

Mark Lynn Lloyd

Some disasters, such as infectious diseases, clearly require a veterinary component, but less obvious veterinary issues result from catastrophic scenarios. Captive wildlife facility (CWF) veterinarians are also integral components of institutional management. As such, their contribution may be equally important. Beyond the CWF borders, veterinary staff may play a critical role as advisors to federal mission support teams, the USDA, and the local emergency medical services (EMS) as well. This role serves the community as well as captive animal welfare in a disaster. Familiarity with the incident command system (ICS) facilitates this opportunity.

CWF veterinary considerations are key components in any wildlife institutional disaster plan. This brief overview provides general planning concepts for veterinary professionals and potential solutions to common disaster scenarios. A risk-based approach will build a comprehensive, institution-specific veterinary disaster plan. Some of the best sources for plan development are veterinary colleagues and existing institutional protocols.[1]

PLANNING

Assessing the Risks When Developing an Institutional Disaster Plan

When developing this type of plan, the following stages need to be implemented:
1. Assess risks.
2. Generate a needs list.
3. Create a plan.
4. Train to the plan.
5. Implement the response plan.
6. Recover and reassess risks.

Considerations in Institutional Risk Assessment

- What are the geographic location risks (e.g., natural disasters, transportation and storage facilities, terrorist targets)?
- What are the species-specific animal health risks (e.g., disease susceptibility, environmental limitations, fragility)?
- What are the species-specific public liabilities (e.g., dangerous animals, zoonotic vectors, and reservoirs)?
- What are the structural risks and liabilities at the facility (e.g., building and enclosure integrity, life support, environmental controls)?
- What are the liabilities for both staff and collection sheltered in place (e.g., potable water, billeting capability, emergency resource cache)?
- Regardless of captive wildlife, what are the human health risks and liabilities (e.g., institutional security, on-site hazardous materials, escape options)?

Plume Effect Prediction and Risk Assessment

Plume effect is the progression or movement away from a relatively unitary point source that expands as it moves away from that point source to spread over a logarithmically larger area as distance from the source increases. Common examples include smoke from a single fire in the wind, distribution of contaminated water over a delta, or possibly the expansion of a disease pathogen from an infection reservoir. Plume effects can be unidirectional as with the prevailing wind or watershed, or may expand circumferentially such as volcanic ash without prevailing wind distortion.

Some disasters allow preparation because they are predictable or delayed, but may have a severe onset and subsequent calculable geographic distribution. The plume effect can affect vast areas, but direction and speed may be determined by local meteorologists. Plume effects can be involved in nuclear radiation dispersal, chemical release, smoke, and liquid contaminants such as petroleum products. Plume effects can be airborne or waterborne.

A chlorine transport train wreck in northern West Virginia may plume into the National Zoo on prevailing winds, or a western Gulf of Mexico oil spill may plume into large areas of the western Floridian coast and affect facilities such as Mote Marine Laboratories. Coastal aquatic animal facilities such as Mote Marine Laboratory are often dependent upon open ocean water circulation, rather than closed systems of water filtration and recirculation. This places them at significantly increased risk if oceanic contaminants exist. Wildfires and smoke contamination are difficult to foresee, but plume expansion prediction is important to risk assessment pre-event. The plume effect can expand the devastation, or may mitigate the contamination by dilution as it spreads.

Naturally occurring epizootics, epidemics, or zoonotic outbreaks can follow similar expansion patterns based on vector dispersal, reservoir ranges, or environmental conditions. When prediction is possible, advanced preparations may also be possible.

Facility Infrastructure

Although veterinary staff are seldom responsible for the comprehensive institutional plan, their role as advisor and contributor is critical to any plan. Water and power are highly vulnerable systems and frequently compromised. Often, human potable water uses under normal circumstances can range from human consumption to animal consumption to cage cleaning. However, when potable water is limited or lost, planned nonpotable water collection may be possible for uses other than human consumption.

Power loss will disable infrastructure at many levels. Potable wells and water recirculation systems may be affected. Veterinary facilities are critical infrastructures and may best be served by redundant disaster resources. Separate dedicated veterinary facility generators and fuel reserves are prudent. Individual building water treatment and filtration systems are readily available and of moderate cost. Sanitation for limited volumes of human potable water may even be achieved for a small veterinary staff with inexpensive travel or camping filters. Iodine or chlorine disinfection costs pennies per gallon and may be the final backup solution to ensure that the veterinary staff have sufficient water reserves.

Key power-dependent systems include lighting, medical supply refrigeration, carcass storage, and heating, ventilating, and air conditioning (HVAC) systems. CWF veterinarians should mitigate each vulnerable system within an inclusive veterinary facility disaster plan. Stockpiled medical supplies should be selected for minimally labile products and expiration dates rotated. Heat-stable antibiotics and anesthetics should be selected for disaster storage. However, some critical medical supplies may still require refrigeration. Vaccines such as tetanus, disease-specific inoculations, and some pharmaceuticals require refrigeration.

A small, emergency, low-wattage electric refrigerator may suffice for critical labile items when electricity is limited or generated intermittently. Refrigeration units may be cooled when power is available and then kept tightly closed when power is offline. This applies to necropsy freezers and food refrigeration as well. Top-loading chest-type units retain cold air even when open briefly; upright units immediately lose the cold air when the door is opened or not securely closed or sealed.

Most sport coolers are only effective when ice (or a frozen alternative) is available. Regional infrastructure failure may eliminate ice availability. Some sport coolers may use 12-V automobile cigarette lighters for refrigeration, but vehicular power may be limited as well. Recreational vehicle (RV) refrigerators may use propane or other fuel sources. Acquiring a privately owned RV on temporary loan may provide refrigeration, a restroom, and overnight housing.

Veterinary Facility Design Considerations

The veterinary hospital and quarantine design must consider disaster mitigation. Specific considerations based on risk assessment will vary with every locality and building code. However, a few common concerns exist for many scenarios. Critical systems locations are often based solely on ergonomics or design convenience. Basements are frequently used for electrical boxes, necropsy freezers, refrigerators, generators, and water system controls. Flooding immediately inactivates basement service equipment and system controls, just as a hurricane storm surge did in a coastal Mississippi aquarium in hurricane Katrina. Alternative locations should be considered for any vulnerable systems in construction or remodeling.

Outdoor compressed gas tanks and other weather-proof items avoid loss of valuable indoor hospital space. However, severe environmental conditions may place these at risk. Buoyant compressed gas tanks may float and avulse critical connections. They must be physically anchored, beyond reliance on their own gravity.

Light fixture selection is often based on efficiency and variable construction codes. Additional criteria considered for veterinary hospital disaster preparation might include waterproof designs, backup photovoltaic power sources, and low-voltage lighting. Some emergency lighting fixtures are detachable and rechargeable.

Fuel

Fuel of any type becomes an immediate concern in many disasters. Preparation for a predictable event other than fire, such as weather, plume dispersal (dispersal of effluent in water or aerosolized emissions), or flooding may include filling every veterinary vehicle, every compressed gas cylinder, and every fuel storage container. Some large facilities may use on-site vehicle fuel reserve tanks. Although tanks are frequently buried they should be located on the highest ground to mitigate fuel contamination with water and ground water contamination with fuel.

Fire may uniquely require the opposite preparations. Fire may damage service breakers or result in an explosive situation with outdoor gas or liquid fuel containers unless placed safely behind a nonflammable insulating wall, such as hollow block. Safe fuel removal from outdoor tanks well in advance of an inevitable fire will greatly diminish explosive risk. Some fuels such as propane may be simply and safely exhausted under fire department instructions.

Fuel is one of the most likely resources to be stolen or commandeered. Regional infrastructure recovery may not occur until long after a disaster strikes. Immediate restrictions on fuel consumption may be prudent, even if a rapid recovery is expected. Facility vehicular use, HVAC settings, and consumptive activities such as personal hygiene, and redundant lighting, should be very conservative until regional infrastructure recovery is complete. High-output electrical generators consume fuel reserves quickly. In Houston, TX, pursuant to a major coastal hurricane, several weeks were required before electricity was uniformly available. Generating electricity 24 hours/day, every day, depletes fuel reserves

rapidly. Few facilities have sufficient fuel storage to meet an extended recovery. Intermittent power generation may extend fuel reserves.

Refrigeration units retain "cold" best if filled with thermally dense items, even if the items do not require refrigeration. For example, a nearly empty (air filled) refrigerator loses all the cold air immediately when opened; a refrigerator filled with full water bottles retains almost all the thermal reserves within the bottles when opened.

ADMINISTRATIVE PREPARATION AND DISASTER RESPONSE

Veterinary administrative preparation and disaster response mirror those of the greater facility, with additional considerations and redundancy to ensure veterinary staff support. Animal medical, Drug Enforcement Administration (DEA), pharmaceutical, and other critical records require off-site backup. Any human resource (HR) information retained within the department requires protection as well.

Veterinary staff members are as likely to be victims themselves as any other regional resident. Their personal, financial, and professional needs continue or expand. Simple payroll capability is essential to staff recovery, but requires HR contingency plans. Electronic fund transfers may be offline, but physical paper checks or remote banking may alleviate the dilemma. The staff's familial needs may increase during emergency declarations. Schools and child care are frequently the first to be cancelled in many disasters, immediately stranding parental veterinary departmental employees at home. One Texas zoo used its education department postdisaster to temporarily assist parental staff with child care; otherwise, many staff members might have been absent.

Destruction of residences may require staff or family relocation. Employee transportation to and from the CWF may be difficult, dangerous, or impossible. On-site temporary veterinary staff billeting may allow a viable alternative. If no space is available within the veterinary buildings, a loaned RV or a modified education department bus on-site may be used. Numerous zoological staff remained on zoo grounds post–Hurricane Katrina at one Louisiana zoo because egress was strictly limited.

The veterinary hospital disaster pack should include not only veterinary resources, but a small stockpile of sanitary human supplies accordingly. The closest hospital and/or EMS should also be clearly identified in the disaster plan and posted. A list of alternatives is also prudent as the closest facility may be affected equally to the CWF.

Hazardous Materials

Hazardous materials from supply storage must be clearly identified for responders. Many hazardous substances are required to placard hazard identification codes, risk-type symbols (e.g., corrosive, caustic, flammable) and color codes.[5] However, the placard may not be immediately obvious to responders. A posted list should be available for staff and responders near the building entry. Even low-risk materials such as fertilizer, ammonia, bleach, film developer, or cleaning supplies may become dangerous when dispersed or combined.

Posted Information

Information selection for posting should be based on the most critical information for veterinary staff and key facts for outside responders entering the facility. Posted quick references should be near the entrance and clearly identified. Some critical information may include the following: local veterinary facilities, human hospital/EMS location, directions, and map, locations of hazardous materials and material safety data sheets thereof, multiple human escape routes, staff reunion sites outside the facility, remote phone communications contact, management contact numbers, doses and safety sheets for drugs, and an updated hospitalized species and locations list.

INCIDENT COMMAND SYSTEM

The veterinary management structure within the CWF is usually well established in advance of a disaster. However, it may not mirror the ICS functional units. To integrate seamlessly into a disaster response, staff must be familiar with the mechanics and terminology of the ICS.[5] Every management staff should undergo ICS training. It is available on line free of charge and eligible for continuing education credits through the Federal Emergency Management Agency (FEMA).

ICS was developed in the 1970s by the fire service after devastating California wildfires. Since the early 1990s, it has been incorporated into almost all federal responses (e.g., 9/11, hurricanes, fires, avian influenza). Today, it is used uniformly by almost every state and local law enforcement, fire responders, and emergency agencies. Federal agencies such as FEMA, U.S.

Department of Homeland Security (DHS), U.S. Department of Agriculture (USDA), and National Disaster Medical System (NDMS) all use ICS.[6]

ICS chain of command and functional units may be adapted reliably to any event. The purposes of ICS are the following: (1) span of command and control (2) ensure responder safety; (3) achieve tactical objectives; (4) manage resources efficiently; and (5) integrate all response agencies for any response.

Key Concepts

The ICS maximum manageable span of control is three to seven direct reporting section supervisors. Four functional management modules exist under the ICS structure. They are administrative (anything to do with human resources and documentation), logistics (anything to do with nonhuman resource acquisition, transport, and management), operations (objective accomplishment), and planning and training.[5]

Human safety is the first operational objective; therefore, safety officers lie outside the chain of command as command advisors. They alone have the authority to block a command decision, which is frequently difficult for commanders to accept. Various subject matter experts (SMEs) may be used for command guidance for any subject and also lie outside the direct chain of command.

Engaging the External Responder Command Structure

Captive wildlife facility staff veterinarians should be incorporated outside the facility as SMEs for the responsible response agencies. Ideally, the wildlife SME should be at each daily briefing or conference. Veterinarians must find out where and when the daily disaster responder briefings are held. Comprehensive wildlife expertise at the regional decision table is the most effective means to acquire resources and limit intrusive outside interference. A veterinarian is an excellent institutional choice to serve as SME, particularly in a disease outbreak, but serving as such may be a time-consuming luxury for solo practitioners.

Inclusion or invitation to serve as an SME requires knowledge and persistence. Veterinary SMEs provide an exceptional resource for responders unfamiliar with wildlife issues. Response agencies will be reluctant to allow any individual at the table without a strong grasp of the ICS system. The first request to provide a veterinary wildlife SME from the facility should occur as soon as the response authority agency is identified (e.g., FEMA, state EMS). The request should be in the form of an offer to serve the greater community welfare as it related to the CWF, rather than implying that outside responders may be inadequate. The request should be made as high on the chain of command as possible and use any existing relationships to acquire it. If the facility has a municipal connection, the office of the mayor, governor, or fire or EMS chief may be an excellent direct contact.

VETERINARY LOGISTICAL CONSIDERATIONS

Veterinary logistics may piggyback with general institutional resources. However, veterinary resource acquisition and security may require specialized considerations and may require outside professional assistance from colleagues. Resource selection reflects the nature of the highest risk disasters, but infrastructural limitations are often similar. A plan should anticipate limitations of transportation, communication, thermoregulation, moisture, and power and fuel. Veterinary resource caches should reflect these potential constraints. Wide-thermal rangestable pharmaceuticals such as quinolones, macrolides, and aminoglycosides are far superior for storage than heat-labile pharmaceuticals such as penicillin G. Sufficient portable waterproof containers for the veterinary resource cache should be acquired well in advance of a disaster, before local stocks are depleted.

Resource Acquisition and Commandeering

A close relationship with response authorities, frequent communications, and clear written requests are the key to resource acquisition through local responders. Municipalities and many governmental agencies frequently have fuel stores accessible with credentialing. Municipal, state, and government-associated CWFs may have the opportunity to acquire existing government or commandeered resources. Fuel from abandoned service stations is sometimes commandeered though a governmental emergency declaration.

However, a CWF may also find itself on the other end of disaster declaration commandeering. Resources may be legally taken for agendas deemed to be of greater importance by controlling authorities. Fuel may be commandeered for humanitarian missions such as human hospital operations, as they were from a Gulf

Coast zoological institution after Hurricane Katrina. Resource theft or civil unrest may require 24-hour veterinary hospital security as well.

Resource transportation may be the rate-limiting step in acquisition. Even physically open roads may still be blocked by law enforcement or militia. Mandatory human evacuations are accompanied by road closures by authorities with weapons, excluding looters and preventing early return. If CWF transport vehicles leave, they may be unable to return without proof of authority. Prior to departure, CWF transporters must acquire the appropriate credentials and permission to return. Similarly, vendor delivery vehicles may require credentialing.

Preexisting contractual agreements from commercial transporters and distributors should be part of a complete plan. The contract should provide for immediate action on request in a disaster situation. This includes animal transporters, veterinary supplies, and animal nutrition products. A predetermined drop shipment list may be established with a distributer based on the veterinary risk assessment.

There are few experienced and dependable wildlife transporters. Emergency evacuation of numerous animals simultaneously may necessitate innovative alternatives. Circus animal transport vehicles may augment available commercial transporters. Some agricultural animal transport vehicles may be modified for many wildlife species. Swine trucks may be well constructed as pigs may be strong and destructive. With minimal modification, swine transport crates may accommodate relatively large animals, including some carnivores. However, animals may require anesthesia to load and unload if existing chutes are not appropriate. Every transport vehicle should be visually inspected by the veterinary staff.

Most wildlife veterinarians are eager to assist conservation partners. An integrated disaster plan between wildlife facilities places experienced peers in a position to assist sister institutions effectively and rapidly. Wildlife-specific veterinary resources are backed up by experienced colleagues. Anesthetics, wildlife professionals, and capture and transport equipment may be readily loaned in a disaster. A preexisting written mutual aid agreement is far superior to frantic attempts after communication systems are compromised.

Planning should include designation of multiple veterinary staff escape and/or animal evacuation routes. Any individual route may be compromised, and may rapidly change mid-disaster. Similarly, one or more predetermined reunion locations should be established. At least one designated remote contact number, such as a partner institution, provides a viable veterinary staff communication nexus should direct communication with the CWF be eliminated.

Hard-line telephones (land lines) are the most reliable form of phone communication. Satellite telephones may be difficult to use and may be expensive, but are a valuable alternative in a disaster. Cellular and satellite telephones still require a power source; basic land lines do not. Expect cellular telephone services to be lost, even without tower destruction, because they are quickly overloaded. Text messages require a miniscule band width and may work well, even in lieu of cellular auditory transmissions. CWF veterinary hospitals should maintain several communication options.

Small volumes of potable water may be obtained by several means for emergency veterinary staff consumption. Inexpensive 0.2-μm mechanical filters easily remove protozoa and most bacteria. Finer filters with activated charcoal remove all pathogens and chemicals as well. Irradiated and chemical sterilization may be accomplished inexpensively with units designed for travelers. Chemical sterilization may also be used for larger volumes of water. Sodium hypochlorite, 5.25%, 1 tbsp/gallon, or premeasured iodine tablets may sanitize clear water and kill most pathogens. However, they may only oxidize other chemical contaminants.

Conservation of human nonpotable water may also be required. Sewage service is unreliable in many disasters. Not wasting stored water for flush toilets will extend the supply for animal consumption and cleaning requirements. A dedicated veterinary department emergency chemical toilet may ensure that the veterinary staff gets the first chance at it in a disaster.

OPERATIONAL CONSIDERATIONS

Infectious Disease Disasters

Operational objectives are delineated based on the disaster type and the CWF species vulnerabilities. Catastrophic biologic agent introduction is considered one of the simplest and most likely terrorist stratagems.[3] Many USDA reportable diseases are well established in animal populations internationally. Foot-and-mouth disease pathogens may be readily obtained from many sources, easily smuggled into the country, and disseminated.

Agricultural epizootics may be one of the most economically devastating disasters because of the interruption of the human and animal food chains. Consumer boycott, gratuitous destruction of animal products, and unemployment in the processing industry send ripple effects through the food distribution and consumption industries. These are the primary driving forces for decisive and sometimes dramatic government actions. Such decisions have the intent of immediate outbreak extinction. Mass and indiscriminate euthanasia is a common tool, without consideration for conservation status, relative pathogen resistance, or pathogen barriers. CWF veterinarians provide a source of information for intelligent risk management with regard to wildlife conservation in the face of an epizootic.

Veterinarians must not only consider epizootic and zoonotic pathogens, but also epidemics that may also affect CWF operations. Epizootic pathogens engage the USDA–Animal and Plant Health Inspection Service (APHIS) depopulation procedures, particularly those of significant agricultural impact, such as foot-and-mouth disease, Newcastle disease, and African swine fever (ASF).

The veterinary staff has several critical roles in a disease disaster.[2] Ensuring the sequestration of the vulnerable and reservoir collection species from pathogen exposure may mitigate USDA interference. Animal collection protection from USDA intervention may require the veterinary staff to maintain a reverse quarantine isolation plan. Small CWFs may not maintain a permanent quarantine facility and even the most modern facilities have limited space. Additional institutional space may need to be commandeered. Holding facilities outside the veterinary department may be required.

The degree to which wildlife is physically separated must be based on the disease life cycle. Veterinarians must be in control of these issues. Pathogens requiring direct contact with bodily fluids may be quarantined in open air enclosures. Those for which a vertebrate intermediate host exists, such as avian flu or *Yersinia* spp., may require exclusion of small birds and mammals. Intermediate flying arthropod vectors and airborne pathogens or toxins are the most difficult and may require positive pressure air flow exclusion systems.

CWF veterinarians should play a key role as subject matter experts to the outside response agencies. Species that are potential victims or reservoirs must be defined by an appropriate wildlife veterinarian. The relative vulnerability of endemic wildlife species may be outside the expertise of those making depopulation or testing decisions. Exotic wildlife are most often beyond the scope of agricultural veterinary proficiency.

Federal and state agricultural authorities may be naïve concerning the susceptibility of wildlife to specific epizootics or zoonotics. Many exotic diseases are readily transported to the United States. ASF resulted in a more than 45,000 swine depopulation in the Russian Rostov region in September 2009. If a CWF is within the eradication zone of an ASF outbreak, USDA intervention may be unavoidable. For example, a CWF veterinarian may need to inform their federal response colleagues about whether peccaries may be ASF reservoirs to ensure an appropriate USDA approach.

USDA intervention, testing, or depopulation decisions may be based on whether California condors are most likely a Newcastle disease sentinel species versus a reservoir, as occurred during a California outbreak in 2004. If considered a sentinel species, minimal poultry risk exists and USDA intervention may be avoided. However, if condors are potential reservoirs, USDA testing or euthanasia may be compulsory. One southern California zoo closed their aviary to visitors to minimize potential mechanical vectors, such as shoes of those who might have had contact with game cocks, a Newcastle disease reservoir.

Informed CWF veterinarians may avoid indiscriminate depopulation of valuable collection animals by overzealous responders. Depopulation zones and disease survey areas are intended to eradicate all reservoirs and victims within. The depopulation zone diameter varies based on disease epizootiology. However, it may also consider the range of free-ranging vectors and such dispersal agents as prevailing winds and hydrology. Typical depopulation zone radii are 1 to 5 miles, and the diameter of a circumscribed survey area is 1 to 10 miles beyond the depopulation zone. However, a CWF veterinarian may not know the size of the depopulation zone until an outbreak.

Low-pathogenic avian influenza in the Shenandoah Valley in 2002 used a 1-mile depopulation zone around any positive tracheal swab test farm and a survey testing zone of at least 10 miles. This event resulted in the euthanasia of 4.7 million poultry in one summer. More severe diseases such as foot-and-mouth may result in vastly extended depopulation zones as well as disinfection of substrates or inanimate surfaces. Wildlife veterinarians must be prepared to defend specific collection species within the facility. Veterinarians may mitigate unnecessary collection interference by sharing specific disease information with response authorities with a comprehensive reverse quarantine plan.

Inclusion in a federal or state mission support team (MST) may avoid devastation of valuable or endangered genetic founder collection animals. Obtaining this position should be a high priority for CWF veterinarians.

Political, EMS, and municipal contacts should be used by CWF management to obtain that position for their veterinarians. Those relationships should be built established before a disastrous event, starting with the most local contacts. Once a disaster is predicted, the response pandemonium will limit access to those who make decisions.

Sequelae of Infections

Infectious diseases may also be secondary to a noninfectious disaster. Common sequelae are defined by the disaster, exposure, duration, and species. In most flood zones, septic water contamination is ensured. Metropolitan water treatment plants overflow and urban well systems are inundated with foul contaminants. Assume coliform contamination in any flooding situation. Gastrointestinal illness may be the immediate result of sewage, but sepsis may ensue.

Even nonseptic water or chronic wet substrates may macerate skin, enhancing vulnerability to dermal disease, such as necrotic pododermatitis. Water-dependent vector population explosions increase pathogen exposure. Moist conditions promote masses of hydrophilic organisms such as fungi. Mold spores, such as airborne *Aspergillus*, are highly pathogenic to some species. Animal relocation may be required.

Environmental Contamination

Risk assessment with veterinary input identifies most likely environmental disaster scenarios. For example, burn therapy planning is obvious when fire risk exists, but more deaths occur from smoke inhalation. Evacuation or sequestration of the most smoke-sensitive animals into air recirculation enclosures may be the best preventive action. Based on elevated municipal smoke particulate reports, one central California zoo smoke protocol sequesters California condors indoors because of their smoke sensitivity and conservation status. If the particulate pollution count rises further, evacuation plans are preestablished, including transport crates, documentation, and interzoo recipient agreements for immediate evacuation, as required. At the same institution, an orangutan with chronic air sacculitis is sequestered in a positive pressure building, regardless of individual studbook value, because of the existing respiratory compromise. CWF veterinarians must be directly involved in relative susceptibility determination.

Environmental contamination risk assessment also requires investigation of local and regional storage and transport routes and most likely contaminants, as well as wind and water directional inclination. Primary exposure therapy and decontamination resource requirements may then be determined. Mass petroleum spills often come to mind because of historical events, but risk assessment should include all potential contaminants.

Captive wild birds are more sensitive to toxic gases than mammals. Endangered aviary species may require a preplanned immediate sequestration or evacuation. Mandatory human evacuation is required at levels toxic to mammals, preventing collection relocation. Exposure to chlorine and nitrates are common examples of why CWF veterinary preparations must assess the risk of likely contaminants.

Dissolved nitrate salt from a flooded industrial unit resulted in the mass death of goats near Tirupur, India, in 2009.[7] Nitrates are used extensively in the United States for fertilizer and vast agricultural storage units exist on large farms upstream, as well as in supplier storage facilities. Rumen-absorbed nitrate causes lethal methemoglobinemia between 400 and 800 ppm (mg/liter) of water. Identifying nitrate storage and transport facilities and information about directional hydrology are critical to a complete risk assessment.

Captive wild ruminants are equally susceptible. Caustic and corrosive chlorine is transported in considerable quantities by rail in the United States and lethal chlorine gas is dispersed widely via plume on derailment. In January 2005, three tankers of a freight train derailed near Graniteville, South California, immediately releasing 46 tons of chlorine and 14 more tons over the next 72 hours, exposing the town of 7000 to chlorine gas. Emergency treatment of 525 people was required, 72 were hospitalized, and 8 died.[4]

Even with only a threat of catastrophe, mandatory human evacuation may significantly affect captive wildlife care. The entire central area of Morehead City, North Carolina, was evacuated on January 11, 2010. Several large dockside storage tanks of the highly explosive pentaerythritol trinitrate (PETN), the same explosive used by the Christmas Day bomber (2009), had become compromised. No warning was given. Law enforcement required immediate evacuation, without notice.

Salination via marine water inundation may have equally lethal effects for many fresh water aquatic species. Fresh water flooding may similarly affect marine species. Risk assessment includes coastal and flood plain proximity and must be reflected in veterinary disaster plans.

The distance from storage facilities, water, and railways and prevailing wind direction are important risk assessment criteria. Veterinary input is critical to a complete risk assessment and identification of potential victims. Local EMS and fire officials should be able to provide regional hazardous material storage and risk information.

Trauma

Preparation for specific traumatic injuries may be difficult because of the potential scenario diversity. Windborne and waterborne debris are the most common causes of traumatic injury. Wind itself is seldom injurious, but flying debris at 100 mph may injure and damage caging, even if rated to withstand winds of 100 mph. Water itself is far less hazardous than flood debris. Damaged caging and postevent wreckage in enclosures create risk long after the initial event. Pedal puncture injuries are common, so secondary anaerobic sepsis such as tetanus and gangrene must be considered. Additional cached vaccine stocks may be required. Other common regional weather risks include exposure to prolonged severe cold or heat. Minimal frostbite and subsequent necrosis become life-threatening, even to hardy hoofstock and temperate birds.

Animal Escape and Intrusion

Preparation for potential escape or enclosure compromise affects veterinary planning based on collection size and species. In some unusual cases, escaped animals may return—for example, escaped marine mammals returned to a flooded Mississippi aquarium after Hurricane Katrina. Few veterinary departments maintain sufficient anesthetics for a mass or mandatory collection evacuation or capture. Preparation for a disaster may include obtaining greater volumes of general anesthetics or preexisting written inter-institutional sharing agreements.

Darting supplies, particularly those that involve an explosive charge, may need to be stockpiled before an event. Exposure to water may inactivate the charges in capture darts or ammunition. Waterproof and humidity-proof storage is essential for both. Lethal force may be required for large carnivores or hoofstock to ensure human safety. A structural integrity evaluation of an enclosure should be conducted as soon as it is safe after any destructive event.

The less damaged the facility, the more appealing the refuge may be to displaced, free-ranging wildlife, feral domestic animals, and/or humans. Wildlife invasion should be anticipated, particularly local species, which may require additional physical or chemical capture equipment.

REFERENCES

1. American Association of Zookeepers: Crisis Management, 2010 (http://aazk.org/shop/ publications/aazk-crisis-management-cd/).
2. AmericanVeterinary Medical Association: Animal Health, Disaster Preparedness, 2010 (http://www.avma.org/disaster/default.asp).
3. Centers for Disease Control and Prevention: Emergency Preparedness and Response: Bioterrorism, 2010 (http://emergency.cdc.gov/bioterrorism).
4. David Van Sickle: Chlorine gas, 2010 (http://davidvansickle.com/chlorine).
5. Federal Emergency Management Agency: National Incident Management System, 2010 (http://training.fema.gov/IS/NIMS.asp).
6. Homeland Security Response Network: Emergency Response Guidebook, 2008 (http://www.phmsa.dot.gov/staticfiles/PHMSA/DownloadableFiles/Files/erg2008_eng.pdf).
7. The Hindu: Death of goats due to consumption of nitrate dissolved water: TNPCB, 2009 (http://hindu.com/2009/10/21/stories/2009102154960500.htm).

CHAPTER 7

Guidelines for the Management of Zoonotic Diseases

Donald L. Janssen

Most zoo clinicians have at one time or another encountered a case in which they diagnosed a zoonotic disease. For the purposes on this chapter, a zoonotic disease is defined as any infectious disease that may be readily transmitted between animals and humans. When a serious zoonotic disease is identified, there often is an urgent demand for action without having the time to think things through. In contrast, a subtle zoonotic disease incident may be completely overlooked, and no specific action may be taken. In either case, we may fail to handle the situation in the best interest of the health and safety of animals, employees, or visitors.

To focus our efforts, it may be useful to ask several key questions, including the following:

- What circumstances should trigger a zoonotic disease investigation and response?
- Who is responsible for making decisions about public health implications?
- Who should we notify and what do we say?
- Do we need to report to government regulators?
- What do the caretakers of the animal need to know?
- Do we need to isolate the animal and, if so, what procedures should we implement?
- How do we handle contaminated waste?
- How do we manage the medical care of the infected animal?

This chapter suggests how to answer these questions in a systematic way when dealing with zoonotic disease occurrences in a zoo setting.

SYSTEMATIC PROCESS

Without a plan in place for handling these situations properly, there is a real risk of mishandling them. The consequences of mishandling may be significant. The implications to the animal, its caretakers, the public, the institution, and our professional reputations may quickly become overwhelming.

Failure to respond properly may lead to unnecessary human and animal illness or, in contrast, an overreaction to perceived risks. Other animals in contact with the infected animal may be put at risk. Public health may be compromised through unnecessary contact and exposure of disease agents to employees and guests. A zoonotic disease outbreak could affect the reputation of the institution, leading to public concern and adverse economic consequences. Media attention may become misdirected. Even our professional reputation could be damaged by improperly handling the many issues that come up when a zoonotic disease is identified.

The risk of all these undesirable consequences occurring may be reduced by setting up a systematic process ahead of time (Box 7-1). As a first step, it is important to look for triggers to the process so that we do not overlook the occurrence of a zoonotic disease.

Identifying Triggers

The diagnosis or suspicion of a zoonotic disease in an animal or human contact should trigger the process to

BOX 7-1	Steps in Managing a Zoonotic Disease Case

1. Trigger—zoonotic disease identified
2. Notifications—notify and educate stakeholders
3. Infection control
   a. Animal isolation
   b. Waste management
4. Regulatory reporting
5. Medical management

begin. Often, the specific trigger is a test result (e.g., a culture) reported from the laboratory. Another trigger may be the results of a postmortem examination that provide evidence of a zoonotic disease, either confirmed or suspected. A more unusual trigger could be an employee, volunteer, or guest who is diagnosed with an infectious disease that could have been acquired from contact with animals in the collection.

Once triggered, a systematic approach should be implemented. There are several ways in which this could be approached. In my practice, a zoonotic disease occurrence triggers each of the following steps: (1) notifying stakeholders; (2) isolating the animal from others; (3) managing the contaminated waste from the animals; (4) reporting to authorities, if appropriate; and (5) treating the animal or otherwise managing the clinical illness, if present. All these steps are important, but key steps that need emphasis may be different in each case.

Notify Stakeholders

Once the process is triggered, the most urgent step is to notify the appropriate internal stakeholders involved in the care of the animal and the occupational health care provider for the facility. It may seem desirable to keep the situation quiet and avoid overreaction and unnecessary attention to the situation. Approaching the problem that way, however, is almost always a mistake. It is critical that employees be informed so that they may take proper precautions and report signs and symptoms of disease that they may be experiencing. It is useful to provide a written disease fact sheet to all stakeholders to remind them of the signs and symptoms. Well-written fact sheets on many zoonotic diseases are readily available in books, pamphlets, and online.[1,2]

Isolate the Animal

This is the first of two important infection control steps. The veterinary and animal care staffs should determine whether it is appropriate to isolate the infected animal and/or the facility in which it is located. The decision should be based on evaluating risks and feasibility. A quick risk assessment may be performed based on the severity and contagiousness of the disease. This should be balanced against the feasibility of performing the isolation safely and effectively. Isolation should be done in the case of an animal housed in a public contact setting.[6]

As in quarantine, separate tools and equipment should be used. A footbath may be helpful to reduce

the spread of contamination and to remind workers of the isolation entry control point. In addition, this is a good opportunity to remind staff of the importance of proper hygiene (especially hand washing) and the use of appropriate personal protective equipment, and how to implement them.

Waste Handling

This is the second step critical for infection control. Instruct the animal care staff on proper waste disposal procedures, including disposal of bedding, to avoid spreading contamination. Dispose of contaminated waste through a sanitary sewer, if possible. Follow local and regional regulations for the disposal of biomedical wastes. Provide proper disinfection of premises using disinfection best practices.[4]

Report to Regulatory Authorities

Some zoonotic diseases are reportable to regional public health and veterinary authorities. Reportable diseases vary with the region, and public agencies have different criteria for what is reportable. Before such issues arise, it is helpful to develop a rapport with local public health departments. To keep alert to trends, it may be useful to develop an internal mechanism to track the zoonotic diseases that occur in your facility over time.

Medical Management

If indicated, treat the animal with appropriate antimicrobials and perform follow-up diagnostics as appropriate. Be sure to establish criteria for case resolution and an endpoint for patient and facility isolation. (e.g., test negative and/or clinically normal).

SAMPLE ZOONOSIS SCENARIOS

The following scenarios, based loosely on actual cases, provide examples of how this process might be used in real-life situations. In each scenario, all steps are addressed, but each example highlights steps of key importance for that particular case.

Shigellosis in a Mother-Reared Infant Gorilla

The trigger to action in this case was the combination of suspicious clinical signs (diarrhea and general illness) along with the eventual positive fecal culture for *Shigella* sp. The key step in this case was to notify the keepers caring for the infant and the occupational health provider. A fact sheet from the Centers for Disease Control and Prevention (CDC) about shigellosis, including signs, symptoms, and method of transmission, was provided to the animal care staff. Isolation of the animal was not feasible nor was it required because the risk of disease transmission to the keeper staff and public was low. The low risk was a result of primate biosafety precautions that were already in place as standard operating procedures for primate areas. Reporting to regulatory authorities was not required, but the case was added to an internal tracking log to aid in following trends. The animal was treated with antibiotics. The endpoint of the process was determined to be the resolution of clinical signs, not necessarily a negative follow-up fecal culture.

Methicillin-Resistant *Staphylococcus aureus* in a Hand-Reared Elephant Calf

The trigger to action in this case was the presence of pustular skin lesions in an elephant calf and its caretakers from which methicillin-resistant *Staphylococcus aureus* (MRSA) was isolated in culture.[3,5] A major effort was made to notify and educate caretakers about the disease and how to avoid being infected. In this case, the key steps centered on infection control—that is, animal isolation and waste management. The calf was isolated from unnecessary contact with staff and other animals. Elephant care staff wore personal protective equipment such as gloves, disposable coveralls, and rubber boots. Footbaths were placed in strategic areas, creating an isolation zone around the animal. Waste, especially contaminated bedding, was managed carefully, and the premises and surfaces were thoroughly disinfected. Discussions were begun with local public health authorities who were instrumental in providing authoritative, unbiased information to staff and the public. The calf's medical condition was managed with appropriate antibiotics and the lesions quickly resolved, although the calf did not survive for other reasons. Employees who developed lesions consistent with MRSA were also treated, and all were resolved.

Interactive Lorikeet Aviary

The trigger to action in this case was a *Chlamydophila*-positive polymerase chain reaction (PCR) laboratory report from samples collected during routine flock surveillance. None of the birds in the large flock had shown evidence of disease. As a first priority, keepers and the occupational health provider were notified, and disease-specific educational materials were provided to those caring for the birds. For infection control, the birds that were PCR-positive were isolated at the hospital, and the exhibit was temporarily closed. Waste material was hosed into drains that went into the sewer. Additionally, the concrete substrate, perches, railings, and other surfaces were disinfected. Because this was a reportable disease in the region, the key step in this case was quickly reporting to public health officials, who were helpful in advising how to proceed with isolation and treatment procedures. With their agreement, all birds were started on treatment in their food for 45 days.[7] The exhibit was reopened after 7 days of treatment, with good compliance. Birds hospitalized were released following treatment and documentation of PCR-negative samples. Routine surveillance of the birds continues to assess ongoing disease risks.

CONCLUSIONS

The consequences of mishandling a zoonotic disease occurrence may be enormous. A systematic process will help avoid mistakes and failures to act when a zoonotic disease is identified. Furthermore, a well thought-out process helps these situations to be handled consistently and professionally.

Acknowledgment

I would like to acknowledge the collaborative contributions that were provided by the Collection Health Staff of the Zoological Society of San Diego in the creation of this chapter.

REFERENCES

1. Center for Food Security and Public Health: Zoonotic Diseases—Fact Sheets. 2010 (http://www.cfsph.iastate.edu/Infection_Control/zoonotic-disease-information-for-producers.php).
2. Centers for Disease Control and Prevention (CDC): Healthy Pets Healthy People. 2010 (http://www.cdc.gov/healthypets/browse_by_diseases.htm).
3. Centers for Disease Control and Prevention (CDC): Methicillin-resistant Staphylococcus aureus skin infections from an elephant calf—San Diego, California, 2008. MMWR Morb Mortal Wkly Rep 58:194–198, 2009.
4. Dvorak G: Disinfection 101. 2005 (http://www.cfsph.iastate.edu/BRM/resources/ Disinfectants/Disinfection101Feb2005.pdf).

5. Janssen DL, Lamberski N, Donovan T, et al: Methicillin-resistant Staphylococcus aureus infection in an African elephant (Loxodonta africana) calf and caretakers. In American Association of Zoo Veterinarians: 2009 Proceedings AAZV-AAWV Joint Conference, Yulee, Fla, 2009, American Association of Zoo Veterinarians, pp 200–201.

6. Miller RE: AZA Policy for Animal Contact with the General Public. 1997 (http://www.aza.org/animal-contact-policy).

7. National Association of State Public Health Veterinarians (NASPHV): Compendium of Measures to Control *Chlamydophila psittaci* Infection Among Humans (Psittacosis) and Pet Birds (Avian Chlamydiosis). 2010 (http://www.nasphv.org/Documents/Psittacosis.pdf).

CHAPTER 8

Integrated Pest Management

Jennifer N. Langan

Pests, including insects, rodents, nuisance birds, and certain mammals, are common in zoos because of the ready availability of food, water, and shelter. Control of pests is a critical aspect of preventive medicine at zoological parks. Pests may be vectors or reservoirs of disease that may adversely affect zoo animals and guests. Pests may also significantly degrade buildings, exhibits, and the esthetic quality of the park. They have an economic impact by damaging facilities, preying on collection animals, introducing disease, and consuming animal diets. Developing a pest management program is key to controlling pests in a zoological setting and is required for licensed animal facilities (Animal Welfare Act; 7 U.S.C. s/s 2131 et seq [http://campusvet.wsu. edu/iacuc/pdfs/awapdf.pdf]).

The most successful vermin control strategies in zoological facilities include integrated pest management (IPM), which involves analysis of the pest and attempts to use the safest approach to control the population, in keeping with environmental concerns.[5,26] IPM uses regular monitoring to determine if and when control measures are needed. This pest management approach takes into account the biology of the target pests and the effects of any control methods on the pests, animal collection, employees, and visitors to manipulate natural processes for maximal effectiveness.

The goal of IPM is to reduce pest numbers to an acceptable level through methods that are safe for a zoo's animal collection and least disruptive to the park's environment. A comprehensive program should define the scope and magnitude of the problem, identify appropriate expertise, define a safe and effective plan, implement the program, regularly reevaluate the results of the program, and make improvements when necessary. Communication among animal care staff, pest control staff, animal and facilities managers, and veterinary staff is essential to the success of an IPM program.[5]

The pest species is usually identified by animal care staff or guests. Animal care staff, managers, and pest control officers discuss how to use the most effective, least toxic, and appropriate control measures; plans are reviewed by management and approved with veterinary input prior to being implemented.

IPM uses a combination of control measures for effective pest control, including exclusion, habitat management, sanitation, removal (trapping, baiting, relocation, or euthanasia), and repellents. These control measures may be divided into indirect and direct suppression tactics to control pests. Indirect suppression is focused on education and prevention, whereas direct suppression implements trapping and eliminating pest species.

INDIRECT SUPPRESSION

Although each pest species varies in its preference for food, water, and shelter, preventing and decreasing access to these essentials has been shown to provide the best long-term effects with pest management. A study evaluating the efficacy of different pest management strategies has shown that mechanical alterations to buildings, restricting access to nutrients and shelter for pests, and education, in association with regular chemical treatments, is more effective than repeated pesticide application alone.[17] This same observation has been supported by Collins and Powell,[5] who described indirect suppression (e.g., modifying exhibits, changing human behavior, educating staff) as being the most important strategy for long-term pest control as part of IPM within a zoological park. Nonanimal areas, particularly those used for storage, are areas frequently underemphasized in a zoo's IPM program, but are equally as important to maintain and inspect, because they often contribute to pest harborage.

Educating staff, especially animal care and maintenance staff, is the first line of defense against pests, because they work in locations in the zoo where evidence of a pest problem is likely to be first noted. They are responsible for cleaning and sanitation in their respective areas. They may alert pest control staff if they identify signs of pest infestation, prepare areas for treatment, and move animals as necessary. Working within their areas of responsibility, they remove dead and dying pests, maintain and monitor bait stations, and set traps as supplied and recommended by pest control staff. Communication and appropriate logs to document pest reports and control measures should be recorded by staff so that managers and pest control officers may review and respond to changing needs for pest control.

Zoo management has the responsibility to educate, encourage, and provide the means for animal care and maintenance staff to maintain sanitation and structural integrity in the park. All zoo employees have the responsibility to promote the health and well-being of the animal collection and should be encouraged to do their part to reduce pest contamination and infestation in their areas. Sanitation standards should be maintained throughout the zoo, including concession, administrative, and education facilities and should ensure that refuse (e.g., garbage, recycling, compost) is inaccessible to pests.

Sanitation and maintenance guidelines as they pertain to the care and well-being of zoo animals have been established by the U.S. Department of Agriculture (USDA) Animal and Plant Health Inspection Service (APHIS) through the Animal Welfare Act. The maintenance of an effective program for the control of insects, birds, and rodents in animal areas and the main commissary storage areas is the legal obligation of USDA-licensed facilities. USDA inspections identify areas of institutional noncompliance and encourage compliance through the education and cooperation of zoo personnel. Simulated USDA inspections in zoo units have proven to be helpful for achieving compliance with pest control goals through staff education.[5]

DIRECT SUPPRESSION

The direct suppression or mechanical control of pests varies based on the species and location of the infestation and should always include a multisystem approach to ensure the most effective pest management. Direct control measures of IPM often include: exclusion, baiting, repellents, trapping, removal, euthanasia, and relocation. Taxa-specific control options, including exclusion recommendations, chemical control measures, and natural remedies for specific species, are presented in Tables 8-1 and 8-2.

Exclusion

Exclusion and habitat management may be the most important control mechanism to eliminate or prevent pests, but are extremely difficult in zoological parks because of naturalistic exhibits, long periods of indoor and outdoor access, temperate to tropical climates throughout most buildings, and aging infrastructure in many zoos. When exclusion is an option, physical barriers such as fencing are often the first point to deter entry of pests. Other control measures include eliminating areas for pests to find shelter indoors and outside, trimming trees and plantings away from the perimeters of buildings, and preventing access to burrows for mammals and perching structures for nuisance birds. Eliminating or preventing access to harborages indoors such as false ceilings, hollow walls, and gaps around piping and electrical wires is especially important for insect and rodent control.[26]

Baiting

Baiting should be undertaken with caution and may only be effective at reducing pest populations when incorporated into a multifaceted and IPM plan. Baiting used alone will not be sufficient to reduce or eliminate a pest infestation.[17] This method of direct pest suppression is most appropriate when pest numbers are high or there is a concern about infectious disease exposure to the animal collection, staff, or guests. Zoological parks present unique challenges for pest control compared with residential settings because additional efforts must be made to protect collection animals and nontarget species. The biggest concern with the use of toxic bait is untargeted and secondary toxicity, in which animals other than the intended pest (e.g., small mammals, birds) consume bait directly or consume pest species that have consumed toxic bait.

Accidental primary and secondary toxicity have been documented in association with pest control efforts in zoological parks. Unintentional primary toxicity has been reported to affect multiple nontarget wildlife species such as ground squirrels, chipmunks, voles, waterfowl, and passerines commonly found on zoo grounds.[3,16,27] Primary toxicity in collection animals is rare but has been associated with rodent control efforts.[9]

TABLE 8-1 Vertebrate Pest Control

Species	Physical Control	Chemical Control
Rodents: mice (deer, harvest, house, meadow, white-footed mice, cotton), rat (Norway, roof, wood)	Exclusion: Remove food sources and shelter, identify entry sites (sprinkle nontoxic powder [flour, chalk, talcum] around suspect holes), plug active exit and entry sites (>0.6 cm with 18- to 22-gauge wire hardware cloth), maintain door sweeps on all exterior doors, screen drains, place guards along pipes and wires, prune trees and shrubs to maintain a gap of ≥1 m between foliage and ledges and rooftops, prune ground cover and shrubs along buildings to expose lower 45 cm of trunk. Trapping: Inside buildings, along edges; check traps twice daily (snap traps, live traps, glue boards), bait traps (peanut butter, cheese, cotton) before setting trigger.	Baiting Anticoagulants *First generation:* Warfarin Diphacinone Chlorophacinone *Second generation:* Brodifacoum Bromadiolone Single-dose toxins Zinc phosphide Vitamin D3 Outdoor Bait Stations Protecta Rat Depot Bait Safe
Ground squirrels, moles, gophers	See rodent exclusion methods. Prevent access to food. Trapping: Underground live traps	Baiting not recommended, high risk of secondary toxicity Repellents: moth balls/flakes (naphthalene), Bitrex, thiram, ammonium soaps applied to vegetation
Tree squirrels	See rodent exclusion methods. Exclusion: Use sheet metal bands on trees, close external openings to buildings, use plastic tubes on wires, set up squirrel-proof bird feeders. Live trapping	Repellents: moth balls/flakes (naphthalene), Ropel Spray, capsaicin, polybutenes
Rabbits	Netting, electric fencing, live traps, tree wrap	Repellents: Hinder Deer & Rabbit Repellent, National Scent, Ropel Spray, Green Screen, Getaway
Opossums and skunks	Exclusion, live trapping, and removal; seal off burrows (Safeguard, Tomahawk, Havahart)	Not recommended
Raccoons	Exclusion: Maintain roofs (replace loose shingles, repair holes near eaves of the roof), limit roof access (trim trees, shrubs), prevent access to chimneys (commercial spark arrestor cap of sheet metal and hardware cloth over top of chimney, heavy screen wire securely over opening); use garbage cans with tight-fitting lids. Live trapping: Bait traps (Safeguard, Tomahawk, Havahart) q48h (crisp bacon, fish, fresh vegetables, cat food, chicken parts and entrails, corn, sardines); set multiple traps in many locations, especially close to den; check traps twice a day; trap, release, relocate based on wildlife regulations; sterilization, culling	Not recommended
Bats	Exclusion and removal: One-way door over entry, exit holes; bat eviction valve; fine mesh (≤1.25 cm) over entry and exit sites; seal gaps of ≥0.6 × 3.8 cm and openings ≥1.6 × 2.2 cm; copper mesh hole filler; netting; bat, swallow, and woodpecker kits for home-made bat check valve; fill open spaces with fiberglass insulation; use sticky repellents around entry, exit site; supply a bat house for roosting.	Repellents: Moth flakes (naphthalene)
Carnivores: Bobcats, cats (feral, domestic), coyotes, dogs, foxes, mountain lions	Exclusion, trapping, and removal for small cats, dogs, and foxes	Immobilization through remote injection and removal for coyotes, dogs, and large cats

Continued

TABLE 8-1	Vertebrate Pest Control—cont'd	
Species	Physical Control	Chemical Control
Deer	Buffer zones that extend ≥365 m from cover or woodlands; plant diversionary plots of alfalfa, clover; plant-resistant ornamental foliage; deer exclusion fencing; wire cylinder tree guards; reproductive control (PZP vaccine, surgical sterilization); cull via hunting	Chemical repellents: Human hair, hot sauce, predator scents, blood meal, egg solids (Deer Away)
Birds: Canada geese, crows, ducks, European starlings, egrets, herons, house sparrows, pigeons, raptors	Habitat modification: Prune trees; net off roosting sites and over exhibits (mesh <2-cm openings); eliminate overhangs and ledges from buildings; nest destruction every 10-14 days; mechanical repellents to prevent roosting (wire prongs, sheet metal spikes placed along ledges or under eaves). Live trap: Rotate sites (Tomahawk) Deterrents: Alarms and detonators (distress calls to deter Canada geese, electric shock, flashing light, reflective tape) Repellents: Balloons, gel, kites, sticky repellent, adhesive	Repellents: Ropel, Bird Proof Gel/Liquid, 4-The-Bird Repellent

Secondary toxicity from consuming rodents poisoned with second-generation rodenticides (e.g., brodifacoum) has occurred primarily in carnivorous birds (e.g., raptors, turkey vultures, kookaburra, Von der Decken's hornbill, small mammals).[3,27] Secondary toxicity has also occurred in granivorous birds via consumption of food contaminated by cockroaches transporting rodenticides. Additional specific chemical toxicities in wildlife have been thoroughly reviewed.[10,22]

Over time, and with continuous application, pests may develop resistance to toxic agents used as bait, making them less effective or ineffective. The best-known example involves coumarin-based rodenticides, which inhibit the coagulation cascade and result in death. Coumarin-based rodenticides have been used as pest control agents for over 5 decades and constant exposure has led to selection of resistant individuals. Research has revealed the genetic point of mutation, which is the basis of resistance.[23] Consequently, if rodenticide-resistant rodent populations are established, newer control methods will need to be developed. Incorporating multimodal IPM may reduce the likelihood of resistant populations developing.

Any chemical control strategy should be used in conjunction with the pest's natural biology to minimize the risks for nontarget animals and the environment. As part of this effort, bait stations should be designed to target a specific pest species so that the bait must be consumed for the pest to leave the station, and so that little to no toxin may be carried out. Bait stations should be numbered, secured far enough outside animal

enclosures to prevent exposure to the toxin, and carefully monitored to see whether their placement is appropriate and effective.

Repellents

Repellents (e.g., noise, light, smell) are safer than baiting, but may be less effective and require more staff time, because frequent or repeated applications are often necessary. Many species become acclimated to repellents, after which they lose their impact to deter pests. Natural products and deterrents (without toxic or dangerous compounds) have been gaining popularity and offer IPM plans additional resources for managing pests. There are numerous recommendations and products (e.g., pheromones) available that apply natural pest control strategies, but little referred literature is available to validate their efficacy or to compare the cost-benefit ratio to traditional suppression efforts using chemicals and trapping for control. Some examples of nontoxic and natural pest control products are included in Tables 8-1 and 8-2.

Trapping

Trapping involves live and lethal capture methods of controlling problem species in an IPM program. Live trapping allows for removal, translocation, and humane euthanasia of pest species. Euthanasia of wild animals is generally regulated by federal, state, or municipal laws and a zoo's IPM plan should be in accordance with

TABLE 8-2	Invertebrate Pest Control		
Insect	**Physical Control**	**Chemical Control**	**Natural Remedies**
Ants	Remove attractants (food, water), keep counters free of crumbs, remove water sources (drips, soaking dishes), high-performance vacuum, heat treatment, sticky barrier, solar-powered ant trap (for fire ants), Teflon barrier, tree wrap	Baits (abamectin, fenoxycarb, hydramethylnon, methoprene, pyriproxyfen, spinosad, sulfluramid), fipronil, botanic sprays, borate-based insecticides, diatomaceous earth with pyrethrin, insecticidal soap, pyrethrin, garlic repellant spray, silica aerogel with pyrethrin	Deterrents: Baby powder, cayenne pepper, coffee grounds, yarn soaked in citrus oil, mint leaves, cloves, low-wattage light in areas of most activity can disrupt foraging patterns Instant grits, rice: Taken back to queen, expand when eaten result in death
Bees	Bee swarm traps, pheromone lure, spray, varroa mite trap, remove colonies (consult local bee keeper), remove nest after colony is removed, caulk or repair entrance hole to prevent further infestation	Boric acid, diatomaceous earth with pyrethrin, insecticidal soap, pyrethrin, resmethrin plus components that freeze wasps, silica aerogel with pyrethrin	Essential oils, plant oils (mint oil)
Cockroaches	Sanitation and exclusion, reduce food and water sources, store food in insect-proof containers, tight lids on garbage cans, increase ventilation where condensation develops, vacuum cracks, crevices to remove food and debris, eliminate hiding places, caulk holes and entry spaces, traps (glue board)	Baits: Abamectin dust, spray or gel bait, borate-based bait, fipronil, hydramethylnon, indoxacarb, imidacloprid Dusts: Diatomaceous earth, hydroprene insect growth regulators (IGRs), pyrethrin, silica aerogel with pyrethrin	Deterrents: Bay leaves, cayenne, catnip sash, (1 quart water and 2 tbsp tobacco sauce, spray problem areas)
Flies (blow, deer face, flesh, horse, house)	Screening, traps, sticky trap, tape, black light and electrocution traps	Botanic fly repellents, pyrethrin, diatomaceous earth with pyrethrin, silica aerogel with pyrethrin	Crushed mint, bay leaves, cloves, and eucalyptus wrapped in cheesecloth square, sweet basil and clover, Pine-Sol
Mosquitoes	Eliminate standing water, change water (e.g., bird baths) once/wk or more, clean debris from rain gutters, drain, fill temporary pools of water with dirt, move animals inside during at dawn and dusk, maintain screens, replace outdoor lights with yellow bug lights, stock bodies of water with fish species that feed on larvae.	Larvicides: Bacterial insecticides (*Bacillus thuringiensis* serovar *israelensis*, *B. sphaericus*), methoprene, organophosphate insecticide (temephos), others (mineral oils, monomolecular films, oils—films disperse as thin layer on water surface, causes larvae and pupae to drown) Controlling adult mosquitoes: Malathion, naled, permethrin, resmethrin, synthetic pyrethroids (sumithrin), DEET repellent	Repellents: Eucalyptus oil, Bite Blocker with 2% soybean oil, fresh basil hung in netting bag, citronella, neem oil, one part garlic juice mixed with five parts water, Thai lemon grass
Mollusks, slugs, snails	Barriers and exclusion devices, copper snail barrier, traps (Slug Saloon, traps with barley, rice yeast bait)	Insecticidal soap with pyrethrin Baits: Metaldehyde, iron phosphate	

Continued

TABLE 8-2	Invertebrate Pest Control—cont'd		
Insect	Physical Control	Chemical Control	Natural Remedies
Yellow jackets and wasps	Habitat alteration, clean garbage cans regularly, fit them with tight lids, empty cans, dumpsters daily prior to periods of heavy traffic, clean drink dispensing machines, screen food dispensing stations, put trash cans away from food-dispensing windows, caulk holes, and entry spaces in siding, traps.	Insecticide: Treat ground, aerial nests after dark; wear protective bee suit; use pressurized liquid spray, aerosol; plug entrance hole with dusted steel wool, copper gauze; dust plug and area around entrance; cut aerial nests down and seal in plastic bag; use insecticides (boric acid), diatomaceous earth with pyrethrin, insecticidal soap, pyrethrin, silica aerogel with pyrethrin	Essential oils, mint oil

appropriate legislation. Permits may be granted by federal and state wildlife agencies on a case by case basis to control specific species (e.g., oiling waterfowl eggs to control the numbers of Canada geese) in a park. Public sentiment toward some species may also preclude more aggressive control means (e.g., hunting or shooting deer on zoo property). Educating zoo staff, the public, and local communities about the necessity of pest control and euthanasia is vitally important to a successful pest control campaign and should incorporate public relations staff when possible. Most zoos also have associations with local animal shelters and animal control officers as part of managing domestic or feral dogs and cats collected from zoo grounds.

Lethal trapping is preferred over baiting for the removal of vertebrate pests because of the risks of secondary and nontarget toxicity, except in cases of severe rodent overpopulation.[2,26] To be effective, traps must be placed and monitored regularly, which is labor-intensive and costly and is generally only effective when used with appropriate exclusion measures. Snap traps are commonly used for rodents, whereas most other species are live-trapped (see Tables 8-1 and 8-2). Consult with local pest control, animal control specialists, and/or wildlife biologists prior to embarking on a planned trapping program to ensure the greatest success.

One benefit of trapping and removing pest species as part of an IPM plan in a zoo has been potentially reducing the risk of infectious and zoonotic diseases in the park.[1,15,24] Disease surveillance programs designed to collect blood and tissue from pests in association with an IPM program may be a valuable tool to identify emerging disease trends that could present a risk to animal and human health. Zoos should have protocols in place to allow collection of biologic materials from pests for the purposes of disease investigation, surveillance-based risk assessment, and veterinary recommendations. Pests known to carry infectious and zoonotic diseases should be evaluated for evidence of disease via gross necropsy and histopathologic examination. If pest species are anesthetized prior to euthanasia, serum may be collected for banking to allow for retrospective disease investigations.

If individual animals are translocated or rereleased onto zoo grounds, individual animal identification should be pursued by standard methods, such as ear tagging, tattooing, or transponder placement. Vaccination against infectious disease before release has also been implemented as a strategy to lessen the risk of contagious disease transmission (e.g., canine distemper virus [CDV], rabies) to a zoo's animal collection. It is important to conduct such prevention programs in coordination with local wildlife officials when handling and altering wildlife, because these activities may be regulated by county, state, or federal authorities.

INFECTIOUS DISEASE POTENTIAL
Rodents

Many common pest species may carry or act as vectors of diseases that could cause significant morbidity and mortality to a zoo's animal collection, staff, and visitors. Rodents have been involved with transmission of many bacterial and viral diseases of concern, including leptospirosis, salmonellosis, plague, Lyme disease, lymphocytic choriomeningitis virus (LCMV), encephalomyocarditis virus (EMCV), and hantavirus infection.

Rodents have also played a role in the transmission of parasitic diseases. Toxoplasmosis outbreaks in captive collections have been documented in marsupials, lemurs, and New World monkeys, in which ingestion of cat feces, intermediate hosts (e.g., mice, birds), and cockroaches contaminated with cat feces have been suspected routes of exposure.[4] These diseases and many others associated with rodents are zoonotic and appropriate personal protective gear is recommended when working in close contact with feral rodents.

Small Mammals

Small mammals, including skunks, foxes, raccoons, and coyotes, may act as vectors of rabies. Pest management programs to prevent rabies from these species should be developed in conjunction with local wildlife regulations and may include relocation, euthanasia or vaccination programs to control exposure of the animal collection to rabies. Raccoons and domestic dogs prey on zoo species and may carry CDV and rabies, both of which pose significant risk to a zoo's animal collection. Repeated cycles of CDV infection in raccoon populations have resulted in the development of more lethal lineages and viral resistance to vaccination.[19] Large exotic felids have been shown to develop titers to CDV when cyclic distemper outbreaks were documented in local raccoon populations.[20] Other collections have experienced mortality in zoo felids from CDV transmitted by pest species.[1] *Baylisascaris procyonis* is a zoonotic roundworm of raccoons, which has been documented to cause mortality in a large variety of zoo species, including primates, ratites, and psitticines.[13,18,28] Infection is associated with a wide range of clinical signs but often includes neurologic disease.

Feral dog and cat populations are becoming an increasing problem in the United States and may endanger collection animals by transmitting diseases such as parvovirus, calicivirus, and feline leukemia virus (FeLV). Fatal feline panleukopenia virus (parvovirus) and feline calicivirus infections in zoo felids have been linked to exposure to feral cats.[7,14] Evidence of FeLV infection and FeLV-induced disease has been documented in captive nondomestic felids and has also been linked to feral domestic cats.[12,25]

Opossums, commonly found on zoo grounds in North America, are the reservoir for the protozoan parasites *Sarcocystis neurona* and *S. falcatula*. *S. neurona* is the most important cause of equine protozoal myeloencephalitis (EPM) and causes EPM-like disease in other mammals, including cats, mink, raccoons, skunks, sea otters, and Pacific harbor seals.[8,21] *S. falcatula* causes severe disease or death in Old World psittacines infected with this coccidian. Infection results when animals consume opossum feces, contaminated food, or cockroaches that have consumed or are contaminated with opossum feces. Prevention is the key to controlling *Sarcocystis* spp. infections in zoological collections. Opossums must be excluded from animal enclosures and food storage areas. This may be done by elevating bird cages off the ground, using an electric wire fence around the facility, and using dogs for biologic control of opossums.[11]

Deer

Deer cause marked damage to landscaping and have the potential to transmit disease to collection animals. Tuberculosis *(Mycobacterium bovis)*, Johne disease (*M. avium* subsp. *paratuberculosis*) and chronic wasting disease are endemic in different wild deer populations and have the potential to cause disease in collection animals. Exclusion with appropriate fencing and depopulation are effective control measures, but may be difficult to maintain because of cost and public sentiment, respectively.

Birds

Free-ranging avian species expose captive birds to numerous infectious diseases, prey on collection animals, and may be a danger to zoo visitors (e.g., aggressive, nest-protective Canada geese). Feral birds have been implicated in the introduction of *M. avium*, *Chlamydophila psittaci*, *Salmonella* spp., *Mycoplasma* spp., Newcastle disease, and avian influenza to birds held in zoological collections. Exclusion and good sanitation may significantly decrease the risk of exposure to disease and predation by avian species.

Insects

Insects are implicated as vectors of disease spread for many infectious agents. They play an important role in the amplification of disease (e.g., mosquitoes and flavivirus), transmit fecal borne pathogens (e.g., *Salmonella* spp., *Escherichia coli* O157:H7, flies), act as vectors of disease (e.g., fleas and plague, mosquitoes and dirofilariasis) and may be intermediate hosts (e.g., snails and schistosomiasis). Cockroaches are prolific zoo pests found worldwide. Control requires significant financial cost and staff resources. Ongoing IPM for insects may help prevent disease such as parasitic infections linked to the consumption of cockroaches (*Gongylonema* spp. infections in *Callimico goeldii*).

REGULATION OF PEST MANAGEMENT PRACTICES

An IPM program should be the responsibility of senior management staff that is knowledgeable about pest management principles, animal health and disease, state and federal wildlife regulations, and legal aspects of pesticide use. The Environmental Protection Agency (EPA) regulates the use of many pesticides used for pest control in zoos. Local and state regulations may further restrict the use of these products by licensed and/or certified individuals. All activities, particularly the application of pesticides, should be logged and tracked as part of a zoo's IPM program. Lack of appropriate zoo-wide pest control, inadequate documentation, and unapproved use of pest control products, without a certified applicator on site, has led to citations by the Association of Zoos and Aquariums (AZA) during reaccreditation inspections and investigation by the local state Department of Agriculture for illegal use of rodenticides.[6]

Some states require certified applicators to distribute rodent baits, insect growth regulators, spray wasps/bees, treat standing water for mosquitoes, and topical ectoparasite products. Topical pesticides commonly used to control fleas, ticks, and flies in veterinary medicine (e.g., imidacloprid, fipronil, fly sprays) may also be regulated pesticides and require a veterinary prescription or pest control log to accompany these products in certain states.[6] To become a certified pesticide applicator, an individual must complete training and an examination administered by the state or local authority that enforces the EPA regulations on pesticides (Federal Insecticide, Fungicide, Rodenticide Act: 7 U.S.C. s/s 136 et seq., as amended [http://agriculture.senate.gov/Legislation/Compilations/ Fifra/FIFRA.pdf]). This certification allows the person to purchase and apply restricted use pesticides.

CONCLUSIONS

IPM programs may be effective at reducing infectious disease, preventing contamination of food, and improving exhibit maintenance and appearance. Successful pest management has been achieved at zoological parks with comprehensive IPM programs.[5,6] Care should be exercised to select the most suitable products or chemicals to minimize the hazards to nontarget animals. Ensuring that accidental poisoning does not occur in an animal collection is a significant challenge and requires the cooperation of pest management experts and animal care and facilities staff, as well as veterinary oversight.

Acknowledgments

I would like to thank Drs. Debbie Evans and Kimberly Mayer for their assistance with literature review and Drs. Meehan and Adkesson for manuscript review for this chapter.

REFERENCES

1. Appel MJ, Yates RA, Foley GL, et al: Canine distemper epizootic in lions, tigers, and leopards in North America. J Vet Diagn Invest 6:277–288, 1994.
2. Bennett GW, Owens JM, Corrigan RM, et al: Truman's scientific guide to pest management operations, 6th ed, Duluth, Minn, 2003, Purdue University Press.
3. Borst GH, Counotte GH: Shortfalls using second-generation anticoagulant rodenticides. J Zoo Wildl Med 33:85, 2002.
4. Carme B, Ajzenberg D, Demar M, et al: Outbreaks of toxoplasmosis in a captive breeding colony of squirrel monkeys. Vet Parasitol 163:132–135, 2009.
5. Collins D, Powell D: Applied pest control at Woodland Park Zoological Gardens. Proc Am Assoc Zoo Vet 290–295, 1996.
6. Denver M: Evolution of a pest control program at the Maryland Zoo in Baltimore. Proc Am Assoc Zoo Vet 77–78, 2008.
7. Duarte MD, Barros SC, Henriques M, et al: Fatal infection with feline panleukopenia virus in two captive wild carnivores (*Panthera tigris* and *Panthera leo*). J Zoo Wildl Med 40:354–359, 2009.
8. Dubey JP, Lindsay DS, Saville WJA, et al: A review of *Sarcocystis neurona* and equine protozoal myeloencephalitis. Vet Parasitol 95:89–131, 2001.
9. Enquist K, Montali R: Aluminum phosphide toxicosis in two red pandas. Proc Am Assoc Zoo Vet 135–136, 2003.
10. Fowler ME: Toxicities in exotic and zoo animals. Vet Clin North Am 5:685–698, 1978.
11. Godoy SN, DePaula CD, Cubas ZS, et al: Occurrence of *Sarcocystis falcatula* in captive psitticine birds in Brazil. J Avian Med Surg 23:18–23, 2009.
12. Guimaraes AM, Brandão PE, de Moraes W, et al: Survey of feline leukemia virus and feline coronavirus in captive neotropical wild felids from southern Brazil. J Zoo Wildl Med 40:360–364, 2009.
13. Hanley CS, Simmons HA, Wallace RS, et al: Visceral and presumptive neural baylisascariasis in orangutan (*Pongo pygmaeus*). J Zoo Wildl Med 57:553–557, 2006.
14. Harrison TM, Sikarskie J, Kruger J, et al: Systemic calicivirus epidemic in captive exotic felids. J Zoo Wildl Med 38:292–299, 2007.
15. Hillyer EVM, Anderson MP, Greiner EC, et al: An outbreak of sarcocystis in a collection of psittacines. J Zoo Wildl Med 22:434–445, 1991.
16. James SB, Raphael BL, Cook RA: Brodifacoum toxicity and treatment in a white-winged wood duck (*Cairina scutulata*). J Zoo Wildl Med 29:324–327, 1998.
17. Kass D, McKelvey W, Carlton E, et al: Effectiveness of an integrated pest management intervention in controlling cockroaches, mice, and allergens in New York City public housing. Environ Health Persp 117:1219–1225, 2009.

18. Kazacos KR, Fitzgerald SD: *Baylisascaris procyonis* as a cause of cerebral spinal nematodiasis in ratites. J Zoo Wildl Med 22:460–465, 1991.

19. Lednicky JA, Dubach J, Kinsel MJ, et al: Genetically distant American canine distemper virus lineages have recently caused epizootics with somewhat different characteristics in raccoons living around a large suburban zoo in the USA. Virol J 1:1–14, 2004.

20. Meehan TP, Hungerford LL, Smith CL: Risk factors for canine distemper virus seropositivity in zoo cats. Proc Am Assoc Zoo Vet 133–134, 1998.

21. Mylniczenko ND, Kearns KS, Melli AC: Diagnosis and treatment of *Sarcocystis neurona* in a captive harbor seal *(Phoca vitulina)*. J Zoo Wildl Med 39:228–235, 2008.

22. Plumlee KH: Toxicant use in the zoo environment. J Zoo Wildl Med 28:20–27, 1997.

23. Rost S, Pelz HJ, Menzel S, et al: Novel mutations in the VKORC1 gene of wild rats and mice—a response to 50 years of selection pressure by warfarin? BMC Genet 10:4, 2009.

24. Scanga CA, Holmes KV, Montali RJ: Serological evidence of infection with lymphocytic choriomeningitis virus, the agent of callitrichid hepatitis, in primates in zoos, primate research centers and a natural reserve. J Zoo Wildl Med 24:469–474, 1993.

25. Sleeman JM, Keane JM, Johnson JS, et al: Feline leukemia virus in a captive bobcat. J Wildl Dis 37:194–200, 2001.

26. Spelman LH: Vermin control. In Fowler ME, Miller ER, editors: Zoo and Wild animal medicine, 4th ed, Philadelphia, 1999, W.B. Saunders, pp 114–120.

27. Stone WB, Okoniewski JC, Stedelin JR: Poisoning of wildlife with anticoagulant rodenticides in New York. J Wildl Dis 35:187–193, 1999.

28. Wolf K, Lock B, Carpenter J, Garner M: *Baylisascaris procyonis* infection in a Moluccan cockatoo *(Cacatua moluccensis)*. J Avian Med Surg 21:220–225, 2007.

CHAPTER 9

Noninvasive Techniques to Assess Health and Ecology of Wildlife Populations

Ursula Bechert

The use and varied applications of molecular technologies has rapidly expanded over the past 20 years, transforming how veterinarians and researchers diagnose, treat, learn about, manage, and conserve wildlife, including elusive and less well-known species. Medically, the word *noninvasive* has been used to describe diagnostic procedures that do not involve penetrating the skin or organism with an incision or an injection. In this chapter, noninvasive techniques are defined to include the collection of samples without the need for immobilization (e.g., skin samples collected by remotely fired biopsy darts).

There are many advantages to noninvasive assessments using samples such as hair, feathers, feces, urine, saliva, regurgitated material, sloughed skin, or even museum specimens. Analyzing urine or feces to evaluate endocrine function without animal capture, restraint, and/or anesthesia minimizes stress and provides a broader measure of endocrine status over a period of hours to days when compared with point in time measures obtained from blood samples. Data collected from fecal hormone and genetic analyses and then overlaid by sample location data may provide information about home ranges, animal movements, stress levels, and habitat use,[24] as well as gender and gender ratios. Hair may be analyzed to yield much information about the following: occurrence, distribution, and relative abundance of populations; aspects of population genetics, niche, or diet; detection of rare species; and identification of individuals for wildlife management and forensic purposes.[18] Skin samples may be used to create stress response profiles, which may serve as early indicators of health risks.[2]

Given the growing number of analytic tests that may be performed with single samples, it may be tempting to include a broad range of parameters in analyses and then derive meaning from the results. However, it is the research question and experimental design, not the analytic tools used, that will produce meaningful results. Why, what type of, and how data should be collected are key questions that need to be addressed when designing a study. Molecular tools may then be applied thoughtfully to answer important questions.

This chapter describes collection methods as well as DNA- and non–DNA-based analytic procedures used to study the reproductive status, nutritional state, genetic characteristics, and general health of free-ranging wildlife. Methods to collect and store samples are covered separately because single samples may often be used in several analytic techniques, and field and laboratory research activities are often conducted by different individuals. This brief overview provides the reader with enough basic information to understand and apply noninvasive analytic tools currently available for wildlife field research.

SAMPLE COLLECTION AND STORAGE METHODS

The tradeoffs and benefits of working with different samples and analytic techniques must be weighed against research objectives and priorities. Frequently, a variety of samples and analytic approaches may be combined to answer research questions in greater depth or provide a broader understanding of wildlife population health (Table 9-1). Through the collection of hair or fecal samples, large remote areas may be surveyed, several population metrics may be calculated, and collection costs are minimal. In some cases, collections must be made noninvasively to avoid sampling bias. The types of samples and collection methods used will vary depending on the species, study objectives, and environmental conditions. For example, hair is collected relatively easily

TABLE 9-1 Overview of Biologic Samples, Study Applications, Basic Analytic Techniques, and Collection and Storage Methods*

Sample	Study Application	Analytic Technique	Collection	Storage
Hair	Occurrence and distribution of populations	mtDNA to identify species using various methods	Baited or passive devices	Dry and keep in paper envelopes ± desiccant
	Population structure, size, or abundance	Microsatellites to identify individuals	Hair follicles using capture-recapture methods	
	Relationships of species with habitat and environmental factors	Datasets overlaid with collection sites using GIS	Hair follicles using grid-based strategy	
	Nutritional status	Stable isotope and element analysis	Hair shafts	
Feces	Occurrence and distribution of populations	mtDNA to identify species using various methods	Scat detection using dogs	Dry and store with desiccant, freeze, or saturate in buffer solution
	Population structure, size, or abundance	Microsatellites to identify individuals	Capture-recapture methods	
	Relationships of species with habitat and environmental factors	Data sets overlaid with collection sites using GIS	Grid-based strategy	
	Nutritional status	Various nutrition and genetic assays based on objectives	Preferably within 24 hr of defecation; examine grossly	Dry and store in Ziploc bag or freeze
	Stress level	Glucocorticoids quantified by EIA, ELISA, HPLC	Noninvasive collection required	Freeze-dry, extract, store in Na azide or ethanol, freeze; or use C18 cartridges
	Reproductive status	Steroid hormones quantified by EIA, ELISA, HPLC		
	Viruses and bacteria	Microbiologic and biochemical tests; depends on study objectives	Preferably within 24 hr of defecation; examine grossly	Depends on study objectives
	Gastrointestinal parasites	Fecal flotation; microscopic examinations		
	Predation	Microsatellites to identify individuals	Examine grossly for rough identification of content	Dry and store predator and prey DNA samples separately in Ziploc bags
Urine	Reproductive status	Steroid hormones quantified by EIA, ELISA, HPLC	Special collection devices or extraction from substrate	Freeze
	Stress level	Glucocorticoids quantified by EIA, ELISA, HPLC		Freeze
	Urinary function	Urinalysis; metabonomic applications using NMR or other technique	Clean catch required	
	Genetic makeup	Depends on study objectives		Filter paper absorption, 10% ethanol, or freeze
Skin	Stress level	Immunohistochemistry; stress response profiling	Remotely fired biopsy dart	10% Formalin
	Genetic makeup	Depends on study objectives		70%-100% Ethanol, with desiccant, or saturate in buffer
Saliva	Forensic identification	Microsatellites to identify individuals	Swabs from bite wounds	Air-dry, keep in paper envelope, freeze

See text for details and limitations.

and may be stored for long periods of time but contains smaller amounts of DNA compared with fecal samples. On the other hand, chemical inhibitors present in feces may restrict the amplification of DNA.[18]

Hair

Determining the occurrence and distribution of populations is a common goal of hair collection studies, and hair may be used to answer questions about population genetics and structure when DNA quality is high. However, estimating population size or abundance via hair collection surveys is not as effective because it depends on reliable individual identification based on nuclear DNA analysis, and collection methods may not be efficient enough to provide a sufficient capture-recapture sample size. Population trends may be estimated by repeatedly monitoring occupancy if detection probability may be determined, and these data may guide wildlife management decisions (e.g., documenting wildlife use of highway crossing structures). Evaluating relationships of species with habitat and human variables using grid-based sampling, combined with identification of individuals through genotyping, is possible,[1] and hair samples may be analyzed in nutritional studies as well.

The best source of DNA is follicles, which are more frequently present on plucked as compared with shed hair,[10] although hair shafts may provide useful DNA contributed by saliva, dander, or other adherent tissue.[26] Hair should be collected within 3 to 4 weeks of deposit for the best genotyping results because ultraviolet light and moisture degrade DNA over time. Hair may be collected opportunistically or with sampling devices, which may be passive or baited. Passive devices collect hair during normal behavior and include hair-snagging devices mounted on natural rub objects (e.g., on trees for bears) or along travel routes (e.g., barbed wire strands for badgers). Baited sampling devices include food or scent lures to attract animals to collection sites. Catch structures should be designed to minimize collection of hair from multiple individuals or species, and variables such as animal behavior, movement, concentrations, and collection intervals should contribute to design strategies. Hair should be stored dried in small paper envelopes or vials with silica gel desiccant until it is analyzed.

Feces

A single fecal sample may provide information about reproductive status, genetic makeup, stress, viruses, internal parasites, predation, and diet. Noninvasive capture-recapture survey techniques may be adapted to estimate population size by supplementing detection data with genetic analyses of hair or scat samples, indigestible plastic chips recovered in scat, or cameras to identify individuals.[20] Capture-recapture methods through scat collection may be successful if the target population is not of extremely low density, sampling methods have a high rate of detection and low level of sampling bias, population size does not change between collection periods, and accurate identification of individuals is possible.[14] Collection of fecal samples may be greatly facilitated by the use of dogs that have been trained specifically to search for wildlife scats.[24] Dogs may even be trained to distinguish individual animals by their scat. However, detection rates may vary among dog-handler teams, making proper training and a study design that allows for estimation and correction of detectability highly important. Thorough mixing of a fecal sample prior to collecting a subsample will help ensure reliable results because corticosteroids and their metabolites may be unevenly distributed in feces.[15]

There are several ways that fecal samples may be stored, depending on the analyses to be performed. For endocrine assessment, sodium azide or other preservatives such as ethanol may be mixed with feces to prevent bacterial growth because bacteria and their enzymes will degrade steroid metabolites in a few hours. Alternatively, fecal samples may be stored frozen at –20° C for preferably no longer than 90 to 120 days prior to extraction and analysis.[13] A field-based extraction and storage technique using C18 cartridges (Varian, Walnut Creek, Calif) makes it possible to store samples at ambient temperatures for up to 2 weeks before freezing or analysis.[3]

Fecal samples collected for genetic studies can be stored using various techniques, such as drying and storing in 70% to 100% ethyl alcohol or in a desiccant, freezing at –20° C, or saturation and storage in a buffer solution. Hydrolysis, oxidation, UV radiation, alkylation, and structural damage from freeze-thaw cycles are the primary activities that may damage DNA; storage techniques are aimed to minimize these effects. Efficacy of storage techniques vary widely from one study to the next, depending on different species and their diets, environmental conditions, and protocols used in the field and laboratory. Conducting pilot studies to test storage and extraction methods, and performing extractions shortly after collection, will help minimize the deterioration of DNA in fecal samples.

For nutritional studies, fecal samples should ideally be collected within 24 hours of defecation, and indicators may include degree of wetness and lack of insect damage. Dietary components may be determined by gross physical examination of fecal samples as well as laboratory analysis to determine diet preferences of various species, assess nutrient content, and monitor forage quality. Molecular tools have forensic applications as well—for example, in areas in which predation on livestock is suspected.[8] For carnivore species, scats may be air-dried on sterile paper, prey remains examined grossly for rough identification and subsequent DNA analysis, and bile powder separated to identify predator species. Dried samples should be stored in Ziploc bags in a dark, dry location until DNA extraction. Fecal samples from herbivores should be dried at 80° C for 48 hours, ground into a fine powder, and then stored frozen until time of analysis.

Routine collection and storage of fecal samples for health diagnostics will vary, depending on the tests to be performed. Gastrointestinal parasites and viral or bacterial infections may be detected using various diagnostic tools, including fecal flotation and sedimentation tests, cultures, and genetic techniques.

Urine

Urine samples, like fecal samples, may be used for endocrine evaluations and genetic analyses.[12] Urinary DNA is easier to extract and analyze than fecal DNA; however, potential gender-specific differences in urination behavior may affect estimation of population size and gender ratios. Urine samples may be collected from captive wildlife housed in exhibits with concrete flooring and may also be extracted from natural substrates such as snow or sand.[16] Simple collection devices may also be devised (e.g., containers mounted on the end of sticks to catch urine from arboreal primates). Although collection of urine samples in the field may occasionally be challenging compared with fecal samples, urine requires no further processing before being assayed in the laboratory and may be preserved by absorption onto filter paper, mixing with 10% ethanol for storage at room temperature for up to 12 weeks, or freezing indefinitely.[18]

Skin

Full-thickness epidermal skin samples may be collected from some animals with the use of remotely fired biopsy darts. The dart weight, size and shape of the biopsy tip,

barb style, tail piece, and whether an embedded telemetry device is needed are all factors that contribute to the design of darts for use in different species, terrain, and environmental conditions. Skin samples are usually preserved in 10% formalin for immunohistochemistry and histologic studies but, for DNA analysis, should be placed in 70% to 100% ethyl alcohol, stored with a desiccant, frozen at –20° C, or saturated and stored in a buffer solution.

Saliva

Saliva has been used for determination of blood glucose and plasma steroid hormone concentrations, as well as detection of several diseases. Salivary concentrations of testosterone, 17β-estradiol, and cortisol correlate best with blood levels 20 to 40 minutes prior to collection in humans and sheep. Samples of saliva may be collected using a bulb, which requires some animal handling but, compared with venipuncture, these minimally invasive techniques are less stressful. Salivary DNA may be recovered from carcass bite wounds to identify the species, gender, and individual identity of the predator.[26] For genetic testing, swab samples should be air-dried for 24 hours, sealed in a paper envelope, and stored in a plastic bag at –20° C until they are analyzed.

Supplementary Observational Techniques

Behavioral observations, track surveys, images from remote cameras, and movements monitored via radio or satellite telemetry units may augment data acquired from field samples and help validate assays. Surveys of tracks in mud or dust may assess the presence and distribution of animals in remote or relatively inaccessible areas (e.g., aerial track survey), but determination of relative abundance requires identification of individual animals. Natural sign surveys have been documented for numerous animals and may be affected by adjacent habitat characteristics and environmental conditions. Population size may be estimated when the probability of scat detection is known; this depends on an understanding of the rates of scat decomposition and defecation,[14] especially when search areas cannot be cleared of scat (as by a snowstorm) prior to surveying.

Various cameras, motion sensors, and triggers may be used to collect information about different species noninvasively, even those that are very shy. Use of camera traps requires knowledge of an animal's natural history and the technical function of remote cameras.

Cameras triggered by pressure pads may exclude smaller bodied, nontarget species and may only operate within precise triggering distances. Active infrared (AIR) sensors detect motion when a narrow pulsing beam of light energy is broken by any object, whereas passive infrared (PIR) sensors have a broad or narrow detection area but only detect moving objects that differ in temperature from the environment.

Once animals have been fitted with radio or satellite telemetry units, these devices may be used to locate animals during key life stages (e.g., denning bears), access carcasses to document causes of mortality, and learn about habitat use based on movement and survival and mortality rates. These data may be combined with information obtained from the analyses of biologic samples collected noninvasively in the field to provide a more comprehensive understanding of the biology and ecology of certain species.

ANALYTIC TECHNIQUES AND APPLICATIONS

Genetic, endocrine, and nutritional analyses, disease diagnostics, and metabolic profiling with associated analytic laboratory techniques will briefly be described in this section. A basic understanding of these tools and how they have been used in research and veterinary health applications, as well as their capabilities and limitations, will help inform research design and wildlife health management strategies.

Genetic Analyses

DNA-based sampling and analytic techniques have been used to address research objectives related to abundance, occupancy, hybridization, paternity and relatedness, diet assessment, population genetics, community relationships, and spatial organization in various species, most often using hair or fecal samples.[23]

A basic technique commonly used to initiate genetic analyses is the polymerase chain reaction (PCR), which is a method to amplify a portion of the genome so that small amounts of DNA may be detected and sections may be visualized on an electrophoresis gel (Fig. 9-1). In this process, DNA strands are denatured in a thermal cycler and then forward and reverse primers are used to identify sections of the genome to be copied. Primers may be derived from mitochondrial or nuclear genomes of an organism. Mitochondrial DNA (mtDNA) is less variable within a species as compared with nuclear DNA

and may be used to determine species, whereas nuclear DNA is needed to differentiate individuals within a population. Microsatellites are a class of nuclear DNA primers commonly used for conducting population genetic analyses because they are highly variable in almost all vertebrates, alleles from both chromosome pairs in diploid organisms are recognized, heterozygous and homozygous individuals may be distinguished, and they conform to many population genetic models.[18]

Different analytic techniques may be used to identify species using mtDNA. A region of the genome may be sequenced and then matched through a national database. A DNA barcode may be created using a standardized region of the mtDNA or a restriction enzyme test may generate DNA fragments, which are then separated by gel electrophoresis to create unique patterns (restriction maps) for individual species. Most identification of species is based on mitochondrial DNA, which is more durable than nuclear DNA because it is protected from enzymatic action within the cell.[9] A greater number of microsatellites is needed for small and inbred populations because genetic variation is less.[22]

Gender determinations typically are made using one of three genes: (1) the *sex*-determining *r*egion *Y* (SRY) gene is present only on the male Y chromosome; (2) genes in the zinc finger region of X and Y chromosomes are of variable length; and (3) the amelogenin gene is of variable length in X and Y chromosomes.

Various genotyping errors may occur that may either overestimate or underestimate abundance or identify individuals inaccurately.[22] Genetic errors may be identified and dealt with in several ways. Genotyping consistency may be ensured by analyzing each locus up to seven times; however, this may be expensive and requires more DNA. The amount of DNA present in each sample may be quantified so that estimates may be made of the optimal number of times that each sample should be analyzed to eliminate errors. Other techniques use computer algorithms to estimate genotype reliability, detect genotyping errors, and assess the number of loci needed to provide enough power to achieve the study's objectives.

Endocrine Analyses

Fecal or urinary hormone analysis has become increasingly popular as a noninvasive way to monitor endocrine function in various mammalian and avian species.[13,19,25] Noninvasive collection methods do not affect endocrine research results, which is important because anesthesia has been associated with a decline

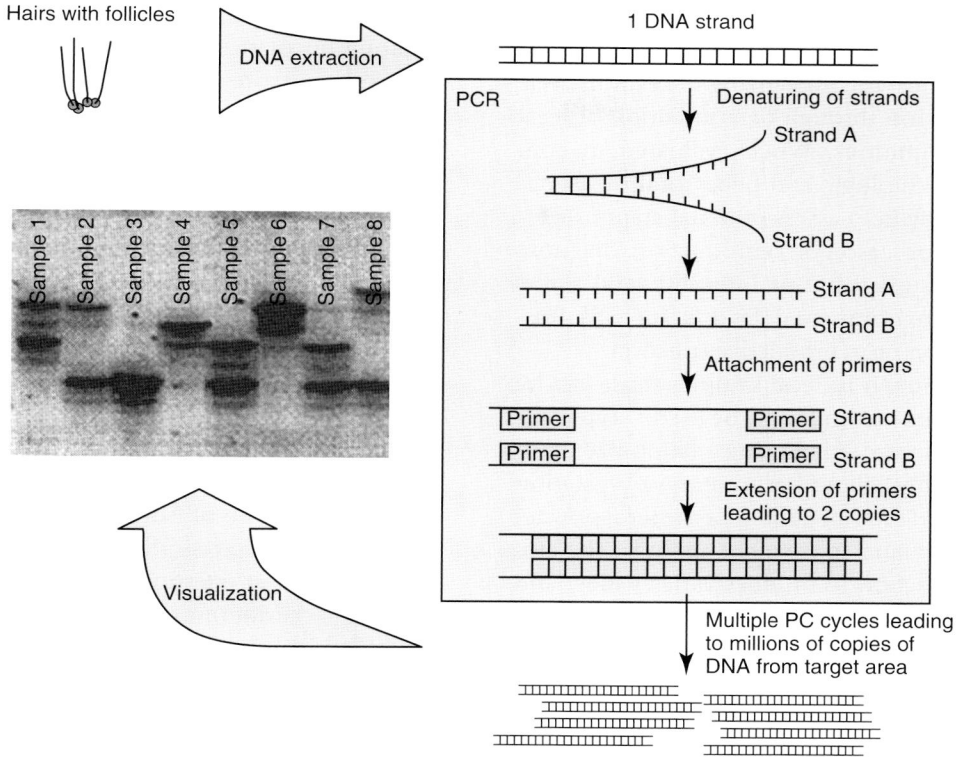

Hairs with follicles

DNA extraction

1 DNA strand

PCR

Denaturing of strands

Strand A

Strand B

Strand A
Strand B

Attachment of primers

Primer | Primer | Strand A
Primer | Primer | Strand B

Extension of primers
leading to 2 copies

Multiple PC cycles leading
to millions of copies of
DNA from target area

Visualization

Sample 1 Sample 2 Sample 3 Sample 4 Sample 5 Sample 6 Sample 7 Sample 8

Figure 9-1

Schematic illustration of the process of deriving individual identification from hair samples. This process begins with DNA extraction, which produces DNA strands. Next, a particular region of the DNA is amplified using (in this case) microsatellite primers and the polymerase chain reaction (PCR). The PCR process involves three major steps: (1) the denaturing of the double-stranded DNA molecule; (2) the attachment of primers at a particular locus in the genome; and (3) the extension of these primers to produce a copy of the original locus. After multiple PCR cycles, millions—if not billions—of copies of the region are created, and may then be visualized on an electrophoresis gel. This gel image shows eight Canada lynx samples evaluated at one microsatellite locus. Even with one locus, multiple individuals may already be discerned, but samples 5 and 7 produce the same banding pattern at this locus. Ultimately, when additional loci were run, these two samples were determined to be from different individuals. *(From Long RA, MacKay P, Zielinski WJ, et al [eds]: Noninvasive survey methods for carnivores. Washington DC, Island Press, 2008, p 241.)*

in testosterone secretion in some species and handling likely affects concentrations of corticosteroids in stress-related studies.[13] Endocrine status determined by fecal or urine hormone analysis may be evaluated over an extended period of time instead of a single point in time, so much larger data sets may be generated. Because circulating glucocorticoid levels may increase rapidly in response to handling—within 2 minutes for birds and small mammals—fecal glucocorticoid levels represent a more meaningful and accurate assessment of stress over time. Additionally, the diurnal fluctuation in glucocorticoid levels appears to be attenuated in fecal samples, making it a more reliable indictor of stress than point in time blood glucocorticoid concentrations.

Different species metabolize hormones to varying degrees (e.g., only 7% of glucocorticoid metabolites are excreted in the feces of pigs compared with 86% in cats).[17] Fecal concentrations of glucocorticoids may also vary naturally based on nutritional status, gut transit time, reproductive life history, gender, pregnancy, seasonal cycles, and many other adaptive physiologic states. Therefore, elevated concentrations of glucocorticoids alone do not necessarily indicate elevated levels of stress and must be evaluated in concert with other physiologic and environmental factors.

Ideally, endocrine profiles may be matched with other types of physiologic or behavioral data to strengthen the interpretation of results. For example, reproductive activity may be assessed noninvasively by observing behaviors during estrus, mating, and parturition and simultaneously characterizing the estrous cycle and length of gestation through determination of fecal progestagen concentrations. When evaluated in conjunction with other biologic and behavioral measures, this information may help assess pubertal status, determine the influence of season on reproduction, diagnose possible causes of subfertility or infertility, and assess the influence of environmental factors such as husbandry and nutrition on reproductive function.

Hormones quantified in fecal samples must first be extracted, and various methods may be used.[13] Typically, frozen samples are freeze-dried using a lyophilizer, pulverized and sifted through a filter to remove vegetation and other debris, and then an aliquot of the fecal powder is used for extraction and subsequent analysis. The efficacy of various extraction techniques varies widely and is measured by evaluating the recovery of labeled steroids. Fecal steroid hormones may be quantified using enzyme immunoassay (EIA), enzyme-linked immunoassay (ELISA), or radioimmunoassay (RIA). ELISA was developed in 1970 and the early 1980s marked a steady divergence in the use of ELISA versus RIA according to the number of publications using these terms. However, immunoassay-based tests using antibodies cannot identify and quantify all individual metabolites in a sample. For this purpose, high-performance liquid chromatography (HPLC) is used to separate immunoreactive hormone metabolites and characterize endocrine profiles further.[19]

Validation of fecal sampling and storage procedures should be performed for different species and to ensure that endocrine data have not been altered by postdefecation metabolization and breakdown.[18] Appropriate biochemical and physiologic validations of fecal steroid hormone assays should also be reported. Biochemical validations include demonstration of parallelism using serially diluted fecal extracts against standard curves, quantitative recovery of exogenous hormone added to fecal samples prior to extraction, assay precision involving both intra-assay and interassay coefficients of variation, and treatments in which additional hormone administered by injection may be detected in fecal samples postadministration. Physiologic validation is not routinely done but is important, and helps indicate that both direct stimulation of the endocrine axis (e.g., adrenocorticotropin stimulation demonstrates an increase in corticosteroids detected in feces) and meaningful in situ hormone levels may be detected by the assay. Augmenting laboratory findings with supplementary information, such as matching estrogen hormone fluctuations with behavioral signs of estrus, may help ensure that results are physiologically relevant.

Nutritional Analyses

Questions about ecologic niche and differences in diet between and within species may be answered through stable isotope and elemental analysis of various samples. For example, stable isotope analysis of hair has demonstrated that one population of brown bears fed primarily on salmon whereas another at higher elevations fed on berries. All biologically active elements exist in several different isotopic forms, of which two or more are stable. The ratio of isotope forms may be altered by biologic and geophysical processes, and these differences may answer questions about the diet and ecology of animals. Furthermore, set rates of growth make it possible to identify recent geographic histories through isotopic analysis. For example, the ratio of ^{18}O to ^{16}O in the shells of a clam species has been used to assess the historical extent of a river delta estuary prior to the construction of upstream dams.[6] The main elements used in isotope ecologic analyses are carbon, nitrogen, oxygen, hydrogen, and sulfur.

Fecal samples may be used to infer dietary preferences and assess nutrient content in various species. Acid digests are typically performed on processed plant and/or herbivore fecal samples in preparation for analysis by atomic absorption spectroscopy to determine element content, and fecal nitrogen levels indicate dietary protein intake. Remains of prey in feces and predator DNA from sloughed gastrointestinal cells or bile powder may be analyzed to study carnivore diets.

Disease Diagnostics

Biologic samples collected noninvasively may be analyzed to learn about disease transmission and dynamics and inform treatment and management decisions. Wildlife diseases may serve as indicators of pollution or degradation of ecosystems. Movements of wildlife prompted by environmental changes such as global warming may lead to movement of pathogens into susceptible host populations; most pathogens that cause human and animal diseases may infect and be transmitted by more than one host species. Diagnostic molecular assays may be used as effective noninvasive health monitoring tools in wildlife populations by detecting broad host pathogens actively shed in fecal material and applying geographic information system (GIS) technology and spatial data analysis to evaluate regional disease exposure risks. Additionally, consumed prey in carnivore feces may be detected, which is of interest because certain prey species may increase the disease exposure risk to carnivores.

Some routine clinical tests currently used to diagnose disease often rely on single disease biomarkers (e.g., prostate-specific antigen [PSA]), which are not specific enough and are inappropriate when a number of factors are involved.[7] These unique proteins are usually originally identified by mass spectrometry (MS) and then used to develop an ELISA-based platform to screen multiple samples for the presence of the biomarker. However, success in discovery of novel diagnostic biomarkers has been remarkably poor for two reasons: (1) valuable biomarkers that are expressed at low abundances are not routinely detected using current technology; and (2) physiologic variability of the clinical sample obtained (e.g., urine, serum, plasma) makes the identification of a unique biomarker challenging. The measurement of a panel of identified biomarkers for a particular disease state may dramatically increase overall diagnostic accuracy.

Metabolic Profiling

The idea that biologic fluids reflect the health of an individual has been around for a long time. Urine charts were used in the middle ages to link the colors, tastes, and smells of urine to various medical conditions that were metabolic in origin. By the mid-1980s, nuclear magnetic resonance (NMR) spectroscopy was sensitive enough to identify metabolites in unmodified biologic fluids, which led to the discovery that altered metabolite profiles are caused by certain diseases or by adverse side effects to drugs. The metabolome has been defined as "the qualitative and quantitative collection of all low molecular weight molecules (metabolites) present in a cell that are participants in general metabolic reactions and that are required for the maintenance, growth and normal function of a cell."[11] In the past decade, metabolomics has become increasingly popular because of the ability to measure multiple metabolites directly from complex biologic systems with excellent accuracy and precision. Another advantage of analyzing the metabolome is that the downstream product of gene expression more appropriately reflects cell function and takes environmental effects into account. Metabolite markers have diagnostic and therapeutic

applications, but may also be used in research to facilitate understanding of the causes of disease processes and develop new drug targets. An example of a metabolomics application is described and illustrated in Figure 9-2.

MS is the most widely applied technology in metabolomics, because it provides a blend of rapid qualitative and quantitative analyses with the ability to identify metabolites. MS studies usually require metabolites to be separated from the biologic fluid before detection, typically by using HPLC. NMR is the only detection technique that does not rely on separation of the analytes, and therefore the sample may be recovered for further analyses. ^{1}H-NMR spectroscopy is the most sensitive and most commonly used—all types of small molecule metabolites may be measured simultaneously and biologic samples require no special treatment prior to analysis (Fig. 9-3). Many other analytic techniques may be used to quantify metabolites, including Fourier transform infrared (FTIR) spectroscopy, Fourier transform ion cyclotron resonance MS, and Raman spectroscopy.[7]

Metabonomics became used more widely when it was realized that pattern recognition methods, also known as chemometrics or multivariate statistical analysis, could help interpret the complex data sets that result from these studies.[21] Unsupervised methods, such as principal components analysis, are used to reduce data complexity and look at natural differences and similarities among data sets by clustering them into groups using scatter plots. Supervised methods, such as partial least squares, are techniques for sample classification using calibrated models.

FUTURE NONINVASIVE TOOLS AND CHALLENGES

Veterinary medicine typically adapts new technologies to further its own medical and conservation goals relevant to a wide variety of wildlife species. In the future, technologies will evolve further to provide advanced treatment and management options in addition to current diagnostic and research applications.

Remote camera technologies are constantly improving through the use of digital high-capacity memory cards, silent shutter mechanisms, and infrared illumination. Advances to enhance weatherproofing, incorporate the ability to download images remotely, and install automated baiting mechanisms will likely represent the next generation of cameras.

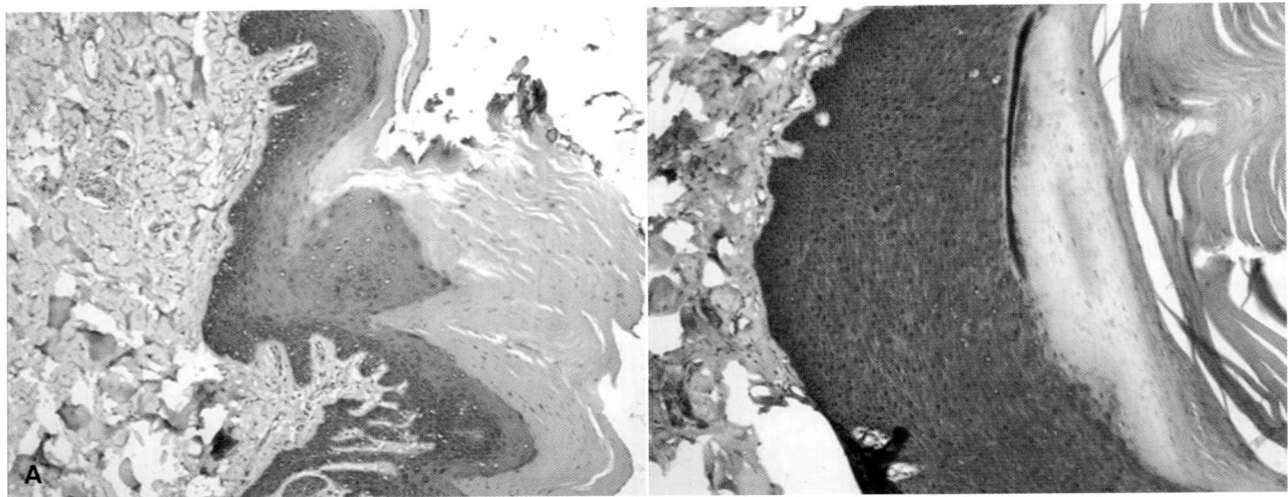

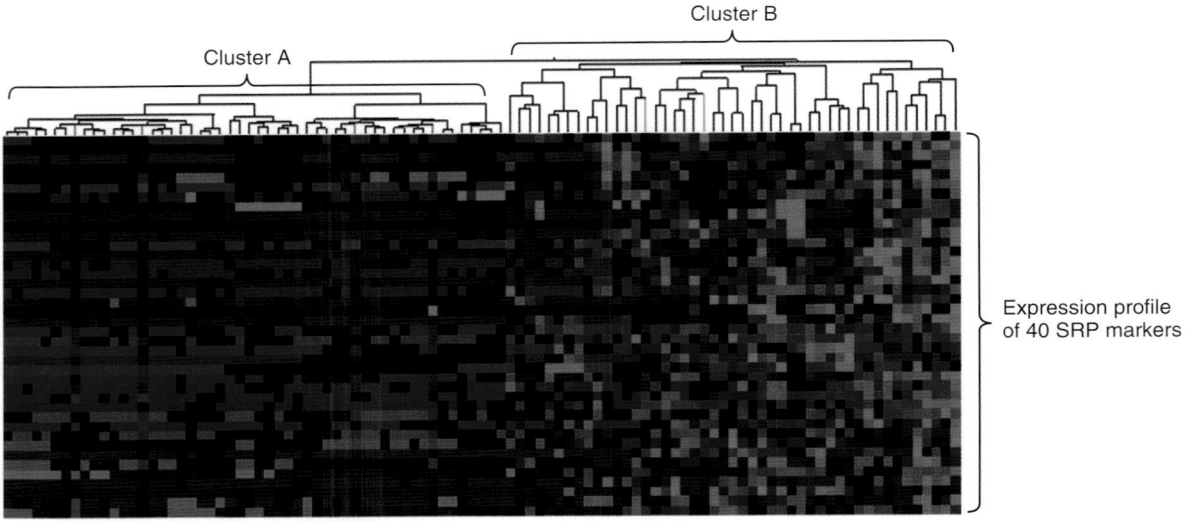

Forty individual SRP markers were measured in skin samples (n = 99) from nine species of mammals (humans, four species of dolphin, three species of whales):
• Physiologically stressed (diseased, injured, extreme environmental conditions); n = 46
• Not stressed (healthy controls), n = 47 and African elephants.
• Physiologically stressed (diseased); n = 2
• Not stressed (healthy controls); n = 4.
Measurements were normalized relative to the average marker level in controls and log-transformed. Relatedness between expression profiles of SRP markers was analyzed using hierarchic clustering (Ward method, geometric x scale). The green-black-red color scheme indicates increasing marker levels. Similar profiles are in clusters. SRP expression profiles of control and stressed subjects are in separate clusters (A and B) demonstrating accurate diagnosis of stress.

Figure 9-2

Stress response profiling (SRP) may be used to assess chronic stress in free-ranging African elephants by measuring expressed levels of multiple stress response proteins in skin biopsy samples using immunohistochemical staining and image analysis. The effects of stress occur on a cellular level and are characterized by a range of responses mediated by the endocrine, immune, and nervous systems. Examples of SRP biomarkers include cyclooxygenase 2, heat shock proteins 40, 60, and 90, interleukin (IL)-6, IL-8, IL-10 and IL-12, ferritin, and glucocorticoid receptors. The general SRP pattern is conserved across many mammalian species, gender, age, and a broad range of stressors. Principal components analysis is initially used to determine which SRP biomarkers are most stress-sensitive, based on several stress response pathways. *A,* Immunohistochemical stained epidermal skin samples are subject to computerized image analysis. *B,* Variations in staining intensity are then used to create profiles through hierarchic clustering to discriminate between physiologically stressed and unstressed individuals. A large number of specimens may be processed simultaneously using a high-throughput adaptation of SRP profiling. Recognition of elevated cellular stress using SRP profiling may serve as an early warning of compromised health and as a guide for monitoring the impact of conservation and management strategies. *(From Bechert U, Southern S: Unpublished data.)*

Control

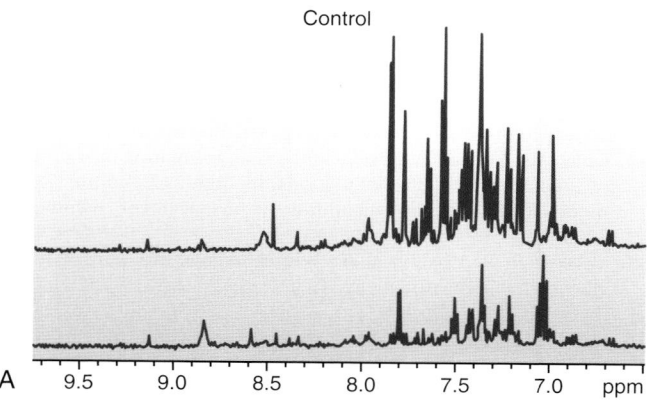

Interstitial cystitis

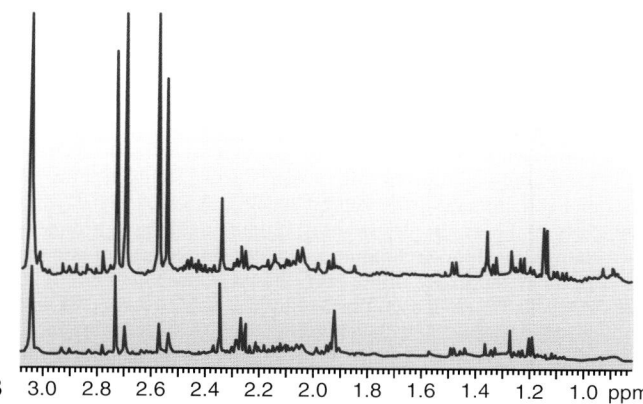

Bacterial cystitis

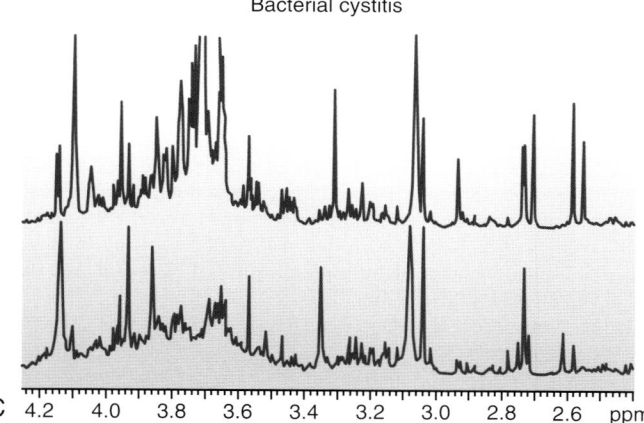

Figure 9-3

Comparison of ¹H-NMR spectra of urine samples obtained from normal controls **(A)**, interstitial cystitis patients **(B)**, and bacterial cystitis patients **(C)**. *(From Van QN, Klose JR, Lucas DA, et al: The use of urine proteomic and metabonomic patterns for the diagnosis of interstitial cystitis and bacterial cystitis. Dis Markers 2003-2004;19:175.)*

We will see more advances in gene technologies and an increase in the types and numbers of DNA-based applications. Microarrays are becoming more popular and allow hundreds of loci to be examined at one time so that specific physiologic functions, such as immune and stress responses, may be explored. Single-nucleotide polymorphisms may eventually replace microsatellites because they are more common throughout the genome and presumably provide data with absolute scores, facilitating comparisons among studies with the same species.[18] Landscape genetics is an emerging field that links genetic structure to landscape features and enables the study of population fragmentation, functional connectivity, and animal movements.[5]

The number of publications including the terms *Raman, FTIR,* or *near-infrared (NIR) spectroscopy* in conjunction with *cancer* increased fivefold between 2000 and 2005, indicating the growing level of interest in these analytic tools.[7] As more in-depth understanding of disease progression becomes realized, it will become possible to generate qualitative and quantitative predictions from infrared and Raman spectroscopies, leading to the potential ability to detect the stage of progression of a particular disease (e.g., cancer) and not just its presence or absence. Optical technology is rapidly developing and instruments are already available commercially as portable, hand-held, and microdevices. These include infrared filtometers and infrared and Raman mobile microspectrometers. Future field assays will allow samples to be analyzed instantaneously, eliminating the need for time-consuming storage and processing methods, which could potentially alter results.

Metabolome-wide association studies, which identify relationships between metabolic profiles and disease risks for individuals and populations, will be the next big step in metabonomics. Genetically based, personalized medicine strategies make sense, but progress in this field has been disappointing because of genome complexity and the fact that most major diseases are strongly influenced by the environment and other external factors. However, individual metabolic profiles may eventually guide treatment strategies. Future challenges revolve around ways to interpret data generated in the field of metabolomics correctly. High-throughput experiments are being conducted to discover biomarker metabolites that may discriminate between apparently matched case and control samples with some level of certainty; however, only about 10% of papers in the field of metabolomics mention any statistical treatment.[4] Key challenges to overcome include bias introduced by confounding variables, inadequate sample size and statistical power, excessive false discovery rate because of multiple hypotheses testing, inappropriate choice of particular numeric methods, and inadequate validation. It is extremely important that prevalence be taken into account because a biomarker test for a disease with a low prevalence is likely to have many more false-positives than a disease characterized by higher prevalence. The recent number of publications specifically addressing these challenges is encouraging.

Acknowledgment

I thank Cynthia Chapman for the time she took to edit this chapter.

REFERENCES

1. Apps CD, McLellan BN, Woods JG, et al: Estimating grizzly bear distribution and abundance relative to habitat and human influence. J Wildl Manage 68:138–152, 2004.
2. Bechert U, Southern S: Monitoring environmental stress in African elephants through molecular analysis of stress-activated proteins, In Proceedings of the American Association of Zoo Veterinarians, 2002, Yulee, Fla, 2002, AAZV, pp 269–273.
3. Beehner JC, Whitten PL: Modifications of a field method for fecal steroid analysis in baboons. Physiol Behav 82:269–277, 2004.
4. Broadhurst DI, Kell DB: Statistical strategies for avoiding false discoveries in metabolomics and related experiments. Metabolomics 2:171–196, 2006.
5. Cushman SA, McKelvey KS, Hayden J, et al: Gene flow in complex landscapes: testing multiple hypotheses with causal modeling. Am Nat 168:486–499, 2006.
6. Dickin AP: Radiogenic isotope geology, New York, 2005, Cambridge University Press.
7. Ellis DI, Dunn WB, Griffin JL, et al: Metabolic fingerprinting as a diagnostic tool. Pharmacogenomics 8:1243–1266, 2007.
8. Farrell LE, Roman J, Sunquist ME: Dietary separation of sympatric carnivores identified by molecular analysis of scats. Mol Ecol 9:1583–1590, 2000.
9. Foran DR: Relative degradation of nuclear and mitochondrial DNA: an experimental approach. J Forensic Sci 51:766–770, 2006.
10. Goosens B, Waits LP, Taberlet P: Plucked hair samples as a source of DNA: reliability of dinucleotide microsatellite genotyping. Mol Ecol 7:1237–1241, 1998.
11. Harrigan GG, Goodacre R: Metabolic profiling: its role in biomarker discovery and gene function analysis, London, 2003, Kluwer Academic.
12. Hausknecht R, Gula R, Pirga B, et al: Urine—a source for noninvasive genetic monitoring in wildlife. Mol Ecol Notes 7:208–212, 2007.
13. Keay JM, Singh J, Gaunt MC, et al: Fecal glucocorticoids and their metabolites as indicators of stress in various mammalian species: a literature review. J Zoo Wildl Med 37:234–244, 2006.
14. Lancia RA, Kendall WL, Pollock KH, et al: Estimating the number of animals in wildlife populations. In Braun CE, editor: Techniques for wildlife investigations and management, Baltimore, 2005, Port City Press, pp 106–153.
15. Millspaugh JJ, Washburn BE: Within-sample variation of fecal glucocorticoid measurements. Gen Comp Endocrinol 132:21–26, 2003.
16. Monfort SL: Endocrine measures of reproduction and stress in wild populations. In Wildt DE, Holt W, Pickard NA, editors: Reproduction and integrated conservation science, Cambridge, England, 2003, Cambridge University Press, pp 147–165.
17. Palme R, Rettenbacher S, Touma C, et al: Comparative aspects regarding metabolism, excretion, and noninvasive measurement in fecal samples. N Y Acad Sci 1040:162–171, 2005.
18. Schwartz MK, Monfort SL: Genetic and endocrine tools for carnivore surveys. In Long RA, MacKay P, Zielinski WJ, et al, editors: Noninvasive survey methods for carnivores, Washington, DC, 2008, Island Press, pp 238–262.
19. Schwarzenberger F, Mostl E, Palme R, et al: Faecal steroid analysis for noninvasive monitoring of reproductive status in farm, wild and zoo animals. Anim Reprod Sci 42:515–526, 1996.
20. Silvy AJ, Lopez RR, Peterson MJ: Wildlife marking techniques. In Braun CE, editor: Techniques for wildlife investigations and management, Baltimore, 2005, Port City Press, pp 339–375.
21. Valafar F: Pattern recognition techniques in microarray data analysis. N Y Acad Sci 980:41–64, 2002.
22. Waits JL, Luikart G, Taberlet P: Estimating the probability of identity among genotypes in natural populations: cautions and guidelines. Mol Ecol 10:249–256, 2001.
23. Waits LP, Paetkau D: Noninvasive genetic sampling tools for wildlife biologists: a review of applications and recommendations for accurate data collection. J Wildl Manage 69:1419–1433, 2005.
24. Wasser SK, Davenport B, Ramage ER, et al: Scat detection dogs in wildlife research and management: applications to grizzly and black bears in the Yellowhead ecosystem, Alberta, Canada. J Zool 82:475–492, 2004.
25. Wasser SK, Hunt KE, Brown JL, et al: A generalized fecal glucocorticoid assay for use in a diverse array of nondomestic mammalian and avian species. Gen Comp Endocrinol 120:260–275, 2000.
26. Williams CL, Blejwas K, Johnson JJ, et al: A coyote in sheep's clothing: predator identification from saliva. Wildl Soc Bull 31:926–932, 2003.

CHAPTER 10

Culture and Media Shifts: Challenges and Opportunities for Veterinarians

Jill Allread and Robert Hilsenroth

In an age of high-speed communications, social media, and citizen journalists, professionals cannot underestimate the influence of communications on their job and on public perception of their work. Veterinarians who work in a public wildlife agency or in an institution with animals on public display increasingly are required to use their communication skills to navigate societal changes regarding animals and their relation to humans. Heightened public interest in animals and their welfare is leading to veterinarians in zoos, aquariums, and wildlife management being increasingly called on to talk publicly about animal welfare issues, animal care practices, and veterinary treatment.

Today, institutions are calling on their veterinarians to be key spokespersons with print, broadcast, and even social media, such as in web blogs or in videos on YouTube, on topics that include animal deaths, which until the 1990s were generally not of interest to the media. Veterinarians are being interviewed by reporters, many of whom are more closely scrutinizing the care and welfare of zoo and aquarium animals. This interest is in part to the result of national and international campaigns and other efforts by animal rights organizations working to establish legal rights for animals, and who oppose animals being used by humans. For most of these groups, animal use includes keeping animals in zoos and aquariums; managing wildlife populations; using animals in research, livestock production; hunting and fishing; and people using animal-based products such as food, clothing, or animal products for cultural uses.

For decades, the public has generally assumed that animals in accredited zoos and aquariums have a high quality of life. More than 180 million people visit Association of Zoos and Aquarium (AZA)–accredited zoos and aquariums annually,[3] and attendance and public support for these institutions remains strong. Societal attitudes, however, are rapidly changing. They have been influenced by a growing number of animal rights organizations formed since the1980s and the expansion of animal law and its influence on changing the status of animals in society. These changes have contributed to more scrutiny by the media and questions by the public about animal care and management in zoos and aquariums and about the human, and humane, management of wildlife populations. These shifts are changing the role of veterinarians working in these specialty areas.

This chapter provides insights into culture changes that will continue to require veterinary professionals not only to be excellent practitioners but to be highly effective communicators. It examines some of the influences behind changing public attitudes about the role of animals and their relationship to humans in a rapidly urbanizing society, and identifies opportunities for zoo and wildlife veterinarians to be proactive when addressing issues that reinforce their expertise and leadership role in animal care. Later in the chapter, we also provide specific tips and tactics that enable veterinarians to strengthen their own communication skills and to be an effective and valued resource for the media and public.

CULTURAL ISSUES AND CHANGES

Animals Elicit Emotion

Most people love animals. In fact, 62% of all American households (71.1 million)[1] have pets, compared with only 46% of households having children younger than 18 years at home.[9] Pet owners annually spend $45.5 billion on their pets and almost 50% of them consider the animals living with them to be members of their family. It's not surprising, then, that animals elicit such strong emotional responses. With increasing public interest in animals and broader promotion of animal rights activism, the relationship between humans and animals has been experiencing one of its most significant shifts in the last 50 years.

Media already are responding to the increasing public interest in animals. For example, Animal Planet Channel features many programs, including "Meerkat Manor," "Petfinder," and "Animal Cops," and the popular network show "Funniest Pets and People," enjoys growing audiences and sponsor support. There are hundreds of pet magazines and publications, pet websites, blogs, and Facebook fan pages, and many newspapers publish pet advice columns that offer advice, local events for pets, animal stories, and pet finder resources.

From Farm to Family

In the last 40 years, America's agricultural-based society has drastically shifted to a predominantly urbanized society. With less than 2% of the U.S. population involved in farming today, and most people three to four generations removed from the farm, a significant detachment has evolved regarding the role of farm animals.[6] People are much less likely to have experienced animals being raised on a farm, primarily for food products. Few children living in cities today think about a live chicken when ordering chicken nuggets from a menu.

The changing perceptions regarding the status of animals in society have created vastly differing views, ranging from the extremes of close companion to consumption or exploitation to education. They have also affected public opinions about animal management, including displaying animals in zoos, aquariums or wildlife parks, and managing populations of animals (e.g., wild horse management, wolf reintroductions, deer culling) on public-owned lands. The discussion also arises, and is covered by the media, when urban living and wildlife conflict, such as when coyotes threaten people's pets, raccoons take over attics or, even the case when a 150-pound cougar was shot in a Chicago neighborhood alleyway in April 2008.[5] As a result, animal-related controversies arise.

Also, the attention of animal rights groups and the media are more focused on any issues related to animals, including the following: agribusiness, including dairy, eggs and meat production; fur and leather use, from fashion to footballs; research, including cosmetics and pharmaceutical product testing; education, including

biology classes using animal specimens for dissection; fishing and hunting; pet stores; dog and cat breeders and purebred competitions; and circuses, rodeos, and even grocery stores. For example, some food producers now seek the "Certified Humane Raised and Handled" labels, which indicate that the animal involved was raised humanely and without a diet that includes antibiotics or hormones. The program is managed by the Humane Farm Animal Care (HFAC) group, a national nonprofit organization dedicated to improving the lives of farm animals by certifying their humane treatment. It is supported by more than 36 animal-focused organizations, including the American Society for the Prevention of Cruelty to Animals (ASPCA), and the Humane Society of the United States.[4]

Lawyers for Animals

Animal law is one of the fastest growing segments of law practice in North America. It includes efforts to ensure the welfare, and in some cases the legal rights, of animals by establishing new case law through the courts and legislation. In many cases, an individual or group seeks court rulings to establish legal standing for animals, similar to the rights afforded a person.

Animal law encompasses companion animals, wildlife, animals used in entertainment, animals raised for food, and animals used in research. Animal law permeates and affects most traditional areas of the law, including tort, contract, criminal, and constitutional law, and in just a few years it has shown how animal law activities are now an established part of contemporary American and Western culture.

Law schools in North America have responded to the interest. As many as 116 of 180 law schools now offer animal law courses or programs. which is 10 times as many as just 10 years ago. This in turn increases the amount of litigation involving how animals are treated and their legal standing by law; it can encompass veterinary malpractice, animal custody cases, and trusts for companion animals. High-profile cases, such as Leona Helmsley leaving a $12 million inheritance to her dog Trouble, has raised awareness that 39 states allow pet owners to endow pet trusts.

Few will argue that cruelty to animals is unacceptable; however, it has only been in the last 10 years that states began passing stricter animal cruelty laws, including felony animal cruelty laws in 42 states. The high-profile conviction of National Football League quarterback Michael Vick for participating in illegal dog fighting is an example of the intensified protection of animals by laws and the counts. Attorney Michael Socarras told the Association of American Medical Colleges that "there is a very important shift underway in the manner in which many people in law schools and in the legal profession think about animals. This shift has not yet reached popular opinion. However, in [the United States], social change has and may occur through the courts, which in many instances do not operate as democratic institutions. Therefore, the evolution in elite legal opinion is extremely significant."[7]

Celebrity Influence

Once seen as often too extreme in their views—that animals deserve the same rights as humans—animal rights groups, such as People for the Ethical Treatment of Animals (PETA), are using strategic communications and creative projects to gain more broad recognition from the public and media as animal advocates. PETA's often edgy campaigns—for example, going naked to oppose wearing fur—draw media and public attention, and they successfully use the social media to enlist and mobilize a wide range of supporters who share their beliefs. For example, following the death of a high-profile elephant, some zoos received hundreds of e-mail messages generated by PETA followers requesting that the zoo close its elephant program within hours of the animal's death. PETA and In Defense of Animals (IDA) both have national campaigns that include websites, public programs, and dedicated staff working at removing elephants from zoos permanently.

Celebrities, with their strong influence particularly on young people in their teens and 20s, play an influential role in animal rights issues. Pamela Anderson is frequently a spokeswoman for PETA's antifur campaign. Former "The Price is Right" star Bob Barker, who in 2010 donated $5 million to Sea Shepherd Conservation Society to fight whaling, as well as $1 million to stop pigeon shoots in Pennsylvania, has consistently made $1 million grants to numerous U.S. law schools, including Harvard, Stanford, University of Virginia, and Northwestern University, for the establishment of animal law programs. Noted animal lawyer and former Animal Legal Defense Fund president Steven M. Wise says that Barker, with his direct donations, has the right idea regarding how to change the status of animals in society rapidly. Wise taught the first animal law course at Harvard Law School and wrote the seminal animal rights book, *Rattling the Cage: Toward Legal Rights for Animals*.[8]

VETERINARIANS IN THE SPOTLIGHT

The cultural shifts affecting the status and legal standing of animals directly affects how zoo and wildlife veterinarians and their institutions must talk about the management of animals in their care. Zoos and agencies have become more proactive in telling their story to the public, which includes articulating and demonstrating their expertise, training, and commitment to the well-being of animals. Most zoos recognize that their institution's reputation could be seriously damaged if it allows a critic to tell the zoo's story instead of a zoo spokesperson. In some cases, an investigation by the media may create a crisis, not just for an institution, but for an entire industry. For example, shortly after *The Washington Post* launched a series of investigative stories in 2003 examining animal deaths and animal husbandry, health, and care at the Smithsonian Institution's National Zoological Park (National Zoo), media in cities around the country began looking more closely at animal care in zoos and aquariums in their communities.

The U.S. Freedom of Information Act (FOIA)[10] provides for access to public records, and an FOIA request is frequently used by animal rights groups to obtain access to animal health records in publicly managed zoos. When the National Zoo story attracted national news coverage, reporters around the country began making FOIA requests seeking detailed information about the cause or circumstance surrounding any zoo animal deaths, including necropsy reports and treatment records. Questions are often asked of zoo veterinarians regarding animal deaths and their age at death. Zoo veterinarians are called on as key spokespersons to help the media and public better understand the level of care of zoo and aquarium animals.

Most zoos have been surprised by the intense media interest in animal deaths. Until the 1990s, zoos and aquariums had not proactively publicized most animal deaths on the assumption that the public understood that all animals, like all humans, die at some point. Suddenly, some zoos found the media inquiring about every zoo animal death, almost as if every animal death might be considered suspicious. Zoos have since become more proactive in talking about all animals' circle of life, including death, and demonstrating to the media and public the extraordinary care and expertise that they provide for animals in their care.

The same is true for government agencies charged with animal population management. For example, the media extensively covered the planning and subsequent protest by the Humane Society of the United States of the National Oceanic and Atmospheric Administration (NOAA) Fisheries intention to cull up to 85 California sea lions a year for 5 years in the Columbia River at Bonneville Dam. This is where they gather annually to feed on the spring Chinook salmon, predation that was causing significant negative impact on the salmon population.[2] Veterinarians and other animal experts played a role in telling this complex story to the media.

With training, credentials, and experience, veterinarians will have an increasingly important voice in public and media discussions about the care of animals and wildlife. At no time has it been more critical for veterinarians working in zoo and aquarium animal and wildlife management agencies to be trained and prepared as effective communicators.

Working With the Media is Essential

The job of a reporter, whether working for newspaper, radio, television, or online, is to gather and report the news. Unless on special assignment, most reporters come to work not knowing what they will be researching and reporting on during their work day. News directors make assignments, and the reporter's job is to gather the facts and develop a news story.

Reporters have much expertise in collecting information and producing the stories that we read, hear, or see, but they often know little about the animals that zoo and wildlife veterinarians treat. They must rely on the information that the zoo or wildlife veterinarian provides to deliver the news accurately. It is important to remember that reporters attempt to represent the public when seeking information that is of interest to them.

If the zoo or wildlife veterinarian establishes himself or herself as an expert (which they are), then he or she may build a good working relationship with reporters. Once that relationship is established, the media will seek a veterinarian for accurate information. They will understand that what veterinarians have to say is science-based rather than emotion-based. Over time, the media may help disseminate an institution's key messages and will be open to hearing an institution's side of the story when the news may not be so good.

Establish a Relationship With Media

The media will not know about the extraordinary animal stories happening in zoos or concerning wildlife unless someone informs them. Begin building a relationship with reporters by offering interesting, truthful, and informative news stories. Be sure to work with the institution's public relations or communications staff, and make sure that supervisors are informed and have approved the outreach. Keep in mind that most of what a veterinarian does may seem mundane to those in the profession, but to the general public, zoo and aquarium veterinarians perform modern medical miracles to care for and extend the life of exotic animals. News releases are the preferred method to get the media's attention, and a follow-up phone call or two usually helps. Don't be discouraged when your releases are ignored, but chances are that sooner or later, a reporter or editor will be interested in covering a story.

Develop and strengthen a reputation for newsworthy information and for knowing about current issues. Stay current about zoo and wildlife news by reading articles, watching newscasts, and listening to radio reports, especially when the news involves species in your collection. Stay in contact with colleagues to exchange information and to stay informed. Ask friends who are not in the zoo and wildlife field to be vigilant for news that might be of interest to the public. Ask staff to do the same.

Most zoo and wildlife veterinarians have access to animals, and animal stories are great visual stories for television and newspapers. Let the media know that you have these resources and are willing to talk about a story. Those in the media need sources that are knowledgeable, credible, accessible, and quotable (sound bites). Also, expect any videotaped stories to end up on the Internet, either on the news station's website or on YouTube. This means that it will be accessible for a long time, so prepare your messages before going on videotape.

Learn to speak the language that reporters need to hear, which is clear, concise, and factual. Veterinarians are highly trained and have an impressive vocabulary, but if the listener, viewer, or reader cannot understand what is being said, the point of the interview is lost. Use language and terms that everyone can understand. For example, we all know that it's an abdomen, but to most people, it's a belly—so call it a belly.

Pitch stories that might be important to the viewers, listeners, and readers in the local area. The media is attracted to stories that tie in with the public they serve. There might be a new diabetes diagnostic and treatment center set up at the local hospital—are any zoo animals under treatment for diabetes? A local sports figure might suffer a fracture that requires extensive orthopedic procedures—has a zoo animal had a similar fracture repair that could be discussed? Urban wildlife encounters happen all the time, such as when coyotes and even cougars show up in the middle of a city. This is a good time to tell the animal's side of the story and deliver a key message about human and wild animal relationships. Each story helps establish veterinarians as trained, knowledgeable animal experts.

When offering a story to the media, make sure that the story fits the medium. A radio station probably is not interested in great visual opportunities, and television stations usually aren't interested unless there are great visual opportunities. Newspapers like stories that may be accompanied by a photograph, and photographs of nondomestic animals are popular.

It is advisable to remain flexible and respect deadlines to earn respect with the media. It helps to understand that what might be an important story to a zoo veterinarian might not be as important to the local media if there is an unexpected snowstorm or other breaking news develops. See if they could do the story another time. If the reporter is relying on you for a story, it is imperative that you cooperate and respect deadlines. If a reporter comes back to the newsroom empty-handed because you weren't available when needed, you probably will not get another chance with that reporter or that newsroom.

Ask questions about the story and make sure that you have addressed them prior to talking about an animal issue. These could include the following:

- Who is affected by the story?
- What is the story about?
- When is it happening?
- Where is it happening?
- Why is it happening?
- Why is it important?
- How does it affect the public?

The Hot Seat

With increasing attention on animal care and welfare in zoos and aquariums, and on public lands, it is likely that the media will contact your institution to talk about what could be perceived as bad news. The truth is that bad things, like the unexpected death of a high-profile animal, do happen, and it is human nature to want to know what happened. Use this as a time to educate an interested public. Veterinarians can provide factual medical information to help educate the public not only about a particular animal, but also to address points about the important work that zoos and aquariums do for species around the globe. However, be prepared.

When the media call for information, an institution first must determine who is the most qualified person to do the interview. Look at the issue from the point of view of the public, think about what questions might be on their minds, and then select a spokesperson. Issues such as disease, illness, or trauma are definitely veterinary issues, and it would be best to have a veterinarian do the interview. Issues involving general husbandry, management, enclosure design, or financing would be assigned to others with expertise in those areas. It is not advisable for a veterinarian to do the interview if the issue does not involve veterinary medicine.

In most cases, the angle of the story will be obvious. If an anesthetized animal dies during a routine physical examination, the public will want to know what went wrong. Or, perhaps there is a collection of rare water fowl in a natural enclosure, and after years of attempted breeding there are finally some offspring. You schedule a surgery to render the chicks flightless—the media might want to know why you are intentionally maiming these rare creatures. Or, a hiker is killed by a free-ranging mountain lion in your jurisdiction and the public wants the animal killed; questions will arise concerning this situation.

Be aware, however, that during an interview, or even prior to an interview, the reporter might take a different angle to the story. Prepare the best that you can, and try to think of all the angles that the story might involve.

Prepare for the Interview

Always prepare for an interview. Take some time, clear your mind, go some place where you won't be disturbed, and review key messages and facts about the interview topic.

Anticipate questions. Write down all the questions that you can think of that a layperson might want to know about the situation. You should come up with a pretty significant list. It might also help to ask staff members to do the same, and then give you their lists as soon as they're done. Make sure that you write down the questions that might make you squirm.

Formulate answers. Read each question and think of a short answer. Be precise, and don't elaborate. Make sure that your answers are actually responses to the questions being asked.

Memorize key messages.

- What good news might come from this incident?
- What would you like to say that educates the public about the importance of what you are doing?

- Does your institution have a list of key messages that it would like disseminated?

Think of bridges.

- What could you add to your answers that will bridge to your key messages?
- Which ones lend them to a natural link to a key message?

Here's an example. An animal is anesthetized for a preshipment examination prior to shipping to another institution for breeding purposes. It dies during the procedure. The question is "What did you do when the animal had a bad reaction to the anesthetic?" You answer by saying that "We recognized the reaction very quickly and began all necessary emergency procedures." The bridge is that the good news is that this is very rare. The key message point is that without procedures such as this one, which are necessary for translocation of these animals, this species might become extinct.

Here's another example. An institution supplements some of its carnivores' diets with a commercially available pet food that has been recalled because it was found to be tainted with a potentially fatal ingredient. The question is "How will you prevent your animals from getting sick or dying?" You answer by saying that "We've temporarily removed this ingredient from our menu and tested all the animals who had received it for any signs of toxicity, and none appeared." The bridge is "Our staff nutritionist is evaluating other sources for the essential ingredients." The key message point is "Our medical health team will continually monitor animals that might have eaten this diet in the past and are prepared to treat them in case something shows up."

Practice, practice, practice. You might only have ten minutes left, but stand up, talk out loud to yourself so you can hear your answers, and practice answering in short sentences. It's all right to have some "uhs and ums" in your answers. The public expects you to be human and will respect hearing about the passion veterinarians have for doing what is best for animals.

Practice in advance. It might be a good idea to occasionally sit down with staff, think up some "bad news" scenarios, and go through the exercise of thinking of questions, answers, bridges, and key messages. It may even help to role play with one of you being a reporter and another being the interviewee. You may be surprised how easy it is to turn bad news into good news if you give it a try. Finally, make sure that you get professional media training when you see it offered.

Prepare to Carry a Global Message

Zoo and wildlife veterinarians have a deepening responsibility and opportunity to communicate not only about the animals in their care, but also about animal species trying to survive in a rapidly changing world. Today's world is facing mass species extinctions and loss of biodiversity. This is not the first time in history that this has happened, but to our knowledge, past mass extinctions were caused by natural events, such as asteroids hitting the planet or an ice age advancing. This mass extinction is being caused by people, and only people will be able to slow or stop it. Many veterinarians doing zoo or wildlife work are making great strides in understanding the problems and helping create solutions, but it does no good for a small number of people to do this work and not communicate it to the rest of the world and motivate them for action. Veterinarians can communicate messages to the public by effectively communicating with the media.

CONCLUSION

Veterinary medicine and the care of zoo and aquarium animals and wildlife will continue to evolve, just as societal norms regarding our relationship with animals evolves. Even our vocabulary reflects a division of perspectives. For example, animal rights groups refer to "captive" or "imprisoned" animals living in zoos, but zoos refer to the "animals in their care" and raise awareness of their demonstrated commitment to animal conservation globally. Although people with both viewpoints care about animals, they have vastly differing views on how that advocacy and care should translate into ensuring animals' well-being. We have yet to see where the evolution of the status or rights of animals will eventually go in society:

- Will people own pets or will they be guardians of companion animals?
- Will pets or farm animals or zoo animals have standing in court and be guaranteed certain rights, like humans?
- How will these changes affect veterinary medicine and veterinarians?

Although it is too soon to predict the answers, we may assume that these rapid changes will have significant, long-term effects on how animals are treated by society, and veterinarians who are well-prepared spokespersons will have a voice in helping society navigate these questions.

REFERENCES

1. American Pet Products Association: Pet Ownership, 2009–2010 (http://www.americanpetproducts.org/press_industrytrends.asp).
2. National Oceanic and Atmospheric Administration (NOAA) Fisheries: Permanent Removal of California Sea Lions at Bonneville Dam, March 2008 (http://www.nwr.noaa.gov/Marine-Mammals/Seals-and-Sea-Lions/upload/Sec-120-Bonneville.pdf).
3. Association of Zoos and Aquariums: Visitor Demographics, 2009 (http://www.aza.org/Membership/detail.aspx?id=2967&terms=annual+zoo+attendance).
4. Certified Humane: Raised and Handled, 2010 (http://www.certifiedhumane.org).
5. Manier J, Shah T: Cops kill cougar on North Side: neighborhood stunned as animal cornered, shot in back alley. Chicago Tribune, April 15, 2008.
6. Dairy Farming Today: Media Center, 2010 (http://www.dairyfarmingtoday.org/DairyFarmingToday/Learn-More/Media-Center).
7. A-R News: 'Personhood' redefined: animal rights strategy gets at the essence of being human (http://lists.envirolink.org/pipermail/ar-news/Week-of-Mon-20031124/011299.html).
8. Wise SM: Rattling the cage: Toward legal rights for animals. Cambridge, 2000, Mass, Perseus.
9. U.S. Census: Current population survey, February 2009.
10. U.S. Department of State: Freedom of Information Act, 2010 (http://www.state.gov.m/a/ips).

CHAPTER II

Dangerous Animal Crisis Management

Hayley Weston Murphy

Working with exotic and wild animals is always a dangerous business. No matter how careful and conscientious the staff of the institution, animals will always try to escape, and some will succeed. Being well prepared for such events may make the difference between success and failure, and may even mean the difference between life and death. Many zoos and animal facilities have well-written and comprehensive dangerous animal escape protocols and measures in place to try to prevent adverse events involving dangerous animals from occurring. Such plans should be developed with the input of all relevant personnel, including veterinary staff, animal care staff, supervisors, maintenance, security and facility personnel, and top administration. It is recognized that even strict adherence to these protocols may not prevent the occurrence of events involving dangerous animals and potential human contact. Therefore, zoological institutions need to have a schedule of regular review and training in place to fully implement a well-rounded plan for crisis management involving dangerous animals.

RISK MANAGEMENT

The Association of Zoos and Aquariums (AZA) defines risk management as a plan in which areas of potential risk for injury and/or harm to the visiting public and employees, as well as ways for prevention of such injury and/or harm, are identified.[2] Each zoological institution needs to do a periodic risk assessment on every exhibit that houses and displays animals. Even nondangerous animals may pose a threat to local flora and fauna if they escape. Reviews of containment structures, holding areas, standard operating procedures (SOPs), and emergency response protocols need to be done on a schedule, just like any other preventive maintenance schedule in the facility. Things to consider when doing such

reviews include animal collection changes, such as new species or changing individuals within an exhibit (e.g., animals maturing to full size and strength, new group compositions), physical facilities needing repairs and updates, staff changes, and changing standards because of events at other zoological institutions. Growing complacent with existing facilities and protocols may be a costly mistake. An employees' committee should be appointed to implement the risk management plan, identify areas of potential risk, and review previous incidents. This committee should be made up of a cross section of staff from many areas of the zoo, with differing expertise. The committee needs to meet on a regular documented basis and also be available for review and critique of any adverse events and/or practice drills as they occur. Whenever injuries result from any incident, a written account outlining the cause of the incident, how the injury was handled, and a description of any resulting changes to the safety procedures or the physical facility must be prepared and maintained.

Facilities

Most injuries to people involving captive wildlife occur because of one of two factors, human error or facility flaws and/or mechanical failures. It is imperative to establish a cooperative, inclusive design team whenever new exhibits and/or new species are added to a facility. This team should take into account current species standards, as well as the composition of collections and possible future needs. A review of current events both in the facility and in similar facilities may reveal potential problems that could be corrected before becoming an issue at the zoo. When doing facility reviews, particular attention must be given to shift doors, gates, staff access points, staff and animal visibility, and exhibit barrier dimensions and construction. Visual access to all animal holding areas and shifting areas should be reviewed to try to eliminate areas with blind shifting or access to areas that cannot be visualized. If staff cannot see where an animal is at all times without putting themselves in danger, the facility should review how to minimize the risks (e.g., incorporate two-person shifting protocols, develop an alert system when entering areas that may be blind). All service exit doors must be clearly marked and in good working order, and all locks and shift doors must be maintained at all times in good working order.

Facility review should also take into account possible overhanging plants, dead trees or compromised trees in exhibits, older mesh or fencing, or potential for other changes that could lead to an animal being able to breach containment. Public barriers to exhibits provide the first line of defense in protecting the public from the animals. Inspection and immediate repair of any public barriers also needs to be part of facility maintenance plans. Any breach of public barriers should be documented so that if recurring issues involving one particular area develop, it may be addressed in a timely manner. Some solutions include increasing the height or distance of the barrier, planting thorny or irritating plants between the barrier and exhibit, or installing alarm systems that notify staff if a breach occurs. Obviously, if a person gets all the way into an exhibit with an animal, all responses should follow the predetermined dangerous animal response and recovery plan.

All areas housing venomous animals or animals that pose a serious threat of catastrophic injury and/or death must be equipped with appropriate alarm systems and/or have protocols and procedures in place that will notify staff in the event of an injury, attack, or escape from the enclosure. These systems and procedures must be routinely checked to ensure proper functionality, and periodic drills must be conducted to ensure that appropriate staff members are notified. Alarm systems may be elaborate notification systems such as panic buttons, radio alert systems, or loudspeaker activation, or may be as simple as fog horns or blinking lights that can be activated in emergencies. Whichever system is used, it is critical to make sure that it is operational, staff knows what activation means, staff members are aware of how to use system, and the alarm may reach intended responders. For example, activating a fog horn inside a building that cannot be heard outside the holding area may not be useful as an alert system. All containment areas must be maintained and inspected on a predetermined schedule. All fencing should be closely examined daily before animals are placed into exhibits. Perimeter fencing should be separate from all exhibit fencing or other enclosures and be of good quality and construction. All facilities must be enclosed by a perimeter fence at least 8 feet high or by a viable barrier.[2] The fence must leave no gaps anywhere, including gates that would allow entry to the grounds by feral or wild animals or permit the egress of a collection animal in the event of an escape from a primary enclosure. Although these requirements are sufficient for trying to prevent escapes or entry through the fence, most zoo animals that may be considered dangerous could easily scale an 8-foot fence. A goal during any escape is to keep the animal on zoo grounds, avoid contact with the perimeter fence, and prevent animal escape outside the property.

Communication

The key to success with any plan is good communication and practice. Staff should always be reassured to err on the side of safety. It is better to inform staff that a dangerous animal is out and have it be false than to wait and lose precious time in responding. Areas of concern that have been noted in many zoological institutions after adverse animal events include repeated interpersonal conflict, ineffective and inappropriate communication, and poor staff morale leading up to the incident. Personality conflict, significant differences in opinion, and an inability to work together in a productive manner undoubtedly contribute to poor performance and poor team mentality.[8] In the case of dangerous animal escapes, this could lead to tragic outcomes and must be addressed by management as part of a comprehensive risk management plan. Some tools to try to address poor communications and morale issues include regular staff meetings, using consultants who may be able to act as team builders and negotiators, and encouraging professional development. When developing a response team, all these factors should be taken into account by management to try to avoid interpersonal conflict that might result in carelessness and unprofessional behavior.

PUBLIC RELATIONS

Incidents involving zoo animals may not only be potentially physically costly to the institution in terms of injury and loss of life, both animal and human, but may also be a public relations (PR) nightmare and cost the zoo goodwill and income from the local community. The development of strategies designed to guarantee communication among the administrative, veterinary and animal care, and public relations staff is critical and should be elucidated via an institutional emergency contingency plan for each AZA-accredited institution.[2] This plan could include press release templates and specific local media contacts who are assured to handle the release in a responsible manner. In addition, ongoing communication should be maintained with local and state public health and veterinary officials. In case of a human injury, preexisting relationships with media outlets, as well as public health officials, will be critical to follow-up communications. A geographically separate place, away from the incident command center (see later), should be predesignated for the press and zoo's press spokesperson. Most in the media will want to speak to someone with animal or event knowledge; however, this might be hard to balance because most of these people may be involved in the response. It is a good idea in this case to have the communications coordinator also remember to update the PR representative periodically. Once the incident is resolved, having predesignated key staff member(s) as spokespeople to deal with the press is a good idea. This person needs to go through an immediate incident debriefing before speaking to the press so that facts will be presented concisely and accurately. It helps to send designated staff to some PR and crisis communication training sessions beforehand so that they have the tools to be able to effective communicators. This will be invaluable in preserving community relationships and support in the aftermath of an incident.

Planning the Response (see Chapter 11)

Dangerous animal response and recovery plans should be in place and designated personnel well trained and rehearsed before any event occurs. All staff should have a role and know what that role is, even if it is to stay in one place and not respond. Every situation will be unique. It is impossible to write a plan that will address every situation that might arise. A well thought-out plan does, however, provide guidelines and best practices that can be used in most situations and modified as needed. Detailed plans need to outline all aspects of the response to an animal escape or emergency involving a dangerous animal. Plans should include details on chemical immobilization, lethal weapons, communications and public relations, protection of public and employees, and incident command structures (see later). These plans need to be reviewed on a regular basis and also reviewed after each incident and/or drill to see if areas of improvement could be made. Any time

plans are changed, staff must review and sign off on those changes. All staff needs to be familiar with the overall plan for response in the event of an emergency involving an animal, but it also helps to break the plan down into smaller subsections that are area and/or job specific. By doing this, people are not as overwhelmed by the potential lengthy procedures outlined in the facility plan and may concentrate on their specific role. This may help in maintaining training and compliance with required reviews of the plan across all staffing levels. It is advisable to have assistance from contractors, volunteers, interns, and visiting scientists who could review at least the portion of the plan that would pertain to the area of the facility in which they will be working.

ANIMAL CARE STAFF

Animal care (AC) staff training and compliance with policies and standard operating procedures are critical and should be the first step in prevention of an incident involving dangerous animals. AC staff needs to be trained and supervised until they have acquired an appropriate level of proficiency and are following zoo policies reliably. If an animal care staff member believes for some reason that they cannot perform to this standard, they should be able to discuss this with their supervisor freely, and without negative consequence, and alternate work plans should be considered. If a supervisor thinks that an AC staff member cannot perform to the standard of safe operations at any given time, mechanisms need to be in place for that person to be moved out of that job until a solution is found. At no time should anyone work with dangerous animals if there is any doubt that they cannot perform safely and up to standards. This work performance assessment should include the number of close calls that have occurred. Identifying and examining close calls may indicate areas of weakness and concern before dangerous situations occur and should not be ignored. The facility design and maintenance reviews are critical, but there also need to be mechanisms in place for SOP review in all animal areas. A predetermined review schedule allows for review and revision of SOPs based on current needs of the staff and facility and does not rely on what worked in the past.

This is the time to encourage staff participation and open communications. These events are always stressful, whether or not an injury occurs, and bringing in crisis counselors for all staff after an incident may save the zoo time and money in the long term. Staff will need to have their emotional needs addressed promptly and some individuals may need long-term follow-up.[6]

EMERGENCY MEDICAL RESPONSE

In incidents involving dangerous animals, serious injuries and even fatalities may occur. In some facilities, especially those with venomous animals on grounds, maintaining their own emergency medical technicians (EMTs) on staff might help mitigate these circumstances. Many facilities cannot justify this, however, and in those cases, designating staff to be trained in emergency medical response, as well as working closely with local EMTs, ambulance services, and emergency rooms may be invaluable.[3] First-aid kits offering treatment options for a wide array of injuries should be maintained in multiple locations throughout a facility and staff should know how to access them. Training ahead of time should also extend to local emergency room staff and emergency responders ; it should include instruction on chemical immobilization agents that the zoo might use and on venomous animal responses that may be needed. Thus, in case of an accidental human drug exposure or envenomation, emergency room personnel will be familiar with those agents and possible lifesaving measures may be initiated. A laminated booklet of all drug package inserts should be kept in an easily identifiable container that accompanies the drugs to the scene of any emergency. If accidental human exposure should occur, this container should accompany the victim to the emergency room.

Drills

Facilities need to schedule emergency drills regularly to ensure that the staff know their duties and responsibilities. These drills should involve all appropriate staff for the emergency situation being drilled, as well as consideration to involving potential outside partners such as police, fire, and emergency medical personnel. Area-specific drills, as well as zoo-wide drills with and without the public present, may identify weaknesses in training and plans before an actual emergency arises. These drills need to be recorded and evaluated to ensure that procedures are being followed, staff training is effective, and what is learned is used to correct and/or improve the response procedures. Records of these drills must be maintained and improvements in procedures duly noted whenever they are identified. Making a recording of drills with times noted for acknowledgment and response to the emergency may be beneficial

when reviewing the training exercise. This is also a good idea during an actual event for later debriefing and analysis purposes. Drills may and should include many different scenarios, including animals breaching containment, animals loose in secondary containment, and people in an area with animals. Differing environmental conditions may also be an issue so drills should take place in sunlight and in other scenarios, such as after dark, winter, and summer. Deficiencies in equipment and ability to respond in varying conditions may be highlighted and corrected this way. In any drill or actual incident, a debriefing of all involved should be mandatory so that lessons may be learned and procedures modified as needed.

Incident Command

During stressful events and emergency responses, there is always the potential for conflicts regarding decision-making authority. Variables are hard to predict and include rapidly changing scenarios, individuals under extreme stress, and potential for life-threatening conditions to develop quickly. There are many ways in which institutions can plan for these conditions; the most important part is advanced planning and designation of protocols that are put into place during any event. It is important to have a designated chain of command in place before situations arise. All plans need to have some flexibility built into them to account for staff availability and situational problems that might occur. When developing emergency response plans, it is critical to consider which outside agencies could become involved in emergencies at the facility.

Today, because cell phones and access to the Internet are widely available, there may be times when outside agencies are notified of a problem in the facility before facility managers or AC staff know that an event is occurring.[7] Developing memorandum of understanding (MOU) documentation ahead of time may help determine which agency will respond, where they will report, who will be in charge, and the system of communication that will be used. The MOU needs to outline the role of emergency responders and law enforcement clearly. Details should be specified about when and how law enforcement respond and how they will interact with and help zoo staff in the response. Areas of command, roles, and liability should be clearly delineated. Confidence in each other's ability to respond rationally and appropriately to emergency situations may be attained by including local emergency responders in emergency drills at the zoo. It might also be

BOX 11-1   Incident Command System Overview

The incident command system (ICS) is a standardized, on-scene, all-hazards incident management approach that involves the following:
- Allows for the integration of facilities, equipment, personnel, procedures, and communications operating within a common organizational structure
- Enables a coordinated response among various jurisdictions and functional agencies, both public and private
- Establishes common processes for planning and managing resources

An ICS is flexible and may be used for incidents of any type, scope, and complexity. An ICS allows its users to adopt an integrated organizational structure to match the complexities and demands of single or multiple incidents.

An ICS is used by all levels of government—federal, state, tribal, and local—and by many nongovernmental organizations and the private sector. It is also applicable across disciplines and is typically structured to facilitate activities in five major functional areas: command, operations, planning, logistics, and finance-administration. All the functional areas may be used, based on the incident needs. Intelligence and investigations is an optional sixth functional area that is activated on a case by case basis.

As a system, an ICS is extremely useful—not only does it provide an organizational structure for incident management, but it also guides the process for planning, building, and adapting that structure. Using an ICS for every incident or planned event helps hone and maintain skills needed for large-scale incidents.

Adapted from Federal Emergency Management Agency: Incident Command System (ICS), 2010 (http://www.fema.gov/emergency/ nims/IncidentCommandSystem.shtm).

helpful—to provide a good experience and build confidence in outside partners—to invite them to observe routine procedures involving dangerous animals and to observe and play a part in dangerous animal response team training. Training in incident command and national communication is available from the Federal Emergency Management Agency.[5]

It is highly recommended to train critical staff at the facility in the same training courses used by responding agencies (Box 11-1). Various means of communication, including a walkie-talkie, pager, cell phone (and/or smart phone), intercom, telephone, alarm, or other electronic device, need to be interchangeable between the zoo responders and responding agencies. One way

to do this is to have a few staff members designated as communication responders. They would have the preassigned role of communicating with outside agencies, be familiar with all available communication tools, and respond to command central as soon as possible. In this way, the zoo staff representative would carry the zoos' communication system device and then communicate to and from the police and/or emergency responder about what is happening during the event. This ensures a more efficient means of communication between both agencies. Predesignating an incident command center and staff is important for event coordination. This area should be well known to emergency responders from all potential areas and should be where people and equipment can gather safely and efficiently. Personnel who report to the incident command center will include the zoo's incident commander and possibly a communication officer(s) and logistics officer and the police or fire incident commanders. Key responder identification should be predesignated and can be used so that zoo staff can gain immediate access in case of an emergency. This should include identification such as color coded ID badges, specific vest etc, that will allow zoo staff access through such points as police barricades or staff gates and make them easily identifiable as a zoo responder. In the case of individuals who are designated to carry dart guns or weapons, making them easily identifiable to outside agencies and possibly to other shooters may even be lifesaving.

Chemical Immobilization

If an animal cannot safely be manipulated into an appropriate holding area using such tools as shifting equipment, press boards, or nets, and if human safety may be secured without the need for lethal force, the next preferable option is chemical immobilization. All facilities that house dangerous animals should have a plan that addresses chemical immobilization in emergency situations. These plans should be developed by the veterinary team and designed to maximize safety for animals and humans. Drug selection and dosages used in uncontrolled circumstances may be different from the choices that veterinary staff would make to anesthetize the same species in close confinement under controlled circumstances. Depending on the size and composition of the animal collection, it may be useful to cross-train staff members involved in emergency response procedures involving chemical immobilization and dart projectors, dosages, and applications.

Relying on the veterinary staff to be there and available for every situation, every day of the year, may not always be feasible or realistic. Staff training for chemical immobilization should include principles of safety (a loaded dart gun should be treated just like a loaded weapon), anesthesia and darting, and loading and shooting darts and guidelines for approach of darted animals, redosing and reversal, aftercare, and accidental human exposure to narcotics. This training may be facilitated by the veterinary staff or outsourced to a private agency, such as Safe-Capture International.[1] Ideally, the types of drugs and drug dosages specified for emergency chemical response use one or two drug combinations, may be volume-restricted for ease of dart loading, do not include any class 2 narcotics under the U.S. Controlled Substance Act, and may be used at dosages high enough to try to shorten induction times.[1,11]

Once an animal has been successfully immobilized, it should undergo a veterinary examination and be moved into an appropriate holding facility as soon as possible. No drug should be reversed until the animal may be safely contained. Developing drug immobilization cards to include species and ideal drugs to use in uncontrolled circumstances, and that may be available to staff in emergency areas and with equipment, is critical. These cards should include information pertaining to differences in size among adult, juveniles, male, and female animals and need to be reviewed periodically and updated as needed for new drugs, protocols, and new species. Staff needs to be familiar with these cards, how to use them, and know when the information is changed. Many emergency darting protocols will include the use of federally controlled drugs that legally require documentation of use. It is advisable to have an agreement between local drug enforcement agencies (DEAs) and the facility noting that the use of controlled substances is allowed under these circumstances and under veterinary advisement in emergency situations.

Good records and drug log books may be maintained by adding a waterproof marker and labels to emergency equipment. All darts need to be labeled with the name of drug they contain and the amount. Darts may be prenumbered and logged before being placed in response equipment so that after an emergency darting, an inventory can be taken to determine how many darts were fired and whether they are all accounted for. It may be useful to color-code the darting equipment so that different darting systems are used properly. Institutions need to have a written formal procedure in place and

available to the AC staff about the use of animal drugs for emergency animal immobilization in case a veterinarian is not on zoo grounds. Such procedures should include at least the following:

- Those persons authorized to administer animal drugs
- Situations in which they are to be used
- Location of animal drugs
- Emergency procedures in case of accidental human exposure

Human drug exposure kits should be assembled and maintained and accompany the drugs to any dangerous animal event. Kit contents and procedures to follow until appropriate medical help arrives should be documented and reviewed by trained human medical staff. Capture equipment must be maintained in good working order and available to authorized trained personnel at all times. Periodic review of the equipment should be carried out, including scheduled maintenance of equipment, review of new equipment and/or updates available, and inventory of available emergency darting supplies. Documentation tracking practice sessions of each staff member trained in dangerous animal recovery and chemical immobilization needs to be in place. These records should detail who trained, when, and on what equipment. A minimum standard of practice should be established and personnel who cannot maintain this should be removed from the emergency response team. All controlled substances must be stored in an approved securely locked container.

LETHAL FORCE

In any adverse event involving an animal in a zoo or captive setting, safeguarding human health and well-being is always the first priority. Many zoos keep animals that could attack and kill humans faster than they could be chemically immobilized and every institution needs to have a plan for using lethal force in these cases. This is an act of last resort when human life is in imminent danger and the animal cannot be sedated quickly enough to prevent serious injury or death. In several cases, the lives of emergency responders and bystanders have been placed at risk by an inappropriate use of firearms while attempting to resolve such events.[3]

Zoos historically have varied in their approaches to lethal weapons and staff training.[4] Some facilities choose to train zoo staff and keep appropriate firearms on grounds, whereas other facilities prefer to allow local law enforcement agencies to respond if lethal weapons are required. Appropriate equipment, training, and certification, as well as insurance and liability coverage for lethal weapons staff, is necessary if a zoo wants to maintain its own lethal weapon response team. Staff needs to be certified to predetermined levels to obtain access to the weapons. Selection for a lethal weapons team varies; it may be based on previous weapons training, hunting experience, managerial level, and ability to remain calm and committed to training. Many zoos are located in urban areas where shooting a high-powered weapon may have disastrous consequences. Recommendations of how to fire a weapon safely and appropriately will vary, depending on weapon size, ammunition choice, animal size and strength, shooter skill, and surrounding backdrop. Some zoos opt to use the local police department and, although police officers are highly trained and qualified, they may lack the experience, knowledge, and weapons to deal with large dangerous animals. One of the best reference sources for these situations might be local big game hunters. They may have the experience and weaponry needed to help zoo staff and law enforcement in developing appropriate lethal weapon responses to all animals in the collection.[9]

The zoo veterinarian also needs to be involved with designating and training the lethal weapons team, especially when training in efficient and humane methods of swiftly ending life and lessening the potential for any needless suffering. Before obtaining a weapon, current local statutes should be reviewed to ascertain gun control legislation, as well as the extent of liability for staff members on the shooting team. This is especially important if a dangerous animal escapes from the zoo grounds and must be pursued beyond the zoo's perimeter fence. It is advisable to have written authorization from local law enforcement agencies regarding when, where, and in what circumstances designated zoo staff may use lethal weapons. Part of the training for lethal weapons responders, whether they are zoo staff, law enforcement officers, or a combination of both, should be walk-through drills and training exercises on zoo grounds, where variables may be taken into consideration. As with chemical immobilization, availability of drug cards, protocols, and lethal weapons cards for each species considered to be dangerous enough to warrant the potential use of lethal weapons is advisable. These cards may contain information such as where to shoot an animal to quickly kill it, which type of weapon and ammunition to use, ricochet potential, backdrop considerations, and alternate weapons choices. Firearms

discharge forms and ammunitions tracking are also effective tools for documentation in emergency use of weapons. All weapons staff training needs to be well documented and any staff member who cannot maintain established levels of training and marksmanship should be removed from the team. Some excellent aids for developing weapons protocols have been developed by Okimoto[9] and Piwonka and Kaemmerer.[10] Another aspect of training, both for chemical immobilization and the use of lethal force, is training responders to be familiar with the animal's natural behavior and stress responses. The basic factors affecting animal behavior should be emphasized, and learning about primary signs of aggression and the fight-or-flight response can be critical in avoiding animal and human injury and death.

CONCLUSIONS

As zoo professionals, one of the most dreaded potential career-related events is the escape of or human injury or death from a dangerous animal in our care. The value of having well thought-out and documented procedures, well-trained staff, documented practice drills, and reviews of deficiencies may make the difference between a successful outcome and a tragic one. It is a challenge to address all issues that might arise in advance completely, but a comprehensive plan with trained and dedicated staff should provide for flexibility in response to any situation or circumstance that may arise. It is important to have a chain of command in place for any given situation, and that this is clear to all participants.

REFERENCES

1. Amass KD, Drew M: Chemical immobilization of animals: Technical field notes 2006, Mt. Horeb, Wisc, 2006, Safe-Capture International.
2. Association of Zoos & Aquariums: The accreditation standards and related policies, 2010 edition (http://www.aza.org/accred-materials/.html).
3. Baker WK, Jr: The veterinary role as first responder to a medical emergency in a crisis management situation. J Am Assoc Zoo Keepers 34:497–501, 2007.
4. Beetem D: Firearms use and training in AZA institutions. J Am Assoc Zoo Keepers 34:569–583, 2007.
5. Federal Emergency Management Agency: Incident Command System (ICS), 2010 (http://www.fema.gov/emergency/nims/IncidentCommandSystem.shtm).
6. Fitzgerald L, Sanchez G, Pratte J: Critical incident stress management: a proven tool for addressing staff needs after a traumatic event. J Am Assoc Zoo Keepers 34:502–505, 2007.
7. Kaemmerer K, Piwonka N: Developing a program for dangerous animal emergencies: procedures for animal escape, unauthorized

person in with dangerous animals, and unified command system. J Am Assoc Zoo Keepers 34:506–512, 2007.

8. Miller DS: A tiger (Panthera tigris) attack on a keeper: A veterinarian's perspective. Presented at the AAZV/AAWV/ARAV/NAZWV Joint Conference, Orlando, Fla, 2001.

9. Okimoto B: Lethal weapons: A veterinarian's perspective. Presented at the AAZV/AAWV/ARAV/NAZWV Joint Conference, Orlando, Fla, 2001.

10. Piwonka N, Kaemmerer K: Developing a weapons team for dangerous animal emergencies: Organization and training. J Am Assoc Zoo Keepers 34:480–487, 2007.

11. U.S. Department of Justice, Drug Enforcement Administration, Office of Diversion Control: Section 1308: Schedules Of Controlled Substances, 2010 (http://www.deadiversion.usdoj.gov/21cfr/cfr/2108cfrt.htm).

CHAPTER 12

Sustainable Practices for Zoological Veterinary Medicine

Gretchen E. Kaufman and Gwendolyn Griffith

Habitat loss, degradation of air and water resources, and global climate change all threaten the ecosystems we depend on and the health that we seek to protect. In veterinary medicine and in ecosystem health, the priority rule has long been to first do no harm. As environmental impacts grow in severity, it has become imperative that veterinary medicine apply this principle to reduce our own impact on how we build and operate veterinary facilities and how we offer leadership and education in our communities.

Veterinarians have a strong appreciation for the link between environment and health; many of the diseases and problems we work on are rooted in the environment of our patients. In the zoo setting, environmental awareness is further heightened through a commitment to conservation. The zoo community is increasingly calling for the need to preserve ecosystem health and seek sustainable solutions that protect wildlife and wild places, but is also looking for ways to adopt green practices within their own institutions. This was recently demonstrated by the launch of the Association of Zoos and Aquariums (AZA) climate initiative[3] and the formation of the AZA Green Scientific Advisory Group. The zoo can strengthen its mission to educate the public toward conservation and protection of biodiversity by adopting sustainable practices in their own operations and serving as a model in their own communities.

Medical practice, human and veterinary, has a significant environmental impact through its buildings and grounds, use of disposable products and hazardous chemicals (including drugs), and energy-intensive technologies. Fortunately, opportunities exist for reducing a veterinary hospital clinic's environmental footprint, ranging from greening an existing facility to starting from the ground up. Targeted improvements can be made by the following:

- Making structural changes to an existing hospital building that maximize energy and water efficiency and provide a healthier environment for patients and staff
- Realigning waste contracts to make sure that hospital waste is minimized and is being handled responsibly
- Installing systems or buying power from renewable energy providers
- Taking care to purchase environmentally responsible products whenever possible
- Changing the culture of the staff to be more conscious of their daily choices and practices
- Building or renovating facilities to be Leadership in Energy and Environmental Design (LEED)–certified buildings.

This chapter will introduce some basic approaches for reducing the environmental footprint of a zoo hospital, from everyday routines to operations management to green buildings. At the end of the chapter, two green zoo hospitals are noted as examples of what can be done.

STRATEGIES FOR ENVIRONMENTALLY RESPONSIBLE VETERINARY PRACTICE

Engage Everyone in the Process

Developing successful strategies for greening the daily performance of a veterinary clinic includes not only identifying areas to implement changes, but also changing the culture in the clinic. The success of any initiatives that involve change depends on the cooperation and enthusiasm of the people who implement it. Including staff in a collaborative approach to green initiatives makes them part of the solution and aligns the institutional mission with their own personal goals and commitments to a sustainable future. Integrity of purpose comes when institutional commitments match those being asked of staff and are supportive of healthy lifestyles, such as providing a secure bicycle rack to promote biking to work, providing discounts for public transportation, and providing zoo logo reusable mugs and water bottles for the office kitchen. Incentive programs, such as award recognition programs and green competitions designed by staff, can provide valuable incentives that generate a positive team spirit.

Reduce, Reuse, Recycle

The mantra to reduce, reuse, recycle wherever possible, can form the foundation for greening veterinary practice. The greatest impact can be achieved through the first approach, reduce. Reducing consumption of goods and resources and reducing waste not only produces significant environmental benefits, but also provides obvious economic advantages.

Reduce
Consumption
By reducing consumption of a given product, the following will automatically be decreased:
- The need for natural resources used in extraction and manufacture of that product, including water
- Toxic byproducts released into the environment during the manufacture of products
- Toxic health effects experienced by workers involved with the manufacture of products
- Packaging and shipping materials needed to get the product to the veterinary clinic
- Energy required to manufacture and ship the product
- Amount of waste produced after the product is used, including any toxic waste involved in its disposal or degradation

Consumption should be reduced by systematically evaluating what the veterinary clinic uses. One way to identify excessive consumption involves conducting a trash audit that documents everything that leaves the clinic, both in the trash and recycling, and identifying where needless waste is occurring. This will reveal sensible institutional choices that encourage buying less and using more reusable products. The process can be repeated once a year to document progress or identify new items to focus on.

In most cases, shipping and packaging materials make up most of the solid waste found in a trash audit, such as cardboard, plastic wrap, and polystyrene peanuts or forms. Reducing packaging can be a challenge, but can be addressed from several angles. Buying frequently used items in bulk and reusing packaging for subsequent shipments are two options. Another option is to pressure suppliers to use less packaging or at least use environmentally friendly packing materials for shipment of their products, such as recyclable air-filled plastic bags, 100% recycled cardboard boxes and molded forms, shredded paper, newspaper, or cornstarch peanuts instead of polystyrene. In some cases, distributors will take their packaging back to reuse for other customers. If they need help, refer them to the Sustainable Packaging Coalition.[14]

Water
Reducing water usage is a key area to address. Most international experts believe that a global water shortage will rapidly become one of the most serious issues facing our planet. The world water crisis will affect the availability of clean drinkable water (affecting health directly), water for irrigation in agriculture (affecting our food supply), and water to sustain natural ecosystems everywhere. Americans consume more water per capita than any other nation[16] and take for granted our ready and seemingly unlimited sources of fresh water right out of the tap. Because global climate change will affect water quality and availability, unconscious overconsumption must be corrected through technology, policy, and individual choices and actions.

In a veterinary practice, using water-efficient washing machines and dishwashers,[20] low-flow toilets, and taking care not to leave faucets and hoses running are a good place to start. Installing a water catchment system on the clinic roof that delivers water into barrels for landscaping and hosing down outdoor areas is another fairly simple option. Reducing water consumption will also decrease the water bill, water heating bill, and resulting waste water or sewer bills.

Energy
Reducing energy use and switching to renewable energy sources is another important strategy to address. Simple actions such as turning off lights, using more efficient Energy Star–rated appliances and electrical devices, disconnecting standby settings, lowering or raising the thermostat a few degrees, replacing or insulating windows and doors, purchasing green power,[16] and encouraging staff to bike or walk to work all have obvious benefits, from decreasing the negative impacts of fossil fuel–dependent energy systems (e.g., oil extraction and oil spills, costly delivery) to keeping down costs in an escalating market. At the outset, building a new clinic with energy conservation in mind is the best

way to maximize energy efficiency, but retrofitting existing buildings is effective and worthwhile.

Waste

Reducing waste is a key strategy to a more environmentally responsible veterinary practice and is achieved by reducing consumption of materials (see earlier). It also means carefully selecting materials that must end up in the waste or recycling stream, and making sure that waste is properly taken care of after it leaves the hospital. Medical solid waste is dumped in a landfill or incinerated. In the landfill, there are issues with land use, soil contamination from chemicals and heavy metals, and runoff or groundwater contamination that threatens water supply and freshwater ecosystems. Medical waste constitutes one of the leading sources of dioxin, mercury, lead, and other pollutants that end up in the environment from incineration,[7,18] and incineration requires significant energy to burn the trash.

Over 6600 tons of waste are generated daily by American hospitals, but only about 15% of that waste is considered hazardous.[11] Biohazardous waste is expensive to handle, so careful disposal of hazardous materials, including drugs, will result in significant savings. Drugs that are poured down the drain and enter the sewer or municipal water system may not be removed by water treatment systems and have been documented in natural bodies of water. The American Veterinary Medical Association has developed best management practices for pharmaceutical disposal.[2] Although the contribution to medical waste from zoo veterinary hospitals is not significant compared with the human health care industry, veterinary practices nationwide should play a role in providing sustainable health care.

Reuse

Options to reuse materials in a veterinary hospital setting can be challenging, especially because we are often dealing with hazardous waste and infectious organisms. The strategy in this case is to look for reusable substitutes for disposable items that never become contaminated or that can be sterilized before reuse. In some cases, it may appear that disposable items are less expensive than reusable ones, but this may not be true after factoring in the hidden costs beyond the purchase price for these items including disposal cost and packaging, occupational health cost, liability cost, environmental consequences, and warehouse cost. Common and inexpensive (or free) reusable items to seek out include newspaper bedding, stainless steel food and water bowls, refillable spray bottles and squirt bottles and other refillable products, and reusable staff kitchen materials.

Certain mildly soiled items can be resterilized, such as syringes and surgical instruments. Reusing items that need some processing, must take into account the added costs of labor to clean, repackage, and resterilize the product, as well as the environmental costs of water and energy used in processing. In addition, some forms of chemical sterilization used to resterilize materials are actually harmful to human health (e.g., glutaraldehyde, ethylene oxide).

Switching to cloth drapes, linens, and gowns may be preferable to using polyester single-use products because cloth is more absorbent and more comfortable. Some manufacturers are now marketing organic cotton gowns, which reduce the environmental impacts of growing cotton.

Recycle

Recycling saves energy, water, and natural resources. The more we recycle, the less impact is also felt from extraction and manufacturing but, if efforts are initially made to reduce and reuse, then there will be even less to recycle. Recycling does involve some energy to transport and handle the materials and may also use water to clean materials. Not everything is recyclable, because commercialized recycling is dependent on a viable market for the recycled product. These markets are growing and making an effort to buy as many recycled products as possible will help build and sustain new markets.

Usually, recycling requires some cooperation and retraining from your staff. Items may have to be sorted to comply with recycler needs, or different items may be handled by different vendors or recyclers. Make it as easy as possible for staff to comply with recycling requirements. Involve them in deciding where to place collection bins and make it very clear what can and cannot be recycled with the use of appropriate signage. Provide multiple convenient receptacles wherever possible. Some suggestions to facilitate good recycling compliance include the following:

- Color-code your sorted recycling (e.g., blue for paper, green for plastic and metal, grey for trash).
- Clearly label bins and provide unambiguous information on acceptable items.
- Place paper recycling bins next to copy machines, at every desk, in the medical records room.

- Place plastic, metal, and glass recycling bins in human and animal food preparation areas.
- Make sure that a sink is easily accessible for rinsing materials, if required by the recycler.
- Place plastic and glass recycling bins in surgery preparation areas for acceptable packaging materials.
- Create a convenient institutional process for collecting and storing recyclables until pickup by recycling vendors.

Make Good Product Choices

There is a wide range of medical products that a veterinary practice uses in daily activities. Careful evaluation of these products can lead to more responsible choices that decrease the environmental footprint of the practice and help push the manufacturing and distribution stream to be more environmentally friendly. There are resources to help select products and follow principles of environmentally preferable purchasing. Some resources are listed at the end of this chapter, with additional information at Greenvetpractice.com,[6] based on research conducted at the Tufts Cummings School of Veterinary Medicine.

Products should be evaluated based on a number of criteria, including the principles of reduce, reuse, and recycle, but should also take a cradle to cradle[9] or life cycle assessment[17] view to appreciate their impact and cost to the environment fully.

In conducting research on any specific product, the following questions should be asked:

- What is the product made from?
- How is the product made?
- Can the product be reused?
- Can the product be recycled or composted?
- How is the product shipped?
- How is the product disposed of?
- Is the product user-friendly?
- What is the cost?
- Are there alternatives, and how does the product compare?

It is important to determine the composition of the product to assess whether the manufacture and disposal of that item would present a problem. In many cases, reading the label or reviewing the product's website will provide this information. However, in some cases a special request to the manufacturer will have to be pursued. For example, a plastic-type product made of vinyl or polyvinylchloride (PVC) involves the production of dioxin and other persistent organic pollutants during manufacture and disposal (incineration). PVC-based products also often include plasticizers to make the item soft and pliable, but these are also harmful to the environment and health because they contain phthalates, which are potent endocrine disruptors. A consequence of this analysis would be to avoid products made from PVC and seek out more environmentally friendly plastics, such as polypropylene. In some cases, items can be resterilized and reused. This has obvious benefits in product supply savings and from the standpoint of production and disposal of less waste.

Product assessment is not as difficult as it appears. Most medical products are made of similar materials, and they can often be evaluated quickly and simply by knowing the positive and negative attributes of the basic materials used in these products. See Box 12-1 and refer to GreenVetPractice[6] for analysis and recommendations for alternatives to common products used in veterinary practice.

As part of a hospital's greening strategy, an inventory should be conducted of everything that the hospital or clinic uses. The inventory can be done as an exercise by going from room to room or by analyzing purchasing records. All items should be evaluated as noted and more harmful products can be targeted for substitution or altered handling, as shown for a treatment room in Table 12-1. This sort of exercise could be conducted on an annual basis to document improvement and pinpoint new areas to be addressed.

Make Green Technology Choices

Technology in business and in veterinary medicine has brought incredible advantages and tools, from financial and patient records management to communications to advanced diagnostics, such as digital radiography. Most of these tools are also fundamentally more environmentally sustainable than their predecessors. However, all these tools use electricity and contribute to an operation's overall carbon footprint. It is important to consider the specific energy profile of any equipment intended for purchase to understand how and where discarded equipment will be handled and to use existing equipment responsibly and efficiently to minimize energy use. When buying new products, check the EPA's Energy Star and WaterSense guide to products to find the ones that are most efficient.[20,21]

Power-saving management options should be selected for all computers and monitors during use. It should be noted that energy is consumed even in standby or sleep settings, so computers and other

BOX 12-1	Basic Materials Found in Medical Products*

Bleach
Cellulose
Chlorhexiderm
Cotton
Detergents
Disinfectants
Ethylene vinyl acetate
Glass
Glutaraldehyde
Heavy metals
Hydrogen peroxide
Isoprene
Isopropyl alcohol
Latex
Natural rubber
Nitrile rubber
Nylon
Plasticizers
Plastics
Polyester
Polyethylene
Polypropylene
Polystyrene
Polyurethane
Polyvinyl chloride
Povidone iodine
Rayon
Silicone
Sodium nitrate
Steel
Teflon
Vinyl
Wood
Zinc sulfate

The analysis of these materials can be found at http://www. greenvetpractice.com.

BOX 12-2	Sustainable Community Elements

- Smart growth planning
- Good development site choices
- Better site design
- Sustainable building design
- Sustainable landscape design
- Good construction practices
- Post construction performance
- Protective maintenance practices

monitors use significant more energy than flat screen liquid crystal display (LCD) monitors and should be considered for replacement.

Care must be taken when replacing computers, printers, and other technology equipment to make sure that it is recycled or disposed of properly. Computers contain heavy metals, flame retardants, and other toxic chemicals that are hazardous to human and environmental health. Many recyclers and universal waste haulers ship their technology overseas, where environmental regulations are lax. Try to find a responsible computer and equipment recycler, or see whether the manufacturer is part of a take back program.[5]

LOW-IMPACT BUILDINGS, GROUNDS, AND FACILITY OPERATIONS

Elements of care for our built environment follow the principles of sustainability for smart growth planning, low-impact development, green building, and green operations. These principles should be applied at every stage, from regional to community to the individual site and building (Box 12-2).

Choices About Where to Build

For the least impact on our natural resources, new development and buildings should be located according to a few simple smart growth guidelines. These are particularly important when siting a new zoological park but can also apply to new buildings within its boundaries.

1. Buildings need to be located out of the flood plain and away from steep slopes. Leaving flood plains undeveloped protects critical habitat, prevents structural flood damage, and reduces the severity of floods when they do occur. Steep slopes should also be left in their natural state to prevent storm water damage and protect wildlife habitats.

electronic equipment not required to operate continuously for 24 hours daily should be turned off when not in use for more than 1 hour. Smart strips can be used to stop phantom power use, even in equipment that is turned off. These strips allow several devices to be shut off when the central controlling machine is turned off. Removing phantom power use can save 5% to 10% or more of the total electricity bill, which can be hundreds of dollars every month. If the veterinary clinic does limited printing—a good target to reduce paper and ink—consider an inkjet printer, which uses 90% less energy than laser printers. Older cathode ray tube (CRT)

TABLE 12-1 Sample Hospital Inventory Analysis—Treatment Room*

Item	Composition	Reuse, Recycle Options	ENVIRONMENTAL IMPACT		Alternatives	Recommendations
			Production	Disposal		
Bandaging	Plastic, latex	None	Possible DEHP, dioxin	General waste	Non-PVC	Use prudently, prefer non-PVC product
Cast padding	Cotton	None	Significant pesticide use	General waste	Organic cotton	Use prudently, prefer organic cotton if available
Cotton balls	Cotton	None	Significant pesticide use	Biohazard or general waste	Organic cotton	Use prudently, prefer organic cotton if available
Cotton-tipped applicators	Cotton, wood	None	Significant pesticide use	Biohazard or general waste	Organic cotton	Use prudently, prefer organic cotton if available
Feeding tubes	Plastic	Reuse, recycle	Possible DEHP, dioxin	General waste, recyclable	Non-PVC	Prefer polyethylene or polypropylene product, sterilize and reuse
Fluid bags	PVC	Limited	DEHP use, dioxin release	General waste, recyclable	Non-PVC fluid bags (polyethylene or EVA)	Prefer non-PVC product, recycle
	Polyethylene, polypropylene	Recycle	None noted	General waste, recyclable	None	No alternative necessary, recycle
Gauze bandage, sponge	Cotton	None	Significant pesticide use	Biohazard or general waste	Organic cotton	Use prudently, prefer organic cotton if available
Gloves (latex)	Latex	None	None noted	Biohazard or general waste, biodegradable	None	Use prudently
Gloves (nitrile)	Nitrile	None	Acrylonitrile exposure	Biohazard or general waste, nonbiodegradable	Latex	Limit use to handling dangerous chemicals, seek alternative
Infusion set	Plastic	Recycle	Possible DEHP, dioxin	Biohazard waste	Non-PVC	Prefer polyethylene or polypropylene product
IV catheters	Plastic	Recycle	Possible DEHP, dioxin	Biohazard waste	Non-PVC	Prefer polyethylene or polypropylene product
IV extension set	Plastic	Recycle	Possible DEHP, dioxin	Biohazard waste	Non-PVC	Prefer polyethylene or polypropylene product
Needles	Plastic, steel	None	Air and water pollution, possible DEHP	Biohazard waste	Non-PVC hub	Use prudently, prefer polyethylene or polypropylene hub
Syringes	Plastic	Reuse, recycle	Possible DEHP, dioxin	Biohazard or general waste, recyclable if uncontaminated	Non-PVC	Use prudently, prefer polyethylene or polypropylene product

DEHP, *Di(2-ethylhexyl) phthalate;* EVA, *ethylene vinyl acetate.*
See more room inventories at GreenVetPractice.com.

2. Ideally, buildings should be 100 feet or more away from stream banks with an undisturbed vegetated stream bank zone (riparian zone) that serves to filter and clean storm water, protect stream water quality, shade the water to keep it cool, provide leaf litter for the aquatic food chain, offer habitat for terrestrial and aquatic life, and provide biologic corridors for species mobility and population dynamics.

3. New buildings or redevelopment sites should be located where human infrastructure already exists with connections to, for example, existing roads, public transit, water lines, and sewers, power lines. This prevents sprawl, reduces the environmental impact, and saves significant costs for the developer, building owner, and community.

Choices for Designing and Developing a Site

Using low-impact development principles benefits the landowner, environment, and entire community. There are several resources available that indicate the principles of low-impact development, including the 22 principles of better site design from the Center for Watershed Protection,[4] the principles of conservation design from the Low Impact Development Center,[8] and the newest guidance from the Sustainable Sites Initiative (SITES) of the American Society of Landscape Architects.[1] All focus on the green infrastructure approach to reduce impervious surface area, maximize habitat and green space, and mimic the natural predevelopment hydrology of the site. The common key guidelines include the following:

1. At the regional or community scale, new development sites can aim to enhance and integrate with regional green infrastructure elements, such as greenways, parks, riparian zones, and biologic corridors.

2. At the development site scale, such as the zoological park campus, it is critical to build with the smallest building footprint possible, including keeping the percentage of impervious cover from roofs, roads, and parking lots to a minimum while leaving maximum tree canopy and natural green space.

3. At the individual building and landscape scale, using green infrastructure practices will also help reduce building impacts. These are natural or designed elements that function more like nature

and help the site mimic the natural hydrologic function and ecologic services that the site had before it was built on. This means preserving existing trees, restoring tree canopy, and reducing impervious surfaces with practices such as pervious concrete or pervious pavers for parking areas, green roofs to slow and filter rainfall, and encouraging rainfall infiltration with rain gardens, bioswales, and bioinfiltration zones. These elements help manage storm water runoff, enhance habitat and aesthetics, and can save on maintenance and storm water fees.

4. The landscape features for the finished site should also mimic nature where possible. Native and drought-tolerant species with low maintenance requirements are the starting point. This includes minimizing turf grass and maximizing trees, plants, and native grasses that have deep root systems. Also, avoid irrigation when possible, use ultraefficient drip irrigation where necessary, and use minimal chemical inputs, such as mowing, fertilizers, pesticides, and herbicides. An emphasis on restoring rich, healthy soils with ample organic material is also important.

Choices for Building Design, Construction, and Maintenance

Using green building principles brings many benefits, including cost savings, energy and water savings, improved air and water quality, improved indoor air quality and patient health, and enhanced employee health, retention, and job performance. There are several established green building programs that guide the builder to achieve maximal environmental performance and provide third-party certification for green building practices. These programs include the basic U.S. Environmental Protection Agency (EPA) Energy Star[21] for buildings to the Leadership in Energy and Environmental Design (LEED) program of the U.S. Green Building Council (USGBC).[22] The LEED program demands leadership in high-performance buildings to achieve certification at the certified, silver, gold, or platinum level. Always at the cutting edge, LEED is moving now into restorative building practices that go beyond zero impact into the realm of improving air and water quality as part of a building's function.

All the national, regional and local green building programs operate on a point system and allow for multiple levels of achievement based on site selection and design, energy efficiency, water efficiency, indoor environmental quality, storm water management, materials and resources, waste management, and education and operations (Box 12-3).

Site Selection and Design
Points are awarded for choosing and designing sites according to the principles of smart growth and low-impact development described earlier.

Energy Efficiency
The efficient use of energy and production of renewable energy are the cornerstones of green building. According to the U.S. Department of Energy, buildings consume 37% of the energy and 68% of the electricity produced in the United States each year. Production of energy from fossil fuels, especially coal, is one of the greatest of all environmental stressors to our ecosystems through air pollution, water pollution, and greenhouse gases causing global climate change. Nuclear power and hydroelectric power also carry serious environmental impacts.

Energy efficiency in a building begins with minimizing energy needs. For lighting, this is done by maximizing daylight in the building, thus reducing lighting requirements during the day and benefiting occupants with the natural light spectrum, which improves mood, job performance, and overall employee health and retention. It is also important to use high-efficiency T5 fluorescent lighting fixtures, compact fluorescent bulbs, or better yet, light-emitting diode (LED) lights throughout the facility.

For heating and cooling, energy efficiency is designed with optimal sealing of the building envelope and duct system; maximum insulation of floors, walls, and ceiling; and correct sizing of high-efficiency heating, ventilating, and air conditioning (HVAC) units. With well-sealed and insulated buildings, there can be significant savings in the size of the HVAC unit needed at construction and in utility bill savings over time. A high-performance building can save 50% or more on heating and cooling costs, depending on occupants' behavior. Behavior choices include turning off lights and electronic equipment, limiting hot water use, and using programmable thermostats. Use of photovoltaic solar panels for electricity production further reduces energy use and costs from the electricity grid and, in some cases actually generates income, through buy-back systems by utility providers. Use of ground-source heat pump geothermal systems is also a high-efficiency choice for heating and cooling a building. Although expensive to install, geothermal systems can drastically reduce operational costs and be paid for in 5 to 7 years or less through cost savings.

Water Efficiency
The efficient use of water resources involves both indoor and outdoor conservation measures. According to the USGBC, approximately 340 billion gallons of U.S. fresh water are withdrawn each day from rivers, streams, and reservoirs for human use. Of this, almost 65% is discharged back into the rivers after use or treatment. This does not include the vast amounts of water also withdrawn from underground aquifers, which cannot be quickly replenished. In some parts of the United States, water levels in the aquifers have dropped more than 100 feet since the 1940s.

Water efficiency also saves the vast amounts of energy it takes to provide potable water from municipal systems. An estimated 10% to 20% of total energy use in the United States is devoted to collecting, cleaning, distributing, and then recleaning potable water in our communities. This makes water efficiency one of the top energy-saving measures that people can use.[13]

Outdoors the goal is to reduce water use for landscaping by 50% and ideally not use any potable water for irrigation where possible. Many innovative technologies now exist through rain water harvesting methods, so that captured rain can be the primary landscape water in some parts of the country. In arid climates, drought-tolerant native plants should be used so that irrigation is not required. Ultraefficient drip irrigation with soil moisture and weather sensors also limits water use. A high-efficiency irrigation unit can save hundreds of thousands of gallons of water each year for even modestly sized sites over conventional irrigation practices.

Indoor water efficiency in commercial buildings can reduce water use by 30% or more using technology and behavior by occupants. Use of WaterSense appliances[20] will save 20% or more in most cases. These can be found at comparable prices for a number of items, such as faucets, showers heads, toilets, dishwashers, and washing machines. In particular, the newer front-loading washing machines are highly efficient, saving 50% or more water and energy. There are also recirculating pumps that prevent waste water from going down the drain while waiting for warm water at the faucet. In public buildings, use of waterless urinals or ultraefficient 1-pint urinals can save up to 40,000 gallons/year or more for each urinal unit. Dual-flush toilets also significantly reduce toilet water use.

Water reuse systems can also be installed for building use. Gray water systems can send gray water from showers, sinks, and washing machines into a holding tank for a second use for irrigation, thus drastically saving on potable water and energy use.

For a controlled facility such as a zoological park, one especially low-impact water practice that could double as an educational exhibit would be to set up a biologic filtering process to clean on-site waste water using a constructed wetland system. In this case, some or all waste water is filtered using natural biologic processes that mimic wetland conditions. An extensive series of tanks or ponds is used for slow water filtration and restoration to potable conditions before release into a stream or on-site reuse. There are commercial systems that can be designed to treat whatever water system requirements a building, or even a large development site, might need.

Indoor Environmental Quality

It is estimated that Americans spend 90% or more of their time indoors. This means almost constant exposure to indoor air pollutants in the form of outgassing from various synthetic materials or chemical compounds. Their effects may contribute to the 17 million people who have asthma or the 40 million with allergies. In a very well-sealed and insulated building, adherence to the use of safer materials and practices becomes all the more important. Studies have shown that careful attention to indoor environmental quality results in 15% to 20% improvements in worker health and productivity, thus saving on the most important expense related to doing business.

Preventing indoor air pollution is much easier than expensive retrofitting later, so designing for optimal indoor air quality is an important step. First, specify materials with little or no harmful outgassing chemicals. This includes carefully choosing such items as paints, adhesives, construction materials, composite woods, furniture, carpets, and flooring composed of zero volatile organic compounds (VOCs) or other toxic

materials, such as urea formaldehyde. Fortunately, these materials are now comparable in cost to standard materials. Thousands of products are rated for their air quality impact by the Green Guard system (http://www.greenguard.org). Air emissions can also be reduced by staging construction steps to allow off-gassing time, protecting air handling equipment during the construction process, and increasing the ventilation rates and ratios of filtered air in the HVAC system. Finally, moisture management is critical to avoid mold and mildew issues in any building.

Storm Water Management

Effective handling of rainfall runoff lets a site treat storm water as a resource instead of a waste product. Use of green infrastructure features as described earlier can provide affordable functionality and aesthetic qualities to any building site. It also helps support watershed health by promoting aquifer recharge, flood avoidance, and water quality protection.

Good soil conditions are another important consideration for low-impact landscaping and storm water management. Natural soil is a dynamic living system that can absorb and hold moisture and support a healthy landscape. However, during typical construction, the topsoil is stripped off and the remaining soil is severely compacted and degraded in terms of organic content and soil life. It is important to restore soil conditions back to health using composted materials and natural life promoters ,such as compost tea and organic enrichment. This ultimately reduces landscape maintenance needs and helps hold rainfall on the site.

Materials and Resources

Materials management is an important aspect of reducing building impacts. Harvesting, manufacturing, and transporting building materials can affect habitats, reduce air and water quality, and deplete natural resources. Construction waste usually takes up 40% or more of the total waste stream in the United States and as much as 70% of total landfill space. The LEED system allows for a default value of approximately 45% of total costs for the estimated cost of construction materials on a construction project. Thus, savings on materials brings significant benefits to the builder, occupant, local community, and environment.

Reuse of existing buildings or materials is the most effective conservation measure possible. Second is design and building practices that conserve materials used. For example, advanced framing methods reduce the use of wood for on-site construction. Prefabricated panel wall systems reduce materials use even further through off-site manufacturing techniques. It is also beneficial to use recycled content materials and locally sourced materials, preferably within a 500-mile radius, whenever possible. The management of construction waste with maximum reuse or recycling of materials can cut landfill waste materials by 70% or more.

Waste Management

In addition to construction waste management, it is important to design and operate a building for maximum waste reduction practices (see earlier). Designing for easy collection, storage, and transporting of recycled materials is important for compliance with recycling goals. Limiting storage space can also discourage over-buying products. Responsibility for what ends up in the waste stream belongs with the veterinary hospital and it is important to select waste disposal contracts carefully.

Education and Operations

Once a building has been well designed and constructed for maximum efficiency, it becomes important for those using, cleaning, and maintaining the building to understand how its systems work. Each building needs to have a customized operations and maintenance manual that clearly explains how systems are to be operated. In addition, a training program for all staff should be used at least once annually to be sure that everyone is well briefed on proper energy, water, and waste procedures. This also applies to cleaning practices to strike a balance between disinfection needs and avoiding toxic cleaning products.

In addition to individual green building achievements, there are also opportunities to excel with larger scale green building, such as the LEED for Neighborhood Development (LEED-ND) program. This emphasizes the total site development picture, with a focus on smart growth and sustainable site design.

Getting started on the construction of a green building begins with education about the options and processes through various educational venues. It is a wise practice to take a 1- or 2-day review course on a green building program such as LEED as a starting point. Then, find a highly experienced design team that can guide you through the process for retrofitting or new construction. The best way to be sure of high-performance achievement is to seek certification under one of the green building programs. However, significant green building achievements can be accomplished by following these efficiency and quality principles without going through the actual certification process.

When seeking LEED certification, the use of a LEED facilitator is extremely helpful to be sure that the extensive documentation required is carried out properly. Building commissioning is also highly recommended to assist in the construction review process.

When upgrading an existing building, start by analyzing the carbon footprint of the building and take measures for energy and water efficiency to reduce the carbon emissions of the facility. Often, simple measures, such as upgrading insulation, envelope and duct sealing, better windows and doors, and operational changes can make significant improvements for modest costs.

In summary, the design, construction, and operations of green buildings and grounds of a zoo hospital is an opportunity to reduce environmental impact significantly, save on costs, benefit the health of patients, and greatly enhance the health and productivity of staff. It is a significant commitment to undertake but much worthwhile for the triple bottom line of social, economic, and environmental benefits over the long term.

PROFILES OF TWO GREEN ZOO HOSPITALS

Palm Beach Zoo Animal Care Complex

In April 2009, the Palm Beach Zoo dedicated their Melvin J. and Claire Levine Animal Care Complex, including the Salvatore M. Zeitlin Animal Hospital (Fig. 12-1). This building is certified by the USGBC as a LEED gold facility. During construction, the project made concerted efforts to minimize soil erosion and prevent waterway sedimentation. They maintained 20% of the site as open space and landscaped with native plants. They sourced local construction materials where possible and managed to recycle 75% of all construction waste. Of the wood-based materials used in the building, 50% were Forest Stewardship Council (FSC–certified and low-VOC products were used whenever possible, including adhesives, sealants, paints, coatings, carpeting, and wood products.

They are saving water through the use of water-efficient fixtures inside the building, and outside through the installation of an efficient irrigation system, matched by the selection of drought-tolerant plants. Installation of permeable walkways and parking areas helps minimize storm water runoff and soil erosion.

Energy management included the installation of 80 photovoltaic solar panels on the roof of the building, covering approximately 2000 square feet and providing 31,397 kilowatt-hours (kWh) of emissions-free power

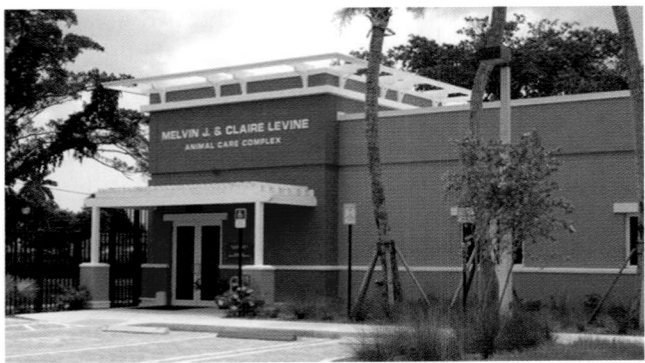

Figure 12-1

Claire Levine Animal Care Complex, Palm Beach Zoo, Palm Beach, Florida. *(Courtesy of Kristen Cytacki.)*

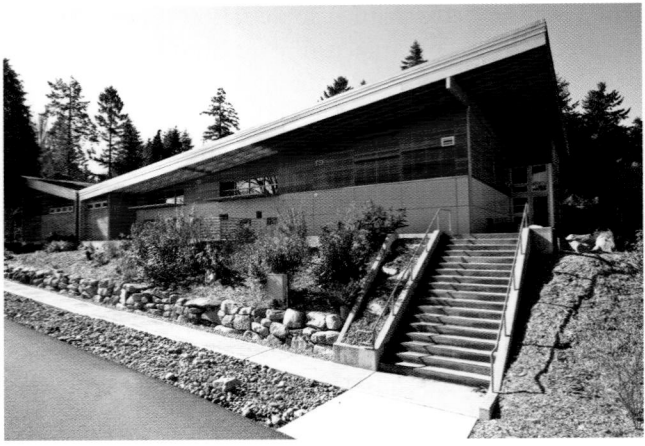

Figure 12-2

Animal health care facility, Point Defiance Zoo and Aquarium, Tacoma, Washington.

annually. During peak usage, the solar panels offset 13% of the buildings' energy use and the zoo purchases green power to offset at least 35% of the buildings' electricity needs. Additional energy savings are made through careful design of the building envelope and superefficient HVAC and lighting systems. Printing and copying have been consolidated, thermostats are on timers, and most lights, except in animal areas, use motion detectors.

In addition to recycling of paper, cardboard, metal, plastic, and glass materials, they purchase recycled products (all signage, and paper) and seek out green companies for furniture. They use digital radiography, thus avoiding issues with film and toxic chemicals, and house their own computer server to support imaging and electronic medical records. The hospital uses only green cleaning products, is designed to minimize light pollution, and has adopted a low environmental impact pest management policy. Zoo staff takes advantage of preferred parking spots for low-emission, energy-efficient vehicles as well as designated bicycle storage areas and shower facilities for bicycle e-riders.

To use their example as a teaching tool and demonstrate their commitment to conservation, the public areas of the building include educational materials about the green features of the building. In addition, the zoo's website includes a link to a real-time energy meter for the public to view.[10,10a]

Point Defiance Zoo and Aquarium Animal Health Care Facility

The Point Defiance Zoo's Animal Health Care Facility was also designed to serve as a community education

tool to promote sustainable building (Fig. 12-2). It is considered an off-exhibit exhibit, and sustainable aspects were designed to be apparent and to communicate this important aspect of the zoo's mission. LEED certification was not formalized because of the short timeline and limited budget available to design and build the facility, but they worked closely with their architect to follow and incorporate LEED and other sustainable design standards. Existing structures at the zoo were used for portions of the new facility and efficient functional design was the focus. The building form, with its butterfly green roof, elegantly integrates the structure into the park setting while allowing natural light and ventilation to be maximized in the areas needed to create healthy environments for animals and staff. Low- and zero-VOC interior finishes add to the indoor environmental quality strategies. Energy savings have been gained through the use of radiant heating and solar panels for heating domestic water and minimizing the need for artificial light by using occupancy sensors and maximizing daylight. Water quality and efficiency measures were accomplished by reducing storm water runoff and promoting infiltration, collecting rain water from the roof for irrigation use, and using low-flow plumbing fixtures. Other green features include the use of recycled glass cullet as site fill and perimeter drainage-ballast for the green roof, recycled aggregate and high-volume fly ash content to reduce CO_2 emissions in the concrete, a 100% postconsumer recycled plastic grid for the gravel paving system in the drive, sustainably harvested FSC redwood siding, and recyclable cement board siding. They also installed countertops made from compressed recycled sunflower seed hulls (Dakota Burl) and recycled scrap from the factory. Researching costs and availability of materials, balancing decisions for the greatest impact, and securing donations have ensured a successful sustainable building.[12]

REFERENCES

1. American Society of Landscape Architects: Advocacy: Sustainable Design, 2010 (http://www.asla.org/ContentDetail.aspx?id=23122).
2. American Veterinary Medical Association: Best Management Practices for Pharmaceutical Disposal, 2010 (http://www.avma.org/issues/policy/pharmaceutical_disposal.asp).
3. Association of Zoos and Aquariums: Reducing Climate Impacts on Wildlife and Wild Habitats, 2010 (http://www.aza.org/Conservation/detail.aspx?id=12645&terms=climate+initiative).
4. Center for Watershed Protection: Better Site Design: A Handbook for Changing Development Rules in Your Community, 2010 (http://www.cwp.org/categoryblog/101-better-site-design-.html).
5. Electronics Takeback Coalition: Responsible Recycling, 2010 (http://www.computertakeback.com/responsible_recycling/index.cfm).
6. GreenVetPractice: Greening Your Practice, 2010 (http://greenvetpractice.com/index.htm).
7. Healthcare Without Harm: Issues: Waste Management, 2010 (http://www.noharm.org/us_canada/issues/waste).
8. Low-Impact Development Center: Low-Impact Development Design Strategies: An Integrated Design Approach, 1999 (http://www.lowimpactdevelopment.org/pubs/LID_National_Manual.pdf).
9. McDonough W, Braungart M: Cradle to Cradle: Remaking the Way We Make Things, 2006 (www.mcdonough.com/cradle_to_cradle.htm).
10. Palm Beach Zoo: The Melvin J. and Claire Levine Animal Care Complex: Home of the Nation's First LEED Certified Zoo Animal Hospital, 2009 (http://www.palmbeachzoo.org/pdf/press/2009-04-22-acc-leed-fact-sheet.pdf).
10a. Michele Miller, personal communication.
11. Practice Greenhealth: Waste Management, 2008 (http://practicegreenhealth.org/educate/operations/waste).
12. Reed H: Personal communication, 2010.
13. River Network: Water-Energy Toolkit: Understanding the Carbon Footprint of Your Water Us, 2010 (http://www.rivernetwork.org/resource-library/water-energy-toolkit-understanding-carbon-footprint-your-water-use).
14. Sustainable Packaging Coalition: (http://www.sustainablepackaging.org), 2010.
15. United Nations Development Programme: Human Development Report 2006: Beyond Scarcity: Power, Poverty and the Global Water Crisis, 2006 (http://hdr.undp.org/en/reports/global/hdr2006).
16. U.S. Environmental Protection Agency: Green Power Partnership, 2010 (http://www.epa.gov/grnpower).
17. U.S. Environmental Protection Agency: Life-Cycle Assessment (LCA), 2010 (http://www.epa.gov/nrmrl/lcaccess).
18. U.S. Environmental Protection Agency: Locating and Estimating Air Emissions from Sources of Dioxins and Furans, 1997 (http://www.epa.gov/ttnchie1/le/dioxin.pdf).
19. U.S. Environmental Protection Agency: The Economics of Low-Impact Development: A Literature Review, 2007 (http://www.epa.gov/region8/water/stormwater/pdf/LID_Economics_Literature_Review.pdf).
20. U.S. Environmental Protection Agency: WaterSense, 2010 (http://www.epa.gov/watersense).
21. U.S. Environmental Protection Agency–U.S. Department of Energy: Energy Star Program, 2010 (http://www.energystar.gov).
22. U.S. Green Building Council: Leadership in Energy and Environmental Design (LEED), 2010 (http://www.usgbc.org/DisplayPage.aspx?CategoryID=19).

ADDITIONAL RESOURCES FOR GREENING VETERINARY PRACTICE

Green Guide for Health Care (http://www.gghc.org), 2010.
Healthcare Without Harm (http://www.noharm.org), 2010.
Healthier Hospitals Initiative: Improving Sustainability and Safety in Healthcare (http://www.healthierhospitals.org), 2010.
Practice Greenhealth (http://practicegreenhealth.org), 2008.
Sustainable Hospitals (http://www.sustainablehospitals.org/cgi-bin/DB_Index.cgi), 2000.
U.S. Environmental Protection Agency: Environmentally Preferable Purchasing (EPP) (http://www.epa.gov/epp), 2010.
U.S. Environmental Protection Agency: Managing Wet Weather with Green Infrastructure (http://cfpub.epa.gov/npdes/home.cfm?program_id=298), 2010.
U.S. Green Building Council: LEED for Healthcare (http://www.usgbc.org/DisplayPage.aspx?CMSPageID=1765), 2010.

CHAPTER 13

Anthrax in Free-Ranging Wildlife

Roy G. Bengis

Anthrax is an infectious, frequently fatal disease of domestic and wild animals and humans, caused by the gram-positive, nonmotile, endospore-forming bacterium, *Bacillus anthracis*. Anthrax is one of the oldest infectious diseases known to humans, and the biblical fifth and sixth plague, that first affected livestock and then humans were probably anthrax. From earliest historical records up until the development of an effective vaccine midway through the 20th century, anthrax was one of the foremost causes of uncontrolled mortality in cattle, sheep, goats, horses, and pigs worldwide.[22] A sharp decline in anthrax outbreaks occurred in livestock during the 1930 to 1980 era as a result of successful national vaccination programs in many parts of the globe, as well as the subsequent advent of antibiotics. More recently, however, a resurgence of this disease in livestock has been reported in some regions, where complacency and a false sense of security have derailed vaccination programs. Some animal health regulators have become forgetful of the environmental resilience of this organism, its endemic persistence, and circulation in certain wildlife-dominated ecosystems.

The life history of *B. anthracis* differs markedly from most other pathogenic bacteria in that its replication and persistence appear to depend on extreme virulence and acute death of its hosts, where after it survives as a highly resistant spore during prolonged periods outside a host.[3] Anthrax is an internationally reportable disease and, in 2009, the OIE (World Organization for Animal Health) reported that anthrax was still present in most countries of Africa and Asia, a number of European countries, certain countries and areas of North, Central, and South America, and certain areas of Australia. Many outbreaks of anthrax in wildlife go undetected and unreported because of surveillance inadequacies and the difficulties associated with disease monitoring in free-ranging wildlife.

RECORDED WILDLIFE HOST RANGE

Anthrax is a multispecies disease that can infect mammals of most taxonomic groupings. Ruminants and hindgut digesters are the most susceptible. Carnivores and primates (including humans) are more resistant to infection, and ostriches are the only avian species in which natural infection has been regularly reported. Carcass scavengers are generally highly resistant to anthrax.

Hugh-Jones and de Vos have listed a range of wild felids, canids, ursids, viverids, and mustelids that have been reported to have died of anthrax in zoological gardens. These deaths were most commonly associated with the inadvertent feeding of anthrax-infected carcasses, meat, or bone meal to exhibited animals. They also listed 4 free-ranging perissodactylids, 24 artiodactylids, 9 carnivore, and 2 primate species confirmed with natural infection in southern Africa.[12]

On a broader geographic scale, Cormack Gates and colleagues[3] have also listed 23 free-ranging bovids and 6 cervid species confirmed to have died of anthrax, as well as several free-ranging zebra and rhinoceros species, Asian and African elephants, 17 free-ranging carnivores, and 2 free-ranging primate species worldwide.

BIO-ECOLOGIC CONSIDERATIONS

Organism and Sources of Infection

During the interoutbreak periods, the anthrax bacterium survives in the environment as a highly resistant spore. Anthrax spores survive best in alkaline soils that are rich in calcium and have a relatively high moisture and organic content. The characteristics of dormancy and resistance to environmental factors displayed by these spores are a function of their structure, especially their hydrophobic exosporium and spore coat. The low water content of the spore confers resistance to heat and ultraviolet light.[16] Calcium cations appear to participate in maintaining dormancy, as well as in the germination process. In combination with dipicolinic acid (DPA), calcium forms an extensive salt lattice that effectively immobilizes enzymes, DNA, and other metabolically active components in the core, maintaining metabolic dormancy and conferring heat resistance to core components.[9]

These spores can survive for years in the environment and, under optimal conditions, some spores may survive for decades or even centuries. Although *B. anthracis* appears to be a relatively monomorphic species, recent progress using molecular techniques to determine phylogenetic relationships of isolates from various global locations has enabled a broad separation of isolates into two major clonal groups, referred to as A and B. The A and B2 branch isolates are distributed worldwide, and the B1 branch is found only in southern Africa.

After entering the host's body, germination appears to be triggered by moisture and warmth, as well as the presence of L-alanine in the blood serum. After germination has occurred, the vegetative bacilli undergo exponential replication, resulting in septicemia; it is the bacterial exotoxins that cause the pathology that results in the death of the animal (see later, "Pathogenesis").

A common misconception about *B. anthracis* is that vegetative cells (bacilli) require the presence of atmospheric oxygen for sporulation to occur. In all *Bacillus* species, sporulation is a response to low nutrient conditions or dehydration, which effectively limits the diffusion of nutrients to the bacillus. The anaerobic conditions within a carcass prevent the anthrax bacilli from replicating or sporulating, even though they are in a nutrient-rich medium. In addition, putrefactive anaerobic bacteria from the gastrointestinal tract start to decompose the carcass rapidly. The vegetative form of *B. anthracis* are susceptible to competition from other microbes and, if putrefactive organisms reach them before the carcass is opened, they are quickly eliminated.[23,25] In nature however, carcasses are rarely left intact long enough for putrefaction to eliminate all the vegetative anthrax bacilli. Instead, opening the carcass helps disperse vegetative *B. anthracis* into aerobic microenvironments where, either through metabolic activity or dehydration, nutrients become limited and sporulation can proceed.[2] Pools of blood and tissue fluids, under aerobic conditions around the carcass site, favor

sporulation. Many of these spores remain at the site of the dead animal, but some may be dispersed by water runoff, wind, and scavengers. Following sporulation, the cycle of environmental dormancy of the organism repeats itself.

Pathogenesis

It is well established that *B. anthracis* is not a highly invasive organism. Research results from many sources indicate that LD_{50} values for anthrax challenge are much higher by the oral or inhalation routes than via the parental route. However, once the anthrax spore has entered the mammalian body and germinated, it undergoes exponential replication within regional nodes, and then passes via the lymphatic vessels into the bloodstream. Bacilli that have entered the bloodstream are taken up in other parts of the reticuloendothelial system, particularly the spleen, to establish secondary centers of infection and proliferation.[17] The vegetative anthrax bacilli produce a lethal combination of exotoxins, responsible for the severe clinical signs and postmortem lesions seen in anthrax. The toxin complex consists of two separate protein toxins, designated edema factor (EF) and lethal factor (LF), and a cell receptor–binding protein called protective antigen (PA).[11,13] The toxin complex acts to reduce phagocytosis, increase capillary permeability, and damage blood-clotting mechanisms. The net effect produces massive edema (including the lungs and brain), hemorrhage, renal failure, and terminal hypoxia.

Various wildlife species have differing sensitivity to these exotoxins, reflected in the terminal bacteremial counts seen in the blood. Lower sensitivity to exotoxins requires higher terminal bacteremic counts to kill the animal, and vice versa.

ROUTES OF INFECTION, TRANSMISSION, AND SEASONALITY

Anthrax outbreaks are commonly associated with low-lying depressions and rock land seep areas with high moisture content, high organic content, and an alkaline pH. Successive cycles of flood runoff and evaporation appear to concentrate the anthrax spores in these depressions, which may be referred to as concentrator areas.[7] With the seasonal decrease in water levels in these concentrator areas, the resident wildlife using this water source may be increasingly exposed to higher concentrations of accumulated spores.

In addition, water and wind erosion may expose spores hidden in the soil column or may expose carcass remnants of previous anthrax victims. Alternatively, spores may be brought to the surface by large- or small-scale seismic events.

Transmission of anthrax relies on the ingestion of infected spores or parental inoculation of spores. Ingestion of spores is generally associated with drinking from a contaminated water source or ingesting contaminated grazing, browse, flesh, or bones; oral infection is probably the most common route of infection in wild animals. In predators and porcines, edematous lesions generally develop in the oral and pharyngeal areas, whereas in domestic and wild ruminants, necrohemorrhagic lesions develop in Peyer's patches or segmental regions of the small intestine, eventually progressing to septicemia.[14,15] Osteophagia by pregnant or lactating animals, or animals on rangeland with phosphate-deficient soil, is an important mechanism of infection in certain regions.

Anthrax may also penetrate broken skin or mucous membranes, and this route of infection is most commonly seen in humans who have handled anthrax-infected animal products. The animal equivalent is infection of subcutaneous tissues, generally as a result of mechanical transmission by contaminated mouthparts of biting insects. Cellulitis characterized by subcutaneous swellings is particularly common in equines. In addition, in carnivores, the massive facial and oral edema and necrosis is thought to be caused by penetration of oral or pharyngeal mucous membranes by bone spicules while chewing the bones of infected carcasses (Fig. 13-1). Following percutaneous penetration, the spores germinate and give rise to a small edematous area containing capsulated vegetative bacilli. The lesion then progresses in size, macrophages and fibrin deposits appear, lymphatics dilate, and fragmentation of connective tissue occurs, with increasing edema.[4] Phagocytosis appears minimal, and the infection then progresses into a lymphangitis followed by lymphadenitis. If the infection is not halted at this stage, it may become systemic and result in fatal septicemia.

Inhalation infection is probably the least common route of infection in free-ranging wild animals living in the open air because the natural anthrax spores tend to clump together with surrounding organic material and are not easily aerosolized. However, experimental infections have demonstrated that the spores do not germinate in the airways, but are phagocytosed by mobile macrophages, which then migrate to the

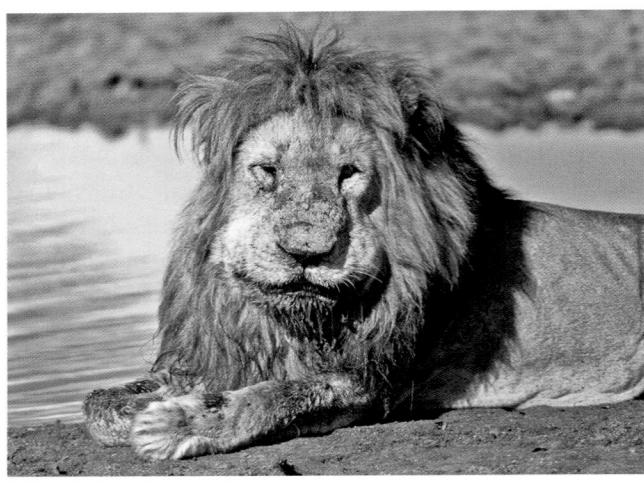

Figure 13-1

Male lion with severe facial swelling caused by anthrax infection. *(Courtesy DF Keet.)*

tracheobronchial lymph node.[10] Germination begins once the infected macrophages have arrived in the lymph node, and the vegetative cells freed from the phagocytes then proliferate, causing severe lymphadenopathy and rapid septicemia.[20] Inhalation anthrax generally has a very rapid fatal course.

During an anthrax outbreak, each successive victim may become an additional source of infection. Transmission modes from the infected carcass or bacteremic animals to the surrounding population at risk will vary in different environments with their associated species and potential vectors. Anthrax spores may directly contaminate pasture or water in close proximity to the carcass. In addition, anthrax bacilli and spores from a carcass may also be dispersed by water runoff, scavenging birds, and carnivorous mammals. Vegetative anthrax bacilli do not survive the digestive processes of carnivorous birds and mammals, but the hardy anthrax spores pass through the gastrointestinal tract unscathed and can contaminate distal sites indirectly.

Browse contamination occurs through the agency of nonbiting necrophilic flies, which feed on the body fluids of infected carcasses and then alight on nearby vegetation, depositing infectious vomit and fecal droplets on the leaves. This is an important transmission mode in ecosystems that are well populated by browsing antelope. In addition, a whole range of hematophagous biting flies have been implicated in the mechanical transmission of anthrax infection. In conclusion, the anthrax transmission mode will depend on environmental variables, host species, and vector mixes.

Anthrax in North American Wildlife

In northern Canada (Alberta and northwestern territories), regular outbreaks of anthrax were recorded between 1962 and 2001 in wood bison *(Bison bison)*. These outbreaks generally occurred during the hot, dry summer months, and part of this period (August to September) coincides with the wood bison rut. Rutting behavior of bison bulls, such as wallowing, dirt digging with their horns, and dust rolling is thought to increase the chance of exposure to anthrax spores by ingestion or inhalation greatly. The wallowing pits that are annually reused tend to become larger over time, and may serve as spore concentrator areas. In northern Canada, this late summer period is also frequently associated with an increased number of tabanid flies, which may also be involved in the mechanical transmission of infection. The only sympatric species recorded to have died of anthrax during these outbreaks were the occasional moose *(Alces alces)* and a few black bears *(Ursus americanus)*. Mammalian and avian scavengers are thought to play a role in dispersal of spores.

Parts of southwest Texas (Val Verde, Uvalde, and Webb counties) have a historic presence of endemic anthrax. This region has shallow, lime-rich, humus soils overlying limestone, which is ideal for anthrax spore survival. This endemic state is periodically punctuated with epidemic flare-ups during hot, dry summer weather, usually following heavy spring and early summer rains. These outbreaks frequently involve white-tailed deer *(Odocoelius virginianus)* and unvaccinated cattle, and mortalities can be spectacular. Biting flies, locally called charbon flies, are thought to be important in propagating the epidemic by mechanical transmission of anthrax bacilli from bacteremic animals, resulting in centrifugal spread of infection.[12]

Anthrax in Wildlife in Sub-Saharan Africa

In the various sub-Saharan African countries that regularly report anthrax in free-ranging wildlife, a range of wild herbivore species emerge as important epidemiologic role players in the various habitats, landscapes, and ecozones.

In the southeastern subtropical savannahs of South Africa and Zimbabwe, anthrax is a multispecies disease, with mortalities recorded in 36 wild species. However, analysis of the outbreaks in this ecosystem has shown that greater kudu *(Tragelaphus strepsiceros)* are the most important anthrax host, and that contamination of natural browse by blowflies *(Chrysomyia* and *Lucilia*

spp.) is the most important transmission mode during these anthrax epidemics. Kudu carcasses are totally overrepresented in the carcass counts during outbreaks, which is illustrated by the fact that in the Kruger National Park, where this species constitute only 3.7% of the total large ungulate population, during four anthrax outbreaks between 1990 to 1999 they represented 42% to 62% of the anthrax-positive carcasses found.[1] In addition, the fact that kudu develop very high-terminal bacteremias and have thin skins that are easily opened up by most scavengers, makes kudu an important anthrax amplifier in this ecosystem.[6] Nyala *(Tragelaphus angasi)*, another browsing antelope, are also frequently infected during outbreaks in the localities where they occur.

During these outbreaks, significant mortalities were also reported in African buffalo *(Syncerus caffer)*, waterbuck *(Kobus ellipsiprymnusc)*, zebra *(Equus burchelli)*, impala *(Aepyceros melampus)*, and Roan antelope *(Hippotragus taurinus)*, all of which are mainly grazers, and transmission of infection to these species is probably via infected water or contaminated grazing. These outbreaks generally occur in the dry winter season or dry climatic cycles, and appear to be linked to an absolute or relative overabundance of key wildlife species, and to be stress-related to resource competition.

In the more arid southern African savannahs of Botswana and Namibia, elephants *(Loxodonta africana)*, African buffaloes, zebras, and springbok *(Antedorcas marsupialis)* are important role players, and transmission appears once again to be mainly via infected water or grazing related to dry season resource stress and population clustering. The situation in Etosha National Park in northern Namibia is unique in that anthrax is endemic in this park and cases are confirmed in most years. In addition, this park has temporal clustering of cases in elephants at the end of dry season, followed by a summer (wet season) outbreak in plains ungulates such as zebra, wildebeest *(Connochaetes taurinus)*, and springbok, probably related to contamination of grazing by carcasses or contamination of rain pools by wading vultures.[8,17]

The Northern Cape Province of South Africa also has certain anthrax-endemic areas. However, in contrast to the rest of southern Africa, anthrax outbreaks in this Province are generally wet summer season phenomena, with disease propagation typically linked to huge buildups of biting flies *(Hippobosca* spp.), and mechanical transmission from bacteremic animals.

In the Zambian Luangwa river system and the Ugandan Great Lakes, the key species affected by anthrax are hippopotami *(Hippopotamus amphibius)* and African buffaloes. Once again, population overabundance and resource stress generally precede outbreaks, and transmission appears to be mainly via contaminated water and grazing, although biting flies may play some role with hippopotami.

Anthrax has also been sporadically reported in buffalo and impala in Tanzania, in Grevy's zebra (*E. greyvi*) in northern Kenya and in lesser kudu (*Tragelaphus imberbis*) in Ethiopia.

Anthrax in European Wildlife

Anthrax in northeastern Europe has been most regularly documented in reindeer (*Rangifer tarandus*). Hematophagous flies are thought to be the most important transmission mode.

Anthrax in Asian Wildlife

Anthrax in Asian wildlife has been reported in water buffalo (*Bubalus bubalus*), sambar deer (*Cervus unicolor*), Asian elephants (*Elephas maximumus*) and Indian rhinoceros (*Rhinoceros unicornis*). Transmission appears to be mainly related to the ingestion of contaminated water or vegetation.

OTHER EPIDEMIOLOGIC DETERMINANTS
Gender Predilection

In most outbreaks of anthrax in wildlife, no significant gender predilection could be detected. An exception to this observation has been recorded in wood bison in northern Canada and African buffalo in South Africa, where a gender bias of anthrax infection toward adult males has been detected. This is thought to be linked to the similar wallowing and mud-digging behavior shown by bulls of these two species.

Age Predilection

Generally, there is no age predilection seen in anthrax outbreaks, except that young animals tend to be spared. This is probably linked to the fact that little of the fluid and nutrient requirements of unweaned animals are obtained from the environment.

Patterns of Disease

The general pattern seen in anthrax endemic regions is that of sporadic cases occurring on an irregular basis,

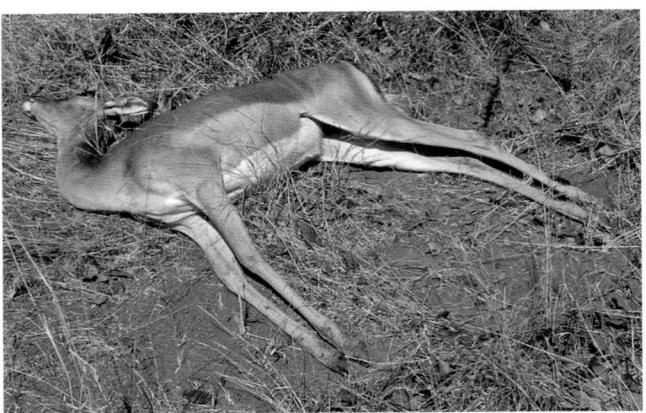

Figure 13-2

Typical posture of the carcass of a wild ruminant (impala) that has died of anthrax.

with some form of seasonal pattern. These sporadic events are interspersed with periodic outbreak clusters or even propagating epidemics.[5] The propagating epidemics are generally linked to densities or concentrations of preferred host species in the system. These propagating epidemics are generally self-limiting and tend to follow a normal epidemic curve pattern. A feature of dry season outbreaks in southern Africa is that these outbreaks or epidemics are dramatically terminated by the onset of the summer rains.

CLINICAL SIGNS

Anthrax may present as a peracute or acute disease in ruminants. Clinical signs include disorientation, ataxia, respiratory distress, and apoplectic seizures, followed by acute death. The victims are generally in good body condition and carcasses frequently demonstrate opisthotonus, with extensor rigidity of the forelimbs (Fig. 13-2). In equines and porcines, abdominal pain (colic) is frequently evident, and there may be diarrhea. Cutaneous and localized swellings, which may be present at various anatomic sites, are also common in these two taxa.

Although predators in general are less susceptible to infection by *B. anthracis*, they are however, at high risk because of massive exposure when they feed on infected carcasses, ingesting billions of organisms. Anthrax infection has been documented in lions (*Panthera leo*), leopards (*P. pardus*), jackals (*Canis mesomelas*), and even wild dogs (*Lycaon pictus*) during epidemics in Southern Africa. Most lions present grossly swollen heads caused by massive cellulitis of the head and oral structures (see

Fig. 13-1). Clinical cases in predators are generally more common during the early phases of an epidemic in a new locality. If predators survive their first few exposures to anthrax, they appear to develop a strong immunity. Most predators in anthrax endemic areas appear to become totally resistant.[24]

Cheetah *(Acinonyx jubatus)* however, appear to represent an unusual group among carnivores in relation to anthrax. Significant anthrax–associated mortalities in cheetah have been recorded in Namibia, and this appears to be related to the fact that cheetah rarely scavenge and do not get the same opportunities to build up acquired immunity.[18]

Postmortem and Gross Pathology

Generally, postmortem rigor mortis is incomplete or absent, and rapid bloating occurs. Blood-stained fluid may exude from one or more body orifices. Petechiae and ecchymoses are often present in unpigmented or hairless areas of the skin. The blood is dark and tarry and frequently does not clot.[12] The principle macroscopic lesions seen in septicemic anthrax in herbivores are widespread edema, hemorrhage, and necrosis.[15]

Splenomegaly, with typical currant jelly appearance of the red pulp, as well as hemorrhagic and edematous lymph nodes are a common finding. There is frequently excessive amounts of free blood-tinged fluid in the body cavities and numerous petechiae and ecchymoses are present on serosal surfaces. Extensive pulmonary and mediastinal edema is a common finding.

In lions and leopards, the lesions vary in severity and are frequently localized to the subcutaneous tissues of the head, oral cavity, and regional lymph nodes. The changes may vary from localized glossitis or stomatitis to extensive necrotic cellulitis of the lips and face, resulting in severe edema and swelling of the head (see Fig. 13-1).

Histopathology

Microscopic findings in generalized cases are dominated by the presence of large numbers of anthrax bacilli in blood and most other tissues. Necrotic lesions are invariably associated with tissue invasion by the bacteria. Edema and extravasation of blood is a common finding in many organs and there is loss of splenic and lymph node architecture, plus flooding of these organs with erythrocytes.[21]

LABORATORY AND DIFFERENTIAL DIAGNOSIS

It is important to remember that *B. anthracis* is not highly infectious and that humans are moderately resistant. Nonetheless, biosafety level 2 laboratory practices, containment equipment, and facilities are appropriate for routine laboratory diagnostic tests.

When a suspect animal anthrax case is detected, the carcass should not be opened. A blood smear should be taken from the pinna of the ear, tip of the tail, or any superficial vein. In older carcasses (2 days or more), or carcasses that have been reduced to skeleton and skin, the coronary band and hoof lamellae offer an excellent site to locate a drop of blood that also has minimum putrefactive contamination (Fig. 13-3). Always make at least two smears, one for differential staining and in case one inadvertently gets broken. Allow the smears to air-dry, place in a slide-holding container, or wrap in tissue paper or a small paper data sheet. Record all information regarding the carcass, including global positioning system (GPS) coordinates if possible.

Laboratory Diagnosis

Blood and Tissue Smear Examination
Generally, blood smears are fixed with 95% to 100% methanol or by heating and then staining with Gram, McFadyean, malachite green, or Giemsa stain (differential staining) or Ziehl-Neelsen stain (spores).[19] Many field laboratories routinely use Giemsa stain because to

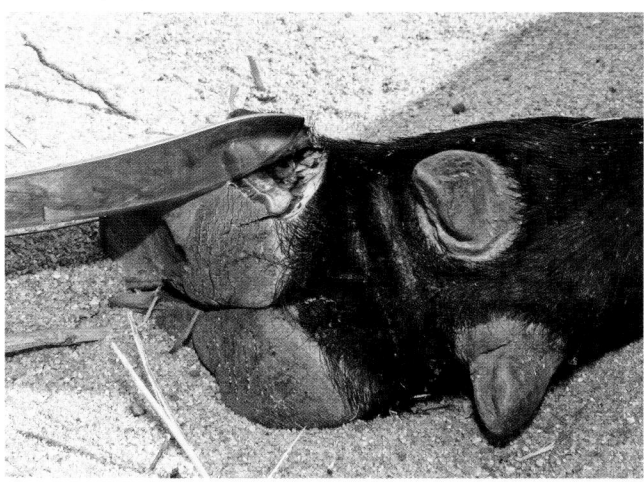

Figure 13-3

Technique for obtaining a blood smear from the coronary band and hoof lamellae from putrefied or consumed carcasses.

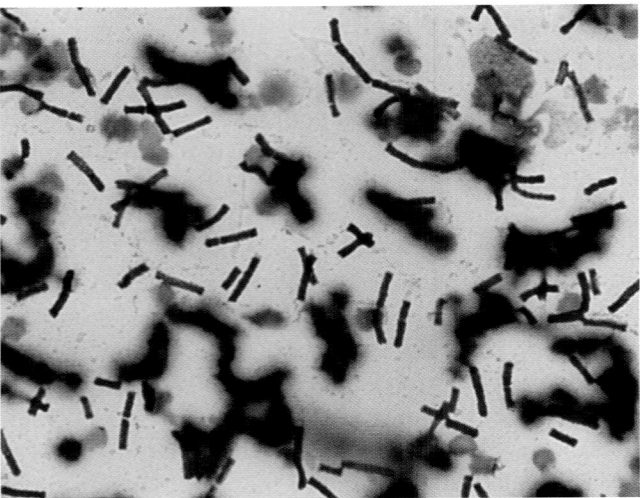

Figure 13-4

High-terminal anthrax bacteremia in the blood smear of a greater kudu (Giemsa stain, ×1000).

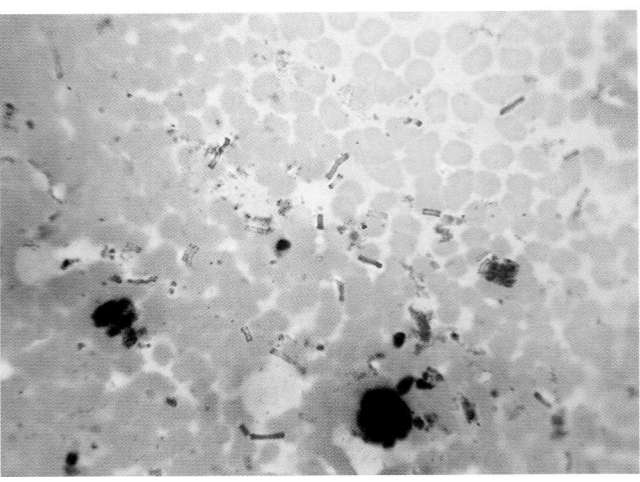

Figure 13-5

Anthrax "ghost" cells in a blood smear from a putrefying carcass (Giemsa stain, ×1000). *(Courtesy EH Dekker.)*

the experienced eye, postmortem putrefactive organisms and anthrax bacilli can be microscopically differentiated on appearance as a result of stain color uptake, size, shape, and chain formation. In blood smears from herbivores, the anthrax bacilli appear cylindric, with flattened ends, are monomorphic, stain a deep magenta color, endospores are not visible, and bacilli generally occur singly or in short chains. Certain species such as greater kudu have high-terminal bacteremias (Fig. 13-4), whereas African buffalo generally have low-terminal bacteremias. In addition, when using Giemsa stain on smears from putrefied carcasses, the capsular remnants of dead anthrax bacilli appear as pink outlines of the bacillus, frequently referred to as ghost cells (Fig. 13-5). Putrefactive bacilli, on the other hand, have rounded ends, generally stain deep purple with Giemsa, vary in size and thickness, may form long chains, and may produce polar or equatorial spores that are greater in diameter than the parent bacterial cell. In lions, anthrax bacilli may not be detectable in peripheral blood smears, but are frequently detectable in smears of the edema fluid from the head tissues.

Culture and Phage Typing

Culture of tissues is used to confirm the identity of the bacilli seen in blood or impression smears, and is also used to confirm the presence of anthrax spores in old animal tissue specimens (frequently bones or dried skin) or environmental samples. Specimens for anthrax culture are placed in a water bath heated to 62°C to 65°C for 15 to 30 minutes to kill all vegetative bacteria,

and heat shock any spores present. Only spore-formers survive this procedure; these include bacteria of the genera *Bacillus* and *Clostridium*. The specimen is then aerobically cultured on selective media, such as polymyxin, lysosome, EDTA, and thallous acetate (PLET) and total serum bile acids (TSBA). *Clostridium* spp. are anaerobes and are thus eliminated by aerobic culture. Thus, the colonies that grow on these selective media are mostly bacteria of the genus *Bacillus*. After overnight incubation, *B. anthracis* colonies are white, with a frosted glass appearance, may exhibit some tailing, and are exceptionally tenacious when teased with an inoculating loop. Suspect colonies are then subcultured on blood–tryptose agar and identification is then confirmed by assessing whether the colonies are hemolytic (*B. anthracis* is nonhemolytic) and checking for penicillin and phage sensitivity.[19]

Serologic Testing

The Ascoli precipitin test is an old test, developed in 1911 to supply rapid retrospective evidence of anthrax infection in an animal product. It was designed to detect *B. anthracis* antigens in the tissues of animals and their byproducts. The test makes use of commercially prepared serum, harvested from hyperimmunized rabbits, which reacts with the boiled filtrate of the suspect tissues in a test tube, and a line of precipitation develops at the antigen-antibody interface.

With the specter of bioterrorism becoming increasingly apparent, military research has developed a rapid handheld immunochromatographic device for detecting the presence of *B. anthracis* protective antigen, as well as a rapid handheld enzyme-linked immunosorbent assay (ELISA) kit for on-site diagnosis.

Molecular Techniques
Various molecular techniques have been developed for detecting *B. anthracis* DNA in specimens. These tests make use of the polymerase chain reaction using different primer systems to detect various *B. anthracis* genes, such as capsular (capB) and protective antigen (pagA) genes. Commercial kits for a range of sample types have become available. Nucleotide sequencing is important for strain typing and molecular epidemiologic studies.

Differential Diagnosis

In wild herbivores, anthrax must be differentiated from other conditions that cause sudden death. Common differential diagnoses are the various clostridial infections of herbivores, which also cause acute death and may show gram-positive rod-shaped bacteria in blood or organ smears.

Other conditions that should be considered are lightning strikes, cyanobacterial intoxications, acute plant poisonings, acute organic or inorganic poisonings, and snake bite. In wild carnivores, differential diagnoses include other acute infections or envenomations that may cause localized swellings (e.g., insect stings, snake bite).

DOMESTIC ANIMAL AND VETERINARY PUBLIC HEALTH CONCERNS

In areas in which anthrax is endemic in wildlife, or in which there is an active anthrax outbreak, the organisms may be transmitted from this source to livestock by means of water runoff and dispersal by birds and other carrion feeders and necrophilic flies, as well as biting insects.

During an anthrax outbreak in wildlife, it is important to embark on a mass vaccination campaign that targets the livestock at immediate risk. Multimedia public awareness campaigns are important, and local communities should be informed of the disease outbreak, disease prevention in livestock, and zoonotic risk and warned not to handle or consume animal carcasses. People should be encouraged to report carcasses, and carcass disposal should be efficiently addressed.

Anthrax is an important zoonotic disease and the World Health Organization (WHO) estimates between 20,000 and 100,000 human cases/year globally. In remote areas, local medical clinics or rural hospitals should be informed and reminded of the clinical presentations of anthrax in humans.

Cutaneous anthrax accounts for 95% of human cases reported. It is characterized by an initially pruritic lesion that progresses to vesiculation, plus surrounding edema. The vesicle ruptures, revealing a black necrotic center, which is painless. There is regional lymph adenopathy and low-grade fever. If left untreated, 20% of cases will progress to severe systemic and potentially fatal infection.

Enteric anthrax is more common in rural areas of the developing world, where carcasses are considered a windfall by protein-starved people. Edema, ulceration and hemorrhage occur in the gastrointestinal tract, which results in symptoms such as acute diarrhea, nausea, vomiting, and abdominal pain, which may progress to hematemesis, bloody diarrhea, and acute abdomen, followed by shock and death.

Inhalation anthrax was historically an occupational disease of wool sorters handling the skins or wool of infected sheep within the confines of a sorting shed in the 18th to 20th centuries. It has more recently been described in musicians playing drums that were covered with skins sourced from anthrax carcasses. However, with the exception of deliberate release or bioterrorism events, inhalation anthrax is probably the least common presentation of this disease. Radiologically, human patients show little evidence of pneumonia but do have signs of pleural effusion, hilar lymphadenopathy, and mediastinal widening.

CONTROL AND TREATMENT
Control Measures
Vaccination
The mainstay for control of anthrax in domestic livestock is vaccination using the noncapsulating strain 34F of *B. anthracis* (commonly known as the Sterne spore vaccine) in combination with various adjuvants.[22] This is an inexpensive and highly effective method of maintaining herd immunity in livestock, but needs to be repeated annually. Care should be taken when using these vaccines in caprines and llamas, because these species may develop severe reactions.

Vaccination of wildlife has been practiced from ground vehicles, hides, or helicopter platforms. This requires remote injection by means of drop out darts or biodegradable ballistic implant projectiles (in thin-skinned species). These techniques are useful for solitary or small group species such as larger antelope, rhinoceroses, and large predators. Another technique relies on mass capture of herd animals in a capture corral, followed by inoculation using multidose hand-held or pole syringes from the sides of an exit chute. These techniques can be highly effective, but are time-consuming and prohibitively expensive, and the need to repeat annually is daunting. There is, therefore, a definite need for the development of an effective oral vaccine for ranched and habituated wildlife, which can be delivered by means of water or feed.

Carcass Disposal

The primary source of environmental contamination by anthrax spores is the carcass of an animal that has died of anthrax. To minimize sporulation, carcasses should not be opened and should preferably be disposed of intact. Effective disposal options include incineration, rendering (not practical for free-ranging wildlife), or burial. Incineration can be effected by means of local fossil fuels, inflammable chemicals (e.g., napalm), down-directed blow torches, or portable incinerators. Burial is not ideal and is labor-intensive without earth-moving equipment, and spores will tend to surface again at a later date. Carcasses should be buried to a depth of at least 2 m, and one part chloride of lime should be mixed with three parts of soil during the filling of the grave to accelerate lysis of the carcass tissues and reduce the survival of spores.[19]

It is an important concept that keeping carcasses intact until significant putrefaction has occurred will theoretically kill most vegetative anthrax bacilli and reduce the opportunity to sporulate. Thus, making the carcass unattractive to scavengers will reduce the number of carcasses that are opened. In Canada, 5% formaldehyde sprayed on and around the carcass was found to be an effective deterrent for scavengers and had the positive spinoff of disinfecting the surrounding contaminated soil.[12]

Another relatively new but unproven technique that has promise relies on simply making the carcass inaccessible to invertebrate, avian, and small mammalian scavengers for an adequate period of time to allow putrefaction to proceed to an advanced state and eliminate most anthrax bacilli. This entails the covering or wrapping of the carcass in thick agricultural plastic sheeting or placing the carcass into purpose-built body bags and leaving these carcasses in situ to decompose for several days, depending on environmental temperatures. At a later stage, the carcass remnants can then be buried or incinerated at a central site. This technique

may only be practical for use in animals up to the size of a large antelope, but it is important to remember that these thin-skinned animals are also those species with high-terminal bacteremias, which are opened relatively easily by small scavengers.

Other Control Techniques

In regions in which invertebrates have been shown to be epidemiologically important, such as biting fly transmission or environmental contamination by necrophilic flies, targeted control of these insects may be attempted.

In certain habitats in which hot spots have been identified during an anthrax outbreak, range land burning may be considered as a method of reducing transmission and mortality. The rationale behind this intervention is that by burning the hot spot area, the fire destroys many spores on the vegetation, kills many invertebrate vectors, makes mammals disperse from the area, and then makes the area unattractive to herbivores for a varying period. This technique has been effectively used in certain African savannah systems in which anthrax has a winter–dry season pattern.[1]

Treatment

B. anthracis is susceptible to most antibiotics; however, because of the peracute nature of anthrax disease in herbivores, by the time the victims show clinical signs, it is usually too late to treat with antibiotics. In carnivores, however, anthrax has a less acute course and, during outbreaks in southern Africa, lions and leopards with typical clinical signs (e.g., swollen faces and lips), have been successfully treated with megadoses of long acting penicillin.

Prophylactic treatment may also be indicated prior to moving animals out of an outbreak zone. These animals can then be vaccinated at destination after a minimum of 14 days from the date of antibiotic administration. Antibiotics and vaccine should never be given together.

CONCLUSION

With the greater part of the life cycle of *B. anthracis* occurring as a dormant, highly resistant spore in the environment, accepting that surveillance and monitoring for infection in free-ranging wildlife is by nature difficult, and knowing that prevention and treatment are unlikely to succeed with current technology, we can expect that anthrax outbreaks in wildlife will continue to occur sporadically in many regions of the globe in the future.

REFERENCES

1. Bengis RG: Anthrax everywhere. Orlando, Florida, 2010 January, Presented at the North American Veterinary Conference, pp 16–20.
2. Choquette LPE: Anthrax. In Davis JW, Karstadt LH, Trainer DO, editors: Infectious diseases of wild mammals. Ames, Iowa, 1970, Iowa State University Press, pp 256–266.
3. Cormack Gates C, Elkin B, Dragon D: Anthrax. In Williams ES, Barker IK, editors: Infectious diseases of wild mammals, 3rd ed, Ames, Iowa, 2000, Iowa State University Press, pp 396–412.
4. Cromatie WJ, Bloom WL, Watson DW: Studies on infection with Bacillus anthracis. 1. A histopathological study of skin lesions produced by B. anthracis in susceptible and resistant animal species. J Infect Dis 80:1–13, 1947.
5. de Vos V, Bryden HB: Anthrax in the Kruger National Park: Temporal and spatial patterns of disease occurrence. Salisbury Med Bull 87(special suppl):26–30, 1996.
6. de Vos V, Turnbull PC: Anthrax. In Coetzer JAW, Tustin RC, editors: Infectious diseases of livestock, 2nd ed, Oxford, 2004, Oxford University Press, pp 1788–1818.
7. Dragon PC, Rennie RP: The ecology of anthrax spores: Tough but not invincible. Can Vet J 36:295–301, 1995.
8. Ebedes H: Anthrax epizootics in Etosha National Park. Madoqua 10:99–118, 1976.
9. Gould GW: Mechanisms of resistance and dormancy. In Hurst A, Gould GW, editors: The bacterial spore, Toronto, 1984, Academic Press, pp 173–209.
10. Henderson DW, Peacock S, Belton FC: Observations on the prophylaxis of experimental pulmonary anthrax in the monkey. J Hyg 54:28–36, 1956.
11. Hoover DL, Friedlander AM, Rogers LC, et al: Anthrax edema toxin differentially regulates lipopolysaccharide-induced monocyte production of tumor necrosis factor alpha and interleukin-6 by increasing intracellular cyclic AMP. Infect Immun 62:4432–4439, 1994.
12. Hugh-Jones ME, de Vos V: Anthrax and wildlife. Rev Sci Tech 21:359–383, 2002.
13. Ianaco-Connors LC, Schmaljohn CS, Dalrymple JM: Expression of the Bacillus anthracis protective antigen gene by baculovirus and vaccinia virus recombinants. Infect Immun 58:366–372, 1990.
14. Jackson FC, Wright GG, Armstrong J: Immunization of cattle against experimental anthrax, with alum precipitated protective antigen or spore vaccine. Am J Vet Res 18:771–777, 1957.
15. Kriek NPJ, de Vos V: Species differences in the pathology of wildlife in the Kruger National Park, South Africa. Salisbury Med Bull 87(special suppl):82, 1996.
16. Koshikawa T, Tamazaki M, Yoshimi M: Surface hydrophobicity of spores of Bacillus spp. J Gen Microbiol 135:2717–2722, 1989.
17. Lindeque PM, Turnbull PCB: Ecology and epidemiology of anthrax in Etosha National Park, Namibia. Onderstepoort J Vet Res 61:71–83, 1994.
18. Lindeque PMK, Nowell K, Preisser T, et al: Anthrax in wild cheetahs in Etosha National Park, Namibia. In Proceedings of the ARC-Onderstepoort OIE International Congress with WHO-cosponsorship on anthrax, brucellosis, CBPP, clostridial and mycobacterial diseases. South Africa, 1998 August, Bergen-Dal, Kruger National Park, pp 9–15.
19. Turnbull PC (exec ed): Anthrax in Humans and Animals, 4th ed, 2008 (http://www.who.int/csr/resources/publications/anthrax_webs.pdf).
20. Ross JM: The pathogenesis of anthrax following the administration of spores by the respiratory route. J Pathol Bacteriol 73:485–494, 1957.
21. Smith HA, Jones TC: Diseases due to simple bacteria (anthrax). In Smith HA, Jones TC, editors: Veterinary pathology, 3rd ed, Philadelphia, 1966, Lea and Febiger, pp 463–466.
22. Sterne M: The use of anthrax vaccines prepared from avirulent (uncapsulated) variants of Bacillus anthracis. Onderstepoort J Vet Sci An Ind 13:307–312, 1939.
23. Sterne M: Anthrax. In Stableforth AW, Galloway IA, editors: Infectious diseases of animals: diseases due to Bacteria. New York, 1959, Academic Press, pp 16–52.
24. Turnbull PC: Serology and anthrax in humans, livestock and Etosha National Park wildlife. Epidemiol Infect 108:299–313, 1992.
25. Turnbull PC, Carman JA, Lindeque PM, et al: Further progress in understanding anthrax in Etosha National Park. Madoqua 16:93–104, 1989.

CHAPTER 14

Cyanobacterial Biointoxication in Free-Ranging Wildlife

Peter E. Buss and Roy G. Bengis

The phylum Cyanobacteria (blue-green algae) is large and diverse, containing over 1000 species of oxyphototrophs.[12] Prehistoric evidence suggests that photosynthetic cyanobacteria existed in shallow seas 3.8 billion years ago and were responsible for changing atmospheric water vapor, carbon dioxide, and nitrogen to the oxygen-dominated atmosphere of today. This evolutionary leap allowed development of higher multicellular life forms. Anaerobic bacteria, which had previously dominated the planet for over 1000 million years, were relegated to isolated areas devoid of oxygen.[9] Because of their capacity for aerobic and anaerobic photosynthesis, cyanobacteria are able to thrive in a variety of habitats. In eutrophic surface water, they may multiply rapidly and form intense blooms.[18] With global warming and increased eutrophication of certain water bodies, some cyanobacteria have significantly expanded their geographic ranges and have adapted to previously unsuitable environmental conditions.[14]

Cyanobacteria produce a large variety of biologically active organic compounds, many of which are toxic. These biotoxins are responsible for intermittent but frequently repeated intoxication events, affecting both wild and domestic animals. Toxins include microcystins, nodularin, anatoxins, saxitoxins, cylindrospermopsins, lyngbyatoxin a, and aplysiatoxins.[2] They may be classified into five functional groups: hepatotoxins, neurotoxins, cytotoxins, dermatotoxins, and irritant toxins. These cell-based toxins may be released in high concentrations, with cell lysis.[18] The most toxic freshwater cyanobacteria are *Microcystis*, *Anabaena*, and *Panktothrix* spp. (Table 14-1); the most commonly produced toxins are microcystins.[8] The microcystins include seven cyclic aminopeptide hepatotoxins, with 65 structural isoforms currently described.[3,7] The most common form is microcystin-LR, with the two variable L-amino acids being leucine (L) and arginine (R).[9] Most microcystins have an LD_{50} of 60 to 70 μg/kg when administered intraperitoneally in mice.[4] Microcystins cause hepatic cellular disruption, leading to sinusoid destruction and intrahepatic bleeding, with fatal hemorrhagic shock. Nodularin is a cyclic pentapeptide with a structure closely related to that of the microcystins and with similar hepatotoxic effects mediated through the potent inhibition of protein phosphatases. The alkaloid toxins are anatoxin, saxitoxins, cylindrospermopsin, and lyngbyatoxin a. Anatoxins function as depolarizing neuromuscular blocking agents in higher vertebrates. The toxins are not affected by acetylcholinesterase, resulting in excessive stimulation of muscle cells, followed by fatigue and paralysis. There is no known antidote and death is usually attributed to respiratory arrest. Saxitoxins are similarly neurotoxic; death is caused by muscle paralysis and respiratory arrest in mammals. Nerve cells are affected through inhibition of the opening of voltage-gated Na^+ channels. Cylindrospermopsin is an irreversible inhibitor of protein biosynthesis, primarily affecting the liver, along with other major organs. Lyngbyatoxin a, a highly inflammatory toxin, is also a strong tumor promoter through activation of protein kinase C. Aplysiatoxins are commonly known for their dermatotoxic effects and cause inflammation of the skin. They are also potent tumor promoters.

FACTORS CONTRIBUTING TO GROWTH AND TOXICITY OF CYANOBACTERIAL BLOOMS

The toxicity of a cyanobacteria bloom is influenced by a number of factors, including temperature, pH, light intensity, organic nutrients, and age of algal cells.[8] Changes in toxin content occur on temporal and spatial scales. This probably reflects alterations in species and

TABLE 14-1	List of Known Cyanobacteria and Toxins Produced
Genus	**Toxins Produced**
Anabaena	Anatoxins, microcystins, saxitoxins
Anabaenopsis	Microcystins
Aphanizomenon	Saxitoxins, cylindrospermopsins
Cylindrospermopsis	Cylindrospermopsins, saxitoxins
Hapalosiphon	Microcystins
Lyngbya	Aplysiatoxins, lyngbyatoxin a
Microcystis	Microcystins
Nodularia	Nodularin
Nostoc	Microcystins
Phormidium (Oscillatoria)	Anatoxin
Planktothrix (Oscillatoria)	Anatoxins, aplysiatoxins, microcystins, saxitoxins
Schizothrix	Aplysiatoxins
Trichodesmium	Yet to be identified
Umezakia	Cylindrospermopsin

Adapted from Cyanosite: Cyanobacterial toxins, 2010 (http://www-cyanosite.bio.purdue.edu/cyanotox/toxiccyanos.html).

strain composition, with variations in toxins related to changes in environmental conditions influencing growth of the organism. At low winter temperatures, growth of Microcystis spp. may be negligible, but a sustainable viable population persists until temperatures start rising again. Growth of Microcystis aeruginosa is reported to be severely limited below 15° C, with optimal growth at 25° C to 32° C. However, maximal toxin production occurs at approximately 20° C. At temperatures of 32° C and 36° C, toxicity in cell culture was 1.6 and 4 times less than Microcystis spp. cultured at 28° C, suggesting that the level of toxicity is not correlated with greatest growth rate. Temperature changes are also reported to induce changes in peptide composition and concentration of toxins.[11] The ability of cyanobacteria to grow at higher temperatures gives them a competitive advantage over other phytoplankton species, such as diatoms and green algae. Warming of surface waters also increases vertical stratification of water bodies, reducing vertical mixing. With increased global temperature trends, this is occurring earlier in spring and persisting until later in autumn, which increases the growth period for cyanobacteria.[14] At favorable light intensities, M. aeruginosa will undergo an initial lag phase of 5 days, followed by an exponential growth phase of approximately 11 days. As light intensity increases, growth rate declines. Gas vacuole content and buoyancy of the cells are also influenced by light intensity, initially increasing as the brightness increases and then decreasing. Buoyancy is regulated by a complex relationship between light and composition changes in protein-to-carbohydrate ratios within the cyanobacterial cells. This characteristic is important in the pathogenesis of toxicosis because most animals drink from the surface of water bodies. Blooms of Microcystis spp. and increased microcystin concentrations have been associated with eutrophication, characterized by higher water nitrogen-to-phosphorus ratios. These are often caused by addition of nutrients derived from human wastes from mining, industrial, and forestry activities, as well as sewerage, or the input of fertilizers or animal wastes from intensive farming. Availability of Zn^{2+} and Fe^{2+} is also reported to influence to toxin yields because Fe^{2+} is required for nitrogen assimilation, respiration, and chlorophyll synthesis.

TOXICITY IN ANIMAL SPECIES

Blooms caused by various cyanobacteria species have been associated with mortalities in fish, turtle, birds, and mammals worldwide. Bivalves are able to ingest cyanobacteria toxins by filtering water containing cyanobacteria for their food. Contradictory reports have suggested that they may promote toxic blooms through passing live Microcystis spp. in their pseudofeces or reduce blooms by ingesting the Microcystis spp., clearing the water of the organism. Several bivalves have been shown to be able to accumulate and store toxins, with relative resistance to the toxin themselves. Crayfish tolerate and grow well on Microcystis spp. Toxins accumulate in the intestines and hepatopancreas, with no apparent harmful effects. Because of the bioaccumulation of cyanotoxins, including microcystin, nodularin, and saxitoxin in these invertebrates, they are potential sources of these toxins for the animals and humans that consume them.[18] It should be stated however, that evidence that supports the transfer of microcystins within the food web and biomagnification of the toxin is currently limited. Variations occur in these two processes depending on the toxin involved, and efforts to determine the effects of cyanotoxins in aquatic food webs are frequently complicated by a multitude of stress factors that occur concurrently during blooms.[4]

Mass mortalities of fish have been linked to the secretion of microcystins in association with algal blooms. Potential contributing factors include low water level, high water temperature, high pH, high ammonium concentration, low dissolved oxygen concentration, and the presence of other toxin-producing microorganisms.[4,7] Fish are exposed to toxins during feeding or when toxins pass over their gills during breathing. In early life stages of fish, microcystins interfere with developmental processes and organ function. These include alterations in time to hatching of embryos and dose-dependent decreases in survival and growth rates of juveniles. The most pronounced effects are poor yolk resorption, small head, curved body and tail, hepatobiliary abnormalities, alterations to hepatocytes, and cardiac problems. Chronic toxic effects are hypothesized to be caused by increased energy demands required by the detoxification systems in these life stages.

In adult fish, the main organs affected by microcystins are the kidneys and liver with pathology similar to that described for mammals, including a loss of liver structure resulting in necrosis and loss of function.[18] The toxin binds protein phosphatases 1 and 2A, which causes an increase in reactive oxygen species in hepatocytes, leading to oxidant shock and cell necrosis.[7] Nodularin is reported to have similar hepatotoxic effects in fish. Epithelial cells of the gills undergo cellular degeneration and necrosis. Gill cell chloride ion pumps may be disrupted affecting osmotic balance. Cardiac effects from environmentally relevant microcystin concentrations include increased heart rate, stroke volume, and cardiac output. Variations in sensitivity to the toxin have been demonstrated among different species of fish. This may be related to selective feeding of toxic or nontoxic strains of *Microcystis*, duration of digestion, and the number of lysed cells releasing toxins. Species native to eutrophic habitats are generally more resistant than those found in oligotrophic habitats. It has been demonstrated that cyanobacterial hepatotoxins may accumulate in fish tissue, especially the liver and, to a lesser extent, in muscle and viscera. These may be transferred up the food web, constituting a risk to piscivorous birds, animals, and humans that consume these fish.

In recent years, there have been reports of mass mortalities of lesser flamingos in East Africa—30,000 birds at Lake Bogoria, Kenya in 2000 and at Lake Embagai, Tanzania, 800 birds died during 2003. During 2004, deaths of large numbers of birds occurred in two alkaline lakes, Big Momela and Manyara, Tanzania, with 15,000 reported fatalities at Lake Manyara during a 2-month period. The cause of these deaths is presumed to be the consumption of the cyanobacterium *Arthrospira fusiformis*. This is an important natural food item for these birds and, until recently, was considered a nontoxic species. *A. fusiformis* has recently been shown to produce microcystins and anatoxin a.[6] Birds intoxicated with anatoxin a develop symptoms of staggering, muscle fasciculation, hyperpnea, cyanosis, paralysis, hyperesthesia, opisthotonus, convulsions, and death caused by respiratory failure.[3,18] A number of theories have been proposed for the pathogenesis relating to these flamingo deaths, including the existence of toxic and nontoxic strains of *A. fusiformis*, changes in environmental conditions that allow this strain to become toxic, toxin level variations through the lifespan of the organism, and cellular concentration in the water column.

In South Africa, cyanobacterial blooms are an increasing problem in freshwater bodies. This is predominantly caused by progressive eutrophication but has been influenced by the general trend of increasing environmental temperatures in the Southern Hemisphere since the 1950s.[13]

Cyanobacterial blooms on a water body are frequently variable in a spatial context, with patches of high and low concentrations of the algal elements. Winds push the floating cyanobacteria cells so that they accumulate on the leeward shore of water bodies and tend to leave the windward shore free of cyanobacteria.[16] Gas vacuoles of hollow proteinaceous vesicles filled with air facilitate buoyancy regulation in cyanobacteria, allowing them to access near-surface light energy and the more nutrient-rich deeper waters.[6] It has been observed that cattle, sheep, goats, and wildlife will consume this concentrated scum of *M. aeruginosa*, although they have the option of avoiding these denser portions of the bloom. Laboratory mice will preferentially consume dense cultures of this harmful cyanobacteria rather than limpid water. The reasons for this preferential selection have not been determined, but the mice did not appear to differentiate between toxic and nontoxic strains of the cyanobacteria. The mice reportedly had to consume up to 90% of the lethal dose before any measurable adverse effects were manifested.

Clinical Signs and Treatment

Susceptibility to cyanobacteria toxins varies in domestic species. Anatoxins most often affect pigs and dogs, with waterfowl susceptible and ruminants relatively resistant.

The quantity of toxin consumed influences onset and duration of clinical symptoms, from peracute to chronic. In peracute cases, hepatotoxins result in death within hours, frequently without any premonitory signs. Acutely to subacutely affected animals have symptoms associated with liver damage, including icterus and hepatogenic photosensitization. Other symptoms include vomiting, lethargy, ruminal stasis, constipation, and diarrhea. Death usually occurs in 1 to 2 weeks. Chronic cases usually result from the ingestion of sublethal doses over a prolonged period and typical symptoms are emaciation, inappetence, and chronic photosensitivity, with alopecia. In severe cases, hepatic enzyme levels may be elevated and coagulation parameters altered, with hyperbilirubinemia and hypoglycemia present. Treatment of hepatotoxicity is symptomatic and supportive,[3] although implementation in free-ranging wildlife may be challenging. Many species do not adapt well to captivity or being restrained to allow administration of treatment regimens.

Diagnosis

Diagnosis of poisoning caused by cyanobacteria depends on a history of exposure to cyanobacteria or bloom consumption, clinical findings, gross pathologic lesions and histopathology, identification of cyanobacteria in water, and identification and quantification of toxin in the water.[3] Examination of a wet sample preparation collected from the suspect water body or obtained from the gastrointestinal tract of the affected animal is the first step in determining an initial diagnosis, based on colony and/or cell morphology of the cyanobacterium involved.[17] To determine specific algal identification, a number of molecular biological techniques are used to determine DNA base ratios, DNA-DNA hybridization, and gene sequencing. More recently, amplified fragment length polymorphisms have been used to identify genetic diversity within strains of cyanobacteria, including *M. aeruginosa*.[12] The degree of hepatotoxicity may be evaluated using an enzyme-linked immunosorbent assay, protein phosphatase inhibition assay, or mouse bioassay. The use of animal cell cultures, such as rat or African sharptooth catfish hepatocytes, is a possible alternative for in vivo testing in mice.[8] High-performance liquid chromatography may be used in identification and quantification of hepatotoxins and neurotoxins. Thin layer chromatography, fast atom bombardment mass spectrometry, gas chromatography–mass spectrometry, and liquid chromatography–mass spectrometry have also been used.[10]

KRUGER NATIONAL PARK: A CASE STUDY

In 2005, a major algal bloom occurred in two artificial impoundments in the southeastern region of Kruger National Park. These blooms occurred following a very dry summer season and an abnormally warm autumn and early winter. River levels were low and intraspecific competition in the deeper pools of the rivers had driven large numbers of hippopotami *(Hippopotamus amphibius)* into several artificial impoundments in the nearby vicinity. These impoundments are generally constructed to stabilize surface water resources for the wildlife during the dry winter season. The water levels in both impoundments were dropping and they both supported high concentrations of hippopotami, which are thought to have been, at least in part, the cause of high levels of nitrogen- and phosphate-rich organic matter in the form of urine and fecal matter deposited in the water. These large amphibious mammals also physically stir up thick layers of rich organic sediment, which is the major repository of these nutrients.[8] In addition, these impoundments also result in stagnation of the drainage systems, which are unable to flush naturally.

These dammed water bodies developed a bright green discoloration of the upper strata of the water column, as well as a surface scum layer characteristic of an algae bloom (Fig. 14-1). Water samples taken from these dams showed the dominant presence of *Microcystis* spp.

A total of 52 mammalian carcasses were found clustered around the dams in a typical point source pattern

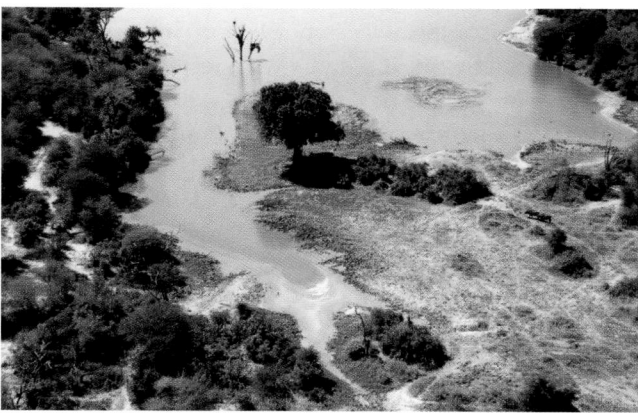

Figure 14-1

Aerial view showing the bright green discoloration of a dam in the Kruger National Park caused by a cyanobacterial bloom.

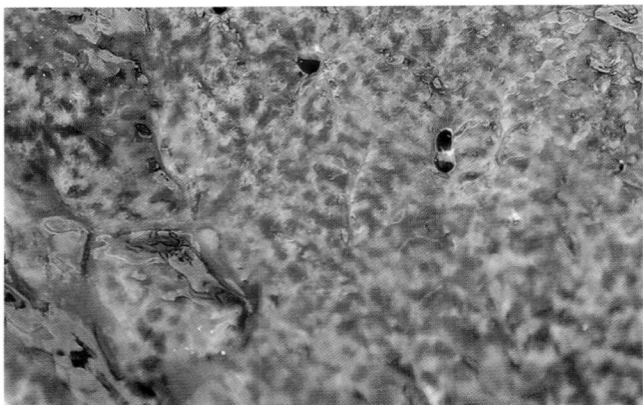

Figure 14-2

Surface of the liver from a zebra that died following ingestion of water affected by a *Microcystis* sp. bloom.

and the deaths were believed to be associated with the algal blooms. This multispecies event included 7 white rhinoceros (*Ceratotherium simum*), 2 lions (*Panthera leo*), 2 cheetahs (*Acinonyx jubatus*), 9 zebras (*Equus burchelli*), 23 wildebeest (*Connochaetes taurinus*), 1 hippopotamus (*Hippopotamus amphibious*), 1 giraffe (*Giraffa camelopardalis*), 1 warthog (*Phacochoerus aethiopicus*), and 1 kudu (*Tragelaphus strepsiceros*). Most of the carcasses were already a few days old when discovered, and were in an advanced stage of putrefaction or had already been fed on by vultures and other scavengers, leaving only a mummified skeleton covered by dried skin. A fresh zebra carcass was found and necropsy demonstrated acute hepatic swelling, with mottled orange and brown discoloration, petechiation, icterus, and acute pulmonary edema on macropathology (Fig. 14-2). A diffuse hepatic necrosis, compatible with a diagnosis of cyanobacterial poisoning, was reported on histopathology. Water samples from the dams were tested by means of a diagnostic mouse bioassay, with follow-up histopathology on the mouse organs, and confirmed the presence of microcystin toxins.

In June 2007, a second cluster of mortalities was reported in the same region of the Kruger National Park, during similar climatic conditions and, once again, white rhinoceroses, zebras, and wildebeest were overrepresented in the carcass count (22 carcasses).[8,13] On necropsy, a pregnant zebra showed a typical mottled coppery orange and brown friable liver, with rounded edges with subcapsular petechiation; the fetal liver was similar in appearance, suggesting that the cyanobacterial toxin crossed the placental barrier. There was blood-tinged fluid in the abdominal cavity and severe

pulmonary edema. Hemorrhages were present in the subcutaneous tissues, fascial planes and serosal surfaces. A mediastinal hematoma was present, and there were diffuse sub-endocardial ecchymoses.[1] Histopathology confirmed that death was caused by liver and respiratory failure. The gross pathology findings in a young adult white rhinoceros bull were similar (Fig. 14-3A). The liver was enlarged, with rounded edges, extremely friable, and dark reddish brown in color. The parenchyma was jelly-like in consistency, with apparent loss of structure (see Fig. 14-3B). The lungs were moist, with areas of hemorrhage and areas of atelectasis. There were numerous hemorrhages affecting serosal surfaces throughout the body and severe hemorrhaging in large areas of the subepicardial and endocardial tissues of both ventricles (see Fig. 14-3C). Histopathology indicated extensive disruption of the hepatic architecture caused by a massive hepatocyte necrosis, resulting in acute liver failure.[5] The average water surface temperature for both these events ranged from 19° C to 21° C, and both events occurred in the fall and early winter. It is interesting to speculate why certain species, including elephants (*Loxodonta africana*), buffalo (*Syncerus caffer*), and hippopotami were underrepresented in the carcass counts although they also frequented the affected dams. Some possibilities are that they are more resistant to the microcystin toxins, they wade out past the scum line and drink water that is not as heavily loaded with organisms as water at the edges, or avoid drinking from the leeward side of the dams, where rafting of the algae scum occurs following windy periods.[1] White rhino rhinoceruses, zebras, and wildebeest are not wading species and generally approach their water points from the downwind side.

CONTROL OF CYANOBACTERIAL BLOOMS

The control of cyanobacteria blooms on natural water bodies frequented by wildlife may be challenging. Treatment of large water bodies is often expensive and impractical. Application of chemical controls resulting in cell lysis may release large amounts of toxin into the water, making it unsuitable for consumption for 2 to 3 weeks before biodegradation commences.[11] Frequently, it is not possible to control the various environmental factors (e.g., water temperature, pH, eutrophication) promoting the bloom formation. Most commonly used algicides are copper sulfate, diquat (Reglone A, JR Johnson Supply, Roseville, Minn), simazine aluminum

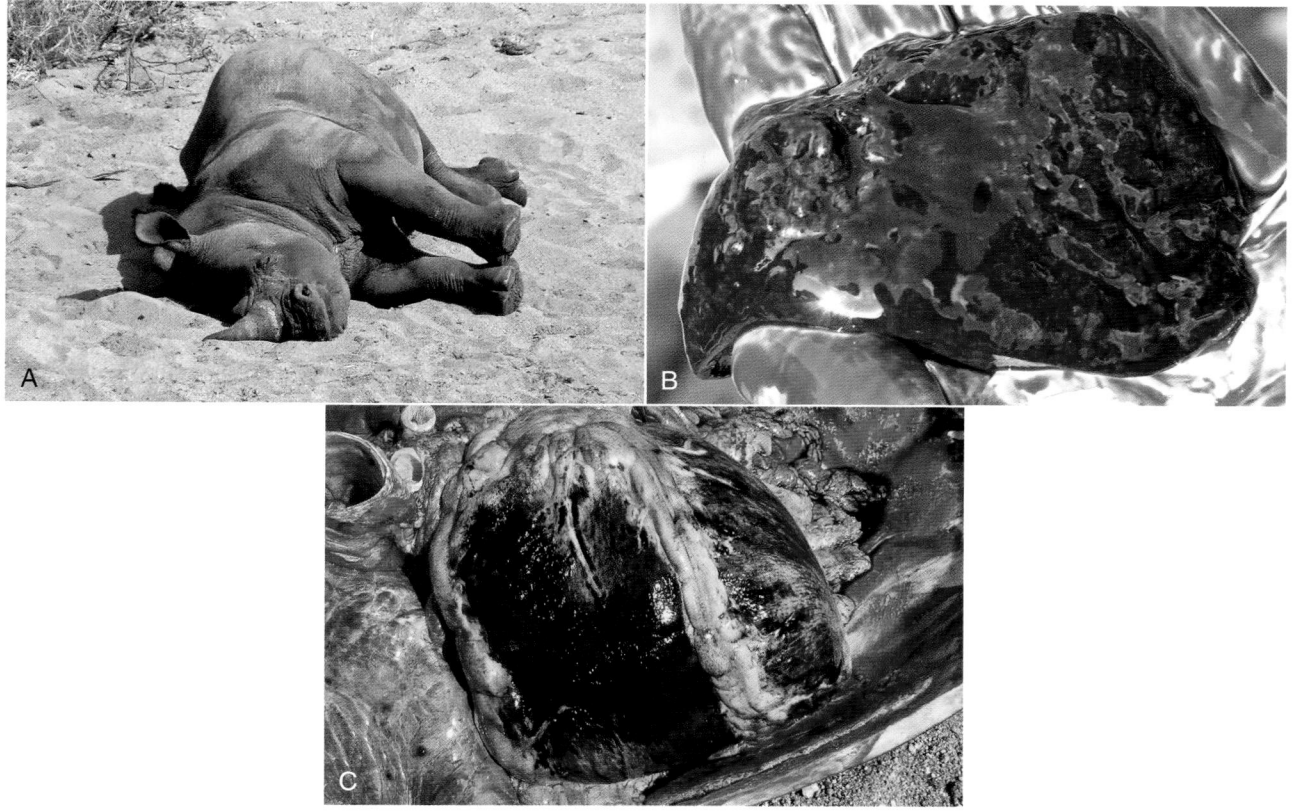

Figure 14-3

A, Subadult male white rhinoceros shortly after it died from the hepatotoxic effects of mycrocystin. **B,** Severe disruption of the normal hepatic architecture, jelly-like in consistency. **C,** Severe hemorrhaging into the subepicardial tissues of both ventricles.

sulfate (alum), and lime. Alum and lime remove phosphorus from the water. The other chemicals disrupt cell functions, including new cell wall synthesis, photosynthesis, and other enzymatic reactions.[15] Copper is reported to be an effective algicide in natural waters for the control of cyanobacteria. Copper concentrations required to decrease growth rates or cause cell death depend on cyanobacteria concentrations. The resulting cell lysis releases intracellular toxins into the surrounding water, making it hazardous for use by animals. This problem also occurs with the use of diquat and simazine and, to a lesser degree, with the use of lime.

It must be appreciated that it is difficult to fence off water bodies temporarily in African multispecies systems that support large populations of ungulates and pachyderms. Both alum and lime cause coagulation of the cyanobacteria, resulting in flocculation, and represent a more favorable method of control because of minimal toxin release in farm dams or lakes, but in situations in which hippopotami are present, their activities will stir up and reactivate the sludge.[15] Decomposing barley

straw or hay has been reported to be effective in reducing the growth of cyanobacteria. Chemicals released during the decomposition are suspected to result in an inhibitory effect.[11] Several bacterial agents causing lysis of cyanobacteria have been isolated and characterized but have only been tested on laboratory-cultured cyanobacteria. Studies on the application of biocontrol agents are limited. Before bacterial biocontrol agents are applied to freshwater systems, information must be available on the antialgal activity against target species, the effects on other organisms in the system, and the prediction of algal dynamics after removal of target algae. *Bacillus cereus* in floating biodegradable plastic carriers was an effective in situ control of natural floating *Microcystis* blooms, eliminating 99% of floating cyanobacteria in 4 days. Reducing phosphorus concentration as a means of eutrophication management has been proposed as a possible method of control. This is easier to achieve than reducing nitrogen levels because there is no atmospheric source of phosphorus that is bioavailable. Significantly less phosphorus than nitrogen needs to be removed to have an equivalent reduction in cyanobacteria growth. The chemical removal of phosphorus has been tried with various agents, including alum, ferric salts, ferric aluminium sulphate, clay particles, and lime, with limited degrees of success. Some of these substances will rerelease phosphorus under certain conditions of pH and anoxia, whereas others are toxic. Lanthanum, a rare earth element, incorporated with bentonite to overcome its potential toxicity, has experimentally shown promise in reducing phosphorus levels in the water body and sediment, without affecting pH and nitrate concentrations. This has resulted in reduced cyanobacterial growth and prevented onset of an algal bloom.

The use of floating booms or curtain devices may effectively prevent rafted cyanobacteria from reaching the shoreline and has been successfully used in small farm dams. This technique, however, is doomed to failure with large hippopotamus and crocodile populations living in the water body and large wading pachyderms, such as elephants, visiting the water body for drinking purposes.[1]

CONCLUSION

Cyanobacteria present a potential toxic threat to vertebrate species that use natural water sources for drinking. Eutrophication and water temperature, along with other factors, play an important role in determining algal blooms. Cyanobacterial toxicity should be included in the differential diagnosis of mass mortalities in wildlife associated with natural water bodies. In conservation areas with free-ranging wildlife, the only long-term solution to regular cyanobacterial events may be to improve the flow and flushing of the aquatic system, address the source of eutrophication, or drain the impoundment and physically remove the accumulated nutrient-rich organic sludge.

REFERENCES

1. Bengis RG, Govender D, Keet DF: Multi-species mortality events related to cyanobacteroial bio-intoxication in the Kruger National Park. In Proceedings of the 4th Veterinary and Paraveterinary Congress, South Africa, 7–11 July, 2008, Sun City.
2. Cyanosite: Cyanobacterial toxins, 2010 (http://www-cyanosite.bio.purdue.edu/cyanotox/toxiccyanos.html).
3. Gous T: Cyanobacterial (blue-green algal) poisoning of livestock with special reference to South Africa. Elsenburg J 1:17–27, 1999.
4. Ibelings BW, Bruning K, De Jonge J, et al: Distribution of microcystins in a lake foodweb: No evidence for biomagnification. Microb Ecol 49:487–500, 2004.
5. Lane E: Personal communication, 2010.
6. Lugomela C, Pratap HB, Mgaya YD: Cyanobacteria blooms—a possible cause of mass mortality of lesser flamingos in Lake Manyara and Lake Big Momela, Tanzania. Harmful Algae 5:534–541, 2006.
7. Malbrouck C, Kestemont P: Effects of microcystins on fish. Environ Toxicol Chem 25:72–86, 2006.
8. Masango MG, Myburgh JG, Labuschagne L, et al: Assessment of *Microcystis* bloom toxicity associated with wildlife mortality in the Kruger National Park, South Africa. J Wildl Dis 46:95–102, 2010.
9. McCarthy T, Rubridge B: The Story Of Earth and Life: A Southern African Perspective on a 4.6-Billion-Year Journey. Cape Town, 2005, Struik Publishers.
10. Msagati TAM, Siame BA, Shushu DD: Evaluation of methods for the isolation, detection and quantification of cyanobacterial hepatotoxins. Aquat Toxicol 78:382–397, 2006.
11. Oberholster PJ, Botha A-M, Grobbelaar JU: *Microcystis aeruginosa:* Source of toxic microcystins in drinking water. Afr J Biotechnol 3:159–168, 2004.
12. Oberholster PJ, Botha A-M, Muller K, et al: Assessment of the genetic diversity of geographically unrelated *Microcystis aeruginosa* strains using amplified fragment length polymorphisms (AFLPs). Afr J Biotechnol 4:389–399, 2005.
13. Oberholster PJ, Botha A-M, Myburgh J: Linking climate change and progressive eutrophication to incidents of clustered animal mortalities in different geographical regions of South Africa. Afr J Biotechnol 8:5825–5832, 2009.
14. Paerl HW, Huisman J: Blooms like it hot. Science 320:57–58, 2008.
15. Pocock G: Phosphorus limitation as a method of cyanobacterial bloom control, PhD thesis, Pretoria, 2008, University of Pretoria (http://upetd.up.ac.za/thesis/available/etd-05302009-120841).
16. Rodas VL, Costas E: Preference of mice to consume *Microcystis aeruginosa* (toxin-producing cyanobacteria): A possible explanation for numerous fatalities of livestock and wildlife. Res Vet Sci 67:107–110, 1999.
17. Van Halderen A, Harding WR, Wessels JC, et al: Cyanobacteria (blue-green algae) poisoning of livestock in the Western Cape Province of South Africa. J S Afr Vet Assoc 66:260–264, 1995.
18. Wiegand C, Pflugmacher S: Ecotoxicological effects of selected cyanobacterial secondary metabolites: A short review. Toxicol Appl Pharmacol 203:201–218, 2005.

CHAPTER 15

Children's Zoo Medicine: Zoonoses

Stephanie B. James

This chapter is a general overview of common zoonotic diseases, diseases that may be transmitted from animal to human that are seen in children's zoo and education animals. Although zoonotic disease is a concern for all areas of the zoo, it is most worrisome in areas in which the public has direct contact with the collection animals. The Association of Zoo and Aquariums has guidelines regarding the risk of disease transmission in animal contact areas developed over 10 years ago that still apply today.[4] Topics discussed in this chapter are the responsibilities of the zoo veterinarian, general zoonotic disease transmission and prevention, and the most common zoonotic diseases found in children's zoo and education animals, including discussion of the clinical signs, diagnostic modalities, and the means or mode of disease transmission. The material in this chapter should be regarded as a general overview of those diseases; the reader is encouraged to contact further sources for additional details and treatment options. The diseases presented in this chapter should in no way be considered the only diseases of concern because new zoonotic diseases and modes of transmission are continually being discovered.

RESPONSIBILITIES OF THE ZOO VETERINARIAN

The responsibilities of the zoo veterinarian as they relate to zoonotic diseases are varied. He or she needs to diagnose, prevent, and treat, where indicated, zoonotic diseases in animals, thereby minimizing the transmission of these diseases to people. The zoo veterinarian is required to know which zoonotic diseases require reporting in their state and which regulatory authorities need to be informed. He or she is responsible for educating the zoo staff, including volunteers, part-time and full-time keepers, and managers, with special emphasis toward those who work with the animals in question. The zoo veterinarian should also be involved in exhibit and hand washing station design, and have input into the development of signage for contact animal areas. All these considerations will help decrease zoonotic disease transmission to the zoo visitor.

It is important for zoo veterinarians to develop a relationship with their U.S. Department of Agriculture (USDA) veterinarian and with local public health officials and resources, because at some time there will be concern that the animals at the zoo caused a disease in the zoo visitor and a good relationship with regulatory officials is beneficial when these situations arise.

ZOONOTIC DISEASE TRANSMISSION AND PREVENTION

First, and most important, sick animals should be removed from exhibit or taken off education programs. As a result, an ill animal is usually not the source of zoonotic disease because they are usually not exposed to the public. Thus, removal of the animal is a necessary but not sufficient enough step to prevent the transmission of disease. The difficulty for the veterinarian lies in the prevention of disease transmission from asymptomatic animals.

Transmission of zoonotic organisms from animal to person may occur through direct or indirect contact. Direct transmission includes contact with an animal's mouth, saliva, contaminated coat, or feces. Indirect transmission includes contact with a contaminated environment, water, or food sources. Transmission may occur through ingestion, referred to throughout this chapter as fecal-oral, or through aerosol or skin contact.[16]

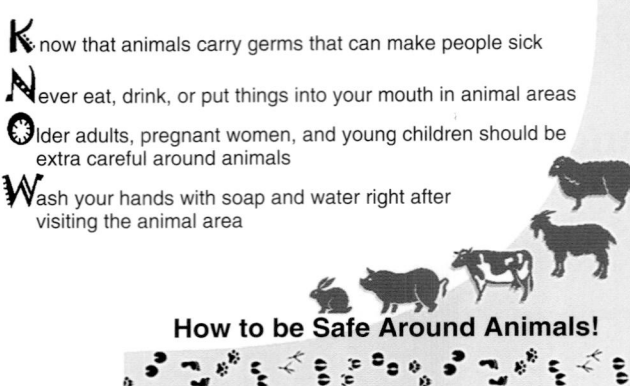

Know that animals carry germs that can make people sick

Never eat, drink, or put things into your mouth in animal areas

Older adults, pregnant women, and young children should be extra careful around animals

Wash your hands with soap and water right after visiting the animal area

How to be Safe Around Animals!

Figure 15-1

Educational poster for contact animal exhibits. *(Centers for Disease Control and Prevention: MMWR 58 (RR-5): 1-21, 2009, http://www.nasphv.org/Documents/AnimalsInPublicSettings. pdf).*

Directions for Washing Hands

HOW

- Wet hands with running water
- Place soap into palms
- Rub together to make a lather
- Scrub hands vigorously for 20 seconds
- Rinse soap off hands
- Dry hands with disposable paper towels, not on clothing

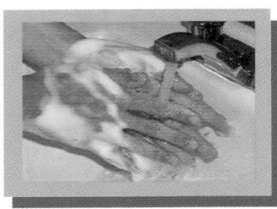

WHEN

After going to the toilet

Upon exiting animal areas

Before eating

Before preparing foods

After removing soiled clothes or shoes

Figure 15-2

Hand washing poster for contact animal exhibits. *(Centers for Disease Control and Prevention: MMWR 58 (RR-5): 1-21, 2009, http://www.nasphv.org/Documents/AnimalsInPublicSettings. pdf).*

In animals, zoonotic organisms may be carried asymptomatically, making it impossible to determine when the animal is infected and infective. Zoonotic organisms may only be shed intermittently in the feces or through respiratory secretions, making it difficult to diagnose infectivity, and it may be impossible to clear animals of zoonotic organisms. Therefore, prevention of zoonotic disease transmission to the public is of utmost importance. The cornerstones of prevention are education of the staff and public, appropriate hand hygiene facilities (hand washing and hand sanitizer stations), appropriate exhibit design, and clear signage (Figs. 15-1 and 15-2). A retrospective study of hygiene and zoonotic disease transmission[1] has found that hand hygiene education is the most important factor in the prevention of disease transmission. The study showed that nonantibacterial soap is more protective than antibacterial soap and that benzylalkonium chloride–based hand sanitizers are more protective than alcohol-based hand sanitizers for the prevention of respiratory disease. Therefore, the recommendation to wash hands immediately after leaving an animal exhibit is the most important step to reduce and prevent disease transmission.[17]

Prevention of zoonotic disease transmission is the same for all diseases discussed in this chapter and, as noted, is of the utmost importance for public health. Education of staff and public, hand washing and hand sanitizer use immediately after contacting the animal, signage, and exhibit design (including exhibits away from food sources, appropriate individual drainage systems, and one-way traffic flow) are the basic preventive principles that apply throughout this chapter.

RUMINANTS

Bacterial Diseases

Enteric Bacterial Disease

This group of animals is usually asymptomatic carriers of enteric bacterial pathogens and will shed these organisms intermittently, contaminating the environment.[16] At this time, laboratory testing is limited and culturing fecal specimens in an attempt to identify, screen, and remove infected asymptomatic animals may reduce the risk of transmission but cannot eliminate it. Antimicrobial treatment also does not eliminate the infection, does not prevent shedding, and cannot protect against reinfection; it may even prolong shedding and contribute to antimicrobial resistance.

Escherichia coli *O157:H7 Infection*

E. coli is a gram-negative, motile or nonmotile, facultatively anaerobic bacillus of the family Enterobacteriaceae. This discussion will focus on the enterohemorrhagic *E. coli* O157:H7, which is most commonly a food-borne pathogen but has been observed in petting zoos and farms. *E. coli* O157:H7 is part of the normal flora of ruminant livestock,[6] with cattle being a major source of infection but sheep, goats, deer, and New World camelids are also asymptomatic carriers. Clinical signs are usually inapparent in adults and only rarely are clinical signs associated with disease in neonatal calves.[21] The organism is shed in the feces, with shedding higher in the summer months, leading to more outbreaks from May to November. Any change in feed, feeding practice, or any stress that disturbs the normal intestinal flora could promote transient colonization with *E. coli* O157:H7, resulting in increased shedding. Diagnosis is difficult because the organism is part of the normal intestinal microflora and because fecal shedding is transient and intermittent. Transmission occurs via the fecal-oral route (e.g., contact with manure-contaminated hair coats, contact with environmental structures contaminated with feces).

Salmonella *Infection*

Salmonella spp. is a gram-negative, motile, facultatively anaerobic bacteria of the Enterobacteriaceae family. Clinical signs in children's zoo ruminants range from asymptomatic carriers in adults to diarrhea and sepsis in kids, lambs, fawns, and calves. *Salmonella* spp. may also cause abortions, especially in sheep and goats, but does not appear to be a major problem in New World camelids.[8] Ruminants may be latent carriers—bacteria lodge in the lymph nodes or tonsils so that the organism is not shed in the feces—or they may be passive carriers and shed *Salmonella* spp. intermittently in the feces, contaminating the environment. Latent carriers may become active shedders during times of stress.[20] Diagnosis in ill animals is via fecal culture but it may not be possible to identify asymptomatic carriers. Transmission is via the fecal-oral route, similar to *E. coli*.

Campylobacter *Infection*

Campylobacter jejuni and *C. fetus* are curved, non–spore-forming, gram-negative, microaerophilic bacteria. *C. jejuni* is carried asymptomatically in ruminants and *C. fetus* is the most significant cause of abortion in sheep. Clinical signs in sheep include late-term abortions, stillbirths, and weak lambs. Ewes abort and then become immune but some may become persistently infected and shed the organism in feces. Diagnosis from ewes is by culture of the organism from placenta, fetal abomasal contents, and maternal vaginal discharge. Diagnosis of *C. jejuni* is through fecal culture but the organism maybe a normal inhabitant and be shed intermittently. Transmission to humans is through handling aborted fetuses or fecal-oral.[15]

Nonenteric Bacteria of Zoonotic Concern

The following bacterial diseases are of zoonotic concern or have the potential for zoonotic transmission. Overall, these are not as problematic for the veterinarian and are not as much a concern for disease transmission as the enteric diseases.

Tuberculosis

Tuberculosis is a term that encompasses various diseases caused by bacteria of the *Mycobacterium tuberculosis* complex, including *M. tuberculosis*, *M. bovis*, and *M. africanum*, with *M. bovis* being the most common cause of human tuberculosis attributable to animals.[12] All ruminants are susceptible to mycobacterial diseases and New World camelids appear to be very susceptible.[8] Animals may be asymptomatic for long periods before clinical signs of enlarged lymph nodes, wasting, or emaciation become apparent. Diagnosis is via acid-fast staining of tissues, tissue culture, and the tuberculin skin test. The intradermal skin test may not be effective or practical for use in all species, but has been accepted by the USDA for identification of *M. bovis* in cattle, bison, goats, and captive cervids. Other diagnostic methods rely on the cellular immune response and are performed in vitro (e.g., lymphocyte blastogenic assays or interferon gamma tests), with results comparable to those obtained with intradermal tests. Mycobacterial culture is still considered to be the gold standard diagnostic test. Transmission of the disease is via aerosol or ingestion but may be spread through the contamination of cuts and abrasions. Mycobacteria are viable for several months in feces or in animal carcasses.

Q Fever

The causative agent of Q fever is *Coxiella burnetii*, a gram-negative coccobacillus. Clinical signs in cattle, sheep, and goats range from asymptomatic carriers to animals with mild fevers and abortion. Diagnosis is based on placental findings, serology, and isolation of the organism. Transmission is via inhalation, handling contaminated animals, and contact with contaminated body fluids.[14] This organism is mostly problematic for institutions with indoor birthing exhibits.

Other Nonenteric Bacteria

The following organisms have the ability to cause disease in humans but the risk of transmission from animals is low. *Leptospira interrogans* and its serovars infect cattle, sheep, goats, deer, and New World camelids. Clinical signs range from asymptomatic to abortions, anorexia, and sepsis (especially in neonates), with signs of intravascular hemolysis. Diagnosis may be made by changes in laboratory values (e.g., anemia, hyperbilirubinemia, hemoglobinuria, hemoglobinemia), identifying spirochetes on dark field microscopy of urine or plasma, or rising antibody titers. Transmission occurs by contact with infected urine, aborted tissues, contaminated ponds and water sources, and other body fluids.[15] *Listeria monocytogenes* occurs equally in sheep, goat, cattle, and New World camelids. Clinical signs include depression and anorexia, which progress to more complex neurologic signs, including facial and vestibular lesions. There are no specific diagnostic tests. *Listeria* may be shed by sick, recovering, or clinically normal animals in milk and feces for long periods.[8] This is usually a food-borne pathogen but may be transmitted through the fecal-oral route. Brucellosis is caused by *Brucella melitensis* in goats and sheep and *B. abortus* in cattle. It is not considered a major disease of New World camelids but is a problem in reindeer. Abortion is the most common clinical sign but ruminants may also present with mastitis, lameness, and/or orchitis.[9] Diagnosis is made primarily by serology. Transmission is via contact with infected materials through breaks in the skin, ingestion, or inhalation. *Chlamydophila psittaci* is found in sheep, goats, and cattle and may cause abortion, pneumonia, keratoconjunctivitis, epididymitis, and polyarthritis.[7] Diagnosis is through culture of the organism and serology. Transmission is fecal-oral or through contact with infected placentas, but the mammalian forms of *Chlamydiophila* do not appear to be as zoonotic as avian strains.

Viral Diseases

Rabies

Rabies, a lyssavirus, may infect all mammals. Ruminants and New World camelids display a variety of clinical signs, including depression, anorexia, nystagmus, muscle tremors, lameness, ataxia, and posterior paresis. These animals rarely exhibit the aggressive forms of rabies and the disease will usually progress as an ascending paralysis. Fortunately, New World camelids are not able to spit when suffering from rabies.[8] Diagnosis is via direct fluorescent antibody testing on the brain of a suspect case. Rabies always needs to be included on a rule-out list in an animal with neurologic signs. Transmission to people is via a bite or saliva from infected

animals that gets into an open wound.[16] All animals demonstrating neurologic signs should immediately be removed from animal contact areas.

Orf: Contagious Pustular Dermatitis, Sore Mouth, Contagious Ecthyma

Orf is caused by a parapoxvirus and is found in sheep, goats, New World camelids, and reindeer.[3,8] Clinical signs include proliferative crusting lesions usually involving the mucocutaneous junctions of the nose and mouth but may also occur on the feet, teats, and genitalia. These lesions may persist for months but are usually self-limiting. Diagnosis is by physical examination and histopathologic identification of the virus in tissues. The virus is hardy in the environment and in scabs. Transmission is via direct contact with an infected animal, a recently vaccinated animal, or through the environment. It should be noted that a nonattenuated, live virus vaccine that has been developed to create a controlled flock outbreak may cause clinical disease in humans if there is accidental exposure to the lesions of a vaccinated animal.

Fungal Diseases

Dermatophytosis: Ringworm, Lumpy Wool, Club Lamb Fungus

Dermatophytosis caused by *Trichophyton verrucosum, T. gypseum, T. mentagrophytes,* or *Microsporum canis* may be found in all ruminants and New World camelids in children's zoos. Animals may be asymptomatic carriers or display clinical signs of the typical circular lesions of alopecia on the face and ears, with or without pruritis. Diagnosis is via Wood's lamp, skin, and hair cultures. Microscopic examination of hairs taken from the periphery of the lesion and prepared with 10% KOH solution is a quick diagnostic test that may be done on site. Transmission is through direct or indirect contact, because organisms remain viable in crusts and hairs for years in the environment.[3]

Parasitic Diseases

Cryptosporidiosis

Cryptosporidium parvum, a protozoal parasite, may be carried asymptomatically in adult ruminants and New World camelids and may cause diarrhea in young animals. Diagnosis is by fecal examination but asymptomatic animals will shed the organism intermittently, making diagnosis difficult. The organism may be persistent in the environment. Transmission is fecal-oral.[13]

See Chapter 73 for further information regarding this zoonotic disease.

Giardiasis

Giardia is a protozoal parasite that is commonly seen in 2- to 4-week-old sheep and goats. Clinical signs include a self-limiting transient diarrhea but animals may shed cysts for long periods. Diagnosis is via fecal examination. Transmission is via the fecal-oral route.

EQUIDS

Equids do not appear to be a major source of zoonotic disease for the zoo visitor. Preventive measures previously discussed should still be followed when interacting with these animals.

RABBITS

Bacterial Disease

Pasteurella multocida Infection

Pasteurella multocida, a gram-negative, nonmotile coccobacillus, causes snuffles in rabbits and may be considered a zoonotic disease. Clinical signs include purulent nasal discharge, coughing, and sneezing. Diagnosis is by deep nasal cultures, polymerase chain reaction (PCR) assay, and paired serology. Transmission is via aerosol or fomites.[24] Veterinarians should be aware of the zoonotic potential of this disease, but any sick rabbit should not be used in programs.

Salmonella Infection

Salmonella spp. is not common in rabbits and may cause high morbidity and mortality. Animals usually become septic and die quickly. Transmission is via the fecal-oral route.

Viral Diseases

Rabies

Rabbits may carry rabies but should not be housed in an area where they are in contact with wild mammals. Clinical signs include depression, weakness, and paralysis.[24] Diagnosis and transmission are as described for ruminants.

Fungal Diseases

Ringworm

Ringworm caused by *Trichophyton mentagrophytes* and *Microsporum canis* infects rabbits. Clinical signs include crusty dry lesions that may or may not be pruritic. Diagnosis is via skin scrape and KOH preparation[24] and culture. Transmission is through contact with the infected animal.

Parasitic Diseases

Encephalitozoon cuniculi Infection

Encephalitozoon cuniculi is an intracellular protozoal parasite that affects rabbits in multiple ways. Clinical signs depend on the involvement of specific organ systems. If the nervous system is affected, animals will present with signs relating to the central nervous system such as ataxia, head tilt, or vestibular signs.[24] If the protozoa affects the kidneys, animals are generally asymptomatic because renal function is not usually impaired, and ocular infection may result in uveitis and cataracts. Diagnosis is by physical examination, complete blood count, serum biochemistry, and serology. Transmission to people is via contaminated urine but organisms may be shed intermittently and the protozoa is long-lived (up to 1 month) in the environment.

Ectoparasite Infection

Cheyletiella parasitovorax is a nonburrowing mite found on rabbits. The clinical signs include pruritis, large flakes of white scales, alopecia, and oily dermatitis.[24] Diagnosis is via skin scrape. Transmission is through direct contact.

RODENTS: MICE, RATS, HAMSTERS, GERBILS

Bacterial Diseases

Salmonella Infection

Salmonella enteriditis and S. typhimurium are the most common Salmonella serotypes recovered from rodents and one of the most important zoonosis in gerbils. Animals may be asymptomatic or show signs of anorexia, weight loss, enteritis, lymphadenopathy, or septicemia. Transmission is direct (fecal-oral).[10,17]

Viral Diseases

Lymphocytic choriomeningitis virus, an arenavirus, may be carried by rodents. Rodents may be asymptomatic or show signs of weight loss, tremors, convulsions, or photophobia. Diagnosis is via serology. Transmission is through exposure to contaminated feces or urine or through a bite.[17] All rodents are susceptible to rabies but should not be maintained in an area in which they are in contact with wild animals.[10]

Fungal Diseases

Fungal diseases of rodents are rare but animals may be infected with *Trichophyton* and *Microsporum* spp., with clinical signs ranging from none to typical signs of ringworm, including pruritis and areas of scaly alopecia.[10] Diagnosis is via skin scrape and KOH preparation, culture, and Wood's lamp. Transmission is through direct contact or contact with fomites.

Parasitic Diseases

Cryptosporidium parvum is rare in rodents but because this parasite is not host-specific, rodents may be infected. Diagnosis is via fecal examination and transmission is via the fecal-oral route.[10] *Giardia* spp. (e.g., *Giardia lamblia, G. mesocricetus, G. muris*) infect the hamster and gerbil and animals may be asymptomatic or present with diarrhea. Diagnosis is via fecal examination and the organism may be transmitted to humans via the fecal-oral route. Hymenolepiasis is caused by the cestode *Hymenolepis nana* or *H. diminuta*. Clinical signs are usually not apparent and diagnosis is via fecal samples. Transmission is via the fecal-oral route.

Other Zoonotic Diseases in Rodents

Other zoonotic diseases in rodents are of minor significance and include but are not limited to *Acinetobacter* spp., dermatophytosis,[10] *Streptobacillus moniliformis, Spirillum minus*, the cause of rat bite fever, *Streptococcus pneumonia, Leptospira interrogans*, and hantavirus. *Yersinia pestis*, the causative agent of plague, is not a clinical disease observed in zoos but is problematic in wild rodents.[17]

Allergic reactions to the dander and urine of rodents is always possible[10] and, although not a zoonotic disease per se, must be kept in mind when the public is working with and handling rodents.

HEDGEHOGS
Bacterial Diseases

Salmonella serotype Tilene is a pathogen of hedgehogs. Clinical signs include anorexia, diarrhea, and weight loss but hedgehogs may also be asymptomatic carriers. Diagnosis is through fecal culture. Transmission occurs via direct and indirect contact.[19] Hedgehogs may also carry *Salmonella typhimurium, S. enteriditis, Yersinia pseudotuberculosis, Y. pestis, Mycobacterium marinum*, or *M. avium intracellulare* but these are not major sources of zoonotic disease. Antibodies to *Coxiella burnetii, Chlamydophila* spp., and *Leptospira* spp. have also been isolated from hedgehogs.

Viral Diseases

There are not many viral diseases of hedgehogs. They are susceptible to rabies[19] and a human herpesvirus was confirmed in a single African pygmy hedgehog with clinical signs of acute posterior paresis. It is unclear at this time if this is a zoonotic disease in hedgehogs.

Fungal Diseases

Dermatophytosis caused by *Trichophyton mentagrophytes* var. *erinacei* and *Microsporum* spp., may be carried asymptomatically, or may cause a nonpruritic, dry, scaly skin with bald patches and spine loss. Diagnosis is as described earlier. Transmission is via direct contact.[19]

Parasitic Diseases

Cryptosporidiosis has been diagnosed in a juvenile hedgehog.[19] Its zoonotic potential is unknown.

CHINCHILLAS

Overall, chinchillas represent a low zoonotic risk.[18] Diseases of concern include *E. coli, Salmonella* spp., dermatophyte, and protozoal infections (e.g., *Giardia* spp., *Cryptosporidium parvum*), all of which have the potential to be transmitted to humans.

FERRETS

Ferrets may carry, both symptomatically and asymptomatically, numerous diseases that are considered zoonotic. Transmission of disease from the ferret to people, however, has only been documented for a few organisms (e.g., orthomyxoviruses).

Ferrets may be infected with *Salmonella* spp., *Listeria* spp., *Mycobacterium* spp., *Leptospira* spp., *Campylobacter* spp., rabies, *Microsporum canis, Trichophyton gypseum, Giardia* spp., *Cryptosporidium parvum*, and/or scabies (*Sarcoptes scabiei*),[25] all of which are potential zoonotic diseases. Influenza A and B, orthomyxoviruses, cause respiratory disease in ferrets similar to that in humans. Diagnosis is via an enzyme-linked immunosorbent assay (ELISA) for rapid diagnosis. Transmission between ferret and people is through aerosolization and the disease is usually diagnosed in the ferret after the owner has been ill.

BIRDS

Bacterial Diseases

Chlamydophila Infection

Chlamydophila psittaci, an obligate intracellular bacteria, has been isolated from approximately 100 bird species and is most commonly identified in psittacines but may be found with some regularity in pigeons, canaries, and finches.[22] Clinical signs in birds are not easily distinguishable from other systemic illnesses and include lethargy, anorexia, ruffled feathers, serous or mucopurulent ocular or nasal discharge, diarrhea, and the production of green to yellow-green urates. Some birds may be asymptomatic and shed the organism intermittently in the feces and nasal secretions. Shedding may be activated by stress factors, including relocation, shipping, crowding, chilling, and breeding. Diagnosis is via culture of clinical specimens, detection of antigen with immunofluorescence, paired serology, or identification of Chlamydiaceae in macrophages or through ELISA, PCR, or fluorescent antibody tests on feces, cloacal swabs, or respiratory tract and ocular exudates. Transmission is usually by inhalation of dried feces or respiratory secretions of infected birds, nose to beak contact, and handling infected feathers and tissues.

Salmonella Infection

Salmonella spp. may colonize the gastrointestinal tract of birds. Several serotypes are found in birds with *S. gallinarum*, *S. pullorum*, and *S. typhimurium* found in galliformes and *S. typhimurium* infecting wild and pet birds. Birds with *Salmonella* may be symptomatic or asymptomatic and the organism is shed in the feces. Diagnosis in birds, as in mammals, is via fecal culture.[5] Transmission is via the fecal-oral route.

Campylobacter Infection

Campylobacter jejuni infects poultry and wild and pet birds. Clinical signs include lethargy, anorexia, weight loss, and yellow diarrhea. Healthy birds of many species, particularly poultry, have a high rate of intestinal infection and may shed the organism in the feces.[5] Diagnosis is through fecal culture. Transmission is via the fecal-oral route.

Yersinia Infection

Yersinia pseudotuberculosis and *Y. enterocolitica* are gram-negative coccobacilli belonging to the Enterobacteriaceae family. These pathogens are of much greater importance in birds than mammals, with *Y. pseudotuberculosis* more prevalent than *Y. enterocolitica*. Canaries and toucans appear more susceptible to these organisms than other species.[5] Clinical signs are nonspecific but include peracute mortality. Diagnosis is via necropsy findings and cultures of the liver and spleen, and transmission is via the fecal-oral route.

Other Bacterial Diseases of Minor Zoonotic Importance

Pasturella multocida, *Erysipelothrix rhusiopathiae*, *Coxiella brunetii*, *E. coli*, and *Listeria monocytogenes*[5] are all found in birds put present a low zoonotic risk. Mycobacteriosis, consisting of *Mycobacterium avium*, *M. intracellulare*, and *M. scrofulaceum*, has been reported in all types of birds and is not considered a major zoonotic pathogen.

Viral Diseases

Influenza

Influenza viruses are orthomyxoviruses and consist of three types, categorized as A, B, and C. Type A, the most important zoonotic agents, have been associated with recent widespread epidemics and pandemics,[5] and all subtypes of influenza A virus (e.g., H5N1, H7N7, H9N2) may be isolated from captive birds, along with waterfowl and migrating birds. Clinical signs in birds range from asymptomatic to multisystemic disease.[2] Diagnosis is through serologic testing and virus isolation from tracheal swabs, cloacal swabs, and fecal samples. Infected birds may shed the virus in respiratory secretions, conjunctiva, and feces and transmission is through inhalation and from environmental sources.

Newcastle Disease

Newcastle disease, avian paramyxovirus 1, is very prevalent in poultry, ostriches, and pigeons. Psittacines also appear to be highly susceptible to the virus.[5] Clinical signs range from none to respiratory disease, green diarrhea, muscle tremors, circling, paralysis, and swelling of tissues of the neck and eyes. Diagnosis is via serology and necropsy. Transmission is via the fecal-oral route or via aerosolization.

Fungal Diseases

Histoplasmosis

Histoplasma capsulatum, although not a clinical problem in birds, is found in soil enriched with avian feces in the Ohio and Mississippi valleys. The organism is transmitted by the inhalation of airborne spores from the soil. Birds are mechanical vectors, transporting the fungi from place to place.[5]

Cryptococcosis

Cryptococcus neoformans is also not a disease of birds, but is commonly found in soil contaminated with pigeon feces, especially under roosting sites. Transmission is via inhalation of the spores and less commonly by direct contact with the skin. Prevention of the disease should include limiting exposure to areas contaminated with pigeon feces.[5]

Parasitic Diseases

In general, parasitic diseases in birds present a very low zoonotic risk. *Ornithonyssus* spp. and *Dermanyssus* spp. are both mites found on birds that may cause pruritis and anemia. Mites are large enough to be seen on the bird and transmission is via contact with an infected animal. *Cryptosporidium* spp. has been found in birds but there have been no reports of avian cryptosporidiosis infecting man. Birds are usually asymptomatic and fecal shedding is probably low.[5] *Giardia* spp. may infect birds asymptomatically or with signs related to enteritis. They have been found in numerous species but there is no documentation of transmission from birds to humans.

REPTILES

Bacterial Diseases

Salmonella Infection

Salmonella spp. are common in reptiles and animals are usually asymptomatic. Fecal shedding of the organism is intermittent, making diagnosis via repeated fecal, cloacal, and water samples useful but not conclusive in identifying carriers. Transmission is via the fecal-oral route.[11]

Aeromonas Infection

Aeromonas spp., a gram-negative bacteria found in fish, frogs, and reptiles, has been cultured from clinically healthy reptiles. Diagnosis is through culture of the mouth or feces. Transmission may occur by direct contact (water in open wounds, injuries, or from bites or scratches inflicted by the reptile living in a contaminated environment)[11] or via the fecal-oral route.

Mycobacterium Infection

Mycobacterium marinum, M. avium, and *M. tuberculosis* have all been diagnosed in reptiles. Clinical signs include granulomatous and nongranulomatous lesions in different body systems. Definitive diagnosis is via cultures of the lesions. Transmission is by direct contact (scratches, bites) or through aerosolization.[11]

Other Bacteria of Minor Zoonotic Significance

Other bacteria that may be found in reptiles include *Campylobacter jejuni* and *C. fetus. C. fetus* was identified in an asymptomatic box turtle. The organism was diagnosed through fecal culture, suggesting that turtles may be reservoirs of *Campylobacter.*[11] *Citrobacter* spp., *Enterobacter* spp., *Klebsiella* spp., *Proteus* spp., *Serratia* spp., *Erysipelothrix rhusiopathiae, Yersinia enterocolitica, Y. pseudotuberculosis,* and *Pseudomonas* spp. have all been identified in reptiles. Transmission is through direct contact after scratches or bite wounds, inhalation, or ingestion.

Viral Diseases

Reptiles are reservoir hosts to Western equine encephalitis (WEE) and West Nile virus (WNV). The viremia in snakes (WEE) and alligators (WNV) is cyclic and may be significant enough to infect the vector (mosquitoes) for both diseases, but the role of reptiles in the epidemiology of these diseases is unknown.[11]

Fungal Diseases

Zygomycoses (e.g., phycomycosis, mucormycosis, entomophthoromycosis) are ubiquitous saprophytes. All are common inhabitants of the gastrointestinal tract of reptiles and are common in decomposing organic material. Transmission is via inhalation, ingestion, inoculation, or contamination of the skin with spores. *Mucor* spp., *Aspergillus* spp., *Candida* spp., and *Trichosporon* spp. have all been isolated from reptiles and the possibility of zoonotic transmission exists, although it has never been documented.[11]

Parasitic Diseases

Cryptosporidium is carried asymptomatically by reptiles. At this time, there is no documented evidence that reptilian cryptosporidiosis is zoonotic.[11] Pentastomes are primitive arthropods that may infect reptiles, especially wild-caught animals. Clinical signs range from none to parasites being identified in the mouth of the reptile. Transmission occurs through handling infected reptiles and then placing contaminated hands in the mouth. *Ophionyssus natricis*, the snake mite, does not cause disease in humans, but may bite. This ectoparasite has been documented to transmit *Aeromonas hydrophilus*.

AMPHIBIANS

Amphibians have been shown to carry a number of zoonotic pathogens asymptomatically. These include *Leptospira* spp., *Listeria monocytogenes*, *Edwardsiella* spp., and *Yersinia enterocolitica*. *Mycobacterium* spp. (e.g., *M. chelonei*, *M. fortuitum*, *M. xenopi*) may cause dermal lesions in amphibians and *Chlamydophila psittaci* may cause amphibian mortalities. All these organisms have zoonotic potential.[23] Amphibians also carry *Salmonella* spp. asymptomatically and recently (end of 2009) have been indicated in the cause of clinical disease in young children who housed frogs at home. It is therefore necessary to practice the same preventive measures outlined at the beginning of this chapter when handling amphibians.

2009 H1N1 INFLUENZA

At the time this chapter was written, 2009 H1N1 influenza had been diagnosed in swine, ferrets, cats, cheetahs, turkeys, and dogs, with all animals appearing to acquire the disease from an infected person with which they had aerosol contact. As of December 2009, there had been no reported cases of transmission from animals to humans in zoological settings. At this time, animal collections do not present a concern for public health.

CONCLUSION

Zoonotic disease transmission from children's zoo and education animals to the zoo visitor is always a risk. However, with proper quarantine procedures for newly acquired animals, well-designed education programs for the staff and zoo visitor, appropriate signage and exhibit design, and well-placed hand sanitizing and hand washing stations, this risk is greatly diminished. The visitor experience is greatly enhanced by direct contact with appropriate species and, with the precautions outlined in this chapter, this experience can be safe and rewarding.

REFERENCES

1. Aiello AE, Coulborn RM, Perez V, et al: Effect of hand hygiene on infectious disease risk in the community setting: A meta-analysis. Am J Publ Health 98:1372–1381, 2008.
2. American Veterinary Medical Association: Backgrounder: Avian influenza, 2010 (www.avma.org/public_health/influenza/avinf_bgnd.asp).
3. Anderson DE, Rings DM, Pugh DG: Diseases of the integumentary system. In Pugh DG, editor: Sheep and Goat Medicine. Philadelphia, 2002, WB Saunders, pp 197–222.
4. Association of Zoos and Aquariums: Advisory to AZA Members Regarding Type A Influenza H1N1 Virus, 2009 (http://www.aza.org/h1n1-advisory).
5. Carpenter JW, Gentz EJ: Zoonotic diseases of avian origin. In Altman RB, Clubb SL, Dorrestein GM, et al. editors: Avian Medicine and Surgery. Philadelphia, 1997, WB Saunders, pp 350–363.
6. Centers for Disease Control and Prevention: Outbreaks of *Escherichia coli* O157:H7 associated with petting zoos—North Carolina, Florida, and Arizona, 2004–2005 (http://www.cdc.gov/mmwr/preview/mmwrhtml/mm5450a1.htm).
7. Eidson M: Psittacosis/avian chlamydiosis. J Vet Med Assoc 221:1710–1712, 2002.
8. Fowler M: Infectious diseases. In Fowler ME, editor: Medicine and Surgery of South American Camelids. Ames, Iowa, 1998, Iowa State University Press, pp 148–194.
9. Glynn MK, Lynn TV: Brucellosis. J Vet Med Assoc 233:900–908, 2008.
10. Heatley JJ, Harris MC: Hamsters and gerbils. In Mitchell MM, Tully TN, editors: Manual of Exotic Pet Practice. St. Louis, 2009, Saunders Elsevier, pp 406–432.
11. Johnson-Delaney CA: Reptile zoonoses and threats to public health. In Mader DR, editor: Reptile Medicine and Surgery. St. Louis, 2006, Saunders/Elsevier, pp 1017–1030.
12. Kaneene JB, Thoen CO: Tuberculosis. J Am Vet Med Assoc 224:685–691, 2004.
13. LeJeune JT, Davis MA: Outbreaks of zoonotic entries disease associated with animal exhibits. J Am Vet Med Assoc 224:1440–1445, 2004.
14. McQuiston JM, Childs JM, Thompson HA: Q Fever. J Am Vet Med Assoc 221:796–799, 2002.
15. Mobini S, Heath AM, Pugh DG: Theriogenology of sheep and goats. In Pugh DG, editor: Sheep and Goat Medicine. Philadelphia, 2002, WB Saunders, pp 129–186.
16. National Association of State Public Health Veterinarians: Compendium of Measures to Prevent Disease Associated with Animals in Public Settings, 2009 (http://www.nasphv.org/Documents/AnimalsInPublicSettings.pdf).
17. Pickering LK, Marano N, Bocchini JA, et al: Exposure to nontraditional pets at home and to animals in public settings: Risks to children. Pediatrics 122:876–886, 2008.
18. Riggs SM, Mitchell MA: Chinchillas. In Mitchell MM, Tully TN, editors: Manual of Exotic Pet Practice. St. Louis, 2009, Saunders Elsevier, pp 474–492.
19. Riley PY, Chomel BB: Hedgehog zoonoses. Emerg Infect Dis 11:1–5, 2005.
20. Sanchez S, Hofacre CL, Lee MD, et al: Animal sources of salmonellosis in humans. J Am Vet Med Assoc 221:492–497, 2002.
21. Sanchez S, Lee MD, Harmon BG, et al: Animal issues associated with *Escherichia coli* O157:H7. J Am Vet Med Assoc 221:1122–1126, 2002.

22. Smith KA, Campbell CT, Murphy J, et al: National Association of State Public Health Veterinarians: Compendium of measures to control Chlamydophila psittaci infection among humans (psittacosis) and pet birds (avian chlamydiosis), 2009 (http://www.nasphv.org/Documents/Psittacosis.pdf).

23. Taylor SK: Bacterial diseases. In Wright KM, Whitaker BR, editors: Amphibian Medicine and Captive Husbandry. Malabar, India, 2001, Krieger, pp 159–179.

24. Vennen KM, Mitchell MM: Rabbits. In Mitchell MM, Tully TN, editors: Manual of Exotic Pet Practice. St. Louis, 2009, Saunders Elsevier, pp 374–405.

25. Wolf TM: Ferrets. In Mitchell MM, Tully TN, editors: Manual of Exotic Pet Practice. St. Louis, 2009, Saunders Elsevier, pp 345–374.

CHAPTER 16

AAZV Guidelines for Zoo and Aquarium Veterinary Medical Programs and Veterinary Hospitals

Thomas P. Meehan

The American Association of Zoo Veterinarians (AAZV) has developed guidelines for veterinary medical programs and hospitals in zoos and aquariums. The purpose of these guidelines is to assist institutions and veterinarians in the development and evaluation of programs of veterinary care. They are intended to serve as an adjunct to the requirements of the U.S. Department of Agriculture (USDA) for regulating licensed animal exhibitors. The Animal Welfare Act of 1966 and subsequent amendments require that zoos and aquariums in the United States employ an attending veterinarian to ensure certain minimal standards of veterinary care. Whether this attending veterinarian is a full-time employee of the institution or is a part-time contractor, the Animal Welfare Regulations state that licensed exhibitors "shall assure that the attending veterinarian has appropriate authority to ensure the provision of adequate veterinary care and to oversee the adequacy of other aspects of animal care and use."[3]

The guidelines recommend that the veterinarian be an active participant in the institution's management team. They also recommend that additional technical and administrative staff be employed in support of the veterinary care program depending on the size of the institution and animal collection.

The Association of Zoos and Aquariums (AZA) also references these guidelines in the evaluation of accredited institutions. The AZA Accreditation Standards (2010) state that "the institution should adopt the guidelines for medical programs developed by the American Association of Zoo Veterinarians."[4]

VETERINARY CARE

The program of veterinary care must emphasize disease prevention. The animals should be observed on a daily basis and have any signs of illness or injury reported promptly so that the need for veterinary attention may be evaluated. Animals that die in the collection should receive a complete necropsy. Veterinary coverage must be available 24 hours a day, 7 days a week, for any zoo or aquarium.

Staff and Personnel

The veterinarian responsible for the zoo or aquarium must be familiar with the staff and the animal collection. They are also responsible for the development and supervision of long-term preventive medicine programs. The veterinarian must also arrange for the availability of other suitable veterinary coverage when they are unavailable. Although it is preferable to have the services of a full-time veterinarian, this is not warranted by some institutions based on their size. The services of a part-time veterinarian must be covered by an appropriate contractual arrangement.

Any zoo or aquarium in which a part-time veterinarian provides veterinary coverage must have one staff person who serves as the veterinary program coordinator and supervises this program under the direction of the veterinarian. This veterinary program coordinator serves as the main point of communication with the veterinarian regarding medical issues and maintains oversight of medical records, treatments, preventive medicine program, and medical facilities. The veterinary program coordinator may be a keeper, curator, or hospital or clinic manager. Ideally, this person should be a licensed veterinary technician or animal health technician.

Adequate support staff are also required to establish and maintain the veterinary programs and facilities. These would include support in the areas of husbandry, technical, and clerical support. In a large zoo or aquarium, these tasks may be covered by personnel dedicated to each of these areas, such as keepers, veterinary technicians, and administrative support. Although individual personnel in each of these areas may not be required by smaller institutions, it is important that each of these tasks be assigned to specific personnel.

The staff responsible for veterinary care must be familiar with the principles of infection control, the risks associated with chemicals used in the facility, and other aspects of personnel safety, including the appropriate use of personal protective equipment (PPE). Staff should also be aware of potential hazards associated with handling dangerous animals (e.g., bites, envenomation, scratches).[2] Facilities that have macaque species should have a bite and scratch emergency protocol in place because of the risk of infection from herpes B virus.

Veterinary Program

Medical and surgical care must be provided to all the animals in a zoo or aquarium collection, and this care must meet or exceed contemporary practice standards for zoos and aquariums.[2] Those responsible for providing medical care and treatments must be supervised by qualified staff and those treatments performed by or in consultation with the veterinarian. The use of medications must be done in accordance with federal, state, and local regulations. Drugs used on fish must be administered in a manner to prevent contamination of water supplies and introduction into the human food chain. In the United States, these drugs should be administered in accordance with the U.S. Food and Drug Administration agreement with the AZA regarding the use of animal drugs.[4]

Veterinary staff must have diagnostic laboratory support available as an aid in disease diagnostics. It is recommended that minimal diagnostic capabilities be available on site for the performance of fecal parasite examinations and diagnostic cytology of blood or other specimens. Consultation with veterinary pathologists should be available for diagnostic support to the clinician.

All zoos and aquariums must have access to appropriate surgical facilities, anesthesia, and monitoring equipment. This must be available on site for minor procedures. Fully equipped sterile surgery may not be necessary on site based on the size of the institution and type of collection, but these facilities must be available. In emergencies, minor treatment areas should be available that can be adapted for use as sterile surgery sites. Postoperative care must be provided, ideally at the zoo

or aquarium, even when procedures may have been performed off site.

There should be an area set aside in the institution for minor treatments and procedures. An on-site pharmacy or drug storage area must be provided that meets regulatory standards for the drugs in use (e.g., appropriate safes for narcotics). Medications dispensed should be accompanied by complete prescriptions and the staff responsible for dispensing and administering the drugs must be trained on their proper handling. In the case of drugs for chemical restraint, emergency procedures must be in place to deal with incidents of accidental exposure.

Animals that die in the institution and wild or feral animals found dead on grounds should be subject to postmortem examination. This examination should be performed as soon as possible and no longer than 24 hours after death. There should be adequate facilities for carcass storage and postmortem examination that are physically separate from other storage and animal treatment areas. Histologic examination should be performed if the cause of death is not evident on gross examination and, ideally, on all mortalities. If species management programs such as species survival plans (SSPs) have necropsy protocols, these should be followed.

Complete medical records must be maintained under the direction of the veterinarian. These should indicate any veterinary attention, including treatments, prescriptions, surgical procedures, and laboratory findings. Ideally, these should be computerized records and must be duplicated and stored in secondary locations or otherwise protected from the effects of fire, flood, or other incidents. Disease and mortality trends should be reviewed to identify the need for changes in husbandry or preventive medicine programs.

A preventive medicine program should be developed in every zoo or aquarium. This should include quarantine, parasite surveillance and control procedures, immunization, infectious disease screening, dental prophylaxis and periodic review of diets, husbandry techniques, and vermin control.[2] The quarantine protocols should be under the direction of veterinary staff and strictly enforced.

The quarantine procedures are in place to protect the animal collection from the introduction of infectious diseases. A physical or visual examination with appropriate testing should be performed on all animals prior to shipment. The length of quarantine, types of tests performed prior to shipment or during quarantine, and degree of separation from other animals in the collection are determined by the type of animal being moved, particular species needs, and history of the collections at the sending and receiving institutions. The typical length of quarantine is at least 30 days but may be extended based on a particular species requirements or findings during the quarantine period. Quarantined animals should be held in a facility separate from the rest of the collection and serviced by personnel who are exclusive to that area or service that area at the end of the day. Clothing and utensils used by personnel servicing quarantine should not be used in any other areas, and infection control techniques should be in place to maximize the separation of the animals in quarantine from those in the collection. Special considerations may be needed for species that cannot be isolated because of unique needs or environmental requirements. Large or specialized animals such as elephants or marine mammals may need to be housed close to collection animals because of the inability to dedicate separate facilities for the quarantine of that species. For these animals, protocols need to emphasize press shipment testing, the greatest degree of isolation possible, and reduction of direct physical contact. Fish and aquatic invertebrates may be quarantined in groups or as individuals. Although there are limitations in the scope and availability of diagnostics tests for these species, quarantine protocols should rely on taxon-specific risk assessments tailored to the needs of the species involved.[2]

The preventive medicine program should include a program of parasite control developed by the veterinarian. This should include the routine parasite monitoring of individual animals or groups. The timing of the examinations and the need for routine treatment will be determined by the needs of the individual species, their housing, and their history.

The types of immunization needed for the animals in a zoo or aquarium collection are determined by the veterinarian based on the needs of the species and the history of the disease in the collection and surrounding area. SSPs may also have recommendations for the immunization of managed populations.

A program of disease surveillance through diagnostic screening should be set up, depending on the history of a disease in the area, the collection, or government regulations. The veterinarian should work with staff to determine the need for routine examinations of particular animals in the collection. SSPs and taxon advisory groups (TAGs) may be consulted for recommendations regarding the need for routine testing, such as tuberculosis testing of primates or physical examinations.

The veterinarian should be knowledgeable about zoonotic disease that could affect the collection animals, personnel, or visiting public.[2] The veterinarian should work with Human Resources and animal management staff at the institution to address issues of zoonotic disease, including the training of staff on zoonotic disease risks. A preventive health program should be set up for staff in consultation with physicians knowledgeable about infectious diseases and occupational health. Veterinarians should work in cooperation with animal management staff to assess the risk of zoonotic disease transmission in all areas that allow public contact with the animal collection, plan preventive measures, and train staff in contact areas. For further information, the National Association of State Public Health Veterinarians (NASPHV) has developed measures to prevent disease associated with animals in a public setting.[5]

Management

In addition to issues of veterinary medical and surgical care, there are a number of other zoological management decisions that must involve the veterinarian working with other staff, such as curators or nutritionists. These include animal shipments, nutrition, husbandry, pest controls and euthanasia.

The veterinarian is responsible for the preshipment examination and provision of the Certificate of Veterinary Inspection, as well as ensuring that regulatory testing is completed. The veterinarian is also responsible for determining that the methods for shipment ensure the safe transportation of the specimens.

The nutrition program should include regularly scheduled review of dietary husbandry practices, including laboratory analysis of feed items. Diets should be evaluated for appropriateness for the species and life stages involved. The provision of appropriate diets as well as the safe handling and storage of feeds should be monitored by veterinary staff or a qualified staff nutritionist.

Methods used for the cleaning and disinfection of animal exhibits should be developed in consultation with veterinary staff. A formal program of integrated pest management should be in place at each institution and reviewed by veterinary staff.

The zoo or aquarium must have a policy on euthanasia that addresses the decision making process, as well as the methods for humane euthanasia.[2] Animals should be euthanized in accordance with the most current guidelines.[1]

VETERINARY FACILITIES

All zoos and aquariums should have an on-site veterinary facility. An on-site facility allows for the isolation of animals receiving medical care and facilitates observation and treatment of sick and injured animals. The size of the facility and its components will depend on the size and type of animal collection. The facility should be designed with input from the veterinary staff, with the assistance of individuals knowledgeable about animal hospital facility design.[2]

The facility should have designated areas for examination and treatment, sterile surgery, necropsy, animal holding, laboratory, biologic sample storage, radiology, pharmaceutical storage including, when necessary, a safe for controlled drugs that meets the standards set by the U.S. Drug Enforcement Administration (DEA), animal food preparation and/or storage areas, equipment storage areas, and a staff locker-room with showers and restroom facilities. Capture and restraint equipment, anesthetic equipment, autoclave, and basic surgical equipment should be stored in the hospital. Radiology equipment should be of appropriate size and power for the animal collection, and its installation must meet local and state regulations.[2]

The design of the hospital facility should take into consideration the need for sanitation and disinfection of contaminated areas, the segregation of animal and staff areas, and mechanical systems that minimize cross contamination. Adequate storage and support areas should be accommodated in the design.

Some zoos and aquariums may not require a full on-site hospital facility based on the size of the collection and veterinary needs. If an off-site facility is used for major medical procedures, it should be close to the zoo or aquarium and provide adequate facilities to meet the needs of the species in the collection. There should be areas available at the zoo or aquarium for minor treatments, emergency procedures, and postoperative care.

REFERENCES

1. American Association of Zoo Veterinarians (AAZV), Baer CK, editor: Guidelines for Euthanasia of Nondomestic Animals. Lawrence, Kansas, 2006, American Association of Zoo Veterinarians.
2. American Association of Zoo Veterinarians: Guidelines for Zoo and Aquarium Veterinary Medical Programs and Hospitals, 1998 (http://www.aazv.org/associations/6442/files/zoo_aquarium_vet_med_guidelines.pdf).
3. Animal and Plant Health Inspection Service: Animal Welfare Regulations, 2008 (http://www.aphis.usda.gov/animal_welfare/downloads/awr/awr.pdf).
4. Association of Zoos and Aquariums: The Accreditation Standards and Related Policies, 2010 (http://www.aza.org/uploadedFiles/Accreditation/Microsoft%20Word%20-%202010%20Accred%20Standards.pdf).
5. National Association of State Public Health Veterinarians: Compendium of Measures to Prevent Disease Associated with Animals in Public Settings, 2009 (http://www.nasphv.org/Documents/AnimalsInPublicSettings.pdf).

CHAPTER 17

Fundamentals of Zoo Animal Surgery

Rui I. Bernardino

Zoo animal surgery is based on surgical techniques applied to domestic animals and humans. Although technically based on general surgical principles, zoo animal surgery is a specific field because of the wide anatomic and physiologic diversity. Therefore, it requires understanding of surgical procedures as a whole and anatomic and physiologic knowledge of the species involved. It is important for the surgeon to have the opportunity of using necropsies to become familiar with the tissues and anatomy, thus recording the organs' dimensions and topography. This will provide as much information as possible for the actual procedure. Developing practical knowledge is particularly important when compared with other fields of human and veterinary medicine.

Considering surgery as a therapeutic option requires prompt diagnosis, which is one of the main difficulties, particularly because many zoo animal species tend not to show clinical signs. Recent developments in complementary diagnostic methods and their application to zoo animal medicine have helped in facing this difficulty.

Because the demand for zoo animal surgeries is occasional and of a varied nature, in most cases surgeons hone their skills by performing frequent surgeries on domestic species. This approach may hinder a surgeon's preparedness to meet zoo animals' needs fully. It is often necessary to adapt not only to the limitations that will be presented in this chapter, but also to particular anatomic and physiologic features. These adaptations lead to altered techniques used in other fields. Being ready to adjust techniques means also being aware of the different options available to surgery as a whole. Zoo animal surgery is, undoubtedly, a challenging field.

This chapter will summarize the conceptual details of zoo animal surgery and note some of the basic techniques and preparations available for the purpose.

CASE-BASED APPROACH

Zoo animal surgery varies greatly and offers little repetition. Occasionally, it is possible to have surgical indications for almost any of the procedures performed in humans and domestic animals. Nevertheless, we may regard surgery caused by trauma (e.g., resolving perforations, reconstructive plastic surgery, orthopedic surgery) as the most frequently encountered, along with diagnostic and therapeutic laparotomy, particularly for the reproductive system. Surgical dentistry is also common in this field.

SURGICAL FACILITIES AND EQUIPMENT

One of the main characteristics of zoo animal surgery is the wide diversity of procedures and therefore the different materials and equipment that may be necessary. In practice, it is impossible to predict all the surgical equipment and instruments that may be needed. A recommended approach might be to start with basic materials and equipment used in more common surgeries, eventually getting to the point at which more particular items, such as orthopedic or laparoscopic equipment, are mandatory and require specific resources and well-trained staff.

Surgical Area

It would be beneficial to have two surgery rooms, one for small and another one for large animals, because of specific requirements in regard to equipment, surgical tables, and annexed rooms (Fig. 17-1). The surgical area must follow general standards in terms of security, patient and staff circulation, clean and comfortable environment, and proper organization, as described in literature reports.[9,12,14] A video recording system is of

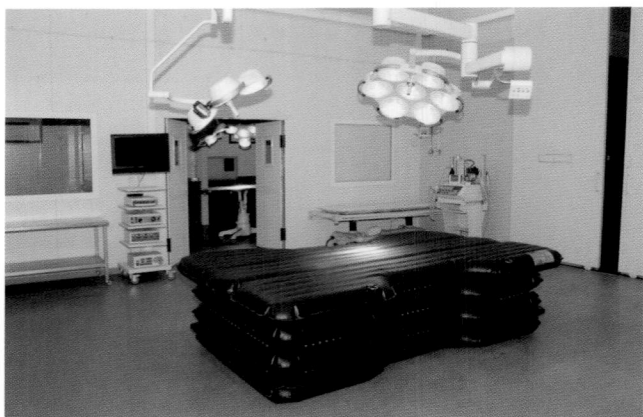

Figure 17-1

Large animal surgical room at the Lisbon Zoo Hospital.

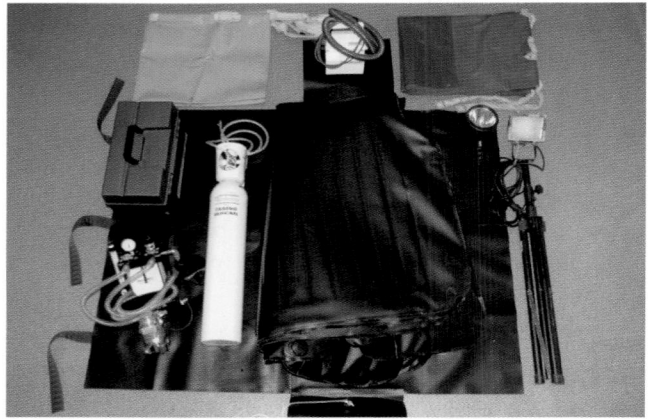

Figure 17-2

Field zoo animal surgery portable equipment, lights, anesthesia device, oxygen tank, transport stretchers, and inflatable surgical table.

TABLE 17-1	Basic Microsurgery Pack for Delicate Surgery*
Quantity	Instrument
4	Baby mosquito hemostats, curved and straight, 3.75 inches (95 mm)
2	Hemostatic clips
1	Adson tissue forceps, 4.75 inches (120 mm)
1	Iris forceps
1	Microscalpel blade handle, 5.5 inches (135 mm)
1 each	Stevens tenotomy scissors, curved and straight
1	Iris scissor, straight
1	Castroviejo needle holder
10	Sterile cotton-tipped applicators
10	Gauze swabs, 0.8 × 0.8 inch (20 × 20 mm)

Binocular magnification loupes, 2.5 to 5×.

particular interest in these procedures as a means of documentation and sharing information.

With the increasing sophistication of surgical techniques and instrumentation available today, surgeries outside a proper surgical facility are becoming less common.[14] Nevertheless, occasionally, field surgery is still the option for zoo animals. This is the prevailing choice for large mammals or patients requiring short-duration anesthesia, or even for quick patient anesthetic recovery in an enclosure. In these circumstances, it is useful to have additional portable equipment available—namely, a good light, anesthesia device, oxygen tank, transport stretcher, and adequate surgical tables (e.g., inflatable systems; Fig. 17-2).

In the perioperative period, being able to use nurseries and animal isolation facilities is essential to monitor the patient more suitably. However, this may not always be a valid option; it might involve isolating a member of a group for a period of time long enough to alter its social structure.

Surgical Instrumentation

Accesses, structures, and target tissues vary enormously, so a considerable range of materials must be available. One may consider three basic and relevant instrument packs:

- Microsurgery pack for very small patients or structures (Table 17-1)
- Surgery instrument pack for small- to medium-sized animals, the most commonly used (Table 17-2)
- Surgery instrument pack for large animals (Table 17-3)

These packs are the basis for any type of surgery and must be complemented whenever necessary, according to the specific intervention. Electrocautery and portable suction units are examples of valuable and accessible equipment that should be included. Moreover, a diversity of retractors is necessary; the most widely used and recommended are Senn and Farabeuf retractors and self-retaining retractors such as Gelpi, Weitlaner, Finochietto, Balfour, and Lone Star retractors. Lid retractors used for laparotomy in very small animals or handheld retractors with sharp prongs for handling very thick abdominal walls may be an option.

In recent years, technologic advances have led to unprecedented access to new surgical equipment.

TABLE 17-2	Basic Pack for Small- to Medium-Sized Animals
Quantity	**Instrument**
3	Halstead mosquito hemostats, curved and straight, 5 inches (125 mm)
4	Kelly forceps, curved, 5.5 inches (140 mm)
4	Rochester-Pean forceps, curved, 7.25 inches (185 mm)
1	Rat-toothed forceps, 5.75 inches (145 mm)
1	Brown-Adson tissue forceps, 4.75 inches (120 mm)
2	Allis tissue forceps, 6 inches (150 mm)
1 each	Scalpel handles, No. 3 and 4
1	Metzenbaum scissors, curved, 7 inches (180 mm)
1	Metzenbaum scissors, straight, 7 inches (180 mm)
1	Mayo scissors, curved, 6.5 inches (165 mm)
1	Mayo-Hegar, Olsen-Hegar or Mathieu needle holder, 7 inches (180 mm)
1	Suture scissors
4	Towel forceps (Backhaus), 5.25 inches (135 mm)
1	Saline bowl
10	Gauze swabs, 4 × 4 inches (100 × 100 mm)

TABLE 17-3	Basic Pack for Large Animals
Quantity	**Instrument**
2	Halsted mosquito hemostats
6	Kelly forceps
2	Kocher-Ochsner forceps
2	Rochester-Pean forceps
3	Rat-toothed forceps
1	Brown-Adson tissue forceps
2	Allis-Thoms tissue forceps, 8 inches (200 mm)
1	Scalpel handle, No. 4
1	Metzenbaum scissors, straight, 8 inches (200 mm)
1	Mayo scissors, curved, 8.25 inches (210 mm)
1	Mayo scissors, straight, 8 inches(200 mm)
1	Mayo-Hegar, Olsen-Hegar, or Mathieu needle holder, 8 inches (200 mm)
1	Suture scissors
6	Roeder towel forceps
1	Saline bowl
50	Gauze swabs, 8 × 8 inches (200 × 200 mm)

Although high prices normally delay the integration of newly developed equipment in veterinary medicine, it becomes more affordable over time. Nevertheless, surgeons must become familiar with equipment before its practical application, acknowledging its advantages and its potential limitations. The use of equipment such as stapling devices, surgical lasers, and recently developed vessel sealing systems has become increasingly more common. When used correctly, this equipment has proven its value. Stapling devices may decrease the time of surgery needed for anastomoses and ligations and may also minimize the associated contamination. LigaSure (Covidien, Mansfield, Mass), a modern bipolar vessel sealing system, and Ultracision (Ethicon, Somerville, NJ), a system of ultrasound energy–based shears, are more efficient methods of coagulation when compared with monopolar and bipolar electrocoagulation.[7]

Suture Materials

Taking required adaptations into account, selecting suture materials should comply with general standards for other species.[3,4] Personal experience is also useful because there are few guidelines regarding zoo species. The wide range of patients requires a variety of available suture materials and sizes. It is important for surgeons to be familiar with the materials they use, which limits the types of sutures available.

SURGICAL PROCEDURES AND TECHNIQUES

The surgery's success may only be ascertained after the postoperative period, and it is traced prior to the intervention itself (preoperative period). These surgical periods are very specific for different zoo species (Box 17-1).

As noted, when performing surgery, specific anatomic and physiologic features and behavioral aspects must be taken into account. The higher probability of suture line breakdown with partial or complete wound dehiscence in some zoo animal species will influence the surgical technique (Box 17-2).

Laparoscopic surgery is also becoming increasingly used in this field. Among other advantages, it prevents major surgical wound dehiscence, because of small port incisions, when compared with conventional surgery. In spite of its benefits, laparoscopic surgery is not indicated for all procedures and requires training and frequent practice.

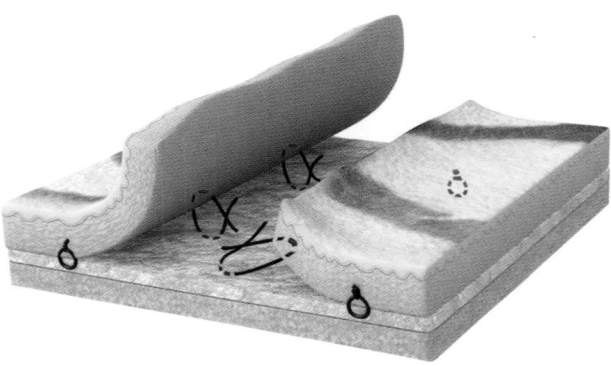

Figure 17-3

Surgical wound in a tiger (in an inaccessible area)—approximation suture. Anchoring and walking sutures used for apposition of the wound deep tissue distribute tension and reduce dead space, thus minimizing tension across the skin closure.

Approximation Sutures and Dead Space Obliteration

Approximation suture is fundamental in most cases for closing tissues, which is important to diminish the tension on the wound suture and to reduce dead space beneath it. In zoo animals, this is true for the following:

- The use of drains to obliterate dead spaces is more limited because of difficulties arising from postoperative maintenance and monitoring, and their removal may imply a second anesthesia.
- The force applied by the panniculus muscle and thick skin is challenging in some species, such as larger felines, thus increasing the tension over the suture line.

- It may be impossible to use bandages. The need for a protective effect and the tension supported in the suture line must be overcome by using alternative techniques.

Tension distribution and dead space obliteration may be achieved through anchoring sutures placed in the subcutaneous space or by using a variation, which approximates skin edges—walking sutures. With this technique, it is possible to advance the skin edges after undermining the skin around the defect, hence diminishing the tension in the suture line. Tension distribution is particularly important in species with considerable skin thickness (Fig. 17-3). The obliteration of dead space prevents the formation of seroma and facilitates rapid healing.

Whenever the use of drains is indicated but not feasible, the only solution is to leave an open space. Ideally, this open space should be in the dependent part of the wound to enable its drainage. Nevertheless, the use of drains should not be neglected in cases in which this is possible.

Closure Techniques

In conventional zoo animal surgery, one of the main concerns arises when closing the wound because of recurrent wound suture dehiscence. The excessive tension is particularly important, so some of the following techniques may be considered.

Despite the lack of references to tension lines in the skin of these species, it is essential to keep the orientation of these lines when suturing (running parallel to them, whenever possible). Skin tension lines described for humans and domestic animals must be used as a reference.[2,5,11] Actually, tension line orientation may be identified by manipulating the tissue while observing its resistance in various directions and by viewing the incision's acquired form during the cutting procedure; for example, when making a circular incision, observe which axis increases in size.

Precautions must be taken with external knots, drains, or protective bandages, particularly for felines (licking and nibbling behaviors) and primate species whose grooming behavior may be a problem. Isolating the patient may be a solution, provided that the suture area is inaccessible to the animal itself. Prolonged isolation periods must be avoided when dealing with hierarchized groups, because isolation may alter the hierarchy and make reintegration in the group more problematic. In these cases, the use of intradermal sutures may be the best technical solution. Stainless steel sutures may also be used, although they will require removal. In large species and for large incisions, the suture must be divided into smaller sections, thus preventing total suture loss in cases of wound dehiscence and therefore increasing its resistance. The fact that intradermal sutures are not suitable for supporting high tension in wound surgical edges should not be disregarded. In primate species, which may be isolated and for whom autogrooming is not a major problem, sutures with external knots may be an option.

In some cases in which specific anatomic characteristics require the use of tension distribution techniques, the stress in the suture line is still substantial. In these situations, tension sutures may be an option used, not only on their own, but also in combination with

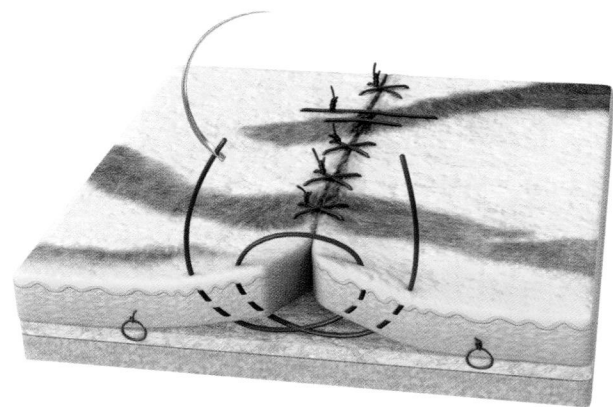

Figure 17-4

Surgical wound in a tiger (in an inaccessible area)—skin suture. Application of far near–near far suture in combination with an interrupted cruciate suture. This combination is particularly suitable to redistribute tension across the wound edges once each of those patterns has four anchor points.

appositional patterns. These sutures may be used by judiciously interspersing with other patterns (e.g., vertical mattress sutures), as referred, while taking precautions not to damage the blood supply to the suture line, placing the tension sutures well away from the skin edges.[3]

Tubing or gauze may be incorporated into mattress sutures to form a quilled or stent suture to further disperse pressure forces on the skin.[10]

The near and far suture pattern used in combination with appositional patterns provides higher tensile strength than either a simple interrupted or mattress pattern and also provides good tissue apposition without eversion of skin edges, which may be an issue in species with a thick dermis—for example, in large felines, tension sutures or the referred combination may be extremely useful, provided that it is in an inaccessible area for the animal and kept isolated during cicatrization (Fig. 17-4). Closing wounds under tension should always be performed with caution.[2]

In group-living animals, if skin suture with external knots is selected and a second anesthesia is not practical, a nonabsorbable monofilament suture must be used. Using this type of suture will lead to minor tissue reaction and, consequently, a less reactive surgical wound. This may be the option for antelopes (Fig. 17-5).

Perioperative Medication

The surgical outcome also depends on proper perioperative medication. This chapter does not include

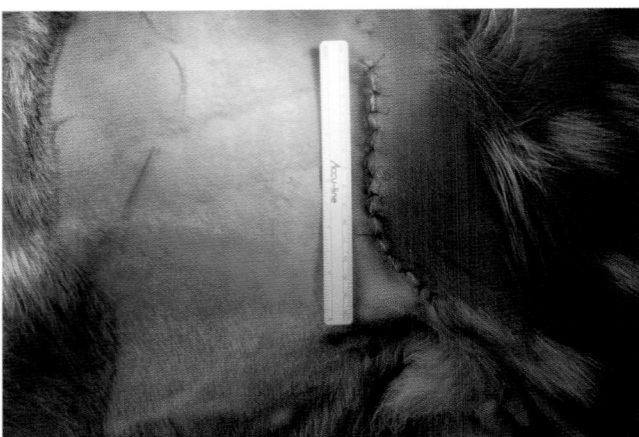

Figure 17-5

Tension suture used to close a flank laparotomy incision in a nyala *(Tragelaphus angasii)*. The closing suture used was a monofilament polyamide 0 (4 mm).

medication indications or the respective analysis, although the subject is covered in detail by a wide range of literature pertaining to the various branches of surgery.[1,8,13,15]

Tissues must have an appropriate antibiotic concentration at the time of surgery, thereby boosting the efficiency of preventing bacterial colonization, which is one of the aims of aseptic surgery.[13] In a significant number of cases, we must proceed to surgery directly, whereby intravenous administration is preferable because of its fast action in the target tissues.

Analgesia is justified to prevent discomfort and pain after a surgical intervention in the postoperative period, because these factors may also contribute to potential wound suture dehiscence. Moreover, analgesia provides the patient with greater comfort and a faster return to normal function. Analgesic requirements should be anticipated and incorporated into each patient's anesthetic management.[6] Tranquilization may also be important to reduce anxiety in the perioperative period.

Administration of drugs in restraint cages during the postoperative period must be avoided, particularly in cases of torso sutures. Because of skin's mobility over the torso, the fastened bars, by immobilizing the skin, place greater stress over the suture, even in areas not in direct contact with the bars, particularly when the animal performs small movements. I have observed cases of skin wound dehiscence on ventral and other lines in patients kept in restraining cages for treatment after surgery (e.g., large felines).

CONCLUSION

There is little opportunity to evolve technically while operating merely on zoo animals. Surgeons are responsible for monitoring developments in the various fields of surgery and any resources that may be applied through suitable adaptation, in addition to performing surgeries on a regular basis. Having the opportunity to perform surgery in other species may be valuable for achieving those goals.

As a zoo veterinarian, one cannot overlook specific knowledge about the anatomy, physiology, and specific behaviors of zoo animals as an essential contribution for one's practice as a zoo surgeon. The work performed at zoos has improved immensely by the development of multidisciplinary teams that integrate members of several fields, such as human medicine and veterinary universities, research institutions, hospitals, and private clinics. The fact that these participants normally do not perform this work on a regular basis often leads to a situation whereby acquired knowledge is not reported and published, and thus is not shared within the scientific community. Because zoo animal surgical practices are so varied and irregular, it is relevant to disclose the respective information and to have an increasing number of surgeons who sustain a particular interest in this challenging field.

REFERENCES

1. Anaya DA, Dellinger EP: Surgical infections and choice of antibiotics. In Townsend Jr CM, Beauchamp RD, Evers BM, editors: Sabiston Textbook of Surgery: The Biological Basis of Modern Surgical Practice, ed 17, Philadelphia, 2004, Saunders Elsevier, pp 257–282.
2. Bailey JV: Principles of reconstructive surgery. In Auer JA, Stick JA, editors: Equine Surgery, ed 3, St. Louis, 2006, Saunders Elsevier, pp 254–268.
3. Blackford LW, Blackford JT: Suture materials and patterns. In Auer JA, Stick JA, editors: Equine Surgery, ed 3, St. Louis, 2006, Saunders Elsevier, pp 187–202.
4. Boothe HW: Suture materials, tissue adhesives, staplers, and ligating clips. In Slatter D, editor: Textbook of Small Animal Surgery, ed 3, Philadelphia, 2003, WB Saunders, pp 235–244.
5. Burns JL, Blackwell S: Plastic surgery. In Townsend Jr CM, Beauchamp RD, Evers BM, editors: Sabiston Textbook of Surgery: The Biological Basis of Modern Surgical Practice, ed 17, Philadelphia, 2004, Saunders Elsevier, pp 2181–2203.
6. Carroll GL: Treatment of perioperative pain. In Fossum TW, Hedlund CS, Hulse DA, et al, editors: Small Animal Surgery, ed 2, St. Louis, 2002, Mosby, pp 93–102.
7. Diamantis T, Kontos M, Arvelakis A, et al: Comparison of monopolar electrocoagulation, bipolar electrocoagulation, Ultracision, and Ligasure. Surg Today 36:908–913, 2006.
8. Dunning D: Surgical wound infections and the use of antimicrobials. In Slatter D, editor: Textbook of Small Animal Surgery, ed 3, Philadelphia, 2003, WB Saunders, pp 113–122.

9. Hobson HP: Surgical facilities and equipment. In Slatter D, editor: Textbook of Small Animal Surgery, ed 3, Philadelphia, 2003, WB Saunders, pp 179–185.

10. Knecht CD, Allen AR, Williams DJ, et al: Suture patterns. In Knecht CD, Allen AR, Williams DJ, et al, editors: Fundamental Techniques in Veterinary Surgery, ed 3, Philadelphia, 1987, WB Saunders, pp 55–71.

11. Mayhew P: Tension-relieving techniques and local skin flaps. In Williams J, Moores A, editors: BSAVA Manual of Canine and Feline Wound Management and Reconstruction, ed 2, Gloucestershire, England, 2009, British Small Animal Veterinary Association, pp 69–99.

12. Seim III HB: Surgical facilities, equipment, and personnel. In Fossum TW, Hedlund CS, Hulse DA, et al, editors: Small Animal Surgery, ed 2, St. Louis, 2002, Mosby, pp 11–14.

13. Seim III HB, Fossum TW: Surgical infections and antibiotic selection. In Fossum TW, Hedlund CS, Hulse DA, et al, editors: Small Animal Surgery, ed 2, St. Louis, 2002, Mosby, pp 60–68.

14. Stick JA: Preparation of the surgical patient, the surgery facility, and the operating team. In Auer JA, Stick JA, editors: Equine Surgery, ed 3, St. Louis, 2006, Saunders Elsevier, pp 123–134.

15. Waguespack RW, Burba DJ, Moore RM: Surgical site infection and the use of antimicrobials. In Auer JA, Stick JA, editors: Equine Surgery, ed 3, St. Louis, 2006, Saunders Elsevier, pp 70–87.

CHAPTER 18

Emerging Diseases at the Interface of People, Domestic Animals, and Wildlife*

Robert A. Cook and William B. Karesh

Increasingly, diseases are moving among people, domestic animals, and wildlife, creating concerns about food safety, public health, and wildlife conservation.[49] Some of these diseases have existed for millennia, whereas others are emerging or reemerging, gaining the ability to jump between species and overloading traditional methods of disease surveillance and prevention. In a list of 1407 human pathogens, 58% are known to be zoonotic; 177 are categorized as emerging or reemerging, and zoonotic pathogens are twice as likely to be in this category as nonzoonotic pathogens.[100]

The impact on human populations may be significant. The 2004 Joint United Nations (UN) Program on HIV/AIDS report on the global epidemic stated that mortality from human immunodeficiency virus (HIV) exceeded 20 million people in the 20 years since first diagnosed in 1980. HIV-1 and HIV-2 were introduced into humans through separate cross-species transmission of simian immunodeficiency virus. HIV-1 is believed to have arisen through transmission from chimpanzees and HIV-2 from sooty mangabeys (Cercocebus atys).[40]

Wildlife species under severe environmental pressure are threatened by extinction from the spread of novel pathogens. Chytridiomycosis, caused by Batrachochytrium dendrobatidis, has been implicated in the massive mortality and global decline in a variety of amphibian species.[45] International trade is thought to play a key role in the worldwide dissemination of this disease.[27,60]

Livestock production and market access to animal protein have been increasingly threatened by the emergence of disease. Since 1992, the economic damages from livestock diseases alone has totalled more than $60 billion. Outbreaks of bovine spongiform encephalopathy, foot-and-mouth disease, avian influenza, rinderpest, and other diseases have prompted governments to impose trade embargoes and to mandate animal culling with increasing frequency. In 2003, the UN Food and Agricultural Organization (FAO) reported that one third of global meat trade was subject to embargoes because of disease outbreaks.[2]

The increase in infectious diseases may be linked to anthropogenic pressures of an urbanizing world, overall population growth, altered land use and agricultural practices, deforestation, global travel and commerce, microbial adaptation, and a weakened public health infrastructure. To forecast and respond proactively to the complex changes that influence the health of people, domestic animals, and wildlife, we must consider the driving forces that are affecting or will likely affect our world.

Globalization is the dominant international system that has made the world an increasingly integrated place, resulting in both threats and opportunities.[30] The global movement of people, animals, and their products has had profound effects on wildlife, livestock, and public health through the unchecked legal and illegal trade in exotic pets and bush meat. Human population increases and the desire for improved standards of living promote have intensified agricultural practices, pollution of air and water, and the unsustainable use of natural resources. There is little evidence to date that climate change has played a significant role in the resurgence of infectious disease. However, many believe that soon global climate change will be responsible for regional climate alterations that affect physical and biologic systems.[68]

---

*Please note that this chapter is reprinted from Fowler ME, Miller RE, eds: Zoo and Wild Animal Medicine, ed 6, St Louis, 2008, Elsevier. The editors believe that this chapter is complementary to the chapters in this volume on epidemiology, the wildlife-livestock interface, the role of veterinarians in conservation programs, and wildlife disease ecology.

These critical driving forces of globalization, human population increases with intensified agriculture, and global climate change provide a structure on which to consider exemplar emerging infectious diseases that imperil the future of humanity and animal life.

HUNTING, PETS, AND GLOBALIZED TRADE IN WILDLIFE

The local hunting of wildlife or bush meat is an ancient practice that forms the fabric of community culture at the rural wildlife interface (Fig. 18-1). Although these fundamental practices have always posed a cross-species disease risk to the local community, they have been mitigated through cultural practices. Ecologic changes, as created by increased human population density, forest fragmentation via road building, and rural development, alter the relationships of pathogens to hosts.[70] These changes, along with increased human movement and the globalized trade in animals for food and pets, facilitate rapid movement to distant sites and greater human-pathogen contact.[99]

The World Trade Organization's 2005 statistics note that in 2004 the global merchandise trade rose by 21% to 8.9 trillion U.S. dollars, with agriculture accounting for $783 billion. There is no breakdown of the share of trade in wildlife, but each year an estimated 350 million live plants and wild animals are shipped globally.[12] The poorly regulated wildlife component of global trade facilitates infections via microbial travel[46] at scales that not only cause human disease outbreaks, but also threaten livestock, international trade, rural livelihoods, native wildlife populations, and the health of ecosystems.[42]

Surveys of live wildlife from markets in Guangzhou, China, included masked palm civets (*Paguma* spp.), ferret badgers (*Melogale* spp.), barking deer (*Muntiacus* spp.), wild boar *(Sus)* spp., hedgehogs (family Erinaceidae), foxes (*Vulpes* spp.), squirrels (family Sciuridae), bamboo rats (*Cannomys* spp.), gerbils (*Rhombomys* spp.), various species of snakes, and endangered leopard cats (*Felis* spp.), as well as domestic dogs, cats, and rabbits.[3] Following the 2003 severe acute respiratory syndrome (SARS) outbreak, 838,500 wild animals were reportedly confiscated from the markets in Guangzhou, China.[7]

Daily, wild birds and reptiles flow through trading centers, where they are in contact with dozens of other species before being shipped to other markets, sold locally, or freed back to the wild as part of religious customs or because they are unwanted pets. In a single market in North Sulawesi, Indonesia, up to 90,000 mammals are sold per year.[22] In a survey conducted at a market in Thailand over 25 weekends, more than 70,000 birds of 276 species were sold[81] (Fig. 18-2). In lieu of precise trade data, a conservative estimate is that in Asia alone, tens of millions of wild animals are shipped regionally and globally for food, pets, or use in traditional medicine every year.

The global movement of animals for the pet trade is estimated to be a multibillion-dollar industry (Fig. 18-3). Between November 1994 and January 1995, U.S. Department of Agriculture (USDA) personnel inspected 349 reptile import shipments with a total of 117,690

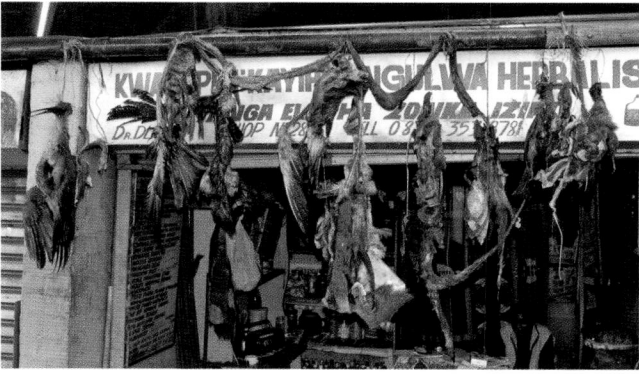

Figure 18-1

South African market with bushmeat for sale. *(Courtesy RA Cook.)*

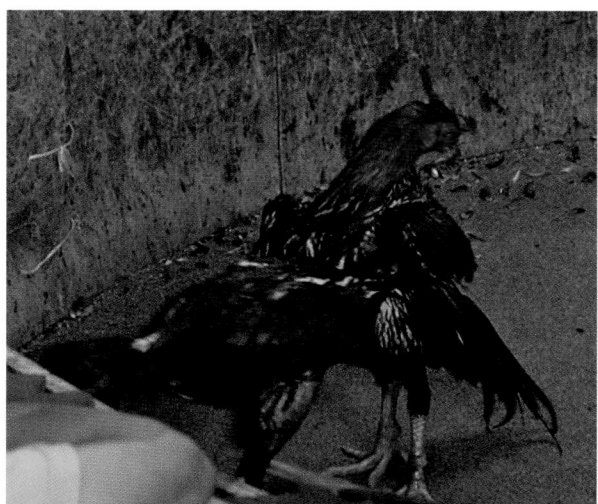

Figure 18-2

Cock fighting in a Thailand wet market. *(Courtesy RA Cook.)*

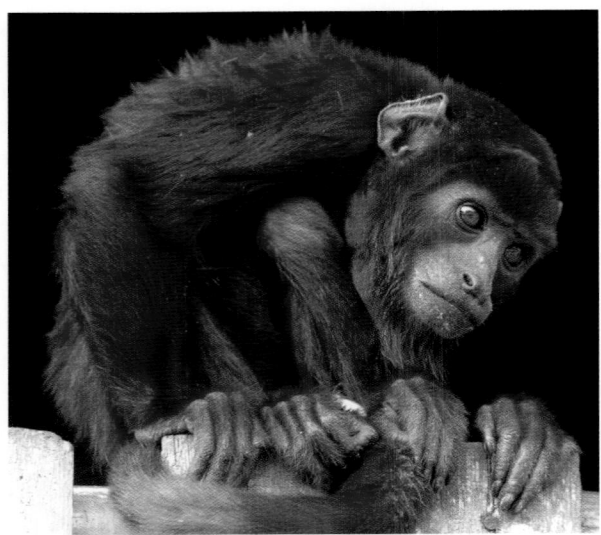

Figure 18-3

Pet howler monkey. *(Courtesy RA Cook.)*

animals originating from 22 countries. Ticks were removed from one or more animals in each of 97 shipments. Infested shipments included 54,376 animals in total.[13]

The estimate for trade and local and regional consumption of bushmeat in central Africa alone is over 1 billion kg/year,[96] and estimates for consumption in the Amazon basin range from 67 to 164 million kg annually.[72] In central Africa, the majority of wild animals harvested are small mammals (including small antelope and primates), birds, and reptiles. Assuming an average body weight of 5 kg results in a conservative estimate of 200 million animals in central Africa and 12 to 35 million in the Amazon basin. The increasingly global scope of this trade, coupled with rapid modern transportation and the reality that markets serve as network nodes rather than as product endpoints, dramatically increases the movement and potential cross-species transmission of the infectious agents that every animal naturally hosts.

Monkeypox

Monkeypox is a rare, viral, smallpox-like disease from central and western Africa that was first diagnosed in laboratory primates in 1958. The first human cases were reported in 1970 in Africa. An outbreak in the Democratic Republic of Congo in 1997 was reported to have infected 88 people, with three deaths, all in children younger than 3 years.[39]

In late May and early June 2003, the first cases of a febrile rash illness in people were reported from Wisconsin, Illinois, and Indiana. Most affected people had been in close contact with recently purchased ill prairie dogs *(Cynonys ludovicianus)* that had been held with a recent shipment of African rodents. The African rodents that spread the disease had been legally shipped from Ghana to the United States in April 2003 for the pet trade. The shipment included a number of species, and studies indicated that two rope squirrels *(Funisciurus)*, a Gambian rat *(Cricetomys)*, and three dormice *(Dryomys)* were carrying the monkeypox virus.[34] By early July, 71 nonfatal human cases from six states were reported to the Centers for Disease Control and Prevention (CDC).[10] Before this event, nonendangered rodents from Africa were legally shipped into the United States for the pet trade with no regulatory controls. Subsequently, restrictions were placed on U.S. importation of African rodents.

Severe Acute Respiratory Syndrome

SARS was first recognized as a newly emerging human disease in November 2002 in Guangdong Province, China.[93] Symptoms included high fever, respiratory illness progressing to pneumonia, in some cases diarrhea, and death. The disease first spread to Hong Kong and thereafter across five continents and 25 countries via infected people.[71] In April 2003, a new coronavirus was discovered to be the causative agent. In July 2003, the World Health Organization (WHO) listed the number of probable SARS cases in humans at 8437, with 813 deaths.[8] Evidence of viral infection, often without signs, was also detected in palm civets *(Paguma)* farmed in the region.[33] The initial suggestion of a link between civets and SARS led to a government directive to cull more than 10,000 masked palm civets in the province despite the ambiguity of the disease link.[9] Later, viral evidence was also detected in raccoon dogs *(Nyctereutes)* and ferret badgers *(Melogale)*, as well as domestic cats. It now appears that the palm civet served as an artificial market-induced host or amplification host, along with a number of other possible species. Subsequent studies determined that three species of horseshoe bat *(Rhinolophus)*[28] were found to be the natural reservoir host for closely related SARS-like coronaviruses.[51,56]

Bats have been found to be reservoir hosts for a number of viral pathogens, including Lyssa, Nipha,[101] Hedra, and Ebola viruses. Their role in emerging disease spread appears to be significant.

Ebola Hemorrhagic Fever

Ebola hemorrhagic fever (Ebola) is named after the river in the Democratic Republic of Congo (DRC, formerly Zaire), where it was first identified. Chimpanzees and humans share 98% of their DNA, and gorillas and humans share 97%.[80] Therefore, bush meat in the form of nonhuman primates poses a particularly high risk of cross-species infection into humans. The first three known outbreaks of Ebola occurred between 1976 and 1979 in DRC and Sudan. Between 2000 and 2004, five human Ebola outbreaks were documented in western central Africa. Epidemiologic studies indicated that these outbreaks resulted from multiple introductions of virus from infected animal sources. The index cases were mainly hunters, and all were infected while handling dead animals, including gorilla *(Gorilla)*, chimpanzee *(Pan troglodytes)*, and duiker *(Cephalophus)*.[53] Thereafter, outbreaks spread quickly among people, especially through caregivers, and were documented to almost wipe out entire villages.[31,52] In people, the symptoms are referable to multiple organ effects, with internal and external hemorrhaging. The Zaire subtype of Ebola virus has been known to have a case-fatality rate of almost 90%, and the Sudan subtype has a rate of approximately 50%.[82]

Ebola has been linked to declines in western equatorial Africa great ape populations. There is evidence that other forest animals, such as the duiker, are also affected.[53] Data do not exist on total numbers of nonhuman primates and duikers that have died of the disease, but it is believed that Ebola rivals hunting as the major threat to ape populations.[92] For some time, the natural reservoir host remained elusive.[75] Bats were long postulated as a potential reservoir host, as recently confirmed in three species of fruit bat.[54]

The movement of nonhuman primates for use in biomedical research has also proved to be a source for the spread of Ebola-related viruses. In 1989, a closely related simian hemorrhagic fever was diagnosed in Reston, Virginia, in imported cynomolgus monkeys from the Philippines that died during quarantine. Named Ebola Reston, the disease was later found not to cause human disease.[62]

EFFECT OF HUMAN POPULATION GROWTH ON AGRICULTURAL PRACTICES

By July 2005, the world had an estimated 6.5 billion human inhabitants, 380 million more than in 2000.

About 95% of all population growth is occurring in the developing world and 5% in the developed world. By 2050, it is estimated that the world population will increase by 2.6 billion.[6] For the 50 years preceding 2000, agriculture focused on meeting the food, feed, and fiber needs of a growing human population. In the next 50 years, the challenge will be not only feeding an expanding human population, but also doing so in a world of declining resources, including water and arable land.[47]

Large-scale agriculture is susceptible to outbreaks of disease. The 1983-1984 poultry epidemic of highly pathogenic avian influenza in the northeast United States caused markets to drop by $349 million during the 6-month period of the disease.[18] The economic impacts of the Nipah virus outbreak in Malaysia in 1997-1998 was estimated to cost $350 to $400 million, whereas the 2001 foot-and-mouth disease outbreak in England and Europe was estimated to have cost markets almost $30 billion (U.S. dollars).[66] In the developed world, agribusiness and government commitments to quality farm practices and rigorous health inspection have created a predominantly safe food supply. To provide food animal protein at the levels required, the industry has moved toward more intensive practices that increase productivity through selective breeding for desirable market traits and large-scale biosecure facilities. These characteristics may also leave operations vulnerable to the introduction and rapid spread of pathogens via errant contact with wildlife or the global movement of animals and products from areas that do not practice similar levels of biosecurity.

Developing country livestock practices are highly different. Often, livestock share space with people in and around the home. The rearing of ducks in Asia is an efficient system in which domestic ducks and geese are given access to recently harvested rice paddies. This allows wild waterfowl and domestic species to mix, but creates an environment conducive to the cross-species spread of pathogens.

Transmissible Spongiform Encephalopathies

The transmissible spongiform encephalopathies include chronic wasting disease of cervids, scrapie of sheep, bovine spongiform encephalopathy (BSE) of cattle, and Creutzfeldt-Jakob disease (CJD) of humans. They are caused by pathogenic prions, which are transmissible particles devoid of a nucleic acid genome and composed of a modified isoform of normal prion protein.[77] These prion proteins are extremely resistant to inactivation by ultraviolet light, ionizing radiation, steam sterilization, and almost all forms of traditional disinfection.

High-volume food production needs prompted the livestock industry to begin feeding ruminant protein to cattle, possibly derived from scrapie-infected sheep. It is believed that this practice led to the outbreak of BSE in the United Kingdom, which then spread to continental Europe, Canada and, more recently, the United States. It was likely through the ingestion of prion-infected meat from cattle that a new emerging disease of people was discovered in 1996, variant Creutzfeldt-Jakob disease (vCJD).

From October 1996 to November 2002, 129 cases of vCJD were reported in the United Kingdom, 6 in France, and 1 each in Canada, Ireland, Italy, and the United States.[11] The World Organization for Animal Health (OIE) has listed more than 184,296 cases of BSE in UK cattle alone as of September 2005. As confirmed, 13 species of zoo animals, including Bovidae and Felidae, have died as a result of infection with the BSE agent.[25]

Chronic wasting disease (CWD) is a prion disease of wild and farmed cervids in North America.[97] It was first recognized in a research herd of mule deer (Odocoileus hemionus) in Colorado in 1967. In 1985, it was diagnosed first in elk (Cervus elaphus) and then in mule deer in a limited region of Colorado. It is believed that the increase in deer and elk farming and the movement of animals for that industry in the United States and Canada provided a means for spread. It has since been diagnosed in multiple states and regions both in captive and free-ranging cervids. Conversion of human prion protein by CWD-associated prions has been demonstrated in an in vitro cell-free experiment[15] but, to date, investigations have not identified evidence for CWD transmission to humans.[14]

Avian Influenza

Avian influenza is an infectious disease of birds caused by type A strains of the influenza virus. Wild birds, predominantly ducks, geese, and shore birds, are the reservoir species for the low-pathogenic strains of avian influenza A virus (LPAI) in nature.[95] In these species, it does not usually cause illness. The virus is subtyped on the basis of the antigenic properties of hemagglutinin (HA, or H) and neuraminidase (NA, or N) glycoproteins; 16 HA and 9 NA subtypes have been demonstrated. Viruses containing subtypes H5 and H7 have been observed to become highly pathogenic avian influenza (HPAI) in poultry. HPAI has been isolated primarily from commercially raised birds, including chickens, turkeys, quail, guinea fowl, and ostrich (Struthio camelus). Influenza A viruses of the H5 and H7 subtypes have also been detected in a variety of mammals, including humans. The H5N1 influenza A viruses have been detected in birds, pigs, cats, leopards, tigers,[44] and people in Asia.[64]

Live bird markets that sell a wide variety of domestic and wild bird species to the public provide the perfect conditions for genetic mixing and spread of flu viruses.[94] In addition, traditional poultry livestock practices that bring people into close contact with domestic fowl and promote the mixing of wild and domestic waterfowl also provide opportunities for domestic wildlife viral exchange and spread into humans. Such an occurrence may have been the cause of the avian flu (H5N1) outbreak in Hong Kong in 1997 and again in late 2003-2004 throughout Asia. Once established in poultry in Asia, a combination of intensive production methods and high-volume poultry movement, in addition to poor sanitation and hygiene, allowed the disease to spread.

In 2005, the H5N1 HPAI was isolated from migratory waterfowl on Quinghai Lake, China,[21] and from a wild whooper swan in Mongolia.[1] However, it remains unclear whether migratory waterfowl are effective carriers of the disease or rapidly succumb to the infection before they spread the disease, as may have happened in Mongolia. Calls for mass culling of wild birds have been countered by conservation groups and the FAO.[4]

Of greater concern should be the global trade in domestic and wild birds. An illegal shipment of two crested hawk-eagles (Spizaetus nipalensis), smuggled into Europe from Thailand, was seized at the Brussels International Airport in October 2004. Both birds appeared clinically normal, and both were positive for the H5N1 HPAI.[91]

The threat posed by avian influenza goes beyond the food supply to becoming a lethal virus that is easily spread among people, a global pandemic. Such a scenario portends grave risk to the economies of nations and to the health of people. The report of the U.S. National Intelligence Council identified a global pandemic as the single most important threat to the global economy.[38] As of December 2005, WHO confirmed 142 human cases, with 74 resulting in death. These tragic statistics pale compared with the greater human disease threat. Genetic reassortment of the H5N1 precursor viruses that caused the initial human outbreak in Hong Kong in 1997 may be traced to outbreaks in poultry in China and seven other east Asian countries between

2003 and early 2004. This same virus has been fatal to humans in the region.[55] The fear is that the H5N1 viruses will gain the ability to spread efficiently among people, causing a global pandemic.

There is good reason for concern. In the 20th century, there have been three global pandemics, all believed to have originated from birds.[73] The most severe was the 1918 Spanish influenza pandemic virus (H1N1), which was estimated to have killed 20 to 50 million people worldwide. Pandemic influenza may originate through at least two mechanisms: (1) reassortment between an animal virus and a human virus that yields a new virus; and (2) direct spread and adaptation of a virus from animals to humans.[16] The characterization of the reconstructed 1918 Spanish influenza pandemic virus[84] showed that the direct spread and adaptation of the avian influenza virus caused the pandemic.

GLOBAL CLIMATE CHANGE

Projections using emissions scenarios based on a range of climate models have suggested an increase in global average surface temperature of 1.4° C to 5.8° C over the period of 1990 to 2100. This projected rate of warming would be unprecedented, based on at least the last 10,000 years.[68] The health of people and animals may be affected by an increase in the frequency and severity of climate extremes (e.g., storms, floods, heat waves) and climate-induced changes in the geographic distribution and biologic behavior of arthropod vector–borne[26] and rodent-borne infectious disease.[61] Climatic factors such as increased temperature, increased or decreased precipitation, and sea level rise may all have an impact on the emergence or reemergence of infectious diseases.

Climate plays a critical role in the maintenance of vector species as well as pathogens. Studies have suggested that warming will enhance transmission intensity and extend the distribution of certain vector-borne diseases.[69,78] The complexity of ecologic systems and human-induced changes to the environment make it difficult to establish definitive links between predicted climate-induced changes and emerging arthropod vector–borne and rodent-borne diseases. However, there are a number of diseases to consider as candidates.

Arthropod Vector–Borne Diseases

Vector organisms, such as mosquitoes and ticks, transport pathogens from an infected individual or its wastes to susceptible individuals, their food, or immediate surroundings. Climate alterations may affect the distribution of vector species, changing their range because of altered conditions for breeding and feeding. Temperature may also affect survival rates of both the pathogen and the vector organism, further influencing disease transmission. The range of the major arthropod vector–borne zoonotic pathogens includes both parasitic and viral diseases. Parasitic organisms spread by vectors include malaria (*Plasmodium*), Chagas' disease (*Trypanosoma cruzi*), Lyme disease (*Borrelia burgdorferi*), and leishmaniasis (*Leishmania*). The vector-spread arboviruses include organisms in the family Flaviviridae (e.g., St. Louis encephalitis, dengue fever, yellow fever, West Nile virus), Bunyaviridae (e.g., La Crosse virus), and Togaviridae (e.g., eastern, western, and Venezuelan equine encephalitis).

Lyme Disease

Lyme disease is transmitted primarily by the deer tick, *Ixodes scapularis*. It is the most common vector-borne disease of people in the United States[36] and is perpetuated in a life cycle that involves rodent reservoir hosts, such as white-footed mice (*Peromyscus leucopus*) in eastern North America and *Apodemus* mice in Eurasia. Lyme disease spirochetes have been shown to infect a diverse number of mammals and birds, but not all have been shown to serve as competent hosts.[79] Symptoms in humans may include erythema migrans in approximately 50% of patients, and signs in both humans and other mammals may include fever, lameness, listlessness, anorexia, lymphadenopathy, and joint swelling. Other signs referable to affected systems may include reproductive difficulties and arthritides.

The dilution effect model suggests that the loss of the diversity of vertebrate reservoir hosts caused by anthropogenic forces may increase the spread of Lyme disease. As habitats are degraded, the diversity of potential hosts decreases. Many members of this diverse group of potential tick hosts are less competent as Lyme disease reservoirs. These species-poor communities tend to have low levels of those species that are less competent as reservoir hosts and high levels of the most competent disease reservoir, the white-footed mouse (*P. leucopus*).[58]

The influence of climate change on the distribution of *I. scapularis* and the spread of Lyme disease in North America has been modeled.[19] Projections suggest that the range of the tick will extend into Canada. In addition, as a disease primarily carried by rodents, climate change may further affect the distribution of Lyme disease by altering the range of the rodent hosts.

West Nile Virus

West Nile virus (WNV) was first isolated from the blood of a febrile woman in the West Nile district of Uganda in 1937.[83] Thereafter, it was isolated from ill people, birds, and mosquitoes in Egypt during the early 1950s. WNV is recognized as the most widespread of the flaviviruses, with geographic distribution in Africa and Eurasia.[37] The disease entered the Western Hemisphere in New York in 1999, with deaths observed in humans, horses, and many species of wild birds, although primarily corvids. The virus subsequently has spread across North America[74] and into tropical America and the Carribbean.[48,50]

WNV presentation varies with the species and may range from no signs to death, with the typical illness including encephalitis and fever. The CDC Division of Vector-Borne Disease notes that more than 284 species of birds and domestic and wild mammals have been affected.

Although bird-feeding species of mosquito are the principal vectors, WNV has been isolated from numerous additional species of mosquito, as well as from ticks.[37] Global climate change alterations that include warmer temperatures with higher humidity would favor the increase in abundance and distribution of the mosquito vectors.[78]

Dengue Fever

Dengue fever (DF) is caused by one of four closely related but antigenically distinct virus serotypes of the genus *Flavivirus*.[35] It is the most common vector-borne disease of humans, infecting an estimated 50 million people in tropical and subtropical regions of the world each year.[89] In humans, symptoms of DF may range from inapparent to a mild influenza-like illness to an immune-mediated hemorrhagic fever that may be fatal if untreated.[85]

Dengue viruses are transmitted between people or between monkeys through mosquitoes of the genus *Aedes*. Estimates are that the zoonotic transfer of dengue from monkeys to sustained human transmission occurred between 125 and 320 years ago.[89] DF is endemic in approximately 100 countries in southeast Asia, Africa, the western Pacific, the Americas, Africa, and the eastern Mediterranean.[20]

The reasons for the global emergence of DF are multifactorial; they include ineffective mosquito control, major urbanization shifts in demographics, and unimpeded international travel, which allows people to move the virus into new population centers. However, climate change is also implicated as a potential future factor;

modeling studies project that a warming of 2° C by 2100 will result in a net increase in the potential latitudinal and altitudinal range of DF and an increase in duration of the transmission season in temperate locations.[61]

Rodent-Borne Diseases

Rodent-borne diseases spread from species to species through contact with rodent urine, feces, or other body fluids. Climate change factors that may expand the range and increase the reproductive potential of rodent populations include increased rainfall, warmer temperatures, and climatic extremes.

Leptospirosis

Leptospirosis is a reemerging zoonotic disease of global importance that occurs in urban settings of industrialized and developing countries,[17] as well as in rural environments worldwide. It affects domestic livestock,[43] alternative livestock,[59] and free-ranging[90] and captive[57] wild mammals, including marine mammals.[23] Both rodents and dogs are important vectors[63] in the urban and agricultural setting. The transmission of leptospirosis occurs most often through contact with water contaminated by urine from infected shedders.

Leptospirosis is caused by a filamentous spiral bacterium that has a predilection for renal tubules. In humans, the disease symptoms may range from subclinical to epidemic leptospirosis, associated with pulmonary hemorrhage, renal failure, and jaundice. In domestic animals, as well as captive and free-ranging wildlife, the animals may appear clinically normal or may present with disease signs referable to renal and reproductive tract infection. In captive wildlife, leptospirosis is often an insidious infection that may result in chronic renal disease and high rates of reproductive failure.

Rodent populations in temperate and tropical climates may serve as the reservoir host for domestic and wild animals as well as human infection. Outbreaks of human disease are often associated with increases in rodent populations after heavy rainfall or during floods.[65,88]

Hantavirus

Hantaviruses (genus *Hantavirus*) cause two major clinical syndromes of people in different areas of the world. Hemorrhagic fever with renal syndrome is seen in Asia and Europe, whereas a pulmonary syndrome is described in the Americas.[76] Hantavirus is a zoonotic virus of rodents and has emerged as a human pathogen as a result of human-induced landscape alterations and climatic changes influencing population dynamics of the rodent reservoir hosts.[98]

Outbreaks of disease may be associated with weather that promotes rapid increases in the rodent population, which may vary seasonally and annually.[32] A study of the relationship between climate and the prevalence of hantavirus pulmonary syndrome in Arizona, New Mexico, Colorado, and Utah regions found an increase in rodents was associated with increased precipitation patterns during the 1992-1993 El Niño. An outbreak of hantavirus pulmonary syndrome occurred in this region during 1993.[29]

INTEGRATED APPROACH TO WORLD HEALTH: ONE WORLD, ONE HEALTH

The dramatic increase in emerging disease outbreaks and the growing number of diseases moving between species indicate that traditional approaches to disease management, currently segregated into human, livestock, and wildlife health, are not effective. In addition to the suffering and death, these diseases result in billions of dollars spent on reacting to outbreaks that would be more efficiently spent on prevention. We must seek to be proactive, prevent rather than react, and control global movement of people and animals more thoughtfully. To devise sound solutions, we must develop a unified approach that incorporates the knowledge and experience of broad areas of science and health. This approach must be flexible to respond to novel threats, adaptive to react to changing situations, distributive to monitor change at the global scale, and inclusive to learn from the varied experience of human, domestic animal, and livestock disease knowledge.[24] In short, a one health approach is needed.[5,41,67] Although this concept is centuries old, the application is new; there is only one health for people, domestic animals, and wildlife.

Changing the Global Perspective

Society has not yet fully adapted to the changes brought on by globalization. Multilateral organizations are responsible for public health (WHO) and livestock health (FAO, OIE), but there is no similar umbrella organization to bring together the worldwide focus on wildlife health. Until such a body is formed, wildlife will continue to be a footnote to human and domestic animal health perspectives and will continue

to be the surprise critical variable in emerging disease spread.

The World Trade Organization (WTO) and other appropriate international bodies must start requiring governments to regulate the health aspects of international trade better in wild and domestic animals. Individual nations must implement and enforce laws to prevent the spread of diseases within their borders. It is clear that trade and the consumption of wildlife have led to global health disasters; governments must therefore make greater efforts to reduce and properly regulate the wildlife trade internationally, regionally, and locally.

Role of Zoo and Wildlife Health Professionals

The complexity of the emerging disease and health issues that humanity confronts at the interface of people, domestic animals, and wildlife requires a multidisciplinary approach to problem solving. Zoo and wildlife health professionals have the unique comparative systems perspective that is essential to the multidisciplinary team. Surveillance for the emergence of new diseases is a critical component of a sound approach to disease mitigation, control, and prevention. For example, the veterinary health professionals from zoos of the Association of Zoos and Aquariums (AZA) participate in reporting systems for tuberculosis monitoring in hoofstock[86] and a national surveillance system for WNV in zoological institutions.[87] This is a significant first step, but it must be followed by expanded efforts for broader disease surveillance on a global scale.

To be effective, the profession must establish collaborative and communications links with public health and domestic animal health agencies, diagnostic centers, human and veterinary medical facilities, and university-based health research institutions. New public-private partnerships must be fostered with the corporate sector. The multinational industries best understand the threat to global supply chains, economies, and the health of their employees and the consuming public. Overall, zoo and wildlife health professionals must become active participants and advocates for a broader view of health.

REFERENCES

1. Anonymous: Avian flu, H5N1, identified in Wild Mongolian birds, 2005 (http://news.mongabay.com/2005/0818-wcs_flu.html).
2. Anonymous: Thinking ahead: The business significance of an avian influenza pandemic, 2005 (http://www.bio-era.net).

3. Anonymous: Species list, Asia Animals Foundation, 2005 (https:www.animalsasia.orgindex.php?module=6&menupos=2&submenupos=5&lg=en).

4. Anonymous: Avian flu: No need to kill wild birds; better biosecurity measures are essential for safer poultry production, Food and Agricultural Organization of the United Nations, 2004 (http://www.fao.org/newsroom/en/news/2004/48287/index.html).

5. Anonymous: One World One Health Symposium, Rockefeller University, 2004 (http://www.oneworldonehealth.org).

6. Anonymous: World Population 2004, United Nations Department of Economic and Social Affairs, 2004 (http://www.unpopulation.org).

7. Anonymous: Animals suffer in war on SARS, British Broadcasting Corporation, 2003 (http://news.bbc.co.uk/l/low/world/asia-pacific/2989479.stm).

8. Anonymous: Cumulative number of reported probable cases of SARS, World Health Organization Communicable Disease Surveillance and Response, 2003 (http://www.who.int/csr/sars/country/2003 07 11/ en).

9. Anonymous: Human SARS virus not identical to civet virus, The Scientist, 2003 (http://www.the-scientist.com).

10. Anonymous: Update: Multistate outbreak of monkeypox—Illinois, Indiana, Kansas, Missouri, Ohio, and Wisconsin, 2003 (http://www.cdc.gov/mmwr/preview/ mmwrhtml/mm5227a5.htm).

11. Anonymous: Variant Creutzfeldt-Jakob disease, World Health Organization, 2002 (http://www.who.int/mediacentre/factsheets/fs180/en/print.html).

12 Anonymous: Souvenir alert highlights deadly trade in endangered species, World Wildlife Fund–United Kingdom, 2001 (http://www.wwf.org.uk/news/scotland/n_0000000409.asp).

13. Anonymous: Report of the committee on Public Health and Environmental Quality, United States Animal Health Association, Proceedings of the USAHA Ninety-Ninth Annual Meeting, Reno, Nevada, 1995, pp 471–480.

14. Belay ED, Gambetti P, Schonberger LB, et al: Creutzfeldt-Jakob disease in unusually young patients who consumed venison. Arch Neurol 58:1673–1678, 2001.

15. Belay ED, Maddox RA, Williams ES, et al: Chronic wasting disease and potential transmission to humans. J Emerg Infect Dis 10:977–984, 2004.

16. Belshe RB: The origins of pandemic influenza: Lessons from the 1918 virus. N Engl J Med 353:2209–2211, 2005.

17. Bharti AR, Nally JE, Ricaldi JN, et al: Leptospirosis: A zoonotic disease of global importance. Lancet Infect Dis 3:757–771, 2003.

18. Brown C: Vulnerabilities in agriculture. J Vet Med Educ 30:227–229, 2003.

19. Brownstein JS, Holford TR, Fish D: Effect of climate change on Lyme disease risk in North America. EcoHealth 2:38–46, 2005.

20. Calisher CH: Persistent emergence of dengue. J Emerg Infect Dis 11:738–739, 2005.

21. Chen H, Smith GJ, Zhang SY, et al: Avian flu: H5N1 virus outbreak in migratory waterfowl. Nature 436:191–192, 2005.

22. Clayton LM, Milner-Gulland EJ: The trade in wildlife in North Sulawesi, Indonesia. In Robinson JG, Bennett EL, editors: Hunting for Sustainability in Tropical Forests. New York, 2000, Columbia University Press, pp 473–498.

23. Colegrove KM, Lowenstine LJ, Gulland FM: Leptospirosis in northern elephant seals (Mirounga angustirostris) stranded along the California coast. J Wildl Dis 41:426–430, 2005.

24. Cook RA, Karesh WB: Ebola, SARS, and other diseases that imperil people and animals. In Guynup S, editor: State of the Wild. Washington, DC, 2005, Island Press, pp 131–138.

25. Cunningham AA, Kirkwood JK, Dawson M, et al: Bovine spongiform encephalopathy infectivity in greater kudu (Tragelaphus strepsiceros). J Emerg Infect Dis 10:1044–1049, 2004.

26. Daszak P, Cunningham AA. Hyatt AD: Emerging infectious diseases of wildlife: Threats to biodiversity and human health. Science 287:443–449, 2000.

27. Daszak P, Strieby A, Cunningham AA, et al: Experimental evidence that the bullfrog (Rana catesbeiana) is a potential carrier of chytridiomycosis, an emerging fungal disease of amphibians. Herpetol J 14:201–207, 2004.

28. Dobson AP: What links bats to emerging infectious diseases? Science 310:628–629, 2005.

29. Engelthaler DM, Mosley DG, Cheek JE, et al: Climatic and environmental patterns associated with hantavirus pulmonary syndrome, Four Corners Region, United States. J Emerg Infect Dis 5:87–94, 1999.

30. Friedman TL: The Lexus and the Olive Tree. New York, 2000, Anchor Books, pp 7–8.

31. Geisbert TW, Pushko P, Anderson K, et al: Evaluation in nonhuman primates of vaccines against Ebola virus. J Emerg Infect Dis 8:503–507, 2002.

32. Glass G, Cheek J, Patz JA, et al: Predicting high risk areas for hantavirus pulmonary syndrome with remotely sensed data: The Four Corners outbreak, 1993. J Emerg Infect Dis 6:238–247, 2000.

33. Guan Y, Zheng BJ, He YQ, et al: Isolation and characterization of viruses related to the SARS coronavirus from animals in Southern China. Science 302:276–278, 2003.

34. Guarner J, Johnson BJ, Paddock CD, et al, Veterinary Monkeypox Virus Working Group: Monkeypox transmission and pathogenesis in prairie dogs. J Emerg Infect Dis 10:426–431, 2004.

35. Gubler DJ, Clark GG: Dengue/dengue hemorrhagic fever: The emergence of a global health problem. J Emerg Infect Dis 1:55–57, 1995.

36. Guerra M, Walker E, Jones C, et al: Predicting the risk of Lyme disease: Habitat suitability for Ixodes scapularis in the north central United States. J Emerg Infect Dis 8:289–297, 2002.

37. Hubalek Z, Halouzka J: West Nile fever: Reemerging mosquito-borne viral disease in Europe. J Emerg Infect Dis 5:643–650, 1999.

38. Hutchings RL: Mapping the Global Future: Report of the National Intelligence Council's 2020 Project, GOP Stock 041-015-0024-6. Washington, DC, 2004, US Government Printing Office.

39. Hutin YJF, Williams RJ, Malfait P, et al: Outbreak of human monkeypox, Democratic Republic of Congo, 1996 to 1997. J Emerg Infect Dis 7:434–438, 2001.

40. Kalish ML, Wolfe ND, Ndongmo CB, et al: Central African hunters exposed to simian immunodeficiency virus. J Emerg Infect Dis 11:1928–1930, 2005.

41. Karesh WB, Cook RA: The human-animal link. Foreign Affairs 84:38–50, 2005.

42. Karesh WB, Cook RA, Bennett EL, Newcomb J: Wildlife trade and global disease emergence. J Emerg Infect Dis 11:1000–1002, 2005.

43. Karesh WB, Uhart MM, Dierenfeld ES, et al: Health evaluation of free-ranging guanaco (Lama guanicoe). J Zoo Wildl Med 29:134–141, 1998.

44. Keawcharoen J, Oraveerakul K, Kuiken T, et al: Avian influenza in tigers and leopards. J Emerg Infect Dis 10:2189–2191, 2004.

45. Kiesecker JM, Belden LK, Shea K, Rubbo MJ: Amphibian decline and emerging disease. Am Scientist 92:138–147, 2004.

46. Kimball AM, Plotkin BJ, Harrison TA, Pautlet NF: Trade-related infections: Global traffic and microbial travel. EcoHealth 39–49, 2004.

47. Kishore GM, Shewmaker C: Biotechnology: Enhancing human nutrition in developing and developed worlds. Proc Natl Acad Sci U S A 96:5968–5972, 1999.

48. Komar O, Robbins MB, Klenk K, et al: West Nile virus transmission in resident birds, Dominican Republic. J Emerg Infect Dis 9:1299–1302, 2003.

49. Kuiken T, Leighton FA, Fouchier RAM, et al: Pathogen surveillance in animals. Science 309:1680–1681, 2005.

50. Lanciotti RS, Roehrig JT, Beubel V, et al: Origin of West Nile virus responsible for an outbreak of encephalitis in the northeastern United States. Science 286:2333–2337, 1999.

51. Lau SKP, Woo PCY, Li KSM, et al: Severe acute respiratory syndrome coronavirus-like virus in Chinese horseshoe bats. Proc Natl Acad Sci U S A 102(39):14040–14045, 2005.

52. Le Guenno B, Formenty P, Wyers M, et al: Isolation and partial characterization of a new strain of Ebola virus. Lancet 345:1271–1274, 1995.

53. Leroy EM, Rouquet P, Formently P, et al: Multiple Ebola virus transmission events and rapid decline of central African wildlife. Science 16:298–299, 2004.

54. Leroy EM, Kumulungui B, Pourrut X, et al: Fruit bats as reservoirs of Ebola virus. Nature 438:575–576, 2005.

55. Li KS, Guan Y, Wang J, et al: Genesis of highly pathogenic and potentially pandemic H5N1 influenza virus in Eastern Asia. Nature 430:209–213, 2004.

56. Li W, Shi Z, Yu M, et al: Bats are natural reservoirs of SARS-like coronaviruses. Science 310:676–679, 2005.

57. Lilenbaum W, Varges R, Moraes IA, et al: Leptospiral antibodies in captive lion tamarins (Leontopithecus sp.). Vet J 169:462–464, 2005.

58. LoGiudice K, Ostfeld RS, Schmidt KA, Keesing F: The ecology of infectious disease: Effects of host diversity and community composition on Lyme disease risk. Proc Natl Acad Sci U S A 110:567–571, 2003.

59. Machintosh C, Haigh JC, Griffin F: Bacterial diseases of farmed deer and bison. Rev Sci Tech 21:249–263, 2002.

60. Mazzoni R, Cunningham AA, Daszak P, et al: Emerging pathogen of wild amphibians in frogs (Rana catesbeiana) farmed for international trade. J Emerg Infect Dis 9:995–998, 2003.

61. McCarthy JJ, Canziani OF, Leary NA, et al: Climate change 2001: Impacts, adaptation, and vulnerability. In Contribution of Working Group II to Third Assessment Report of Intergovernmental Panel on Climate Change. New York, 2001, Cambridge University Press.

62. Miranda ME, Ksiazek TG, Retuya TJ, et al: Epidemiology of Ebola (subtype Reston) virus in the Philippines, 1996. J Infect Dis 179(Suppl. 1):115–119, 1999.

63. Montes AS, Dimas JS, Preciado Rodriguez FJ: Rats and dogs: Important vectors of leptospirosis in agricultural areas in Ciudad Guzman, Jalisco. Rev Cubana Med Trop 54:21–23, 2002.

64. Munster VJ, Wallensten A, Baas C, et al: Mallards and highly pathogenic avian influenza ancestral viruses, northern Europe. J Emerg Infect Dis 11:1545–1551, 2005.

65. Narita M, Fujitani S, Haake DA, Paterson DL: Leptospirosis after recreational exposure to water in Yaeyama Islands, Japan. Am J Trop Med Hyg 73:652–656, 2005.

66. Newcomb J: Economic risks associated with an influenza pandemic: Testimony before the US Senate Committee on Foreign Relations, 9 Nov 2005 (http://bio-era.net/Asset/iu_files/Bio-era%20Research%20Reports/Final_testimony_1108_clean.pdf).

67. Osofsky SA, Koch RA, Kock MD, et al: Building support for protected areas using a "one health" perspective. In McNeely JA, editor: Friends for Life: New Partners in Support of Protected Areas, Gland, Switzerland, IUCN, 2005, World Conservation Union, pp 65–80.

68. Pachauri RK: Address by the Chairman of the Intergovernmental Panel on Climate Change at the High Level Segment. Presented at the 11th Conference of the Parties of the United Nations Framework Convention on Climate Change and 1st Conference of the Parties to the Kyoto Protocol, 2005 (http://www.ipcc.ch/press/sp-07122005.htm).

69. Patz JA, Epstein PR, Burke TA, Balbus JM: Global climate change and emerging infectious diseases. JAMA 275:217–223, 1996.

70. Patz JA, Graczyk TK, Geller N, Vittor A: Effects of environmental change on emerging parasitic disease. Int J Parasitol 30:1395–1405, 2000.

71. Peiris JSM, Guan Y: Confronting SARS: A view from Hong Kong. Trans R Soc Lond Biol Sci 359:1075–1079, 2004.

72. Peres CA: Effects of subsistence hunting on vertebrate community structure in Amazonian forests. In Robinson JG, Bennett EL, editors: Hunting for Sustainability in Tropical Forests, New York, 2000, Columbia University Press, pp 168–198.

73. Perez DR, Sorrell EM, Donis RO: Avian influenza: An omnipresent pandemic threat. Pediatr Infect Dis J 24(Suppl):S208–S216, 2005.

74. Petersen LR, Marfin AA, Gubler DJ: West Nile virus. JAMA 290:524–528, 2003.

75. Peterson AT, Bauer JT, Mills JN: Ecological and geographic distribution of filovirus disease. J Emerg Infect Dis 10:40–47, 2004.

76. Pini N, Levis S, Calderon G, et al: Hantavirus infection in humans and rodents, northwestern Argentina. J Emerg Infect Dis 9:1070–1076, 2003.

77. Prusiner SB: Prions. Proc Natl Acad Sci U S A 95:13363–13383, 1998.

78. Reeves WC, Hardy JL, Reisen WK, Milby MM: Potential effect of global warming on mosquito-borne arboviruses. J Med Entomol 31:323–332, 1994.

79. Richter D, Spielman A, Komar N, Matuschka F: Competence of American robins as reservoir hosts for Lyme disease spirochetes. J Emerg Infect Dis 6:133–138, 2000.

80. Ridley M: Genome: The Autobiography of a Species in 23 Chapters. New York, 1999, Harper Collins, p 28.

81. Round PD: Bangkok Bird Club survey of the bird and mammal trade in the Bangkok Weekend Market. Natl Hist Bull Siam Soc 38:1–43, 1990.

82. Sanchez A, Ksiazek TG, Rollin PE, et al: Reemergence of Ebola virus in Africa. J Emerg Infect Dis 1:96–97, 1995.

83. Smithburn KC, Hughes TP, Burke AW, Paul JH: A neurotropic virus isolated from the blood of a native of Uganda. Am J Trop Med Hyg 20:471–492, 1940.

84. Taubenberger JK, Reid AH, Lourens RM, et al: Characterization of the 1918 influenza virus polymerase genes. Nature 437:889–893, 2005.

85. Thu HM, Lowry K, Myint TT, et al: Myanmar dengue outbreak associated with displacement of serotypes 2, 3, and 4 by dengue 1. J Emerg Infect Dis 10:593–597, 2004.

86. Travis DA, Barbiers RB, Ziccardi MH: An overview of the National Zoological Tuberculosis Monitoring System for Hoofstock. Presented at the Annual Proceedings of the American Association of Zoo Veterinarians (AAZV), Minneapolis, 2003.

87. Travis DA, McNamara T, Glaser A, et al: A national surveillance system for West Nile virus in zoological institutions. In Proceedings of the National Emerging Infectious Disease Conference, Atlanta, 2002. p 69.

88. Trevejo RT, Rigau-Perez JG, Ashford DA, et al: Epidemic leptospirosis associated with pulmonary hemorrhage—Nicaragua, 1995. J Infect Dis 178:1457–1463, 1998.

89. Twiddy SS, Holmes EC, Rambaut A: Inferring the rate and time-scale of dengue virus evolution. Mol Biol Evol 20:122–129, 2003.

90. Uhart MM, Vila AR, Beade MS, et al: Health evaluation of pampas deer (Ozotoceros bezoarticus) at Campos del Tuyu Wildlife Reserve, Argentina. J Wildl Dis 39:887–893, 2003.

91. Van Born S, Thomas I, Hanquet G, et al: Highly pathogenic H5N1 influenza virus in smuggled Thai eagles, Belgium. J Emerg Infect Dis 11:702–705, 2005.

92. Walsh PD, Abernethy KA, Bermejo M, et al: Catastrophic ape declines in western equatorial Africa. Nature 422:611–614, 2003.

93. Wang JT, Chang SC: Severe acute respiratory syndrome. Curr Opin Infect Dis 17:143–148, 2004.

94. Webster RG: Influenza: an emerging disease. J Emerg Infect Dis 4:436–441, 1998.

95. Webster RG, Bean WJ, Gorman OT, et al: Evolution and ecology of influenza A viruses. Microbiol Rev 56:152–179, 1992.

96. Wilkie DS, Carpenter JF: Bushmeat hunting in the Congo Basin: An assessment of impacts and options for mitigation. Biodiversity Conservation 8:927–955, 1999.

97. Williams ES, Miller MW, Kreeger TJ, et al: Chronic wasting disease of deer and elk: A review with recommendations for management. J Wildl Manage 66: 551–563, 2002.

98. Williams ES, Yuill T, Artois M, et al: Emerging infectious diseases in wildlife. Rev Sci Tech 21:139–157, 2002.

99. Wolfe ND, Daszak P, Kilpatrick AM, Burke DS: Bushmeat hunting, deforestation, and prediction of zoonotic disease emergence. J Emerg Infect Dis 11:1822–1827, 2005.

100. Woolhouse MEJ, Gowtage-Sequeria S: Host range and emerging and reemerging pathogens. J Emerg Infect Dis 11:1842–1847, 2005.

101. Yob JM, Field H, Rashdi AM, et al: Nipah virus infection in bats (order Chiroptera) in Peninsular Malaysia. J Emerg Infect Dis 7:439–441, 2001.

CHAPTER 19

Depth of Anesthesia Monitoring by Bispectral Analysis in Zoo Animals

Jean-Michel Hatt and Olga Martin Jurado

General anesthesia is required in zoological medicine for a variety of reasons, including painful (e.g., surgery) and nonpainful interventions (e.g., radiographic examination). Typically, induction will be achieved via an injectable anesthetic, alone or as a combination. In addition to achieving analgesia and hypnosis, anesthesia in zoological medicine aims at the safe immobilization of the patient over a determined time period. Recovery time is expected to be quick, especially under field conditions, and safe both for the animal and the personnel involved. Monitoring of the patient under general anesthesia is done by a variety of tests. Some of these evaluate hemodynamic functions and autonomic nervous responses, such as heart rate, respiratory rate, blood pressure, and oxygen saturation. Others are intended to measure the depth of anesthesia (DoA) with respect to the degree of hypnosis and analgesia, including measurement of the patient's reactions to nonphysiologic positions such as dorsal recumbency (righting reflex), corneal and pupillary reflexes, and toe pinch stimulation.

In human medicine, DoA measurement is of special importance to avoid occurrence of awareness—that is, the postoperative recollection of events occurring during general anesthesia. In a recent review, incidences of awareness up to 0.2% in adults and up to 0.8% in children were reported.[3]

In veterinary medicine, the role of awareness cannot be assessed because animals cannot report their postanesthetic experiences. Measurement of DoA is nevertheless of interest from an animal welfare point of view. In zoological medicine, DoA monitoring is of further interest from a personnel and equipment safety point of view. However, the reliability of a stimulation test with regard to the large number of species encountered by the clinician in zoological medicine is at best adequate in relation to safety.

For safety reasons, often a lower than necessary DoA will be chosen, which only prolongs recovery but increases the dose-dependent cardiopulmonary impairment, resulting in an increase of postanesthetic morbidity and mortality. This is reflected by the high anesthetic- and sedative-related risk of death, which ranges in small mammals from 1.4% to 3.6%, in birds from 1.8% to 16.3%, and in reptiles it is 1.5%, compared with dogs and cats (0.1% to 0.2%) and humans (0.02% to 0.01%[2]). In wildlife anesthesia, mortalities up to 3% have been reported and it was proposed that mortalities above 2% should not be acceptable.[1]

Established DoA monitors include the bispectral index (BIS, Aspect Medical Systems, Norwood, Mass), the Narcotrend index (Narcotrend Monitor, Schiller AG, Baar, Switzerland), and the state entropy (SE) and response entropy (RE), derived from the spectral entropy from the electroencephalogram (EEG; M-Entropy module, GE Healthcare, Helsinki, Finland).

These monitors process the level of corticocerebral activation measured by analog EEGs into a signal that reflects the DoA. The most widely used monitor is the BIS, which in 2004 was used in approximately 34% of all hospital operating rooms in the United States and 78% of teaching institutions, and had a worldwide installation base of over 25,000 units.[8] Numerous studies have investigated the BIS. An Internet search on the term *bispectral index anesthesia* in August 2010 produced over 138,000 results, including a report on the use of the BIS in animals, including the dog, cat, horse, and goat.[9]

Just like any monitor, the BIS offers possibilities but also has limitations, especially with respect to various drugs. The transposition from a single-species environment such as human medicine to the multitude of species encountered in zoological medicine needs to be done with appropriate care, as with pulse oximetry.

147

In this chapter, we review the data from studies with BIS measurement in animals and include data on non-domestic animals obtained from studies that were carried out in our laboratory.

BISPECTRAL ANALYSIS METHODOLOGY

Bispectral analysis is based on a complex statistical evaluation of human electroencephalographic data that was developed to obtain an index of the level of hypnosis. It uses a Fourier transform, an operation that transforms one complex-valued function of a real variable into another, such as time into frequency. The BIS value is represented as a dimensionless value from 0 (cortical silence) to 100 (awake) (Fig. 19-1). In humans, an optimal degree of general anesthesia is defined as that associated with a BIS within the range of 40 to 60.

In 1996, the U.S. Food and Drug Administration approved the BIS monitor as an accepted measure of the hypnotic effect of anesthetics and sedative drugs in humans. Since its introduction, BIS monitoring has gained increasing popularity in daily anesthesia practice. However, the current evidence indicates various cases of paradoxical BIS changes and inaccurate readings, which also need to be to be taken into consideration when applying the BIS in veterinary medicine (Table 19-1).[4,6]

TECHNIQUE AND OPTIMUM SETTING

The equipment includes a monitor, a digital signal processing cable, and three electrodes with sensors. Newer models include four sensors. It is important to note that the algorithm has been constantly adapted from one model to the other. Therefore, every BIS system will yield different values and the anesthetist needs to be familiar with the system that is being used to interpret changes in values adequately. As with the use of pulse oximetry in zoo animals, the most valuable types of information are the trends indicated by the BIS.

The monitor is available as stand-alone system or as an add-on module for most comprehensive patient monitoring systems. Our studies were performed with an A-2000-XP Platform Bispectral Index Monitoring System (Aspect Medical Systems). The sensors were fitted with 24-gauge needles to allow subcutaneous placement instead of the need to shave or pluck the areas, even in small animals. The impedances for sensors 1 and 3 and for sensor 2 were always <7.5 kΩ and <30 kΩ, respectively. Figure 19-2 graphically displays the location of the sensors.

Based on the system we used, the different results are displayed in Figure 19-3. The main value is the BIS value, ranging from 0 (flatline or isoelectric EEG) to 100 (awake), which is displayed every 5 seconds. This represents the mean of the maximum and minimum indices of the last 15 or 30 seconds. This smoothing rate needs to be selected in the main menu. In cases of high interference, a longer smoothing rate (30 seconds) is chosen.

An important additional value is the suppression ratio (SR), which is the proportion of signals over the last 63-second period for which the electroencephalographic signals are considered to be suppressed or inactive (flatline). It ranges from 0 (no suppression) to 100 (maximal suppression, or isoelectric EEG). Therefore, the lower the value, the better the signal.

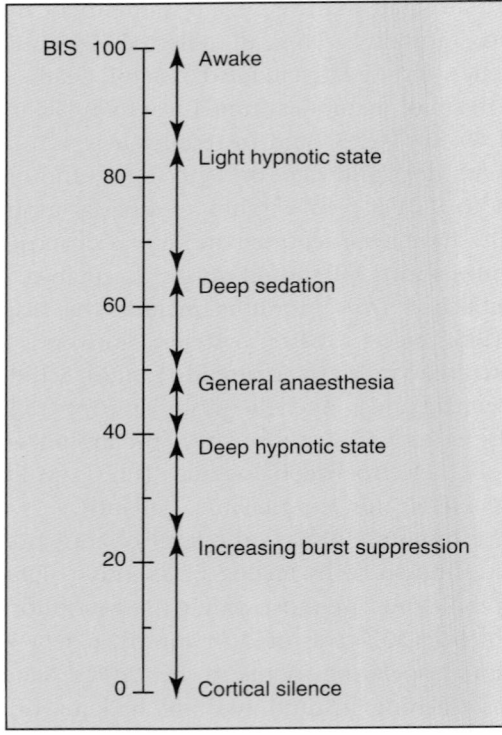

Figure 19-1

The bispectral index (BIS) scale is a dimensionless scale from 0 (flatline) to 100 (awake). We used the A-2000-XP Platform Bispectral Index Monitoring System (Aspect Medical Systems, Norwood, Mass). BIS values of 65 to 85 have been recommended for a light hypnotic state, whereas values of 50 to 65 for deep sedation and values of 40 to 50 for general anesthesia are used. BIS values from 40 to 25 have been seen to produce a deep hypnotic state and, with the BIS less than 25, cortical suppression becomes more and more manifest. *(From Martin Jurado O: Determination of the Anaesthesia Depth in Chickens with Bispectral Index [BIS]. Ph.D. Thesis, University of Zurich, Zurich, 2008.)*

TABLE 19-1 Effect of Various Factors on Bispectral Index Monitoring in Humans and Horses

Effect	BIS Model	BIS Change	Explanation
Anesthetic Agent			
Ketamine	A-1050, A-2000	Paradoxical BIS ↑	β waves ↑, δ waves ↓
Detomidine + butorphanol	A-1000	BIS ↓	In horses
Isoflurane	A-1000	Paradoxical BIS ↑	α, β waves ↑
Halothane	BIS-XP, A-1000	High BIS	Different cortical effect
Clinical Condition			
Warming blanket	A-1000, A-2000	BIS ↑	Air vibration
Hypoglycemia	A-2000, BIS-XP	BIS ↓	δ, θ waves ↑, α waves ↓
Hypovolemia		BIS ↓	Cerebral perfusion ↓
Hypothermia	A-1050, A-1000	BIS ↓	Isoflurane enhancement, propofol enhancement
Brain death	A-2000	BIS 0	Isoelectricity
Neuromuscular blocking drugs	A-1000, A-2000	BIS ↓	Alleviating electromyogram artifact

Data from Dahaba AA: Different conditions that could result in the bispectral index indicating an incorrect hypnotic state. Anaesth Analg 101:765-773, 2005; and Haga HA, Dolvik NI: Evaluation of the bispectral index as an indicator of degree of central nervous system depression in isoflurane-anaesthetized horses. Am J Vet Res 63:438-442, 2002.

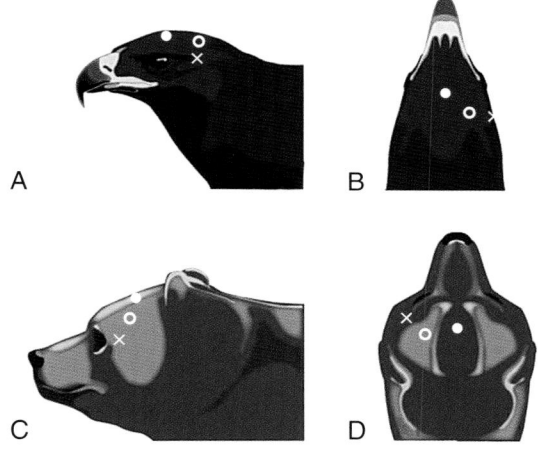

Figure 19-2

Placement of sensors for bispectral index monitoring in a bird (**A, B**) and mammal (**C, D**). Sensor 1 *(dot)* is placed between the eyes in the frontal area. Sensor 2 *(circle)* is placed over the temporal musculature. Sensor 3 *(X)* is placed immediately caudal to the eye angle. *(Courtesy Jeanne Peter, Institute of Veterinary Anatomy, University of Zurich, Zurich, Switzerland.)*

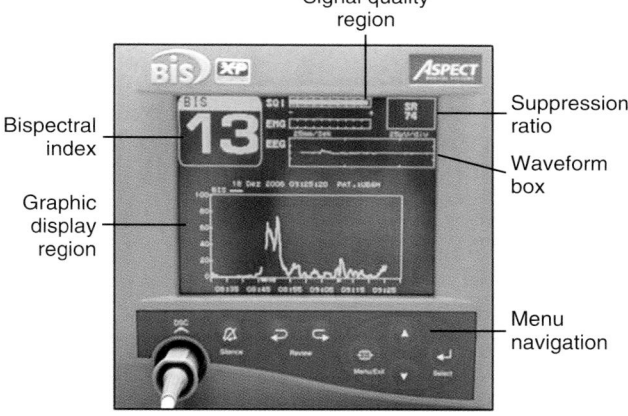

Figure 19-3

Bispectral index monitor. *(A-2000-XP Platform Bispectral Index Monitoring System, Aspect Medical Systems, Norwood, Mass.)*

The quality of the EEG signal is evaluated by combining the signal quality index (SQI) and electromyography (EMG) variables. The SQI is calculated on the basis of impedance data, artifacts, and other variables. It is scaled from 0 (no quality) to 100 (maximal quality). An electromyogram is also scaled from 0 (minimal) to 100 (maximal) and indicates the power in the high-frequency range, as well as muscle activity. Interference control is typically achieved by rejecting SQI values under 50% and/or electromyographic values over 50%. The electroencephalographic signal display works with a preset sweep rate of 25 mm/second and a scale of 25 μV/division.

REPTILES

The determination of the DoA in reptiles is challenging, as shown in the following examples. The electrical activity of the cortex of Hermann's tortoises *(Testudo*

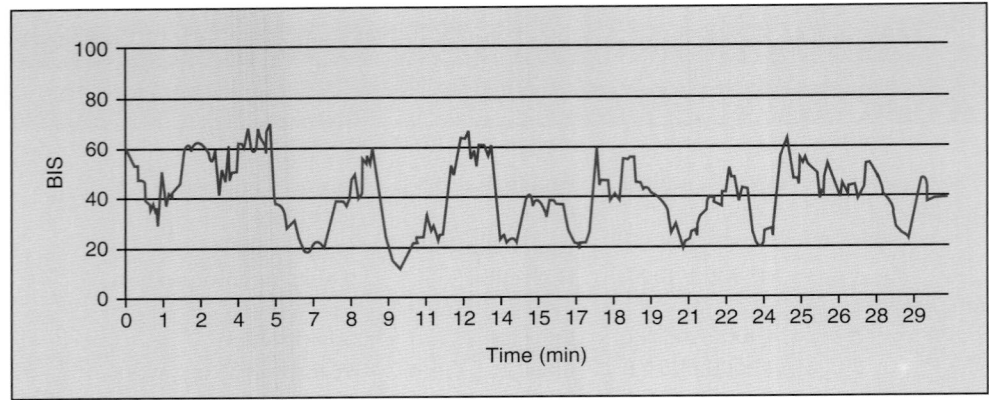

Figure 19-4

Bispectral index values of a Hermann's tortoise *(Testudo hermanni)* during 30 minutes of the intraoperative period, from incision (T0) to the end of the surgery (T30).

hermanni) undergoing anesthesia for soft tissue surgery was evaluated. Following premedication with midazolam (2 mg/kg), butorphanol (0.4 mg/kg), and carprofen (4 mg/kg), anesthesia was induced with intravenous propofol to effect (5-10 mg/kg) and it was maintained with a 1.7% ± 0.7% expiratory fraction of isoflurane. An example of intraoperative BIS recordings is shown in Figure 19-4. In a total of seven Hermann's tortoises, the BIS was able to display the electrical activity of the cortex during anesthesia—patterns of deep suppression (SR, 80; BIS, 15) combined with bursts of cerebral cortex activation (SR, 0; BIS, 60). This wide fluctuation has been described as a safety mechanism developed to avoid brain damage during brumation in conscious, anoxia-tolerant freshwater turtles and Hermann's tortoises.[5,12] Based on these experiences, the BIS does not seem a helpful adjunct to monitor the depth of anesthesia in chelonians.

The electrical activities of the brain of anesthetized snakes *(Boa constrictor)* and green iguanas *(Iguana iguana)* have also been monitored with BIS. The first BIS values after induction of anesthesia with intravenous propofol were 70 to 90. In the following minutes and coinciding with isoflurane administration, thus increasing the depth of anesthesia, BIS values decreased to 20 to 30. Depending on titration of isoflurane during the maintenance of anesthesia, BIS values ranged from 30 to 50. Extubation occurred when the animal was considered to be able to breathe spontaneously or when movements of the limbs or the head were observed. In every case, the BIS at this time point ranged from 60 to 85. We found that extubation of the trachea based on the BIS value (BIS ≥ 60) could safely be performed.

However, very close monitoring of the patient is nevertheless recommended.

The bispectral index has been found to be a very useful tool when performing anesthesia in a venomous lizard. During a coelioscopic procedure for gender determination, the bispectral index was continuously monitored in a Gila monster *(Heloderma suspectum)*. The mean values of BIS and SR for the 25-minute isoflurane anesthesia were 25 ± 10 and 53 ± 25, respectively. No evident signs of awareness or light plane of anesthesia were observed (i.e., presence of movement, increased respiratory or heart rate).

The reason for the lower BIS in the Gila monster versus the iguana and the boa is unknown. It may be hypothesized that venomous or varanid species, to which beaded lizards are related, may undergo deeper planes of anesthesia.

In a specific example, the relevance of the BIS during cardiopulmonary resuscitation was assessed during the anesthetic procedure of an adult bearded dragon *(Pogona vitticeps)* undergoing elective neutering. After premedication with butorphanol (0.4 mg/kg) and meloxicam (0.05 mg/kg), anesthesia was induced with propofol to effect (0.5 mg/kg) and maintained with isoflurane. Intravenous access in the cephalic vein was available. The heart rate (HR) was monitored by Doppler ultrasonography and the respiratory rate (RR) was monitored by counting the excursions of the coelomic cavity. Temperature was maintained with an electric heat blanket. After induction of anesthesia, HR was 44 beats/min, RR was 6 breaths/min, the BIS was 40 and SR was 2. Twenty minutes after induction of anesthesia, the patient moved (HR, 44 beats/min; RR, 4 breaths/min; BIS, 77; SR, 0).

Fifteen minutes later, cardiorespiratory arrest occurred; the BIS was 80 and the SR was 0, perhaps related to the unpredictable shunting ability of reptiles. In the following 5 minutes, the surgery was finished while anesthesia was discontinued, ventilation was assisted, heart massage was performed, and aggressive intravenous emergency therapy was administered (atropine, 0.01 mg/kg; epinephrine, 0.02 mg/kg; doxapram, 5 mg/kg). The mean values of BIS and SR were 90 and 0. Based on BIS (55 ± 18) and SR (13 ± 13) values, the resuscitation effort continued over 20 minutes, although no cardiorespiratory improvements were observed. Within the following 5 minutes, the BIS mean value increased to 90 ± 1 (SR, 0), the heart started to beat (HR, 44 beats/min) and the patient was able to breathe spontaneously (RR, 4 breaths/min). Extubation of the trachea was performed and the patient recovered from anesthesia.

To evaluate the validity of the BIS in bearded dragons, the euthanasia of another patient was monitored. Ten minutes after euthanasia, the BIS decreased to 3 and the SR to 100.

BIRDS

The bispectral index has been successfully validated in the avian species using chickens *(Gallus gallus)* as experimental models.[10,13] Median (range) BIS values during anesthesia were 1.75, 1.50, 1.25, 1.00, and 0.75 and the mean anesthetic concentrations of isoflurane were 25% (15% to 35%), 35% (25% to 45%), 35% (20% to 50%), 40% (25% to 55%), and 50% (35% to 65%), respectively. The median BIS value at extubation was 70 ± 9. Blood pressure changed with end-tidal isoflurane concentrations, whereas the heart rate did not.

Based on this validation study, the BIS has been further used in clinical avian patients as additional monitoring to assess the degree of hypnosis. Satisfactory results have been obtained in a large variety of orders, such as Anseriformes, Ciconiiformes, Psittaciformes, Falconiformes, and Strigiformes.

In an interesting case, the BIS was able to uncover feigning death behavior in a red kite *(Milvus milvus)* during recovery from isoflurane anesthesia.[11] The bispectral index ranged from 44 to 57 during maintenance of isoflurane anesthesia and, at the moment of extubation of the trachea, the BIS was 59. The index rose up to 85 in 1 minute while the kite remained immobile in sternal recumbence. The bird was perched, keeping the upright position. Whereas behavioral or cardiorespiratory variables remained unchanged, the BIS revealed that the bird had regained consciousness.

MAMMALS

The anesthesia of three gelada baboons *(Theropithecus gelada)* for a general examination, tuberculin testing, and radiographic examination were monitored with the BIS. An adequate degree of hypnosis to approach the geladas was achieved after a combination of intramuscular ketamine (5 mg/kg) and medetomidine (0.07 mg/kg) was administered. During the following 15 minutes, manipulations were carried out without episodes of apparent consciousness while the BIS ranged from 30 to 65. Following reversal with atipamezole, the BIS increased to 97 in the following 8 minutes, coinciding with eye blinking and twitching of facial muscles.

Future anesthetic episodes in geladas will benefit from additional monitoring with the BIS because it would increase patient and staff safety (e.g., administration of additional anesthetic drugs before slight movement occurs). The device was able to display a highly accurate state of hypnosis in the presented cases reliably. Similar results were obtained in an orangutan *(Pongo pygmaeus)* anesthetized with intramuscular ketamine (5 mg/kg) and xylazine (3 mg/kg).

Four adult spectacled bears *(Tremarctos ornatus)* were anesthetized with tiletamine and zolazepam (1.1 to 1.7 mg/kg), and medetomidine (0.06 to 0.1 mg/kg). Three of the bears underwent ultrasonographic examination, skin biopsy, and blood sampling. One spectacled bear was anesthetized, followed by euthanasia. The monitoring of the BIS in the first three bears did not contribute to obtaining more information about the degree of hypnosis, likely because of the effects of tiletamine on the brain activity. The BIS values of were always ≥65. In the bear that was euthanized, 10 minutes after administration of the lethal dose the BIS decreased to 5 (minimum, 0 to maximum, 20) and SR increased to 95 (minimum, 50 to maximum, 100). Although the BIS was not able to monitor a reliable state of hypnosis in bears anesthetized with tiletamine, zolazepam, and medetomidine, the decrease of the BIS to 5 in the euthanized bear shows that the BIS may be a reliable indicator of anesthesia depth with a different drug combination in spectacled bears.

A European otter *(Lutra lutra)* was anaesthetized for a surgical intervention with intramuscular ketamine (15 mg/kg) and midazolam (0.5 mg/kg). Maintenance of anesthesia was performed with isoflurane and ventilation was controlled using intermittent positive pressure ventilation. Intraoperative monitoring included arterial blood pressure, pulse oximetry, capnography, and BIS. The first BIS value (50) was obtained 1 hour after induction of anesthesia (end-tidal isoflurane of 0.6%) coinciding with the beginning of the surgery. During the entire surgery (20 minutes), the BIS ranged between 40 and 65. The last BIS value after discontinuation of anesthesia was 74.

The bispectral index has been successfully used to monitor interhemispheric asymmetry in the dolphin species *Tursiops truncatus*.[7] The BIS device was found to be sensitive to the unihemispheric daze of the dolphin, which further encourages the use of this noninvasive monitor to study electroencephalographic changes during sleep and anesthesia in humans.

An adult Eastern black rhinoceros *(Diceros bicornis michaeli)* was anesthetized with intramuscular etorphine (6.7 µg/kg), butorphanol (6 µg/kg), and detomidine (10 µg/kg) for a general examination. The bispectral index was used to monitor the cortical electrical activity of the rhinoceros during the 2-hour procedure. During the entire period, the BIS ranged from 85 to 97. We hypothesized that the effect of etorphine in the brain is responsible for the BIS values.

A BIS reading of 95 could also be obtained in an awake Asian elephant *(Elephas maximus)* by applying the commercial sensors onto the skin.

CONCLUSIONS

BIS readings may be obtained in a large variety of mammals, birds, and reptiles. An exception may be tortoises because of the occurrence of fluctutations between deep sedation and bursts of cerebral cortex activation. Modification of sensors to allow the subcutaneous application of needles appears important to avoid the need to shave or pluck animals and to monitor small species, which have a skull that is smaller than the human skull. The use of ketamine and etorphine may result in paradoxically elevated BIS values, but this may not be generalized and the effect may be dose-dependent. Although there seems to be some indication that a BIS value between 40 and 60 coincides with a deep degree of hypnosis, there is variation.

Nevertheless, an upward trend will indicate that the animal is regaining consciousness; a decrease of the BIS with an increase of SR is a critical sign and must warn the anesthetist of a potentially life-threatening condition. The interpretation of the BIS value is similar to the use of pulse oximetry, in which trends rather than absolute values are important to evaluate the patient's condition. Therefore, it may be concluded that BIS monitoring may be beneficial in zoo animal medicine with respect to early recovery in dangerous species and early recognition of life-threatening conditions. Further studies are needed to evaluate the BIS, especially in relation to the use of different anesthetic agents.

Acknowledgments

We would like to thank Rainer Vogt and Thomas Wiestner for the modification of the BIS electrodes.

REFERENCES

1. Arnemo JM, Ahlqvist P, Andersen R, et al: Risk of capture-related mortality in large free-ranging mammals: Experiences from Scandinavia. Wildl Biol 12:109–113, 2009.
2. Brodbelt DC, Blissitt KJ, MHammond RA, et al: The risk of death: The confidential inquiry into perioperative small animal fatalities. Vet Anaesth Analg 35:365–373, 2008.
3. Bruhn J, Myles PS, Sneyd R, et al: Depth of anaesthesia monitoring: What's available, what's validated and what's next? Br J Anaesth 97:85–94, 2006.
4. Dahaba AA: Different conditions that could result in the bispectral index indicating an incorrect hypnotic state. Anaesth Analg 101:765–773, 2005.
5. Fernandes JA, Lutz PL, Tannenbaum A, et al: Electroencephalogram activity in the anoxic turtle brain. Am J Physiol Regul Integr Comp Physiol 273:R911–R919, 1997.
6. Haga HA, Dolvik NI: Evaluation of the bispectral index as an indicator of degree of central nervous system depression in isoflurane-anaesthetized horses. Am J Vet Res 63:438–442, 2002.
7. Howard RS, Finneran JJ, Ridgway SH: Bispectral index monitoring of unihemispheric effects in dolphins. Anesth Analg 103:626–632, 2006.
8. Johansen JW: Update on bispectral index monitoring. Best Pract Res Clin Anaesth 20:81–99, 2006.
9. March PA, Muir WW: Bispectral analysis of the electroencephalogram: A review of its development and use in anesthesia. Vet Anaesth Analg 32:241–255, 2005.
10. Martin Jurado O: Determination of the Anaesthesia Depth in Chickens with Bispectral Index (BIS). Ph.D. Thesis, University of Zurich, Zurich, 2008.
11. Martin Jurado O, Simova-Curd S, Bettschart-Wolfensberger R, et al: Bispectral index reveals death feigning behavior in a red kite (Milvus milvus). J Avian Med Surg (in press).
12. Martin Jurado O, Vogt R, Eulenberger U, et al: Electrical activity of the brain in tortoises during brumation monitored with bispectral index (BIS). Presented at the Annual Meeting of the American Association of Zoo Veterinarians, Knoxville, Tennessee, October 2007.
13. Martin-Jurado O, Vogt R, Kutter A, et al: Effect of inhalation of isoflurane at endtidal concentrations greater than, equal to, and less than the minimum anesthetic concentration on bispectral index in chickens. Am J Vet Res 69:1254–1261, 2008.

CHAPTER 20

Approaching Health Problems at the Wildlife–Domestic Animal Interface

Jonna A.K. Mazet and Christine K. Johnson

Contact between domestic animals and wildlife is an increasing conservation health challenge, with livestock and pets that accompany our burgeoning human population sharing shrinking habitat and limited water resources with wild animals. When domestic and wild animals are in close proximity, diseases may have severe impacts on biodiversity, population health, and even human health and livelihoods. Pathogens that may readily cross species boundaries and cause disease pose a special conservation challenge for susceptible wildlife populations, especially those that have decreased to critically low numbers of individuals and are at risk of extinction. The complex linkages among domestic animal, wildlife, and human health and behavior necessitate a transdisciplinary or One Health approach to disease investigations, with the most productive studies being aimed at environmental interfaces at which pathogen transmission across species is likely to occur.

Unfortunately, traditional wildlife health and conservation studies have often targeted a single species or pathogen, without regard for the complexity of the ecosystem drivers of disease. This approach has tended toward identification of only one portion of the problem, resulting in a dearth of adequate solutions that could effectively address complex problems. In addition, the role of wildlife reservoirs in emerging infectious diseases of humans is now posing a potential threat to conservation, because some managers responsible for the protection of public health will not be concerned about the fate of wild animals or protection of the habitat that is essential for their survival.

Veterinarians are trained to evaluate problems from a systems approach, taking into consideration the complexity of interacting factors when solving the health problem of an individual animal or population. Therefore, veterinarians are ideally suited to work in multidisciplinary teams to solve the often multifactorial health problems that affect the conservation of wild animals. Although the specific consideration of the interactions among animals, people, and the environment is a relatively recent addition to most curricula, veterinarians have always been leaders in the zoonotic disease field. With the widely recognized paradigm shift to management of disease and natural resources with a One Health approach, the new veterinary graduate is now aware that explosive human population growth and environmental changes have resulted in increased numbers of wild animals living in close contact with livestock and people, increasing the potential for pathogen transmission. Unfortunately, this increased contact, together with changes in land use and climate, may also alter the inherent ecologic balance between pathogens and their hosts, with unanticipated consequences.

One solution to disease and conservation at the wild-domestic animal interface is the implementation of a proactive approach—addressing potential pathogen transmission and the resulting disease transmission before a volatile problem occurs. A wildlife disease surveillance and response strategy that is measurable, adaptive, and responsive is critical for detecting and monitoring cross-species disease transmission, especially zoonotic pathogens that account for most emerging infectious diseases in people, such as influenza and West Nile virus.[15] In fact, more than 75% of these emerging zoonoses are the result of wildlife origin pathogens.[6] Another useful tool for improving the efficiencies of surveillance efforts at wild-domestic animal disease hot spots is the use of important sentinel species. This approach facilitates the improvement of infectious disease models, resulting in higher quality field studies and more specifically targeted molecular diagnostics, and eventually in more effective conservation management strategies (Fig. 20-1).

153

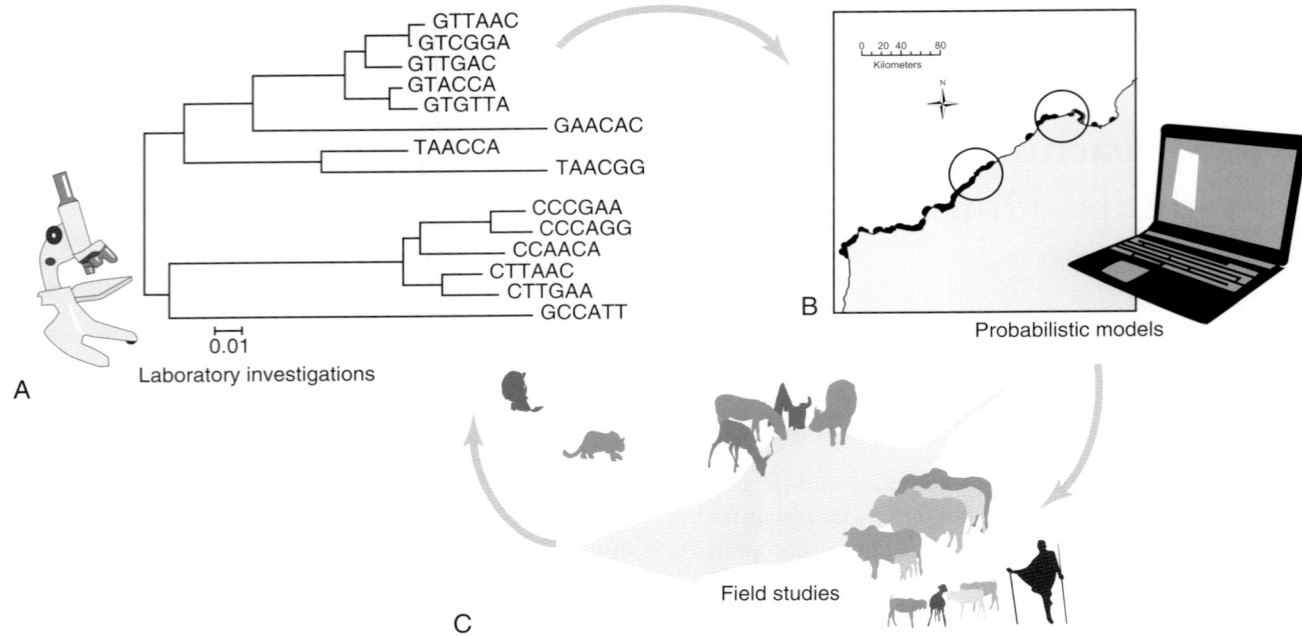

Figure 20-1

Basic strategy for disease investigations at the wild-domestic animal interface. **A,** Intense field studies of domestic animals and free-ranging wild animals to identify pathogens and integrate health and disease indices with observations of individual animal behavior, foraging preferences, and contact. **B,** Laboratory investigations to detect and characterize pathogens and associate pathogen presence with disease. **C,** Modeling of disease dynamics to understand key relationships, target further study, and evaluate management options. *(Graphic artist credit: A. Kent.)*

SPECIAL CONSIDERATIONS AT THE WILD-DOMESTIC ANIMAL INTERFACE

Unlike highly pathogenic, single-host pathogens that are often not sustainable in very small wild animal populations, multihost pathogens may be maintained by a reservoir host if there is recruitment of susceptible individuals in the population.[8] Domestic animal populations, such as livestock herds and feral dog packs and cat colonies, may be able to maintain domestic animal pathogens that are infectious to wildlife and provide a continuous supply of immunologically naive young individuals. Domestic animal populations are capable of being infected with pathogens of wildlife origin if herd health is not maintained through good disease prevention practices. Therefore, domestic animal populations may be able to serve as a reservoir for wildlife pathogens. Similarly, wildlife populations may carry pathogens that do not cause clinical disease in the wild animal host but may cause significant problems to health and productivity in domestic animals at ecological interfaces likely to facilitate transmission. Thus, domestic and wild animal populations may be important sources of pathogens capable of crossing into nearby susceptible animal populations, resulting in spillover and spillback of pathogens of concern.

After centuries of study, pathogens that commonly have an impact on domestic animal health and production are well recognized, and disease surveillance is generally established for these pathogens in many countries that depend economically on livestock production and trade. Diagnostic tests have been developed for use in domestic animal species and, in areas with available resources, surveillance is implemented along with vaccine and other preventive strategies to control disease. If wild animals are suspected to be a source of pathogen spillover into livestock populations, targeted disease-specific surveillance may be initiated in implicated wildlife species. Despite the development of the wildlife disease field, relatively little is known regarding overall health status and disease problems in free-ranging wild animal populations, many of which have direct and regular contact with domestic animal species. Understandably, special considerations must be made when evaluating disease occurrence and pathogen prevalence in wild animal populations, especially because most diagnostic tests available have been developed for domestic animals and not optimized or validated for other species.

In the United States, we have developed comprehensive wildlife health monitoring programs most commonly for threatened and endangered species listed by the Endangered Species Act (ESA) of 1973. The federal wildlife agency, the U.S. Fish and Wildlife Service, authorizes recovery actions and species management based on available science. Ideally, relevant stakeholders, including state wildlife and natural resource management agencies and those representing domestic animal interests and protection of food safety and trade, are directly involved in scientific research and surveillance planning to develop applied study goals and ensure that investigations are likely to inform management. Once study goals are identified, collaborations with experts in relevant scientific disciplines are critical to ensure adequate study design and best practice protocols that can produce high-quality data capable of informing policy and practice. Because of the many special private and governmental interests involved in disease transmission issues at the wild-domestic animal interface, particularly well-designed investigations are needed that can produce scientifically supported inferences and interventions. These should appropriately characterize uncertainty and be rigorous enough to face peer review and criticism that are often a normal part of the process allowing policy makers and managers to implement change at this high-profile interface.

BOX 20-1	Ten Steps for Health Studies of Disease Emergence in Wild Animal Populations at Complex Interfaces*

1. Identify key problems in the population and stakeholders involved in the main issues.
2. Recognize as many of the interacting components of the system as initially possible, including the socioeconomic context.
3. Conduct detailed necropsies with histopathology to characterize disease problems.
4. Commence laboratory characterization of pathogens using molecular techniques.
5. Conduct targeted wild animal captures with health screening, serologic studies, and telemetry and field-based observations.
6. Integrate detailed health and behavioral studies to understand determinants of disease by identifying individual animal and population characteristics associated with disease occurrence.
7. Evaluate temporal and spatial patterns and environmental factors associated with disease occurrence.
8. Develop dynamic models to understand key relationships, characterize uncertainty, and evaluate management options.
9. Translate key findings and recommend interventions and preventive actions to inform management.
10. Carry out continued monitoring to the assess success of policy actions, evaluate new hypotheses, and identify newly emerging determinants of disease in the system.

This is an example of a consistent approach that may be useful in efficiently designing comprehensive health studies at the wild animal–domestic animal interface.

APPROACHING NOVEL WILDLIFE DISEASE PROBLEMS

For wildlife disease studies to result in justifiable and implementable interventions, we suggest a strategic combination of field studies to identify pathogens and their sources, molecular diagnostics for appropriate characterization, and dynamic modeling of the system and potential interventions using a modern risk-based approach. As depicted in Figure 20-1, the modeling helps target and improve field studies, and the data from field studies and molecular diagnostics iteratively improve the risk-based models and recommended interventions.

In many cases, a disease investigation will be the first scientific endeavor to characterize and address an emerging health problem affecting conservation. In these cases, a consistent and measurable process is useful for efficiently designing the approach without falling into a trap of following hunches or leads that may not be at the root of the problem. An example of an approach for comprehensive health studies at the wild-domestic animal interface that may be applied consistently is illustrated in Box 20-1. Slight variations of this approach have been applied successfully in multiple situations in developed and developing country contexts. The following sections provide specific examples for both— identification and mitigation of a disease threat in the threatened sea otter population in California, and the effect of water restriction on zoonotic disease transmission at the domestic-wild animal interface in the Ruaha ecosystem, Tanzania.

MULTIDISCIPLINARY SEA OTTER RESEARCH STRATEGY IN CALIFORNIA

Sea otters *(Enhydra lutris)* have been designated as a federally listed threatened species in California and Alaska because these subpopulations have shown limited or sporadic recovery since overhunting decimated their numbers along the Pacific Rim during the height of the fur trade in the 18th and 19th centuries. Infectious disease and limited prey resources are two key interacting factors impeding recovery of southern sea otters *(Enhydra lutris neries)* in California.[5] Septic peritonitis caused by migration of acanthocephalan parasites and protozoal encephalitis caused by *Sarcocystis neurona* and *Toxoplasma gondii* have been reported as common infectious diseases detected in sea otter carcasses found beach-cast along the California coast.[7,10,16]

Toxoplasma gondii is a ubiquitous, apicomplexan, protozoal parasite with a complex multihost life cycle and an infective oocyst life stage that may persist in the environment. This pathogen may infect all warm-blooded vertebrates, including humans, but domestic and wild felids are the only known definitive hosts for *T. gondii.*[3] The unusually high frequency of *T. gondii* exposure and infection in marine mammals has been a fascinating puzzle, considering the terrestrial nature of all recognized definitive hosts. A wide range of marine mammals has been reported with infections, and these species vary markedly in habitat and prey preference.[9,12] Sea otters and most marine mammals do not consume known intermediate hosts for *T. gondii.* Whereas the processes promoting these infections in marine mammals are undoubtedly complex, *T. gondii* is a multihost pathogen widely recognized for its ability to spill over into susceptible wild animal populations, and it is likely that this pathogen has emerged in sea otters from cats and wild felids.[2]

Research efforts that are underway to uncover the processes promoting *T. gondii* infections in marine animals are an example of the type of large collaborative multidisciplinary efforts needed to understand the transmission and impact of a domestic species pathogen on a threatened wildlife population. The breadth of sea otter research activities engaged in this issue have been made possible by the involvement and collaboration of key federal and state wildlife management agencies, including the California Department of Fish and Game, the U.S. Geological Survey, and several large universities with specific expertise in parasitology, pathology, epidemiology, and animal ecology.

As is most often necessary when initiating health investigations in wild animal populations, basic health screening was initiated for opportunistically sampled live, free-ranging, California and Alaskan sea otters to establish normal health parameter reference ranges and evaluate exposure to a host of possible pathogens that might cause disease in this species. Initial health assessments and baseline disease exposure information provides an historical context of past exposure patterns that may be useful for understanding future disease events. These efforts also identify potential disease issues and provide a focus for disease investigations. This initial effort in sea otters resulted in the first report of a high prevalence (35%) of *T. gondii* exposure among 77 California otters sampled between 1995 and 2000.[4] Seroprevalence, calculated as the number of individuals with serologic evidence of past exposure to a pathogen divided by the number of individuals sampled, may provide insight into the frequency of pathogen exposure during a specified period of time, provided that adequate numbers of individuals are sampled that are representative of the overall population. It is often necessary to calculate age-specific seroprevalence for each age class sampled and evaluate differences by other population characteristics of interest to understand patterns in pathogen exposure better. Furthermore, patterns in pathogen exposure may change quickly, and it is critical to update measures of seroprevalence for pathogens of interest. Seroprevalence studies have identified geographic areas with high levels of *T. gondii* seroprevalence and determined that adult otters were more likely to be seropositive to *T. gondii.* This is likely because this parasite produces tissue cysts that cause lifelong infection and longer lived individuals are more likely to have had opportunities to be exposed to the parasite.[2,11]

Positive serologic results are not directly indicative of disease status in the individual, nor are they an accurate measure of pathogen impact on population health. If pathogens produce a lasting antibody that is detected by a serologic test, evidence of past exposure may be common in adult age classes, particularly to pathogens that do not cause severe disease. At the population level, seroprevalence for highly virulent pathogens may be exceedingly low or even zero for infections that are almost always fatal. The necessary context for interpreting seroprevalence, which may have an inverse relationship with disease severity, may only be made by accompanying field observations and pathology studies of naturally infected individuals found dead and recovered quickly for a comprehensive necropsy before postmortem autolysis (usually 24 to 72 hours). A large stranding network in California facilitated recovery of beach-cast sea otters for decades, but *T. gondii*–related disease in otters could be characterized only when a significant investment was made to involve veterinary pathologists who conduct detailed necropsies that included histologic examination of brain tissue. *Toxoplasma gondii* infection was confirmed in dead stranded otters by immunohistochemistry and culture and isolation of live parasites. Most critically, parasite isolation from infected sea otters enabled mouse bioassay and molecular analysis; this included polymerase chain reaction (PCR) assay and sequencing to confirm the presence of *T. gondii* and not a related pathogen that might cross-react on serologic assays.[1,12,13] Advanced molecular techniques have now differentiated among *T. gondii* subtypes, or genotypes, infecting sea otters, which may facilitate tracking of pathogen spillover from domestic cat and wild felid sources. Laboratory studies have also greatly facilitated validation of the indirect fluorescent antibody test (IFAT) for use in sea otters. By comparing serologic titers to immunohistochemistry and cell culture results, a cutoff was established that maximized sensitivity and specificity to detect *T. gondii* infection in sea otters.

Detailed necropsies also enabled characterization of histologic lesions associated with *T. gondii* cysts in brain tissue so that toxoplasmosis could be evaluated for its role as a primary contributing cause of death in sea otters. Collaboration with facilities that rehabilitate live-stranded sea otters has enhanced interpretation of pathology data by allowing the pathologist to correlate the brain lesions accompanying toxoplasmosis in dead animals with clinical signs observed in those same animals when alive. Once case definition criteria were corroborated, epidemiologic risk factor analyses were used to describe the distribution of *T. gondii* cases among California otters and evaluate associations between *T. gondii* infection and more proximate causes of mortality, such as fatal shark-inflicted wounds.[7]

Armed with a more clearly defined problem of pathogen spillover into this susceptible and threatened wildlife species, research activities have expanded to include field studies of *T. gondii* distribution and shedding in domestic cats and wild felids in geographic regions with demonstrated high risk for sea otters. Follow-up health investigations in sea otters have developed into long-term longitudinal studies of live animals needed to refine our understanding of the behavioral and ecologic risk factors promoting *T. gondii* infection in this population. Modern advances in telemetry technology have permitted a direct view into the behavioral complexity of wild animals by improving our ability to observe individual animal movements, foraging activities, contact with domestic animals, habitat usage, and potentially high-risk behaviors. When detailed tracking studies are combined with health and survival indices, these longitudinal studies may identify specific high-risk behaviors that are associated with pathogen exposure. Just as longitudinal studies of people have advanced public health, disease models in sea otters have been used to evaluate a wide array of behavioral traits and movement patterns for their association with *T. gondii* infection. Modeling efforts have revealed that *T. gondii* infection in otters is related to the use of specific habitats, which has further refined our assessment of geographic hot spots for pathogen pollution.[5] High rates of infection were also identified in sea otters foraging on low-quality prey types, suggesting that increasing rates of protozoal infection in this population may be caused in part by the foraging strategies that have developed to cope with increasingly scarce food resources along coastal California.

Identifying geographic hot spots and high-risk prey species through modeling has allowed improvement of targeted sea otter monitoring and studies evaluating potential environmental interventions to decrease pathogen pollution of the coastal ecosystem. These studies included the development of surrogate microspheres for *T. gondii* that may now be used in environmental monitoring and evaluation of best practices in the wetlands to reduce environmental loading from terrestrial sources of *T. gondii*. In addition, these studies informed more complex watershed modeling to evaluate where interventions in storm water and feral cat management would make the most difference in reducing sea otter and other marine species exposure. Finally, more intensive molecular typing of *T. gondii* strains from terrestrial and marine hosts has allowed the evaluation of the parasite's life cycle and opened windows into the pathogen's evolution and ecology, which will no doubt lead to more discovery and effective interventions. Finally, sea otters are now being used as important sentinel species for coastal pathogen pollution and to monitor the effects of land use and climate change on the near-shore marine environment.

PROACTIVE APPROACH TO A DEVELOPING COUNTRY WILDLIFE HEALTH PROBLEM: HEALTH FOR ANIMALS AND LIVELIHOOD IMPROVEMENT PROJECT

Nowhere in the world are health effects on people and animals more important than in the developing world, where the dependence on natural resources is paramount. Water resources are perhaps most crucial, because humans and animals depend on safe water for health and survival and sources of clean water are dwindling because of demands from agriculture and climate change. As water becomes scarce, animals and people are squeezed into smaller areas. Contact among infected animals then increases, facilitating pathogen transmission. Water scarcity also means that people and animals use the same water sources for drinking and bathing, which results in serious contamination of drinking water and increased risk of sharing diseases. The risk of pathogen transmission puts wildlife at risk in two important ways: (1) diseases, such as rabies and distemper, may directly threaten lives of individuals and the survival of threatened and endangered populations; and (2) the potential for pathogens, such as *Mycobacterium bovis*, to spill over between livestock and wildlife reservoirs and affect livestock and human health has put people at odds with wildlife conservation, making wildlife a target for culling or illegal hunting.

In the Ruaha ecosystem of Tanzania, a sprawling conservation area larger than 45,000 km², as many as 12,000 elephants *(Loxodonta africana)* roam along with Africa's third largest population of critically endangered African wild dogs *(Lycaon pictus)*.[14] Livestock are widespread, abundant, and central to traditional natural resource management in and around the villages bordering Ruaha National Park and the buffering wildlife management area. Unfortunately, livestock-dependent households relying on the sale of animals and animal products for their livelihoods are among the poorest in the nation, and local poverty fuels the demand for illegal wildlife hunting for meat, a known driver for disease emergence.[17] The role of diseases, such as bovine tuberculosis (BTB) and brucellosis, in this region has only just begun to be characterized. Therefore, these diseases became important foci for the Health for Animals and Livelihood Improvement (HALI) Project because of their risk to both wildlife and livestock, as well as the potential for transmission to people in the area, many of whom are also infected with HIV/AIDS.

Additional priorities for HALI were determined through stakeholder meetings and informal interviews with affected pastoralist communities. In the end, HALI was invited to work in the region by its diverse communities, including multiple levels of government, nonprofit organizations, and academic institutions. The community consensus was that disease was affecting a significant proportion of the community and its biodiversity because of pathogen-contaminated water supplies and livestock and wildlife contact. Accordingly, the HALI project began assessing the impact of the interactions between water and animal disease in the Ruaha ecosystem by simultaneously investigating the medical, biophysical, socioeconomic, and policy issues driving the system.

The ongoing HALI multilevel approach began with seasonal testing of wildlife, livestock, and their water sources for pathogens and disease. Environmental monitoring of water quality, availability, and use was also critical for characterizing the interacting components of the system, in addition to assessing wildlife population health and demography. In the rural and poverty-driven Ruaha system, evaluating livestock and human disease impacts on livelihoods was critical. Socioeconomic evaluation was accomplished by examining land and water use impacts on daily workloads and village economies through detailed household surveys and health and economic diaries. Social and economic drivers play a role in the success of every wildlife health study. In the developing context, wildlife health and survival must not be viewed as more worthy of investment than human health and community well-being. Therefore, even if a wildlife disease is identified as a major threat to biodiversity or population survival, it must be addressed in a way that is compatible with community needs. For example in the Ruaha system, the HALI project was especially interested in BTB and its effects on wildlife, livestock, and human health. However, because BTB is an underrecognized human disease, the project also focused on rabies. Rabies was a well-recognized human disease in the region, as well as an important threat to wild animal health, especially that of the African wild dog. By recognizing the desires of the community who invited the project staff to work in the region and improve rabies education, HALI gained the trust and respect of participating households, improving the quality of BTB and other disease research. The involvement of the community—stakeholders—cannot be overstated, because HALI's operations could only be successful with their support and invitation. Without such invitation, conservation projects fight an uphill battle in developing communities and risk a lack of stability and sustainability.

The HALI project has now identified bovine tuberculosis and brucellosis in livestock and wildlife in the Ruaha ecosystem and is using this information to identify geographic areas with varying water availability, in which the risk of transmission among wildlife, livestock, and people may be high. In addition, zoonotic *Salmonella, Shigella, Vibrio, Camplybacter, Cryptosporidium,* and *Giardia* spp. have all been isolated from multiple water sources used by people and frequented by livestock and wildlife. Advanced molecular techniques are being used to characterize strains of pathogens identified to evaluate the disease dynamics more fully, including reservoir and spillover hosts. These data are being used to examine spatial and temporal associations between landscape factors and disease and to identify risk factors that may be mitigated to reduce transmission and diminish the impacts of disease. Detailed models of water availability and quality, and their effects on disease status, are now helping identify target regions for additional interventions.

Survey findings from the beginning of the HALI project have also indicated that more than two thirds of participating pastoral households do not believe that illness in their families could be contracted from livestock, and almost 50% believe the same of wildlife. Furthermore, when the HALI project began working in this region, 75% of households did not consider sharing water sources with livestock or wildlife to be a health risk, illustrating the need for effective community education. Therefore, a targeted zoonotic disease educational campaign began with community outreach events, such as movie nights and radio programs, and targeted household education where disease exposure had been identified. Additionally, the project has introduced new diagnostic techniques for disease detection and pathogen characterization at the Veterinary Faculty in the collaborating Sokoine University of Agriculture (SUA). Through community outreach and SUA, HALI is training Tanzanians of all education levels about zoonotic disease. Education and outreach at the natural resource manager and lawmaker levels will enable informed health and environmental policy interventions to continue to address and mitigate the impacts of diseases of people, wildlife, and livestock in the Ruaha ecosystem.

Mitigating complex ecosystem health problems like the ones described requires identification of implementable and sustainable solutions. Because disease transmission between domestic and wild animals may

place communities and conservationists at odds, approaches to solving these problems need to be framed in a neutral context to encourage participation. In developing and developed countries, the main obstacles to implementing change remain human behavior and tradition. Although strong science is an excellent foundation on which to base recommendations, interventions may succeed only if stakeholders are involved in the characterization of the problem and are willing to make the tradeoffs necessary to balance the needs of people and wildlife.

EMERGING DISEASES: A NEW CHALLENGE FOR WILDLIFE HEALTH PROFESSIONALS WORKING AT LIVESTOCK AND HUMAN INTERFACES

Human and domestic animal contact with wild animals may drive the emergence of zoonoses that pose a threat to global health. Critical interfaces promoting zoonotic diseases of wildlife origin occur when diverse pools of wildlife pathogens come into direct and sustained contact with humans or their domestic animals. Efforts to recognize and control zoonotic disease are underway in resource-rich countries but, until recently, fewer scientific resources to identify emerging infectious disease have been allocated to countries in which pathogens are most likely to emerge. A challenge has been posed to today's wildlife health professionals—design SMART (strategic, measurable, adaptive, responsive, targeted) wildlife disease surveillance and health studies that may detect disease outbreaks, forecast disease emergence, and identify key ecosystem drivers that increase disease risk. Such surveillance and health studies will not only greatly advance our understanding of emerging infectious diseases that threaten humans, but could also enable the development of sustainable wild animal disease surveillance and preventive strategies to protect biodiversity.

Acknowledgments

Unfortunately, authorship constraints limited the level of participation we could solicit from our excellent collaborators. Therefore, we gratefully thank the following for years of productive discussion and intellectual contribution to these projects and the One Health discipline: Alonso Aguirre, Jack Ames, James Bodkin, Walter Boyce, David Bunn, David Casper, Deana Clifford, Patricia Conrad, Peter Coppolillo, Peter Daszak, Erin Dodd,

James Estes, Jonathan Epstein, Jon Erickson, Joseph Fair, Ian Gardner, Kirsten Gilardi, Martin Gilbert, Tracey Goldstein, Frances Gulland, Michael Harris, David Jessup, Damien Joly, William Karesh, Rudovick Kazwala, Michel Masozera, Ann Melli, Melissa Miller, Woutrina Miller, Stephen Morse, Michael Murray, Andrea Packham, Harrison Sadiki, Kristine Smith, Julie Stewart, M. Tim Tinker, Marcela Uhart, Nathan Wolfe, and Michael Ziccardi.

REFERENCES

1. Cole RA, Lindsay DS, Howe DK, et al: Biological and molecular characterizations of *Toxoplasma gondii* strains obtained from southern sea otters *(Enhydra lutris nereis)*. J Parasitol 86:526–530, 2000.
2. Conrad PA, Miller MA, Kreuder C, et al: Transmission of *Toxoplasma:* Clues from the study of sea otters as sentinels of *Toxoplasma gondii* flow into the marine environment. Int J Parasitoly 35:1155–1168, 2005.
3. Dubey J: Advances in the life cycle of *Toxoplasma gondii*. Int J Parasitol 28:1019–1024, 1998.
4. Hanni KD, Mazet JA, Gulland FM, et al: Clinical pathology and assessment of pathogen exposure in southern and Alaskan sea otters. J Wildl Dis 39:837–850, 2003.
5. Johnson CK, Tinker MT, Estes JA, et al: Prey choice and habitat use drive sea otter pathogen exposure in a resource-limited coastal system. Proc Natl Acad Sci U S A 106:2242–2247, 2009.
6. Jones KE, Patel NG, Levy MA, et al: Global trends in emerging infectious diseases. Nature 451:990–993, 2008.
7. Kreuder C, Miller MA, Jessup DA, et al: Patterns of mortality in southern sea otters *(Enhydra lutris nereis)* from 1998–2001. J Wildl Dis 39:495–509, 2003.
8. McCallum H, Dobson A: Detecting disease and parasite threats to endangered species and ecosystems. Trends Ecol Evol 10:190–194, 1995.
9. Miller MA: Tissue cyst-forming coccidia of marine mammals. In Fowler ME, Miller RE, editors: Zoo and wild animal medicine. Current Therapy, ed 6, Philadelphia, 2008, WB Saunders, pp 319–340.
10. Miller MA, Crosbie PR, Sverlow K, et al: Isolation and characterization of *Sarcocystis* from brain tissue of a free-living southern sea otter *(Enhydra lutris nereis)* with fatal meningoencephalitis. Parasitol Res 87:252–257, 2001.
11. Miller MA, Gardner IA, Kreuder C, et al: Coastal freshwater runoff is a risk factor for *Toxoplasma gondii* infection of sea otters *(Enhydra lutris nereis)*. Int J Parasitol 32:997–1006, 2002.
12. Miller MA, Gardner IA, Packham A, et al: Evaluation of indirect fluorescent antibody test (IFAT) for demonstration of antibodies to *Toxoplasma gondii* in the sea otter *(Enhydra lutris)*. J Parasitol 88:594–599, 2002.
13. Miller MA, Grigg ME, Kreuder C, et al: An unusual genotype of *Toxoplasma gondii* is common in California sea otters *(Enhydra lutris nereis)* and is a cause of mortality. Int J Parasitol 34:275–284, 2004.
14. Ray JC, Hunter L, Zigouris J: Setting conservation and research priorities for larger African carnivores, 2005 (http://www.catsg.org/cheetah/05_library/5_3_publications/R/Ray_et_al_2005_Conservation_priorities_for_larger_African_carnivores.pdf).
15. Taylor LH, Latham SM, Woolhouse MEJ: Risk factors for human disease emergence. Philos Trans R Soc Biol Sci 356:983–989, 2001.
16. Thomas NJ, Cole RA: The risk of disease and threats to the wild population. Endangered Species Update 13:23–27, 1996.
17. Wolfe N, Daszak P, Kilpatrick AM, Burke DS: Bushmeat hunting: Deforestation, and prediction of zoonotic disease emergence. Emerg Infect Dis 11:1822–1827, 2005.

Wildlife Disease Ecology: What Can Zoo and Wildlife Veterinarians Learn from this Discipline?

Sonia M. Hernandez and Michael J. Yabsley

It is not the strongest of the species that survives, nor the most intelligent that survives. It is the one that is the most adaptable to change.

Charles Darwin

HISTORY OF DEVELOPMENT OF WILDLIFE DISEASE ECOLOGY

Ecology emerged in the late 19th century as a mathematical interdisciplinary study of the distribution and abundance of organisms and their and interactions with other organisms and the environment. It is distinguished from natural history, which is the descriptive study of organisms. Ecology is also the examination of ecosystems. Ecosystems describe the web of relations among organisms at different scales of organization. It is important to note that "ecology" is not synonymous with environmentalism or conservation. Ecology envelops closely related disciplines such as physiology, evolution, genetics, and behavior. Some leading themes of ecology include the organism's life processes that explain adaptations, the distribution and abundance of organisms and the mechanisms for such distributions, the movement of energy through living communities, the successional development of ecosystems, and the abundance and distribution of biodiversity in the context of the environment. There are many practical applications of ecology, such as wetland and natural resource management, city planning (urban ecology), community health, and economics, and it even provides a conceptual framework for understanding and researching human social interaction (human ecology). Because ecologists often undertake long-term observations of particular systems, and because profound changes have taken place in those systems, many ecologists are conservationists, many conservation applications stem from ecologic studies, and these studies have shaped the field of conservation biology and, by extension, conservation medicine.

With few exceptions, the field of ecology largely ignored disease and its effect on populations, communities, and ecosystems until fairly recently; this only changed as a result of mathematical models designed by May and Anderson in the 1970s, which were syntheses between parasitology and population biology.[2] These earlier models were significant because they presented the effect of pathogens on hosts and populations as another density-dependent mechanism driving populations toward equilibrium or keeping populations from exponential growth, and were analogous to predator-prey models. Disease ecology focuses on understanding how infectious diseases spread through and affect host populations and how hosts and pathogens react and evolve in response to one another; thus, it borrows principles from epidemiology and evolutionary biology. More recent events that advanced disease ecology forward were the Isaac Newton Institute meeting which resulted in one of the first disease ecology texts, soon followed by others such as *The Ecology of Wildlife Diseases,*[12] *Disease Ecology: Community Structure and Pathogen Dynamics*[3] and, most recently, *Infectious Disease Ecology: Effects of Ecosystems on Disease and of Disease on Ecosystems.*[21] With the development of each text, the theory of disease ecology has been increasingly supported by empirical data with applied objectives.

PRINCIPLES OF DISEASE ECOLOGY

As noted, ecology is firmly rooted in mathematics and mathematical models have allowed generalizations to explain a multitude of population dynamics. Here, we very simply review the backbone of the earlier compartmental models, termed *SIR models*, which form the foundation of disease ecology and stem from a set of differential equations.

Let x = the number of *susceptible* individuals, y = the number of individuals who are *infected*, and z = the number of individuals who have *recovered* (SIR). All these compartments are fractions of the total population, or N. For simplicity, we will assume in this model that all recovered individuals retain immunity but do not pass it on to their offspring, although more recent models have been adapted to represent more realistic scenarios, such as reinfection. Susceptible individuals enter the population through birth (immigration is not considered here). Instantaneous birth rate is represented by b and, if it is the same for all three types of individuals in the population, the number of new susceptible individuals added to the population may be represented as b(x + y + z). The number of susceptible individuals in a population may be reduced by infection or death. Contact between an infected and susceptible individual may or may not result in transmission; the rate at which individuals are infected (thus, have moved from the susceptible pool and into the infected compartment) is represented as βxy, where β is a constant termed the *transmission coefficient*, and which, roughly speaking, takes into account that the probability of contact between an infected and susceptible individual results in infection. This is somewhat analogous to predator-prey models, in which predators have to come into close contact to eat prey, and not every predatory event results in a kill.

Individuals may also leave the susceptible pool by dying; mortality is represented as d. Thus, an equation for the instantaneous rate of change of the susceptible proportion of the population is given by the following:

$$dx/dt = b(x + y + z) - \beta xy - dx$$

This equation states that the rate of change in the number of susceptible individual—dx/dt—in the population is equal to the total number of individual added to the population by birth in all three of the possible host conditions (SIR; b[x + y + z]), decreased by the number of susceptible individuals infected (βxy) and number of susceptible individuals dying (dx). Additionally, we assign D to represent the death rate of the infected group because it is reasonable to assume that the infection portion of the population will have a higher death rate than the other portions. Thus, the infection portion may be given by the following:

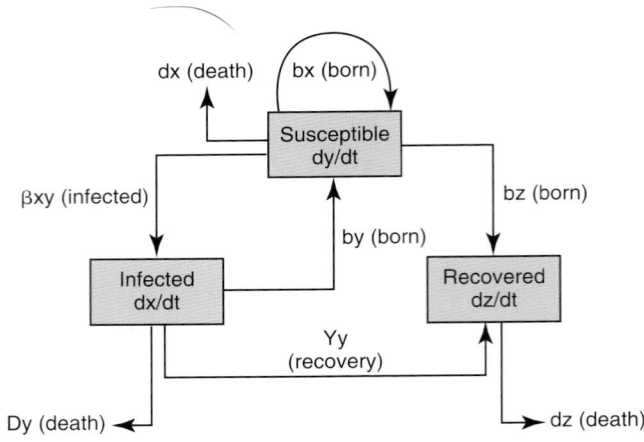

Figure 21-1

Relationships among susceptible, infected, and recovered individuals in an infection model. (*Modified from Ricklefs RE, Miller GL: Ecology, ed 4, New York, 2000, WH Freeman.*)

$$dy/dt = \beta xy - (D + Y)y$$

This equation simply says that the instantaneous rate of change of the number of infected in the population, dy/dt, is increased by the rate of infection (βxy) and decreased by the death and recovery ([D + Y]y). The rate of change in the number of recovered individuals is the rate of recovery, Yy, which adds individuals to the recovered group minus the rate of death of recovered individuals, dz,

$$dz/dt = Yy - dz$$

as illustrated in Figure 21-1.[23] These equations may then be rearranged to determine the threshold value of infection.

At the center of the SIR models is R_0, which is defined as the number of secondary cases produced per initial infection. If $R_0 > 1$, then a pathogen will be successful in that the introduction of a single infectious individual into a wholly susceptible population will result in sufficient secondary cases to allow the pathogen to persist. However, if $R_0 < 1$, the infection will die out, even when a small number of secondary cases develop. It is assumed that a population threshold exists below which R_0 is <1 because of the size and/or density of the population, because size and density increase per capita contact rates among individuals. R_0 has been calculated for a variety of host-pathogen situations and has proven useful for predicting the course of a pathogen through a population, such as louping ill virus in red grouse populations or host (fox) density required for rabies persistence.

SIGNIFICANCE OF DISEASE ECOLOGY FOR ZOO AND WILDLIFE VETERINARIANS

Most zoo and wildlife veterinarians are involved in some aspect of disease investigation. Wildlife disease investigation developed firstly as a descriptive science—the who, what, where, when and why of epidemiology—as a response to a need for management, particularly in response to public health concerns.[28] Most wildlife disease investigation stems from visible mortality events, or epizootics. Wildlife disease specialists are traditionally trained through veterinary medicine and/or master's or doctoral programs in wildlife disease, pathology, virology, microbiology, or related sciences. These disciplines, when applied to the field of wildlife disease investigation, adhere strictly to the principles of epidemiology. More recently, wildlife disease investigation has become more experimental in nature. Ultimately, epidemiologists and wildlife disease specialists share the common goal of limiting or managing diseases, which sometimes moves beyond concentrating on the host-pathogen situation and involves environmental modifications. Currently, however, wildlife disease investigation has also grown to involve questions that bring it more closely to disease ecology, such as the influence of disease on population dynamics, the effects of chronic and more subtle diseases on the fitness of hosts, and the effects of diseases on small isolated populations (what we call the "so what"). It is this latter stretching of traditional epidemiology and merging with the principles of wildlife biology and ecology that comprise the future of the science of wildlife disease investigation. For the last 10 years, the number of presentations dealing with pathogens and disease at the annual conference of the Ecological Society of America has grown exponentially and, equally, disease ecology sessions have been found at the Wildlife Disease Association meetings consistently for the last 5 years. At the center of these two disciplines, traditional wildlife disease investigation and wildlife disease ecology, stands conservation medicine. The American Association of Zoo Veterinarians and the Wildlife Disease Association have both had sessions and journal sections consistently dedicated specifically to conservation medicine for the last 5 to 8 years. Conservation medicine, truly multidisciplinary, offers both groups a common ground of interest and is a field to which both zoo and wildlife veterinarians are actively contributing.

Therefore, we strongly believe that any veterinarian involved in wildlife disease investigation and conservation medicine will greatly benefit from understanding basic disease ecology principles and from reviewing the body of literature that this discipline has to offer. Given the ease with which literature searches are now available, it is logistically simple to peruse a number of disease-related publications.* To save time and effort, busy veterinarians may use automated online search and alert systems such as PubCrawler, a free alerting service that scans daily updates to the PubMed and GenBank databases and alerts users of the current contents of Medline and GenBank by listing new articles that match their customized research interests.

POPULATION EFFECTS OF DISEASE

Veterinarians are well trained in recognizing, identifying, diagnosing, and treating diseases in individual animals. Although herd health is paramount to some aspects of veterinary medicine, the potential population effects of pathogens are at the core of disease ecology because they may explain some cycling in population numbers. For example, one of the best-recognized empirical studies demonstrating population cycles driven by disease was by Dobson and Hudson[4] on red grouse (*Lagopus lagopus scoticus*) in northern England, whereby infection with *Trichostrongylus tenuis* was shown to have negative effects on grouse fecundity, leading to population cycles that were not explained by other factors such as climatic effects or food availability. This is a simple but elegant article detailing the experimental treatment of isolated red grouse populations with antiparasitics, which demonstrated the significant attenuation of grouse population cycles in treated grouse and put the effects of parasites on populations on the map.[11]

The science of ecology has explored the effects of parasites and pathogens on host populations in other ways, such as through the hypothesis that assumes that parasites alter male secondary sexual characteristics and that females choose less parasitized males as a way to select males that may have resistance genes that can be passed on to her offspring.[23] Again, experiments with a lekking species, the sage grouse (*Centrocercus* spp.), were able to demonstrate that males infected with avian malaria attended less frequently, bred later in the

*These include the *Journal of Ecology, Frontiers in Ecology, Ecological Applications, Ecological Monographs, Ecology Letters, Journal of Animal Ecology, Public Library of Science (PLOS) Biology, PLoS ONE, Journal of Applied Ecology, Emerging Infectious Diseases, Proceedings of the Royal Society of London B (Biology), Conservation Biology, Proceedings of the National Academy of Sciences of the United States of America,* and *EcoHealth.*

breeding season than healthy males, and mated with less fit females.[13] Ecologic studies have also been useful to tease out complexities such as the relationship between environmental factors and infection, expression of clinical disease, or severity of disease in populations. The expression of clinical mycoplasmosis in desert tortoises and mortalities of lions caused by coinfection with canine distemper and *Babesia* spp. positively correlated with periods of drought illustrate these complexities. Additionally, chicks of sage thrashers (*Oreoscoptes montanus*) that were parasitized with blowfly larvae grew and fledged at the same rate as nonparasitized chicks during years with average precipitation, whereas significant differences in offspring survival and fledging success occurred in years with adverse climatic conditions.[10] These subtleties in the effects of pathogens on individuals that are translated to population effects are largely being examined by disease ecologists and will likely revolutionize our thinking about disease in wild animals.

CURRENT THEMES IN DISEASE ECOLOGY

Here we review some of the themes in current disease ecology research that we believe are applicable and interesting to veterinarians. This is not an exhaustive list because this field is growing rapidly and new themes are likely to emerge, particularly those that overlap heavily with conservation and public health objectives.

Effect of Host Diversity on Disease Dynamics

Pathogens use a wide range of transmission schemes, directly from one host to another, indirectly through contaminated food or water, through ingestion of infected prey, or via biologic or mechanical transmission by arthropod vectors. In addition, most pathogens have defined hosts that they are capable of infecting. Alterations in a community, vertebrate or invertebrate, may alter the transmission of pathogens.

One of the best examples of how community vertebrate diversity alters this transmission risk is the relationship of *Borrelia burgdorferi*, the causative agent of Lyme disease in humans, and the diversity of potential tick hosts for *Borrelia*, which includes mammals, birds, and reptiles.[17] In the eastern United States, *B. burgdorferi* is transmitted by the black-legged tick (*Ixodes scapularis*)

and is maintained in nature by various rodent reservoir hosts, but the white-footed mouse (*Peromyscus leucopus*) is the principal reservoir. This dilution effect model shows that as vertebrate host diversity increases, the likelihood of ticks becoming infected with *B. burgdorferi* decreases because these other hosts, which are less reservoir-competent for *B. burgdorferi* compared with the white-footed mouse, serve as an alternative blood meal for *I. scapularis*. The model predicts that if white-footed mice are the only hosts that are providing blood meals to *I. scapularis* nymphs, then the prevalence of *B. burgdorferi* would exceed 90%. As specific hosts are removed from the community, the prevalence of *B. burgdorferi* in ticks changes, depending on the reservoir competence of that particular host. For example, the prevalence of *B. burgdorferi*–infected ticks decreases dramatically in a relatively intact system, including white-footed mice, chipmunks, white-tailed deer, raccoons, opossums, skunks, short-tailed shrews, *Sorex* shrews, tree squirrels, and four species of ground nesting birds. However, some species are more important dilution hosts. For *B. burgdorferi*, gray and red squirrels are the least competent hosts for the bacteria but serve as common hosts for the ticks, thus contributing significantly to the dilution effect. Interestingly, even when white-footed mice are removed from the community, other hosts, such as shrews, may be rescue hosts, because they serve as important reservoirs, are infested with large numbers of ticks, and may occur at high densities. Importantly, this model has also been validated using long-term field data.

Although the *B. burgdorferi*–vertebrate host diversity transmission relationship is one of the most studied examples, there are numerous others, including flea-borne *Bartonella* spp. infections in Irish rodents, tick-borne encephalitis in rodents in Europe, and tick-borne louping ill virus in red grouse (*Lagopus lagopus scoticus*) in England. Evidence is increasing that the transmission of some directly transmitted pathogens, such as hantavirus in rodents, may be altered in complex communities, possibly because of changes in behavior (e.g., interspecies interactions).[24] Currently, conflicting evidence exists for a dilution effect and West Nile virus as avian hosts.[18] It has been suggested that non–vector-borne parasites may also respond to community diversity changes. For example, *Myxobolus cerebralis* have used *Tubifex* worms as intermediate hosts, but it has recently been recognized that cryptic species of *Tubifex*, some of which are resistant to infection, may dilute infection. Additionally, reproductive success of the trematode *Ribeiroia ondatrae* is lower in communities in which tree frogs are present because fewer metacercariae are transmitted to their final host.

Diseases of Keystone Species and Conservation

Because a keystone species plays a critical role in maintaining an ecosystem, a disease process that affects it will have a significant impact on the entire community. Southern sea otters *(Enhydra lutris nereis)* were one of the first organisms described as a keystone species because of the dramatic effect they have on kelp communities.[16] In areas in which sea otters are abundant, the kelp communities are diverse and healthy because of the predation of sea urchins by sea otters. If left unchecked by sea otters, sea urchins will overgraze the kelp that provides habitat for spawning fish, which will lead to declines in fish species. This relationship is so strong that monitoring kelp forest ecosystems may be used as a measurement of sea otter recovery. In recent years, southern sea otters have experienced declines, and up to 40% to 63% of mortalities are related to parasitic, bacterial, fungal, or other possible infectious diseases.[15] Many of these diseases are related to anthropogenic change such as the introduction of *Toxoplasma gondii* and *Sarcocystis neurona* by two species exotic to California, domestic cats and Virginia opossums *(Didelphis virginiana)*. Acanthocelphalan peritonitis caused by *Profilicollis* spp. is more common in otters that are forced to forage on sand crabs *(Emerita analoga)* present in sandy habitats. Sea otters that feed on abalone, which are concentrated in resource-abundant ecosystems, have a lower risk of contracting many of these parasites. Currently, the recovery of the southern sea otter is hampered by many non–disease-related threats (e.g., trauma, domoic acid intoxication, gunshot, gill net drowning, oiling) and disease-related issues (e.g., fungal and bacterial pneumonia and sepsis, plus the diseases noted). Processes related to increases in the primary cause of mortality—infectious diseases—need to be investigated further.

Several other examples of disease threats to keystone species have been studied including *Ichthyophonus* infection of Chinook salmon *(Oncorhynchus tshawytscha)*, *Mycoplasma*-associated upper respiratory disease in gopher tortoises *(Gopherus polyphemus)*, and plague in black-tailed prairie dogs *(Cynomys ludovicianus)*. Black-tailed prairie dogs are a keystone species in the prairie ecosystems of the western United States. By digging burrows, they provide habitats for numerous species, including tiger salamanders, rattlesnakes, and burrowing owls. Also, they alter water availability for grasslands and serve as the primary prey item for the endangered black-footed ferret. In addition, they may alter the community composition of other rodents and their associated flea communities, which in turn may alter disease dynamics among the various rodents. Prairie dogs are highly susceptible to sylvatic plague *(Yersinia pestis)* and experience almost 100% morality, whereas other species of rodents (e.g., certain species of *Microtus* and *Peromyscus*) may serve as reservoirs.[3] Because prairie dogs may alter rodent and flea communities, they may actually facilitate transmission of plague, which could lead to outbreaks. Clearly, decreases in keystone species, related to disease or other factors, would significantly alter community structure and ecosystem function.

Exotic or Invasive Species and Disease

Exotic or invasive species may have significant effects on ecosystems. Often, these species do well in their introduced range because of a combination of escape from natural predators and release from natural parasites or pathogens. The loss of parasites or pathogens could simply be related to the initial introduction of few hosts, which will not harbor all possible pathogens, or the initial density of hosts is too low to sustain transmission of directly transmitted organisms. Parasites with complex life cycles may lack required intermediate hosts or vectors to complete their life cycle. These phenomena have been well-studied; examples include the release of invasive European slugs from parasitic nematodes, *Wolbachia* in Argentine ants *(Linepithema humile)*, and parasitic castrators of European green crabs *(Carcinus maenas)*. Importantly, exotic species may introduce exotic pathogens that might be important to the health of native wildlife, domestic animals, or humans. These introductions have had devastating effects on some native ecosystems, such as the introduction of avian malaria *(Plasmodium relictum)* to Hawaiian birds, *Myxobolus cerebralis* to North American salmonids, exotic parasites to native Hawaiian fishes, and *Toxoplasma gondii* to numerous species and locations by domestic cats.[15] Conversely, introduced species may pick up pathogens from their introduced range that may or may not cause significant disease (e.g., *Mycoplasma gallisepticum*) in introduced populations of eastern house finches *(Carpodacus mexicanus)*.[19] Collectively, these examples illustrate that exotic species are often successful related to their escape from natural diseases, but may represent significant risks themselves because of the introduction of novel diseases to native fauna.

Disease and Ecosystem Function

Ecosystem function, the processes and interactive relationships that occur within an ecosystem—and their alteration from normal—is currently a significant topic in ecology and conservation literature. In conservation, the concept of ecosystem function is being promoted as a way to attribute value to specific ecosystem processes for the benefit of humans (e.g., clean water as a consequence of reforestation). Some have suggested that a healthy ecosystem is one that in addition to being biodiverse and resilient, supports important ecologic functions, resists colonization by invasive species, and has a low degree and frequency of disease events.[5] This latter part is highly controversial and difficult to measure. Nevertheless, there is interest in investigating this hypothesis and it has gained momentum in the parlance of the general public, public health, and ecologic studies.[14]

Because ecosystem processes are affected by the biota in those ecosystems, it follows that factors that affect those organisms, such as disease, might have significant consequences for the overall function of the system. The disease ecology literature has borrowed methods from the field of disturbance ecology, which aims to predict the type and magnitude of ecosystem function that a pathogen will have; however, most examples apply to plant pathogens[6] or to keystone species (see earlier).

One clear empirical example in animals involves chytridiomycosis, which has resulted in catastrophic amphibian declines worldwide. Much effort has been devoted to documenting amphibian loss of biodiversity as a result of the introduction of this disease. Only recently have examinations of the potential effects of amphibian extinctions on ecosystem function surfaced, such as the long-term integrity of tropical stream quality after amphibian declines. Without tadpoles of stream-breeding amphibians, the primary grazers of algae and other detritus, stream quality measures were poor immediately after an epizootic of chytridiomycosis.[27] Another interesting example of a pathogen disturbing ecosystem integrity involves plague epizootics and prairie dogs, during which a significant number of prairie dog colonies were affected and that translated to attenuated effects on grassland vegetation in Colorado.[8]

Emergent Diseases and Their Management

Traditionally, management of disease outbreaks has involved manipulation of the host or the pathogen, although various manipulations of the environment typically used by wildlife management agencies have been summarized by Wobeser.[28] Holt has used the analysis of community modules to examine the emergence of diseases as a result of a disturbance on interspecific interactions and has specifically proposed that predators, even when "not directly involved in disease transmission, by imposing mortality or modifying prey behavior, may influence disease dynamics."[9] Given the long-standing human history of predator control, their sensitivity to habitat disturbance, and the typical low reproductive rate of vertebrate predators, it is not difficult to find examples in which predator populations have been disturbed and its effects on prey easily quantified. Packer and coworkers[22] have continued to suggest that at its simplest form, removal of predators may release a variety of deleterious prey-pathogen relationships, and several theoretical and empirical studies have supported this theory. The mechanism behind this hypothesis is the predator's ability to alter the abundance and dynamics of single-prey (host) populations. This may also occur in multihost pathogens. One such example would be the effect of apparent competition already occurring between ring-necked pheasants and grey partridges, which have different responses to infection with *Heterakis gallinarum*. To this example, one may add a predator to illustrate the theory mentioned. Ring-necked pheasants do not suffer measurable losses to body condition when infected with *Heterakis* as compared with grey partridge, which are significantly affected by this nematode. Previous data have demonstrated that *H. gallinarum* fecundity and survival is greater in pheasants than in partridges, suggesting that the primary source of nematode infection to wild grey partridges in Scotland is reared pheasants.[25] In this example, apparent competition occurs indirectly between these two species, which are consumed by the same predator. The increase of ring-necked pheasants (i.e., from reduced predation) might cause the decline of grey partridges because the increase in density of pheasants increases *H. gallinarum* in the environment.[26]

CHALLENGES AND FUTURE DIRECTIONS

We believe that the scientific community dedicated to the study of wildlife disease is at the cusp of significant changes. Recurrent reports of the emergence of novel diseases, threats of bioterrorism, socioeconomic importance of some pathogens, increase in international movement of pathogens, and additive effects of a variety of anthropogenic activities, as well as the media attention given to these diseases, have resulted in an upsurge of interest in the study of wildlife disease. As a result, there are more types of scientific researchers involved in this field. This leads to a more diverse group of people, trained in a variety of ways, approaching problems from a range of perspectives and has led to some elegant work, as illustrated by the examples presented. All this activity demonstrates positive growth toward the merging and mixing of the different perspectives that these disciplines may offer. Unfortunately, however, this also means that the different groups, having developed in their own, often insular, environments, can occasionally have trouble communicating at various levels. Already we enjoy the fruit of elegant, multidisciplinary, truly collaborative work; however, from our perspective, there are some growing pains that both fields will need to experience before we may advance further to reach our collaborative potential.

First, as a result of neither preveterinary requirements nor veterinary curriculums including ecology courses, veterinarians may not be familiar with common ecologic terms, principles, and techniques and often have a poor understanding of population and community ecology. Because veterinarians often lack this ecologic background, they tend to underappreciate the value that ecologists can provide to investigations, particularly in regard to quantitative methods, statistical analyses, and measures used to estimate population abundance, occupancy, and dynamics. Aguirre has recently stated that "veterinary curricula are too inflexible to … provide sufficient training to … be effective in the conservation of biodiversity" and recommended "further training in zoology, conservation biology, ecology or a related field in the form of an advanced graduate degree or specialty residency…."[1] Even veterinary colleges that offer a variety of zoological medicine topics lack ecology courses and most available externships are unlikely to provide a sufficient foundation.

Similarly, epidemiologic vocabulary is sometimes misused, and biomedical techniques may be misinterpreted by classically trained ecologists. For example, a growing area of research is using traditional biomedical techniques to estimate stress in wild animals, particularly at the population level. Assumptions and conclusions about the meaning of stress and the consequence of stress levels in wild animal populations are made using techniques that are considered inadequate by

trained pathologists. Additionally, ecologic research by nature tends to identify common trends and generalities that may be applied to multiple systems. In contrast, with regard to pathogens and parasites, details are important; for example, generalities across host species susceptibilities, parasite life cycles, or pathogenesis cannot be made. A strong background in immunology, pathology, and pathogens is often needed to understand these subtleties. And, even when the details about the natural history of a particular pathogen are known, other variables such as differences in habitat, species composition, and climate may significantly alter pathogen dynamics, preventing generalizations from being useful.

These criticisms should not be overemphasized and we believe that, on the whole, these disciplines have much to gain from one another. For example, when keratoconjunctivitis caused by *Mycoplasma gallisepticum* in house finches (*Carpodacus mexicanus*) emerged in the 1990s, an extraordinary amount of work quickly emerged; a search in Web of Science for mycoplasma conjunctivitis–house finches has revealed 49 publications since 1996. Most significantly, many publications delve into the population-level consequences of this emergent disease, its effects on population dynamics (especially between eastern and western populations), and environmental factors related to pathogen transmission and disease development (e.g., as noted by Faustino and associates).[7] Such a surge in information about the ecologic details of this pathogen was possible largely in part because the details of *M. gallisepticum* (the who, what, and why) of this pathogen had been known for decades as a result of its economic importance to poultry. These were quickly extrapolated to house finches through traditional disease investigation methods (e.g., by Luttrell and coworkers[20] and Kollias and colleagues[15]). This has allowed the more intricate ecologic investigations to build on a solid foundation in regard to the natural history of the pathogen, transmission, pathogenesis, and diagnostic methodologies.

Some specific activities that will lead to better understanding and shared respect might be regular attendance and presentation of scientific work in each other's professional organizations' conferences, reading and publishing in journals outside our immediate arena, cross-pollination of editorial boards in pertinent journals, and/or the creation of think tanks that involve a variety of relevant professionals. More inclusive graduate advisory committees or postgraduate clinical training mentors—for example, having a veterinarian sit on the advisory committee of an ecology student or ecologists providing supervision and mentorship to residents undertaking research projects—will prove useful. This has been our approach at the University of Georgia. We hope that our professional organizations will welcome the growth of disease ecology and reach out for these activities and consider other integrative ways for collaboration.

Acknowledgment

We would like to acknowledge Dr. Nicole Gottdenker who actively participated in earlier discussions that framed the content of this chapter.

REFERENCES

1. Aguirre AA: Essential veterinary education in zoological and wildlife medicine: A global perspective. Rev Sci Tech 28:605–610, 2009.
2. Anderson RM, May RM: Regulation and stability of host-parasite population interactions. 1. Regulatory processes. J Anim Ecol 47:219–247, 1978.
3. Collinge SK, Ray C: Disease ecology: Community structure and pathogen dynamics, New York, 2006, Oxford University Press, p 227.
4. Dobson AP, Hudson PJ: Regulation and stability of a free-living host-parasite system-Trichostrongylus tenuis in red grouse. 2. Population Models. J Anim Ecol 61:487–498, 1992.
5. Epstein PR, Dobson A, Vandemeer J: Biodiversity and emerging infectious diseases: Integrating health and ecosystem monitoring. In Grifo F, Rosenthal J, editors: Biodiversity and human health, Washington DC, 1997, Island Press, pp 60–67.
6. Eviner VT, Likens GE: Effects of pathogens on terrestrial ecosystem function. In: Ostfeld RS, Keesing F, Eviner VT, editors: Infectious disease ecology: Effects of ecosystems on disease and of disease on ecosystems. New York, 2008, Princeton University Press, pp 260–283.
7. Faustino CR, Jennelle CS, Connolly V, et al: Mycoplasma gallisepticum infection dynamics in a house finch population: Seasonal variation in survival, encounter and transmission rate. J Anim Ecol 73:651–669, 2004.
8. Hartley LM, Detling JK, Savage LT: Introduced plague lessens the effects of an herbivorous rodent on grassland vegetation. J Appl Ecol 46:861–869, 2009.
9. Holt RD: The community context of disease emergence: Could changes in predation be a key driver? In Ostfeld RS, Keesing F, Eviner V, editors: Infectious disease ecology: Effects of ecosystems on disease and of disease on ecosystems, New York, 2008, Princeton University Press, pp 324–346.
10. Howe FP: Effects of Protocalliphora braueri (Dipetra, Calliphoridae) parasitism and inclement weather on nestlike sage thrashers. J Wildl Dis 28:141–143, 1992.
11. Hudson PJ, Dobson AP, Newborn D: Prevention of population cycles by parasite removal. Science 282:2256–2258, 1998.
12. Hudson PJ, Rizzoli A, Grenfell BT, et al: The ecology of wildlife diseases, New York, 2001, Oxford University Press, p 197.
13. Johnson L, Boyce MS: Female choice of males with low parasite loads in sage grouse. In Loye JE, Zuk M, editors: Bird-parasite interactions: Ecology, evolution and behavior, New York, 1991, Oxford University Press.
14. Johnson PT, Thieltges DW: Diversity, decoys and the dilution effect: How ecological communities affect disease risk. J Exp Biol 213:961–970, 2010.
15. Kollias GV, Sydenstricker KV, Kollias HW, et al: Experimental infection of house finches with Mycoplasma gallisepticum. J Wildl Dis 40:79–86, 2004.
16. Kreuder C, Miller MA, Jessup,DA, et al: Patterns of mortality in southern sea otters (Enhydra lutris nereis) from 1998-2001. J Wildl Dis 39:495–509, 2003.
17. LoGiudice K, Ostfeld RS, Schmidt KA, Keesing F: The ecology of infectious disease: Effects of host diversity and community composition on Lyme disease risk. Proc Natl Acad Sci U S A 100:567–571, 2003.
18. Loss SR, Hamer GL, Walker ED, et al: Avian host community structure and prevalence of West Nile virus in Chicago, Illinois. Oecologia 159:415–424, 2009.
19. Luttrell MP, Fischer JR, Stallknecht DE, et al: Field investigation of Mycoplasma gallisepticum infections in house finches (Carpodacus mexicanus) from Maryland and Georgia. Avian Dis 40:335–341, 1996.
20. Luttrell MP, Stallknecht DE, Kleven SH, et al: Mycoplasma gallisepticum in house finches (Carpodacus mexicanus) and other wild birds associated with poultry production facilities. Avian Dis 45:321–329, 2001.
21. Ostfeld RS, Keesing F, Eviner V, editors: Infectious disease ecology: Effects of ecosystems on disease and of disease on ecosystems, Princeton, NJ, 2008, Princeton University Press, p 506.
22. Packer C, Holt RD, Hudson PJ, et al: Keeping the herds healthy and alert: Implications of predator control for infectious disease. Ecol Lett 6:797–802, 2003.
23. Ricklefs RE, Miller GL: Ecology, ed 4, New York, 2000, WH Freeman.
24. Suzán G, Marcé Giermakowski JT, Mills JN, et al: Experimental evidence for reduced rodent diversity causing increased hantavirus prevalence. PLoS One 4:e5461, 2009.
25. Tompkins DM, Dickson G, Hudson PJ: Parasite-mediated competition between pheasant and grey partridge: A preliminary investigation. Oecologia 119:378–382, 1999.
26. Tompkins DM, Greenman JV, Hudson PJ: Differential impact of a shared nematode parasite on two gamebird hosts: Implications for apparent competition. Parasitology 122:187–193, 2001.
27. Whiles MR, Lips KR, Pringle CM, et al: The effects of amphibian population declines on the structure and function of neotropical stream ecosystems. Frontiers Ecol Environment 4:27–34, 2006.
28. Wobeser GA: Disease in wild animals: Investigation and management, ed 2, Heidelberg, Germany, 2007, Springer.

Aquatic

CHAPTER 22

Medical Management of Rays

Natalie D. Mylniczenko

Of all the elasmobranchs, the charismatic rays have gained immense popularity in the last several years with the increased prevalence of touch pools in zoos and aquaria. The most popular species in contact areas is the cownose ray *(Rhinoptera bonasus)*, followed by the southern stingray *(Dasyatis americana)* and occasionally other species. Outside of these unique exhibit opportunities, rays remain an integral part of elasmobranch collections. Still, little has been published on their medical management.

BIOLOGY, ANATOMY, AND PHYSIOLOGY

Rays inhabit a wide variety of environments, from complete freshwater to gradients of saltwater, including full ocean water. They are euryhaline (wide range of salinity tolerance) or stenohaline (narrow range of salinity tolerance), which may greatly affect husbandry and treatment strategies. There are three classes of rays—those that are strictly saltwater, those that are exclusively freshwater (potamotrygonid species), and those that may live in both.[2] All rays are depressiform, with eyes positioned dorsally, or in some cases laterally, and mouths positioned ventrally. Genders are easily distinguished because males have obvious claspers at the pelvic fins whereas females do not. The skin is covered with placoid scales composed of dentin and enamel. Rays have no teeth but have crushing plates of modified placoid scales embedded in their gums, with differences among species based on prey.[8] As with shark teeth, these plates constantly overturn by moving forward to the edge of the mouth.

Rays have gill slits on their ventral body wall and usually a spiracle (respiratory aperture) on their dorsum. Respiration occurs through active pumping of water over gills by pulling water into the mouth or the spiracles and then bathing the gills; thus, for those species that rest on the bottom, use of the spiracles provides unobstructed respiration, unlike some of their shark counterparts that must continually swim to respirate.[8] Manta rays are unique in that they possess gill rakers, much like the whale shark. The musculoskeletal system is almost completely cartilaginous, with the exception of occasional ossification of the vertebral column. The simple cardiovascular system has one ventricle, one atrium, a sinus venosum, and a conus arteriosis (Fig. 22-1). The heart is separated from the coelom by a rigid pericardium.[16] A renal portal system has been documented. Rays possess no bone marrow, so hematopoiesis occurs via the spleen, Leydig organ, and epigonal organ. The latter two vary greatly in size and contribution of hematopoietic cells per species. Thyroid tissue is present but is disseminated and difficult to identify unless diseased.

The liver is a predominant organ, occupying most of the length and width of the coelom (see Fig. 22-1). It is light tan in color, a reflection of the high lipid content (a natural hepatic lipidosis); lipids make up to 80% of the liver's architecture.[8] The liver contributes significantly to buoyancy because there is no swim bladder. A gallbladder is present that produces bile acids that form alcohol sulfate esters (versus taurine salts in birds and mammals, which are reflected in available bile acid assays). The gastrointestinal tract (Fig. 22-2) is simple, with a distensible esophagus, descending cardiac stomach with pronounced rugae, and ascending pyloric stomach that is connected directly to a spiral colon, also called the spiral valve. The colon varies anatomically with species but typically has copious folds or layers that increase digestive capability. There is a rectum that empties into a cloaca. Unique to elasmobranchs is the rectal gland, which opens into the intestine-rectum area and is involved in the osmoregulation of sodium and chloride ions. Freshwater stingrays have reduced or no

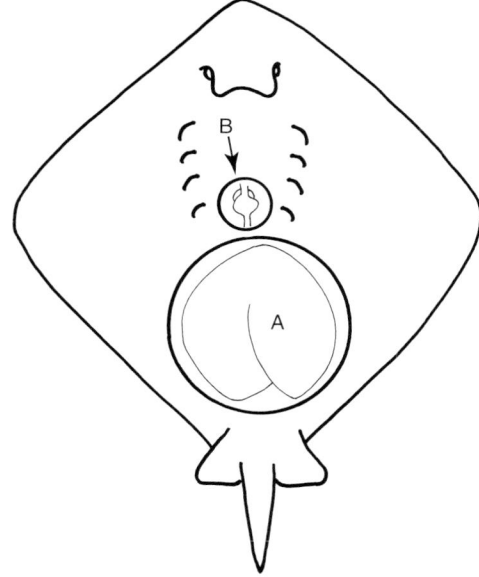

Figure 22-1

General anatomy of the stingray in ventral recumbency. *A,* Location and distribution of the liver. *B,* Location of the heart with the ventricle in the ventral position, superimposing the atrium.

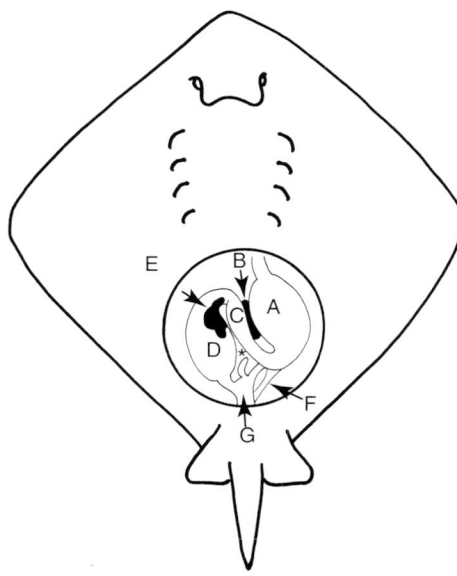

Figure 22-2

General anatomy of the stingray in ventral recumbency with the liver removed. *A,* Descending cardiac stomach. *B,* Spleen. *C,* Ascending pyloric stomach. *D,* Spiral colon (valve). *E,* Pancreas. *F,* Gonadal duct. *G,* Cloaca. *Rectal gland.

functional rectal gland tissue, depending on their water salinity.[2] Coelomic (abdominal) pores, adjacent to cloaca, have a direct connection to the coelomic cavity. Their function is not fully understood but is suspected to regulate electrolytes and maintain osmoregulatory homeostasis.[6] Some clinicians have used these pores for examination of the coelom with a laparoscope or for flushing the coelom; others question this technique because of its suspected regulatory function.

Vision is poor compared to other senses; pupil dilation may be controlled by the animal, unlike in teleosts but compared with mammals' pupillary light reflexes, are slow or difficult to assess when stimulated. Because of pigmentation, the lenses in some species may be slightly opaque.[4] Olfaction and taste are keen sensory abilities. Non–filter-feeding rays mouth objects to determine whether they are edible and they may discriminate between fish types. It may be difficult to distinguish mouthing or crushing of food from actual consumption of food. The ampullae of Lorenzini (mucopolysaccharide-filled electrosensory organs) detect external vibration and low-frequency electrical pulses for the detection of animate versus inanimate objects.[8] Filters and pumps too close to an enclosure may disturb these organs and cause aberrant behavior. A lateral line is present, with a lining of neuromast cells that respond to pressure changes.

All saltwater rays are hyperosmotic to their environment. They have a high urea content in the blood as well as other solutes that increase osmolarity. A specialized protein, trimethylamine *N*-oxide (TMAO), is lighter than seawater and is thought to aid in buoyancy.[8] Freshwater elasmobranchs have a significantly lower urea content; those that are obligate freshwater animals have negligible levels.[2]

Copulation in the rays occurs with the male grasping the female on the wings (usually resulting is some degree of trauma) and then inserting a clasper into the female's cloaca, which transfers sperm from the male. Sperm storage occurs in multiple species with varying durations. Aplacental viviparity occurs with the production of uterine milk, which is absorbed by the embryo. The uterus develops trophonemata; these are villi of the uterine epithelium that secrete histotroph, a rich yellow opaque fluid that feeds the embryos (but should not be mistaken for pyometra). Ray embryos have a yolk sac, but it is absorbed by the time gestation is 75% complete, after which they rely on histotroph for nutrition. Gestation is variable (2 to 12 months) and estimating the birth date may be complicated, given their ability to store sperm for several months.[4,13]

HUSBANDRY AND MANAGEMENT

Water quality parameters and specific exhibit suggestions may be found elsewhere.[13] Special focus will be paid to contact or touch pools because these have gained immense popularity in the last several years. There has been some notoriety associated with these exhibits in the media that has reported on large population declines caused by sudden animal death. In many touch pools, these are related to a life support problem. Most of these pools are shallow and populated beyond optimum carrying capacity. Many of these exhibits are temporary and housed in facilities that do not typically support large aquaria. Specific causes of these events have been attributed to hyperthermia, hypoxia, well water contamination by heavy metals, and inanition caused by poor acclimation. The first two issues may be avoided with alarm systems that broadcast an alert when water quality parameters are out of range. Water sources should be tested for contaminants. Acclimation becomes an issue with recent capture of free-range specimens, usually young animals that need special attention to transition to a captive diet. Using experienced adult animals in these exhibits may avoid this issue; alternately, the animals must be managed throughout this period by offering foods that approximate their wild diet and often by supportive assist feeding. Rarely do these animals suffer from touch-related issues. Although these animals are encouraged to be out and touchable, hiding places should be made available for them. Most will choose to interact because the species chosen are gregarious by nature.

RESTRAINT

Not all rays possess spines or barbs on their tails; for example, *Urogymus* spp. and the manta rays lack barbs and are not venomous.[5] Those that do have spines or barbs are typically gentle but will defend themselves in situations in which they are stepped on or manipulated excessively. Although being abraded or punctured by a stingray barb is dangerous, one should also be cautious of their bites, recalling that these animals crush crustacean prey. The barb or spine of a stingray is cartilaginous and often serrated. Venom on the barbs is not produced by venom glands but by two longitudinal grooves under the barb that contain venom-secreting glandular cells. The spine is covered with epidermis; when a human is punctured, not only is there venom to contend with but pieces of integument and cells remain in the wound, increasing the exposure to microorganisms and venom. The venoms are largely cardiotoxic, although some are neurotoxic as well.

Protocols for managing stingray injuries are recommended.[5] Some institutions will trim the barbs of these animals, which reduces the risk of puncture, but exposure through abrasion is still possible because the base of the barb still contains venom. Barbs are naturally shed two or three times/year; therefore, regrowth may be expected at this interval.[13] Removal of the barb may be done surgically; on occasion, the procedure may result in infection, permanent scarring, or regrowth, sometimes in an abnormal position. In freshwater stingrays, the epidermal bumps around the barb also contain venom. Anecdotally, freshwater stingrays have more potent venom, resulting in a greater pain response in affected humans, although most of these injuries are manageable with analgesics. Placing plastic tubing around the tail and barb will prevent accidental exposure.

Manual restraint is possible, although special precautions should be used, as noted. Tonic-clonic immobilization may be achieved by flipping the animal over until it is in a trancelike state; care should be taken when placing pressure on the coelom, because the liver may fracture. This is much easier with animals that are acclimated to handling; for them, operant condition is a successful tool for rays. Anesthesia should be used in naïve or large specimens and for lengthy procedures. Chemical restraint is usually accomplished by immersion. Injectables are not commonly used and no reports have been published. Most anesthesia is performed via bathing in tricaine methane sulfonate (MS-222), with an equal mass of buffer (bicarbonate), in a variety of concentration ranges, from 60 to 300 ppm (typically at the lower end of that dose range). Animals should be ventilated with a syringe and tubing or a pump delivering water that is slowly and gently flowed over the gills; a rapid current may prevent gas exchange. Recoveries should also be under gentle flow ventilation because this greatly increases the oxygen saturation of the blood rather than the traditional walking of the animal in the water. In a recent study of different immersion anesthetics, 20 ppm eugenol, 15.7 ppm isoeugenol, and 55 to 65 ppm MS-222 were compared in *Daysatis americana*. Minor variations were noted but, overall, all the agents provided adequate anesthesia for short-term immobilizations and minor procedures.[11] An important note when handling gravid females is that abortion may occur with anesthesia or handling, more likely later in gestation. If very late in gestation, it is possible that these pups may be successfully raised.

PHYSICAL EXAMINATION

Routine examinations should include an ocular examination; note that there is large variation in iris shape and there is a normal poor pupillary light response. Gills should be examined by use of a transilluminator or laparoscopic equipment. Because of the size and depth of the gill slit, using a biopsy forceps, such for laparoscopy equipment, facilitates obtaining gill samples. Bleeding does occur and applying pressure for several minutes is important. A cloacal lavage may be used to obtain fecal samples, although because of rapid gastrointestinal (GI) transit time, yields are typically poor if the animal is fasted. Ultrasonography is an important aspect of the physical examination. Cardiac examination of contractility and rhythm provide a good assessment on the animal's stability under anesthesia— weak contractility is an indication to awaken the animal; ultrasonic Doppler may be used but does not provide information about myocontractions. Coelomic ultrasound is important for evaluating the condition of the animal and, in experienced hands, may indicate disease conditions prior to the manifestation of overt clinical signs. Hepatic echotexture should be hyperechoic to mammal livers, reflecting the normal state of lipidosis, and the liver should extend from the cranial coelom to the area just short of the pelvic girdle. A gall bladder is present and the entire GI tract may be scanned (Figs. 22-3 and 22-4). The spleen and pancreas may be visualized in larger specimens. Reproductive organs and embryos may be identified in sexually active and mature animals. Minor amounts of fluid are normal, but there should not be more than a small amount in the caudal coelom.

Blood may be collected from the ventral tail vessel, midline, at a 90-degree angle; the needle must pass firm connective tissue, usually with a distinctive pop. Although cardiac puncture is possible, it is difficult to reach through the cartilage and is not practical. Additionally, there is potential to dilute the sample because of the presence of pericardial fluid.[10] There are few reports on normal reference ranges in rays.[3,12,13] Like other elasmobranchs, they possess unique white blood cells termed *granulocytes*; different nomenclature exists for the different cell types, which may lead to frustration when trying to determine what constitutes normal results. Laboratories familiar with elasmobranch cytology should be used or in-house standards should be prepared and trends observed; explanations of these cell types are found elsewhere.[1,12,13] Overall, they have a low hematocrit (~20% to 25%) and the clinician should not

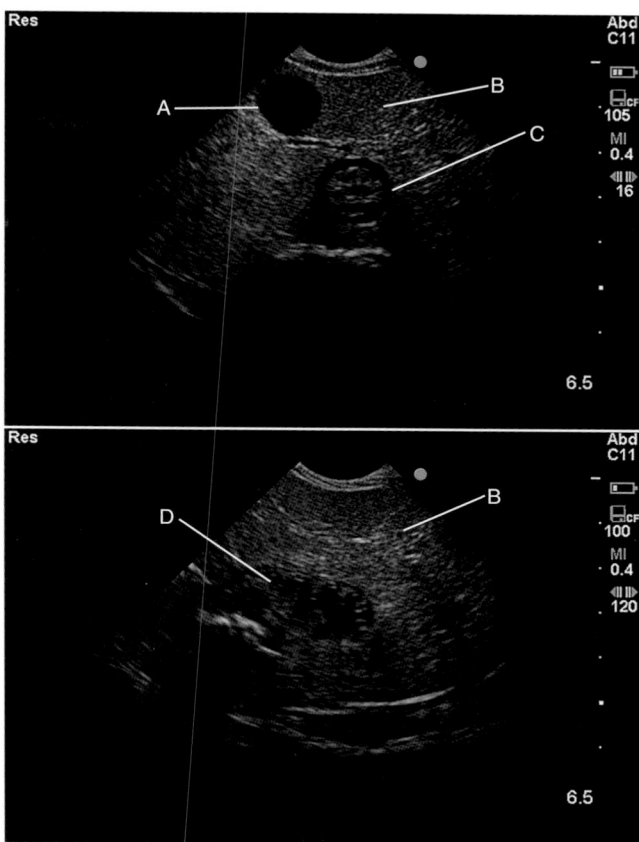

Figure 22-3

Ultrasonographic anatomy of a southern stingray (*Dasyatis americana*). *A,* Gallbladder. *B,* Liver. *C,* Esophagus. *D,* Cardiac stomach.

be alarmed. Serum chemistry results have some marked differences from teleosts. Blood gases are important and should be monitored, if possible, during handling events or long transports using handheld units. Serum blood and blood gas parameters for stingrays are given in Tables 22-1 and 22-2. A recent study[9] examining blood culture status in normal elasmobranchs not only noted 30% normal positive results, but rays showed a higher percentage of normal positives, approaching 50% of the population examined. This is congruent with the results of other studies, in which tissue cultures are also frequently positive, reflecting normal microbial colonization of healthy elasmobranch tissues. Positive blood culture results must be interpreted cautiously and clinicians are encouraged to obtain repeat cultures or use two different sites for simultaneous collection. Cerebrospinal fluid (CSF) aspiration may be easily accomplished while guided by ultrasound because there is moderate fluid surrounding the brain. Coelomic lavage

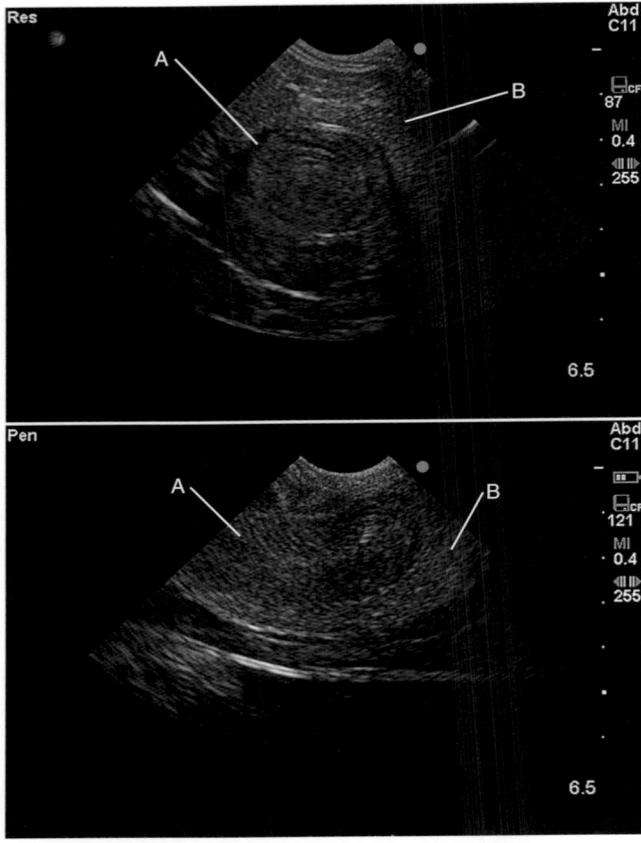

Figure 22-4

Ultrasonographic anatomy of a southern stingray *(Dasyatis americana)*. *A*, Spiral colon (valve) in transverse view (above) and sagittal views (below). *B*, Liver.

TABLE 22-2   Generalized Blood Gas Parameters for Stingrays

Parameter	Saltwater Stingrays	Potamotrygonid Freshwater Stingrays
pH*	7.3-7.6	7.0-7.4
Po_2* (mmol/L)	Highly variable	Highly variable
Sao_2* (%)	>85	>80
Pco_2 (mm Hg)	7-15	7-15
Tco_2 (mmol/L)	4-6	4-8
BE (mmol/L)	−18 to −25	−18 to −25
HCO_3 (mmol/L)	4-6	2-6
Lactate (mmol/L)	<3	<3
Ionized calcium (mmol/L)	>2.50[†]	1.3-2.3

*Corrected temperatures.
[†]Unreadable on most units >2.5 mmol/liter.

TABLE 22-1   Generalized Serum Blood Parameters for Stingrays

Parameter	Saltwater Stingrays	Potamotrygonid Freshwater Stingrays
Blood urea nitrogen (mg/dL)	800-1100	2-10
Sodium (mEq/L)	250-300	170-180
Chloride (mEq/L)	250-300	164-175
Calcium (mg/dL)	15-20	8.5-13.5
Glucose (mg/dL)	20-40	20-40

is a standard diagnostic tool, particularly for cownose rays, to evaluate coccidial burden.[14] Low-level (clinically irrelevant) coccidia may be identified on these lavages, but in stressed and diseased animals the fluid will be copious and thick or opaque, white to green in color, instead of being translucent and thin.

DISEASES

Signs of disease or stress in rays include inappetance or complete anorexia, loss of muscle mass and condition, curling of the disc edges, not burying in the substrate, flashing because of pruritis, and decreased swimming. Often, there are overt signs of trauma to and redness of the fins, as well as erosions. However, sudden death is also seen, with no premonitory signs. Ulcerations are common but may be hard to recognize because most are on the ventrum of the animal and are not seen if the animal is not swimming with its ventral area in view. Color or pallor may also be an indicator of illness, but it should be remembered that animals exposed to sun will actually acquire a suntan, so their indoor counterparts may be considerably lighter. Anorexia or inanition is a problem in recently captured or quarantined animals and in ill animals; it is a common cause of death. Animals lose weight and condition, and their liver becomes smaller and gains a denser echotexture. Recognizing poor body condition is challenging: coelomic fill, wing, or disc muscle thickness and a prominent vertebral column or pelvic girdle are all factors in the assessment. Assist (gavage) feeding these animals is paramount: neither repeat handling nor assist feeding will usually prevent normal eating behavior when the animals are prepared to eat. During this period, live food, whole prey, and offering wide varieties is crucial. Animals may take several weeks before resuming normal feeding.

Trauma is another common issue. It may occur during the breeding season (bites around the disc), may be caused by stereotypy, resulting in ocular and fin damage, and may result in ulcerations of the ventral skin from being on an inappropriate substrate or spending too much time at the bottom of the enclosure.

Bacteria and fungi may be primary and secondary pathogens.[13] In freshwater rays, *Saprolegnia* spp. is a common secondary invader and exacerbates skin ulcers. Septicemia is a typical sequel to nonhealing wounds. Parasites may be commensal or pathogenic. Observing the animal's clinical condition (weight and body condition loss) is important, and identifying the specific organism may be useful in determining its role in disease. Protozoal infections are rare but possible; in general, rays are not very susceptible to primary disease. Trypanosomes have been associated with disease, with leeches as a vector; the leeches themselves may also serve as a pathogen. Intestinal coccidians are of unknown importance. Coelomic *Eimeria* spp. may cause mortality but may be normal in healthy animals.[1] Digenetic trematodes may be found in new imports, but because an intermediate host is necessary to carry out the life cycle, it is rarely a long-term problem. Monogeneans (flukes) are a larger concern because their life cycle is rapid and direct. Some are species-specific but many are not. Some trematodes have haptors made of chitin, which if present are treatable with chitin inhibitors. Gill and skin infestations may cause death in high numbers. Isopods, when noticed, are easily pulled off. Cestodes may be found burrowing under the skin, leaving track marks. Freshwater rays will have infestations of *Argulus* spp.

Reproductive diseases, although not well documented, have been seen at a number of facilities. Pyometra (distinguished from normal histotroph) has been seen in mature females and is a chronic condition that animals seem to be able to tolerate for several months, but to which they may ultimately succumb. Spaying is a challenge as the uterus is intimately associated with the body wall in many species and with chronic disease may also have resultant adhesions, which complicate removal of organs. Dystocia has been reported.[15]

Noninfectious diseases include exposure to toxic fumes from volatile paints and glues during construction or filter repair, GI foreign bodies and associated sequelae, and neoplasia. Although not common, goiter (thyroid hyperplasia) has occasionally occurred, though rays are not as susceptible as shark species. Prevention with iodide supplementation is recommended via commercially prepared elasmobranch vitamins orally or through water supplementation; weekly additions are necessary because there is a rapid system consumption rate. Quarantine is mandatory to decrease the incidence of widespread disease in elasmobranch populations.[13] Necropsies should be performed on all animals.

TREATMENT

There are no published reports of pharmacologic testing in rays. Most reports are anectodal[13] or extrapolated from shark species, and the reader is directed to these references. In situations in which fluid therapy is warranted, elasmobranch Ringer's solution or oral freshwater may be used in saltwater species, whereas freshwater rays may benefit from fluids derived for teleosts.[7]

Although copper, formalin, and ivermectin have been used for parasite control in various ray species with no ill effects, these drugs are generally not used because of mortalities associated with them. Organophosphates carry the same caution. Osmotic baths may be very useful and, in freshwater rays, have no negative side effects, particularly with long-term immersion in a low- saline solution (2 to 5 ppt); with some saltwater species, caution should be exercised based on the tolerance of varying saline levels. Fenbendazole may be used but, as with many other species, morbidity and mortality have been seen at doses higher than 25 mg/kg. Praziquantel and diflubenzaron (Dimilin) combined are effective for managing monogeneans with haptors. Osmotic baths may be helpful, but stenohaline species may be very sensitive and, in some anecdotal accounts, have succumbed to osmoregularity imbalance. Other considerations for parasitic treatment should include biologic control with cleaner wrasses and shrimps.

Assist-feeding animals is a common treatment; a gruel may be made up and gavaged at 2% to 5% body weight (ensure passage past the esophageal sphincter). If regurgitation occurs, the gill cavity must be flushed or else the gills will become coated and respiration will be hampered. The following recipe is suggested, which may be frozen and aliquotted: 800 g mackerel or herring fillets, 100 g shrimp with shells but without tails, two sheets of nori seaweed, 100 mL of a concentrated high-calorie liquid diet and dietary supplement (Stat; PRN Pharmacal, Pensacola, Fla), and cod liver or salmon oil ground to a smooth pastelike consistency. Avoid using carbohydrate sources, which are common in many prepared gruel feeds. Consider adding elasmobranch vitamins for long-term care.

ZOONOTIC DISEASES

There is minimal risk of disease with contact animals. Humans who are sensitive to saltwater or fish mucus may suffer a reaction to touching these animals. Marine bacterial *Vibrio* spp. are always a concern, but in these animals, punctures or abrasions are the highest risk factor.

Acknowledgment

The author would like to extend thanks to Don Neiffer, Lisa Naples, and Kevin Maxson for their input into the material in this chapter.

REFERENCES

1. Arnold JE: Hematology of the sandbar shark, carcharhinus plumbeus: Standardization of complete blood count techniques for elasmobranchs. Vet Clin Pathol 34:115–123, 2005.
2. Ballantyne JS, Robinson JW: Freshwater elasmobranchs: A review of their physiology and biochemistry. J Comp Physiol B 180:475–493, 2010.
3. Cain DK, Harms CA, Segars: Plasma biochemistry reference values of wild-caught southern stingrays (dasyatis americana). J Zoo Wildl Med 35:471–476, 2004.
4. Carrier JC, Musick JA, Heithaus MR: Biology of sharks and their relatives, Boca Raton, Fla, 2004, CRC Press.
5. Diaz JH: The epidemiology, evaluation, and management of stingray injuries. J La State Med So 159:198–204, 2007.
6. Dobbie JW: From philosopher to fish: The comparative anatomy of the peritoneal cavity as an excretory organ and its significant for peritoneal dialysis in man. Perit Dial Int 8:3–6, 1988.
7. Greenwell MG, Sherrill J, Clayton LA: Osmoregulation in fish. Mechanisms and clinical implications. Vet Clin North Am Exot Anim Pract 6:169–189, 2003.
8. Hamlett W: Sharks, skates, and rays: The biology of elasmobranch fishes, Baltimore, 1999, Johns Hopkins University Press.
9. Mylniczenko ND, Harris B, Wilborn RE, et al: Blood culture results from healthy captive and free-range elasmobranchs. J Aquat Anim Health 19:159–167, 2007.
10. Neiffer D: Personal communication, March 3, 2010.
11. Neiffer DL, Nolan EC, Wilson A: Comparison of three immersion agents (tricaine methanesulfonate, aqui-s[iso-eugenol], and eugenol) for short duration immobilization of captive southern stingrays (dasyatis americana) from an open water system in the Bahamas. Proc Am Assoc Zoo Vet 2009.
12. Semeniuk CAD, Bourgeon S, Smith SL, et al: Hematological differences between stingrays at tourist and non-visited sites. Biol Cons 142:1818–1829, 2009.
13. Smith M, Warmolts D, Thoney D, Hueter R, editors: The elasmobranch husbandry manual: Captive care of sharks, rays, and their relatives, 2004 (http://www.flyingsharks.eu/literature/Census_of_Elasmobranchs_in_Public_Aquaria.pdf).
14. Stamper MA, Lewbart G, Barrington P, et al: Eimeria southwelli infection associated with high mortality of cownose rays. J Aquat Anim Health 10:264–270, 1998.
15. Stamper MA, Lewbart GA, Wrangell A: Manually induced parturition of two yellow spotted stingrays (urolophus jamaicensis) with dystocias. In (editors): Proceedings of the American Association of Zoo Veterinarians and the American Association of Wildlife Veterinarians Joint Conference. 1998:366–367.
16. Stoskopf MK: Fish medicine, Philadelphia, 1993, WB Saunders.

CHAPTER 23

Basic Water Quality Evaluation for Zoo Veterinarians

M. Andrew Stamper and Kent J. Semmen

Of the various marine organisms, only marine mammals have specific government enforced regulations. The Animal and Plant Health Inspection Service (APHIS) has water quality standards for coliform count, pH, chemical additives, and salinity. Although these are the only taxa and parameters that are regulated, all other organisms need specific requirements. The first step in understanding these elaborate processes is to appreciate the complexities of water chemistries and some of the more advanced techniques to keep the parameters within acceptable biologic limits. Although it is easy to focus on one parameter that is out of range, it is imperative that the clinician examine each chemical in context with the bigger picture of chemistries. For example, temperature and pH greatly influence other values, such as ammonia levels. Determining only selected chemistry values may give the veterinarian a partial view and false impression of the situation, possibly resulting in improper action. Parameters for all aquatic animals other than mammals and birds include specific basic measurements, such as temperature, pH, dissolved oxygen (DO), ammonia, nitrite, and nitrate levels, salinity (conductivity), hardness, and alkalinity, but there are also more detailed analyses that may need to be carried out if these parameters are within normal limits (see Chapter 25). These may include oxidation-reduction potential (ORP), total organics, metals, and organic contaminants, which may involve more specialized equipment, such as mass spectrophotometers, total organic carbon analyzers, and ORP analyzers. These are not readily found in the zoo setting, so reference laboratories may need to be used.

This chapter is intended to be a primer. Most discussions will focus on marine systems because of their complexity, but variations with freshwater will be highlighted. Many studies of aquatics have been presented in the literature but most do not mention water quality in significant detail. Tables 23-1 and 23-22 and Figure 23-1 provide basic information about recognizing water quality–related health issues and how to address these problems. For more information on general water quality,* we recommend studies by Spotte,[16] Clesceri and colleagues,[4] and Mohan and Aiken.[13]

WATER PARAMETERS AND TESTING

Sample Collection

Accurate water analysis begins with proper sampling protocol. Consideration of contamination issues and water collection technique standardization are critically important for accurate results. For more information on techniques, see the study of Clesceri and associates.[4] When faced with an unknown water quality condition, always save water prior to changing the situation. Approximately 500 mL of water should be frozen for further chemical analysis if first-round diagnostics do not answer the question. Other more elaborate preservation methods are necessary for longer storage periods and are specific to the types of analyses to be conducted. Check the analyzer manuals for these preservation techniques.

Test Methods

Test methods that are commonly used in the zoo and aquarium industry include colorimetric, titrimetric, electrometric, nephelometric, and thermometric methods. A variety of test kits are available; some use test strips, some use wet reagents, and others use dry

*For species-specific information, see references 3, 5, 6, 8, 9, 11, 14, 15, 18, 22, and 23.

TABLE 23-1 Water Parameters and Their Dynamic Relationships With Water and Health

Parameter	General Range	Environmental Cofactors*	Symptoms	System Management	Comments
Temperature	22°-28°C		±12°C: Shock causing paralysis of the respiratory and cardiac muscles; may cause bloat, loss of balance, and death from undigested food gas formation or ammonia autointoxication and death; parameters affected—metabolism, gas exchange, pathogens, drug kinetics	Adjust heating and cooling systems, circulation; may need to add bagged (sealed) ice to cool down or use appropriate heaters; slow water change also helpful	
pH	6.5-8.5 FW; 7.8-8.4 SW	Alkalinity, H_2S, NH_3, cyanides, heavy metals	Increased skin and gill mucus; extremes cause skin and gill hemorrhaging	Check for alkaline substances from groundwater makeup or runoff; monitor acid rain or runoff; and check for overactive biofiltration	Species-dependent (e.g., some freshwater fish require low pH)
Alkalinity	75-200 mg/liter FW; >175 mg/liter SW	CO_2, pH, hardness	Affects stability of pH (see above)	Check for alkaline substances from groundwater makeup or runoff; monitor acid rain or runoff; and check for overactive biofiltration/ photosynthesis	Affects toxicity of metals
Calcium hardness	63-250 mg/liter FW	CO_2, pH, alkalinity	Low hardness leads to physiologic stress caused by blood sodium and potassium deficiencies affecting heart, nerve, and muscle function, which may lead to death.	Monitor assimilation by high biologic loading†; check for soft or hard water input; monitor for mineral dissolution or precipitation	High hardness may affect hatchability of fish eggs (e.g., tetras).
Ammonia (NH_3)	<0.05 mg/liter	pH, temp, DO, CO_2	Restlessness or agitation, irregular or increased respiration, congregation at surface, lose equilibrium, muscle spasms, lateral recumbency, open mouth and opercula flaring, body surface pale, followed by death	Monitor biofiltration, circulation, gas exchange	Outdoor systems typically have organic loading from terrestrial sources; dependent on pH.
Nitrite (NO_2^-)	<0.10 mg/liter	O_2, temp, Cl^-, K^+, Na^+, Ca^+	Methemoglobin >50% total hemoglobin; torpid, loses orientation, nonreactive to stimuli	See above, but if NH_3 is low, biofilter stage 2 not established or inhibited by environmental stressor (i.e., temp., pH or salinity shock, copper, chlorine, etc)	Marine organisms generally more tolerant; symptoms reversible by reductase; NaCl competes with nitrite uptake

Parameter	Acceptable level	Related parameters	Clinical signs	Management	Comments
Nitrate (NO_3^-)	<100 mg/liter	Phosphate, iron	Eutrophication with excessive growth of algae and plants; secondary effects on fish	Denitrification and photosynthetic activity not well established, managed, or inhibited	Some marine invertebrates may be less tolerant.
Salinity (osmolality)	30-35 ppt SW		Osmotic stress, inability of fish to control internal osmotic pressure; followed by death	Monitor sea salt makeup system, evaporation control (Check for uncontrolled freshwater input from rain, irrigation system, leaky pipe)	
Chlorine, active	<0.03 mg/liter	Organic load, ammonia, pH	Restlessness, jumping out of the water, muscle tetanus, lateral recumbency, spasmic movement of the mouth, fins and tail, buccal spasms hinder respiration, suffocation, and death	Neutralize with thiosulfate; water changes	
Total bacteria	<100,000 CFUs/100 mL	Temp, nitrate, phosphate, organic load	Outbreak of saprophytic bacterial diseases, such as furunculosis (FW; Aeromonas salmonicida), columnaris (FW), vibriosis (SW)	Check for organic pollution of makeup water, poor mechanical filtration, inadequate, poorly maintained or malfunctioning disinfection equipment	Some bacterial pathogens may survive up to 1 wk in tap water; balanced microbial community competes with pathogens.
Supersaturation with dissolved gas	<10% more than barometric pressure (mm Hg)	Barometric pressure, temp, DO	Bubbles block capillaries; dorsal and caudal fins may be affected, with bubbles visible between fin rays; epidermal and other tissue distal to occlusions then become necrotic; death may occur as result of blockage of major arteries; resembles the bends that deep sea divers may experience when they return to surface	Gas exchange components (aeration may be cause or solution), check plumbing design and integrity, flow rate, and/or mixing (to prevent thermoclines)	Deep aquariums offer depth compensation pressure, which may be calculated,

Continued

TABLE 23-1 Water Parameters and Their Dynamic Relationships With Water and Health—cont'd

Parameter	General Range	Environmental Cofactors*	Symptoms	System Management	Comments
Hydrogen sulfide (H_2S)	<0.4 mg/liter	pH, temp, DO	Gill damage, increased opercular movement, respiratory arrest, death	Could be a problem with asset management, including inadequate mechanical filter maintenance, leading to organic particulate buildup in system niches; could have poor system flow leading to excessive anaerobic pockets, or inadequate aeration, gas exchange, and/or poor denitrification filter management	Oxygen converts H_2S to nontoxic form.
Copper	<0.001 mg/liter	pH, alkalinity, TOC	Heavy breathing, potential gasping for air at water surface, excessive body and gill mucous, followed by death	Check for overdosing of copper, ectoparasite treatment, algicide contamination, contaminated makeup water, copper oxidation in system, condensation from copper air lines, contaminated runoff, synergy with other metals	Activated carbon has limited removal efficacy in high pH water; organics may be protective.
Iron II (soluble compounds)	<0.1 mg/liter	DO, pH, temp	Asphyxiation leading to death from ferrous iron compounds and associated iron-related bacteria coating and damaging respiratory epithelium, resulting in gross appearance of clear or brown tufts protruding from gills	Check for contaminated makeup water, iron oxidation in system, condensation from rusty surfaces over system, contaminated runoff	Iron may be limiting algae nutrients in seawater systems.

FW, Fresh water; SW, saltwater; temp, temperature; TOC, total organic carbon.

*Defined as other parameters that affect the level of physiologic stress inflicted when this parameter is out of range (listed in order of importance).

†Bio-organic loading includes all organic inputs to the system plus the total organism bioloading, which increases total respiration and ammonia production and excretion.

TABLE 23-2 Water Quality Emergencies

Emergency Kit Item	Event	Instructions
Chemical Treatment		
Sodium thiosulfate solution (0.2 g/mL)*	Total Cl > 0.05 mg/L	One drop/gallon treats 0.95 mg/L
AmQuel solution (0.6 g/mL)*	NH_3-N > 0.50 mg/L	1 mL/gallon treats 1 mg/L
Zeolite ammonia remover	NH_3-N > 0.50 mg/L in a freshwater system	5.7 g (1 tsp)/gallon treats 1 mg/L
Sodium chloride	NO_2-N > 1.00 mg/L in a freshwater system	11 g (2 tsp)/gallon
1:6 baking soda–soda ash buffer*	pH > 0.3 below acceptable level	Add 2 tsp/gallon, then as needed
pH-decreasing powder	pH > 0.3 above acceptable level	Follow directions on bottle
Granulated activated carbon (GAC)*	Toxic levels of heavy metals, Cl, ozone, medications, pesticides, organic contaminants, unknown toxins	Use 454 g (1 lb)/200 gallons (GAC)
Hydrogen peroxide (3%)	DO < 2 mg/liter	Use 5 mL/gallon
Equipment		
Water weld	System leak in tank or pipe	Makes repairs under water in minutes
Portable canister filter	To use with GAC or zeolite	Filter water for toxic substances
AC/DC air pump(s) with air stones, air tubing, diffuser stones	Poor gas exchange caused by power outage	Aerate(s) system
Scuba tank with air line regulator	Same as above	Same as above
Appropriate transport containers, system nets, and holding tanks with adequate life support to accommodate all system animals	To rescue fish from major system failure or a water contamination event	Transport fish to the holding system
Reserve system water for a 100% water change	Major water contamination or loss	Replace or change out system water

reagents. Although the test strips are handy for quick checks, they are not as reliable as kits that use dry and wet reagents or bench top analyzers. Before acquiring a kit, make sure that it contains reagents that have expiration dates. For detailed explanations of these tests, see report by Clesceri and coworkers.[4]

WATER QUALITY PARAMETERS AND ANALYTIC TESTING FOR MARINE ANIMALS

Temperature

Most fish are poikilothermic. A poikilothermic organism's enzymes are developed to work within its preferred temperature range, so temperatures outside their optimal range have deleterious effects. Fish have some capability to regulate their body temperature through behavioral thermoregulation by the use of sun, shade, currents and thermoclines. However, this is difficult to achieve in artificial settings and makes it more important to be sensitive to temperature in aquarium settings. The metabolic rate of fish is closely correlated to the water temperature—the higher the water temperature (i.e., the closer to optimum values within the normal range), the higher the metabolism. This generalization applies particularly to warm water fish. Cold water fish, such as salmonids, whitefish, or burbot, have a different type of metabolism; their metabolic rate may continue at comparatively low temperatures, whereas at high water temperatures, usually above 20° C, they become less active and consume less food.

Water temperature also has a great influence on the initiation and course of a number of fish diseases. The immune system of most fish species studied has an optimum performance at water temperatures of approximately 15° C. At the other extreme, low temperatures slow metabolism, depress the immune response, and

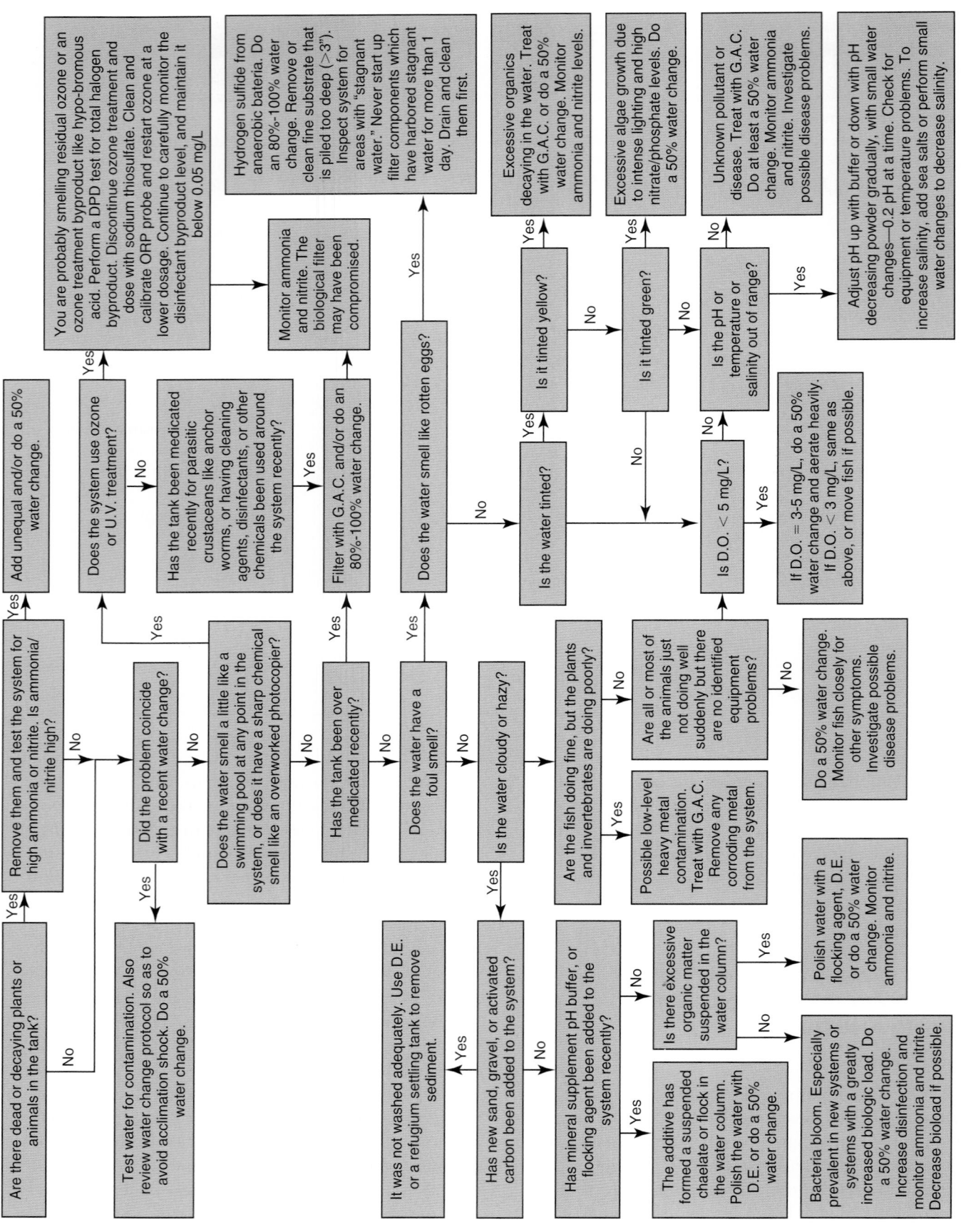

Figure 23-1

Algorithm for trouble-shooting water challenges. *DE,* Diatomaceous earth; *GAC,* granulated activated carbon.

impair digestion. Poikilothermic organisms tend to be more severely affected in terms of physiologic stress by rapid temperature fluctuations rather than by large gradual changes within acceptable limits for the species. Temperature changes should be gradual, ideally no more than 2° C/hr.[19] As a general rule, high temperatures also promote more rapid growth and reproduction of parasites and bacteria.

Dissolved Oxygen

DO may be measured with an electrode system wherein the dissolved oxygen reacts at the cathode, producing a measurable electrochemical effect. DO is more soluble at lower temperatures and salinities. Every aquarium system has a certain demand for oxygen that is created by the life that is present, known as biologic oxygen demand (BOD). The BOD is high when a large amount of organic matter is present that serves as food for bacteria and other microorganisms. The nitrifying bacteria that live in the biologic filter are aerobic and, as such, they are also adversely affected by DO lower than 2 mg/liter.[7] It is important to note that oxygen may be the principal factor limiting biologic filter efficiency, and that its carrying capacity may be increased by almost 30% by using prefiltration techniques to remove gross and dissolved organics, thereby reducing the oxygen consumed in filtration.[12] It is also important to make sure that the air supply is safe. Some operations have air intakes that may be in another building and pumped throughout an aquarium. Always examine the area for potential exhaust intake. Diesel exhaust or even a smoking area within the vicinity of the intake may be lethal to fish and would be difficult to detect with the usual testing methods in a zoo or aquarium. This would also apply to pesticides or painting that might be done in the area.

Carbon Dioxide

Just as in terrestrial animals, excessive carbon dioxide may affect the erythrocyte's ability to deliver oxygen to the cell. Low DO exacerbates this effect. Carbon dioxide is more soluble in water than oxygen; however, increasing water temperature and salinity decreases CO_2 solubility. Typically, carbon dioxide is high in well water and, if not gassed off before entering a system, the carbon dioxide in well water may affect oxygen delivery and also decrease water pH. In recirculating systems poorly designed for gas exchange, the carbon dioxide from respiration may accumulate to the point that toxicity occurs. A packed column (or degassing column) is an efficient and low-cost method of providing gas exchange. In ponds, the pH may vary over 1.5 units during the diurnal cycle because of both fish and plant respiration.[20] Phytoplankton is a significant contributor to overall carbon dioxide level, especially in a pond setting. A high CO_2 level commonly occurs during transport of fishes. Fishes transported in bags are subjected to a high CO_2 level, especially if packed in high density. Similarly, hauling tanks, if tightly closed, may prevent CO_2 from being gassed off, even if the water is vigorously aerated with oxygen.

Conductivity and Salinity

Conductivity measures the ability of a solution to conduct an electric current between two electrodes. In solution, the current flows by ion transport. With an increasing amount of ions present in the liquid, the liquid will have a higher conductivity. The various salts and minerals dissolved in aquarium water are reasonably uniform in their contribution to conductivity. Therefore, conductivity serves as an indicator of total dissolved solids in freshwater and salinity in seawater.

Marine and estuarine fish need not only NaCl but all the micronutrients on which natural sea water is based. There are approximately 78 inorganic elements composing seawater.[2] Salt mixtures may be bought premixed or formulas may be made up, as described in various texts. Salinity of marine fish will depend on their native environment, with estuarine fish being more adaptive to salinity changes. Marine system enclosures exposed to the elements have evaporative and dilution effects (rain and deck hosing), creating fluctuations that need to be carefully monitored. The smaller the enclosure and the larger the surface area, the greater the variation. Salinity may be measured indirectly with a salinometer (refractometer), conductivity meter, or hydrometer, which is a flotation device with a metric scale to measure the depth at which the indicator floats in the sample. The scale is usually in specific gravity units or mg/liter salinity at a specific temperature. The specific gravity of seawater decreases as water temperature increases. The true specific gravity of seawater at 35 ppt is 1.026. For safety's sake, glass hydrometers (e.g., glass thermometers) are best used in hydrometer cylinders rather than in the aquarium. Refractometers measure the amount of light refraction through a sample film of water on a scale that converts to specific gravity and/or salinity. Some have automatic temperature compensation and some are manual. Refractometers depend on background lighting and operator judgment for accuracy.

Recommended Salinity Concentrations

Salinity concentrations recommended for marine mammal water is 22 ppt or higher; other studies have suggested keeping the salinity between 15 and 36 ppt. Even though most marine mammals may withstand freshwater for short periods of time, salts are needed for periods longer than 1 or 2 days. AHPIS now requires that primary enclosure pools be salinized for marine mammals requiring saltwater (all marine mammals, excluding polar bears and Lake Baikal seals). There has been speculation that magnesium is important for skin health, but we could not find documentation to this effect.

Although marine mammals are maintained in waters of four generic types, including freshwater, brine (sodium chloride dissolved in tap water), artificial seawater (some or all of the major ions dissolved in tap water), and seawater, we recommend only a full-constituent natural or artificial sea salt—with the exception of polar bears and Lake Baikal seals.[17]

NITROGEN CYCLE
Total Ammonia Nitrogen

The primary source of ammonia is the protein metabolism of the fish. Ammonia is the primary waste product and it is passively excreted across the gills. A lesser amount is excreted in feces and urine. Uneaten food and decomposing organic matter are also sources of ammonia. Total ammonia nitrogen (TAN) consists of two forms, ionized ammonia (NH_4^+; ammonium ion) and un-ionized ammonia (NH_3). Un-ionized ammonia (UIA) is 100 times more toxic than ionized ammonia. At a pH of 7.0, most of the TAN is present as ionized ammonia. As pH and temperature increase, the percentage of TAN that is UIA increases. Because ammonia toxicity is primarily associated with UIA, the veterinarian must know the pH and temperature of the water to determine how much TAN is un-ionized ammonia accurately. These relationships may be found in easily accessible charts. An UIA level of 0.05 mg/liter causes gill damage and reduced growth; as the level of UIA increases, mortality may result.

Total ammonia nitrogen may be measured in two ways, the ammonia salicylate and Nessler methods.

Seawater may be analyzed by the Nessler method by adding 1.0 mL of mineral stabilizer to the sample before analysis. The mineral stabilizer complexes the high magnesium concentrations found in sea water, but the sensitivity of the test is reduced by 30% because of the high chloride concentration. The ammonia salicylate method is more reliable. Water treated with formalin or one of the ammonia locking compounds (e.g., AmQuel, Foster & Smith, Rhinelander, Wisc; Ammo-Lock, Mars Fishcare, Chalfont, Pa) will have a falsely elevated TAN level when using the Nessler method. This reaction does not occur if the ammonia salicylate method is used. It is important to note that the Nessler reagent contains mercury, and water samples treated with this reagent must be disposed of as a hazardous material.

Nitrite

Nitrite is a byproduct of ammonia oxidation produced by the nitrifying bacteria generically known as *Nitrosomonas*, but in the aquarium, other genera might also be responsible.[10] Nitrite is colorless and odorless, and may result in signs of toxicity at a level as low as 0.10 mg/liter in freshwater. Nitrite binds with hemoglobin and prevents the erythrocyte from delivering oxygen to the cell (methemoglobinemia or brown blood disease). Sensitivities to nitrite are species-dependent and it is important to understand these sensitivities to determine safe levels.

Research has shown that the chloride cells in the fish gills cannot distinguish between nitrite and chloride ions; both are transported across the gill epithelium, so the rate of nitrite uptake depends therefore on the nitrite-to-chloride ratio in the water.[19] In freshwater, the uptake of nitrite at the gill may be blocked by the addition of chloride, either as sodium chloride or calcium chloride, at the rate of 10 mg/liter of chloride for each 1 mg/liter of nitrite ion. Thus, nitrite is usually not an issue in salt water.[19] The mechanisms for this physiology are not completely understood.

Nitrate

Nitrate is the byproduct of nitrite oxidation produced by nitrifying bacteria generically known as *Nitrobactor*. Older literature has stated that nitrate is nontoxic. More recent studies have indicated that nitrate may alter hematologic factors in striped bass at levels as low as 200 mg/liter. Many references cap a safe level at 100 mg/liter. In the natural environment, there are many factors, including vascular plants and bacteria, that convert nitrate to other products.[19] The easiest way to reduce nitrate is to do frequent large water changes or denitrification. For a complete description of denitrification, see Chapter 24.

pH

pH is extremely important to marine fish and invertebrate physiology. Nitrifying bacteria also have an optimum range (6.5 to 9) and do not function below a pH of 6.5. Low pH may also result in the solubilization of heavy metal ions if a source is present in the water. pH has a wide influence on the biochemical reactions of aquatic organisms. Most natural waters have a pH between 6 and 9. The pH of seawater is fairly uniform, approximately 7.5 to 8.3. Most fish have an optimal pH range in which they will thrive. pH decreases over time by the addition of organic acids from animal and bacterial waste products. pH testing must be performed daily for all marine life. The electrometric method for measuring pH offers the best accuracy, ±0.2 pH units or better. Colorimetric methods offer an accuracy of ±0.5 pH units.[4]

Marine Mammals and pH

Its importance with marine mammals is mostly associated with chemical reactions, including sterilizing agents, which are often unpredictable. APHIS specifically requires that pH testing be performed daily for all marine mammals and most facilities keep the pH between 7.2 and 8.4. The one exception are facilities open to natural seawater, which are exempt from daily sampling. In the artificial environment, the best compromise for optimum efficiency of chlorination and natural seawater pH is approximately 7.8.

OTHER PARAMETERS AFFECTING WATER QUALITY

Alkalinity

Alkalinity is the measure of the buffering capacity or acid-neutralizing capacity of a solution. In fish culture waters, alkalinity is determined primarily by bicarbonate, carbonate, and hydroxide ions. The nitrifying bacteria that reside in biologic filters consume bicarbonate at the rate of 7.14 g of alkalinity for each gram of TAN oxidized. Alkalinity must be determined before using copper as a treatment in freshwater systems because it is directly linked to toxicity. The alkalinity level may be decreased by the use of muriatic acid and increased by using a 5:1 ratio of sodium bicarbonate to sodium carbonate.

Hardness

Hardness is the measure of the divalent cations, primarily calcium and magnesium. Freshwater fish constantly lose electrolytes to the water column, and it is easy for them to take up calcium and magnesium as needed for osmoregulation. Hard water may have an adverse effect on hatchability of some fish eggs, especially the fish that originate from soft water, i.e., tetras (family Characidae). Water hardness more than 150 mg/liter minimizes the toxicity of heavy metals. The U.S. Environmental Protection Agency (EPA) has developed guidelines for hardness of natural water: soft, 0 to 75 mg/liter; moderate, 75 to 150 mg/liter; hard, 150 to 300 mg/liter; very hard, ≥300 mg/liter.

Microbial Factors

Because of the complexity of this topic, see Chapter 25 for a more detailed discussion.

BASIC PROCEDURES

Coliform Count

As for current techniques and regulations, coliform count sampling is mandatory when housing marine mammals, but marine fish systems are not monitored. Coliform counts may be determined by the multiple tube fermentation test or the more accurate membrane filter test, which pulls 100 mL of water through a filter membrane placed on a culture medium to determine the number of colony-forming units (CFUs). Water samples should be taken in a consistent way to ensure accuracy. This may be accomplished by adhering to the following protocols.

Samples should be taken at the same place and same time of day, at least 2 to 3 feet below the surface, near the middle of the pool or drain, and before emptying the pool, rather than just after filling. Samples must be processed within 30 hours of collection and refrigerated if not tested within 1 hour. Tests must be performed weekly and counts must not exceed 1000 MPN (most probable number)/100 mL of water. If the count exceeds 1000/100 mL, then two subsequent counts must be taken at 48-hour intervals; all three counts are averaged to determine the accuracy of the first test. If the coliform count is still high, then the conditions are unacceptable and the situation needs to be corrected immediately by changing or sterilizing the water. The water must be retested after either of these options is exercised.[1]

Chemical Sterilization: Chemical Oxidizing Substances

Chemical oxidizing substances include chlorine-based or bromine-based oxidants and ozone, as well as others not discussed in detail here. Chlorine and chloramine are widely used by public municipal water suppliers to deliver safe drinking water to consumers. Typically, chlorine arrives at the consumer's tap at 1.5 to 2.0 mg/liter. However, chlorine at 0.05 mg/liter may be toxic to many fish species. Because of their long-lasting effects, these chemicals need to be carefully monitored to ensure that they stay within safe parameters and should only be used in marine mammal systems that do not house fish. They are regulated by APHIS, which requires daily water tests to ensure that any chemical added does not cause harm or discomfort—higher levels of each oxidant may cause corneal, skin, or respiratory damage. For a complete description of chlorine sterilization, see the EPA manual.[21]

Special Considerations for Birds: Oxidants and Oils

To maintain the waterproofing of aquatic bird feathers, special attention is needed to ensure that the condition of feathers and oils are kept intact. Water should be checked for overall ORP levels, which should be carefully monitored so that plumage health is maintained. We have noted that ORP levels between 300 and 350 mV do not oxidize waterproofing oils or feather structure. Surface skimming should be carried out to prevent exogenous oils from building up and solubilizing natural waterproofing. Cleaning solutions with soaps and surfactants should be used sparingly, and some phytoplankton may produce surfactants that may disrupt water proofing.

REFERENCES

1. Arkush KD: Water quality. In Dierauf LA, Gulland FMD, editors: CRC handbook of marine mammal medicine, ed 2, Boca Raton, Fla, 2001, CRC Press, pp 779–787.
2. Bidwell J, Spotte S: Artificial seawaters, formulas and methods, Boston, 1985, Jones and Bartlett.
3. Cambre RC: Water quality for a waterfowl collection. In Fowler M, Miller R, editors: Zoo and wild animal medicine: Current therapy 4, St. Louis, 1997, WB Saunders, pp 292–299.
4. Clesceri L, Greenberg E, Eaton AD, editors: Standard methods for the examination of water and wastewater, ed 20, Baltimore, 1998, United Book Press, Parts 1000 and 2000.
5. Crainfield MR: Sphenisciformes (penguins). In Fowler M, Miller R, editors: Zoo and wild animal medicine: Current therapy 5, St. Louis, 2003, WB Saunders, pp 103–110.
6. Gage L: Pinnipedia (seals, sea lions, walrus). In Fowler M, Miller R, editors: Zoo and wild animal medicine: Current therapy 5, St. Louis, 1999, WB Saunders, pp 459–475.
7. Garrido JM, van Benthum WAJ, van Loosdrecht MC, et al: Influence of dissolved oxygen concentration on nitrite accumulation in a biofilm airlift suspension reactor. Biotechnol Bioeng 53:168–178, 1997.
8. Geraci JR: Marine mammal husbandry. In Fowler M, Miller R, editors: Zoo and wild animal medicine, ed 2, St. Louis, 1986, WB Saunders, pp 757–760.
9. Harms CA: Fish. In Fowler M, Miller R, editors: Zoo and wild animal medicine: Current therapy 5, St. Louis, 1999, WB Saunders, pp 2–20.
10. Hovanec TA, DeLong EF: Comparative analysis of nitrifying bacteria associated with freshwater and marine aquaria. Appl Environ Microbiol 62:2888–2896, 1996.
11. Loyd M: Crocodilai. In Fowler M, Miller R, editors: Zoo and wild animal medicine: Current therapy 6, St. Louis, 2008, WB Saunders, pp 59–70.
12. Manthie D, Malone R, Kumar S: Elimination of oxygen deficiencies associated with submerged rock filters used in closed, recirculating-aquaculture systems. In: Proceedings of the national symposium on the soft-shelled blue crab fishery, 1985, pp 49–55.
13. Mohan PJ, Aiken A: Water quality and life support systems for large elasmobranch exhibits. In Smith M, Warmolts D, Thoney D, Hueter R, editors: Elasmobranch husbandry manual: Captive care of sharks, rays, and their relatives, Columbus, Ohio, 2004, Biological Survey, pp 69–88.
14. Mylniczenko ND: Caecilians. In Fowler M, Miller R, editors: Zoo and wild animal medicine: Current therapy 5, St. Louis, 2003, WB Saunders, pp 40–45.
15. Reidarson TH: Cetacea (whales, dolphins, porpoises). In Fowler M, Miller R, editors: Zoo and wild animal medicine: Current therapy 5, St. Louis, 2003, WB Saunders, pp 442–459.
16. Spotte S: Captive Seawater fishes: science and technology. New York, 1992, John Wiley and Sons.
17. Spotte S: Sterilization of marine mammal pool waters: theoretical and health considerations. U.S. Department of Agriculture, Animal and Plant Health Inspection Service, Technical Bulletin No. 1797. Washington DC, U.S. Department of Agriculture, 1991.
18. Stoskopf MK, Kennedy-Stoskopf S: Aquatic birds. In Fowler M, Miller R, editors: Zoo and wild animal medicine, ed 2, St. Louis, 1986, WB Saunders, pp 294–313.
19. Svobodova Z, Lloyd R, Machova J, et al: Water quality and fish health. EIFAC technical paper No. 54. Rome, Food and Agriculture Organization of the United Nations, 1993.
20. Tucker CS: Water analysis. In Stoskopf M, editor: Fish medicine, Philadelphia, 1993, WB Saunders, pp 166–197.
21. U.S. Environmental Protection Agency: Alternative disinfectants and oxidants guidance manual, 1999 (http://www.epa.gov/ogwdw000/mdbp/alternative_disinfectants_guidance.pdf).
22. Walsh MT, Bossart GD: Manatee medicine. In Fowler M, Miller R, editors: Zoo and wild animal medicine: Current therapy 4, St. Louis, 1999, WB Saunders, pp 507–516.
23. Whitaker B: Preventive medicine programs for fish. In Fowler M, Miller R, editors: Zoo and wild animal medicine: Current therapy 4, St. Louis, 1999, WB Saunders, pp 163–181.

CHAPTER 24

The Mechanics of Aquarium Water Conditioning

M. Andrew Stamper and Kent J. Semmen

Beyond the fundamental water condition practices such as mechanical and bacterial filtration, there are many techniques used in modern aquarium water systems to ensure clean and safe environments for aquatic life. The art and science of water conditioning is the ultimate preventive medicine challenge for the veterinarian working with aquatic systems. It is imperative that the veterinarian understand the components and chemical, biologic, and physical properties of water conditioning.

The artificial filtration methods used in zoos and aquariums are similar to the ones used in swimming pool, municipal waste water, and drinking water treatment. Better understanding and consideration of natural stabilizing processes may provide more efficient and cost-effective life support for aquatic animals. First, understanding aquatic animal housing water flow systems is critical. Open systems have direct circulation with a natural body of water and do not usually require filtration. Semiclosed systems have basic filtration systems but rely on partial exchanges with an external water body. The third and most complex type of system is the closed system. Because this includes all types of filtration, this chapter will concentrate on this system. Basic marine mammal or bird pools are the simplest closed systems. These afford much more freedom from a water conditioning standpoint because the animals are not dependent on ultraclean water for respiratory needs, as in fish systems (Fig. 24-1). The most complex is the mixed exhibit, in which the fastidious needs of fish and the federal regulations for marine mammals must be addressed. To complicate issues, many exhibits now have people swimming in these systems and thus must meet public health regulations.

The simplest is the basic marine mammal system, which consists of dump and fill. This is based on human swimming pool rules of chlorination and shock chlorination when the parameters are out of acceptable levels. Brine (NaCl) may be used, although many in the industry do not believe that NaCl alone fulfills marine mammal needs. Therefore, a number of institutions use a saline marine mammal mix—$MgSO_4$, $MgCl$, $NaCl$. The next level consists of the use of chlorine and chloramines with filtration to keep the particulate and bacterial loads down to acceptable levels for longer periods, saving on water and salt expenses. The next generation of marine filtration systems includes ozone with chlorine (or) bromine to keep environmental oxidant levels down. From there, foam fractionation and ultraviolet (UV) sterilization may be used. Once biologic filtration is added, the addition of chlorine becomes complicated; it usually is discouraged because chlorine interferes with the establishment and maintenance of a biofilter.

Once fish are added to systems, general oxidant sterilization cannot be used. These systems operate without chlorine and bromine and residual ozone oxidants should maintain an oxidation-reduction potential (ORP) below 350 mV. Systems in which water exchanges are nonexistent or limited need to consider denitrification systems to convert nitrates to nitrogen gas, which is off-gassed. With fish exhibits or mixed taxa exhibits, gas exchange partial pressures need to be considered. Once invertebrates are added, detailed chemistry control is needed but is beyond the scope of this chapter. It is important to recognize that conflicting information is based on varying philosophies between older traditional thoughts verses new ideas of ecologic approaches to water conditioning. For further reading, see studies by Carlson,[3] Overby,[5] Spotte,[6] Van der Toorn,[7] and Watson and Hill,[8] and the website of the Aquatic Animal Life Support Operators (http://aalso.org).

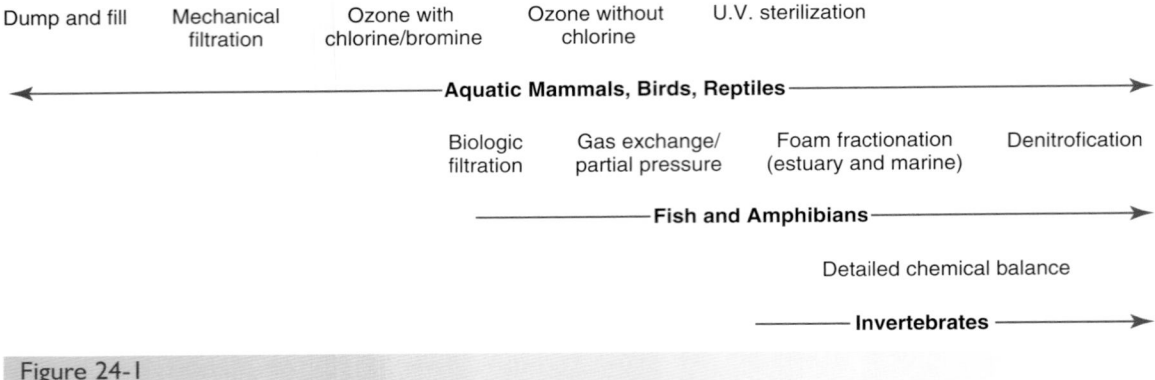

Figure 24-1

Filtration continuum. The left portion of the spectrum is the most basic filtration, and least expensive. Progression to the right indicates more sophisticated conditioning methods, which allow more taxa to be displayed.

TRADITIONAL ROUTES OF WATER CONDITIONING

Traditional methods for organic removal involve surface skimming and bottom drains to remove organic accumulates, followed by physical removal of large particulates via large strainer baskets and/or sand filtration. Foam fractionation uses air through the water column to attract and remove the hydrophobic portions of molecules. Protein waste products are converted to nontoxic chemicals through microbial conversion; other material is then removed through chemical sterilization followed by sidestream or full stream sterilization. If working with a fish system, a gas exchange tower is used to provide aeration and to ensure that gas pressures are equalized.

Gas Exchange and Aeration

The very large surface area–to–volume ratio of most natural aquatic systems allows good gas exchange with the atmosphere. However, most large bodies of water in nature are chemically stratified. Mechanisms such as wave action and surface turbulence from wind help facilitate natural gas exchange. The vast diversity of biologic activity in a natural ecosystem helps maintain the needed balance of dissolved gases. Eutrification of natural systems from inorganic and organic pollution may cause dissolved oxygen depletion from microbial and phytoplankton proliferation. This leads to the die-off of most of the aquatic life in the system.

Maintaining a natural balance of dissolved gases in (artificial) systems is critical to support biologic filtration, maintain plant and animal photosynthesis and respiration, maintain pH, and prevent supersaturation, which may lead to gas bubble disease in fish. The three most critical dissolved gases that require management are N_2, CO_2, and O_2.

The natural ratio to try to maintain is an $O_2/N/CO_2$ ratio of approximately 1:2:4, which are the normal environmental proportions. This ratio is the natural ratio of gases when air is dissolved in water under atmospheric pressure and is adequately maintained when the system water has adequate contact rate with the atmosphere. The actual concentration of these gases depends on atmospheric pressure, water temperature, salinity, pH, and biologic activity.

The primary components used in artificial systems for maintaining adequate gas exchange are air diffuser stones, degas chambers (trickle filters), and venturi injector which uses the negative pressure of the water flowing through plumbing of the exhibit (used on foam fractionators and ozone reactors). Surface skimming devices are also used to remove mostly dissolved organics attracted to the surface of our tanks, which hinder gas exchange there. The larger the surface area–to–volume ratio in a tank, the better the gas exchange that may be maintained.

FILTRATION METHODS
Organic and Bacterial Loads

We believe that there is a fine balance between organic load, bacterial load, color of the water, and health of the animals. Thus, this chapter is organized around how to address organic loads in the context of water management. Mechanical filtration will be discussed, followed by biologic filtration, chemical filtration, sterilization, and gas exchange.

Origin of Filtration Methods

Most of the artificial filtration methods used in aquariums and zoos were adopted from the municipal waste water, drinking water, and swimming pool industries. There is very little in the regard to filtration design and methods that have been developed specifically for aquatic life support on a large scale. Closed recirculating systems are those that are completely dependent on human manipulations to condition the water and sustain life. The heart of most of our filtration systems is natural biologic (bacterial) filtration.

Because there are missing links in artificial systems compared with natural ones, some supplemental mechanical and chemical filtration is also necessary. At our institution, some but not all natural filtration processes in our systems are used, and an incomplete cycling of nutrients results. This causes the accumulation of byproducts from these processes, such as nitrates, phosphates, and some insoluble organics. It is our goal to find ways to complete these natural cycles as much as possible to recycle or eliminate these accumulates from our systems.

Mechanical Filtration

Mechanical filtration is divided into large, medium, fine, and dissolved materials. Large particulates are usually removed via a prefilter, which involves screens such as basket screens in skimmers during surface skimming or large rotating drum screens for the most challenging systems. Medium-sized material is removed by pressure sand filtration or canister filters. Sand filters may use various grades (decreasing in size) of gravel and sand are referred to as mixed bed filters. Water flows through the filter, with large to smaller particulates being removed. Water pressure builds as material gathers in the filters. When the filters reach a predetermined saturation, determined by water pressure, they are backflushed and the filtrate is flushed to sanitary sewer outlets. Canister filters use the same principle but use pleated filters.

Flocculation is a method of using chemicals to bind particulates to make them bigger and easier to remove. It focuses on dissolved organic carbon (DOC). Common flocculants used in freshwater include aluminum sulfate (alum) and natural and synthetic polymers (cationic polyelectrolytes). These act by reducing surface charges on dissolved or suspended particles, thus allowing them to collide and coagulate. They reach their peak effectiveness at pH < 7.5. The true effects on fish and invertebrate

species is not fully known and should be used with caution especially when other techniques are available.

Dissolved organics may also be removed using activated carbon, which has specialized binding sites. As with mechanical filtration, carbon may become saturated and bacteria may use it as a growth surface, which will decrease its efficiency.

Foam Fractionation

A safer alternative is foam fractionation, in which particles are brought together mechanically by causing flow conditions that promote particle collisions. Mucopolysaccharides produced by bacteria and algae stick together, along with other substances, as they collide. Foam fractionation may be accomplished by slowly pushing water (salinity ≥15 ppt) down a column. As this is done, air is injected at the bottom of the column, creating a steady upward stream of very small bubbles. Organic molecules (including the mucopolysaccharides) often have hydrophilic and hydrophobic parts, causing them to collect at air-water interfaces. As they come into contact with the air bubbles, these molecules will collect and form an organic film on the surface of the bubbles. When the bubbles reach the surface, the film stays intact for a period of time, which creates foam. The resulting foam is then skimmed and flushed to a drain, thus removing the organic waste from the system.

Biologic Filtration

In natural systems, it is the role of plants to acquire nutrients continually from the water to build their tissues. It is the role of bacteria to break down organics rapidly enough to supply plants with these needed nutrients. As a result, without human interference, nutrients are typically not accumulated in the water of natural systems.

In artificial systems, plant growth is discouraged. Unnaturally large populations of relatively few species of bacteria (a fraction of the natural biodiversity in nature) are encouraged to convert organic waste products and nitrogenous toxins (ammonia and nitrite) to less toxic waste products, such as nitrate, phosphate, carbon dioxide, and biologically inert organic compounds, which cause the yellowing of aquarium water. These bacteria also compete with the aquarium's fish and invertebrate population for oxygen.

This makes biologic filters very sensitive and fickle to environmental changes. Filter bacteria are simple cells that are not capable of carrying out the complex internal digestive and excretory processes of higher organisms. In the presence of much accumulated organic matter, the bacterial environment becomes acidic, high in CO_2, methane, and ammonia and low in dissolved oxygen (DO), with many bacterial enzymes for organic breakdown. Bacteria use complex organic foods, but have simple nutritional needs (e.g., simple sugars; small amounts of vitamins, amino acids, and micronutrients). Only a small portion of the nitrogen, phosphorus, and sulfur in these foods is used. (The majority of) these become organic wastes and tend to accumulate in the aquarium and become toxic or stressful to other aquatic organisms.[1]

The whole organic cycle is usually represented to the veterinarian in only partial form. It consists of the aerobic conversion of ammonia to nitrate and usually does not consider other organic processes, such as denitrification, which is usually incorporated in plants in natural systems. Organic biodegradation is an aerobic process in which reactions catalyzed by heterotrophic bacteria convert organic waste to inorganic chemical byproducts and reduced organics. Nitrification is an aerobic two-step process in which catalyzed reactions by highly specific genera of nitrifying bacteria convert NH_4^+ to NO_3^{-2}. Denitrification is an anaerobic two-step process whereby reactions catalyzed by specific bacteria reduce NO_3^{-2} and release N_2 as gas from the system. For further details of the denitrification process, see Chapter 25.

Biologic Treatment Trouble Shooting

A large mass of bacteria is needed for biologic treatment of closed recirculated systems. They are living cells containing enzymes that catalyze a wide range of reactions needed for cell maintenance and reproduction. An environment is needed that is conducive to accumulating the cells that can perform the desired reactions. The actual species that establish a system and primarily carry out the desired biologic reactions will vary, based on the environmental conditions provided by the system and the species' competitive edge (e.g., presence of light usually inhibits nitrifying bacteria growth).

Bacterial species have sensitivities to their environment (e.g., sensitivities to extremes in pH, temperature, and/or toxic substances). The space provided for their growth will have to cater to their specific needs, with some degree of stability and protection. This filtration component, which houses the primary bacterial population, is usually known as a bioreactor or biofilter. Inoculating a new system with nitrifying bacteria off the shelf will probably have mixed results because different species will inhabit different systems, depending on the environment, and therefore will not initially result in the complete cycling of the filter. Drastic environmental changes in a system, like switching from freshwater to salt water, will result in the complete reestablishment of the biologic filter. Cells need three types of basic materials—an electron donor, an electron acceptor, and nutrients. The most common limiting factor to biologic filtration is the DO (electron acceptor) concentration in the water. The high rate of biologic filtration used in these systems reduces the amount of dissolved oxygen available to the animals and should not be underestimated. Electron donors such as NH_4^+, Fe^{2+}, Mn^{2+}, NO^{2-}, H_2, H_2S, and HS^- are found in many organic compounds and may limit microbial physiology when restricted. The electron transfer from donor to acceptor is called the energy reaction and is the mechanism whereby cells gain energy. If limitations of electron acceptors or electron donors are present, better biologic filtration will not be accomplished by adding another biologic filter to a system, and a new system will not complete the establishment of adequate bacteria.

Because our waste compounds serve as critical electron donors and/or electron acceptors for cells, the cells will become dependent for life on a consistent supply. Irregular supply or a change in supply feed rate may have major implications on cell population size in the bioreactor. Other nutrients, along with O and H, provide the building blocks for the bacterial cells; the major nutrients are C, N, P, and S. Other critical elements include Ca, Fe, Mn, and Mo. Some of the common limiting nutrients that provide many of these elements are complexes of bicarbonate and phosphate, which need to be monitored closely.

Biofilter by Design

Some important biofiltration design considerations include the following:
- Surface area (should provide 2 to 5 ft^2/gallon)
- Amount of solid buildup
- Gas exchange properties
- Water flow distribution over biofilm
- Packing—how the media compresses within the filter which affects water distribution throughout the filter
- Backwashing requirements
- Uniformity and stability of biofilm populations
- Biomass shearing
- Water channeling—abnormal distribution of water allowing bypassing of the majority of media

TABLE 24-1	Mechanical Filtration and Biofiltration							
Feature	Bead Filter	Pressure Sand Filter	Canister Filter	Fluidized Bed	Underwater Gravel Filter	Foam Filter	Trickle Filter	Biowheel Filter
Surface area	Excellent	Very good*	Excellent*	Excellent	Very good	Excellent	Poor	Excellent
Controlling solids buildup	Dependent on makeup of feces	Excellent	Very good	Excellent	Poor	Poor	Excellent	Very good
Efficient at removing target particle size	Excellent	Excellent	Poor	Poor	Excellent	Poor	Poor	Poor
Gas exchange properties	Poor	Poor	Poor	Poor	Good	Fair	Excellent	Excellent
Water flow distribution	Excellent	Excellent	Good	Excellent	Good	Good	Good	Excellent
Resists packing	Excellent	Excellent	Fair	Excellent	Fair	Excellent	Excellent	Excellent
Maintenance requirements	Excellent	Excellent	Poor	Excellent	Poor	Poor	Excellent	Very good
Stability of biofilm	Excellent	Very good	Very good[†]	Fair	Excellent	Excellent	Excellent	Excellent
Resists biofouling	Excellent	Poor	Excellent	Excellent	Excellent	Excellent	Excellent	Very good
Resists biomass shearing	Very good	Very good	Excellent	Poor	Excellent	Excellent	Excellent	Excellent
Resists channeling	Excellent	Excellent	Fair	Excellent	Fair	Poor	Excellent	Excellent

*Dependent on surface area of medium.
[†]Dependent on management technique.

Each specialized biofiltration option will be discussed; Table 24-1 compares the relative scores of each item. The undergravel filter is probably the best known biologic filter. It is a highly perforated plate, usually extending over the entire bottom area of the tank and supported above it. An appropriate biologic medium, ranging from fine sand to coarse gravel, is retained on top of the plate. Depending on need, many uplift tubes direct water from the space below the plate and draws the water column to or near the surface of the tank. As a result, water is drawn down through the media where the biofilter bacteria reside. In a reverse flow undergravel filter, biologically untreated but mechanically filtered water is introduced underneath the filter plate by the tubes to percolate up through the gravel from the bottom up and into the aquarium. A foam filter is another common biologic filter. Water is drawn through a block of open-celled polyurethane foam (serving as the biologic medium) by an air-driven uplift tube. The block may vary considerably in shape and size,

depending on the size of the system and specific application. A trickle filter uses a container that serves as a tower to hold most of the appropriate biologic filter medium (usually a plastic open medium with a low surface area) above the water line. Water is evenly distributed across the top surface of the medium via a spray bar or through a perforated diffuser plate. It then drips evenly down through the exposed medium, mixing with the air as it contacts it, and eventually collects in a sump below to be pumped back into the system. A biowheel filter, known as a rotating biologic contactor (RBC) in the waste water treatment industry, is a disc or cylinder of rigid biofilter medium positioned half in and half out of the water, with its axis at the surface. It is slowly turned using a system water pump, auxiliary motor, or air-driven rotation disc exposing all surfaces intermittently to water and air. Another biologic filter is a fluidized sand bed filter, a device consisting of a reactor column through which the system water is injected through the bottom into a suitable biologic medium (usually a fine quartz silica sand). The upwelling water column expands the sand bed upward as it passes through it and then exits out the top to return to the system.

Aquarium Ecologic Filtration versus Biologic Filtration

Biologic filtration or bacteriologic filtration is the process described earlier in which unnaturally large populations of many different types of bacteria in the aquarium convert organic waste products. Ecologic filtration is the natural process whereby balanced populations of bacteria, turf algae, phytoplankton, zooplankton, and other microorganisms interact with each other within their specialized physical environment to form an ecosystem that completely cycles and/or removes waste products in the aquarium while enriching the aquarium with oxygen, buffering pH, and balancing water chemistry. The benefits of ecologic filtration are centered around simplicity, stability, and the holistic approach to water conditioning. The traditional chemical and mechanical methods of maintaining water quality in closed systems fall short of duplicating natural environments. Ecologic filtration removes organic and inorganic micropollutants that may be detrimental to the health of the animals, affect the aesthetics of the exhibit, and affect the operation of the system. Compared with other processes that are commonly used for removing similar contaminants (e.g., granulated activated carbon treatment, ozonation, chlorination, ion exchange, micron filtration), ecologic treatment processes are simple to design and operate and usually are inexpensive. They also tend to balance a system naturally rather than destabilize it.[1] In one study an ecologic turf is actually a community of algae containing up to 40 different species of algae/m^2 of microorganisms, including bacteria, fungi, protozoa, and many types of microinvertebrates. In tropical seawater, red and blue-green algae and diatoms tend to dominate. With high-intensity lighting, diatoms will colonize the turf first, followed by the blue green algae. Green and brown algae are always present, but to a lesser degree. Like a grassland community, the algal turf must be continually grazed or it will eventually build up and go through a succession to a less productive macroalgal forest.[1]

A method that emphasizes the use of algal turfs to manage water quality has been termed *algal scrubbing*.[3] This approach focuses on locking nutrients up in an algal biomass outside the exhibit to achieve artificial ecosystem stability. This method is in contrast to the traditional method of relying heavily on bacterial filtration alone to reduce nonliving organics and animal excretions to elemental and ionic accumulates in the water. The algal turf scrubber filtration unit was developed to use the most efficient photosynthetic components of wild ecosystems (primarily algal turfs) in artificial ecosystems, and to concentrate their activity under optimal conditions and outside the aquarium, where aesthetics may be a concern. It consists of a filtration unit installed inline on the aquarium system and lit with high-intensity metal halide or VHO fluorescent lamps in a cycle opposite to that of the main ecosystem. Algal turf scrubbing is also used with natural sunlight to augment treatment during the day. One perceived disadvantage to ecologic filtration is potential harboring of pathogens, however if the system is balanced the robustness and variety of organisms will provide competition and predation of pathogens. Even though speculative, the ecologically enhanced water would likely lead to a healthier environment resulting in increased immune function of the inhabitants of the system.

STERILIZATION AND DISINFECTANTS

Once gross organic material is removed, as well as ammonia and nitrite, other materials such as basic proteins and infectious agents (e.g., bacteria, viruses, fungi) need to be addressed through sterilizing techniques. Sterilization may be characterized in two forms: (1) point contact sterilization, whereby water that is diverted in a sidestream is in continuous contact with a sterilizing agent and then recycled back to the system (inline UV radiation and ozone); and (2) bulk fluid sterilization, which oxidizes organics and kills microorganisms throughout the water system (chlorine). Note that ozone may create residual oxidative products that travel out into the main system and may easily kill fish. Point contact sterilization is subject to engineering constraints (e.g., sidestream configuration, flow rate). To improve water quality, the rate of sidestream treatment must exceed the rate of system contamination (bacterial growth in the region holding the animals). Because of their long-lasting effects, oxidizing chemicals need to be carefully monitored to ensure that they stay within safe parameters and some (e.g., chlorine, bromine) may only be used in systems that do not house fish or invertebrates. They are regulated by the Animal and Plant Health Inspection Service (APHIS), which requires daily water testing to ensure that any chemical added does not cause harm or discomfort (higher levels of each oxidant may cause corneal, skin, or respiratory damage). (For more details, see Arkush[2] and Spotte.[6])

Halogen oxidizers include chlorine- and bromine-based oxidants. Only chlorine will be discussed here, but bromine, formed by the oxidation of bromide which is found in high concentrations in sea water, has similar reactions. Chlorine is probably the most cost effective and well-known sterilizing agent. Efficacy is determined by chlorine concentration, contact time, temperature, pH, number and types of microorganisms, and amount of organic matter. Chlorine is added as a gas or as a salt of sodium or calcium hypochlorite. Chlorine dioxide (ClO_2) is an effective sterilizer but is not frequently used because it is sensitive to temperature, pressure, and light and may be dangerously unstable. Chlorine species reacts with water to form hypochlorous acid (HOCl) and hypochlorite (OCl^-) which are considered forms of free chlorine. HOCl is the superior sterilizing agent (150 to 300 times more effective than OCl^-). The efficacy of sterilization (ratio of HOCl to OCl^-) is dependent on pH (lower pH leads to more HOCl which is the superior oxidant). HOCl reacts with free ammonia to form chloramines—monoamine (NH_2Cl), diamine ($NHCl_2$), and trichloramine (NCl_3), which are persistent oxidants. However, their oxidation potential is much less than free chlorine and chloramines are more irritating. Thus, organic matter increases chlorine demand and decreases efficacy. Combined chlorine is the sum of NH_2Cl, $NHCl_2$, and NCl_3 in the water sample. Total chlorine is the sum of free and combined chlorine. A testing guideline for marine mammal pool water is to test the water twice daily for the concentrations of chlorine and/or other oxidizing agents. Others have recommended that total chlorine be less than 1 ppm and free chlorine be at least 50% of the total.

Chlorine-based oxidants react with organic compounds to produce trihalomethanes (THMs) such as chloroform, which are considered mutagens and carcinogens. These may be removed through aeration and do not result in concentrations that are considered harmful to marine mammals or humans. Chlorination of seawater is more difficult because of the high concentrations of magnesium, iron, and manganese that interfere with proper chlorination. Ozone may be used in combination with chlorine or bromine, which has a synergistic effect and may lower the use of both chemicals. Chlorine is easily neutralized with sodium thiosulfate at 2.6 mg/L treats 0.95 mg/L of total chlorine. Activated carbon will also remove chlorine, but requires frequent replacement. The practice of collecting the water for dissipation of chlorine is not reliable, because

20 hours is required for each 1 mg/liter of chlorine. Chloramine, a stable combination of chlorine and ammonia, is also toxic to fish. To eliminate chlorine, the bond between chlorine and ammonia must first be broken and then each removed separately. There are products available, such as sodium hydroxymethanesulfonate, that neutralize chloramine.

Ozone Disinfection

Ozone has a number of uses in aquarium water treatment, including clarifying the water column by oxidizing the carbon bonds of pigmented organic molecules, oxidizing harmful nitrogenous chemical species such as ammonia and nitrite, controlling disease-causing microorganisms, and reducing turbidity by the process of microflocculation.[4] Ozone is O_3, an allotrope of oxygen that is highly oxidative, which is good for sterilization and water clarification. Ozone is generated by passing high AC voltage across a discharge gap in the presence of O_2. Ozonizers such as UV sterilizers, trickle filters, foam fractionators, and aerators tend to maintain a high ORP. There are four processes for ozone to work safely and efficiently: ozone gas generation, gas to liquid absorption, contact time for reaction, and ozone residual removal. Note that ozone is short-lived, so many of its residuals may be limited by increased contact time in a sidestream contact chamber. Water is then passed through a biofilter and/or activated carbon, UV light, or intense heat to remove residuals. Packed column aeration is another procedure for removing ozone residuals from the water. Postozonated water is trickled down a tower filled with inert material as a fan blows air upward into the tower. Most residuals are volatile compounds and are released at this point into the air. Ozone is unstable and must be generated on site. The big disadvantages of ozone are that its use results in higher equipment and operational costs. There are considerable human health and fire hazards if not handled correctly, so the ambient air ozone concentration in enclosed areas must be monitored. See Chapter 25 for a discussion of its chemical dynamics.

Silver and Copper Sanitation

Silver and copper together create a bactericidal and fungicidal treatment. Thus it is produced by ion generators using a small direct current of a silver or copper bar. Silver-copper is efficient because the ions do not dissolve, so the bactericidal effects may last for months. The technique works best in soft water because electrodes form scale deposits in hard water and a high level of dissolved solids take silver ions out of solution. Chlorine may still be used as an oxidizer but at an 80% dose reduction. Another advantage is that this chemical combination also prevents algae growth. EPA limits are silver, 100 ppb and copper, 1000 ppb.

Ultraviolet Sterilization

UV sterilization uses UV radiation in the 254-nm range to irradiate pathogens and proteinaceous material. The advantage is that there is no residual effect but because it is localized, microbial density in the body of water nearest the animal may not be diminished. This technique is best used in flow-through systems in which the incoming water is irradiated and has limited use in closed and semiclosed systems. The efficiency of UV is fluid and must be continuously monitored. Target organism kill rates must be established. Tubes need to be changed every 6 months and quartz sleeves and wiped down as frequently as daily or weekly to keep up with the system biofouling rate.

Water Conditioning for Marine Bird–Only Systems

Marine birds are frequently kept in freshwater systems to facilitate maintenance with routine water changes and to decrease oxidation demand on disinfectants such as ozone, bromine, or chlorine. This is an option if other marine taxa will not be sharing the exhibit or system water, such as fish, reptiles, or mammals. A system designed this way may be challenging to renovate later if a multitaxa exhibit is desired.

Algae Control

See Chapter 25 for water treatment chemicals used.

HEATING AND CHILLING

Heat exchanger devices are typically used in large aquatic exhibits to maintain temperatures within the exhibit species tolerable range and prevent thermoregulatory stresses from rapid or wide temperature fluctuations for the species being supported. The most efficient placement of a heat exchanger in the water treatment circuit is last in line before returning to the exhibit directly or via a deaeration tower for fish systems. Heat exchangers commonly used include plate, spiral, tubular, and in-vessel types. The most important criteria for selecting a heat exchanger are as follows: (1) sizing it correctly for the temperature range of the species being maintained and the size, flow rate, and thermal characteristics of the system; and (2) selecting one with water-contacting components made of materials that will not contaminate the system (e.g., heavy metals) for which a titanium heat exchanger is usually the best choice, especially for seawater aquariums.

REFERENCES

1. Adey WH, Loveland K: Dynamic aquaria: Building living ecosystems, ed 2, San Diego, 1998, Academic Press.
2. Arkush KD: Water quality. In Dierauf LA, Gulland, FMD, editors: CRC handbook of marine mammal medicine, ed 2, Boca Raton, Fla, 2001, CRC Press, pp 779–787.
3. Carlson BA: Organism responses to rapid change: What aquaria tell us about nature. Am Zool 39:44–55, 1999.
4. Johnson JV: Application of ozone in marine parks and large aquariums. Bull Institut Océanographique Monaco 1:25, 2001.
5. Overby JM: In the aquarium with ozone: A matter of living clearly? Water Cond Purification 44:60–62, 2002.
6. Spotte S: Sterilization of marine mammal pool waters: Theoretical and health considerations. U.S. Department of Agriculture, Animal and Plant Health Inspection Service, Technical Bulletin No. 1797, Washington DC, 1991, U.S. Department of Agriculture.
7. Van der Toorn JD: A biological approach to dolphinarium water purification: I. Theoretical aspects. Aquat Mammals 13:83–92, 1987.
8. Watson CA, Hill JE: Design criteria for recirculating, marine ornamental production systems. Aquacult Engin 34:157–162, 2006.

CHAPTER 25

Advanced Water Quality Evaluation for Zoo Veterinarians

M. Andrew Stamper and Kent J. Semmen

As indicated in the basic water quality chapter (see Chapter 23), conditioning water is much more involved than monitoring and adjusting water for the basic parameters such as temperature, pH, dissolved oxygen (DO), ammonia, nitrite, nitrate, pH, salinity (conductivity), hardness, and alkalinity. This chapter is designed to inform veterinarians, many of whom oversee the water quality laboratories in zoos and aquariums, about the more complex aspects of water conditioning. These may include oxidation-reduction potential, total organics, metals, microbial dynamics, and organic contaminants. Most of the discussion will focus on marine systems because of their complexity, but variations with freshwater will be highlighted. This chapter is intended to be a primer; for more detailed information, see Spotte[24] and Clesceri and colleagues.[5]

WATER PARAMETERS AND TESTING

Sample Collection

One critical source of information for the veterinarian involved in complex water quality testing and condition is found in Clesceri and associates.[5] See Chapter 23 for basic information about collecting water samples.

ADVANCED WATER QUALITY

Dissolved Gases

Partial pressures are extremely important but are underanalyzed in an aquarium setting unless direct gas bubbles are forming on the glass of the aquarium or emboli are observed in the fish. Chronic and/or sublethal levels may cause morbidity and mortality from secondary factors. Partial pressures are measured using a gas tensionometer or saturometer. Baseline pressures are dependent on temperature and salinity and should be analyzed with methods provided in the appropriate literature.[8] Because of its insolubility and biologic unavailability, nitrogen is usually the culprit, but oxygen and carbon dioxide may cause issues in extreme cases. If chronic dissolved gas levels cannot be resolved, fish should be encouraged to swim below the compensation depth, which would prevent bubble formation. This may be accomplished by feeding and shelter strategies that keep them at depth.

Carbon Dioxide

Nitrogen is the most abundant gas in aquatic systems, but oxygen and CO_2 concentrations are the most dynamic because of manipulation by biologic activity. In an ecologically balanced system, oxygen and CO_2 tend to be inversely related in terms of their activity because one is constantly being exchanged for the other between plants or photosynthetic protoctists (e.g., algae, cyanobacteria) and animals, which has resulted in many ocean symbioses; thus, this effectively using light energy to drive chemical equilibria and stability in the system.[1] Probably the most important part that CO_2 plays in the aquarium setting is its role in the carbonate alkalinity system, which controls the pH level and its stability; this system is crucial to maintaining organisms' health. Other factors affecting this system include carbonic acid, carbonate, bicarbonate, and hydrogen ion levels. This is especially true in marine environments, in which animals have adapted to a very stable pH and narrow pH range.

CO_2 reacts with water to form carbonic acid (H_2CO_3), which dissociates to bicarbonate (HCO_3^-) and then carbonate (CO_3^{2-}) and hydrogen ions (H^+), chemically proportioned by temperature, pressure, and salinity equilibria[24]:

$$CO_2 + H_2O \rightleftarrows H_2CO_3 \rightleftarrows H^+ + HCO_3^- \rightleftarrows 2H^+ + CO_3^{2-}$$

Nitrifying and some denitrifying biologic water treatments use autotrophic microorganisms that metabolize the carbon from the carbonate system into biomass and hydrogen ions, driving the alkalinity and pH of the system downward. The mineralizing (biologic processes that convert organic to inorganic substances) and some denitrifying heterotrophic bacteria involved in organic decay in the system metabolize their carbon from biomass and respire CO_2 along with the fish and invertebrates, which easily becomes excessive in a typical aquarium with a high bioloading. Another source of excess CO_2 in systems is from rain water, which usually has at least a moderately acidic pH because of interactions with the atmosphere, even if unpolluted.

Too rapid an input of CO_2 relative to photosynthetic activity and gas exchange in a system results in an accumulation of CO_2 and H_2CO_3, increasing the H^+ concentration and decreasing pH, which may be alleviated with vigorous gas exchange. A simple jar test for this in the laboratory is to stir a water sample from the system vigorously with a vortex while monitoring pH and maintaining system temperature. An increase in pH indicates inadequate gas exchange in the system relative to total CO_2 input. If inadequate gas exchange cannot be easily addressed, the addition of sodium hydroxide (NaOH) to a system may help drive the conversion of excess H_2CO_3 from dissolved CO_2 to bicarbonate:

$$H_2CO_3 + OH^- \rightarrow HCO_3^- + H_2O$$

It also converts bicarbonate into carbonate[13]:

$$HCO_3^- + OH^- \rightarrow CO_3^-$$

Extreme caution must be taken not to overdose with this artificial method, which would result in too great or too rapid a pH change for the animals. We have found that adding it too rapidly to a seawater system by pipe injection may result in the precipitation of calcium carbonate, rapidly giving the exhibit water the appearance of skim milk. A more natural balancing method is to add photosynthesis to the treatment system and/or exhibit with aquatic plants and/or photosynthetic protoctists, although this approach should be in conjunction with adequate gas exchange for good pH balance.

Denitrification

In cases in which water changes are not feasible or at lower levels than desired, denitrification is the process of turning nitrate into nitrogen gas through anaerobic microbial action. An additional carbon source is needed

through the use of methanol or sulfur, which helps facilitate the autotrophic denitrification process in which the carbon issued is from the CO_2. These are complex processes and denitrification should not be attempted without experienced staff because toxic elements may be produced and released into the main water system if the procedure is not performed correctly. It is important to note that our understanding of bacteria in the nitrogen cycle is in its infancy; once more information is gained, we could significantly alter our water-conditioning capabilities. For example, as recently as 2002, it was discovered that bacteria could perform anaerobic ammonium oxidation (anammox) to N_2 gas. These four genera of anammox bacteria were identified as *Brocadia*, *Kuenenia*, *Scalindula*, and *Anammoxoblobus* and are responsible for 24% to 67% of nitrogen loss in marine systems.[9] They may be grown autotrophically with CO_2 as the only carbon source, thus eliminating the complex dependency on several bacterial pathways, including anoxic denitrification using methanol or sulfur. It is currently being applied in industrial use and is highly experimental but could be used in zoo and aquarium settings. We would then not have to depend on complex biologic filtration systems, which are prone to failures.

Phosphates

Phosphate enters natural systems from dissolved inorganic phosphate (DIP) from rock, sediments, and fertilizers, dissolved organic phosphate (DOP) from sewage and organic fertilizers, and particulate organic phosphate (POP) from sediment. Algae readily take up DOP and DIP in the natural environment. Phosphate concentration is normally the primary limiting factor in the bloom of microalgae in freshwater and marine systems, but nitrogen and iron are critical nutrients as well. Sewage and fertilizer contamination may cause phytoplankton blooms in natural systems, with catastrophic toxic effects to resident animals. In aquarium systems, phosphate builds up through the introduction of food into the system. Depending on the type of system, these may be limited through biologic uptake by biologic oxidant demand (BOD), oxidizing bacteria, and precipitation with lime, lanthanum chloride, or aluminum and iron salts.

Sulfur

Sulfur may sometimes be an issue in aquarium settings. Hydrogen sulfide may build up in sediment and improperly maintained filter beds in which anoxic processes may take hold. Sulfur, in moderation, is beneficial for the sulfur cycle. The aim should be not to eliminate sulfur but to keep it minimal to prevent toxicity.

Total Organic Carbon

Total organic carbon (TOC) is an underappreciated component of aquarium chemistry. Organic compounds enter the ambient water from various sources, including influent water, animal waste products, uneaten food, and drift from the air (e.g., pollen, dust):

$$TOC = \text{particulate organic matter (POC)} + \text{dissolved organic matter (DOC)}$$

POC is usually efficiently removed through mechanical filtration and DOC is the fraction of the TOC that passes through a filter of a stipulated pore size of 0.45 μm. Two major components of DOC are humic and fulvic acids, which can color the water and are often discouraged in the aquarium setting. An excessively high TOC level increases oxidant demand, reduces efficacy of sterilization, and creates toxic byproducts. Biologic filtration bacteria reduce POC and DOC by incorporating the carbon when growing and reproducing but, even though this occurs, TOC often overwhelms a system. The easiest way to reduce the TOC level is to change the water, but this may be expensive or impractical, so other steps have been developed to condition the water. Ozone can be regarded as a molecular chainsaw that randomly breaks large molecular chains into smaller ones, with unpredictable ways. The combinations are dependent on water composition and are impossible to predict. Activated carbon efficiently removes TOC. We have speculated that excessive ozone and activated carbon use may lead to manipulations of the TOC level, which has adverse effects on the animal health; for example, head and lateral line disease could result.

Turbidity: Measurement of Particulates in Water

Nephelometric methods are specific to water turbidity measurement. The suspended matter in the sample is measured via a specially designed meter that sends a focused light beam through the water sample. Suspended materials such as solids, dirt, silt, plankton, and bubbles scatter the light, which is measured by a photodiode at a 90-degree angle incident to the light source. The results are expressed in nephelometric turbidity units (NTUs), and are more qualitative than quantitative. Our concern with turbidity is primarily to maintain the viewing clarity of exhibits and to assess the performance of the mechanical filtration.

Heavy Metals

Metals in appropriate amounts are essential for good health. Microelements, for the most part, have a very small therapeutic margin of safety in regard to being too little or too much. It is helpful to know whether a mineral is toxic and/or if it is a heavy metal. Metal toxicity is also profoundly dependent on speciation (bound to various organic carbon materials; this is why chelated copper is less toxic than in its pure form. For more information, see Sorensen.[23]

Volatile Organics

Volatile organic compounds (VOCs) are theoretically a concern around aquatic animals. Regardless of direct exposure to the water surface and absorption, one must always be concerned with the air intake, which is efficient at transferring organics into the water column.

BACTERIA AND ANIMALS

Microbes are everywhere. In every milliliter of surface seawater, there are 0.5 to 1 million bacteria and 10 million viruses.[3] They are on every surface and comprise very complex ecosystems called biofilms. For those who think of biofiltered bacteria as good and pathogens as bad, it is much more complex. Unfortunately, our thinking about the aquatic environment has been biased by our previously limited tool of culturing bacteria. This is unfortunate because current estimates predict that <1% of the bacteria in water may be culturable; this figure may be higher when culturing fish internal organs because their internal environment is compatible with our medical culture technology.

The following are some examples of the important role of bacteria in aquarium systems. Animals use bacteria to fend off bad bacteria through surface competition and antagonism—chemical inhibitors.[4] No animal demonstrates this complex relationship better than corals. Corals are known to harbor an abundance of microbes, with approximately 10 million bacteria/cm[2] of coral surface.[15,20] The mucus layer, along with the bacterial community associated with it, is used as a protective barrier against pathogens by producing antibiotics or simply by occupying the available space.[10] Over 400 strains of surface-associated bacteria from various species of seaweed and invertebrates from Scottish coastal waters have been isolated, and 35% of them produce antimicrobial compounds. This is a much higher proportion than free-living marine isolates or soil bacteria. Corals have the ability to recruit bacteria from the water column, which allows them to adapt to changing environmental conditions. Disease and bleaching in corals are often associated with changes in the composition or activity of the associated microbial community.[19] It has been speculated that coral-associated bacteria also benefit the coral by fixing nitrogen, breaking down waste products, and cycling basic nutrients back to the photosynthetic zooxanthellae.

Similar beneficial effects may be seen in the mucus layer of fish. Studies in blue gills have found that bacterial counts are 1×10^3 cells/mL and that three to seven times more bacteria are present in the mucus layer as compared with the lake water.[11,12] Phylogenetic analysis has demonstrated a great difference between lake water and mucus. Of the isolates from mucus, 60% were gram-positive and could be divided into two major groups. Strains sampled in July were closely related to the genus *Staphylococcus*, whereas strains in November were close to *Mycobacterium*. In contrast, most isolates from the lake water were gram-negative and gram-positives were only found in the November sampling. Almost all mucus isolates (10 of 12 strains) had difficulty growing in lake water culture media, whereas 50% (6 of 12 strains) of the lake water isolates were able to grow in lake water culture media. This helps demonstrate that mucus has an effect on aquatic bacterial communities that become dependent on this environment. These complex relationships should be considered before consideration of antibiotic treatment.

Microbes, Biofilms, and the Water Environment

As noted, microbes are found throughout the water column but are also on every surface and are known as biofilms. Biofilms include organisms beyond bacteria and comprise fungi, algae, protozoans, and metazoans. An intricate ecologic process occurs as various environmental parameters change. These organisms secrete an assortment of chemicals known as extracellular polymeric substances (EPSs), which add to the TOC and are

critical to the health of the water environment.[25] These include mostly lipopolysaccharides but there are also proteins, carbohydrates, and lipids, some of which may have protective properties. The quality and quantity of EPSs are dependent on environmental factors such as pH, salinity, aeration, and temperature; they are completely altered by ozone or are removed by activated carbon.

These substances may be involved with the health of the fish. In salt water systems, fish constantly take in water to stay hydrated. Water, along with the substances in the water, should be thought of as a nutrient source to fish; its importance is not known at this point but should be considered. Conversely, some EPSs may be bad for fish. Adaptations to hostile environments or some pathogenic gram-negative bacteria may produce endotoxins or exotoxins that are lipopolysaccharides and may be very harmful to fish.[2]

New Procedures to Track Bacteria

To increase our understanding of these complex systems, there are several technologies that help better understand bacterial populations and their dynamics. One is fluorescent microscopy, which may directly determine absolute populations of bacteria. Unlike cultures, which only grow the populations that may survive on the media, these are simple counts for absolute abundance and may determine live versus dead bacteria. To determine bacteria types, analysis of microbial DNA extracted from the environment (metagenomic sequencing) is necessary. Metagenomics[21] is a new field combining molecular biology and genetics in an attempt to identify and characterize the genetic material from environmental samples. It is used to examine the diversity, distribution, and ecologic roles of viruses and bacteria in a wide range of environments, including seawater, marine animals, and mucus. These genera (type and relative abundance) may be tracked to see how they fluctuate in the regard to various parameters (e.g., time, temperature, salinity, social interactions in the case of fish and invertebrates). These techniques may be used to help hone culture methods for further identification of specific bacteria. In the case of corals, metagenomics may help provide insight into the stability of bacterial communities associated with corals and, in particular, the effect of transplant restoration efforts on bacterial composition. With that information, we may be able to determine whether culture conditions lead to changes in the composition of coral-associated bacterial communities, which may affect the health and survival of reef communities and the success of restoration efforts. This may also be applied to fish species as well.

OXIDATION-REDUCTION: STERILIZATION VERSUS DISINFECTION

In basic terms, the oxidation-reduction potential (ORP), measured in millivolts, indicates the activity of the oxidizing reactions in the water being measured. Ozone is O_3, an allotrope of oxygen. Ozone may generate a high oxidation potential and is recommended to be greater than 700 mV to sterilize water. ORP levels in marine mammal system may be maintained as high as 500 mV but it is better to keep it below 400 if possible to reduce any potential of irritants. Aquarium ORP levels with fish and/or invertebrates should be maintained between 200 and 350 mV. Levels lower than these indicate an unacceptable accumulation of toxic, reduced organic compounds. Levels higher than this indicate too active an oxidizing environment, with possible damage to delicate plant and animal tissues. ORP levels are dynamic. Overfeeding, lack of water changes, low aeration, poor mechanical filter maintenance, and overstocking all tend to lower the ORP. If ozone is used in fish systems, ORPs should not enter the ambient water above 350 mV. Therefore, the higher ORP levels need to be in a contact area outside the fish holding area. As for reptiles, birds, and mammals, most facilities regulate their water to be free of residual dissolved ozone because this could be detrimental to feathers, fir, skin, eyes, and the respiratory system. O_3 reacts directly with oxidizable compounds; these are any substance that will accept oxygen (e.g., proteins, fatty acids in cell walls). This is a very short-lived process (within seconds) because O_3 is extremely unstable.

The oxidation process is affected by TOC, pH, bicarbonate, and temperature. Products of these oxidation events include free radicals, hydroperoxide species, and unstable ozonide intermediates, which in turn are weaker oxidizers but last longer in the water column. One such product is bromine. O_3 reacts with bromide to yield hypobromous acid (HOBr) and hypobromite (OBr^-). Ozonation is less efficient in the presence of bromide; Br^- may be regenerated from OBr^-, causing catalytic destruction of ozone and increasing ozone demand. OBr^- is a weak persistent oxidant; it reacts with organic materials to produce carcinogenic and mutagenic compounds (e.g., bromoform, formaldehyde) but these are in small concentrations and are not harmful if regulated appropriately. To accomplish this, HOBr is measured and used as an indicator to ensure that ozone oxidation is not excessive; it is kept at a level at which excess HOBr is not produced. The advantages to ozone are that it has extremely high antimicrobial properties compared with chlorine, approximately three times more effective. It destroys POC, which normally decolorizes the water. Some tips for understanding ORP fluxuation include the knowledge that variable results are often obtained with ORP measurement. If two different ORP systems are within a 50-mV agreement, it is acceptable but one should strive for better resolution. ORP is best used for measuring trends rather than taking isolated readings. ORP varies at different areas in an aquarium system and at different points in feeding and lighting cycles. Take readings accordingly for comparison.

For more information, see Chapter 24 and Johnson.[14]

KNOWN EFFECTS OF CHEMICALS ON BIOFILMS

There have been several papers published on the effects of chemicals on the biofilter and this is the most important consideration when adding therapeutic agents to water (Table 25-1).[6,7,16-18,22] It is important to know that most, if not all, of these drug interactions are dose-dependent and affect the biofilter's efficiency to varying degrees; they should not be considered as having an all or nothing relationship. Biofilter efficiency may fluctuate 5% to 10% over a period of several days. Factors that might affect biofilter efficiency include length of treatment, species of bacteria, thickness of the biofilm, hardness, and binding agents such as TOCs. For this reason, it is important not to depend on anecdotal information and even to treat experimental information with speculation. To guard against unpredicted reactions from therapeutic agents, it is important to consider water changes and appropriate dose adjustments. It is advised that the facility maintain a biofarm (isolated cultured bacteria). These may be kept by adding ammonia chloride or sulfate titrated to effect, or clean fish living in the system that provide a more natural ammonia source for the bacteria. Other factors such as phosphate and alkalinity are important to monitor and adjust as needed. These may be used to supplement a struggling biofilter or reestablish a biofilter if a system needs to be sterilized.

BACTERIAL DIGESTION OF CHEMICALS

When controlling an environment like the aquarium industry's current standards, millions of bacterial

TABLE 25-1   Effects of Chemotherapeutic Agents on Biofilters*

	Dose	Nitrosomonas	Nitrobacter	Comments
Ampicillin	Dose dependent 34-136 mg/L	+[a]	+[a]	
Chloramine T	Dose dependent 5-40 mg/L	+[a]	+[a]	
Chloroamphenicol	10-80 mg/L	−[a], +[c]	−[a], +[c]	
Copper II sulphate	1-16 mg/L	−[a], −[b]	−[a], −[b]	
Enrofloxacin	Dose dependent 5-40 mg/L	−[a]	+[a],	Note: Did have a dose dependent effect on Nitorbacter
Erythromycin	Dose dependent 10-80 mg/L	+[a]	+[a]	
Formalin	25 mg/L every other day	−[b], −[e]	−[b], −[e]	
Formalin + Malachite green	25 mg/L + 0.1 mg/L every other day	−[b]	−[b]	
Kanamycine disulphate	Dose dependent 10-80 mg/L	−[a]	−[a]	
Levamisole	Dose dependent 4-32 mg/L	+[a]	+[a]	
Malachite green	2-16 mg/L	−[a], −[b]	−[a], −[b]	
Methylene blue	Dose dependent 1-8 mg/L	+[a], +[b]	+[a], +[b]	
Neomycin sulphate	10-80 mg/L	−[a]	−[a]	
Nitropirinol	50 mg/L	+[c]	+[c]	
Oxytetracyline	50 mg/L; 12.5-75 mg/L (>50 mg/L completely inhibited)	−[c], +[d]	−[c], +[d]	Type of bacteria and experimental conditions
Patassium permaganate	4 mg/L	−[b]	−[b]	
Polymyxin B	Dose dependent 1-8 mg/L	+[a]	+[a]	
Potassium penicillin G	20-160 mg/L	−[a]	−[a]	
Sodium cloride	5,000 mg/L	−[b]	−[b]	
Sulfamerazine	50 mg/L	+[c]	+[c]	
Tetracycline	10-80 mg/L	−[a]	−[a]	
Trimethoprime/Sulphadoxin	40-160 mg/L	−[a]	−[a]	

[a]*Nimenya et al., 1999*
[b]*Collins et al., in 1975 demonstrated that methylene blue at 5 mg/L completely stopped nictification for 16 days whereas therapeutic levels of formalin, malachite green, formalin and malachite green, copper sulfate, potassium permanganate and NaCL (in freshwater) had no effect on nitrification.*
[c]*Collins et al., 1976 found no effect with OTC at 50 mg/L for 26 days. Other chemicals that caused inhibition at 50 mg/L included choloramphenicol, sulfamerazine, nifurpirinol.*
[d]*Klaver, AL, Matthews, RA determined that nitrification was inhibited at all levels of oxyteteracycline (OTC) tested (12.5-75 mg/L). Concentrations of 50-75 mg/L OTC resulted in nearly complete inhibition of nitrification within 7 days.*
[e]*Lars et al. also found nitrification was not impaired in systems treated with formalin on a daily basis as compared to untreated systems. This was repeated by the authors but other anecdotal information indicates there may be complicating variables, as also demonstrated in the OTC that may be cofactors causing biofilter issues.*

species are starved to inactivity. These bacteria, although they may not be obvious, could still exploit any limiting nutrient sources, whether it be ammonia, nitrite, or phosphorus. This also applies to other nutrients that might enter the water. For the most part, therapeutic agents are given to an animal that is placed in a sterile environment once it enters the systemic body, but this is not the case when placed into a body of water. It is important to recognize the impact of microbes on chemicals, especially those with carbon chains that may act in a similar fashion as these nutrients. With the diversity of microbes in a water column, it is possible that one species will have an enzyme to break those chemical chains and use it as a food source. We have seen exponential decay of formalin and praziquantel concentration levels in a treated body of water, which would suggest bacterial digestion of the chemical. This also may be seen when ethanol is introduced as a solvent. Oxygen levels fall quickly and microbial blooms may be seen. Ethanol is a short-chain carbon source that is easily exploited by bacteria, which are carbon-limited. Therefore, it is important to invest in procedures for monitoring chemical concentration when treating animals. It is also important to recognize that there are different microbial communities in various institutions. Interactions with various chemicals will result in different experiences by husbandry staff and clinicians.

REFERENCES

1. Adey WH, Loveland K: Dynamic aquaria: Building living ecosystems, ed 2, San Diego, Calif, 1998, Academic Press.
2. Bhaskar PV, Bhosle NB: Microbial extracellular polymeric substance in marine biogeochemical process. Curr Sci 88:45–53, 2005.
3. Breitbart M, Rohwer F: Here a virus, there a virus, everywhere the same virus? Trends Microbiol 13:278–284, 2005.
4. Burgess JG, Jordan EM, Bregu M, et al: Microbial antagonism: A neglected avenue of natural products research. J Biotechnol 70:27–32, 1999.
5. Clesceri L, Greenberg E, Eaton AD, editors: Standard methods for the examination of water and wastewater, ed 20, Baltimore, 1998, United Book Press, Parts 1000 and 2000.
6. Collins MT, Gratzek JB, Daw DL, Nemetz TG: Effects of parasiticides on nitrification. J Fish Res Board Can 32:2033–2037, 1975.
7. Collins MT, Gratzek JB, Shotts FB, et al: Effects of antibacterial agents on nitrification in an aquatic recirculating system. J Fish Res Board Can 33:215–218, 1976.
8. Fickeisen DH, Scheider MJ, editors: Gas bubble disease: Proceedings of a workshop, Richland, Washington, October 1974 (http://www.archive.org/details/gasbubbledisease00paci).
9. Francis CA, Beman JM, Kuypers MM: New processes and players in the nitrogen cycle: The microbial ecology of anaerobic and archaeal ammonia oxidation. Int Soc Microb Ecol 1:19–27, 2007.
10. Frias-Lopez J, Zerkle AL, Bonheyo GT, et al: Partitioning of bacterial communities between seawater and healthy, black band diseased, and dead coral surfaces. Appl Environ Microbiol 68:2214–2228, 2002.
11. Hashizume T, Obayashi M, Morisaki H: The effect of the surface mucus of bluegills (Lepomis macrochirus) on bacterial activity. Microbes Environ 20:97–103, 2005.
12. Hashizume T, Takai C, Naito M, Morisaki H: Characteristics of the mucus layer on the surface of the bluegill. Microbes Environ 20:69–80, 2005.
13. Holmes-Farley R: Chemistry and the aquarium, 2002 (http://www.advancedaquarist.com/issues/may2002/chem.htm).
14. Johnson JV: Application of ozone in marine parks and large aquariums. Bull Institut Océanographique Monaco 20, 2001.
15. Kellogg CA: Tropical Archaea: Diversity associated with the surface microlayer of corals. Mar Ecol Prog Ser 273:81–88, 2004.
16. Klaver AL, Matthews RA: Effects of oxytetracycline on nitrification in a model aquatic system. Aquaculture 123:237–247, 1994.
17. Pedersen L-F, Pedersen PB, Nielsen JL, Nielsen PH: Long-term/low-dose formalin exposure to small-scale recirculation aquaculture systems. Aquacult Eng 42:1–7, 2010.
18. Nimenya H, Delaunois A, La Duong D, et al: Short-term toxicity of various pharmacological agents on the in vitro nitrification process in a simple closed aquatic system. ATLA 27:121–135, 1999.
19. Pantos O, Cooney RP, Le Tissier MD, et al: The bacterial ecology of a plague-like disease affecting the Caribbean coral Montastrea annularis. Environ Microbiol 5:370–382, 2003.
20. Rohwer F, Seguritan V, Azam F, et al: Diversity and distribution of coral-associated bacteria. Mar Ecol Prog Ser 243:1–10, 2002.
21. Schloss PD, Handelsman J: Metagenomics for studying unculturable microorganisms: Cutting the Gordian knot. Genome Biol 6:229, 2005.
22. Schwartz MF, Bullock GL, Hankins JA, et al: Effects of selected chemotherapeutants on nitrification in fluidized-sand biofilters for cold water fish production. Int J Recirc Aquacult 1:61–81, 2000.
23. Sorensen EM: Metal poisoning in fish, Boca Raton, Fla, 1991, CRC Press.
24. Spotte S: Captive seawater fishes: Science and technology, New York, 1992, John Wiley and Sons.
25. Weiner R, Langille S, Quintero E: Structure, function and immunochemistry of bacterial exopolysaccarides. J Industrial Microbiol 15:339–346, 1995.

CHAPTER 26

Quarantine of Fish and Aquatic Invertebrates in Public Display Aquaria

Catherine Hadfield

Quarantine reduces the risk of introducing infectious diseases into established collections. For fish and aquatic invertebrates, key components are the provision of excellent water quality and a suitable environment, isolation from collection animals, and easy access to allow monitoring, as well as diagnostics and treatments where necessary.[7,11,20] Methods will depend on the needs of the institution, facilities available, species acquired, and condition of the animals. This chapter will focus on quarantine within closed, or recirculating, systems in public display aquaria.

Fish or aquatic invertebrates within a quarantine system are often managed as a group, because they are exposed to the same environmental conditions and pathogens. Regular visual examinations on all members of the group are essential, but diagnostics (e.g., necropsies or hands-on examinations) on a subset of the group are often representative of the whole quarantine system. Treatments are often needed in response to specific pathogens, particularly if they are highly pathogenic or novel to the target population. Prophylactic treatments may also be used, especially with animals that were wild-caught or came from large distributors, or when the target exhibits are large, with diverse species and complex life support systems. It is common in these situations to treat for protozoal ectoparasites in teleosts and for monogeneans in teleosts and elasmobranchs.

Shipments vary from one large specimen to several thousand small fish. Animals may come from other zoos and aquaria or be wild-caught by the institution, but they usually come from distributors. Many common freshwater fish are bred in captivity; the more unusual freshwater species and most marine species are wild-caught. Sources and shipping are not discussed in this chapter but using a reliable source, excellent shipping conditions, and the shortest shipping times will improve quarantine success.

COMMON PROBLEMS

Some of the more common problems seen in quarantine are as follows[7,11,13-16,19]:

- Inappetence or poor body condition: This may be caused by inappropriate collection techniques, prolonged transport, or an unsuitable environment, diet, or social structure.
- Trauma: This may be from transport, restraint, an unsuitable environment, or aggression; compatibility is dependent on the species, size, gender, stocking density, habitat complexity, and feed provision.
- Ammonia toxicity: Quarantine systems are at high risk because they are put through sudden increases in bioload, and some immersion treatments may affect the biologic filtration.
- Viral diseases: Some are common during quarantine, such as lymphocystis, a cosmetic concern that may prohibit animals from going onto exhibit. Some are rare but serious, such as koi herpesvirus.
- Bacterial diseases: These may be primary but are often secondary to other diseases or stressors. Examples include vibriosis and infections caused by *Aeromonas*, *Edwardsiella*, *Yersinia*, and *Flavobacterium* spp.
- Fungal diseases: Oomycete infections are common in freshwater fish secondary to trauma.
- Protozoal ectoparasites: *Ichthyophthirius* and *Chilodonella* spp. in freshwater, and *Cryptocaryon*, *Brooklynella*, *Amyloodinium*, and *Ichthyobodo* spp. in salt water may cause acute mortalities, with few preemptive signs. Several have life stages that are not susceptible to treatment and thus require repeated or long-term treatments (e.g., *Cryptocaryon*, *Ichthyophthirius*, *Amyloodinium* spp.).

- Monogenean ectoparasites: Gyrodactylids are viviparous and may reproduce rapidly, causing acute mortalities. Other families such as the dactylogyrids and capsalids are oviparous and treatment often needs to continue through several life cycles.
- Copepods, leeches, lice: Although not detrimental unless loads are high, these must not be introduced into exhibits because they are particularly hard to eradicate once established.

GENERAL PLANNING

An ideal quarantine area is one isolated from the established collection, such as in a separate building or area, with dedicated staff.[3] If this is not possible, protocols should be in place to prevent cross-contamination (e.g., isolated systems, lids on tanks, separate equipment, hand washing facilities) and the area should have minimal through-traffic.

Fiberglass tanks with viewing windows are ideal for quarantine. Some species require more specialized tanks (e.g., kreisel tanks for jellyfish). In general, smaller systems allow for easier monitoring and access and, in the event of a system-wide issue, fewer animals will be affected. Larger systems tend to have more stable environmental conditions.

For smaller systems, sponge filters are ideal. Larger systems usually include sand filters and biotowers.[13,19] If systems are periodically unoccupied, protocols should exist to maintain biologic filtration, such as routine dosing with ammonium chloride. Undergravel filters (and substrate in general) should be avoided, because parasites and intermediate hosts may collect in substrate. Ultraviolet (UV) filtration may help reduce bacterial and viral load in the water. Ozone is generally not practical in quarantine systems because of the variable bioload. Filters with activated carbon or zeolite clay should be available for adsorption of drugs following immersion treatment. There should be redundancy in the life support equipment in case of failure. Disposal of waste water, in-water medications, and filter media should follow relevant regulations.

The Association of Zoos and Aquariums (AZA)–recommended minimum quarantine duration is 30 days.[3] At the National Aquarium, quarantine for fish not treated for protozoal ectoparasites is a minimum of 90 days; some pathogens have presented up to 65 days into quarantine (e.g., *Amyloodinium* in temperate species).

A wide variety of good-quality foods should be available, including pelleted and flake foods, gel foods (e.g., Mazuri Gel diets), frozen foods (e.g., fish, crustaceans, mollusks), algae sheets, leafy greens, and vegetables.[7] It may be hard to convert some wild-caught animals to a captive diet, and they may not have eaten recently. Most facilities maintain some live foods to encourage food intake, such as brine shrimp, glass shrimp, rotifers, minnows, and mollies. These should be bred in-house or put through a quarantine period.

Plans for cleaning and disinfection of equipment and systems need to be established. Many types of disinfectants are available (e.g., chlorine, iodophors, quaternary ammonium, peroxygen compounds), and these should be rotated routinely.[20]

CONSIDERATIONS PRIOR TO ACQUISITION AND ON ARRIVAL

Prior to Acquisition

Animals should be provisionally allocated to systems based on their environmental requirements (e.g., temperature, pH, salinity, water flow, lighting), their compatibilities, and the target stocking density. Water parameters should not be changed rapidly to accommodate incoming shipments because this damages the biologic filtration. Invertebrates, teleosts, and elasmobranchs should not be quarantined in the same system because this limits treatment options. Juveniles, or any animals considered potentially sensitive to treatments, should not be housed with large groups of other fish. Stocking densities should be kept low to decrease competition and disease transmission. Based on a review of quarantine data, stocking density for freshwater and salt water fish quarantine at the National Aquarium is less than 1.5 inch of fish/U.S. gallon (or 1.5 cm/liter). Some systems should remain available in case groups need to be split.

Prior to the animals' arrival, the water quality should be checked to ensure that it is within the target range. Décor that is suitable for the species should be added, such as plastic plants at the surface for freshwater butterflyfish (*Pantodon* spp.). Gravel or sand may be needed for a few species, such as garden eels (*Gorgasia* spp.). Suitable vinyl nets or stretchers should be available.

Where animals are being acquired from another institution, a history and preshipment examinations should be obtained. Pertinent questions include whether the animals were wild-caught or captive-bred, when they were acquired, any infectious disease concerns, and water quality, diet, and behavioral information. For most shipments, however, the history is limited to the area where the animals were caught or bred.

On Arrival

Most fish and aquatic invertebrates are shipped in clear bags with water and air or oxygen, packed in an insulated container. Larger fish usually have their own transport container and may have continuous aeration and filtration. Over time, transport water shows increased ammonia levels and decreased dissolved oxygen and pH, and will gradually adapt to the ambient temperature. Unless shipping containers are badly fouled or drained, water from the target system should be gradually introduced over 20 to 60 minutes to allow the animals to adapt to the new parameters before they are moved to the new tank (acclimation). They must be closely monitored; acclimation should be shortened if there are any signs of distress (e.g., increased gilling rates, neurologic signs). Low light conditions and minimal noise may be beneficial during acclimation and the first 12 to 24 hours.

It is important to record the shipping conditions, including delays in shipping, bag condition, stocking density, and fouling. Temperature, dissolved oxygen, pH, and total ammonia of the transport water should be recorded. This information helps determine stress levels during shipment, which may affect susceptibility to infectious diseases, and may be used to compare shipping methods.

MONITORING

Regular visual examinations must continue throughout quarantine—subtle changes in behavior and food intake are usually the first signs of impending issues (Box 26-1). Monitoring sheets may be used to track essential data, such as temperature, water quality, food intake,

BOX 26-1	Clinical Signs of Concern During Quarantine

Mortalities
Increased respiratory rate, effort, piping (gasping)
Flashing (rubbing)
Hyperemia, pallor, ulceration of the skin; hyperemic or tattered fins
White spots, black spots, visible parasites
Decreased food intake, inappetence, poor body condition
Abnormal swimming (e.g., whirling, change in swimming speed)
Abnormal behavior (e.g., isolated schooling fish, burrowing fish on the substrate)

mortalities, treatments, and drug levels, when assayed (Fig. 26-1). Water quality should be checked daily until stable and then at increased intervals. It is important to have a set of acceptable water quality parameters and protocols to correct parameters as necessary (Table 26-1).

EXAMINATION AND DIAGNOSTIC PROCEDURES

Necropsies

Dead fish should be removed and necropsied as soon as possible. The priority is to assess food intake and look for infectious diseases that may be of concern to the quarantine or exhibit group. At a minimum, each animal should receive physical examinations, skin scrapes, gill biopsies, an assessment of gastrointestinal (GI) contents, and GI squash preparations. A full necropsy should be done when possible, with tissue impression smears; tissue squash preparations; kidney, liver, or blood cultures; and histopathology. Culture results are dependent on sampling methods and culture conditions. Polymerase chain reaction (PCR) assays are available for some pathogens in commonly cultured species, such as spring viremia of carp. Yanong[21] has provided an excellent review of fish necropsies.

Examination of Live Animals

Live fish showing clinical signs should be examined as soon as possible (see Box 26-1). If premortem diagnostics are limited (e.g., small fish), some affected individuals from the group may be euthanized for diagnostics. Fish are commonly euthanized by immersion with tricaine methanesulfonate (Finquel MS-222; U.S. Food and Drug Administration [FDA]–approved in the United States).[1,21] In groups with no clinical signs, examinations may be considered on a subset of the group (e.g., 2% to 5%) or on the whole group.[7]

Restraint may be manual or chemical, depending on the species, size, and procedure.[17] The most common anesthetic is tricaine methanesulfonate, used at 50 to 120 mg/liter for sedation, buffered in soft water.[6,7,17] Metomidate (Aquacalm) has recently been approved for the sedation of ornamental fish.[17] Many elasmobranchs will show tonic immobility (decreased responsiveness) when placed in ventrodorsal recumbency.[8] Hyperoxygenation of the water (e.g., 110% to 120%) may provide light sedation in elasmobranchs. Various anesthetics have been reported in aquatic invertebrates, such as

Freshwater Fish Quarantine

Arrival date: May 26	Number in	Species	ID number	Number out	Cleared quarantine:
Source: Wild-caught X island	50	Blacknose dace	xxxxxx		By:
System: 12					Destination:
Volume (gal): 400 gallons					

Date May/June	26	27	28	29	30	31	1	2	3	4	5	6	7	8	9	10	11	12	13	14	15	16	17	18	19	20	21	22	23	24
Quarantine day	1	2	3	4	5	6	7	8	9	10	11	12	13	14	15	16	17	18	19	20	21	22	23	24	25	26	27	28	29	30
Temperature (F)																														
pH																														
Salinity (g/L)																														
Total ammonia (mg/L)																														
Water change (%)																														
Food intake (Good, poor, none, fasted)																														
Mortalities																														
Skin scrapes, gill bx																														SS
Fomalin (25 ppm 6 hr)										F		F		F																
Praziquantel (2 ppm 5 d)																	PZ													
Salinity (2-3 ppt continuous)	S	S	S	S	S	S	S	S	S	S	S	S	S	S	S	S	S	S	S	S	S	S	S	S	S	S	S	S	S	S

Comments:

Figure 26-1

Example of a monitoring sheet for fish quarantine.

TABLE 26-1   Examples of Acceptable Water Quality Parameters

Parameter	Salt Water Fish	Salt Water Invertebrates and Corals	Brackish Water	Freshwater	Soft Freshwater
Dissolved oxygen (%)	90-100	90-100	90-100	90-100	90-100
Salinity (g/liter or ppt)	28-35	28-35	12-20	0-1	0
pH	7.8-8.5	7.8-8.5	7.5-8.2	6.5-8.0	5.0-6.5
Ammonia (mg/liter or ppm)	<0.04	<0.04	<0.04	<0.04	<0.04
Nitrite (mg/liter)	<0.2	<0.2	<0.2	<0.2	<0.2
Alkalinity (mg/liter $CaCO_3$)	>200	>200	70-150	15-150	1-15
Calcium (mg/liter)		350-475			

magnesium chloride and ethanol.[11] Whether under manual or chemical restraint, source water must be used and temperature, dissolved oxygen, and ammonia levels must be appropriate. Gloves should be worn to prevent trauma to the animals, exposure to anesthetics, and transmission of zoonoses, such as atypical mycobacteria, *Aeromonas* spp., and *Edwardsiella tarda*.[20]

The following diagnostic modalities may be considered[4,7,14,19,20]:

- Physical examination with assessment of body condition
- Morphometrics (e.g., weight, total length, width, and girth)
- Skin scrapes and gill biopsies examined under direct microscopy
- Fecal examinations. Many fish defecate under chemical restraint or fecal material may be collected by cloacal flush.
- Blood samples from the ventral tail vein (most fish), posterior cardinal vein (elasmobranchs), or branchial vessels (teleosts). Dry heparin is a suitable anticoagulant. A complete blood count should be determined within a few hours using the Natt-Herrick technique, modified for elasmobranchs.[2]
- Hemolymph samples may be collected from the cardiac sinus in many aquatic invertebrates (e.g., horseshoe crabs, crustaceans, cephalopods). For example, they may be used to look for *Hematodinium* in blue crabs (*Callinectes sapidus*).
- Diagnostic imaging, e.g., ultrasonography or radiography. Ultrasonography is especially useful in elasmobranchs to evaluate the liver, GI, and reproductive tract.
- Other species-specific procedures may be used, such as a coelomic flush in cownose rays (*Rhinoptera bonasus*) to look for coccidia (*Eimeria southwalli*).

Individuals may be identified based on external characteristics, fin clips, fin tags (e.g., Floy tags), or intramuscular transponders. Results should be considered in terms of the risk to the quarantine group and the exhibit group; for example, pentastomids are of concern if the fish will be on exhibit with reptiles, the definitive hosts.

TREATMENTS FOR FISH

Unless there is a disease outbreak, most treatments should be delayed until the animals have had 7 to 10 days to recover from shipping and are eating well. There are many considerations before using medications in

---

| BOX 26-2 | Calculations for Medicated Gel Foods |

Determine target dose of medication (e.g., metronidazole, 50 mg/kg PO).
Estimate or calculate gel intake (e.g., 2% body weight/day = 20 g food/kg body weight).
Calculate the dose of medication per kilogram of food (e.g., 50 mg/kg of body weight = 50 mg/20 g of food = 2500 mg/kg of food [wet weight]).
Offer the prepared medicated gel at the target dose (e.g., 40 fish weighing ~5 g each, eating 2% body weight/day, should be given ~4 g of gel).

---

fish.[7,10,12,14-16,18,19] Diseases are often secondary to environmental stressors (e.g., elevated total ammonia, inappropriate pH) and these must be corrected. Other management changes may reduce the need for medications (e.g., decreased stocking density or organic load, altered temperature). Pharmacokinetic data should be followed if available, but doses are often empirical. For immersion treatments, the volume should be calculated accurately and all components of the life support system should be considered (e.g., removal of carbon and UV filtration prior to treatment, potential damage to biologic filtration; see Chapter 23 for further details). For oral and parenteral medications, animals should be dosed accurately based on body weight (Box 26-2). Some species and life stages are sensitive to particular treatments. For novel species, the veterinary, aquaculture, and hobbyist literature should be reviewed. Treating a subset first may be warranted. Institutions should maintain a list of potential drug reactions, including information on doses, species, sizes, overall health, and concurrent stressors. Treatments should be reassessed regularly, and thorough records are essential.

Freshwater and Salt Water Dips

- Target: Ectoparasites
- Route, doses: Short-term immersion (up to 5 minutes) in water of the same pH and temperature as the source water, at 0 g/liter for saltwater fish and 27 to 30 g/liter salinity for freshwater fish. The sediment may be examined under direct microscopy.
- Precautions: If done appropriately under close monitoring, these are usually tolerated by most larger fish, but some are sensitive (e.g., *Corydoras* catfish).

Long-Term, Low-Dose Salinity

- Target: Reduce osmotic stress in freshwater teleosts and reduce uptake of nitrites.[5] This is recommended for freshwater fish quarantine.
- Route, doses: Long-term immersion at low salinity (e.g., 1 to 4 g/liter) for freshwater fish. Salt water, sodium chloride, or a commercial salt mix may be used.
- Precautions: This is generally well tolerated by most fish.

Copper

- Target: Ectoparasitic ciliates and flagellates, with some effect on monogeneans. This is recommended for most larger marine teleosts that were wild-caught or came from large distributors, and that will tolerate the treatment.
- Route: Long-term immersion. It is given as the ionized form (e.g., copper sulfate pentahydrate) or chelated form, which has a wider safety index (e.g., citrated copper sulfate or copper-amine complexes).
- Doses: Effective dose for *Cryptocaryon* is typically 0.18 to 0.20 mg/liter of ionized copper, maintained for 21 days.[10]
- Precautions: Considered toxic to most invertebrates, elasmobranchs, and plants; may be toxic to many teleost species. Be cautious with juveniles and novel species, and avoid rapid increases in ionized copper (e.g., secondary to a decrease in pH or bolus). Because copper is immunosuppressive, it should only be started once the fish are doing well. Use only with alkalinity greater than 50 mg/liter; avoid in freshwater systems. Add the drug slowly (e.g., drip system), gradually increase it to the therapeutic level, and assay ionized copper levels daily. Discontinue treatment if fish show behavioral changes or decreased food intake.[15]

Chloroquine Diphosphate

- Target: Ectoparasitic ciliates and flagellates (especially *Cryptocaryon* and *Amyloodinium*), with some effect on monogeneans and bacteria.
- Route: Long-term immersion.
- Doses: Often 10 mg/liter. Redosing schedules vary; use assays for accurate redosing.
- Precautions: Be cautious with juveniles and novel species; may damage biologic filtration. Tank should be darkened for treatment. Personal protective equipment (PPE) is recommended.

Formalin (37% Formaldehyde)

Some formalin products are FDA-approved in finfish. Malachite green, commonly combined with formalin, is under high regulatory priority and should be avoided.

- Target: Ectoparasitic ciliates and flagellates (especially *Ichthyophthirius*), with dose-dependent effects on monogeneans, water molds, and bacteria. It is recommended for most freshwater teleosts that were wild-caught or came from large distributors, and that will tolerate the treatment.
- Route: Short-term or long-term immersion.
- Doses: Low-dose administration is usually 10 to 25 mg/liter for up to 24 hours (25 mg/liter = 1 mL formalin in 10 U.S. gallons). High-dose therapy may be 100 to 150 mg/liter for 1 hour. Treatments are often repeated (e.g., every other day for three doses).[10,14,19]
- Precautions: Considered potentially toxic to most invertebrates, elasmobranchs, and plants and some scaleless teleosts (e.g., some catfish). Be cautious with juveniles and novel species. Toxicity is increased with open skin lesions, and with low pH and high temperatures. Formalin decreases dissolved oxygen so supplemental aeration must be provided. High doses may damage biologic filtration and increase turbidity. PPE is required.[15]

Praziquantel

- Target: Monogeneans, digenetic trematodes, and cestodes. Immersion treatment with praziquantel is recommended for most fish to treat monogeneans.
- Routes: Short-term or long-term immersion, intramuscular, or oral (e.g., in prey items or medicated gel food [see Box 26-2]).
- Doses: Immersion treatment is usually 2 to 5 mg/liter. Duration varies from hours to days and treatment may be repeated. Using a fine mesh filter or initially dissolving the drug in 95% ethyl alcohol (~1 mL/g praziquantel) helps dissolution. Oral and intramuscular doses vary.[10,14,18]
- Precautions: Generally well tolerated at low to moderate doses.

Organophosphates and Chitin Inhibitors

- Target: Reserved for parasitic infections that cannot be treated by other methods (e.g., some leeches or copepods).

- Route: Short-term immersion using the organophosphate trichlorfon (Dylox) or the chiton inhibitor diflubenzuron (Dimilin).
- Doses: Vary; usually repeated in 7 to 10 days.[10,12,14]
- Precautions: Organophosphates are toxic to most invertebrates and potentially toxic to many species; be very cautious. PPE is required. Chitin inhibitors have a wider safety index for animals that lack chitin. For both medications, disposal of medicated water must be considered.[15]

Fenbendazole or Levamisole

- Target: Gastrointestinal nematodes, with little effect on encysted stages. Levamisole is a potential immune stimulant.[9]
- Routes: Intramuscular or immersion (levamisole), oral (fenbendazole and levamisole).
- Doses: Vary.[10,12,14]
- Precautions: Be cautious with fenbendazole in bottom-feeders, especially temperate species (e.g., rainbow and greenside darters, *Etheostoma* spp.). Levamisole immersion may damage biologic filtration.

Antibiotics

Florfenicol is licensed in the United States for use in ornamental fish; specific oxytetracyclines and potentiated sulfonamides are licensed for use in catfish and salmonids.
- Target: Bacteria.
- Routes: Oral, immersion, intramuscular, or intracoelomic. Ideally, these should be targeted to individuals but, for very small fish, immersion may be the only practical route.
- Doses: Vary.[10,12,14,16,18,19]
- Precautions: These should be used only if there is a high index of suspicion for a bacterial infection. Immersion antibacterials may damage biologic filtration. Disposal of medicated water must be considered.

Vaccines

FDA-licensed inactivated immersion vaccines currently exist for *Vibrio anguillarum*, *Aeromonas salmonicida*, *Yersinia ruckeri*, *Flavobacterium columnare*, and infectious salmon anemia virus. *Vibrio* vaccines have been used by some institutions for syngnathids during quarantine.

TREATMENTS FOR AQUATIC INVERTEBRATES

There is little information available on the significance and treatment of infectious diseases in aquatic invertebrates. However, some pathogens are known to cause high morbidity and mortalities (e.g., *Perkinsus marinus* in oysters), especially when environmental conditions are suboptimal, and invertebrates may be carriers for some fish pathogens. Possible ectoparasite treatments are temperature or salinity changes and metronidazole or milbemycin immersion. Antibiotics that have been used include tetracyclines, chloramphenicol, and enrofloxacin.[11] Treatments should be used with caution.

Clearing Quarantine

Visual or physical examinations, and a review of diagnostic procedures and treatments, should be completed prior to clearing animals from quarantine. If there are no significant health concerns and the animals have passed the minimum quarantine period, they may be cleared.

Assessing Quarantine

It is important to review quarantine protocols regularly. This will include tracking morbidity and mortalities through quarantine (e.g., within the first 24 hours, first week, first month, or subsequently), and reviewing whether any pathogens seen on exhibit could have been avoided through quarantine. Finally, this review should incorporate any changes to the facilities or needs of the institution, such as new exhibits.

REFERENCES

1. American Veterinary Medical Association: AVMA guidelines on euthanasia, 2007 (http://www.avma.org/resources/euthanasia.pdf.)
2. Arnold JE: Hematology of the sandbar shark, *Carcharhinus plumbeus*: Standardization of complete blood count techniques for elasmobranchs. Vet Clin Pathol 34:115–123, 2005.
3. Association of Zoos and Aquariums: The accreditation standards and related policies, 2010 (http://www.aza.org/uploadedFiles/Accreditation/Microsoft%20Word%20-%202010%20Accred%20Standards.pdf).
4. Francis-Floyd R: Clinical examination of fish in private collections. Vet Clin North Am Exot Anim Pract 2:247–264, 1999.
5. Greenwell MG, Sherrill J, Clayton LA: Osmoregulation in fish. Mechanisms and clinical implications. Vet Clin North Am Exot Anim Pract 6:169–189, 2003.
6. Harms CA: Anesthesia in fish. In Fowler ME, Miller RE, editors: Zoo and wild animal medicine: Current therapy, ed 4, Philadelphia, 1999, WB Saunders, pp 158–163.

7. Harms CA: Fish. In Fowler ME, Miller RE, editors: Zoo and wild animal medicine: Current therapy, ed 5, Philadelphia, 2003, WB Saunders, pp 2–20.
8. Henningsen AD: Tonic immobility in twelve elasmobranchs: Use as an aid in captive husbandry. Zoo Biol 13:325–332, 1994.
9. Kumari J, Sahoo PK: Dietary immunostimulants influence specific immune response and resistance of healthy and immunocompromised Asian catfish *Clarias batrachus* to *Aeromonas hydrophila* infection. Dis Aquat Org 70:63–70, 2006.
10. Lewbart GA: Fish. In Carpenter JW, editor: Exotic animal formulary, ed 3, Philadelphia, 2005, WB Saunders, pp 5–29.
11. Lewbart GA: Invertebrate medicine, Ames, Iowa, 2006, Blackwell Scientific.
12. Mashima TY, Lewbart GA: Pet fish formulary. Vet Clin North Am Exot Anim Pract 3:117–130, 2000.
13. Mohan PJ, Aiken A: Water quality and life support systems for large elasmobranch exhibits. In Smith M, Warmolts D, Thoney D, Hueter R, editors: The elasmobranch husbandry manual: Captive care of sharks, rays and their relatives, Columbus, Ohio, 2004, Ohio Biological Survey, pp 69–88.
14. Noga EJ: Fish disease and treatment, ed 2, St Louis, 2000, Mosby.
15. Roberts HF, Palmeiro BS: Toxicology of aquarium fish. Vet Clin North Am Exot Anim Pract 11:359–374, 2008.
16. Roberts HF, Palmeiro BS, Weber ES: Bacterial and parasitic diseases of pet fish. Vet Clin North Am Exot Anim Pract 12:609–638, 2009.
17. Ross LG, Ross B: Anesthetic and sedative techniques for aquatic animals, ed 3, Oxford, 2008, Blackwell Science.
18. Stamper MA, Miller SM, Berzins IK: Pharmacology in elasmobranchs. In Smith M, Warmolts D, Thoney D, Hueter R, editors: The elasmobranch husbandry manual: Captive care of sharks, rays and their relatives, Columbus, Ohio, 2004, Ohio Biological Survey, pp 447–466.
19. Stoskopf MK: Fish medicine, Philadelphia, 1993, WB Saunders.
20. Whitaker BR: Preventative medicine programs for fish. In Fowler ME, Miller RE, editors: Zoo and wild animal medicine: Current therapy, ed 4, Philadelphia, 1999, WB Saunders, pp 163–181.
21. Yanong RP: Necropsy techniques for fish. Semin Avian Exot Pet Med 12:89–105, 2003.

Reptile and Amphibian

Section 3

CHAPTER 27

Behavioral Training of Reptiles for Medical Procedures

Gregory J. Fleming

The words training and enrichment appear to have been lost when used in conjunction with the word reptile or amphibian. Even though enrichment is attempted in many species, reptiles still tend to be kept in small sterile environments. Enriching captive reptiles will allow the animal to exhibit their natural array of behaviors. Similarly, we rarely hear of the word training used in association with reptiles and amphibians. This chapter will focus on training reptiles for veterinary procedures; however, the act of training may also enrich the reptile's life by providing positive enriching environments. When veterinarians hear the word training, we often think of large mammals such as hoof stock or primates that have been trained to allow for passive diagnostic sampling, ultrasound, and radiography. These same techniques may be used to train reptiles and amphibians to assist with medical procedures and to facilitate daily keeper-animal interactions.

ENRICHMENT

Enrichment may be defined as a process for improving or enhancing animal environments and care within the context of their inhabitants' behavioral biology and natural history.[3] It is a dynamic process in which changes to structures and husbandry practices are made with the goals of increasing behavioral choices available to animals and drawing out their species-appropriate behaviors and abilities, thus enhancing animal welfare.

The enrichment framework developed at Disney's Animal Programs provides a process to ensure that the enrichment program meets the needs of the animals and provides them with the opportunity to experience enhanced animal welfare.[1] Animal welfare involves the physical health of the animals (e.g., preventing and treating illnesses and injuries) and their psychologic well-being. As an important aspect of welfare,

an animal's psychologic well-being is influenced by whether it can do the following:

- Perform its highly motivated behaviors
- Respond to environmental conditions using its evolutionary adaptations
- Develop and use its cognitive abilities
- Effectively cope with challenges in its environment

Thus, keeping a snake in a plastic box with newspaper and a water bowl is not sufficient. We should attempt to provide a more complex environment to watch and enjoy the animals that we keep in captivity. Balancing proper husbandry, thermoregulation, and veterinary concerns can become difficult, but it is our obligation to do this for the animals we keep in captivity.

TRAINING

The term *animal training* often conjure up images of a parrot show, side show, or animal act in a circus in which animals have been trained to complete a variety of unnatural acts for our entertainment. Training now has a different context, which includes teaching animals to exhibit a variety of behaviors for husbandry, educational, and entertainment purposes.

Animals continually gather information and respond to it. This process may be described as learning. A similar definition might be that learning is a change in behavior that occurs as the result of practice. Whether we are aware of it or not, as animal caretakers, we influence what is learned by animals in zoos and aquariums. In other words, as caretakers, we are teaching or training our animals all the time. Sometimes, we are aware of what we are teaching or training; we make conscious efforts to train animals to exhibit a variety of behaviors. Sometimes, we influence (train) animals' behavior inadvertently through our actions, husbandry routines, or other stimuli present in the captive environment. In effect, animal care staff is always involved in training and they need to be aware of that. Training is all about associations. The key to an optimal captive environment is to facilitate animals' opportunities to make associations that enhance their well-being.

Setting up a Training Program

A well-planned, consistently delivered training process is critical to the success of any program. To achieve this type of program, many facilities use a framework that is taught in course given by the American Zoo and Aquarium Association (AZA), Managing Animal Enrichment and Training Programs. Steps in this SPIDER model framework include *s*etting goals, *p*lanning, *i*mplementing, *d*ocumenting, *e*valuating, and *r*eadjusting. More information on this process may be found at Disney's Animal Programs: Training Program.[2] It is beneficial to start a training program by determining the overall behavioral goals (i.e., detailing the specific behaviors to be trained). This is the first step in the SPIDER process, setting goals. During this goal development process, it is important to include all parties involved with the management of the animals. This may include meeting with and seeking feedback from keepers, veterinary staff, nutritionist, behavioral husbandry staff, curators, and managers. Goals should be based on the needs of staff. For example, a veterinarian would like a blood sample from the animal. The goals in this case would then be to train an animal to enter a crate and desensitize to a blood draw. The next step is planning; having everyone on the same page, with clearly laid out plans, assignments, and timelines helps facilitate a smooth process. Defining roles and creating clear avenues of communication among all participants is also important. This may be accomplished through regularly scheduled team meetings, a consistent method of documentation, and continual communication among all staff involved in training. Planning also includes creating a training plan, a step by step guide for how trainers are going to shape the behavior. Training plans are meant only to be a guide, a way for the trainer to think through the process he or she starts training an animal. Creating a training plan also creates a historical document for future reference. One way to write a plan is to establish what the final behavior will look like and then break down the behavior into a series of small steps; these small steps are called successive approximations. The next sections will discuss other considerations when starting a program.

Selecting and Shaping Behaviors

It is possible to train reptiles for a variety of behaviors. To select the most effective and appropriate techniques and behaviors for the species, it is necessary to consider the following:
1. The animal's natural history. It is important to consider the animal's predispositions. For example, it may make more sense to ask an arboreal animal to station off the ground/on a perch.
2. The animal's individual history. It is important to consider the early rearing and life experiences of the animal being trained. For example, an animal that is imprinted on humans may be trained substantially differently than a wild-caught animal brought in as an adult.
3. The animal's function or role in your collection. The animal may be in the collection as part of a breeding or education program. The type of training and your level of interactions with that animal may differ, depending on the function that this animal serves in your collection.

When selecting shaping techniques, these factors must be considered, as well as the safety of the staff and animal. Two shaping techniques that work well with reptiles are baiting and targeting. Baiting is when a trainer uses food to lure an animal. Tongs or forceps may be used to hold the food as an extension of the trainer's hand. Targeting may also be used effectively with reptiles. The animal must be previously trained to touch a body part to the target—for example, a crocodilian may be trained to touch the end of its snout to a buoy. Once this behavior is reliable, the target may be a useful tool to get an animal to move from one location to another or into a crate.

Training Area

When beginning a training program, it is best to start training in an area that is safe for the animal care staff and animal. An area in which trainers may have access to the animal safely is usually the night quarters or holding area. Training may also be done in crates, chutes, or even open exhibit areas. Because all facility designs are different, training staff will have to be creative and use the space available. For safe access to an animal for a behavior, such as a blood draw, it is recommended that the animal be trained to enter a crate, which allows safe access to body parts. It is important to remember that a fancy expensive facility is not necessary to accomplish a successful training program—just a creative mind.

Reinforcement

A critical component to positive reinforcement training is finding a reinforcement or reward for which an animal is willing to work. Because reptiles are poikilothermic, environmental temperature and amount of food reinforcement must be considered and may become critical to a training program. Temperature of the animal and animal's environment is critical; it must be within the preferred optimum body temperature (POBT) of that species. The POBT is a range of temperatures that a certain reptile species must reach to maintain normal metabolic and physiologic functions. Once the temperature is in the POBT (i.e., 25° C to 35° C), the reptile should be physiologically able to train.

In most cases, the animal's regular diet may be used for training. Breaking the animal's diet up into smaller portions may provide good opportunities for more training sessions. Even the larger reptiles do not need large portions of reinforcement for each session. Most reptiles do not get fed every day, sometimes going months without feeding, but the animal still seems to retain any training done previously. If you only train crocodiles once a week, they will still retain what they have learned from previous sessions. It has been observed that reptiles learn and make associations very quickly, sometimes after only one reinforcement. Because of this, having a well thought-out plan before training starts is important. However, it should be noted that an animal may easily be reinforced for something that a trainer does not want.

It is helpful to have a bucket containing diet near the trainer so that reinforcement may be easily retrieved and delivered in a timely manner. Delivery of reinforcement may occur by placing the food item on tongs and passing it through the barrier or by tossing meat over or under the barrier. Hand feeding is not recommended. It may be a safety issue for the keeper and may also cause the reptile to become aggressive and focused on the trainer.

Record Keeping

It is important for trainers to keep records of all sessions. Trainers may go back and look for patterns in the information, which helps keep consistency among trainers, and leaves a historical record for others. For examples of documentation methods, see Disney's Animal Programs: Training Program.[2]

CASE STUDIES

The following sections present sample training programs with Nile crocodiles, Komodo dragons, amphibians, and snakes.

Crocodiles

The training program for the Nile crocodiles at Disney's Animal Kingdom is unique in that all 27 animals are housed and managed together. Animal managers identified a need to monitor the physical well-being of this group closely because of the large number of animals being housed together and the potential for less dominant animals to be overwhelmed by their more dominant counterparts. It was determined that none of the adult Nile crocodiles had any previous training and that it was assumed that they had limited intelligence (when compared with a mammal) for complex training.

The first step was to set goals and identify what behavior was needed. The staff began the planning process by working together to create a training plan. The plan was to train the animals to shift on cue. Once the plan was complete, the implementation part of the SPIDER process could begin. In order for all the animals to identify the cue both above and below the water, a pipe was partially submerged in the water while the staff hit the pipe with another pipe. Once the cue was given, the holding gates were opened and all 27 crocodiles shifted as a group into the holding area. The holding area consists of two holding pools and a crate staging pool in which the animals may be separated. It was determined if the crocodile could be trained to walk out of the water and into a crate and hold for some time, this would allow for a close-up inspection by the husbandry and veterinary team.

From the pools, the crocodiles were shift one at a time into a staging pool and a staff member cued the animal into the crate by slapping his or her hand on the top of the crate while the crate door was open. Once the animal entered the crate, the next goal was to allow for physical manipulation of the tail for blood sampling. After the animal entered the crate, the door was closed and PVC poles were placed through the crate and around the animal to restrict its movement (Fig. 27-1). Once the animal was secured, staff and veterinarians could access the animal through several hinged and sliding doors on the crate. The staff was able to examine the animal safely at close range, treat wounds, obtain weights, draw blood, administer medications, and take radiographs as needed. All these procedures could be

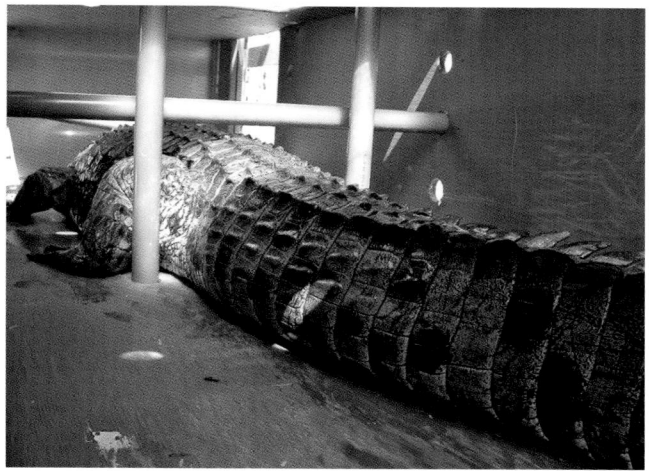

Figure 27-1

An adult Nile crocodile inside the crate. This image was taken though the rear access door on the side of the crate. Once in the crate, PVC restraint poles are placed from the top and sides of the crate to restrict movement of the head and tail. These poles may not be needed in larger crocodiles but allow for a standard crate to be used.

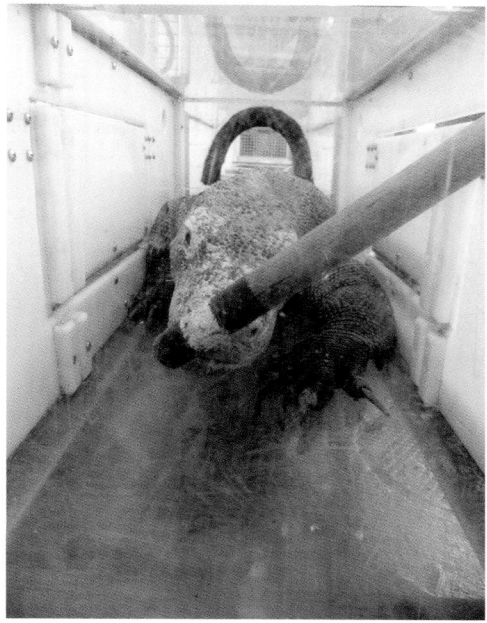

Figure 27-2

A Komodo dragon touching his nose to the target pole in the front of the shift crate.

completed in the holding area without transporting the animal to another location or hospital.

This training program has facilitated a safe working environment for staff and animals while providing medical care opportunities that would ordinarily be impossible without physically capturing and manually restraining the crocodile. Through the records kept during training sessions and meetings to evaluate the training, the staff has learned that even after crocodiles are held in the crate, they do not show any avoidance and will enter the crate the next time that they are asked.

Komodo Dragons

In 1999, Disney's Animal Kingdom began working with two Komodo dragons to shift on and off their exhibits on cue and target by touching their nose to the end of a dowel (Fig. 27-2). Target training has facilitated behaviors such as weighing, front foot nail trim, and crating. Since the inception of the training, the crate was designed to facilitate annual examinations without anesthesia. Historically, the Komodos would have to be anesthetized for annual examinations. Today, because of the training and crate design, the animals are asked to enter the crate and then transported in their crate to the hospital examination area.

Examinations may include obtaining weights and measurements; coelomic palpation and ultrasound;

radiography and blood, oral, and cloacal cultures; and hind foot nail trims if needed. At the hospital, the animals may be asked to target, get into specific positions in the crate, and be restrained in particular positions for procedures. If needed, the crate breaks apart and allows access for abdominal ultrasound, inspection of overall body condition, and other procedures. Once the examinations are complete, the crate and animal are secured and brought back to the holding area and the animal is released into its enclosure. The two male Komodo dragons showed no avoidance to the crate after the examination and would target successfully into the crate within hours of the examination.

Dendrobatid Frogs

Like reptiles, amphibians have been in the category of an animal that is not trainable. At Disney's Animal Kingdom, the animal care staff has developed a training program for several tanks of dendrobatid frogs. The training program began out of a staff member's curiosity to see whether the frogs were capable of associating a sound with feeding and to minimize handling of the frogs. The staff's plan was to pair the sound of a clicker with the animals regular feeding to see whether the frogs would make an association. They wanted to determine if the frogs heard the sound, would they

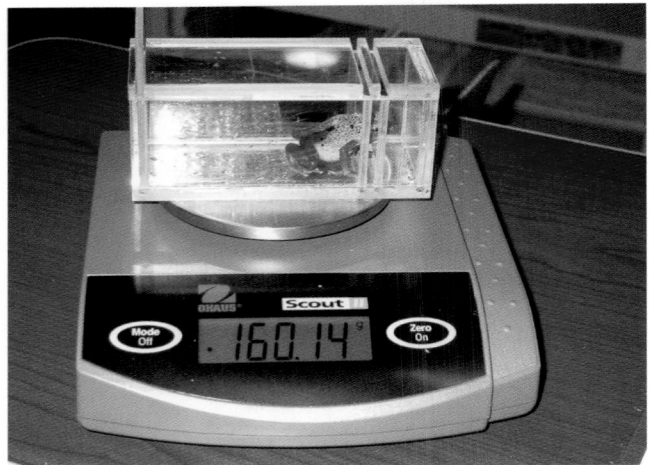

Figure 27-3

A *Dendrobates azureus* (blue poison arrow frog) after it has been cued with a clicker and has entered the shift crate. This is part of a training plan to obtain weekly body weights.

respond and move out of their hiding areas to feed? The frogs quickly responded and would come out after they heard the clicker. After the quick response, the keepers moved on to creating a crate with a small guillotine door at the far end (Fig. 27-3). Once the frog entered the crate, the guillotine was raised and the diet of fruit flies was released. Once the frog entered and received a reward, a door may close behind the frog. The crate may then be placed on a scale to obtain a weight and the frog brought to the hospital for an examination and/or radiography or removed from the enclosure, if needed. This could all be done without the frog being physically handled. The success of this frog training program may only be a hint of the capability of these animals and other amphibians.

Venomous Snakes

The practice of physically removing snakes from their enclosures or exhibits for feeding may often be hazardous for the animal care staff, particularly the handling of venomous snakes. Through training, this practice may now be much safer. Just like other reptiles, snakes may also be conditioned to associate a particular behavior with sounds or vibrations. Several facilities have conditioned their snakes to move from one enclosure to a shift box after they hear or feel a certain sound, such as tapping the side of a box or crate. The snake is then moved to a smaller enclosure for feeding, the door is closed behind the snake, and the snake is moved without

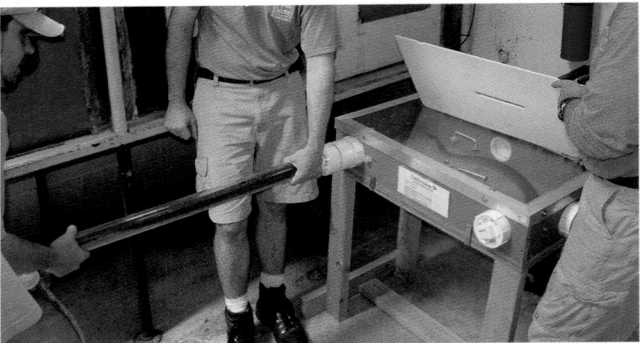

Figure 27-4

A king cobra reentering a shift box after it has entered a handling tube. Once inside the shift box, the snake may then be allowed back into its main enclosure. (*Courtesy Dr. Brad Lock.*)

ever being physically handled. This may also be taken one step further by opening a shift box to allow the snake to go into a handling tube. Once the snake is about one third of its body length into the tube, it is removed from the shift box and the venomous snake may be handled safely (Fig. 27-4). Once the examination is complete, the tube may be reversed to allow the snake to move back into the shift box. This allows for safe handling of venomous snakes.

SUMMARY

This chapter has presented a few examples of how reptiles may be trained to facilitate medical care. These techniques can be applied to various species and sizes of reptiles. It is important to remember that when designing a training program, knowledge of the animals' natural and individual histories are critical to understanding its needs and capabilities. A good partnership between the veterinarians and animal care staff is also crucial to the success of any training program. The responsibility lies with us continually to strive to learn more to care for captive animals better, including reptiles. Training may have a huge impact on an animal's welfare and, although it may require an investment of time and effort, it often pays off in an improved quality of life for the animal.

REFERENCES

1. Disney's Animal Programs: Enrichment Program, 2009 (http://www.animalenrichment.org).
2. Disney's Animal Programs: Training Program, 2010 (http://www.animaltraining.org).
3. Mellen J, Sevenich MacPhee M: Philosophy of environmental enrichment: Past, present, and future. Zoo Biol 20:211–226, 2001.

CHAPTER 28

Diagnosis and Control of Amphibian Chytridiomycosis

Allan P. Pessier

Chytridiomycosis is an emerging infectious disease associated with global amphibian population declines.[8,16,20,38,42] The causative agent, *Batrachochytrium dendrobatidis* (Bd), is a chytrid fungus with a broad host range documented to infect the skin of over 300 different frog and salamander species to date (www.spatialepidemiology.net/bd-maps). Infection with Bd may be subclinical, with minimal skin lesions in some species such as the American bullfrog (*Lithobates catesbeianus*),[13] or cause severe skin disease in highly susceptible neotropical species such as the Panamanian golden frog (*Atelopus zeteki*).[21] Subclinically infected animals are potential sources of infection for more highly susceptible species and may serve as vectors for the introduction of Bd to new geographic regions. There continues to be debate about whether mortality caused by chytridiomycosis results from the introduction of Bd to naïve amphibian populations or whether Bd is a commensal parasite of amphibians that has become virulent as the result of environmental cofactors such as climate change (novel versus endemic pathogen hypothesis).[7,22,23] Supporting evidence for the novel pathogen hypothesis includes demonstration of minimal genetic variation among geographically distinct Bd isolates and ecologic studies that show amphibian mortality and population decline only after the arrival of Bd at new locations.

The impact of chytridiomycosis and Bd infection is not limited to wild amphibian populations. Infection and disease outbreaks are observed in zoo and aquarium collections,[9,25,30,31] laboratory animals,[27] and amphibians in the pet and food trades.[40] Veterinarians who include amphibians in their practice must be able to provide accurate diagnostic testing and treatment for Bd-infected animals and to make recommendations for control and prevention of this disease in amphibian conservation and reintroduction programs.[32] This chapter expands on an overview of amphibian chytridiomycosis presented by Pessier,[29] with an emphasis on new information needed by zoo and wildlife veterinarians for animal management.

CHYTRIDIOMYCOSIS AND AMPHIBIAN SURVIVAL ASSURANCE POPULATIONS

The forward to the 2007 World Conservation Union (IUCN) Amphibian Conservation Action Plan (ACAP) stated that in the last decades of the 20th century, the amphibian extinction rate exceeded the mean extinction rate of the last 350 million years[36] by at least 200 times.[12] These declines are attributable to a multitude of factors, such as habitat loss, climate change, and species exploitation, but many of the most rapidly occurring losses of amphibian biodiversity are associated with chytridiomycosis.[23] Unfortunately, it is possible that many amphibians will become extinct long before the political measures and scientific progress needed to mitigate the declines are implemented. This has resulted in the development of survival assurance populations that bring representatives of imperiled amphibian species into captivity with the goal of establishing healthy and sustainable populations that may be returned to the wild at a later time. The Amphibian Ark (www.amphibianark.org), formed by a cooperative effort of the World Association of Zoos and Aquariums (WAZA), the IUCN Conservation Breeding Specialist Group (CBSG), and the IUCN Amphibian Specialist Group has estimated that over 500 amphibian species could immediately require the type of ex situ intervention represented by survival assurance populations.

Although there are no recognized methods for eliminating or controlling chytridiomycosis in wild amphibian populations or their environments, it has been demonstrated that some amphibian populations that have experienced chytridiomycosis-associated declines subsequently persist at reduced densities with endemic Bd infection.[34] Another encouraging line of research has demonstrated that in some species, colonization of the skin by the bacterium *Janthinobacterium lividum* reduces morbidity and mortality caused by chytridiomycosis.[2,14] These observations require additional investigation, but highlight the possibility that some affected amphibian populations could eventually recover or that methods will be developed to mitigate the effects of infection on wild populations. Furthermore, they provide hope that the creation of survival assurance populations could be a viable conservation strategy for chytridiomycosis-associated population declines.

To maintain healthy and viable assurance populations, the methods used to control chytridiomycosis and other infectious diseases in captive settings have become critically important. A major emphasis has been on improving the biosecurity practices used in zoos and conservation programs to reduce the introduction and transmission of disease to captive animals and to prevent movement of infectious diseases from captive animals to wild amphibian populations as part of reintroduction programs.[30,32] Some of the most important biosecurity practices identified include keeping amphibian survival assurance populations as close as possible to the native range of the species (e.g., the maintenance of Panamanian golden frog assurance populations in Panama), keeping survival assurance populations in long-term isolation from cosmopolitan zoo collections that have species from different parts of the world in close proximity, and use of husbandry protocols that reduce the possibility of transmission of infectious diseases in captive breeding facilities.

CHYTRIDIOMYCOSIS AND THE WORLD ORGANIZATION FOR ANIMAL HEALTH

In 2008, the World Association for Animal Health (OIE) listed two amphibian infectious diseases, chytridiomycosis and ranaviral disease, as notifiable under the Aquatic Animal Health Code.[39] These reporting requirements developed in response to evidence that trade and shipment of amphibians for a variety of purposes have the potential to introduce these significant amphibian pathogens to new locations. Examples of the anthropogenic movement of Bd include exports of African clawed frogs *(Xenopus laevis)* for use in human pregnancy diagnosis and biomedical research,[47] imports of farmed American bullfrogs *(Lithobates catesbeianus)*,[40] and introduction of Bd to a wild population of Mallorcan midwife toads *(Alytes muletensis)* as the result of a captive breeding program.[45]

The implication of the OIE listing of chytridiomycosis for captive amphibian breeding or conservation programs is that the importation of live amphibians will eventually require an official International Aquatic Animal Health Certificate that certifies that animals are free of Bd infection or have been treated in a manner that eliminates infection. Alternatively, infected animals could be imported and quarantined in biosecure facilities for the purpose of creating Bd-specific pathogen-free populations. The regulatory requirements related to Bd, such as OIE reporting and oversight of amphibian import and export, fall to the chief veterinary officer of each country that is a signatory to the OIE (e.g., the U.S. Department of Agriculture's Animal and Plant Health Inspection Service [APHIS]). Details on the OIE requirements related to chytridiomycosis may be found in the Aquatic Animal Health code online (www.oie.int/eng/normes/fcode/en_chapitre_1.8.1.htm).

PATHOGENESIS OF CHYTRIDIOMYCOSIS

Lesions associated with lethal chytridiomycosis in postmetamorphic amphibians are limited to the keratinizing epithelium of the skin. Because the skin is a physiologically important organ for osmoregulation in amphibians, disruption of normal cutaneous function has been frequently cited as a probable cause of death in animals with chytridiomycosis. Recent studies using the White's tree frog *(Litoria caerulea)* as a model species have demonstrated that Bd-infected animals have reduced electrolyte transport across the epidermis, with subsequent terminal hyponatremia and hypokalemia.[44] This suggests that supportive treatment with electrolytes may be helpful for affected animals in clinical settings. Emerging research on the virulence of Bd will examine the roles of the serine protease and fungalysin metallopeptidase gene families, which play a role in the pathogenesis of other fungi.[38] Investigation of the mechanisms of host defense against Bd has focused on antimicrobial peptides produced by the granular glands in amphibian skin, and evidence has suggested that differences in peptide excretion may influence species resistance to chytridiomycosis.[7,37] As noted, other recent research has explored the role of specific cutaneous bacteria such as *J. lividum* that secrete antifungal compounds and function as components of innate cutaneous immunity.[2,14]

DIAGNOSTIC METHODS

The commonly used diagnostic methods for Bd infection either examine samples of the skin microscopically for characteristic fungal organisms (e.g., cytology, histopathology), or use the polymerase chain reaction (PCR) assay to amplify sequences of deoxyribonucleic acid (DNA) specific for Bd.[29] Cytology and histopathology are most useful for the diagnosis of sick animals because large numbers of organisms are usually present and easily detected. In addition, histopathology allows evaluation of the severity of associated skin lesions (e.g., epidermal hyperplasia and hyperkeratosis) and helps determine whether infection was likely to have been clinically significant. In contrast, the PCR-based methods detect much smaller numbers of organisms and are essential for detecting subclinical Bd infections. PCR assays also have the advantage of a requiring a minimally invasive sample (i.e., , skin swabs) for testing. The application of PCR-based diagnostic methods and proper interpretation of PCR results are critical for the control of chytridiomycosis in captive amphibian populations and will be discussed in greater detail.

Polymerase Chain Reaction–Based Methods of Diagnosis

Both conventional and real-time Taqman PCR techniques have been described for the diagnosis of Bd infection and are used in research and commercial diagnostic laboratories.[1,6,15,41] PCR testing is the diagnostic procedure of choice for the following: (1) quarantine screening of new animals that enter collections; (2) surveys of captive or wild amphibian populations for the presence of Bd; (3) evaluating of the success of antifungal treatment of Bd infection; and (4) screening of captive animals prior to reintroduction to the wild or translocation of wild animals.

When properly validated in the laboratory, the Taqman PCR technique has advantages over conventional PCR,[32] including the following:

1. Use of an internal control that alerts the laboratory to the occurrence of PCR inhibition. PCR inhibitors are frequently present in samples taken from amphibian skin and, if not detected, may result in a false-negative test result (e.g., Bd DNA is present in the sample but is not detected by the test).[6,15]
2. Greater analytic sensitivity, which allows for the detection of smaller amounts of Bd DNA. This

is potentially important when screening for low-level subclinical Bd infections.
3. Use of a Bd-specific DNA probe that eliminates the need to confirm positive results by DNA sequencing.

The major disadvantages of the Taqman PCR technique are higher equipment and reagent costs and limited commercial availability in some regions compared with conventional PCR assays.

Sample Collection

A wide variety of different samples has been used to perform Bd PCR assays, including collection of skin swabs, immersion in a water bath, and collection of tissue (e.g., toe clips).[15] The skin swab procedure is most commonly used and is minimally invasive while allowing for sampling of multiple areas of potentially infected skin. Samples are collected with a sterile commercially available applicator stick (swab) applied with a gentle sweeping motion to ventral skin surfaces of the feet, legs, and body. Most sampling protocols call for three to five passes with the swab over each general region of the skin. Because PCR techniques may detect very small amounts of DNA, it is important to avoid cross-contamination of samples from different animals that could cause false-positive test results. Techniques for reducing cross-contamination include the use of a new pair of disposable gloves for every animal and avoiding contact of swabs with surfaces other than the skin of the animal being tested.[24,32,33]

Factors related to sample collection and sample storage may influence the performance and outcome of Bd PCR testing. For instance, a specific fine-tipped rayon swab with a plastic handle (Dryswab Fine Tip MW113, Medical Wire & Equipment, Corsham, Wiltshire, England) is optimal for the recovery of Bd DNA using the Taqman technique.[6,15,32] Other factors that improve recovery of Bd DNA include storage of swab samples dry rather than preservation in an ethanol solution and avoiding exposure of swabs to very high environmental temperatures (>38° C) prior to analysis.[43] Although dry swab samples may be stable at room temperature (23° C) for as long as 18 months after collection, storage under refrigeration (4° C) or freezing (−20° C or below) is suggested if there will be a delay in sample processing.[42] Pooling of samples in the laboratory from multiple animals into a single PCR test reaction has been used as a method for reducing the costs associated with testing large numbers of animals, but may result in reduced test sensitivity when samples from more than five animals are combined. Because of these considerations, the laboratory analyzing samples for Bd PCR should always be consulted for their preferences regarding sample collection and preservation.

Interpretation of Results

Proper interpretation of Bd PCR results is important for making appropriate management decisions and for the success of disease control programs.[32] A positive PCR result means that the test has detected Bd DNA and usually indicates that the animal is infected with Bd. However, false-positive test results may occur from contamination with extraneous Bd DNA, either during sample collection or during sample processing in the laboratory. To avoid false-positive test results, samples should be collected using the techniques noted and laboratories should use procedures and negative controls that prevent and detect incidents of laboratory contamination.

A negative PCR result means that the test has not detected Bd DNA, but does not always indicate that an individual animal is free of Bd infection. Despite the ability of PCR tests to detect very small amounts of Bd DNA, false-negative results sometimes occur in animals with low-level (subclinical) infections or in animals that have recently shed large amounts of infected skin.[15] In some cases, animals with low-level infections will alternately test positive or negative when followed over time with serial PCR tests. Therefore, if it is critical that individual animals are determined to be free of Bd infection (e.g., quarantine), it is not advisable to rely solely on a single PCR test result. In an experimental study, a total of three PCR tests carried out over a 14-day period increased the likelihood of detecting all animals with low-level infections. Obtaining this number of samples outside of a research setting may not be possible because of logistics or finances, and testing decisions may depend on a situational risk assessment (see "Quarantine").

QUARANTINE

Testing of new animals for Bd infection prior to entry into an established collection is strongly recommended as part of the routine quarantine protocol for captive amphibians.[32] The diagnostic methods used to detect Bd infection in quarantine are necropsy examination of any animals that have died and PCR testing of skin swab samples from living animals. A necropsy that includes submission of multiple sections of skin as well as other organs for histopathology may detect characteristic cutaneous lesions of chytridiomycosis while also providing valuable information about other potential

disease problems in the quarantine group. Because subclinical Bd infections are common, skin swab samples for Bd PCR assay should be obtained from living animals in quarantine. PCR testing may not be necessary if the incoming animals originate from established captive populations known to be free of Bd infection (e.g., a specific pathogen-free amphibian population; see later, "Treatment"). As noted, multiple PCR assays may be necessary to ensure that individual animals are free of Bd infection. If this is not possible, then the veterinarian should perform an informal risk assessment to determine a testing strategy. For example, a single PCR test may be adequate for in amphibians originating from captive collections that have a known health history and no recently identified (within 1 year) cases of chytridiomycosis. In contrast, multiple tests are preferable for higher risk situations, such as the following: (1) animals have recently been collected from the wild; (2) animals have been acquired from collections or animal dealers that have an unknown health history; (3) there has been a recent history of chytridiomycosis in the source population; or (4) the established amphibian collection has been determined to be Bd-free or is very valuable and the small risk of introducing Bd with new animals is considered to be unacceptable.

If Bd infection is identified by histopathology or PCR testing, the affected individual or group of animals should be treated with antifungal medication prior to release from quarantine into an established amphibian collection. If one or more animals housed together in a group test positive for Bd by PCR assay, the entire group should be considered Bd-infected, even if some individuals test PCR-negative. Prophylactic treatment of animals with antifungal medication regardless of test results is considered in cases in which PCR testing of animals in quarantine is impossible or if the animals are known to come from a Bd-infected population. Disadvantages of treating amphibians for Bd infection as a routine part of the quarantine period are poor tolerance of treatment by some amphibian species and occasional failure of treatment protocols to clear Bd infection.

TRANSMISSION OF INFECTION AND DISINFECTION

Bd is transmitted by a motile flagellated zoospore that is susceptible to drying (dessication) and heat.[17-19] Often, Bd-infected animals may be housed next to uninfected animals as long as husbandry practices are used that prevent movement of contaminated water, moist substrates, cage decorations or equipment, or infected animals between enclosures. Bd is susceptible to most commonly available disinfectants, including bleach (sodium hypochlorite), quaternary ammonium compounds, ethanol, and potassium peroxymonosulfate (Virkon).[33,46,49] Use of the quaternary ammonium compounds in particular may be useful because of relatively low cost, efficacy in low concentrations, and reduced concerns about environmental toxicity compared with bleach. Surfaces should be thoroughly cleaned to remove organic materials that may inactivate or reduce the efficacy of most disinfectants. Heat might be useful for reducing the risk of transmitting Bd infection by contaminated plants, water, or materials such as wood or soil that are impossible to disinfect by other means.[32] Experimentally, exposure of Bd cultures to 32° C (89.6° F) was effective in 96 hours of exposure and 47° C (116° F) was effective in 30 minutes.

TREATMENT

The ability to treat captive amphibians for chytridiomycosis and to clear animals of subclinical Bd infection safely and successfully has assumed great importance for amphibian conservation programs.[3,32,49] Empirically derived treatment methods have been successful, but variability in treatment efficacy and the inability to tolerate treatment has been observed among different amphibian species and different life stages (e.g., larval and postmetamorphic stages). Inconsistent treatment outcomes, and the need to develop Bd-specific pathogen-free amphibian populations for research and conservation efforts reliably demonstrate a need for controlled experimental trials of treatment efficacy.[4] The availability of PCR-based diagnostic tests has greatly improved the ability to assess treatment success in eliminating Bd infections. PCR testing of animals should begin 2 weeks after the last treatment application to allow animals to shed skin with any remaining Bd DNA or to allow any remaining living Bd organisms to grow to detectable levels. Of the treatment methods described, the azole antifungal drug itraconazole, the antibiotic chloramphenicol, and elevated environmental temperature (heat) are used frequently in amphibian conservation programs or have shown potential for wider application.

Itraconazole

Itraconazole is widely used to treat captive amphibians, ranging from individual infected animals to application in rapid response efforts that rescue animals from wild populations experiencing chytridiomycosis-associated mortality events.[9,10,29,30,32] The original treatment protocol was developed in a small trial of experimentally infected poison dart frogs (*Dendrobates* spp.) and has been subsequently modified, depending on individual veterinary or institutional experience and the availability of treatment components.[26] A commonly used variation places animals into a 5-minute daily bath of 0.01% (100-mg/liter) itraconazole prepared by diluting the commercially available 10-mg/mL oral solution (Sporanox Oral Solution) in amphibian Ringer's solution. When applying the bath treatment, the solution should be periodically agitated to ensure contact of all skin surfaces with medication. Application of the treatment solution by placing animals into plastic bags with a zipper-type closure or into disposable plastic cups has proven to be easier and more cost-effective than placing animals into large, open, treatment containers.

Although for many amphibians the 0.01% itraconazole treatment protocol is well tolerated, there have been observations of suspected treatment-associated morbidity and mortality. These include anorexia, skin irritation after contact with the treatment solution, and unexplained deaths that occur toward the end of a treatment cycle. The reason for adverse treatment outcomes in some cases is unknown, but could include severity of disease prior to treatment, idiosyncratic species or life stage differences, and factors related to the itraconazole formulation, rather than an effect of the drug itself. Acute mass mortality has been observed on several occasions in tadpoles and recently metamorphosed froglets treated with the 0.01% itraconazole protocol, and this dosage regimen should be avoided in these age groups.[4,30] To reduce the potential for treatment-associated morbidity related to the itraconazole formulation, it may be possible to use a lower itraconazole dose. In my experience with chytridiomycosis in colonies of Wyoming toads (*Anaxyrus baxteri*) and White's tree frogs (*Litoria caerulea*), a 0.005% (50-mg/liter) itraconazole bath was well tolerated and appeared to be effective in eliminating Bd infection, as evaluated by post-treatment PCR testing. A recent experimental study using midwife toad tadpoles (*Alytes muletensis*) was apparently effective at much lower doses (0.5 to 1.5 mg/liter); however, this dosage needs to be validated for postmetamorphic animals.[11]

On occasion, itraconazole bath treatments have failed to clear Bd infection when animals were followed by post-treatment PCR testing. In most of these cases, a second course of itraconazole treatment is effective in eliminating infection. Some potential causes for these treatment failures include the following:

1. Following treatment, returning animals to an enclosure that is not free of Bd. The enclosures and cage furniture used during the treatment process should be easily cleaned and disinfected and substrates should be disposable. Rotation of treatment enclosures is suggested—the dirty enclosure from the previous day is set aside for disinfection and animals are returned after treatment to a clean, freshly disinfected enclosure.
2. Failure to agitate the treatment solution during the bath period. This ensures that medication covers all skin surfaces. Agitation of the treatment solution may also be important if the source of itraconazole is a compounded suspension rather than the commercially available oral solution, because the former will often settle to the bottom of the treatment container.

Chloramphenicol

Interestingly, the antibiotic chloramphenicol has been shown to have in vitro and in vivo activity against Bd. The first report of treatment in the frogs *Litoria raniformis* and *L. ewingii* used a continuous (24-hour) 20-mg/liter bath changed daily for 2 to 4 weeks.[28] Treatment was well tolerated in these species as well as in the Archey's frog, *Leiopelma archeyi*.[5] Details on the chloramphenicol treatment protocol may be found online (www.nzfrogs.org/site/nzfrog/files/TreatmentProtocol.pdf). Treatment with chloramphenicol should be validated in other amphibian species before recommendations are made for more widespread use in amphibian conservation programs. The continuous immersion treatment protocol has the most potential for use in totally aquatic amphibian life stages (e.g., tadpoles) or aquatic and semiaquatic species. A focus of any treatment trial should examine the efficacy of shorter treatment times or other alternatives to prolonged baths for medication delivery to terrestrial amphibian species (e.g., toads) that might have problems with osmoregulation and fluid balance when kept continuously in an aquatic environment.

Elevated Temperature

Treatment regimens that use elevated environmental temperatures take advantage of the optimal growth range of Bd between 17° C and 25° C (63° F to 77° F)

and have been successful in clearing Bd infection from several species of frogs.[3,35,48] Experimental treatments have applied heat intermittently (37° C [98.6° F] for 16 hours daily in *Litoria chloris*) or continuously (32° C [89.6° F] for 5 days in *Pseudacris triseriata* and 27° C [80.6° F] for 98 days in *Mixophyes fasciolatus*). As with other treatment methods, heat has not been effective in eliminating Bd infection in all species or situations.[49] Many amphibians will not tolerate prolonged temperature elevation; therefore, the magnitude of any temperature increase and the thermal tolerance of the species selected for treatment should be carefully balanced. Use of elevated environmental temperatures above the optimal growth range for Bd may be a useful adjunct therapy to the administration of antifungal drugs such as itraconazole.

Acknowledgments

The Amphibian Disease Laboratory at the Zoological Society of San Diego is supported by grant LG-25-08-0066, Infectious Disease Control and Bioresource Banking for the Amphibian Extinction Crisis, from the Institute of Museum and Library Services (IMLS). Any views, findings, conclusions, or recommendations expressed in this publication do not necessarily represent those of the IMLS.

REFERENCES

1. Annis SL, Dastoor FP, Ziel H, et al: A DNA-based assay identifies *Batrachochytrium dendrobatidis* in amphibians. J Wildl Dis 40:420–428, 2004.
2. Becker MH, Brucker RM, Schwantes CR, et al: The bacterially produced metabolite violacein is associated with survival of amphibians infected with a lethal fungus. Appl Environ Microbiol 75:6635–6638, 2009.
3. Berger L, Speare R, Hines HB, et al: Effect of season and temperature on mortality in amphibians due to chytridiomycosis. Aust Vet J 82:434–439, 2004.
4. Berger L, Speare R, Pessier AP, et al: Treatment of chytridiomycosis requires urgent clinical trials. Dis Aquat Org published online 10.3354/dao02238, 2010.
5. Bishop PJ, Speare R, Poulter R, et al: Elimination of the amphibian chytrid fungus *Batrachochytrium dendrobatidis* by Archey's frog *Leiopelma archeyi*. Dis Aquat Org 84:9–15, 2009.
6. Boyle DG, Boyle DB, Olsen V, et al: Rapid quantitative detection of chytridiomycosis (*Batrachochytrium dendrobatidis*) in amphibian samples using real-time Taqman PCR assay. Dis Aquat Org 60:141–148, 2004.
7. Davidson C, Benard MF, Shaffer HB, et al: Effects of chytrid and carbaryl exposure on survival, growth and skin peptide defenses in foothill yellow-legged frogs. Environ Sci Technol 41:1771–1776, 2007.
8. Fisher MC, Garner TWJ, Walker SF: Global emergence of *Batrachochytrium dendrobatidis* and amphibian chytridiomycosis in space, time, and host. Annu Rev Microbiol 63:291-310, 2009.

9. Forzan MJ, Gunn H, Scott P: Chytridiomycosis in an aquarium collection of frogs: Diagnosis, treatment and control. J Zoo Wildl Med 39:406–411, 2008.

10. Gagliardo R, Crump P, Griffith E, et al: The principles of rapid response for amphibian conservation using the programmes in Panama as an example. Int Zoo Yb 42:125–135, 2008.

11. Garner TWJ, Garcia G, Carroll B, Fisher MC: Using itraconazole to clear Batrachochytrium dendrobatidis infection and subsequent depigmentation of Alytes muletensis tadpoles. Dis Aquat Org 83:257–260, 2009.

12. Gascon C, Collins JP, Moore RD, et al (eds): Amphibian conservation action plan. Proceedings: IUCN/SSC Amphibian Conservation Summit 2005.

13. Hanselmann R, Rodriguez A, Lampo M, et al: Presence of an emerging pathogen of amphibians in introduced bullfrogs (Rana catesbeiana) in Venezuela. Biol Conserv 120:115–119, 2004.

14. Harris RN, Brucker RM, Walke JB, et al: Skin microbes on frogs prevent morbidity and mortality caused by a lethal skin fungus. ISME J 3:818–824, 2009.

15. Hyatt AD, Boyle DG, Olsen V, et al: Diagnostic assays and sampling protocols for the detection of Batrachochytrium dendrobatidis. Dis Aquat Org 73:175–192, 2007.

16. James TY, Litvintseva AP, Vilgalys R, et al: Rapid global expansion of the fungal disease chytridiomycosis into declining and healthy amphibian populations. PLoS Pathog 5:e1000458, 2009.

17. Johnson ML, Berger L, Phillips L, Speare R: Fungicidal effects of chemical disinfectants, UV light, dessication and heat on the amphibian chytrid Batrachochytrium dendrobatidis. Dis Aquat Org 57:255–260, 2003.

18. Johnson ML, Speare R: Survival of Batrachochytrium dendrobatidis in water: Quarantine and disease control implications. Emerg Infect Dis 9:922–925, 2003.

19. Johnson ML, Speare R: Possible modes of dissemination of the amphibian chytrid Batrachochytrium dendrobatidis in the environment. Dis Aquat Org 65:181–186, 2005.

20. Kilpatrick AM, Briggs CJ, Daszak P: The ecology and impact of chytridiomycosis: An emerging disease of amphibians. Trends Ecol Evolut 25:109–118, 2009.

21. Lips KR, Brem F, Brenes R, et al: Emerging infectious disease and the loss of biodiversity in a neotropical amphibian community. Proc Natl Acad Sci U S A 103:3165–3170, 2006.

22. Lips KR, Diffendorfer J, Mendelson JR, Sears MW: Riding the wave: Reconciling the roles of disease and climate change in amphibian declines. PLoS Biol 6:e72, 2008.

23. Mendelson JR, Lips KR, Gagliardo RW, et al: Confronting amphibian declines and extinctions. Science 313:48, 2006.

24. Mendez D, Webb R, Berger L, Speare R: Survival of the amphibian chytrid fungus Batrachochytrium dendrobatidis on bare hands and gloves: Hygiene implications for amphibian handling. Dis Aquat Org 82:97–104, 2008.

25. Miller DL, Rajeev S, Brookins M, et al: Concurrent infection with Ranavirus, Batrachochytrium dendrobatidis, and Aeromonas in a captive anuran colony. J Zoo Wildl Med 39:445–449, 2008.

26. Nichols DK, Lamirande EW, Pessier AP, et al: Experimental transmission and treatment of cutaneous chytridiomycosis in poison dart frogs. Joint Proc Am Assoc Zoo Vet and Int Assoc Aquat An Med, New Orleans, LA, pp 42-44, 2000.

27. Parker JM, Mikaelian I, Hahn N, Diggs HE: Clinical diagnosis and treatment of epidermal chytridiomycosis in African clawed frogs (xenopus tropicalis). Comp Med 52:265–268, 2002.

28. Poulter RTM, Busby JN, Bishop PJ, et al: Chloramphenicol cures chytridiomycosis. Presented at the amphibian declines and chytridiomycosis: Translating science into urgent action conference, Tempe, Ariz, November 5-7, 2007.

29. Pessier AP: Amphibian chytridiomycosis. In Fowler ME, Miller RE, editors: Zoo and wild animal medicine: Current therapy, ed 6, St. Louis, 2008, Saunders Elsevier, pp 137–143.

30. Pessier AP: Management of disease as a threat to amphibian conservation. Int Zoo Yb 42:30–39, 2008.

31. Pessier AP, Nichols DK, Longcore JE, Fuller MS: Cutaneous chytridiomycosis in poison dart frogs (Dendrobates spp.) and White's tree frogs (Litoria caerulea). J Vet Diagn Invest 11:194–199, 1999.

32. Pessier AP, Mendelson JR, editors: A manual for control of infectious diseases in amphibian survival assurance colonies and reintroduction programs. IUCN/SSC Conservation Breeding Specialist Group: Apple Valley, MN, USA, 2010.

33. Phillott AD, Speare R, Hines HB: Minimising exposure of amphibians to pathogens during field studies. Dis Aquat Org published online 10.335/dao02162, 2010.

34. Retallick RWR, McCallum H, Speare R: Endemic infection of the amphibian chytrid fungus in a frog community post-decline. PloS Biology 2:1965–1971, 2004.

35. Retallick RWR, Miera V: Strain differences in the amphibian chytrid Batrachochytrium dendrobatidis and non-permanent, sublethal effects of infection. Dis Aquat Org 75:201–207, 2007.

36. Roelants K, Gower DJ, Wilkinson M, et al: Global patterns of diversification in the history of modern amphibians. Proc Natl Acad Sci U S A 104:887–892, 2007.

37. Rollins–Smith LA, Conlon JM: Antimicrobial peptide defenses against chytridiomycosis, an emerging infectious disease of amphibian populations. Dev Comp Immunol 29:589–598, 2005.

38. Rosenblum EB, Voyles J, Poorten TJ, Stajich JE: The deadly chytrid fungus: A story of an emerging pathogen. PLoS Pathog 6:1–3, 2010.

39. Schloegel LM, Daszak P, Cunningham AA, et al: Two amphibian diseases, chytridiomycosis and ranaviral disease, are now globally notifiable to the World Organization for Animal Health (OIE): An assessment. Dis Aquat Org published online 10.3354/dao02140, 2010.

40. Schloegel LM, Picco AM, Kilpatrick AM, et al: Magnitude of the US trade in amphibians and presence of Batrachochytrium dendrobatidis and ranavirus infection in imported North American bullfrogs (Rana catesbeiana). Biol Conserv 142:1420–1426, 2009.

41. Skerratt LF, Berger L, Hines HB, et al: Survey protocol for detecting chytridiomycosis in all Australian frog populations. Dis Aquat Org 80:85–94, 2008

42. Skerratt LF, Berger L, Speare R, et al: Spread of chytridiomycosis has caused the rapid global decline and extinction of frogs. EcoHealth 4:125–134, 2007.

43. Van Sluys M, Kriger KM, Phillot AD, et al: Storage of samples at high temperatures reduces the amount of amphibian chytrid fungus Batrachochytrium dendrobatidis DNA detectable by PCR assay. Dis Aquat Org 81:93–97, 2008.

44. Voyles J, Young S, Berger L, et al: Pathogenesis of chytridiomycosis, a cause of catastrophic amphibian declines. Science 326:582–585, 2009.

45. Walker SF, Bosch J, James TY, et al: Invasive pathogens threaten species recovery programs. Curr Biol 18:853–854, 2008.

46. Webb R, Mendez D, Berger L, Speare R: Additional disinfectants effective against the amphibian chytrid fungus Batrachochytrium dendrobatidis. Dis Aquat Org 74:13–16, 2007.

47. Weldon C, du Preez LH, Hyatt AD, et al: Origin of the amphibian chytrid fungus. Emerg Infect Dis 10:2100–2105, 2004.

48. Woodhams DC, Alford RA, Marantelli G: Emerging disease of amphibians cured by elevated body temperature. Dis Aquat Org 55:65–67, 2003.

49. Young S, Berger L, Speare R: Amphibian chytridiomycosis: Strategies for captive management and conservation. Int Zoo Yb 41:1–11, 2007.

CHAPTER 29

Mycobacteriosis in Amphibians

Norin Chai

Mycobacterium species have long been recognized as a significant source of morbidity and mortality in amphibians. This review will underscore important aspects of mycobacterial diseases in amphibians and discuss a recent case of *Mycobacterium liflandii* infection in *Xenopus tropicalis*, a newly described *Mycobacterium* species closely related to *M. ulcerans*.

Mycobacteriosis has a worldwide distribution in humans and animals. The genus *Mycobacterium* comprises 130 species and 11 subspecies. recognized by the list of prokaryotic names with standing in nomenclature (LPSN). These all share the characteristic morphologic features of gram-positive, aerobic, acid- and alcohol-fast bacteria—nonmotile 1- to 10-μm long rods.[7] The pathogenicity of different mycobacteria varies significantly and, for practical purposes, we may differentiate two main groups, the *Mycobacterium tuberculosis* complex and atypical mycobacteria, including the *Mycobacterium avium* complex. The most familiar species is *M. tuberculosis*, the causative agent of human tuberculosis, responsible for the death of over 2 million people each year. Atypical mycobacteria have a very important place in human and animal health as well, especially in immunodepressed hosts.

Mycobacteriosis is the oldest known infectious disease of amphibians, with a history dating back to the latter part of the 19th century. Robert Koch isolated *M. tuberculosis* in 1882. In 1905, Küster reported the first case of amphibian mycobacteriosis in three frogs *(Rana temporaria)*.[12] To our knowledge, only atypical mycobacteria, or MOTT (*m*ycobacteria *o*ther *t*han *M. tuberculosis* complex), have been isolated in amphibians.

EPIDEMIOLOGY

Mycobacteria are ubiquitous in aquatic environments or as soil saprophytes and are found commonly in nature;

they are likely to be seen in most, if not all, amphibian facilities. In that way, the epidemiology of mycobacterial infection in amphibians is different from that seen in birds and mammals—the clinician must always include mycobacteriosis in the differential diagnosis. Mycobacterial disease has been reported among exhibited amphibians and in laboratory models. A review in 2001 described 31 species of amphibians, representing nine families, affected by mycobacteriosis. Since then, this list has likely expanded considerably.[19] An increasingly diverse array of *Mycobacterium* spp. has been isolated from frogs in recent years, supplanting the paradigm of *M. marinum*, *M. fortuitum*, and *M. xenopi* as the only causative agents adequately described. A number of them have been isolated, including *M. abscessus, M. chelonae, M. fortuitum, M. marinum, M. gordonae, M. ranae, M. thamnospheos, Mycobacterium avium, M. xenopi,* and *M. szulgaï.*[2] A newly described *Mycobacterium* species, closely related to *M. ulcerans* and *M. marinum*, has been isolated from *Xenopus tropicalis*.[14] *M. liflandii* is characterized by the presence of insertion sequences IS2404 and IS2606, as well as by the production of the toxin mycolactone. Both mycolactone production and the presence of IS2404 were thought to be restricted to *M. ulcerans*.[18,20] The last part of this chapter will discuss *M. liflandii* in more detail.

Natural transmission of mycobacteria in amphibians is poorly understood. Mycobacteria are ubiquitous in the environment. Water and associated biofilms are natural habitats for many of them, so water-borne transmission seems likely in most amphibians. Vectors must also be considered—borne mycobacteria are known to infect a number of aquatic organisms and survive and replicate in various protozoan hosts.[9] Vertical transmission of mycobacteria has been suggested in fish, but not yet in amphibians.[5] As a rule, it is believed that they infect animals through defects in the integument or by ingestion (contaminated food and water).

Although mycobacteriosis is considered to be precipitated by stress and occurs in immunodepressed host, specific factors leading to disease outbreaks are seldom defined and appear to vary among systems. The initial dose influences disease outcome, as evidenced by a study in the leopard frog *(Rana pipiens)*, in which *M. marinum* produces chronic disease with a low initial innoculum and acute or subacute disease with higher infecting doses. The minimum number of persistent organisms required to stimulate granuloma formation appears to be approximately 10.[4] Furthermore, the study showed that *M. marinum* causes a chronic, granulomatous, nonlethal disease in immunocompetent frogs. However, in experimental frogs immunosuppressed with hydrocortisone, infection results in an acute, fulminant, lethal disease.[17] There have been no reports describing mycobacteriosis associated with large-scale mortality in wild amphibians, although I have studied several large epizootics attributed to the disease in amphibian research facilities.

PATHOGENESIS

Mycobacteria induce granulomatous reactions in human and animal hosts. With the exception of *M. ulcerans* and others, mycolactone-producing mycobacteria (MPM), pathogenic mycobacteria in vertebrates are predominantly intracellular parasites of phagocytes. Several studies in frogs and fishes have suggested that multiple intracellular survival strategies may be used.[8] MPM are unique among mycobacterial pathogens in that they are mainly extracellular and secrete mycolactone. Mycolactone causes apoptosis and necrosis of cultured cells in vitro and inhibits proinflammatory cytokines and phagocytosis. *M. ulcerans* is responsible for the progressive necrotizing skin disease seen in humans afflicted with Buruli ulcer.[10,21] A number of variant mycolactones (A to D) have been identified in *M. ulcerans* from different geographic locations. Mycolactone E is the mycolactone that has been recovered from amphibians with *M. liflandii* infection.[14]

CLINICAL SIGNS AND PATHOLOGY

Mycobacteriosis is predominantly a chronic granulomatous infection. Although insidious chronicity with no clinical signs is the rule, peracute and acute cases may occur, reflecting the heterogeneous biologic behaviour of the various mycobacterial species and the heterogeneity of host responses. Acute disease is generally observed in association with high bacterial loads.

All amphibian tissues may be involved, including skin, visceral organs, musculature, and skeleton (Fig. 29-1). External clinical signs are not pathognomonic and range from some weight loss to cachexia, granulomatous dermatitis, dermal ulceration, pigmentary changes, abnormal behavior, ataxia, and ascites. At necropsy, granulomas are usually observed throughout the whole body, with or without enlargement of visceral organs such as the spleen, kidney, and liver. With the heterogeneity of host responses, significant variation in the size and structural organization of granulomas may be seen, from highly organized lesions with thick epithelioid layers to poorly organized inflammation. Lesions consist of large chronic inflammation areas, composed of concentric layers of epithelioid cells with a discrete spherical form. Diffuse infiltration of activated macrophages and few lymphocytes with central necrosis may be observed.[2] The disease may present as a solitary massive nodule or, more often, as a systemic disease, with granulomas produced in multiple organs or tissues (Fig. 29-2).

DIAGNOSTIC PROCEDURES

Diagnostic procedures carried out in living animals is difficult. Any unexplainable weight loss should be considered to be a potential subclinical mycobacteriosis. An animal suspected to be infected should be isolated and handled with gloves and specific nets until more is known about its infectious status. Laparoscopic examination of the coelomic cavity, using a Hopkins forward oblique 30-degree telescope, 2.7 mm in diameter, may also be conducted under anesthesia[3] (Fig. 29-3). Endoscopic biopsy of enlarged organs or an intracoelomic mass may be performed as well. In all cases, samples for further investigations should be collected from any lesions, skin biopsy or necropsy tissue. Visually affected organs should be removed and samples fixed in 10% buffered neutral formalin for histology with acid-fast staining. Histologic examination can identify disease, and acid-fast staining may reveal the presence of acid-fast bacilli in the tissues (i.e., infection). However, I have seen granulomas with a positive culture but without visible acid-fast bacilli several times (see later). Furthermore, as observed in fish, cryptic infections may exist without evidence of pathology.[9]

The diagnostic process should not be stopped at the histologic level. Samples must also be submitted for culture on liquid and solid media. Cultures are generally incubated at 22° C, 30° C, 37° C, and 42° C

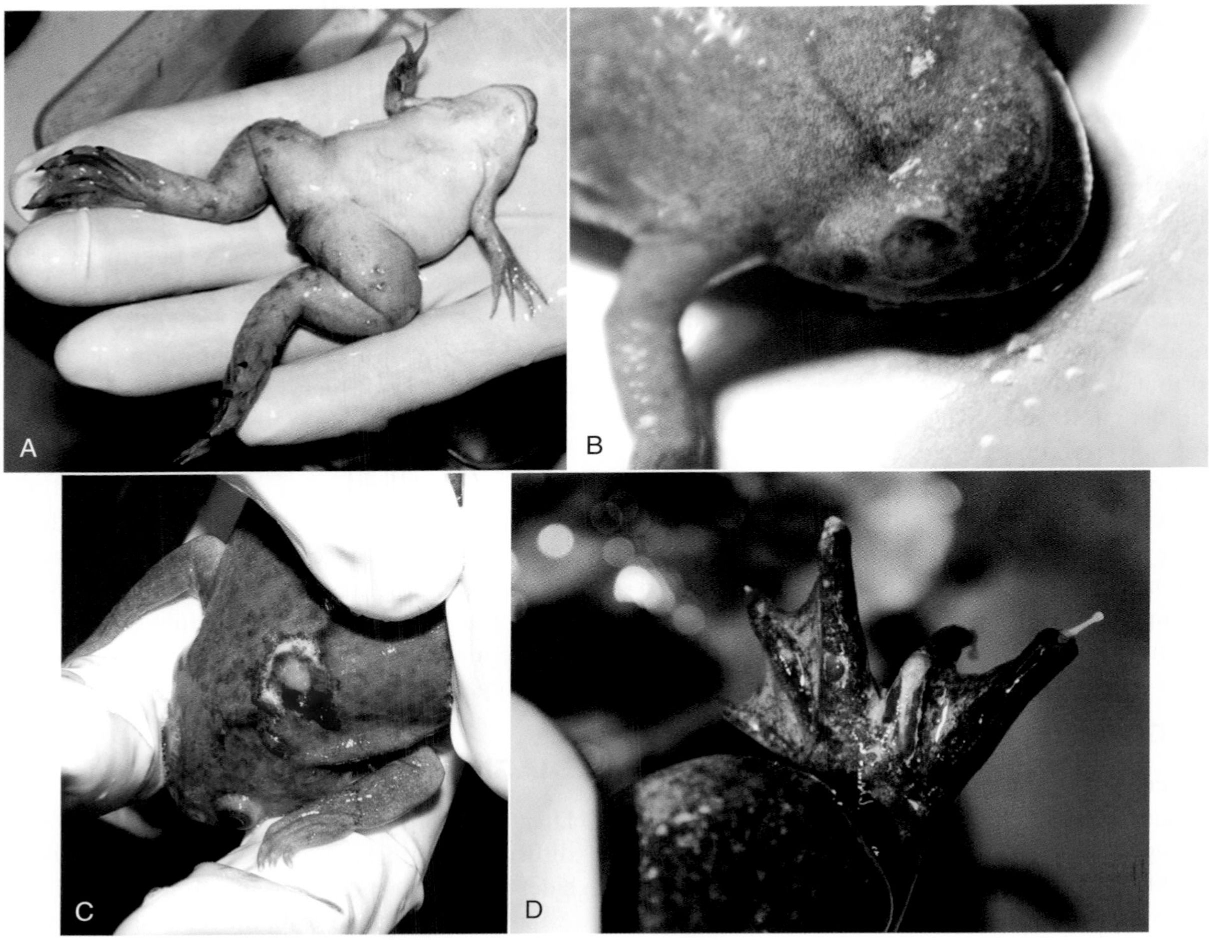

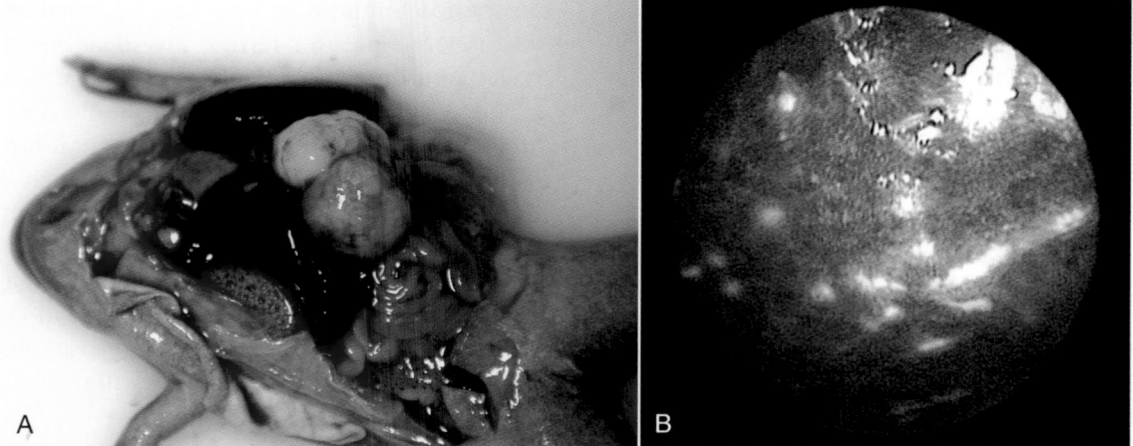

Figure 29-1

Different skin lesions caused by Mycobacteriosis. **A,** Disseminated small granulomas and ulcers. **B,** Single granulomas. **C,** Single large ulcer. **D,** Ulcer with dramatic loss of tissue. *(Courtesy Norin Chai.)*

Figure 29-2

The disease may present as a well-circumscribed surface liver granuloma (**A**) or as a very poorly defined granuloma (**B**). *(Courtesy Norin Chai.)*

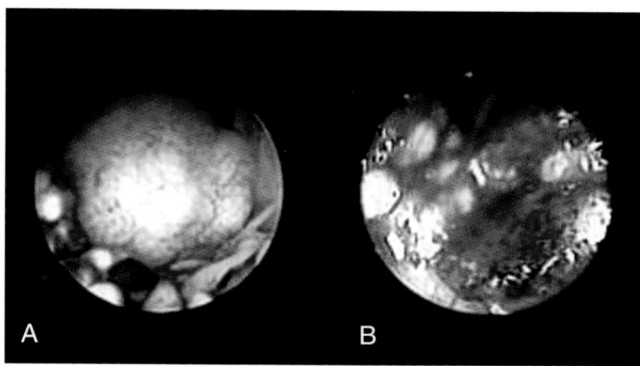

Figure 29-3

A, Single granuloma on the ovaries. **B,** Multiple granulomas in the lungs. These were observed by laparoscopic examination. *(Courtesy Norin Chai.)*

and monitored for growth every 3 days for at least 6 weeks. Interpretation of the results requires careful consideration. It is important to distinguish between mycobacteria simply isolated from amphibians and amphibian-pathogenic mycobacteria. Aseptic isolation from internal organs helps ensure that isolates do not represent contaminants. Isolation of mycobacteria from external sites or from whole-body sampling (in the case of small specimens) is questionable, because isolates could be external contaminants or passively present in ingested matter. Similarly, the presence of mycobacteria in feces from clinically healthy amphibians is unlikely to be significant, given their ubiquitous environmental presence. Aquatic amphibians may ingest bacteria, as I have occasionally found mycobacteria in the digestive tract of some amphibians. Usually, however, bacteriologic examination identifies cultivatable organisms, therefore indicating the presence of infection. A variety of molecular diagnostic methods have been developed for detecting and identifying *Mycobacterium* spp. Species identification is determined by use of the polymerase chain reaction (PCR) amplification of the highly conserved region of the 16S rRNA gene, the 65-kDa heat shock protein (hsp65). The sequences are then compared in the GenBank database to distinguish the species with which the sequence shares the highest nucleotide identity (100%) with the gene encoding 16S rRNA and hsp65.[6] Other gene targets for molecular detection of mycobacteria infecting amphibians include the MPM-associated *IS2404* and *IS2606*. The clinician should always remember that molecular methods detect mycobacterial DNA, but do not indicate whether the bacteria are viable or if disease is present.[9] The gold standard diagnostic process would be the combination

of bacteriology and species identification by molecular techniques, with a careful consideration of the context in which these different tests are applied.

TREATMENT

Currently, there are no widely accepted treatments for mycobacteriosis in amphibians. If antibiotic susceptibility testing on isolates may be performed, using antibiotic therapy runs a significant risk of developing antibiotic resistance and is not recommendded. Furthermore, given the zoonotic potential of the disease, euthanasia is warranted and should be performed. Sodium hypochlorite seems to be an effective sterilizing agent. Ethanol, benzyl-4-chlorophenol and phenylphenol (in some formulations of Lysol), and sodium chlorite have been found to kill *M. marinum* in water rapidly. However, potassium peroxymonosulfate (Virkon S) is ineffective, even after extended contact times.[13]

ZOONOTIC CONSIDERATIONS

The potential for zoonotic transmission of mycobacteria from amphibians to humans has important public health implications, especially in situations involving frequent and prolonged human contact with amphibians in crowded conditions, such as the research setting. Precautions should be taken routinely in the transportation, husbandry, and human contact and handling of these animals. *M. marinum* is a well-known human pathogen, producing granulomatous lesions in skin and peripheral deep tissues, that have repeatedly been described in fishermen and aquarists.[16] *M. szulgai* has been the cause of pulmonary disease. Other *M. szulgai* infections have involved the bursa, tendon sheaths, bones (with osteomyelitis), lymphoid tissues, skin, and eyes.[1,11] *M. fortuitum* and *M. chelonae* are well-known opportunistic human pathogens, especially of immunocompromised persons.[15] Considering the severity of disease caused by *M. ulcerans* infection in humans (Buruli ulcer), the recent discovery of numerous closely related mycolactone-producing mycobacteria is of some concern, although only one case of zoonosis caused by these bacteria has been reported.[4] Other *M. marinum*–like MPM, including *M. liflandii*, have higher temperature tolerance, suggesting that they could survive and replicate in peripheral sites in humans.[14]

As a rule, amphibian mycobacteria should be considered as a possible zoonosis, although confirmed cases of transfer of mycobacteria from amphibians to humans are rare and the significance for public health is unclear. Immunposuppressed individuals are likely to be predisposed to this infection.

EMERGENCE OF *MYCOBACTERIUM LIFLANDII* INFECTION IN *XENOPUS TROPICALIS* IN FRANCE

M. liflandii, an MPM, was identified as the causative agent of epizootic mycobacteriosis in *X. tropicalis* facilities at the University of California and in a Belgian laboratory.[18] It causes an infection with ulcerative and granulomatous dermatitis, visceral granulomas, coelomitis, septicemia, and bloating, resulting in a high death rate.[20] An *M. liflandii* epizootic infection in a French colony of *X. tropicalis* will be described here.

The epizootic appeared 2 weeks after an accidental drop of water temperature from 25° C to 12° C and the interruption of water circulation (general electric breakdown) in the flow-through housing system. Clinical manifestations included ulcerative dermatitis, cachexia, and lethargy, with an average of three deaths daily. *Pseudomonas aeruginosa* was isolated from the frog's skin, a pathogen susceptible to gentamycin or marbofloxacin. Despite a specific treatment with a mix of marbofloxacin and gentamycin, the morbidity and mortality remained high—one death every 3 days. Necropsy and histologic examination of four specimens showed an ulcerative dermatitis and granulomatous hepatosplenic necrosis, with the presence of acid-fast bacilli (AFB). For further examination, 77 animals with *X. tropicalis* infection, with mortality in their tanks reaching 80% in 1 month, were euthanized. Visually affected organs were removed and prepared for histopathologic and microbiologic analysis. From the 77 adults, 77.9% ($n = 60$) were visually affected with ulcers (71.7%), skin discolorations (31.7%), erythema (11.7%), granulomas (5%), and bloating (3.3%) (Fig. 29-4). Of these 60 animals, only 67% showed internal lesions, including in the liver (43%), spleen (36%), and kidneys (12%). Lungs (6%) and ovaries (3% [only one case]) were rarely affected. From 17 animals visually unaffected, 5 (29.4%) showed internal lesions, especially granulomas. Only 60% of the histopathologic evaluations of the visually affected animals with internal lesions showed AFB. In vitro cultures were positive from all the internal lesions after 100 days at 30° C. Species identifications were performed by 16S rRNA and hsp65 gene sequencing. Analysis of a 362-bp hsp65 sequence showed a 100% identity with *M. liflandii* (accession number [AN] AY500839), *M. pseudoshottsii* (AN

DQ987722), or *M. marinum* (AN DQ066746). A similar analysis conducted on a 650-bp 16S rDNA sequence showed a 100% identity with *M. liflandii* (AN AY845224), and 99.9% with *M. pseudoshottsi* (AN AY570988) or *M. marinum* (AN AF456238). Furthermore, positive nested PCR assays were carried out for *IS2404* and *IS2606*. PCR results were also probe-positive for *mlsA*, *mlsB*, and *MUP045*, three mycolactone biosynthesis genes. All together, these methods converged to confirm the identification of an *M. liflandii* isolate.

Zoo technical dysfunction and additive *Pseudomonas* infection may have contributed to the spreading of mycobacterial infection within the colony. In contrast to previous descriptions, the presence of granulomas was not a rule here; bloating and septicemia were also rare.[18,20] Isolation of *M. liflandii* in water sample suggests a possible direct (frog-frog) and indirect (frog-water-frog) transmission. The emerging potential of *M. liflandii* infection through the international trade of *X. tropicalis* enhances the importance of thorough veterinary evaluation. Only MPM that cause disease in humans and animal are isolated.[21] The existence of many silent MPM may not yet have been discovered. The diagnosis of mycobacteriosis in frogs should include genetic analysis, especially of mycolactone biosynthesis genes.

REFERENCES

1. Benator DA, Kan V, Gordin FM: *Mycobacterium szulgai* infection of the lung: Case report and review of an unusual pathogen. Am J Med Sci 313:346–351, 1997.
2. Chai N, Deforges L, Sougakoff W, et al: *Mycobacterium szulgai* infection in a captive population of African clawed frogs *(Xenopus tropicalis)*. J Zoo Wildl Med 37:55–58, 2006.
3. Chai N, De Luze A: Medicine and surgery in amphibians. In Proceedings of the 7th Scientific Meeting of the European Association of Zoo and Wildlife Veterinarians, Leipzig, Germany, 2008, European Association of Zoo and Wildlife Veterinarians, pp 185–188.
4. Chemlal K, Huys G, Laval F, et al: Characterization of an unusual mycobacterium: A possible missing link between *Mycobacterium marinum* and *Mycobacterium ulcerans*. J Clin Microbiol 40:2370–2380, 2002.
5. Chinabut S: Mycobacteriosis and nocardiosis. In Woo PTK, Bruno DW, editors: Fish, diseases and disorders, vol 3, New York, 1999, CABI, pp 319–340.
6. Devulder G, Perrier G, Baty F, Flandrois JP: BIBI, a bioinformatics bacterial identification tool. J Clin Microbiol 41:1785-1787, 2003.
7. Euzéby JP: List of bacterial names with standing in nomenclature: A folder available on the Internet. Int J Syst Bacteriol 47:590–592, 1997.
8. Gauthier DT, Vogelbein WK, Ottinger CA: Ultrastructure of *Mycobacterium marinum* granuloma in striped bass *(Morone saxatilis)*. Dis Aquat Organ 62:121–132, 2004.
9. Gauthier DT, Rhodes MW: Mycobacteriosis in fishes: A review. Vet J 180:33–47, 2009.

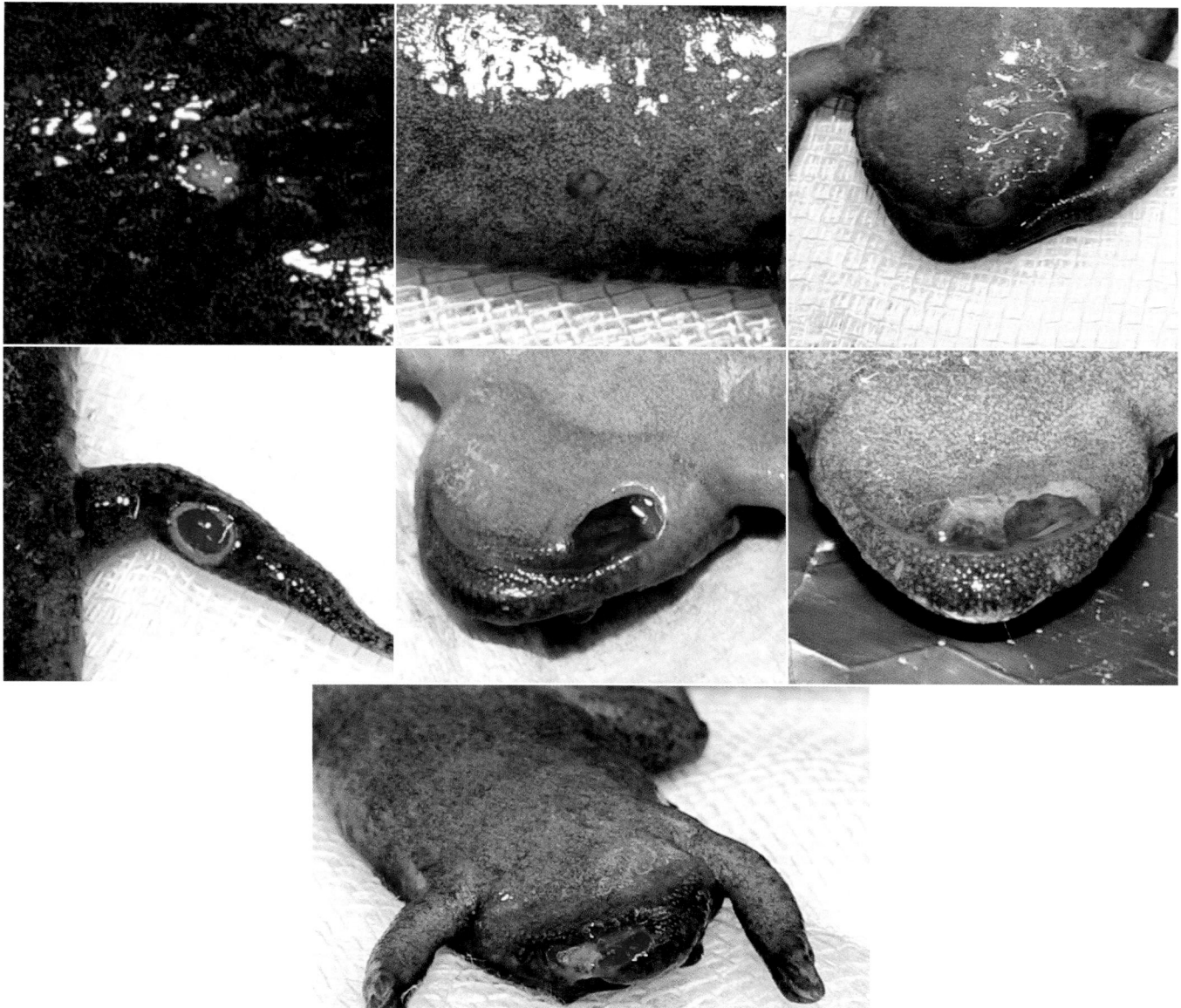

Figure 29-4

Dramatic evolution *of M. liflandii* infection from a simple white dot to a large ulcerative skin necrosis. *(Courtesy Norin Chai.)*

10. George KM, Pascopella L, Welty DM, et al: A *Mycobacterium ulcerans* toxin, mycolactone, causes apoptosis in guinea pig ulcers and tissue culture cells. Infect Immun 68:877–883, 2000.
11. Holmes GP, Bond GB, Fader RC, Fulcher SF: A cluster of cases of *Mycobacterium szulgai* keratitis that occurred after laser-assisted in situ keratomileusis. Clin Infect Dis 34:1039–1046, 2002.
12. Küster E: Über Kaltblütertuberkulose. Münch Med Wochenschr 52:57–59, 1905.
13. Mainous ME, Smith SA: Efficacy of common disinfectants against *Mycobacterium marinum*. J Aquat Anim Health 17:284–288, 2005.
14. Mve-Obiang A, Lee RE, Umstot ES, et al: A newly discovered mycobacterial pathogen isolated from laboratory colonies of *Xenopus* species with lethal infections produces a novel form of mycolactone, the *Mycobacterium ulcerans* macrolide toxin. Infect Immun 73:3307–3312, 2005.
15. Otsuka Y, Fujino T, Mori N, et al: Survey of human immunodeficiency virus (HIV)-seropositive patients with mycobacterial infection in Japan. J Infect 51:364–374, 2005.
16. Petrini B: *Mycobacterium marinum*: Ubiquitous agent of waterborne granulomatous skin infections. Eur J Clin Microbiol Infect Dis 25:609–613, 2006.
17. Ramakrishnan L, Valdivia RH, Mckerrow JJ, et al: *Mycobacterium marinum* causes both long-term subclinical infection and acute disease in the leopard frog *(Rana pipiens)*. Infect Immun 65:767–773, 1997.

18. Schinsky MF, Morey RE, Steigerwalt AG, et al: Taxonomic variation in the *Mycobacterium fortuitum* third biovariant complex: Description of *Mycobacterium boenickei* sp. nov., *Mycobacterium houstonense* sp. nov., *Mycobacterium neworleansense* sp. nov., and *Mycobacterium brisbanense* sp. nov. and recognition of *Mycobacterium porcinum* from human clinical isolates. Int J Syst Evol Microbiol 54:1653–1667, 2004.

19. Suykerbuyk P, Vleminckx K, Pasmans F, et al: *Mycobacterium liflandii* infection in European colony of *Silurana tropicalis*. Emerg Infect Dis 5:743–746, 2007.

20. Taylor SK, Green E, Wright KM, et al: Bacterial diseases. In Wright KM, Whitaker BR, editors: Amphibian medicine and captive husbandry, Malabar, India, 2001, Krieger, pp 159–179.

21. Trott KA, Stacy BA, Lifland BD, et al: Characterization of a Mycobacterium ulcerans–like infection in a colony of African tropical clawed frogs (Xenopus tropicalis). Comp Med 54:309–317, 2004.

CHAPTER 30

Amphibian Viral Diseases

Graham Crawshaw

In earlier editions of this text, viral infections of amphibians received little consideration because they were not considered to be of great clinical importance or were of purely historical significance. In the intervening years, amphibian viruses have been demonstrated to be primary pathogens in both anurans and urodeles. They have been incriminated in morbidity and mortality in wild amphibian populations around the world and likely play a role in the natural ecology of a species, although without having the devastating long-term impact of fungi. Conversely, there have been few reports of viral infections in zoo collections.[7,15] Outbreaks of viral disease in captive animals have principally been reported from commercial frog farms in which the conditions may more closely resemble those in the wild than in the more controlled conditions of zoo collections.[14,16] Excellent papers and reviews on viral infections have been published, but this is a rapidly expanding field.[4,6,9,12,13]

It is not yet possible to quantify the risk of each virus in each species of amphibian. One difficulty lies in the fact that some viruses show persistent but inapparent infection in their natural hosts and yet may be pathogenic to naïve individuals or other species. Susceptibility to a virus, or strain of virus, varies with the species and life stage. Critical periods for infectivity include the time before the larval immune system develops, at metamorphosis while the larval immune system is being modified, and during periods of stress. Metamorphosing individuals are typically most susceptible. Furthermore, with virally induced lymphoid depletion and multiorgan compromise, individual frogs become susceptible to opportunistic pathogens, so it is not always clear which agent is responsible for killing the animal.

It is likely that the relationship between the amphibian hosts and their viruses demonstrate the whole range of outcomes associated with these agents in mammals—complete immunity to infection, infection followed by elimination of the virus and subsequent lifelong immunity, infection with short-lived immunity, persistence of the virus asymptomatically with periodic recrudescence under situations of stress, and overwhelming infection and death.

The most significant and well-studied amphibian viruses belong to the family Iridoviridae (Table 30-1). The taxonomic status of this group is fluid and may be confusing. Iridoviruses have only been isolated from poikilothermic animals and are usually associated with damp or aquatic environments. The host range is variable and there is evidence of transmission across orders or even phyla. The family is currently divided into five genera and several unclassified members. Two genera, *Iridovirus* and *Chloriridovirus*, infect invertebrates such as insects, crustaceans, and mollusks. *Lymphocystivirus* and *Megalocystivirus* infect fish. Those infecting amphibians belong to the genus *Ranavirus*. The term *iridovirus* may denote either a member of the family Iridoviridae or a member of the genus *Iridovirus*.[3]

RANAVIRUSES

Ranaviruses are large (120 to 300 nm), icosahedral, linear, double-stranded DNA viruses. Virus particles may be enveloped (obtained from the plasma membrane) or unenveloped, with viral replication occurring in the cytoplasm or nucleus. Within the genus *Ranavirus*, species and tentative species are named based on the type of disease they induce, the animal from which they were first isolated, or their site of origin.[3]

Ranaviruses have been identified in an increasing number of wild amphibian hosts around the world. The original frog isolates were identified in a study of renal carcinomas in leopard frogs *(Rana pipiens)* but were not associated with any lesions at that time. However,

TABLE 30-1 Summary of Iridoviruses Infecting Amphibians

Name	Comments	Type Species	Related Species or Strains
Family Iridoviridae	Linear, double-stranded DNA genome; infections occur in invertebrates and poikilothermic vertebrates		
Genus *Ranavirus*	Infections occur in fish, reptiles, and amphibians	Frog virus 3 (FV-3)	*Bufo marinus* Venezuelan iridovirus 1, *Lucké triturus* virus 1, tadpole edema virus, tiger frog virus, tadpole virus 2, *Rana catesbeiana* virus X, *Rana temporaria* United Kingdom virus 1, *Bufo bufo* United Kingdom virus
Bohle iridovirus	Isolated from burrowing frogs in Australia		
Rana esculenta ranavirus	Isolated from edible frogs in Europe		
Ambystoma tigrinum virus (ATV)	Isolated from wild and captive salamanders	*Ambystoma tigrinum* virus	*Regina ranavirus, Axolotl ranavirus*

Modified from Chinchar VG, Hyatt A, Miyazaki T, et al: Family Iridoviridae: Poor viral relations no longer, Curr Top Microbiol Immunol 328:123–170, 2009; and OIE (World Organization for Animal Health): Infection with ranavirus, 2008 (http://www.oie.int/aac/eng/Publicat/Cardsenglish/Ranavirus%20card_final.pdf).

disease outbreaks among fish, cultured and wild frogs, and salamanders have since implicated several members of the genus *Ranavirus* as pathogens.[3] There are limited reports of infections in zoo or pet animals but a survey of wild-caught frogs in a zoo collection has shown a high prevalence of ranavirus based on diagnosis by polymerase chain reaction (PCR) assay in live and dead animals.[7] Infection also occurs concurrently with other pathogens, including bacteria and fungi.[15] It is not known whether the paucity of reported cases of infection in captive animals reflects a low viral prevalence or virulence, or the fact that ranavirus infections are not recognized because the clinical and pathologic findings are often nonspecific.[20]

Ranavirus infections are not limited to a single species or taxonomic class of animal. Each virus or viral strain shows a slightly different genomic structure or molecular fingerprint, depending on the location of the isolate or the species in which it was found. Isolation of a ranavirus from a new species of amphibian does not necessarily identify new viral species. At the time of this writing, there are several distinct type species affecting amphibians: frog virus 3 (FV-3), *Ambystoma tigrinum* virus (ATV), Bohle virus, and *Rana esculenta* virus (REIV).[3,17]

In the case of FV-3, the virus has been isolated from amphibians as diverse as midwife toads (*Alytes obstetricans*), Alpine newts (*Mesotriton alpestris cyreni*), common toads (*Bufo bufo*), and common frogs (*Rana temporaria*) in Europe, marine toads (*Bufo marinus*) and the leptodactylid frog *Atelognathus patagonicus* in South America, and American bullfrogs (*Rana catesbeiana*) in North America. In addition, many other species showing a close resemblance to one of the type species have been isolated or identified. Isolates resembling FV-3 have been obtained from anurans worldwide, including gold-striped pond frogs (*Rana plancyi*) in China, *Leptodactylus* spp. in Venezuela, commercial bullfrogs in Uruguay and Brazil, the red-tailed knobby newt (*Tylototriton kweichowensis*), clouded salamander (*Hynobius nebulosus*), red-legged frogs (*Rana aurora*), red efts (*Diemictylus viridescens*), spotted salamanders (*Ambystoma maculatum*), and at least 10 species of plenthodontid salamanders. In many cases, these may be described as ranaviruses or FV-3–like viruses. Further complicating the picture is the fact that some isolates associated with fish and reptiles are also considered to be forms of FV-3. One distinct species, REIV, was isolated from edible frogs (*Pelophylax* kl. *esculentus*) in Europe.

ATV was isolated from tiger salamanders (*Ambystoma tigrinum*). Other species closely related to ATV, such as Regina ranavirus, have been identified in other urodeles, and Axolotl ranavirus was found in a laboratory collection of axolotls (*Ambystoma mexicanum*). In experimental studies, anurans are variably, but generally less, susceptible to infection with ATV-like viruses than urodeles.[24] Bohle iridovirus, a virulent pathogen of the burrowing frog *Lymnodynastes ornatus* in Australia, may be experimentally transmitted to fish and marine toads.

Clinical Effects

Although many of these viruses cause life-threatening infections, subclinical infections also occur.[3,21] Ranaviruses may be transmitted experimentally by injection or by immersion in infected water, and naturally by cohabitation, predation, and wounding. In anurans, viruses such as FV-3 are associated with systemic disease manifested by two major syndromes; the most severe manifestation is one of hemorrhage and edema in internal organs and, in the less acute form, affected animals show erythema, ulceration, or hyperplasia of the skin.[1,5,6] In experimentally infected frogs, those developing the hemorrhagic syndrome died in the acute or peracute stages of the disease within 1 to 2 weeks of infection, whereas frogs with the ulcerative form developed lesions more slowly. These differences may be manifestations of degrees of severity influenced by variations in pathogenicity of the strain of the virus, immunity of the amphibian, route of infection, or weight of viral challenge.

Signs in salamanders are similar. Early lesions include white polyps on the skin of the epidermis that progress to cover most of the body, with progressive hemorrhage and ulceration. The skin may become dark or speckled. Affected animals become lethargic, refuse food, and float near the surface of the water, finally developing loose bloody feces, emesis, anorexia, edema, and cutaneous erosions and ulcers. Death may occur within 48 hours of developing bloody feces.[1,11,19] Progression of the disease may be affected by the ambient temperature. In some experiments, mortality was reduced at elevated temperature, perhaps a result of enhanced immune function; in others, viral replication itself was temperature-dependent.[22]

These syndromes are consistent with descriptions of red-leg, which historically has been regarded as having a primary bacterial (usually *Aeromonas. hydrophila*) cause. Although various bacteria may indeed be responsible,

ranaviruses have also been shown to cause syndromes in which neither the outcome nor progression of the disease was altered by the presence of bacteria, including *A. hydrophila*.[5,6]

Late-stage tadpoles and metamorphs are generally the most susceptible to infection, whereas adults are less frequently affected, a difference likely related to viral virulence and innate or acquired host resistance factors. The high susceptibility of larval stages to ranaviruses has been established in *Xenopus* spp.; however, normal adults of this species are resistant to infection.[21] In other cases, tadpoles as young as 2 weeks of age died while very young tadpoles or those nearing metamorphosis were unaffected.[14] Typically, diseased tadpoles stop feeding, remain at the bottom of a tank, swim abnormally, and appear deformed. Abdominal distension is common because of fluid retention and generalized edema, perhaps reflecting the predilection of the virus for the kidneys. Skin lesions or petechiae may not always be present. Mass mortalities of tadpoles may be seen, with up to 100% of a tank population lost.

Pathologic Findings

Pathologic findings in ranaviral infections mirror the clinical syndromes. FV-3 targets the renal proximal tubular epithelium and erythropoietic tissues, notably in the liver and spleen, and also affects other tissues.* Frogs dying of the hemorrhagic syndrome show an enlarged congested spleen. Petechial or diffuse hemorrhage may be seen on the urinary bladder, testes, intestines, and other viscera. Hemorrhages may also be seen on the skin and in the mouth subcutaneously and in the musculature of the legs, most notably of the hindfeet. Chronic skin ulceration in the absence of internal lesions has also been described. In salamanders, the coelomic cavity often contains clear fluid, with petechiation on the serosal surfaces, edema and hemorrhage in the wall of the stomach, and a mottled liver. Histologically, infected frogs and tadpoles show hemorrhage and necrosis of the hematopoietic tissue (and eventually the parenchyma) of the kidneys, liver, and spleen, with mononuclear infiltrates in later stages of the disease. Fragmentation of melanomacrophages in a wide range of tissues, particularly the liver, was a prominent feature in experimentally infected anurans. Interestingly, infection of splenic lymphocytes was only seen in frogs with hemorrhagic disease and not in those with ulcerative syndrome; hence, it was suggested that infection of the

*References 1, 5, 6, 9, 15, and 21.

spleen is required for frogs to develop hemorrhagic disease. Lesions in salamanders range from foci of degeneration to larger areas of mucosal necrosis and ulceration and hemorrhage in the gastrointestinal tract. Focal or widespread necrosis occurs in the liver in hepatocytes and in associated hematopoietic tissue, intestines, kidneys, and spleen and other lymphoid tissues. Tadpoles show similar lesions but necrosis and an inflammatory response may be limited, particularly in animals dying peracutely.

Large basophilic to amphophilic intracytoplasmic inclusions are typically observed in necrotic areas of the kidney, liver, spleen, lymphoid, and hematopoietic tissues.[1,16,21] In other cases, inclusions may not be seen, even though the virus is associated with the lesions.

Ranaviral infections increase susceptibility to opportunistic pathogens, such as *Aeromonas*, particularly if the normal skin barrier is compromised. It is likely that many deaths attributable to bacteria have an underlying ranavirus infection.

Diagnosis

Although it is currently not possible to treat viral disease in amphibians, identification of the specific agent is important for differential diagnosis and controlling spread to uninfected populations.[4] Diagnosis of ranaviral infections in cases of outbreaks or mortality should be straightforward, although elucidation of primary from secondary pathogens and the role of environmental factors may be more difficult. Diagnosis based on clinical signs alone is not definitive, so a panel of microscopic, serologic, and molecular techniques is required. Pathologic findings may suggest ranaviral infection but, again, these are not specific. The presence of multicentric hemorrhage, along with degeneration and necrosis in hematopoietic tissue of the liver, spleen, and kidney, particularly with the presence of inclusion bodies, should strongly suggest a viral cause. Immunohistochemical staining has been used to identify the presence of ranavirus in specific tissues but the technique is not widely available.[6]

Transmission electron microscopy is capable of classifying the agent as a member of the family Iridoviridae. Viral culture is required to isolate the causative agent. Specimens submitted for bacterial analysis may only result in a diagnosis of *A. hydrophila* when there is an underlying ranavirus cause.[5,16] Ranaviruses grow in a wide variety of cultured fish, amphibian, and mammalian cells, causing a marked cytopathic effect (CPE) and culminating in cell death, likely by apoptosis.

Amphibian-derived viruses grow and cause CPE in fish cell cultures in vitro. Bluegill fry cells (BF-2) and epithelioma papulosum cyprini (EPC) cell lines have been recommended as an international standard for cell culture.

Although sensitive and specific for ranaviruses, viral culture is impractical for large numbers of animals and may not be readily available. Consequently, PCR assay is commonly used to confirm or to rule out *Ranavirus* infection.[4,18] The PCR test is used as both a screening and diagnostic test to identify the genus because the major capsid protein (MCP) of the virus is a highly conserved region of the genome. The most suitable samples for PCR testing are liver, kidney, and skin (if lesions are present). Cloacal or pharyngeal swab, tissue biopsy, and blood samples may also be collected from sick living animals (see later). Conventional PCR testing is highly sensitive and specific for animals dying after experimental infection. However, it may not detect early stages of infection because of the low number of virions present in the animal. Even the methodology of the PCR test may affect the results. In a study of wild-caught but captive frogs, quantitative PCR (qPCR) techniques were more sensitive at detecting viral DNA than conventional PCR.[10] A PCR-positive test indicates that the animal is infected with a ranavirus but further sequence analysis is required to identify the virus to species (e.g., ATV, FV-3, *Bufo bufo* virus). Members of the different viral species are differentiated from each other by various techniques, such as terminal restriction fragment length polymorphism (TRFLP) profiles, virus protein profiles, DNA sequence analysis, and host specificity. Restriction endonuclease (RE) digestion profiling uses the entire viral genomic DNA instead of portions of a single gene to differentiate among iridoviral strains.[24]

Identification of current or previous infection in a live amphibian is more problematic. The ability to screen amphibians for pathogens with the use of nonlethal techniques would be an important advance in the study of amphibian diseases. Serologic testing has been used to identify evidence of previous infection, although this technology is not typically available in diagnostic laboratories.

Clinical infections in live animals have been identified using molecular techniques on tail and toe web clips, and from oral and cloacal swabs, but ranaviral DNA may also be detected in healthy amphibians.[8,25] Ostensibly healthy, and yet infected, adult amphibians have been shown to pass infection to more susceptible juveniles.[7,10] Consideration should be given to culling animals for diagnostic testing on necropsy, which is more sensitive for detecting persistent infections in a group of animals. Interpretation of results is also problematic. A negative test result may be obtained if an animal is truly uninfected, if viremia has yet to be established, or if the sample either contains low levels of virus or the test is unable to detect these low levels. Noninvasive samples, such as tail or toe web clips, may not contain enough virus particles to detect by PCR assay until the animal is showing clinical signs of infection. Neither is a positive result in a healthy animal an accurate predictor that the animal or its contacts will become diseased, but it may be of value in decisions on population management.[20]

Treatment

At this time, chemotherapeutic agents have only been used to treat bacterial pathogens in amphibians. Drugs effective against other viruses have not yet been shown to be efficacious for iridoviral disease. Natural antimicrobial compounds in the skin of amphibians do have antiviral activity, including against FV-3, but these have not been used for therapy or prophylaxis of amphibian viral pathogens.[23] Increasing temperature to the higher end of the preferred temperature range has reduced mortality in a temperate salamander, perhaps by enhancing immune function.[22] Early detection and reduction of exogenous stressors should help infected amphibians clear the virus and ultimately reduce loss.[16]

Viral Transmission and Immunity

There is good evidence that FV-3 and related ranaviruses circulate in a variety of anuran species in the wild and, similarly, strains of ATV or ATV-like ranaviruses are adapted to urodeles. Particular amphibian species have been shown to be susceptible to infection and suffer mortality; however, in similar studies, the same species has been shown to be resistant to infection or pathologic effects. The discrepancy is likely caused by innate or acquired resistance of the experimental host or subtle variations in the pathogenicity of the particular strain of the virus.[24] Following infection with ranavirus, adult clawed frogs (*Xenopus* spp.) produce specific antibodies, are able to eliminate infection within 2 to 3 weeks, and develop long-lasting humoral immunity. Antibody production is boosted further after a secondary exposure. However, immunocompromised clawed frogs succumb to infection. In other species, the

virus persists in adults, which then become a source of infection for tadpoles or metamorphosing individuals of the next generation. In an outbreak of ranaviral disease in a protected captive colony of salamanders, mortality commenced 15 days after the introduction of some newly collected animals and the entire colony had succumbed by day 20.

Ranaviruses are typically transmitted through direct or indirect contact or through cannibalism in the case of salamanders, whose larvae are carnivorous, with siblicidal tendencies. Vertical transmission is considered likely, but has not been documented experimentally. Ranaviruses may persist outside the host for several months, even on dry surfaces, and survive even longer in aquatic environments. Seasonal variations are seen in the prevalence and severity of disease outbreaks in ranaculture systems, with both being greater during the warmer months.

The major concern about ranaviruses in captive amphibian programs is the possibility of a significant mortality in a valuable species or that subclinically infected captive animals could serve as vectors for the introduction of novel viruses into naïve wild populations. Rescue, captive breeding, and reintroduction programs for species such as neotropical anurans and the threatened Wyoming and the Puerto Rican crested toads rely heavily on the presumption that new pathogens are not introduced with repatriated individuals. Isolation of captive populations and avoidance of disseminating infection between institutions are essential for the control of viral disease.

Recommendations for Testing in Quarantine and Control of Ranavirus Infections

At this time, routine testing of living healthy zoo animals in quarantine or preshipment is not recommended.[20] Unlike testing for the amphibian chytrid fungus, the available PCR tests for ranaviruses have not been validated to screen living amphibians for subclinical infection reliably. Laboratories are willing to perform testing, but accurate interpretation of the results may not be straightforward. Data must be viewed with reference to the strengths and limitations of each technique. Without a broad base of knowledge, it is difficult to make recommendations or predictions based on a positive test or negative test result. This is equivalent to attesting the presence or significance of an enteric bacterium based on the culture of a single fecal sample. For the most reliable information on ranaviral status in a group in quarantine, the best samples to submit are tissues collected at necropsy of animals that have died during the quarantine period, regardless of clinical suspicion of virus infection, or those that are culled specifically for disease screening purposes. The health history of the source population should be reviewed for clinical signs or necropsy findings that could suggest ranavirus infection but, at the same time, the equivalent status of the recipient population should be known. Preshipment testing may provide a framework for developing information about the captive population rather than providing a guarantee of pathogen-free status. If suspicious clinical signs or lesions are identified, attempts may be made to confirm or rule out ranavirus infection. Introduction of animals from collections with a recent history of active ranavirus infection should be avoided.

Control of established viral infections in affected collections is difficult, given the limitations in diagnosis and treatment. Isolation of affected and in-contact animals from unexposed individuals, and application of good husbandry and hygiene practices, may reduce the likelihood of transmission or recurrence. Infected amphibians should not be transported into other locations known to be free of ranavirus. Bleach (4%), chlorhexidine (1%), and Virkon-S (1%) for a 1-minute exposure time may be used to disinfect premises and fomites; ozone may be used to sterilize water.[2] Ranavirus vaccines are not currently available for amphibians but low-pathogenic strains have been shown to provide protection against more virulent ones, and vaccines have been developed for related viruses in fish.

Consideration must be given to the value of the affected and at-risk populations with regard to the need for generalized or selective culling of exposed individuals. Recognizing the potential threat of ranaviruses to global amphibian biodiversity, the World Organization for Animal Health (OIE) has listed this pathogen as a notifiable disease, requiring proof of ranavirus-negative results before commercial shipment of amphibians.[17] OIE recommends the use of specific pathogen-free (SPF) stocks for the prevention of ranavirus disease in amphibian farms.

Nonlethal sampling has many advantages over lethal sampling, such as the ability to follow an individual animal's infection status over time, and could be used to help assess the risks to amphibians in breeding and conservation programs. By the time a pathogen is identified in a population, it may already have infected a large proportion of available hosts. Unlocking the mysteries of ranavirus epidemiology in amphibians is a complex task. Further work is needed to develop nonlethal diagnostic techniques for viral pathogens that combine high test sensitivity and specificity.[10] Underestimation of the true prevalence of infection, as PCR testing does for early-stage infections, could delay management action and increase the risk of population decline or extinction. Increased screening of dead and living animals in zoo collections is essential to be able to develop a better understanding of the prevalence and significance of ranviral infections in captive populations and recovery programs.

Other Iridoviruses

Iridovirus-like inclusions have also been seen in erythrocytes of wild frogs (frog erythrocytic virus). Based on a study of similar structures in reptiles, they are likely to be nonranaviral members of the Iridoviridae.

OTHER VIRUSES

Antibodies to Japanese encephalitis virus and Western equine encephalitis virus have been found in wild frogs. Experimental infection with Eastern equine encephalitis and West Nile virus has demonstrated low susceptibility of several species of North American frogs, but it is unlikely that these viruses would be of any concern for captive animals.

Herpesviruses

Amphibians are also known to support herpesviruses. Two amphibian herpesviruses have been classified and studied in detail, Ranid herpesvirus 1 (RaHV-1; Lucké tumor herpesvirus) and Ranid herpesvirus 2 (RaHV-2; frog virus 4). Analysis of the genome has shown that RaHV-1 is related to channel catfish virus, and that these amphibian herpesviruses belong to the family Alloherpesviridae, separate from the mammalian α, β, and γ herpesviruses. RaHV-1 is the causative agent of a renal adenocarcinoma occurring in the northern leopard frog, *Rana pipiens*. The virus may be found not only in the primary tumor but also in metastatic cells in the liver, fat body, and bladder. In the host, RaHV-1 replication is promoted by low (hibernation) temperatures but inhibited by warmer temperatures. In contrast, tumor development is enhanced by warm temperature but inhibited by cold. RaHV-1 has not been cultured in cell lines but has been detected by PCR in frog tumors. RaHV-2 was isolated from the urine of a Lucké tumor–bearing frog but was not associated with tumor development. Skin papillomas and gastric tumors in Japanese newts *(Cynops pyrrhogaster)* are also associated with a herpes-like virus.

Adenoviruses

Adenoviruses have recently been classified into three large families, including Atadenoviridae, found in amphibians and reptiles. Frog adenovirus 1 (FAV-1) was originally isolated from a naturally occurring renal tumor in a Northern leopard frog but may also be isolated from healthy wild frogs. The virus could only be grown in turtle heart tissue culture cells; various other cell types from amphibians, reptiles, fish, and mammals were refractory to infection. No clinical or pathologic effects were associated with the virus with the original isolate or in experimentally infected frogs.

Parvoviruses

Two captive spring peepers *(Pseudacris crucifer)* showed degeneration, atrophy, and necrosis of the tongue and limb musculature, with nonsuppurative inflammation and eosinophilic, intranuclear inclusion bodies. Virus-like particles compatible with a parvovirus were seen on electron microscopy but, because further studies were not performed, the significance of this finding could not be established.

Retroviruses

Amphibians have also been shown to harbor retroviruses. An endogenous virus derived from an African clawed toad *(Xenopus laevis)* has been sequenced. The virus, termed *Xen1*, has one of the largest endogenous retroviral genomes described to date, and is most closely related to the ε-retroviruses, which are large, complex, exogenous retroviruses present in walleye fish. Retroviral sequences have also been detected in other amphibians, including caecilians, salamanders, and toads. Hybrid frogs *(Rana nigromaculata* and *Rana plancyi)* developed pancreatic carcinomas in which C-type retrovirus particles were identified by electron microscopy but, although virions were seen in unaffected tissue, a cause and effect were not established.

Caliciviruses

There is a single report of isolation of a calicivirus from an amphibian, Bell's horned frog *(Ceratophrys ornata)*.

No clinical or pathologic syndrome was definitively associated with the agent.

SUMMARY

Infectious agents, environmental factors, and immune system integrity exist in a delicate balance in any species, but perhaps particularly so in amphibians. Viruses have now been shown to be responsible for clinical and pathologic syndromes formerly attributed to bacteria. However, large gaps remain in our knowledge of amphibian viruses. including the pathogenesis and pathogenicity of the various strains, longevity of immunity, factors that trigger viral recrudescence, and whether exposed healthy individuals represent threats to unexposed individuals. Prospective studies on the prevalence of viral infections in captive collections may help fill these gaps and enable more informed decisions to be made in regard to the health management and conservation of amphibians.

REFERENCES

1. Bollinger TK, Mao J, Schock D, et al: Pathology, isolation, and preliminary molecular characterization of a novel iridovirus from tiger salamanders in Saskatchewan. J Wildl Dis 35:413–429, 1999.
2. Bryan LK, Baldwin CA, Gray MJ, et al: Efficacy of select disinfectants at inactivating *Ranavirus*. Dis Aquat Organ 84:89–94, 2009.
3. Chinchar VG, Hyatt A, Miyazaki T, Williams T: Family Iridoviridae: Poor viral relations no longer. Curr Top Microbiol Immunol 328:123–170, 2009.
4. Chinchar VG, Mao JH: Molecular diagnosis of iridovirus infections in cold-blooded animals. Semin Avian Exotic Pet Med 9:27–35, 2000.
5. Cunningham AA, Hyatt AD, Russell P, et al: Emerging epidemic diseases of frogs in Britain are dependent on the source of ranavirus agent and the route of exposure. Epidemiol Infect 135:1200–1212, 2007.
6. Cunningham AA, Tems CA, Russell PH: Immunohistochemical demonstration of *Ranavirus* antigen in the tissues of infected frogs *(Rana temporaria)* with systemic haemorrhagic or cutaneous ulcerative disease. J Comp Pathol 138:3–11, 2008.
7. Driskell EA, Miller DL, Swist SL, et al: PCR detection of *Ranavirus* in adult anurans from the Louisville Zoological Garden. J Zoo Wildl Med 40:559–563, 2009.
8. Gray MJ, Miller DL, Hoverman JT: First report of ranavirus infecting lungless salamanders. Herpetol Rev 40:316–319, 2009.
9. Green DE, Converse KA, Schrader AK: Epizootiology of sixty-four amphibian mortality events in the USA, 1996-2001. Ann N Y Acad Sci 969:323–339, 2002.
10. Greer AL, Collins JP: Sensitivity of a diagnostic test for amphibian *Ranavirus* varies with sampling protocol. J Wildl Dis 43:525–532, 2007.
11. Jancovich JK, Davidson EW, Morado JF, et al: Isolation of a lethal virus from the endangered tiger salamander *Ambystoma tigrinum stebbinsi*. Dis Aquat Org 31:161–167, 1997.
12. Johnson AJ, Wellehan FX: Amphibian virology. Vet Clin North Am Exot Anim Pract 8:53–65, 2005.

13. Mao J, Green DE, Fellers G, et al: Molecular characterization of iridoviruses isolated from sympatric amphibians and fish. Virus Res 63:45–52, 1999.

14. Mazzoni R, de Mesquita AJ, Fleury LFF, et al: Mass mortality associated with a frog virus 3-like Ranavirus infection in farmed tadpoles Rana catesbeiana from Brazil. Dis Aquat Organ 86:181–191, 2009.

15. Miller DL, Rajeev S, Brookins M, et al: Concurrent infection with *Ranavirus, Batrachochytrium dendrobatidis*, and *Aeromonas* in a captive anuran colony. J Zoo Wildl Med 39:445–449 2008.

16. Miller DL, Rajeev S, Gray MJ, et al: Frog virus 3 infection, cultured American bullfrogs, 2007 [letter] (http://www.cdc.gov/eid/content/13/2/342.htm).

17. OIE (World Organization for Animal Health): Infection with ranavirus, 2008 (http://www.oie.int/aac/eng/Publicat/Cardsenglish/Ranavirus%20card_final.pdf).

18. Pallister J, Gould A, Harrison D, et al: Development of real-time PCR assays for the detection and differentiation of Australian and European ranaviruses. J Fish Dis 30:427–438, 2007.

19. Pasmans F, Blahak S, Martel A, et al: Ranavirus-associated mass mortality in imported red-tailed knobby newts *(Tylototriton kweichowensis):* A case report. Vet J 176:257–259, 2008.

20. Pessier AP, Mendelson JR III, editors: A manual for control of infectious diseases in amphibian survival assurance colonies and reintroduction programs, 2010 (http://www.cbsg.org/cbsg/workshopreports/26/amphibian_disease_manual.pdf).

21. Robert J, Abramowitz L, Gantress J, et al: Xenopus laevis: A possible vector of Ranavirus infection. J Wildl Dis 43:645–652, 2007.

22. Rojas S, Richards K, Jancovich JK, Davidson EW: Influence of temperature on Ranavirus infection in larval salamanders Ambystoma tigrinum. Dis Aquat Org 63:95–100, 2005.

23. Rollins-Smith LA: The role of amphibian antimicrobial peptides in protection of amphibians from pathogens linked to global amphibian declines. Biochim Biophys Acta 1788:1593–1599, 2009.

24. Schock DM, Bollinger TK, Chinchar VG, et al: Experimental evidence that amphibian ranaviruses are multi-host pathogens. Copeia 2008:133–143, 2008.

25. St-Amour V, Lesbarreres D: Genetic evidence of *Ranavirus* in toe clips: An alternative to lethal sampling methods. Conserv Genet 8:1247–1250, 2007.

CHAPTER 31

Sea Turtle Rehabilitation

Terry M. Norton and Michael T. Walsh

CONSERVATION STATUS

There are seven living species of sea turtles, including the flatback *(Natator depressus)*, green sea turtle *(Chelonia mydas)*, hawksbill *(Eretmochelys imbricata)*, Kemp's Ridley *(Lepidochelys kempii)*, leatherback *(Dermochelys coriacea)*, loggerhead *(Caretta caretta)*, and olive Ridley *(Lepidochelys olivacea)*.[17] Sea turtles are found in all oceans except for the Arctic. All species of sea turtles residing in U.S. waters are listed as either "threatened" or "endangered" under the Endangered Species Act (ESA).

Significant threats to sea turtle populations include loss of habitat, light pollution, marine debris ingestion or entanglement, contaminant exposure, poaching and legal use of their meat, eggs, and body parts for a variety of purposes, fishery and boat strike mortality, harmful algal blooms, cold stunning, and infectious disease (Fig. 31-1).[17] (See the following websites for further information: http://www.oceana.org/seaturtles; www.seaturtle.org, http://www.widecast.org/Resources/Pubs.html; http://www.nestscertified.org/pdf/Lighting TechReport.pdf.)

TRANSPORT, HISTORY, AND PHYSICAL EXAMINATION

Live stranded sea turtles should be confined in a sturdy container with foam padding and transported in a temperature-controlled vehicle to the closest rehabilitation facility. A thorough history, visual examination, and detailed systematic physical examination should be performed.[23] Digital images may be used to document specific lesions or injuries. Body weight and standardized morphometric measurements should be obtained. A subjective and calculated body condition score (weight/carapace length [CL])[3] should be recorded and then measured serially during rehabilitation. Deep cloacal temperature may be representative of the turtle's recent environmental temperature and is an important parameter to obtain and monitor. A digital, distant laser, thermal monitoring device (Raynger ST, Raytek, Santa Cruz, Calif) directed at the prefemoral area correlates well with core body temperature. Heart rate and rhythm may be assessed with a Doppler probe placed on the skin between the distal cervical region and proximal front flipper. A standardized neurologic examination and workup should be performed if the patient exhibits neurologic signs.[7]

Critical Care Facilities

Debilitated turtles are often dry-docked on a padded surface and kept moist by regular misting and placing Vaseline or water-soluble jelly (K-Y Jelly) on the skin and shell. Another option is to have recirculated, temperature-controlled, filtered water sprayed over the turtle to keep it wet and prevent drowning. Water levels in rehabilitation tanks should be adjustable to accommodate turtles with varying degrees of debilitation. Water temperature should be kept warmer for newly arrived and ill patients (26.5° C to 29.5° C) to improve their immune function and then slowly decreased as the condition improves. Prior to release, the turtle should be acclimated to current ocean temperatures. Sea turtles require specially designed, circular, nonabrasive fiberglass tanks with a filtration system and continuous flow temperature-controlled salt water. The entire life support system should be outside the tank because sea turtles will destroy and ingest almost anything. It is recommended to quarantine new arrivals. Outdoor enclosures with direct and indirect sunlight or full-spectrum lighting with a natural photoperiod are beneficial.

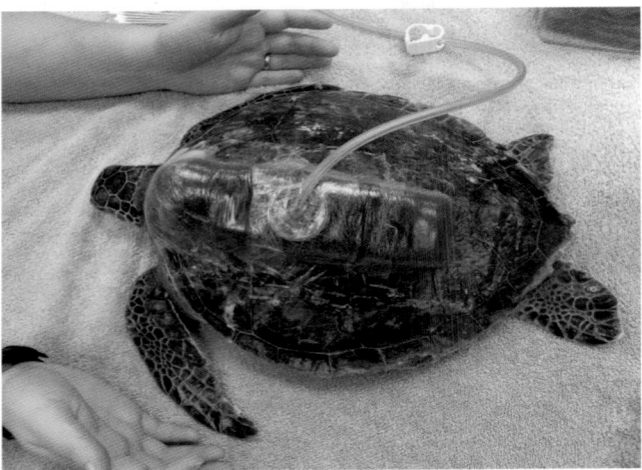

Figure 31-1

Vacuum-assisted closure therapy in a green sea turtle with a boat strike injury.

NUTRITION IN CRITICALLY ILL AND HEALTHY SEA TURTLES

The patient should be well hydrated, have a normal blood glucose level, and some evidence of active gastrointestinal tract (GIT) motility prior to starting oral nutritional support. Begin with smaller volumes and more dilute solutions and steadily increase both to meet the turtle's nutritional requirements. Tube feeding may be a challenge in sea turtles. The volume of material accepted is usually less than predicted because gastric tubes often do not pass into the stomach, increasing the likelihood of regurgitation. A variety of feeding tube sizes and types are used, depending on the size of the turtle. Vegetable oil is used to lubricate the tube. The distance from the beak to the estimated anterior portion of the stomach should be marked on the tube. The patient is placed at a 45-degree incline on a padded board or held in this position in smaller patients to avoid regurgitation. The head and neck should be extended to straighten the esophagus for tube passage, with the head secured by grasping on either side behind the mandible. Steady downward pressure will cause the lower jaw to fatigue and open. A padded speculum is used to keep the mouth open. The turtle is held in this position after tube removal until it swallows to reduce the chances of regurgitation. To avoid possible inhalation, turtles may be placed back in the water to clear the oral cavity of any unwanted material. Esophagostomy tubes are used when necessary. Critical care products (Oxbow Pet Products, Murdock, Neb), fish-based gruels, Ensure (Abbott Laboratories, Abbott Park, Ill), Vital

(Abbott), and Peptomen (Nestle Health Care Nutrition, Minnetonka, Minn) are used alone or in combination for tube feeding depending on the patient's status. An experimental Mazuri tube feeding formula has been developed to replace fish gruels and has shown some promise. Although green turtles are herbivores, they may require a calorie-dense formula when emaciated. Formulas may be supplemented with glucose or honey to maintain adequate blood glucose levels and Pancreazyme (Virbac Animal Health, Fort Worth, Tex) to aid in digestion. Hyperalimentation has been used in selected cases.

Critically ill sea turtles may be fed filleted fish supplemented with calcium until they are defecating regularly. At first, high-protein, low-fat fish, such as smelt or capelin, are good choices; squid and clams take longer to digest and should be avoided initially. Fish may need to be cut into smaller pieces for smaller turtles. Bones, beaks, and chitinous materials may be slowly added back to the diet as the turtle starts defecating more regularly. Holding food in front of the nostrils may help in getting turtles to start eating. Emaciated green turtles may be fed predominantly seafood to improve body condition and then more dark green vegetables may slowly be added. Supplementing the diet with live and fresh-frozen natural prey items is important, especially prior to release back to the wild. Appropriate seafood storage, thawing, and handling protocols should be followed. A fish-based multivitamin containing thiamine (25 mg/kg of fish) and vitamin E (100 IU/kg of fish) should be provided daily. Iron supplementation should be provided and, ideally, based on plasma iron levels. General rules of thumb for the percentage of body weight in food to feed healthy sea turtles are hatchlings, 5%; yearlings, 1.5% to 3%; 2-year-olds, 1.5%; and then approximately 0.8% thereafter. Weight trends and body condition scores should be used for determining the amount to feed. Nutritionally complete gelatin diets are recommended for hatchlings being maintained in captivity for any length of time.[23]

Diagnostic Procedures

An emergency minimum database should consist of a hematocrit, total solids, glucose level and, subsequently, a complete blood count and plasma biochemical panel. A blood sample for culture should be collected before initiating antimicrobial therapy. We recommend taking up to 0.5 to 0.8 mL of blood/100 g body weight in healthy patients and a reduced sample volume for debilitated patients. Lithium or sodium heparin are the anticoagulants of choice, because ethylenediaminetetraacetic acid (EDTA) will cause red blood cell lysis. Plasma is preferred over serum because clot formation is unpredictable and may cause changes in the chemical composition of the sample and the higher volume of plasma obtained.

The preferred blood collection sites in most sea turtle species are the dorsal cervical or occipital sinus.[32] The head and neck should be extended and difficult to bleed turtles (e.g., green turtles) may be positioned with the head directed in a ventral position. The lateral jugular vein is an alternative site for green turtles and the femoral and interdigital vessels are alternatives in leatherbacks.[30] Lymph contamination may occur. Morphologic classification of blood cells[6] and normal reference ranges for complete blood count, clinical chemistry, and plasma electrophoresis for the various sea turtle species have been reported.[4,10,15,21] (See http:// accstr.ufl.edu/blood_chem.htm for ongoing clinical pathology reference values.)

Radiography is an important diagnostic tool used to assess sea turtle patients. Radiopaque materials such as barnacles should be removed from the shell before performing a radiographic study. Anteroposterior and lateral projections using a horizontal x-ray beam and a dorsoventral (DV) view should be performed. Larger turtles may require multiple radiographs to assess the entire coelom from a DV view. Digestive tract radiographic contrast procedures are often necessary to document intestinal obstruction, motility disorders, and foreign bodies. Normal transit times have been established for barium sulfate and nonionic iodinate contrast media.[11] Barium-impregnated polyethylene spheres may be placed in a food item, with subsequent serial radiography to assess gastrointestinal motility. Ultrasonography has been used to evaluate reproductive status and for general diagnostic purposes. Computed tomography (CT) is useful for assessing spinal and head injuries, free air pockets in the coelom, pneumonia, bronchiolar blockage, and internal fibropapillomatosis, although large sea turtles will not fit into most CT chambers. Normal skull CT anatomy has been established in loggerheads.[2] Open magnetic resonance imaging (MRI) is useful for larger sea turtles and normal MRI internal anatomic structures have been established in loggerhead sea turtles.[29] This technology has been used to detect internal fibropapillomas.[9]

Rigid endoscopy has been used for gender determination, evaluation of reproductive activity, exploring the coelomic cavity, organ biopsy for histopathology, and confirming the presence or absence of internal fibropapillomas. The technique has been described by Wyneken J, Mader DR, Weber ES, et al.[32] Rigid and flexible endoscopy may be used to evaluate the cloaca, bladder, and distal GIT and to administer contrast media and enemas into the rectum. Rigid and flexible systems may be used to visualize the location of fish hooks in the esophagus. Flexible endoscopes may be used to evaluate the upper and lower GIT, trachea, bronchi, and anterior lung and for the removal of granulomatous material from the bronchial lumen.

Treatment

As noted, treatment of hypothermia, dehydration, hypoglycemia, and acid-base and electrolyte imbalances should be done in conjunction with starting other therapeutic agents. It is best to keep the sea turtle patient at its preferred optimal temperature zone while on therapy. Culture and sensitivity of various samples should be determined prior to starting antimicrobial therapy whenever possible. The front half of the body should be used for injections, especially when using nephrotoxic drugs. Anaerobic bacteria should be considered when deciding on a therapeutic plan. Several pharmacokinetic studies in sea turtles have significantly advanced treatment capabilities (Table 31-1).[20,23]

Most sea turtles presented for emergency care are dehydrated. Hypoglycemia or hyperglycemia is common, so blood glucose determination is essential for choosing the appropriate fluid therapy. Most crystalloid fluids may be used in sea turtles[23]; however, overhydration is of particular concern in hypoproteinemic patients. Colloidal fluids may be more appropriate in these cases. Whole-blood transfusions using acid citrate dextrose are indicated in cases of acute hemorrhage and life-threatening anemia (5% or less). Fluid therapy, vitamin K, antibiotics, iron supplementation, and other supportive measures are often successful in less severe cases. A purified bovine hemoglobin (Oxyglobin, Dechra Veterinary Products, Overland Park, Kan) has had limited clinical use in sea turtles, with mixed results. Procrit (Epoetin AFA, Centocur Ortho Biotech, Horsham, Pa) has been used in conjunction with iron and nutritional support and has been helpful in treating nonregenerative anemias. Intravenous (IV) or intraosseous (IO) routes of fluid administration allow for rapid rehydration. Ultrasound is helpful for placing IV catheters. Bolus IV fluid therapy via the cervical sinus is often used for initial stabilization. The intracoelomic (IC) route via the inguinal fossa is commonly used for maintenance fluid therapy and allows for crystalloid fluids with up to

TABLE 31-1   Antimicrobials Used in Sea Turtle Patients

Drug	Dosage and Frequency	Comments
Amikacin (A)	2.5-3.0 mg/kg IM q72h	Targets primarily gram-negative bacteria, potentially nephrotoxic
Ceftazidime (C)	20 mg/kg* SC, IM, IV q72h[22]	Same as above but less nephrotoxic
Chloramphenicol	30-50 mg/kg IM q24h; 50 mg/kg PO q24h	Bacteriostatic, aerobic, and anaerobic antibacterial spectrum
Clindamycin	5 mg/kg PO, IM q24h	Anaerobic spectrum; use in combination with A, C, E
Enrofloxacin (E)	5 mg/kg SC/IM q 24-48h*;10-20 mg/kg PO q1wk[20]	Irritating to tissue; dilute when giving Sc
Metronidazole	20 mg/kg PO q24-48h[†]	Anaerobic bacteria, use with A, C, E
Fluconazole (F)	21-mg/kg loading dose,* then 10 mg/kg q5days SC, IV	
Intraconazole	5 mg/kg* PO SID or 15 mg/kg PO q72h	Better choice than F for most common fungal species
Acyclovir	80 mg/kg PO SID[†]	Cutaneous herpesvirus, not FP
Fenbendazole	25 mg/kg SID × 3 days, repeat in 2 wk	Bone marrow suppression
Pyrantel pamoate	10 mg/kg once, repeat in 2 wk	
Praziquantel	25 mg/kg* PO 3× in 1 day[22] or SID × 3 days	Use human form (Biltricide)

*Sea turtle pharmacokinetics.
[†]Other reptiles.

5% dextrose to be given. Subcutaneous fluids are placed in the inguinal fossa, medially in the front limb fossa and ventral neck fold. The oral route of fluid administration should be reserved for use in patients that are mildly dehydrated and maintenance fluid therapy. Placing the turtle in fresh water for 24 hours may be used for rehydration and reduction of epibiotic load. Maintenance fluid rates range from 10 to 25 mL/kg/day.

Physical Restraint, Analgesia, and Anesthesia

Small sea turtles should be grasped on the lateral margins of the shell and the flippers at the shoulder with both hands. Covering the eyes may be helpful for calming some turtles. Larger sea turtles should be firmly grasped on the carapace just caudal to the head with one hand and between the hind flippers with the other. Heavier animals may need numerous personnel or heavy equipment to lift. Healthy sea turtles will try to bite and slap their flippers. Small green turtles are prone to proximal humeral fractures during handling.

Pain may be exhibited by a decreased appetite, depression, or alteration in normal behavior, but is challenging to assess in sea turtles. Nonsteroidal anti-inflammatory drugs such as injectable meloxicam (0.4 mg/kg IM, IV SID for 7 to 10 days, but not absorbed

PO)[8] have been used. Adequate hydration and renal function are important. Opioid drugs have been used in other chelonians for pain control,[27] but further research is needed for sea turtles. Anesthesia or sedation should be used with caution in debilitated patients. Our preference for injectable anesthetics include the following:

1. Dexmedetomidine (D; 50 to 70 µg/kg) in combination with ketamine (K) (5 mg/kg) IM or IV. An opioid such as butorphanol (0.2 mg/kg) may be added for additional analgesia and sedation.
2. Telazol (tiletamine-zolazepam) at 0.05 mg/kg instead of K in combination with D
3. Propofol, 5 to 7 mg/kg IV initial dose, and then half-dose increments for supplementation

Recent deaths and unusually slow recoveries have been reported in small kemps with propofol.[5] It was subsequently determined that some lots of propofol were contaminated with steel which may been ultimately responsible for the problems. All the combinations are useful for relatively noninvasive procedures or for induction of general anesthesia. Intubation and ventilation support are recommended. Inhalant anesthetics are used for invasive or prolonged procedures. Both isoflurane and sevoflurane are used, with some decrease in recovery time noted with sevoflurane. Ventilation and thermoregulatory support should be maintained during the procedure and throughout the recovery period.

Local anesthetics may be used alone or in combination with injectable or inhalation anesthesia. Doppler or ultrasound to detect heart rate, transcutaneous CO_2 monitoring (tcP_{CO_2}), and electrocardiography are the most useful anesthetic monitoring tools.

Surgery

An understanding of normal anatomy is critical in sea turtle medicine and surgery (see the review by Wyneken[31]). The most common surgical approach to the coelomic cavity is the inguinal technique allowing the exteriorization of the intestinal tract from jejunum to colon and access to the female reproductive tract.[12,23,32] The left axillary region has been used to remove gastric foreign bodies. In small greens, the central plastron is not ossified; thus, we have found that a medial incision with two flaps retaining soft tissue integrity laterally for the retention of blood supply provides excellent exposure to the coelom for hook and line removal. Suture patterns should emphasize good apposition because dehiscence is common. Poliglecaperone 25 and polyglyconate are preferred suture materials.[16]

COMMON MEDICAL ISSUES

Drowning

Sea turtles are frequently captured or entangled in nets or fishing lines and may be trapped underwater for extended periods of time. Some turtles may present in a comatose state and recover with cardiopulmonary resuscitation.[23] A marked acidemia and lactic acidosis are common. Once intubated, place the turtle with its head down to drain fluid from the lungs and suction fluid from the endotracheal tube. Limb and head pumping or intermittent positive-pressure ventilation should be performed until the patient is ventilating on its own.

Marine Debris Ingestion

Sea turtles commonly ingest nonbiodegradable materials. Sometimes, these items are passed by the turtle without any problems; however, they may cause irritation, lacerate the GIT, or lead to obstruction and death. Some marine debris such as oil and tar may be found on the skin or shell or may be ingested by the turtle. Fishhooks with a fishing line attached may become anchored in the oral cavity, esophagus, or other parts of the GIT and lead to intestinal plication, intussusception, or coelomitis secondary to hook penetration. A

relatively noninvasive hook removal technique has been used for midesophageal hooks and entails slightly prolapsing the mobile esophageal wall.[24] Dehooking devices are available but involve the risk of tearing the esophagus. Enemas, fluids, petroleum laxatives, and other supportive care may be all that are necessary; however, some cases require surgical intervention.

Biotoxin Ingestion

There have been episodes of mortality in sea turtles associated with brevetoxicosis in Florida[19] and saxitoxins in El Salvador.[25] There have been a number of events in which biotoxins were suspected, although the cause was not determined[19] (see www.georgiaseaturtlecenter.org/blog/wp-content/uploads/2010/02/lndcmeeting synopsis.pdf).

Cold Stunning (Hypothermia)

Hypothermia in sea turtles occurs when the water temperature suddenly drops below 10° C. The turtles lose their ability to swim and dive, and often float to the surface. Secondary complications are common but may not be apparent for several weeks.[23] Electrolyte alterations and metabolic and respiratory acidosis are common.[18] Body temperature and heart rate are used for monitoring treatment progress. Increase the body temperature 3° C/day until it reaches 24° C. Turtles may be warmed up more rapidly if they are fairly responsive. Treatment of open wounds, corneal lesions, and supportive care should be started immediately; antimicrobial therapy is initiated when the turtle's temperature reaches 16° C to 19° C.

Ileus

Gastrointestinal stasis is a common finding in ill sea turtles and should be differentiated from true obstruction. Ileus is precipitated by dehydration, foreign bodies, systemic disease, gastroenterocolitis, and malnutrition. These turtles often develop an impaction by chitinous and shell prey items parts, which is usually resolved with fluids, mineral oil, motility-modifying drugs, enemas, highly absorbable feeding formulas, and low-residue foods.

Buoyancy Disorders

Any condition leading to gas or air accumulation in the intestinal tract, coelomic cavity, or pulmonary disease may cause abnormal buoyancy. A primary diagnosis should be determined. Coelomic free air should be aspirated by tilting the turtle on its side and directing the head ventrally to bring the air pocket up to the inguinal space. An extension set, appropriately sized needle, three-way stopcock, and syringe are used to remove the air. Suction machines have been used in larger turtles. Laparoscopic surgery has been used to repair a lung tear in a sea turtle.[13] Some turtles, especially those with spinal injuries, may remain abnormally buoyant for life.

Fibropapillomatosis

Fibropapillomatosis (FP), caused by a herpesvirus, is the most significant infectious disease affecting sea turtle populations worldwide. Since the mid-1980s, FP has been observed with increased frequency, with a very high local prevalence in some green turtle populations.[14] The disease has been documented in most sea turtle species but is most common and severe in greens. The prevalence of the disease is associated with heavily polluted coastal areas, areas of high human density, agricultural runoff, and/or biotoxin-producing algae.[23] FP-affected turtles may have a depressed immune system. FP may have a presentation ranging from very mild, solitary, wartlike masses on the skin to numerous very large masses covering the skin, shell, eyelids, conjunctiva, and cornea. The disease may impair the turtle's mobility and vision, leading to severe emaciation and eventual death. Internal organs may be affected, which may be identified by radiography, advanced imaging, and laparoscopy. Humane euthanasia is recommended

in these cases. Initial treatment consists of supportive care and antimicrobial therapy. Laser surgery is the preferred surgical modality to remove the tumors. Table 31-2 summarizes the significant infectious and parasitic diseases that have been documented in sea turtles.

Traumatic Injuries and Wound Care

Sea turtles presenting to rehabilitation centers commonly have skin and shell wounds caused by traumas such as boat strikes, shark bites, fishing gear entanglements, entrapment in dredging equipment, dropping on a boat deck after incidental capture, and wounds developing secondary to cold stunning or attached epibionts. Basic principles of wound care, such as débridement and heavy irrigation, should be followed. Waterproof bandaging techniques are commonly used. Topical wound care products used successfully in sea turtles include a variety of silver-containing products, natural honey and sterile honey products (Medihoney, Wound Central, Plainfield, Ill). Products used to pack into deep wounds include silver sulfadiazine cream (Kings Pharmaceutical, Bristol, Tex) mixed with ilex paste (Medcon Biolab Technologies, Grafton, Mass) and honey mixed with honeycomb (Fig. 31-2). Petroleum-impregnated gauze may aid in further waterproofing. A combination of Tegaderm (3M, St. Paul, Minn), waterproof tape, and super glue is used to create a watertight bandage. In areas that are difficult to bandage, suture loops may be placed around the wound with umbilical tape placed through the suture loops and tied together to hold the bandage materials in place. Tricide-Neo

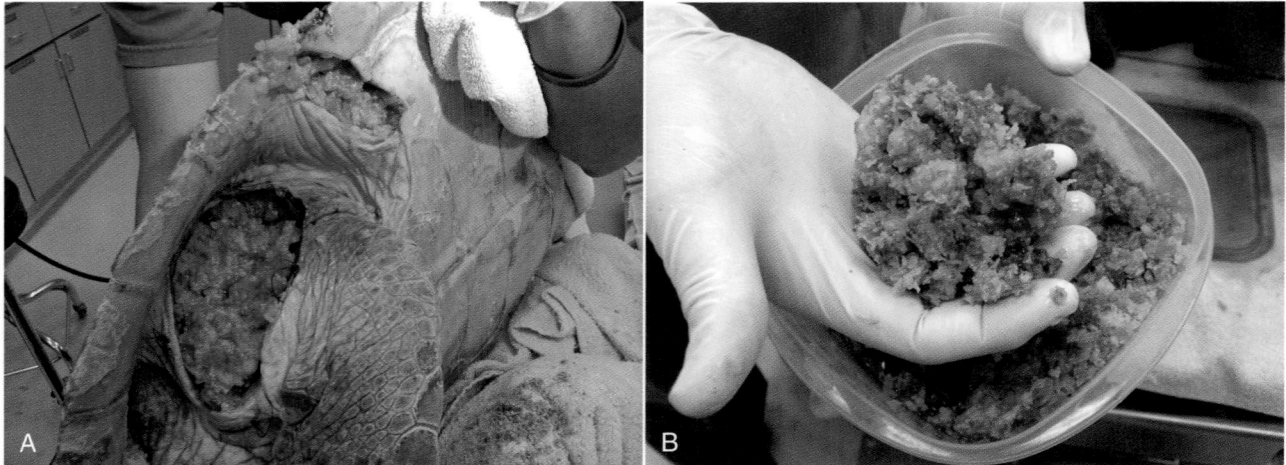

Figure 31-2

Honey and honeycomb used to pack deep propeller wounds in a loggerhead sea turtle.

TABLE 31-2 Selected Infectious Disease Agents and Parasites

Pathogen	Site or Type of Infection	Treatment	Comments
External Parasites, Epibiota			
Barnacles, tunicates, bivalves, algae, leeches, others	Carapace, head, oral cavity	Fresh water soak, manual removal	85 epibionts documented on normal loggerheads
Internal Parasites			
Spirorchidae spp., digenetic trematode	Cardiovascular; eggs to the viscera, arterioles	Praziquantel for adults	Eggs cause foreign body inflammation
Caryospora cheloniae	Large intestine, extraintestinal		High mortality in captive, wild
Eimeria spp., coccidia	Adrenal glands, leatherback		Unknown significance
Anasakis nematode	Gastric ulceration	Fenbendazole	
Lungworms	Loggerheads trachea, main bronchi	Fenbendazole	
Bacteria			
Salmonella	Intestinal tract	Oral antibiotics	Zoonotic
Opportunistic gram-negatives	Granuloma, pneumonia, gastrenterocolitis, septicemia	Antibiotics	
Corynebacterium	Brain		
Chlamydia	Cardiac, hepatic		Captive only
Mycobacterium	Osteomyelitis		Kemp's Ridley predisposed
Nocardia	Osteomyelitis		
Anaerobic bacteria		Antibiotics	
Fungal Agent			
Candida	Gastroenterocolitis	Nystatin, other antifungals	
Aspergillus, Mucor, Geotrichium, Penicillium, Cladosporidium, Rhizopus, Sportrichium, Basidiobolus, Fusarium, Paecilomyces spp.	Osteomyelitis, pneumonia, granulomas	Itraconazole	
Viral Agent			
Herpesvirus	Lung, eye, trachea, skin[28]		
	Loggerhead, genital, respiratory[28]		
	Loggerhead or cutaneous[28]		
	Fibropapilloma		
Papillomavirus	Proliferative dermatitis[22]		

ointment (Koi Depot of San Diego, Lakeside, Calif),[26] Doxirobe gel (Pfizer Animal Health, Exton, Pa), and bone cement impregnated with antibiotics have been used on exposed shell bone and can be maintained in the water without a bandage. A modified vacuum-assisted wound care protocol has been successfully used, with benefits previously described for other species.[1]

REFERENCES

1. Adkesson MJ, Travis EK, Weber MA, Kirby JP, et al: Vacuum-assisted closure for treatment of a deep shell abscess and osteomyelitis in a tortoise. J Am Vet Med Assoc 231:1249–1254, 2007.
2. Arencibia A, Rivero MA, Casal AB, et al: CT and cross-sectional anatomy of the normal head of the loggerhead sea turtle (*Carreta caretta*). Anatom Histol Embryol 34(Suppl 1):3–31, 2005.
3. Bolten AB: Techniques for measuring sea turtles. In Eckert KL, Bjorndal KA, Alberto Abreu Grobois F, Donnelly M, editors: Research and management techniques for the conservation of sea turtles, 1999 (http://www.iucn-mtsg.org/Publications/Tech_Manual/Tech_Manual_en/23-godfrey.pdf).
4. Bolten AB, Bjorndal KA: Blood profiles for a wild population of green turtles (*Chelonia mydas*) in the southern bahamas: size-specific and sex-specific relationships. J Wildl Dis 28:407–413, 1992.
5. Boylan S: Personal communication, 2009.
6. Casal AB, Oros J: Morphologic and cytochemical characteristics of blood cells of juvenile loggerhead sea turtles (*Caretta caretta*). Res Vet Sci 82:158–165, 2007.

7. Chrisman CL, Walsh MT, Meeks JC, et al: Neurologic examination of sea turtles. J Am Vet Med Assoc 211:1043-1047, 1997.
8. Clauss T: Personal communication, 2010.
9. Croft LA, Graham JP, Schaf SA, et al: Evaluation of magnetic resonance imaging for detection of internal tumors in green turtles with cutaneous fibropapillomatosis. J Am Vet Med Assoc 225:1428-1435, 2004.
10. Deem SL, Dierenfeld ES, Sounguet GP, et al: Blood values in free-ranging nesting leatherback sea turtles (Dermochelys coriacea) on the coast of the republic of gabon. J Zoo Wildl Med 37:464-471, 2006.
11. DiBello A, Valastro C, Staffieri F: Contrast radiography of the gastrointestinal tract in sea turtles. Vet Rad and Ultrasound 47:351-354, 2006.
12. Di Bello A, Valastro C, Staffieri F: Surgical approach to the coelomic cavity through the axillary and inguinal regions in sea turtles. J Am Vet Med Assoc 228:922-925, 2006.
13. Dover S: Personal communication, 2004.
14. Foley AM, Schroeder BA, Redlow AE, et al: Fibropapillomatosis in stranded green turtles (Chelonian mydas) from the eastern United States (1980-98): trends and associations with environmental factors. J Wildl Dis 41:29-41, 2005.
15. Gicking J, Foley AM, Har KE, et al: Plasma protein electrophoresis of the atlantic loggerhead sea turtle. J Herpetol Med Surg 14:14-18, 2004.
16. Govett PD, Harms CA, Linder KE, et al: Effect of four different suture materials on the surgical wound healing of loggerhead sea turtles, Caretta caretta. J Herpetol Med Surg 14:6-10, 2004.
17. Gulko D, Eckert K: Sea turtles, an ecological guide, Honolulu, 2004, Mutual Publishing.
18. Innis CJ, Tlusty M, Merigo C, et al: Metabolic and respiratory status of cold-stunned kemp's ridley sea turtles (Lepidochelys kempii). J Comp Physiol B 177:623-630, 2007.
19. Jacobson ER, Homer BL, Stacy BA, et al: Neurological disease in wild loggerhead sea turtles Caretta caretta. Dis Aquat Org 70:139-154, 2006.
20. Jacobson E, Gronwall R, Maxwell L, et al: Plasma concentrations of enrofloxacin after single-dose oral administration in loggerhead sea turtles (Caretta caretta). J Zoo Wildl Med 36:628-634, 2005.
21. Kakizoe Y, Sakaoka K, Kakizoe F, et al: Successive changes of hematologic characteristics and plasma chemistry values of juvenile loggerhead turtles (Caretta caretta). J Zoo Wildl Med 38:77-84, 2007.
22. Manire CA, Stacy BA, Kinsel MJ, et al: Proliferative dermatitis in a loggerhead turtle, Caretta caretta, and a green turtle, Chelonia mydas, associated with novel papillomaviruses. Vet Microbiol 130:227-237, 2008.
23. Norton TM: Chelonian emergency and critical care. Semin Avian Exotic Pet Med 14:106-130, 2005.
24. Parga M, Pont S, Ninou FAI: Ten years removing hooks from accidentally caught wild loggerhead turtles (Caretta caretta) [abstract]. In Proceedings of the Joint Conference of the American Association of Zoo Veterinarians: Wildlife Disease Association, 2004, pp 501-502 (http://www.wildlifedisease.org/Documents/Proceedings/San_Diego_04.pdf).
25. Red tide causes el salvador turtle deaths, 2006 (http://www.seaturtle.org/mtn/archives/mtn113/mtn113p19.shtml).
26. Ritchie B: Personal communication, 2010.
27. Sladky KK, Miletic V, Paul Murphy J, et al: Analgesic efficacy and respiratory effects of butorphanol and morphine in turtles. J Am Vet Med Assoc 230:1356-1362, 2007.
28. Stacy BA, Wellehan JFX, Foley AM, et al: Two herpesviruses associated with disease in wild atlantic loggerhead sea turtles (Caretta caretta). Vet Microbiol 126:63-73, 2008.
29. Valente ALS, Cuenca R, Zamora MA, et al: Sectional anatomic and magnetic resonance imaging features of coelomic structures of loggerhead sea turtles. Am J Vet Res 67:1347-1353, 2006.
30. Wallace BP, George RH: Alternative techniques for obtaining blood samples from leatherback turtles. chelonian Conserv Biol 6:147-149, 2007.
31. Wyneken J: The anatomy of sea turtles, 2001 (http://courses.science.fau.edu/~jwyneken/sta).
32. Wyneken J, Mader DR, Weber ES, et al: Medical care of sea turtles. In Mader DR editor: Reptile medicine and surgery, ed 2, St. Louis, 2006, Elsevier, pp 972-1007.

CHAPTER 32

Reptile and Amphibian Analgesia

Ann Duncan

The last 2 decades have seen improved understanding of the mechanisms of nociception and importance of treating pain in vertebrates of all classes. The treatment of pain has become standard practice in veterinary medicine, because there is a moral imperative to treat pain and alleviation of pain has been found to facilitate anesthetic recovery and healing in animals.[6] At one time, it was assumed that lower vertebrates were less capable of perceiving pain and distress, but the current understanding is that pain perception in these species is likely to be analogous to that in mammals.[11] In a survey of 367 members of the Association of Reptile and Amphibian Veterinarians, 98.4% of respondents stated that they believe that reptiles and amphibians feel pain.[15] Despite this, only 39.5% regularly provided analgesia to their patients. Veterinarians treating reptiles and amphibians have historically used empirical dosing and anecdotal observations to guide treatment of pain. Recently, methods for measuring antinociception have been successfully adapted to amphibians and reptiles, allowing data for these taxonomic groups to expand (Table 32-1). Despite these advances, large gaps remain regarding analgesic efficacy, pharmacokinetics, and toxic side effects for many commonly used analgesics. Although the long-term goal is to develop specific dosages for all classes of reptiles and amphibians, those charged with the care of these animals must make judicious use of current knowledge to treat pain.

PAIN PATHWAYS AND MECHANISMS: THE CASE FOR PAIN

The evidence for pain in reptiles and amphibians is found by the following: (1) behavioral responses to painful stimuli; (2) identification of pain pathways; and (3) demonstration of effective analgesia. It is often difficult to recognize when an animal is in pain, and even more difficult to characterize and measure their pain objectively. Even in the case of human medicine, in which patients are able to provide verbal information, quantification is subjective and may vary among individuals experiencing similar painful stimuli. Characterizing normal versus abnormal behavior and discriminating behaviors indicative of pain are crucial to the understanding of pain in animals. Behavioral responses arising from a finite, overt, painful stimulus, such as a toe pinch or pinprick, may be easier to recognize than behaviors arising from chronic pain. Pain associated with a healing surgical incision or chronic disease process is less likely to stimulate vigorous activity and more likely to cause nonspecific subtle changes, such as inactivity, changes in posture, and loss of appetite. In a clinical setting, it is often this chronic pain that needs to be recognized and treated.

Behaviors arising from pain vary considerably among species. Prey species are more likely to survive if they avoid showing pain-associated behaviors that might attract predation. During examination or observation, these animals are more likely to be stoic and hide signs of discomfort. Alternatively, in predators, you might see aggression in an animal that is normally passive and tractable. Although loss of appetite and increased heart and respiratory rates may be seen in many vertebrates experiencing pain, absence of these changes does not ensure comfort. Amphibians may respond to pain by spending more time in atypical locations in their environment, such as on the ground versus on perching locations or on land versus in water. They may show color changes, postural changes, or flick or wipe at the site of pain. Chelonians may show discomfort by stretching their head and neck in and out of the shell, biting when handled, or closing their eyes. Snakes may become restless, easily startled, or appear agitated during

TABLE 32-1	Dosages According to Analgesia Research Findings		
Species	Agent	Dosage	Comments
Red-eared sliders	Morphine	1.5 mg/kg SC	Effect at 4 hr, lasts 8+ hr
		6.5 mg/kg SC	Effect at 2 hr, lasts 8+ hr
	Buprenorphine	0.075 mg/kg SC	Give in forelimb, lasts 24+ hr
	Tramadol	10 mg/kg PO	Lasts 6-96 hr
		10 mg/kg SC	Lasts 12-48 hr
Green iguanas	Butorphanol	1.5 mg/kg IM	May not provide analgesia for all noxious stimuli
	Ketoprofen	2 mg/kg IM	Lasts >24 hr
	Meloxicam	0.2 mg/kg PO	Effect at 9 hr, lasts 24+ hr
Bearded dragons	Morphine	10-20 mg/kg SC	Effect at 8 hr
Snakes	Butorphanol	20 mg/kg SC	Very high dose, watch for adverse effects (e.g., respiratory depression)
Crocodilians	Morphine	0.3 mg/kg IC	Effect at ½ to 2 hr
Leopard frogs	Morphine	10 mg/kg IC	Effect at ¼ to 1 hr, lasts 12 hr
	Butorphanol	25 mg/kg IC	Effect at ¼ hr, lasts 8-12 hr
	Xylazine	10 mg/kg IC	Effect at ¼ hr, lasts 12- 24 hr
Red-spotted newts	Butorphanol	0.5 mg/liter bath	Continuous, 24 hr/day
	Buprenorphin	50 mg/kg IC	q24h

handling. They may also hold their bodies less coiled at the site of pain or tuck the affected area. Lizards may also show postural changes, including arching the back, head pressing, or tucking the abdomen. They may remain standing or seem to avoid recumbency, close their eyes, or elevate and extend their head. They may also scratch or flick their feet at the affected area or tense their abdomen during palpation.

Pain is the result of exchanges among three major components of the nervous system, the peripheral nerves, spinal cord, and brain. The basic anatomic, physiologic, and biochemical components of pain pathways that exist in mammals also exist in nonmammalian species.[1,8] In amphibians, four distinct afferent nerve fibers have been identified that are analogous to those found in mammals to transmit different types of noxious stimuli.[11] Afferent nerve fibers release neurotransmitters that activate neurons in the spinal cord, which then transmit electrical impulses to the thalamus region of the brain. In humans, the thalamus sends pain messages to three specialized regions of the brain. The somatosensory cortex identifies and localizes pain, the limbic system is responsible for emotional response and the experience of suffering, and the frontal cortex assigns meaning to pain. The limbic and cortical brain may then modulate the nociceptive signal with a number of endogenous substances that may act to increase or

decrease the pain experience. Amphibians and reptiles do not have the well-defined limbic cortex and neocortex typical of later evolved species, and the thalamocortical connections in frogs appear diffuse and poorly organized compared with those of mammals.[9] How these anatomic differences affect the perception of pain is unknown. Research has shown that reptiles and amphibians have similar endogenous mechanisms to modulate pain and that analgesia may be achieved through the use of pharmacologic agents used to treat pain in other species.[1,18,20-22]

DOSING PRINCIPLES AND SIDE EFFECTS

The diversity found within the reptile and amphibian classes is very broad, and analgesia research has been conducted only on a very limited number of species. Drugs with species-specific pharmacokinetic data and proven efficacy should be selected when possible; however, extrapolation is often necessary. As with other classes of drugs, clinicians rely on knowledge of basic physiology to inform empirical dosing. The metabolic rate of reptiles and amphibians is lower than that of mammals and, as poikilotherms, it is critical that they are maintained at their preferred optimum temperature zone during treatment. Dehydration and malnutrition may affect drug absorption and clearance and should be corrected prior to treatment, especially when using potentially nephrotoxic or hepatotoxic drugs. The site of drug administration may also affect pharmacokinetics. It has been shown that a substantial proportion of blood from the hindlimbs of turtles may drain directly to the liver.[7] Consequently, drugs that are extracted by first pass through the liver may have lower systemic availability when injected into the hindlimb, as observed in red-eared sliders being dosed with buprenorphine.[10]

The three major classes of analgesic drugs used in veterinary medicine are opioids, α-adrenergic agonists, and nonsteroidal anti-inflammatory drugs (NSAIDs). It is prudent to monitor for side effects seen in other species and administer all drugs judiciously in animals with concurrent disease. Common side effects seen with opioid administration in mammals include respiratory depression, gastrointestinal hypomotility and sedation, whereas NSAIDs have been associated with gastrointestinal irritation, cardiovascular side effects, platelet inhibition, and renal compromise. Many of these side effects will be more difficult to recognize antemortem in amphibians and reptiles. Postmortem findings will need to be correlated with the clinical use of analgesics. This is an area in which zoological collections could provide valuable information.

Veterinarians are often interested in providing analgesia at the time of anesthesia. Reptiles and amphibians undergoing biopsy, endoscopy, surgical treatment for trauma, or other procedures expected to be painful should be provided with analgesia. In general, it is recommended that analgesia be provided before a painful procedure (preemptive analgesia) to avoid sensitization of the nervous system and amplification of pain. In reptiles and amphibians, analgesics may need to be administered well before a procedure to achieve therapeutic levels. Monitoring anesthetic depth and parameters of cardiovascular and respiratory function may be difficult in amphibians and reptiles. Clinicians may be concerned that administering opioids or α_2 adrenergics will depress cardiovascular or respiratory reflexes, or prolong anesthetic recovery. A study comparing cardiovascular effects and blood gas changes during isoflurane or isoflurane and butorphanol anesthesia in the green iguana has found that preemptive or intraoperative use of butorphanol is unlikely to be detrimental to cardiac function.[12] It is of note that in both study groups, animals were mechanically ventilated during the study and the effects on respiration were not measured. Therefore, more research is needed to determine the affect of providing analgesia at the time of anesthesia.

REPTILE RESEARCH FINDINGS

Chelonia: Turtles and Tortoises

Among neuropeptides, the opioids are the most potent analgesics and are classified according to their receptor subtypes, including mu, delta, and kappa receptors. Few studies have been undertaken to determine which opioid receptor types are involved in analgesia in reptiles. Mu and delta receptors are located throughout the brain in red-eared sliders. The delta receptors are more abundant; however, it is thought that they play a lesser role in antinociception.[18] Butorphanol is considered the most widely administered analgesic in reptiles; therefore, demonstrating efficacy and determining dosages is a priority.[15] Red-eared slider turtles were used in a study to determine the thermal antinociception efficacy of morphine and butorphanol.[19] Morphine administered IM at low (1.5 mg/kg) and high (6.5 mg/kg) doses significantly increased hindlimb withdrawal latencies, showing effects after 2 to 4 hours that lasted at least 8 hours postadministration. The higher dose provided more rapid onset but otherwise similar results. At 24 hours postadministration, some increase in withdrawal latencies remained, but the results were not significant. An unexpected finding was that butorphanol at a dose of 2.8 or 28 mg/kg provided no thermal antinociception in red-eared sliders. Morphine is primarily a mu agonist with delta and kappa activities, and butorphanol is a kappa agonist and mu antagonist. Additional trials using selective agonists for each opioid receptor type have led to the conclusion that in red-eared sliders, thermal antinociception is a result of mu receptor activation.[18] Kappa receptor activation, either with a receptor-selective opioid or with butorphanol, was not found to produce thermal antinociception.

Buprenorphine is a synthetic opioid with partial agonist action at the mu receptor and antagonist actions at the other opioid receptors. In humans, buprenorphine is about 20 to 30 times more potent than morphine as an analgesic, is long-acting, and is associated with less respiratory depression. Plasma levels of 1 ng/mL are associated with effective analgesia in human surgery patients. After administration of 0.05 mg/kg SC, 85% of red-eared slider turtles maintained this target plasma level for 24 hours.[10] Pharmacokinetic data have suggested that this plasma level is expected to be achieved for at least 24 hours after SC administration of a dose of 0.075 mg/kg in the forelimb of red-eared sliders. Injection in the hindlimb provided lower plasma levels, suggesting that there is substantial first-pass metabolism by the liver.

A study was conducted to elucidate the effects of opioid analgesia on respiration. It was determined that both morphine and butorphanol cause respiratory depression in red-eared sliders by decreasing breathing frequency.[19] Tidal volumes were not affected and were actually increased with butorphanol. Ventilatory suppression was more marked and longer lasting with morphine.

The analgesic and respiratory effects of tramadol have also been investigated in the red-eared slider. Tramadol has a dual mechanism of action and provides analgesia by acting at mu opioid receptors and inhibiting the reuptake of norepinephrine and serotonin. Analgesic effects were measured using hindlimb withdrawal latencies to thermal stimuli. Oral doses ranging from 1 to 25 mg/kg and SC doses of 10 and 25 mg/kg were tested.[2] Tramadol, 10 mg/kg PO, increased latencies for 6 to 96 hours after dosing compared with 12 to 48 hours when given subcutaneously. When given by either route at a dose of 25 mg/kg, mouth gaping and muscle flaccidity were seen. Respiratory depression was seen at all oral doses over 5 mg/kg. A pharmacokinetic study of the NSAID meloxicam in red-eared sliders has shown that intramuscular dosing is the most effective way to provide predictable blood levels by avoiding rapid clearance (seen with IV dosing) and secondary peaks (seen with PO dosing).[16]

Sauria: Lizards

Both green iguanas and bearded dragons have been the subject of studies to evaluate the antinociceptive effects of butorphanol. In juvenile green iguanas, response to a thermal stimulus was not significantly different after administration of butorphanol at a dose of 1 mg/kg IM.[4] The same dose provided no isoflurane-sparing effect in mature green iguanas, an effect that has been attributed to analgesic properties of the drug in other species.[12] In bearded dragons, butorphanol doses of 2 and 20 mg/kg and morphine doses of 1 and 5 mg/kg did not alter hindlimb withdrawal responses to a noxious thermal stimulus. However, morphine at both 10 and 20 mg/kg significantly increased latency times compared with baseline responses 8 hours after administration.[17] These doses are high compared with doses used in mammals as well as those found to be efficacious in red-eared sliders. The duration of effect for bearded dragons at the lower dose of 10 mg/kg was less than 24 hours. Different results were seen in a study

using electrostimulation rather than thermal stimulation as the noxious stimuli. A butorphanol dose of 1.5 mg/kg given IM in the green iguana resulted in a significant decrease in tail movement in treated versus control animals.[5]

The pharmacokinetics of a single dose of ketoprofen, an NSAID commonly used in veterinary medicine, has also been studied in the green iguana. Unlike corticosteroids, which inhibit production pathways for many proinflammatory products, NSAIDs impede the synthesis of prostaglandins by inhibiting only cyclooxygenase (COX). Thus far, at least two and possibly three isoenzymes of COX have been identified. In general, drugs with preferential activity against COX-2 are expected to provide more anti-inflammatory and analgesic benefits and have fewer side effects. Because the mechanisms of COX receptor upregulation in reptiles undergoing inflammation are unknown, a nonspecific COX inhibitor such as ketoprofen may have advantages over drugs with COX-2 specificity, such as carprofen, meloxicam, deracoxib, or firocoxib. In the iguana study, 2 mg/kg of ketoprofen was administered both IV and IM and the bioavailability and half-life of the drug were determined.[26] The data revealed that once-daily administration at this dose may be more frequent than is necessary. A similar study in green iguanas looked at the pharmacokinetics of a single dose of 0.2 mg/kg meloxicam given orally and intravenously.[3] Both routes of administration provided blood levels considered to be therapeutic in humans and dogs for 24 hours after administration. With oral dosing, plasma levels did not reach a therapeutic level until 9 hours after administration. The toxic side effects of meloxicam were investigated by dosing green iguanas with 1 or 5 mg/kg PO daily for 12 days. No histologic changes were noted in gastric, hepatic, or renal tissues. Abnormalities in several blood parameters, including pronounced leukocytosis and elevations in total protein and uric acid level, were seen. The doses used to determine side effects were well above those generally used therapeutically. In a separate study, green iguanas were given carprofen (2.0 mg/kg IM) or meloxicam (0.2 mg/kg IM) for 10 days to assess changes to hematologic and biochemical parameters. Those receiving carprofen had higher levels of aspartate aminotransferase (AST) than the control or meloxicam groups; however, all blood parameters were within normal reference ranges after the 10-day trial.[25] Because side effects are a concern when administering any NSAID, using higher doses than necessary should be avoided. More research is needed to establish safe repeat dosing regimens.

Serpentes: Snakes

Compared with the other classes of reptiles, very little is known about analgesia in snakes. Snakes differ from chelonians and lizards in that they show antinociceptive effects in response to butorphanol, but not to morphine. In corn snakes, a butorphanol dose of 20 mg/kg significantly increased thermal withdrawal latencies 8 hours after subcutaneous administration whereas a lower dose of 2 mg/kg had no effect. Morphine doses ranging from 1 to 40 mg/kg SC did not increase withdrawal latencies during the period 2 to 24 hours after administration.[17] The butorphanol dose of 20 mg/kg is significantly higher than that used in other species and further investigation is needed to see whether this dose is associated with respiratory depression or other negative side effects in snakes. For example, red-eared sliders given a much lower dose of 1.5 mg/kg SC butorphanol responded with depressed respiration.[19] The magnitude of the thermal withdrawal latencies seen in the corn snakes were low compared with those seen in red-eared sliders, which may be an indication that snakes process thermal nociception differently than turtles. This could help explain the high incidence of thermal burns seen in snakes housed with malfunctioning hot rocks. A study comparing postoperative physiologic parameters in ball pythons receiving preoperative butorphanol (5 mg/kg) or meloxicam (0.3 mg/kg) showed no significant differences from untreated snakes.[13] The parameters measured in this study are those consistently altered in mammals experiencing pain and include blood pressure, heart rate, blood gas values, and plasma cortisol and catecholamine levels.

Crocodilians: Alligators, Crocodiles, Caimans, and Gharials

Morphine given at even very low doses (0.05 mg/kg) increases hot plate withdrawal latencies in crocodiles.[8] Statistically significant withdrawal latencies were seen in crocodiles at doses 20 times lower than those in studies involving rats and mice, with a maximal effect reached at a dose of 0.3 mg/kg. Response latencies were increased as soon as $\frac{1}{2}$ to 2 hours after intracoelomic (IC) injection. The dose of 0.1 mg/kg did not produce statistically significant latencies in all pain-related behaviors, showing only a weak effect in some animals. In the same study, meperidine (mu receptor agonist) at a dose of 2 mg/kg IC also induced a statistically significant increase in response latencies.

Local analgesia has also been used in crocodilians for the treatment of dental disease.[27] Administration of a mandibular nerve block was facilitated by the use of a nerve locator. The positive electrode of the stimulator was attached to the skin behind the front leg. Then, a needle attached to the negative electrode was placed so that strong movement of the intermandibularis muscle was stimulated and 2% mepivacaine was injected around the nerve. After 2 minutes, current was applied again and, if no muscle movement was seen, nerve block was achieved. This technique is especially useful in species for which nerve anatomy is less familiar.

AMPHIBIAN RESEARCH FINDINGS

Most of the analgesia research conducted in amphibians has used the acetic acid test. In this model, increasing concentrations of glacial acetic acid are applied as a single drop to the dorsal surface of the test subject's thigh or leg.[14] The nociceptive threshold is reached if the animal exhibits a wiping response, a motor reflex in which the subject removes the drop with either hindlimb. Although much work has been done to identify the opioid receptor types responsible for analgesia in amphibians, several questions remain. Regardless of receptor type, the analgesic potency of mu, delta, and kappa opioid pharmaceuticals in amphibians is similar to that seen in mammals, and analgesic efficacy has been demonstrated for many mu and kappa opioids, including morphine, fentanyl, meperidine, and buprenorphine.[20] Most of the opioid agents tested provide dose-dependent analgesia lasting up to 4 hours or longer, but many show a low margin of safety at higher doses.[20] The adrenergic agonists clonidine, epinephrine, norepinephrine, and dexmedetomidine also provide analgesic effects mediated by α_2-adrenergic receptors.[1] In *Rana pipiens*, dexmedetomidine began producing analgesic effect 15 minutes after SC administration, with peak effect at 30 to 60 minutes and a total duration of effect of at least 8 hours. At analgesic doses, the adrenergic agonists were shown to have no effect on righting reflex, corneal reflex, and hindlimb withdrawal reflex. In addition to the opioid receptor agonists and α_2-adrenergic agents, other types of drugs, including antipsychotics (chlorpromazine and haloperidol), a benzodiazepine (chlordiazepoxide), a partial opioid agonist (buprenorphine), and a histamine antagonist (diphenhydramine) were shown to produce moderate to strong analgesic effects.[21]

Morphine has been shown to be an effective analgesic at a dose of 10 mg/kg in frogs.[14] Morphine at this dose was compared with butorphanol, xylazine, and flunixin using acetic acid as the noxious stimulus.[24] All drugs were given IC by injection and were found to provide good analgesia for at least 4 hours. Xylazine (10 mg/kg) provided the best, longest lasting analgesia for duration of 12 to 24 hours. Butorphanol (25 mg/kg) was effective for 8 to 12 hours and flunixin lasted only 2 to 4 hours. None of the treatments affected normal motor behavior, but butorphanol and xylazine treated frogs were calmer and easier to handle.

Local hypothermia was tested as a method of providing analgesia using the acetic acid test.[23] For each frog, one leg was immersed in ice water (6° C) for 10 minutes after applying a tourniquet to maintain regional hypothermia. The analgesic effect was found to be stronger than morphine given 10 mg/kg IC and was partially blocked by opioid antagonists, indicating that the effect is at least in part mediated by opioid receptors.

All the results described for amphibians thus far are derived from the acetic acid test, which uses a chemical stimulus applied cutaneously. One study evaluated behavior in eastern red-spotted newts after bilateral forelimb amputations under anesthesia.[9] The analgesic efficacy of buprenorphine and butorphanol was measured to this more chronic noxious stimulus. Newts undergoing anesthesia but not surgery and given no postoperative analgesia were compared with the experimental group by assessing body posture, food consumption, and response to stimulation. Buprenorphine was administered at a dose of 50 mg/kg given IC after surgery and again at 24 and 48 hours after surgery. Butorphanol was administered by addition to the water at a concentration of 0.5 mg/liter and the activated charcoal filter was removed from the system for the duration of treatment (72 hours). Both methods for providing analgesia significantly promoted the resumption of normal behavior postoperatively. In the experimental group, changes in body posture were noticed for the first 10 minutes after anesthetic recovery and were attributed to delayed onset of analgesia, underscoring the need for interoperative or preemptive dosing of analgesics.

REFERENCES

1. Brenner GM, Klopp AJ, Deason LL, et al: Analgesic potency of alpha adrenergic agents after systemic administration in amphibians. J Phamacol Exp Ther 270:540–545, 1994.
2. Cummings BB, Sladky KK, Johnson SM: Tramadol analgesic and respiratory effects in red-eared slider turtles (Trachemys scripta).

Presented at the Conference of the American Association of Zoo Veterinarians, Tulsa, Okla, October 25–30, 2009.
3. Divers SJ, Papich M, McBride M, et al: Intravenous and oral pharmacokinetics of meloxicam in the green iguana (Iguana iguana). Am J Vet Res 71:1277–1283, 2010.
4. Fleming GJ, Robertson SA: Use of thermal threshold test response to evaluate the antinociceptive effects of butorphanol in juvenile green iguanas (Iguana iguana). Presented at the Conference of the American Association of Zoo Veterinarians, Tampa, Fla, September 19–24, 2006.
5. Greenacre CB, Takle G, Schumacher JP, et al: Comparative antinociception of morphine, butorphanol, and buprenorphine versus saline in the green iguana, Iguana iguana, using electrostimulation. J Herpetol Med Surg 16:88–92, 2006.
6. Hardie EM, Hansen BD, Carroll GS: Behavior after ovariohysterectomy in the dog: What's normal? Appl Anim Behav Sci 51:111–128, 1997.
7. Holz PI, Barker K, Burger JP, et al: The effect of the renal portal system on pharmacokinetic parameters in the red-eared slider (Trachemys scripta elegans). J Zoo Wildl Med 28:378–385, 1997.
8. Kanui TI, Hole K: Morphine and pethidine antinociception in the crocodile. J Vet Pharmacol Therap 15:101–103, 1992.
9. Koeller CA: Comparison of buprenorphine and butorphanol analgesia in the eastern red-spotted newt (Notophthalmus viridescens). J Am Assoc Lab Anim Sci 48:171–175, 2009.
10. Kummrow MS, Tseng F, Hesse L, et al: Pharmacokinetics of buprenorphine after single-dose subcutaneous administration in red-eared sliders (Trachemys scripta elegans). J Zoo Wildl Med 39:590–595, 2008.
11. Machin KL: Amphibian pain and analgesia. J Zoo Wildl Med 30:2–10, 1999.
12. Mosely CA, Dyson D, Smith DA: Minimum alveolar concentration of isoflurane in green iguanas and the effect of butorphanol on minimum alveolar concentration. J Am Vet Med Assoc 222:1559–1564, 2003.
13. Olesen MG, Bertelsen MF, Perry SF, et al: Effects of preoperative administration of butorphanol or meloxicam on physiologic responses to surgery in ball pythons. J Am Vet Med Assoc 233:1883–1888, 2008.
14. Pezalla PC: Morphine-induced analgesia and explosive motor behavior in an amphibian. Brain Res 273:297–305, 1983.
15. Read MR: Evaluation of the use of anesthesia and analgesia in reptiles. J Am Vet Med Assoc 224:547–552, 2004.
16. Rojo-Solis C, Ros-Rodriguez JM, Valls M, et al: Pharmacokinetics of meloxicam (Metacam) after intravenous, intramuscular and oral administration to red-eared slider turtles (Trachemys scripta elegans). Presented at the Conference of the American Association of Zoo Veterinarians, Tulsa, Okla, October 25–30, 2009.
17. Sladky KK, Kinney ME, Johnson SM: Analgesic efficacy of butorphanol and morphine in bearded dragons and corn snakes. J Am Vet Med Assoc 233:267–273, 2008.
18. Sladky KK, Kinney ME, Johnson SM: Effects of opioid receptor activation on thermal antinociception in red-eared slider turtles (Trachemys scripta). Am J Vet Res 70:1072–1078, 2009.
19. Sladky KK, Miletic V, Paul-Murphy J, et al: Analgesic efficacy and respiratory effects of butorphanol and morphine in turtles. J Am Vet Med Assoc 230:1356–1362, 2007.
20. Stevens CW, Klopp AJ, Facello JA: Analgesic potency of mu and kappa opioids after systemic administration in amphibians. J Phamacol Exp Ther 269:1086–1093, 1994.
21. Stevens CW, Maciver DN, Newman LC: Testing and comparison of non-opioid analgesics in amphibians. Contemp Top Lab Anim Sci 40:23–27, 2001.
22. Stoskopf MK: Pain and alalgesia in birds, reptiles, fish and amphibians. Invest Ophthalmol Vis Sci 35:755–780, 1994.

23. Suckow MA, Terril LA, Grigdesby CF, et al: Evaluation of hypothermia-induced analgesia and influence of opioid antagonists in leopard frogs (Rana pipiens). Pharmacol Biochem Behav 63:39–43, 1999.

24. Terril-Robb LA, Suckow MA, Grigdesby CF: Evaluation of the analgesic effects of butorphanol tartarate, xylazine hydrochloride and flunixin meglumine in leopard frogs (Rana pipiens). Contemp Top Lab Anim Sci 35:54–56, 1996.

25. Trnkova S, Knotkova Z, Hrda A, et al: Effect of non-steroidal anti-inflammatory drugs on the blood profile in the green iguana (Iguana iguana). Vet Med 11:507–511, 2007.

26. Tuttle AD, Papich M, Lewbart GA, et al: Pharmacokinetics of ketoprofen in the green iguana (Iguana iguana) following single intravenous and intramuscular injections. J Zoo Wildl Med 37:567–570, 2006.

27. Wellehan JFX, Gunkel CI, Kledzik D, et al: Use of a nerve locator to facilitate administration of mandibular nerve blocks in crocodilians. J Zoo Wildl Med 37:405–408, 2006.

CHAPTER 33

Virology of Nonavian Reptiles: An Update

Jim Wellehan

Reptile virology is a rapidly changing field, with many ongoing exciting discoveries. We are still learning about the diversity of infectious agents in reptiles and the clinical significance of these agents. This chapter is intended solely as an update on recent developments regarding viruses associated with the most significant pathology, and not as an overview. For overviews, the reader is directed to earlier reviews.[11,27]

WHAT IS A REPTILE?

In comparative medicine, we often lack information in a given species, including which infectious agents are present and their clinical significance. When information is lacking in a species, the best model to use is typically the closest relative from which data are available. This requires knowledge of species relationships; many commonly used terms, such as *reptile* or *lizard*, may lead to erroneous understanding of relationships.

A monophyletic group is defined as a group that contains all descendants of a common ancestor. In comparative medicine, understanding what constitutes a monophyletic group is needed to understand relationships and choose appropriate models. Primates constitute a monophyletic group; when the primates, except for humans, are referred to, the term *nonhuman primates* is generally used. This qualification in the term helps the reader understand that a group is being referred to, with the exception of one member.

When the evolution of the terrestrial vertebrates (tetrapods) is examined, the fossil record and far more complete and convincing nucleic acid sequence phylogeny analyses are in agreement on relationships.[9] The earliest divergence among the tetrapods is between the amphibians and amniotes, who are fully terrestrial (Fig. 33-1). The amniotes are then further divided into

mammals and sauropsids. Within the sauropsids, the next group to diverge is the squamate (lizards and snakes)–sphenodontid (tuatara) clade. Following this, the Testudines (turtles) diverged, and the last two major sauropsid groups to diverge were the crocodilians and dinosaurs. The only surviving group of dinosaurs is the birds. This is supported by the fossil record and by sequence data.[23] Although birds themselves constitute a monophyletic group, if birds are not considered as part of the reptiles, then reptiles are not a monophyletic group. What we really mean by reptiles is sauropsids, and birds are a group of reptiles. Crocodilians and birds share a number of medically relevant similarities, including a four-chambered heart with the right aortic arch being the major outflow for oxygenated blood, and lungs with unidirectional rather than tidal air flow.[5] However, the significant differences between birds and crocodilians are also obvious and the clinician needs to be careful not to overextrapolate. The obvious differences between a caiman and sparrow underscore the more cryptic but greater differences between a caiman and monitor lizard.

Another common error is the idea of lizards as a group distinct from snakes. In squamate evolution, the earliest divergence is the geckos, followed by the divergence of the skinks, night lizards, plated lizards, and girdled lizards (Fig. 33-2). The next groups to branch off were the teiids, lacertids, and amphisbaenids and the remaining group, containing snakes, iguanids, agamids, chameleons, monitors, helodermatids, and anguids, is known collectively as the Toxicofera, named for the commonality of the presence of venom glands.[6] Snakes diverge in the middle of the squamates and, if snakes are removed, then lizards are not a monophyletic group. Snakes are a group of lizards and a ball python is a better model for an iguana than a leopard gecko.

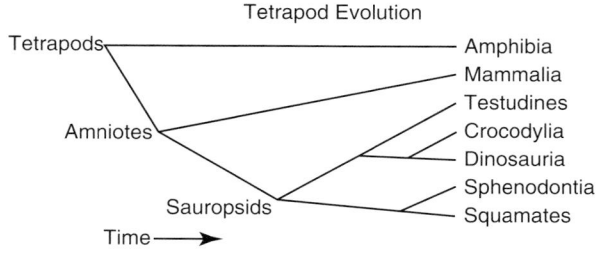

Figure 33-1

Phylogenetic tree of the tetrapods. Branch lengths are not to scale.

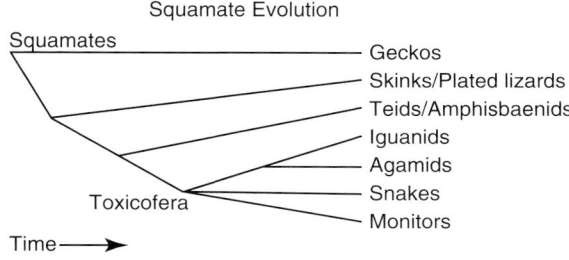

Figure 33-2

Phylogenetic tree of the squamates. Branch lengths are not to scale.

NOVEL VIRUSES

Because reptile virology is still a nascent field, it is not uncommon to find previously unknown viruses. Assessing risk and responding appropriately to the identification of a novel virus requires understanding of context, viral ecology, and evolution. In an ideal situation, we would have information including the results of experimental infection with the virus in a set of animals from the species of concern. This is rarely the case. However, even if it is, it is important to recognize that Koch's postulates represent a concept that should not be over-interpreted. No infectious agent is either a pathogen or not a pathogen. There have been many asymptomatic human Ebola virus infections, and people have died of septicemia caused by *Lactobacillus acidophilus*.[4,14] It is important to correlate infection with clinical patient evaluation and histology before infectious disease is considered as a significant differential. All clinical infectious diseases have multiple contributing factors, including those from the infectious agent, the host, and the environment.

With respect to virus factors affecting infectious disease, even with a novel agent, the biology of a given virus may be used to make clinical predictions. A virus with a lipid envelope will be less stable in the environment than a nonenveloped virus and disinfection protocols should be adjusted accordingly.

Another important viral factor with clinical implications is genome organization; some viruses have segmented genomes. Throughout biology, hybridization is a factor allowing rapid nondetrimental change, allowing species to invade novel habitats.[20] This is considered the main reason for the evolution of sex. Segmentation of viruses, allowing reassortment, is essentially the viral equivalent of sex, providing a hybrid advantage for crossing host species. This has been best studied in the Orthomyxoviridae.

Large biologic differences of significant clinical importance are seen between DNA viruses and RNA viruses. DNA viruses generally replicate more accurately and have proofreading systems for error correction. This enables them to be larger and more complex, and to have a more intricate relationship with the host. A delicate balance such as chronic or latent infection is more commonly seen with DNA viruses. This balance is generally specific to an endemic host and, although infection may be possible in aberrant hosts, aberrant host infections lack balance and are generally rapid in course. This may be associated with significant pathology. As examples, human herpesvirus 1 and Macacine herpesvirus 1 often cause relatively benign cold sore lesions or be asymptomatic in their endemic hosts, which are humans and rhesus macaques, respectively. Infections in aberrant hosts, such as human herpesvirus 1 in a white-handed gibbon or Macacine herpesvirus 1 in a human, result in overwhelming viral encephalitis that is usually fatal and does not generally result in successful further viral transmission. It may actually be advantageous for endemic host populations to be infected with some of these agents, because disease may eliminate competitors and predators, and not the endemic host. DNA viruses do not tend to evolve as rapidly as RNA viruses and are less likely to switch hosts successfully.

Because of lack of proofreading by their polymerases and constant selection by the host immune system, RNA viruses have the fastest mutating genomes found in nature, and tracking evolution of these viruses is highly clinically significant. One recent meta-analysis has found that of the 20 virus families infecting humans, four RNA virus families—Reoviridae, Bunyaviridae, Flaviviridae, and Togaviridae—accounted for more than 50% of emerging and reemerging viruses.[31] Emerging disease is also frequently associated with host switches. The human disease meta-analysis found that 816 of 1407 (58%) are zoonotic and, of human diseases, zoonotic diseases are significantly more likely to be emerging. The simpler nature of smaller RNA viruses and their ability to change rapidly makes them more adaptable to new hosts. This ability to move successfully and rapidly to new hosts removes the selective pressure not to harm the host, and RNA viruses generally tend to result in more explosive epidemiology.

There is generally little that a clinician may do about host factors when dealing with novel viruses, other than to advise avoiding mixing species and resultant aberrant host infections. The areas that the clinician can affect most are environmental factors. Many factors, including but not limited to coinfections, stress, nutritional status, temperature, reproductive status, age, and noninfectious disease processes, all play significant roles in viral disease. Of these, temperature is the area that differs most in nonavian reptiles from what is seen in mammals. Poikilothermy provides the patient with the ability to tolerate a wider range of body temperatures; viruses often tolerate a narrower temperature range, or at least disease may only manifest in a narrower temperature range. Patients with a wide thermal gradient may choose a febrile or other thermal response.[17] Providing appropriate thermal opportunities is often a highly effective therapy.

Adenoviruses

The adenoviruses are large, nonenveloped, DNA viruses. As nonenveloped viruses, they are highly stable in the environment, and disinfection in captive settings is challenging. The characterized adenoviruses of nonavian reptiles fall into two recognized genera, *Atadenovirus* and *Siadenovirus*. Additionally, a number of recently discovered adenoviruses of turtles appear to form a new genus that has yet to be characterized.

The genus *Atadenovirus* is endemic in squamates, although some species have undergone host switches at some point into birds and mammals.[28] These viruses are fairly host-specific and infection is often only seen in the endemic host, in which clinical disease most commonly manifests as hepatitis and enteritis and is most often seen in young animals. Asymptomatic infection is not uncommon. Bearded dragons and king snakes are commonly recognized as clinically affected species.[8] A growing diversity of squamate atadenoviruses is being recognized,[18] and it is likely that most squamate species may have associated atadenovirus species. Persistence appears to be common and, given the environmental stability of adenoviruses, infection tends to become widespread within collections unless highly rigorous biosecurity is practiced. Given the tendency of reptile

breeders to have large collections at high density, acquire reptiles through venues such as trade shows, and practice poor biosecurity, atadenoviruses are ideally suited to become widespread in captive populations. A study of typing of Agamid adenovirus 1 in North American collections has found that different genotypes are widespread across geographically separate collections.[19]

The genus *Siadenovirus* has been associated with the most dramatic pathology of any known virus in tortoises. Sulawesi tortoise adenovirus 1 was associated with necrosis and intranuclear inclusions in the gut, bone marrow, liver, kidneys, spleen, pancreas, gonads, adrenals, and blood vessels, as well as rhinitis and choroid plexitis, in a group of 105 Sulawesi tortoises *(Indotestudo forsteni)*.[21] A group mortality of over 90% was seen. A breach of this virus, with resultant disease, was seen from the initial group into additional tortoise species in the home collection of one caretaker, confirming both pathogenicity and transmissibility of this agent. The high pathogenicity of this agent is not typical of how a large DNA virus behaves in an endemic host, and it is expected that these tortoises were aberrant rather than endemic hosts. Other members of the genus *Siadenovirus* have been found in birds and frogs; bird siadenoviruses tend to be highly pathogenic, and disease has not been studied in frogs. It is not clear which taxa are endemic hosts of the siadenoviruses.

Specific diagnosis of adenoviruses is best accomplished via consensus polymerase chain reaction (PCR) assay and sequencing. Specific therapy of adenoviruses in nonavian reptiles has not been studied. Cidofovir has been found to be affective against adenoviruses in mammals, and further studies on efficacy, safety, and pharmacokinetics in nonavian reptiles are indicated.

Herpesviruses

The herpesviruses are large enveloped DNA viruses. As enveloped viruses, they are less stable in the environment. Herpesviruses are well known for establishing latent infections, and any animal found to be infected with a herpesvirus should be considered to be infected for life. Productive host switches seem to be relatively uncommon, and herpesviruses appear to have evolved along with their hosts over hundreds of millions of years. In humans *(Homo sapiens)*, the best studied single host species, there are eight endemic herpesvirus species. All known herpesviruses of nonavian reptiles are in the subfamily Alphaherpesvirinae. The herpesviruses of the Testudines form a monophyletic cluster consistent with a genus, which has provisionally been called *Chelonivirus.*[3,24] There are approximately 300 extant species in the order Testudines. Given the apparent prevalence of herpesvirus-host codivergence, it is reasonable to hypothesize that the known turtle-tortoise herpesviruses represent a small fraction of cheloniviral diversity.

Among sea turtle herpesviruses, recent developments include the discovery of loggerhead genital-respiratory herpesvirus (LGRV), which is associated with cloacal-genital, tracheal, and eyelid ulcerations, and loggerhead orocutaneous herpesvirus (LOCV), which is associated with tongue ulcerations and hyperkeratotic plaques in the skin.[24] LGRV is clinically similar to lung-eye-trachea virus (LETV) seen in green turtles. LGRV and LETV are genetically distinct but related, and there is some evidence that they may cross-react serologically.

The herpesviruses of tortoises now constitute four published species. Tortoise herpesvirus 1 (THV1) has been found in Russian tortoises *(Agrionemys [Testudo] horsfieldii),* pancake tortoises *(Malacochersus tornieri),* and Greek tortoises *(Testudo graeca),* and appears to be endemic in Russian tortoises. Tortoise herpesvirus 2 (THV2) is found in California desert tortoises. Tortoise herpesvirus 3 (THV3) has been found in a variety of tortoises in the genus *Testudo;* it is unknown which species is the endemic host. Tortoise herpesvirus 4 has been identified in an asymptomatic bowsprit tortoise *(Chersina angulata).*[3] Studies of another herpesvirus of elongated tortoises *(Indotestudo elongata)* remains unpublished, and study of a herpesvirus of red-footed tortoises has been published but never characterized.

The herpesviruses of squamates are even less characterized. Recent reports include a herpesvirus associated with proliferative stomatitis in green tree monitors *(Varanus prasinus),*[29] a herpesvirus associated with papillomatous skin lesions in a green lizard *(Lacerta viridis),*[15] and a herpesvirus associated with multifocal hepatic and enteric necrosis and rapid death in monitor lizards *(Varanus* spp.).[10] The first two reports are consistent with herpesvirus infections in endemic hosts, whereas the last one is typical of an aberrant host infection.

As with any infectious agent, until the reptile herpesvirus of concern is characterized, and all related herpesvirus that may cross-react serologically have been characterized, serodiagnostic procedures for reptile herpesviruses are not very useful clinically. A positive result may mean that there was a humoral immune response to the agent of concern or to a related unknown agent. The clinical differences between human herpesvirus 1 (HHV1, cold sores), human herpesvirus 2 (HHV2, genital herpes), and Macacine herpesvirus 1 (MaHV1,

herpes B) are great, but the genetic distance is minimal. Many antibodies to HHV1, HHV2, and MaHV1 will cross-react. If the existence of a related virus to a given reptile herpesvirus is not known, a virus with significantly different clinical implications may cause false-positive serologic assay results. Additionally, serologic assays are generally not sensitive for herpesviruses, and a significant number of false-negative results may occur.

Specific diagnosis of herpesviruses is best accomplished via consensus PCR assay and sequencing. There are limited data on the pharmacologic therapy of herpesviruses in reptiles. Acyclovir and ganciclovir have limited pharmacokinetic data, but lack safety data and in vivo efficacy data.

Iridoviruses

The iridoviruses are large enveloped DNA viruses, but the envelope is not necessary for infection, rendering them somewhat more stable in the environment. The characterized adenoviruses of nonavian reptiles fall into two recognized genera, *Ranavirus* and *Iridovirus.* Additionally, erythrocytic iridoviruses appear to form a new genus that has yet to be characterized.

The ranaviruses are newly recognized as a significant cause of mortality in testudines, especially eastern box turtles *(Terrapene carolina).*[12] Typical lesions associated with ranaviral disease include necrotizing stomatitis and/or esophagitis, fibrinous and necrotizing splenitis, and multicentric fibrinoid vasculitis.

The genus *Iridovirus* has traditionally been thought of as invertebrate pathogen. However, data suggest that these agents are also capable of infecting squamates. Manifestations seen in infected squamates include weight loss, skin lesions, and keratoconjunctivitis. A squamate isolate has been shown to infect feeder crickets.[25] Further data are needed on these agents as a cause of disease in squamates, but the potential for feeder insects to be a source of viral disease is concerning.

The third group of iridoviruses to infect nonavian reptiles are the erythrocytic iridoviruses. Intracytoplasmic inclusions are seen in erythrocytes. These have been shown to be distinct from other members of the family Iridoviridae at a level consistent with a novel genus.[30] The clinical sign strongly associated with these viruses is anemia, which may be fatal.

Specific diagnosis of iridoviruses is best accomplished via consensus PCR assay and sequencing. Data on pharmacologic therapy of iridoviruses in any species are lacking. Providing appropriate thermal opportunities seems to help in a number of cases.

Reoviruses

The reoviruses are segmented nonenveloped RNA viruses. They are highly stable in the environment, and a recent study evaluating the disinfection of a leopard gecko *(Eublepharus macularius)* reovirus has found that most disinfectants are ineffective, with bleach being the only disinfectant evaluated that worked significantly.[1] As segmented RNA viruses, reoviruses are ideally suited for host switching, and members of the family Reoviridae are found in vertebrates, invertebrates, plants, and fungi. The characterized reoviruses of nonavian reptiles are all in the genus *Orthoreovirus.*[26] Large host jumps and significant pathology appear to be common. It is not uncommon for clinical disease caused by orthoreoviruses to be mistaken for paramyxoviral disease.

Recent reports include a virus first identified in a Mediterranean spur-thighed tortoise *(Testudo graeca)* in Switzerland that was later found to be associated with a high mortality rate and syncytial cell enteropathy and hepatopathy in leopard geckos in a North American collection.[7] A different reovirus was associated with necrotizing hepatitis with hepatocellular syncytia in a rough green snake *(Opheodrys aestivus).*[13]

Specific diagnosis of reoviruses is best accomplished via consensus PCR assay and sequencing. Specific therapy of reoviruses in nonavian reptiles has not been studied. Mycophenolic acid has been found to be affective against avian orthoreoviruses in vitro,[22] and further studies on the efficacy, safety, and pharmacokinetics in nonavian reptiles are indicated.

Paramyxoviruses

The paramyxoviruses are enveloped RNA viruses. As enveloped viruses, they are less stable in the environment. They are relatively simple in organization and contain no genes that are known to be associated with latency. The characterized paramyxoviruses of nonavian reptiles are all in the genus *Ferlavirus,* and have been found in both squamates and tortoises.[16] There is significant diversity that has been identified within the genus.

Paramyxoviruses have been reasonably well known for a comparatively long time in reptile medicine. Many zoo collections routinely test animals in quarantine. The most commonly used serologic test is hemagglutination inhibition (HI). There are three laboratories that perform paramyxovirus HI. They all use different strains in their assays, and one uses two different strains. Only one laboratory has cutoff criteria determined by experimental infections. A recent study has examined a set of 26 samples that were submitted to all the available laboratories and found that their methods do not correlate well with each other.[2] The laboratory using two different strains reported that every sample was positive with both strains, whereas the laboratory with experimentally determined cutoffs found that none were positive.

This underscores several points. First, assays need to be validated. Second, even if appropriate validation is done, running a serologic assay for an entire genus of viruses makes little sense. If you suspect that a mammal patient may have paramyxoviral disease, it is important to decide whether you are looking for rinderpest, measles, or canine distemper, and not to run a single test with the illogical expectation that results will be equivalent, regardless of which virus in the genus *Morbillivirus* is used in the assay. Finally, the reptile humoral response often takes several weeks to manifest. As a small RNA virus, the dynamics of ferlaviral disease are expected to include a relatively rapid course and the patient is either expected to survive or succumb. Evidence of persistent or latent infection in nonavian reptiles is lacking. An animal with a positive titer may well have cleared the infection. The clinician is generally more concerned with whether an infectious agent is present than whether the animal has had a humoral immune response to a prior infection. An animal with a positive titer may actually be beneficial; an animal that has cleared infection may help provide herd immunity. Because of testing limitations, HI results are not easily interpreted in a quarantine situation.

Specific diagnosis of ferlaviruses is best accomplished via consensus PCR assay and sequencing. The polymerase gene has been shown to be the best target for consensus PCR testing.[16] Specific therapy of ferlaviruses in nonavian reptiles has not been studied. Many ferlaviruses appear only to cause disease in a somewhat narrow temperature range, and providing appropriate thermal opportunities is often a highly effective therapy.

REFERENCES

1. Aitken-Palmer C, Wellehan J, Childress AL, et al: Real-time PCR assessment of biosecurity methods for a reptile reovirus. Presented at the Conference of the American Association of Zoo Veterinarians, Tulsa, Okla, October 25-30, 2009.
2. Allender MC, Mitchell MA, Dreslik MJ, et al: Measuring agreement and discord among hemagglutination inhibition assays against different ophidian paramyxovirus strains in the Eastern massasauga *(Sistrurus catenatus catenatus).* J Zoo Wildl Med 39:358–361, 2008.

3. Bicknese EJ, Childress AL, Wellehan JFX: A novel herpesvirus of the proposed genus *Chelonivirus* from an asymptomatic bowsprit tortoise *(Chersina angulata)*. J Zoo Wildl Med 41:353–358, 2010.
4. Cannon JP, Lee TA, Bolanos JT, et al: Pathogenic relevance of Lactobacillus: A retrospective review of over 200 cases. Eur J Clin Microbiol Infect Dis 24:31–40, 2005.
5. Farmer CG, Sanders K: Unidirectional airflow in the lungs of alligators. Science 327:338–340, 2010.
6. Fry BG, Vidal N, Norman JA, et al: Early evolution of the venom system in lizards and snakes. Nature 439:584–588, 2006.
7. Garner MM, Farina LL, Wellehan JFX, et al: Reovirus-associated syncytial cell enteropathy and hepatopathy in leopard geckos, *Eublepharus macularius.* Presented at the Conference of the American Association of Zoo Veterinarians, Tulsa, Okla, October 25–30, 2009.
8. Garner MM, Wellehan JFX, Pearson M, et al: Characterization of enteric infections associated with two novel atadenoviruses in colubrid snakes. J Herpetol Med Surg 18:86–94, 2008.
9. Hugall AF, Foster R, Lee MS: Calibration choice, rate smoothing, and the pattern of tetrapod diversification according to the long nuclear gene RAG-1. System Biol 56:543–563, 2007.
10. Hughes-Hanks JM, Schommer SK, Mitchell WJ, et al: Hepatitis and enteritis caused by a novel herpesvirus in two monitor lizards *(Varanus* spp.). J Vet Diagn Invest 22:295–299, 2010.
11. Jacobson ER, editor: Infectious diseases and pathology of reptiles: Color atlas and text, Boca Raton, 2007, CRC Press.
12. Johnson AJ, Pessier AP, Wellehan JF, et al: Ranavirus infection of free-ranging and captive box turtles and tortoises in the United States. J Wildl Dis 44:851–863, 2008.
13. Landolfi JA, Terio KA, Kinsel MJ, et al: Orthoreovirus infection and concurrent cryptosporidiosis in rough green snakes *(Opheodrys aestivus):* Pathology and identification of a novel orthoreovirus strain via polymerase chain reaction and sequencing. J Vet Diagn Invest 22:37–43, 2010.
14. Leroy EM, Baize S, Volchkov VE, et al: Human asymptomatic Ebola infection and strong inflammatory response. Lancet 355:2210–2215, 2000.
15. Literak I, Robesova B, Majlathova V, et al: Herpesvirus-associated papillomatosis in a green lizard. J Wildl Dis 46:257–261, 2010.
16. Marschang RE, Papp T, Frost JW: Comparison of paramyxovirus isolates from snakes, lizards and a tortoise. Virus Res 144:272–279, 2009.
17. Merchant M, Williams S, Trosclair PL 3rd, et al: Febrile response to infection in the American alligator *(Alligator mississippiensis).* Comp Biochem Physiol A Mol Integr Physiol 148:921–925, 2007.
18. Papp T, Fledelius B, Schmidt V, et al: PCR-sequence characterization of new adenoviruses found in reptiles and the first successful isolation of a lizard adenovirus. Vet Microbiol 134:233–240, 2009.
19. Parkin DB, Archer LL, Childress AL, et al: Genotype differentiation of agamid adenovirus 1 in bearded dragons *(Pogona vitticeps)* in the USA by hexon gene sequence. Infect Genet Evol 9:501–506, 2009.
20. Rieseberg LH, Kim SC, Randell RA, et al: Hybridization and the colonization of novel habitats by annual sunflowers. Genetica 129:149–165, 2007.
21. Rivera S, Wellehan JF Jr, McManamon R, et al: Systemic adenovirus infection in Sulawesi tortoises *(Indotestudo forsteni)* caused by a novel siadenovirus. J Vet Diagn Invest 21:415–426, 2009.
22. Robertson CM, Hermann LL, Coombs KM: Mycophenolic acid inhibits avian reovirus replication. Antiviral Res 64:55–61, 2004.
23. Schweitzer MH, Zheng W, Organ CL, et al: Biomolecular characterization and protein sequences of the Campanian hadrosaur *B. canadensis.* Science 324:626–631, 2009.
24. Stacy BA, Wellehan JF, Foley AM, et al: Two herpesviruses associated with disease in wild Atlantic loggerhead sea turtles *(Caretta caretta).* Vet Microbiol 126:63–73, 2008.
25. Weinmann N, Papp T, Pedro Alves de Matos A, et al: Experimental infection of crickets *(Gryllus bimaculatus)* with an invertebrate iridovirus isolated from a high-casqued chameleon *(Chamaeleo hoehnelii).* J Vet Diagn Invest 19:674–679, 2007.
26. Wellehan JF Jr, Childress AL, Marschang RE, et al: Consensus nested PCR amplification and sequencing of diverse reptilian, avian, and mammalian orthoreoviruses. Vet Microbiol 133:34–42, 2009.
27. Wellehan JF, Johnson AJ: Reptile virology. Vet Clin North Am Exot Anim Pract 8:27–52, 2005.
28. Wellehan JF, Johnson AJ, Harrach B, et al: Detection and analysis of six lizard adenoviruses by consensus primer PCR provides further evidence of a reptilian origin for the atadenoviruses. J Virol 78:13366–13369, 2004.
29. Wellehan JF, Johnson AJ, Latimer KS, et al: Varanid herpesvirus 1: A novel herpesvirus associated with proliferative stomatitis in green tree monitors *(Varanus prasinus).* Vet Microbiol 105:83–92, 2005.
30. Wellehan JF Jr, Strik NI, Stacy BA, et al: Characterization of an erythrocytic virus in the family Iridoviridae from a peninsula ribbon snake *(Thamnophis sauritus sackenii).* Vet Microbiol 131:115–122, 2008.
31. Woolhouse ME, Gowtage-Sequeria S: Host range and emerging and reemerging pathogens. Emerg Infect Dis 11:1842–1847, 2005.

CHAPTER 34

Hellbender Medicine

Randall E. Junge

BIOLOGIC DATA

The hellbender (*Cryptobranchus alleganiesis*) is a large aquatic salamander native to the United States. There are two subspecies; the eastern hellbender (*C. alleganiensis alleganiensis*) is found in the eastern United States from New York to Georgia, extending west through Tennessee and the Ohio River Valley to the Ozarks. The Ozark hellbender (*C. alleganiensis bishopi*) is restricted to the Ozark region of Missouri and Arkansas. Eastern hellbenders are larger (adults up to 70 cm length), with dorsal spotting, uniformly colored lower labium, and papillate elevations in the lateral line canals of the pectoral region. The Ozark subspecies is smaller (30 to 50 cm long) with a dorsal blotching pattern, mottled lower labium, and smooth-surfaced lateral line system in the pectoral region.[15] Hellbenders have small lidless eyes, broad flat heads, and pronounced lateral skin folds. They produce a significant cutaneous mucous layer that is not toxic but may be irritating or noxious to mucous membranes (oral cavity). The hellbender is a habitat specialist dependent on appropriate temperature, dissolved oxygen, water flow, and substrate. They inhabit cold (5° C to 30° C), clear, swift-flowing streams with rocky bottoms. Large rocks must be present for nesting and refuge. Although lungs exist, respiration is almost entirely cutaneous. Hellbenders are long-lived (25 to 30 years and longer). Crayfish make up a large part of the diet, but also included are snails, nymphs, worms, tadpoles, and fish.[12] Hellbenders may be preyed on, especially larvae and juveniles, by fish, turtles, and water snakes, and were historically overharvested by humans for amphibian collectors. Currently, hellbenders are not a federally protected species, but such action is being considered.

Hellbenders are completely aquatic and mostly nocturnal, depending on range and habitat. Gills are present in larval stages, and adults have a singular pair of gill openings. Sexual maturity is reached at approximately 7 years of age. During breeding season (September through November), females often exhibit coelomic distension because of follicular development. Males develop a pericloacal swelling in breeding season, produced by enlargement of glands. Females may produce 300 to 450 eggs, and fertilization is external, unique among North American salamanders.[15] Embryonic development is not precisely known because they have never reproduced in captivity; however, eggs collected in the wild have matured in captivity in approximately 30 days.

Hellbenders in the wild are threatened by stream impoundment, channelization, agricultural runoff (chemical and siltation), disturbances caused by recreational use, and thermal changes.[21] As with amphibians worldwide, populations have declined dramatically in recent years; recent estimates of Ozark populations have suggested a 77% decline.[27]

CAPTIVE HUSBANDRY

Both subspecies of hellbenders are maintained in captivity. Attention must be given to water temperature, flow, and oxygenation, as well as providing an appropriate rocky substrate. Captive diets should mimic wild diets and include crayfish, earthworms, and fish. Routine weight monitoring is important because clinical signs of disease include inappetence, which may be difficult to determine unless regular weights are recorded. In addition, hellbenders have a normal seasonal weight fluctuation that should be monitored to differentiate it from health-related weight changes. Inadequate oxygenation of water may result in hellbenders surfacing frequently to breath or rocking in the water to increase circulation.

INFECTIOUS DISEASES

Two infectious diseases, the fungus *Batrachochytridium dendrobatidis* and ranavirus infection, have been implicated as contributing factors of global amphibian declines.[5,7,18] There are no published reports of ranavirus prevalence in wild populations of hellbenders; however, ongoing research at the University of Tennessee, Knoxville Zoo, and University of Georgia has documented infection. In this study, ranavirus prevalence ranged from 25% to 65% in wild hellbender populations inhabiting two eastern Tennessee watersheds.[22] The occurrence or degree of ranaviral disease or chytridiomycosis in infected individuals is unknown because animals were not collected for necropsy.

Batrachochytridium dendrobatidis (Bd) infection has been detected in captive and wild hellbenders.[3,25] In both populations, Bd has been confirmed by polymerase chain reaction (PCR) assay in hellbenders that were not showing any clinical signs of illness. However, in captive hellbenders that become severely compromised, Bd may have an augmented effect and may contribute to the death of the animal. Bd is most consistently detected by scraping the foot pads, presumably because this site has keratinized epithelium, which the fungus requires for invasion. The ventral aspect of each foot is stroked five times with an appropriate swab (wooden or plastic, depending on the laboratory's preference) and submitted to the laboratory for PCR assay. Comparative testing of swab sites on the body has confirmed that this approach produces the most consistent results.

Saprolegniasis has been reported both in wild[11] and captive[6] hellbenders. This common water mold is most commonly associated with egg mortality. In larvae and adults, infections are usually cutaneous; however it is possible for the fungus to invade into deeper tissues and potentially contribute to death.

Several gastrointestinal parasites have been detected in hellbenders, including the nematodes *Spironoura wardi*, *Zanclophorus variabilis*, *Falcaustra catesbeianae*, *Urodelnema mackini*, and *Kamagainema cingula*,[10] the trematode *Telorchis cryptobranchi*,[24] and the cestodes *Crepidobothrium cryptobranchi* and *Ophiotaenia cryptobranchi*,[24] but none appear to be clinically significant. The leech (*Placobdella cryptobranchii*, previously *Batracobdella cryptobranchii*) is often present on Ozark hellbenders[15] and may be the vector of *Trypanosoma cryptobranchi*.[14] Leeches may be present in large numbers and attachment points may produce small cutaneous wounds. *Trypanosoma cryptobranchi*[19] hemoparasites have been

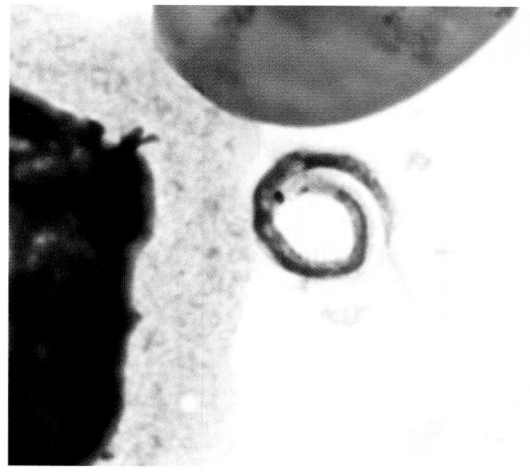

Figure 34-1

Trypanosoma cryptobranchii in a blood smear from an Ozark hellbender (hematoxylin and eosin stain, 40× objective). *(Courtesy J. Merkel.)*

detected in hellbenders; however, the clinical significance is unknown (Fig. 34-1).

NONINFECTIOUS CONDITIONS

Traumatic injuries to digits and appendages appears to be relatively common, presumably from intraspecific aggression and predator injuries. Wild hellbenders are frequently found missing digits or limbs.[11,13,27] In most cases, the animals do not appear to be compromised from these injuries and healing is complete. In captivity, such wounds may occur from intraspecific aggression, trauma, or exhibit materials (rock substrate). On some occasions, distal appendage wounds are difficult to heal, remain open and ulcerated, and local infection of tissues may progress to expose bone. This may be related to the captive environment if bacterial contamination is high, water quality is not correct, or temperature is inappropriate; however, similarly appearing wounds have been reported in wild hellbenders. These lesions are similar to the ulcerative syndrome caused by ranavirus, which results in necrosis of distal digits. They are also similar to a distal limb necrosis resulting in exposed bone; this has been reported in newts associated with *Batrachochytrium* infection.[1] Tissue samples collected from numerous affected hellbenders have been negative for ranavirus. Samples are inconsistently positive for Bd; however, most Bd-positive hellbenders do not have ulcers. The cause and pathogenesis of this condition is not clear. In most cases, antibiotic therapy is required to achieve healing. Antibiotic soaks do not seem to be as therapeutic as injectable treatment regimens. In wounds with protruding bone, surgery is required to obtain healing. Use of recombinant human platelet-derived growth factor becaplermin (Regranex Gel, OMJ Pharmaceuticals, Raritan, NJ) appears to enhance wound healing by causing rapid granulation of wounds, followed by epithelialization.

Nutritional diseases occur commonly in amphibians in captivity because of difficulty mimicking natural diet. These often include inanition, obesity, steatitis, vitamin deficiencies (B and D), and mineral imbalances, including metabolic bone disease.[4] However, none of these diet-related diseases have been documented in hellbenders.

Congenital abnormalities may occur in amphibians because of environmental disturbances during embryonic development. In hellbenders, missing, fused, or supernumerary digits and a bifurcated limb have been documented.[26] In other species of amphibians, this type of defect is attributed to infection with metacercariae[6]; however, the cause in hellbenders has not been defined. It is presumed that more animals with severe abnormalities do not survive. Neoplastic diseases are common in amphibians.[8] In hellbenders, epidermal papilloma, squamous cell carcinoma, Sertoli cell tumor, and a poorly differentiated sarcoma have been documented.[9,11,23]

RESTRAINT AND ANESTHESIA

Physical restraint in hellbenders is complicated by the mucous coating of the skin and the wet environment. Care must be taken not to damage the skin by rough handling. Animals may be placed on a wet cloth towel and then wrapped in the towel for restraint. This protects the animal from rough handling and maintains skin moisture. Hellbenders may be safely and effectively anesthetized with tricaine methanesulfonate (MS-222) at a concentration of 0.025% (250 mg/liter water) buffered to neutral pH with sodium bicarbonate (baking powder). This concentration is lower than that recommended for other aquatic amphibians.[4] In our experience, using the standard amphibian dose (0.05% to 0.1%) results in excessively deep anesthesia and prolonged recovery. Depth of anesthesia is measured by loss of the righting reflex. With the animal in dorsal recumbency, the heartbeat may be visualized and used for monitoring anesthetic level. For surgical procedures, the hellbender is placed on wet towels to maintain moisture. The depth and duration of anesthesia may be controlled by wetting the animal with water from the anesthetic induction bath. At the termination of the procedure, anesthetic recovery is achieved by immersing the hellbender in untreated water. Gently rocking or swaying the animal may facilitate recovery by encouraging gas exchange.

Surgical procedures in hellbenders are similar to those of other species. The coelomic cavity may be entered via a midline or paramidline approach. Avoid the ventral abdominal vein, which runs along the ventral midline on the interior surface of the abdominal musculature. Closure should be in at least two layers. Absorbable suture may dissolve too quickly or carry infection into the site, resulting in dehiscence; therefore, it is recommended to use nylon suture material in the internal and external layers. The paramidline approach has been used for placement of coelomic radiotransmitters. These animals were held for 2 weeks postanesthesia to monitor surgical sites for dehiscence, which is the most common complication of surgery.

Limb amputations may be necessary with some cases of extremity trauma. In cases in which soft tissue injury is extensive and bone is exposed, surgical débridement and closure may be necessary to achieve healing. For limb amputation, it is important that no bone edges are putting pressure on the skin, which will result in dehiscence. Removal of the bone to the joint proximal to the injury is recommended, with closure of soft tissue and skin over the limb end. Small-gauge (2-0 or 3-0) nonabsorbable nylon suture material is preferred to avoid premature dissolution.

DIAGNOSTIC TECHNIQUES

Radiography is useful for examination of the hellbender skeleton and for identifying the contents of the gastrointestinal tract. However, differences in soft tissue scale is small, so organ delineation is difficult. Note that a significant amount of cartilage exists at the joint surfaces of appendages. This may be misinterpreted as evidence of metabolic bone disease (Fig. 34-2).

Coelomic ultrasonography is also a useful imaging modality. Hellbenders may undergo ultrasound in water, which provides excellent wave transmission and improved image quality. Internal organs are well differentiated. Reproductive structures may be identified in mature animals and are relatively easy to locate during breeding season (Fig. 34-3).

Phlebotomy in hellbenders is performed from the caudal vein, located along the ventral aspect of the tail. Animals may be positioned in dorsal recumbency and

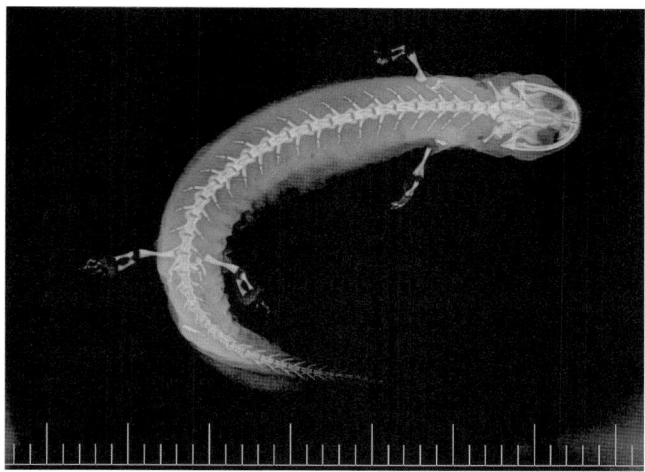

Figure 34-2

Radiograph of an adult hellbender. Note the significant amount of cartilage present at the diaphyseal regions of the longbones. Each hashmark = 1 cm. *(Courtesy R. Junge.)*

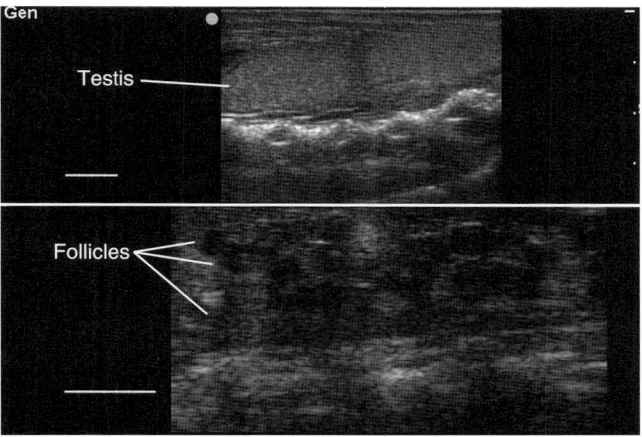

Figure 34-3

Ultrasound image of adult hellbender gonads during the breeding season. The images are longitudinal scans of the caudal coelom. Each bar = 1 cm. *(Courtesy R. Junge.)*

a small-gauge (23- to 25-gauge) needle advanced at the midline to the level of the vertebral column. Alternatively, the animal may be restrained in ventral recumbency and the caudal vein accessed by a lateral approach, advancing the needle from the side to the location ventral to the vertebral column. Normal blood values for captive and wild hellbenders have been published.[17,20]

TREATMENT

Injectable antibiotics are preferred for hellbenders. Topical antibiotic soaks may be useful for prophylaxis or with minor cutaneous infections. Ciprofloxacin soaks (0.01% solution; 10 mg/liter) have been used with apparent positive effects. This antibiotic bath may be used continuously for 10 days. Biologic filters must be removed from the system and a 50% water change carried out every 3 days. However, antibiotic baths should be used only for mild illnesses, because percutaneous absorption may not provide adequate antibiotic levels. Injectable enrofloxacin (10 mg/kg IM every 24 hours), ceftazidime (20 mg/kg IM every 72 hours), amikacin (2.5 mg/kg IM every 72 hours), and pipercillin (100 mg/kg IM every 24 hours) have been used safely and with apparent efficacy in hellbenders. Salt baths (5 to 10 g of salt/liter) for 10 minutes daily may be used as an adjunct treatment because this stimulates the mucous layer and may promote healing. Salt treatment is also effective against some ectoparasites.

There are no specific anthelmentic recommendations for hellbenders. Those recommended for salamanders[4] are probably appropriate, but have not been tested. For analgesia, meloxicam, 0.2 mg/kg IM every 24 hours, has been used, with apparent positive effects.

Antifungal therapy may be necessary for the management of *Batrachochytrium* infections. Itraconazole soaks (0.01% for 5 minutes daily for 11 days) have been recommended[16] and may be useful for low-level infections in uncompromised animals. However, hellbenders that are compromised may require more aggressive therapy to overcome this infection. Oral itraconazole, 5 mg/kg SID for 10 days, has been used, with no apparent negative effects. For compromised patients, especially if cutaneous lesions are present, a multiple treatment regimen yields the best results. For these animals, daily itraconazole soaks and injectable ceftazidime every 72 hours is more effective. Chloramphenicol has been shown to have efficacy against Bd in frogs when used as a bath for 2 to 4 weeks[2]; however, its efficacy in hellbenders has not been tested.

Hyperthermia may also be a useful therapy for Bd.[28] The ideal thermal range for BD is 65° F to 85° F (18° C to 29° C). Elevation of temperatures to 90° F (32° C) for 72 hours effectively kills Bd. Although hellbenders prefer temperatures between 50° F and 70° F (10° C to 21° C), they may tolerate elevated temperatures for a short period of time if they are otherwise healthy, temperatures are elevated slowly, and water oxygenation is maintained. Such treatment has been successful in juvenile hellbenders (3 years old), with concomitant effective treatment of the aquarium. Attempts to heat-treat adults that had cutaneous lesions and possibly bacterial infection was not effective; the animals appeared markedly distressed and compromised, resulting in cessation of the treatment before completion.

Before initiation of heat treatment, hellbenders are pretreated with itraconazole soaks (5 minutes daily for 10 days) and given injectable ceftazidime, 20 mg/kg every 72 hours for three injections to reduce fungal and bacterial load. Water temperature is elevated by 3° F (1.7° C)/day until it reaches 90° F (32° C). Oxygen saturation must be maintained because respiration is compromised at elevated water temperatures. This is accomplished by adding bubblers to the aquarium and reducing the water level to encourage surface respiration. Animals must be monitored carefully and temperatures reduced if animals appear severely stressed or compromised. Animals may abstain from eating at these elevated temperatures, and will roam constantly and rock excessively. Temperature remains at 32° C for 72 hours and then is decreased by 5° F (2.5°C)/day until it reaches the appropriate temperature.

REFERENCES

1. Bovero S, Angelini C, Dogli S, et al: Detection of chytridiomycosis caused by *Batrachochytrium dendrobatidis* in the endangered Sardinian newt *(Euproctus platycephalus)* in southern Sardinia, Italy. J Wildl Dis 44:712–715, 2008.
2. Bishop PJ, Speare R, Poulter R, et al: Elimination of the amphibian chytrid fungus *Batrachochytrium dendrobatidis* by Archey's frog *Leiopelma archeyi*. Dis Aquat Org 84:9–15, 2009.
3. Briggler JT, Larson KA, Irwin KJ: Presence of the amphibian chytrid fungus *(Batrachochytrium dendrobatidis)* on hellbenders *(Cryptobranchus alleganiensis)* in the Ozark Highlands. Herpetol Rev 39:443–444, 2008.
4. Cooper JE: Urodela (Caudata, Urodela). In Fowler ME, Miller RE (eds): Zoo and wild animal medicine, ed 5, Philadelphia, 2003, WB Saunders, pp 33–40.
5. Daszak P, Berger L, Cunningham AA, et al: Emerging infectious diseases and amphibian population declines. Emerg Infect Dis 5:735–748, 1999.
6. Densmore CL, Green DE: Diseases of amphibians. ILAR J 48:235–254, 2007.
7. Green DE, Converse KA, Schrader AK: Epizootiology of sixty-four amphibian morbidity and mortality events in the USA, 1996-2001. Ann N Y Acad Sci 969:323–339, 2002.
8. Green DE, Harshbarger JC: Spontaneous neoplasia. In Wright KM, Whitaker BR (eds): Amphibian medicine and captive husbandry, Malabar, Fla, 2001, Krieger, pp 335–400.
9. Harshbarger JC, Trauth SE: Squamous cell carcinoma upgrade of the epidermal papilloma reported in an Ozark hellbender *(Cryptobranchus alleganiensis bishopi)*. In McKinnell RG, Carlson DL (eds): Proceedings of the 6th International Symposium on Pathology of Reptiles and Amphibians. Saint Paul, Minn, 2002, University of Minnesota Printing Services, pp 43–48.
10. Hasegawa H, Ikeda Y: Helminths from the hellbender, *Cryptobranchus alleganiensis* (Urodela: cryptobranchidae), in Missouri, USA. Comp Parasitol 70:60–65, 2003.
11. Hiler WR, Wheeler BA, Trauth SE: Abnormalities in the Ozark hellbender *(Cryptobranchus alleganiensis bishopi)* in Arkansas: a comparison between two rivers with a historical perspective. J Ark Acad Sci 59:88–94, 2005.
12. Johnson TR: The amphibians and reptiles of Missouri, Jefferson City, Mo, 1992, Department of Conservation.
13. Miller BT, Miller JL: Prevalence of physical abnormalities in Eastern Hellbender *(Cryptobranchus alleganiensis alleganiensis)* populations in Middle Tennessee. Southeastern Naturalist 4:513–520, 2005.
14. Moser WE, Richardson DJ, Wheeler BA, et al: *Placobdella cryptobranchii* (Rhynchobdellida: glossiphoniidae) on *Cryptobranchus alleganiensis bishopi* (Ozark Hellbender) in Arkansas and Missouri. Comp Parasitol 75:98–101, 2008.
15. Nickerson MA, Mays CE: The hellbenders: north American "giant salamanders". Milwaukee, 1972, Milwaukee Public Museum.
16. Nichols DK, Lamirande EW: Successful treatment of chytridiomycosis. Newsletter Colo Coldblooded News 28:1–2, 2001.
17. Normal physiological data values. Apple Valley, Minn, 2002, International Species Inventory System.
18. Pessier AP: Amphibian chytridiomycosis. In Fowler ME, Miller RE (eds): Zoo and wild animal medicine, ed 5, Philadelphia, 2003, WB Saunders, pp 137–143.
19. Roudabush RL, Coatney GR: On some protozoa of reptiles and amphibians. Trans Am Microscop Society 56:291–297, 1937.
20. Solis ME, Bandeff JM, Huang Y: Hematology and serum chemistry of Ozark and eastern hellbenders *(Cryptobranchus alleganiensis)*. Herpetologia 63:285–292, 2007.
21. Solis ME, Liu CC, Nam P, et al: Occurrence of organic chemical in two rivers inhabited by Ozark hellbenders *(Cryptobranchus alleganiensis bishopi)*. Arch Environ Contam Toxicol 53:426–434, 2007.
22. Souza M, Gray M: University of Tennessee; Colclough P, Knoxville Zoo; Debra Miller D, University of Georgia: personal communication, 2010.
23. Trauth SE, Harshbarger CJ, Daniel P, et al: Epidermal papilloma in an Ozark hellbender *(Cryptobranchus alleganiensis bishopi)* from the Spring River of Northern Arkansas. J Ark Acad Sci 56:190–197, 2002.
24. Walton AC: The parasites of the Cryptobranchoidea (Amphibia: caudata). J Parasitol 28:29, 1942.
25. Weiss RB, Wolf TM, Pessier AP, et al: Health assessment of eastern hellbender *(Cryptobranchus alleganiensis alleganiensis)* populations in Ohio and West Virginia. In Proceedings of the American Association of Zoo Veterinarians–American Association of Wildlife Veterinarians Joint Conference, 2009, p 82.
26. Wheeler BA, McCallum ML, Trauth SE, et al: Abnormalities in the Ozark hellbender, *Cryptobranchus alleganiensis bishopi*. J Ark Acad Sci 56:250–252, 2002.
27. Wheeler BA, Prosen E, Mathis A, Wilkinson RF, et al: Population declines of a long-loved salamander: a 20+-year study of hellbenders, *Cryptobranchus alleganiensis*. Biol Conserv 109:151–156, 2003.
28. Woodhams DC, Alford RA, Marantelli G, et al: Emerging disease of amphibians cured by elevated body temperature. Dis Aquat Org 55:65–67, 2003.

Avian

CHAPTER 35

Avian Mycobacterial Disease

Gary Riggs

Mycobacteriosis is an ancient disease that continues to have a major impact in avian collections worldwide. Mycobacterial disease was "discovered" by Koch in 1882, although mycobacterial organisms have been isolated in human remains from 7000 BC and recovered from bison more than 18,000 years old.[10,19,27] A Greek term, *phthisis*, was ascribed to tuberculosis-type lesions in 460 BC and, in the 1020s, a physician, Ibn Sina, in the *Canon of Medicine*, was the first to suggest that the disease caused by mycobacteria could be spread through contact with soil and water. It is these same characteristics that plague avian collections to this day.

By 1882, mycobacterial disease was reported in many avian species in zoological surveys. Reports included Darwin's rhea, common fowl, common peafowl, golden pheasant, grouse, pigeon, partridge, stork, crane, falcon, and eagles.[4] In 1886, Lehman and Neuman discovered what would be known as *Mycobacterium avium*, which was subsequently named based on its pathogenicity in poultry.[12] In 1896, the term *mycobacteria*, or *fungus bacterium*, was introduced, with its name derived from the organism's growth characteristics on liquid media.

Until 1990, most avian mycobacterial infections were attributed to *M. avium* (particularly serotypes 1 and 2). Around that time, however, a new species named *M. genovense* was isolated.[4] It is also an opportunistic environmental mycobacterium, but has proven much more difficult to isolate using standard culture techniques, resulting in underreporting in many cases. Some less common mycobacterial isolates from birds include *M. intracellulare*, *M. fortuitum*, *M. tuberculosis*, *M. gordonae*, *M. nonchromogenicin*, *M. bovis*, and *M. simiae*.[25]

Avian mycobacteriosis is often used synonymously with *Mycobacterium avian* complex (MAC) or with *Mycobacterium avian-intracellulare* complex (MAIC, or MAI) to include a distinct but similar specie,

M. intracellulare. Within *M. avium*, organisms are further divided into four subspecies—*avium*, *silvaticum*, *hominissuis*, and *paratuberculosis*. An international working group has alternatively classified four MAC groups based on the 28 Schaefer serotypes. *M. avium* includes serotypes 1 to 6 and 8 to 11, *M. intercellulare* includes serotypes 7, 12 to 20, 23, and 25, *M. scrofulceum* includes serotype 27 and unclassified mycobacteria serotypes 21, 24, 26, and 28.

The term *mycobacteriosis* may apply to any disease resulting from a mycobacterial infection. It is often used when describing the nontubercle form of mycobacterial disease, a pattern typical of *M. genovense* infections. Similar lesions, as well as tubercle growth (avian tuberculosis; Fig. 35-1), or mixed-type lesions (Fig. 35-2) may occur with MAC infections. All lesion types are capable of shedding organisms.

Mycobacteria are of the order Actinomycetales, family Mycobacteriaceae, and genus *Mycobacterium*. Mycobacteria are intracellular, gram positive, non–spore-forming, aerobic, rod-shaped bacteria that exhibit a lipid-rich waxy cell wall. It is the cell wall that accounts for mycobacterial resistance and increases the difficulty of diagnosis and treatment of mycobacterial disease. This lipid coating also enhances pathogenicity by allowing the organism to persist for long periods, both outside of the host and within the host's endosomal macrophage network.

Structurally, the mycobacterial cell wall is an asymmetric membrane composed of a thin layer of tightly packed long-chain mycolic acids with a diverse array of free lipids (Fig. 35-3). The outer membrane is covalently linked to an arabinoside polysaccharide, which in turn is linked to an underlying layer of peptidoglycan.[14] Additionally, glycopeptidolipids present in the cell wall are believed to be important for the formation of protective environmental biofilms.[11] The high lipid content of

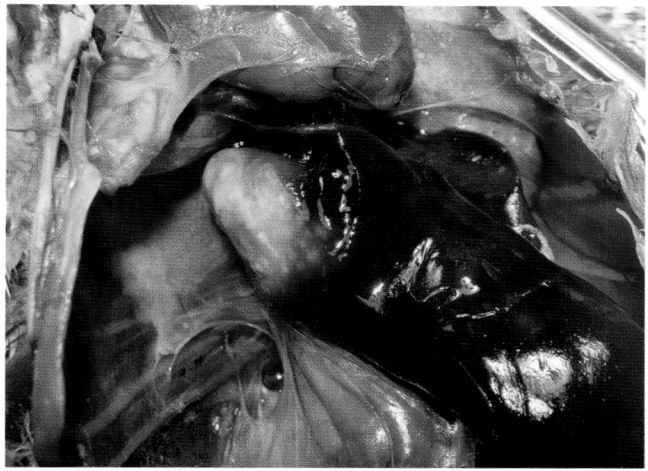

Figure 35-1

Hepatic mycobacterial granuloma.

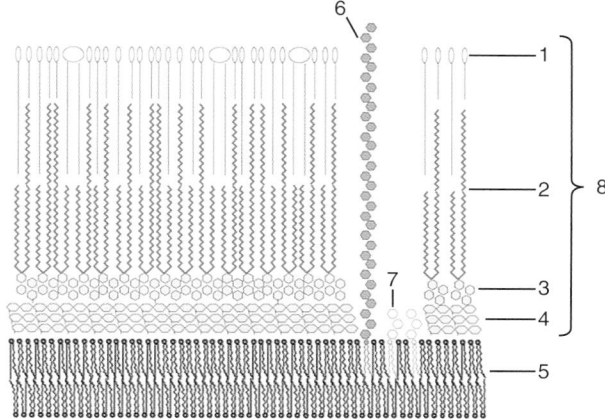

Figure 35-3

Mycobacterial cell wall. *1*, Outer lipids; *2*, mycolic acid; *3*, polysaccharides; *4*, peptidoglycan; *5*, plasma membrane; *6*, lipoarabinomannan; *7*, phosphatidylinositol mannoside; *8*, cell wall skeleton.

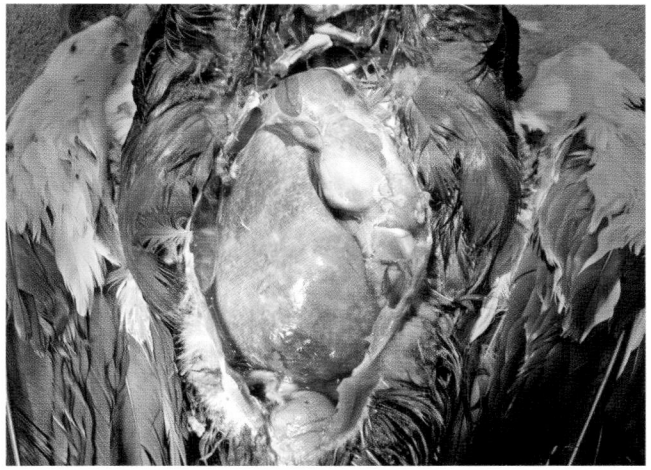

Figure 35-2

Mixed-type mycobacterial infection in a duck.

the cell wall gives mycobacteria the ability to retain basic dyes in an acid-alcohol environment, leading to their acid-fast designation.

SPECIES AFFECTED AND PREVALENCE

Avian mycobacteriosis is a ubiquitous disease in domestic, captive, and wild birds. All birds appear to be susceptible, and no reports of totally resistant species exist. Although diagnosed more commonly in the north temperate zone, avian mycobacterial disease occurs worldwide. Observations by Hejlicek and Treml in 1995 regarding the relative susceptibility of avian species in large collections listed highly susceptible species as domestic fowl, sparrows, pheasants, partridges, and

laughing gulls.[9a] Moderately susceptible species were turkeys and guinea fowl. Moderately resistant birds were reported to be geese and ducks. More highly mycobacteria-resistant species were thought to be pigeons, turtle doves, and rooks.

In general, the disease appears relatively uncommon in individual or small groups of captive held birds. A review of 5345 pet bird necropsies in Switzerland revealed a 3.8% incidence, with *M. genovense* infecting the majority.[4] A recent survey of 23,960 necropsies of captive-held birds in the United States showed that mycobacteria was present in only 1.3% of the cases submitted.[17]

Disease prevalence is even lower, with notable exceptions, in free-ranging wild bird populations. Prevalence in free-ranging North American birds has been reported as less than 1%, which compares to a 0.7% prevalence in a study of 12,000 birds in the Netherlands.[8] A review of 3000 U.S. wild waterfowl necropsies revealed a 0.3% infection rate.[8] Mycobacterial infection in wild raptors is also considered rare and opportunistic.[4] Individual flock history and environmental factors may play a major role in prevalence rates. A free-ranging U.S. whooping crane population was determined to have prevalence rates as high as 39% caused by specific environmental conditions favoring infection and spread.

Avian mycobacterial disease is most common in large flocks of zoological and avicultural collections, although marked prevalence variability occurs. Retrospective avian necropsy reviews from three U.S. zoological institutions have reported 1.2%, 4%, and 24.5%

prevalence rates of mycobacterial disease, respectively.[3,4,26] Husbandry protocols, environmental factors, and the species involved may have a dramatic impact on institutional incidence. In areas of environmental buildup, waterfowl and water birds, which are normally quite resistant in the wild, may be infected in large numbers.

CLINICAL SIGNS

The clinical signs of avian mycobacterial disease vary according to organism species, route of infection (oral, respiratory, or wound), target organ, and chronicity. There are no pathognomonic clinical signs for avian mycobacterial infection. Commonly reported clinical presentations include emaciation with good appetite, abnormal feathers or molt, loss of flock position, diarrhea, dyspnea, abdominal distension, granuloma formation (cutaneous, subcutaneous, and ocular), nervous system symptoms, and lameness. Clinical changes are often subtle until late in the course of disease, with the birds often continuing to eat and behave normally despite marked weight loss.

Differential diagnoses are as varied as the clinical signs but should include any wasting or granulomatous type disease. Differentials include coligranuloma (Hjärre disease), *Yersinia*, *Listeria*, mycosis, avian gastric yeast, pneumonia, parasitism, toxicity, *Salmonella*, neoplasia, and avian Borna virus disease.

DIAGNOSIS AND IMMUNE RESPONSE

A major obstacle in the management of avian mycobacterial disease is the inability to diagnose the disease in its early stages consistently and accurately. As a result, high levels of organism shedding and subsequent environmental buildup may occur from clinically normal individuals.

Hematologic changes most often occur late in the course of mycobacterial disease. When seen, nonspecific changes include heterophilia, monocytosis, hyperfibrinogenemia, thrombocytosis, polychromasia, and anemia.[23] Marked hematologic changes in the form of significant heterophilic leukocytosis often signal the end stage of the disease process and, in some species, may be predictive of a terminal event.[18] Potential serum chemistry alterations include increased hepatic enzyme and bile acid levels, as well as hyperproteinemia, hypoalbuminemia, and hyperglobulinemia. These changes, however, are unreliable and depend on the route of infection and stage of the disease.

Radiology may be effective to help substantiate a diagnosis of mycobacteriosis; however, it is also a nonspecific and inconsistent diagnostic tool. Signs may include organ enlargement, coelomic enlargement, pulmonary nodules and cystic bone lesions. Endoscopic and ultrasonic examinations may be helpful as well, but also suffer from low sensitivity and specificity, particularly in the early stages of infection.[18]

Traditionally, the gold standard for mycobacterial diagnosis has been culture. Culturing the organism, however, is often difficult, time-consuming, and dependent on a sufficient quantity of viable organisms being present (>100 organisms/mL).[4] As a fecal screening test, cultures display low sensitivity and specificity because of environmental contamination issues and unpredictable organism shedding. Automated radiometric liquid culture techniques have improved isolation; however, culture still remains an unreliable screening technique on an individual bird basis.

Acid-fast staining is commonly used as a confirmatory test for swabs and tissues, but is also not an effective means of screening for disease. Accurate acid-fast staining is dependent on the absence of contamination and on the presence of more than 10,000 organisms/mL of sample. Acid-fast fecal screening in one study confirmed only 7% of culture-positive samples.[4]

Other modalities of organism detection have shown higher sensitivity and/or specificity for confirmatory testing, but are also not the answer for screening. DNA probes and polymerase chain reaction (PCR) testing, which may detect the equivalent of a single mycobacterial organism, are the preferred methods of antemortem and postmortem diagnosis of infected tissues and samples. PCR 16s-rRNA gene primers, adapted from *M. bovis* tests, have been very effective in identifying *M. avium* samples.[4] PCR testing has been further used to help differentiate virulent strains using primers such as IS901 insertion sequences.[16] Fecal screening techniques involving PCR technology are hampered by the common issue of unreliable organism shedding. Also, PCR fecal inhibitors and environmental contaminants may negatively affect accuracy. Newer generations of real-time PCR assays, including those targeting 65-kDa heat shock proteins, are being used for improved sample diagnosis. Real-time PCR testing also has demonstrated improved capabilities for quantitative results, with reduced risk of contamination and less sensitivity to inhibitors.

Response to mycobacterial infection is initially controlled by cell-mediated mechanisms but, unfortunately, mycobacteria have evolved many means to evade elimination by the host. Mycobacteria are able to suppress host macrophage production selectively and can block destruction by preventing the normal fusion of phagosomes with lysosomes. Mycobacteria may hide, survive, and even replicate in the host macrophages for years, only to develop into an active infection when the host's immune system is suppressed. Cell-mediated testing, such as the intradermal skin test, used effectively in the commercial poultry industry for flock screening, is unreliable in nondomestic species.[15]

Humoral systems do not seem to play a major protective role and become demonstrable only in the later stages of disease. As noted, humoral responses differ among bird species and display no pathognomonic patterns. Serologic tests such as rapid agglutination testing, enzyme-linked immunosorbent assay (ELISA), and Western blot tests have been used with varying success for flock diagnosis. Western blot analysis, as an example, displayed a sensitivity of 88.24% and specificity of 100% in one study of a known infected population of ring-necked doves.[9] However, results did not correlate with disease severity or stage of infection.

ELISA's have also been developed for use in specific avian populations. Commercial tests are generally unavailable for most exotic species, and the requirement for species-specific antigens makes widespread use of these tests difficult and costly for large mixed collections. To date, ELISA's have not shown an adequate level of sensitivity and specificity in initial disease stages to serve as quarantine screening tests, although specific ELISA's have been used effectively for later stage culling in infected populations.[4] With all serologic testing, best results are seen with flock screening rather than use on the individual level.

Research is ongoing for test development to aid in the early diagnosis of mycobacterial disease. Until a gold standard exists, clinical screening cannot be relied on as the sole management tool.

TREATMENT, SOURCES, PREVENTION, AND CONTROL

Many treatment protocols exist for individual birds. Because of poor prognosis, cost, labor, prolonged treatment requirements, risk of resistance, zoonotic risks, and the difficulty of determining a treatment endpoint, therapy is not generally recommended for collection birds. Treatment plays no role in collection management and disease control.

Vaccination has also not proven to be effective for collection management and limited vaccine trials to this point have not achieved statistical significance.[4] Along with vaccine development complications, it is speculated that excessive environmental exposure to common antigens prior to vaccination may be detrimental to the development of an adequate protective response. Animal models have shown that early exposure to environmental mycobacteria may result in inappropriate priming of the host immune system, possibly resulting in lowered immune response to vaccines and pathogenic strains.[24]

Because of the difficulties of early mycobacterial diagnosis, disease prevention and control for captive birds must focus on environmental and collection planning and monitoring. Outbreaks in free-ranging birds are rare and found most often in species that live in close contact with infected domestic stock, in areas of infected soil, or at collecting points of contaminated water runoff. In captivity, large avian populations under increased stress may result in exaggerated disease incidence. In most surveys of infected collections, waterfowl and water birds are over-represented most, although any species is at risk in a contaminated environment.

Mycobacteria are ubiquitous environmental saprophytes found commonly in marshes, ponds, and rivers at the soil- water interface and are even known to play important roles as nutritional sources in the ecology of some insects.[12] They are routinely isolated from a variety of beddings, soil types, and commercial water sources. Mycobacteria thrive in conditions of low pH, high zinc, high organic content, and increased fulvic and humic acid levels. Their lipid cell walls make mycobacteria extremely resistant to heat and cold. *M. avium* survives above 55° C and may not only survive freezing at −75° C, but may even increase its numbers postfreezing.[13] Mycobacterial organisms are also able to remain viable in soil for up to 4 years using metabolic shutdown mechanisms to survive starvation.[1]

Fecal contamination of the environment by infected shedders is the major means of mycobacterial disease dissemination.[8] Mycobacterial disease is not easily transmitted bird to bird, and environmental reservoirs are usually required for collection outbreaks.[21] Vertical transmission is thought to be unlikely; however, young birds may easily be infected from fecal and soil contamination of the eggs, nest, and environment.

Collection management goals should include all steps possible to minimize mycobacterial buildup in the avian environment. Particular attention should be paid to water sources because mycobacteria may increase exponentially in the nutrient-rich soil-water interfaces. Mycobacteria thrive in water and synthesize polysaccharides containing methylated hexoses; these give the organisms hydrophobic bonds to gas bubbles and surfaces in aquatic environments.[6] The hydrophobic nature and subsequent binding to air bubbles may also markedly increase bird exposures through water aerosolization and dabbling feeding behavior. Additional human sources of aerosolization such as waterfalls, fountains, and hose spraying may increase the number of viable mycobacterial cells per millimeter up to 1000-fold, greatly increasing the risk of respiratory infection in contact birds.[7]

Mycobacterial hydrophobic properties also increase the organism's overall adherence capabilities, making them difficult to remove from environmental surfaces. Simply draining or rinsing ponds or pools will have little chance of removing mycobacteria in surface biofilms. Those organisms not adhered to the pool surface will be attached to suspended particulate matter. Mycobacteria buildup is positively correlated with increased water turbidity, and filtration and reduction of aqueous organic material may be helpful in minimizing environmental contamination and disease risk.

On land, mycobacteria may readily become attached to soil particles via electrostatic van der Waals forces and cell surface hydrophobicity, resulting in strong attachments. These attachments further increase the risk of infection by preventing organisms from settling deeper into the soil. As a result, mycobacteria are retained in the surface layers, where grazing species may be more easily exposed. Additional contamination results when these organisms, attached to surface particles, are washed into environmental water sources. The mycobacterial particle attachment is facilitated by an acid pH in soil and water, making pH one of the few parameters that may be potentially altered to aid in mycobacterial control.[12]

Within water biofilms, mycobacteria may also survive and grow in phagocytic protozoa (*Tetrahymena pyriformis*) and amoeba (*Acanthamoeba polyphaga* and *A. castellanii*).[13] Growth in these common environmental organisms may even increase their virulence by protecting them from antimicrobial agents. Efforts to reduce water biofilm layers are critical to reducing overall mycobacterial levels in the environment.

Insects and invertebrates such as cockroaches, ticks, flies, and earthworms are among the other organisms known to harbor and shed mycobacteria. Small vertebrates may also play a role in disease transmission; pathogenic mycobacteria have been routinely isolated from a variety of wild rodents.

In addition to animals, the environment may be populated by mycobacteria in plants, further increasing the risks for grazing species and contributing to contamination from water runoff. Sphagnum vegetation actually supports mycobacterial growth, creating a heated microenvironment that may markedly enhance organism buildup.[12]

In some cases, however, plants may play a positive role in mycobacterial control. A novel technique for reducing water system mycobacterial buildup uses reed beds as natural biofilters. Drewe and colleagues[5] have reported an adaptation of previous models using wetlands for waste water treatment of an endemic mycobacterial environment. Common reed (*Pragmites australis*) and greater reedmace (*Typha latifolia*) were found to be effective in the eradication of *M. avium* by sedimentation and adsorption onto the reed stems. In their study, effluent PCR analysis was used to demonstrate that near-complete reduction of pathogenic mycobacteria may be achieved downstream from the reed beds. This technique may be especially useful to reduce contamination from endemic areas prior to water release into wildlife or residential waterways.

Mycobacteria are organisms that are resistant to both chemical and ultraviolet (UV) disinfection.[22] They are 700 to 3000 times as resistant to chlorine as *Escherichia coli* and 50 times as resistant to ozone.[13] Among waterborne pathogens, the ultraviolet C (UVC) dose (needed to achieve inactivation) was much higher than levels required for all other pathogenic bacteria studied. Additionally, mycobacteria are capable of high levels of post-UVC exposure repair, further reducing its effectiveness. Therefore, sunlight UVA and UVB irradiation are ineffective in reducing mycobacterial numbers, although substrate drying may be helpful for minimizing organism buildup.

In addition to resistance issues, the use of disinfectants in avian environments may actually be detrimental to mycobacterial control.[7] By destroying nonpathogenic organisms that would ordinarily compete for nutrients, disinfectant use may favor the overgrowth of pathogenic mycobacteria. Because required disinfectant contact times and tuberculocidal conditions are rarely, if ever, met in the field, disinfectants should not be relied on for mycobacterial prevention. Foot baths, commonly used to prevent microbe spread from one avian enclosure to another, may actually only serve to loosen debris and enhance mycobacterial transfer.

Controlling the introduction and buildup of myco-bacteria into a collection through risk management, screening, and culling of collection animals may be effective, but difficult. However, the poultry industry has demonstrated that mycobacterial disease may be nearly totally eliminated when the birds and environment can be controlled absolutely.[23] The strict practices used for the poultry industry, however, are not generally applicable to captive avian collections.

In 2004, an American Zoo and Aquarium Association working group developed a stepwise risk assessment protocol that may be used when analyzing additions to avian collections.[2] The resultant algorithm (Fig. 35-4) is a good working tool for collection managers and also highlights the complexities involved in minimizing mycobacterial risks in large avian populations. Along with risk analysis, minimizing movement of birds in and out of holding areas, frequent health monitoring of the avian collection, and aggressive workup and removal of older birds exhibiting behavioral changes or weight loss may help reduce environmental buildup, thereby reducing disease incidence.

Genetic history may be an important factor to consider as well, because low genetic diversity may increase mycobacterial susceptibility. The nature and number of tubercular lesions in chickens have been linked to individual genetics, and dramatic prevalence increases in some inbred endangered species populations point to genetics as playing a significant role.[18,20,26]

Quarantine of incoming birds is important, but assessment is problematic. A realistic length of quarantine for mycobacterial disease is difficult to determine without sensitive and specific laboratory screening capabilities, and quarantine lengths have been proposed from 30 days to 6 months and beyond. Quarantine length should be extended for as long as is possible for the collection, and should be influenced by the bird's risk analysis, testing, and overall health status.

Of utmost importance in controlling mycobacterial disease is the minimization of stress on the avian collection. Some common stress reduction techniques include reducing bird numbers, segregating incompatible species, optimizing natural behavior (e.g., nonpinioned, multiple perching, adequate hiding areas), optimizing nutrition, and using species comfortable in the environment's temperature, humidity, and substrate ranges.

Design or redesign of avian holding areas to create inhospitable environments for mycobacteria may aid disease control. The elimination of the soil-water interface is of primary importance. Frequent water changes, eliminating nonessential soil and wet areas, increasing the pH of soil and water, and frequent soil change-outs in high population density areas will all be beneficial in minimizing pathogen buildup.

For ponds, using soil-free, cleanable surfaces with particle filtration to decrease turbidity will minimize mycobacterial presence. Pools and water pipes should have routine cleaning schedules to reduce biofilm buildup and water systems should be designed to minimize or eliminate fountains, sprays, and waterfall features near collection birds.

Holding area design should also strive to eliminate water runoff from soil and animal areas into pools or wetlands. If possible, the incorporation of reed bed features for larger connected waterways may be effective for reducing pathogenic mycobacteria in recirculated water systems and improve downstream water quality as well.

ZOONOSIS

Environmental control is important for those servicing, and visitors attending, the avian facility. Although generally of low zoonotic concern, immunsuppressed individuals may experience a significant disease risk in a contaminated environment. Since 1991, MAIC complex has accounted for 96% of mycobacterial infections in AIDS patients, and 50% of HIV-positive patients developed MAIC infections as a terminal event.[4] Staff or visitors contacting a mycobacteria-contaminated environment, particularly if in contact with collection-shared water or water features, could be at increased risk of exposure to potentially pathogenic organisms.

CONSERVATION IMPACT

Mycobacterial infections have had a significant impact on the conservation management of endangered avian species. Complications from infections may be devastating, especially for small breeding populations or for those with the increased stress of a release program. Reduced genetic diversity and the need to maintain older populations may increase mycobacterial prevalence in endangered species collections.

The conservation plan for an endemic infection may be especially difficult. The traditional approach to a severe mycobacterial collection problem involves the culling of the entire contact population and repopulating after environmental changes are made. This approach is not appropriate for most conservation programs. Instead, environmental, husbandry, and screening techniques may need to be modified in

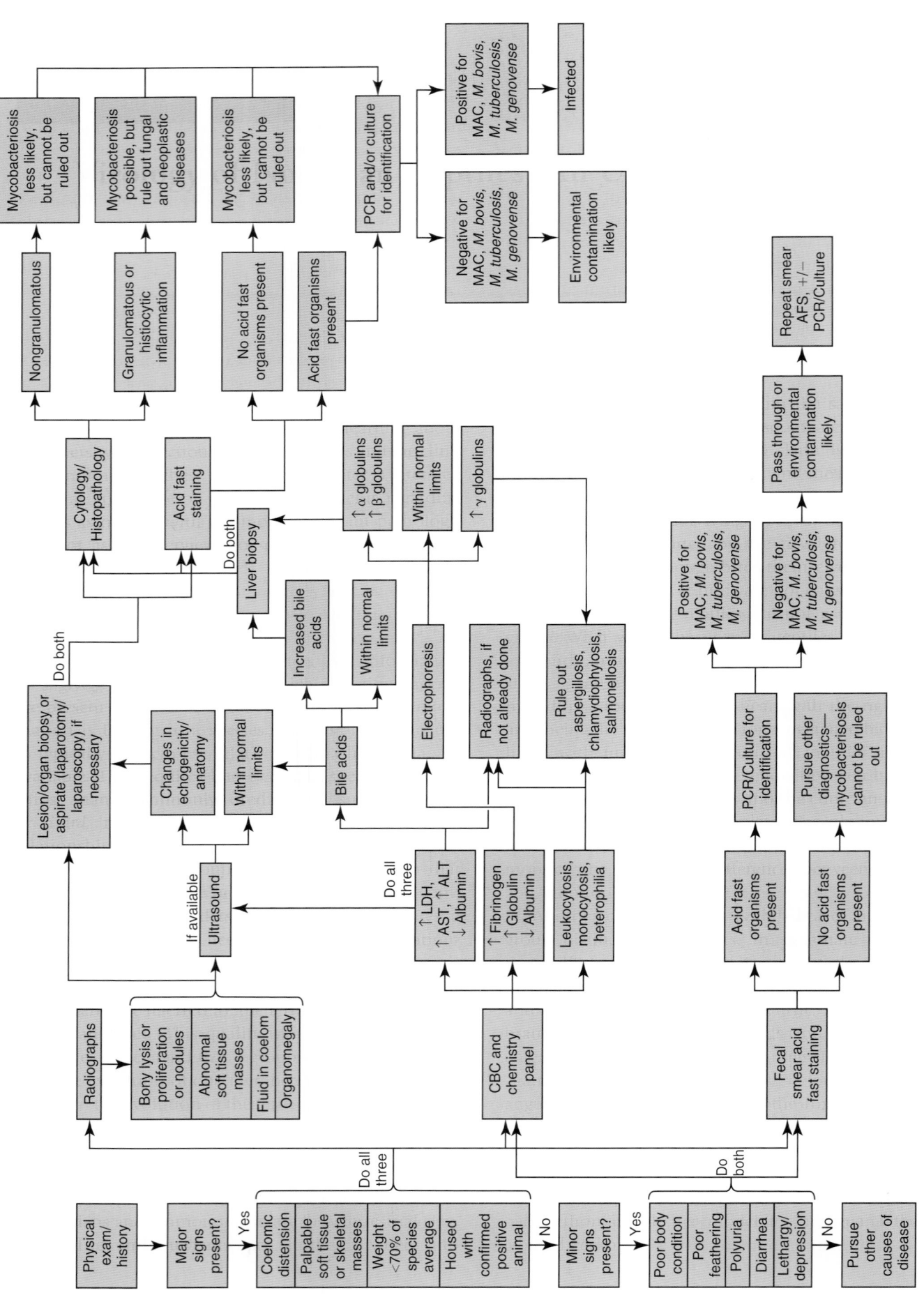

Figure 35-4

Tuberculosis risk analysis tree.

an attempt to produce an isolated disease free sub-population.

An example of this is the white-winged wood duck species survival plan (SSP).[18] Within this program's primary breeding population, there has been an almost 100% death rate by the age of 4 years, with over 95% of the deaths attributed to mycobacterial infection. As a result, the reproductive lifespan of the population is critically reduced and movement of the birds to other collections is affected. Because of low total population numbers and inability to repopulate from an outside source, culling was not an option.

A conservation plan was formulated using an environmental approach to disease control. An isolation facility would be constructed and staffed by personnel servicing only that facility. Strict construction parameters and husbandry controls would be used, including holdings with no soil-water interface, frequent water changes (with biofilm removal), no soil substrate on land, use of artificial perching materials, reduction of specie stressors (nonpinioned, multiple perching, heat and lighting set for natural species requirements), and frequent health monitoring.

The facility was designed to be populated with incubator-raised birds from sources that had experienced minimal historical mycobacterial disease. The eggs used were PCR-tested mycobacteria-negative. Incubation and rearing of the group would be carried out under quarantine conditions, with no soil or other animal contact before moving to the new facility. The future population derived in this manner would then serve as a starter group for eventual repopulation of SSP holding facilities and serve as a control group for further mycobacterial research in this species.

No one protocol will be effective or practical in every conservation situation. Thus, each avian conservation program dealing with mycobacterial issues needs to evaluate their individual risks and options to develop plans suitable to their species and conservation goals.

FUTURE ISSUES

Mycobacterial infection in birds is a ubiquitous problem of varying prevalence and impact. It is an age-old problem and one that is increasing in many collections and wild bird populations because of organism resistance, increased distribution, and difficulty with early and accurate diagnosis. Until a sensitive and specific early antemortem gold standard test emerges, the disease will need to be controlled by the use of aggressive preventive protocols and by carrying out detailed risk analyses for incoming collection birds. Exhibit and holding area designs should incorporate mycobacteria-reducing and stress-reducing features as part of their plans, with the ultimate goal of minimizing any mycobacterial disease impact on the collection.

Acknowledgments

I would like to thank the owners and staff of Sylvan Heights Waterfowl Park and Eco-Center for their support and assistance. Additional thanks go to to Dr. Drury Reavill (Zoo/Exotic Pathology Services) for her survey data.

REFERENCES

1. Archuleta R, Hoppes PY, Primm T: Mycobacterium avium enters a state of metabolic dormancy in response to starvation. Tuberculosis 85:147–158, 2005.
2. AZA/CEF-ASAG Mycobacterial Working Group: personal communication, 2004.
3. Beehler BA: Management of Mycobacterium avium in a mixed species aviary. In Proceedings of the American Association of Zoo Veterinarians, Yulee, Fla, 1990, American Association of Zoo Veterinarians, pp 125–129.
4. Converse K: Avian tuberculosis. In Thomas NJ, Hunter DB, Atkinson CT, editors: Infectious diseases of wild birds, Oxford, 2007, Blackwell, pp 289–302.
5. Drewe JA, Mwangi D, Donoghue HD, Cromie RL: PCR analysis of the presence and location of Mycobacterium avium in a constructed reed bed, with implications for avian tuberculosis control. FEMS Microbiol Ecol 67:320–328, 2009.
6. Empadinhas N, Albuquerque L, Mendes V, et al: Identification of the mycobacterial glucosyl-3-phosphoglycerate synthase. FEMS Microbiol Lett 280:195–202, 2008.
7. Falkinham JO III: Mycobacterial aerosols and respiratory disease. Emerg Infect Dis 9:763–767, 2003.
8. Franson JC, Friend M: Field manual of wildlife diseases, Washington DC, 1999, U.S. Geological Survey.
9. Gray PL, Saggese MD, Phalen DN, et al: Humoral response to mycobacterium avium subsp. avium in naturally infected ring-necked doves (Streptopelia risoria). Vet Immunol Immunopathol 125216–125224, 2008.
9a. Hejlicek K, Treml F: Comparison of the pathogenesis and epizootiologic importance of avian mycobacteriosis in various types of domestic and free-living syntropic birds. Vet Med 40:187–194, 1995.
10. Hershkovitz I, Donoghue MD, Minnikin DE, et al: Electronic journal: detection and molecular characterization of 9000-year-old mycobacterium tuberculosis from a neolithic settlement in the Eastern Mediterranean. PloS One 3:e3426, 2008.
11. Johansen TB, Agdestein A, Olsen I, et al: Biofilm formation by Mycobacterium avium isolates originating from humans, swine and birds. BMC Microbiol 9:159, 2009.
12. Kazda J: The ecology of mycobacteria, Dordrecht, the Netherlands, 2000, Kluwer.
13. LeChevallier MW: Control, treatment and disenfection of mycobacterium avium complex in drinking water. In Pedley S, Bartram J, et al, editors: Pathogenic mycobacteria in water: a guide to public health consequences, monitoring and management, London, 2004, IWA, pp 144–168.

14. Morita YS, Velasquez R, Taig E, et al: Compartmentalization of lipid biosynthesis in mycobacteria. J Biol Chem 280:21645–21652, 2005.
15. OIE (World Organisation for Animal Health): Manual of diagnostic tests and vaccines for terrestrial animals, 2010 (http://www.oie.int/eng/normes/mmanual/a_summry).
16. Pavlik I, Svastova P, Barti J, et al: Relationship between IS901 in the Mycobacterium avium complex strains isolated from birds, animals, humans, and the environment and virulence for poultry. Clin Diagn Lab Immunol 7:212–217, 2000.
17. Reavill D: personal communication, 2009.
18. Riggs GL: White-winged wood duck (Cairina scutulata) species survival plan update. Presented at the American of Zoo Veterinarians—Association of Reptilian and Amphibian Veterinarians Joint Conference Los Angeles, October 11–17, 2008.
19. Rothschild BM, Martin LD, Lev G, et al: Mycobacterium tuberculosis complex DNA from an extinct bison dated 17,000 years before the present. Clin Infect Dis 33:305–311, 2001.
20. Saggese MD, Riggs GL, Tizard I, et al: Gross and microscopic findings and investigation of the aetiopathogenesis of mycobacteriosis in a captive population of white-winged ducks (Cairina scutulata). Avian Pathol 36:415–422, 2007.
21. Schrenzel M, Nicholas M, Witte C, et al: Molecular epidemiology of mycobacterium avium subsp. avium and mycobacterium intracellularity in captive birds. Vet Microbiol 126:122–131, 2008.
22. Shin G, Lee J, Freeman R, et al: Inactivation of mycobacterium avium by UV irradiation. Appl Environ Microbiol 74:7067–7069, 2008.
23. Tell LA, Woods L, Cromie RL: Mycobacteriosis in birds. Rev Sci Tech 20:180–203, 2001.
24. Thom M, Howard C, Villarreal-Ramos B, et al: Consequence of prior exposure to environmental mycobacteria on BCG vaccination and diagnosis of tuberculosis infection. Tuberculosis 88:324–334, 2008.
25. Travis EK, Junge RE, Terrell SP: Infection with Mycobacterium simiae complex in four captive Micronesian kingfishers. J Am Vet Med Assoc 230:1524–1529, 2007.
26. Witte CL, Hungerford LL, Papendick R, et al: Factors associated with mycobacteriosis in captive birds. In Proceedings of the American Association of Zoo Veterinarians, Yulee, Fla, 2007, American Association of Zoo Veterinarians, p 73.
27. Zink AR, Sola C, Reischl U, et al: Molecular identification and characterization of Mycobacterium tuberculosis complex in ancient Egyptian mummies. Int J Osteoarchaeol 14:404–413, 2004.

CHAPTER 36

Feather Follicle Extirpation: Operative Techniques to Prevent Zoo Birds from Flying

Pia Krawinkel

In zoos, birds such as flamingos, pelicans, and waterfowl are ideally exhibited in large areas, often with lakes and islands. In such displays, the birds have to be prevented from escaping. This may be achieved by constructing large free-flight aviaries or by applying different flight restraint methods to the birds. Preventing birds from flying is an important ethical issue and has been discussed extensively, although without satisfying conclusions so far.

However, the method of feather follicle extirpation could be applied to certain bird species without inappropriately influencing their normal behavior because swimming, diving, walking, eating, and maintaining balance during copulation are still possible. Obviously, the problem of maintaining balance is not as challenging for follicle-extirpated birds as it is, for example, for pinioned birds[9] (Box 36-1).

ANATOMY

The skeleton of the wing consists of the humerus, ulna, radius, ossa carpi, and ossa metacarpalia (carpometacarpus) plus three fingers (phalanx proximalis minoris, phalanx proximalis digiti majoris, phalanx distalis digiti majoris; Fig. 36-1). The thumb phalanx, digiti alularis, is located at the os metacarpale majus.

In normal position, with the wing folded, the humerus is resting at the body. Two major muscles are inserting at the humeral bone. The Musculus biceps brachii is responsible for flexion and the M. triceps brachii for the extension of the wing. The pneumatized humeral bone is supplied with air via the saccus clavicularis.

In birds, the ulna and radius run parallel to each other without rotational movement and the ulna is larger than the radius. The carpalia and metacarpalia are joined and reduced to a few bones, such as the carpometacarpus, os carpis ulnare, and os carpi radiale. There are three digits; the thumb (alular digit) may have one or two phalanges and is called the alula. The alula has an important aerodynamic function by capturing the uplifting wind. The second finger (digitis major) has two phalanges. The third finger digit is a minor digit, with only one phalanx. The joints of the wing may only be flexed and extended to obtain a rigid wing. During flight, the main force comes from the distal wing, whereas the proximal region of the wing is providing the uplift.

FEATHERS

Feathers have a cornified epidermis. During growth, the feather is supplied with blood from the follicle. The venous and arterial vessels degenerate once the growth is completed. Therefore, traumatization of newly growing feathers can cause severe blood loss.

The pinion is a contour feather with a hollow shaft and a vane. The shaft consists of the big shaft (rhachis) and the calamus. The vane has plenty of rigid filaments (barbae) in a fan-shaped position. Those carry additional finer filaments (barbulae), which are interconnected with little hooks (hamulus). The umbilicus proximalis is situated at the end of the quill (Fig. 36-2).[1,10]

Feather Follicle

The follicle is a tubular invagination of the epidermis with a papilla of corium at its base, which reaches into the umbilicus of the feather and is equipped with a system of ample blood vessels. The outer follicle sheath is formed by corium and is the base for the feather muscles, Musculi penarum. The inner feather sheath is lined with the epidermis and consists of squamous cells, some dead and some alive.

Historical Methods

- Obliteration of feather follicles: Lack of practical experience
- Tenotomy: Cutting of pectoral muscles (major and minor), coracoid, and (sometimes) deltoid major tendons
- Tenectomy: Removal of portion of extensor of carpometacarpus
- Patagiectomy: Removal of patagial membrane and apposition of radius and humerus
- Functional ankylosis: Fixing ulnar, carpal and metacarpal bones with stainless steel wire

As Acceptable Methods May be Defined

- Brailing: Binding one wing, only as temporary measure
- Feather clipping (temporary)
- Pinioning: Removal of wing tips, removal of hand in juveniles during first week that may result in distress, even if juveniles appear not to suffer much (Pinioning is actually a bone surgery resulting in amputation. Furthermore, this method is officially forbidden in some European countries.)
- Extirpation of feather follicles: Prevents regrowth of flight feathers from which the follicles have been extirpated

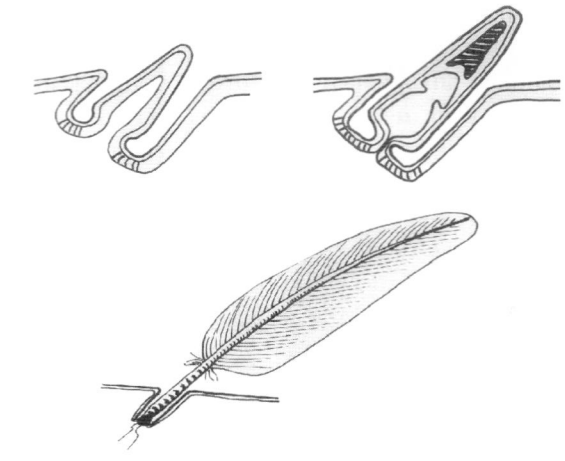

Figure 36-2

Development of a feather.[1,9,10]

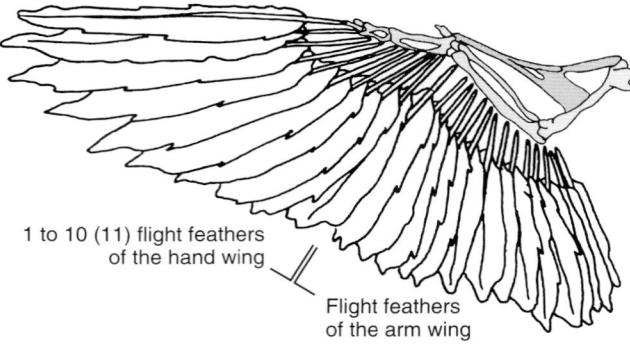

1 to 10 (11) flight feathers of the hand wing

Flight feathers of the arm wing

Figure 36-1

Anatomy of a wing.[1,9,10]

At the point of the calamus is a circular opening, the lower navel umbilicus proximalis inferior, where the corium reaches into the calamus and forms the corium papilla, covered by epidermal cells. This is the area of transition from the live cells of the follicle to the dead epidermal cells of the calamus. Once the growth of the feather is completed, the germinal activity rests until the next regenerative cycle. During the life of a bird, each feather papilla continues to produce feathers.[1,5,10]

Feathers of the Wing

The feathers of a wing are arranged in an overlapping position, anchored by an epidermal collar. This provides a solid but light surface, with an aerodynamic shape. Distal to the carpal joint, the remiges primarii 1 to 6 are attached at the metacarpus and 7 to 11 at the phalanxes. The 11th flight feather is often quite small, attached at the second phalanx of the second digit, called the ranicle.

Most orders have 10 primary flight feathers, grebes, storks and flamingos have 11. However, birds such as ostriches have 16 and cassowaries have 2 or 3 flight feathers on the distal wing.

The number of the secondary flight feathers at the arm (remiges secundarii) varies more and increases depending on the length of the ulna. Hummingbirds and most sparrows have only 10 and albatrosses have 38 to 40.[1]

Unlike the flight feather at the hand, the secondary flight feathers are counted from the carpal joint toward the proximal wing. The spaces between the vaneless quills of the flight feathers are covered by several rows of body feathers (tectrices). The larger body feathers at the carpal area insert distally to the flight feather, whereas the smaller tetrices of the proximal wing insert proximally to the secondary flight feathers. Like the second and third digits, the thumb carries flight and body feathers, which form the alula and influence the flight.[1,10]

Development of a Feather

The corium and epidermis are developing thick layers and develop an elevation at the corium papilla. The epidermis emerges as a quill from the epidermal collar. The sheath is formed by keratinized layers of epidermal tissue. Inside the skin, a feather follicle develops. Mostly active germ cells at its base form a tube, with the pulp inside. The pulp is filled with loose connective tissue, nerves, arteries, and veins. They degenerate during feather maturation and are resorbed later. The keratinized feather sheath dries from the top and breaks off; the vane is slowly released.

Out of the epidermis, cells develop into rows of spiral ledges, which change into keratin and form the rami. The feather shaft forms from parallel ledges. The rames grow out of the feather sheath. The feather unfolds completely and the pulp degenerates. As keratinization proceeds, a hollow shaft develops.[1,5,10]

Molting Season

In general, the molting of the feather occurs once a year—periodic molting. Molting is necessary to guaranty a lifelong supply of healthy, functional feathers. Influenced by weather and mechanical use, the feather is worn and needs to be renewed. Molting enables the bird to adapt to different seasonal periods or to change its appearance completely.

Unlike in mammals, in which the new hair is growing next to the old one, the old feather is slowly pushed out of the follicle by the new feather in birds. The start of the molting depends on nutrition, breeding activity, season, and temperature. Young birds go through various changes of their plumage.

Many birds molt after the hatch of their offspring, stimulated by the decreasing concentration of estrogens and androgens. Some birds molt once a year, whereas others change their feathers during the mating period. Birds that have a camouflage plumage may molt at various times during the year. For example, the grouse molts three times a year. Birds such as ducks and geese are unable to fly during their molt because they lose all flight feathers at the same time. In small birds, the molt takes 3 to 4 months. Some larger birds, such as the eagle or albatross, molt only a few feathers at the time; therefore, the complete replacement may take up to 2 years.

The molt is controlled by the hypothalamus and hypophysis, which release gonadotropin and thyroxine. Thyroxine stimulates the feather follicle and growth of the feather, and androgen and estrogen inhibit the molt.

Progesterone suppresses ovulation and induces a concurrent molt of the feathers. Complications can develop in association with deficient nutrition, causing, for example, hypoproteinemia.

The plumage is connected to follicle muscles inside the follicles. These muscles are controlled by the autonomic nervous system. If a bird is frightened, the muscles relax and all the plumage may be lost. This "fright-or-stress molt" is used to distract predators and offers the bird a chance to escape. Afterward, the feathers will regrow.[1,10]

METHODS OF SURGERY

There are different methods to prevent a bird temporarily or even permanently from flying. Whatever the method used, it has to be taken into consideration that rendering the bird flight-incapable can cause a major impact on the natural behavior of the bird. The legal protection of animals has to be respected and, in some countries, these procedures may require a legal permit.

A bird can be kept from flying until the next molt by unilateral or bilateral trimming of the flight feathers. The same effect can be permanently achieved by follicle extirpation, which destroys the germinal area of the feather. No new feathers will be produced after the next molt. This surgical technique was introduced in 1970 by Gauckler.[5]

The procedure should only be performed on fully grown feathers once follicular activity has ceased. Once the bird has started molting, the germinal tissue cannot be completely extirpated and the residual tissue could induce new feather growth.[5,9]

Not all procedures of electrocauterization of active papillae have been successful and other methods such as laser techniques are being clinically tested.[3]

Anesthesia and Drug Management

The bird is placed in a sternal position with the legs extended to minimize blood pooling, especially in Ciconiiformes.[9] A deep narcosis and analgesia are necessary. Inhalation with isoflurane by means of mask or intubation is the preferred method for the induction of anesthesia (Boxes 36-2 and 36-3).[5,7,8]

The flight (and body) feathers are already removed, and a tourniquet is placed proximal to the surgery field to reduce blood flow and allow a clear visual field. The skin around the surgical area is then disinfected.

There are two different methods of making the incisions to extirpate the feathers (Figs. 36-3 and 36-4).

| BOX 36-2 | Anesthesia and Drug Management[7-9,11] |

Premedication (10-20 min prior to intubation)
0.3-1.0 mg/kg diazepam IM
2.0 mg/kg midazolam IM

Analgesia
1.0-2.0 mg/kg butorphanol IM

Nonsteroidal Anti-Inflammatory Drugs
0.2-0.3 mg/kg meloxicam IM, PO for 1-3 days
2-4 mg/kg carprofen IM for 1-3 days
5-10 mg/kg carprofen PO
1-10 mg/kg flunixin IM[7]

Antibiotics
10-15 mg/kg enrofloxacin IM, PO for 5 days
10 mg/kg marbofloxacin IM, PO for 5 days

| BOX 36-3 | Equipment[5,9] |

Anesthetic machine
Tubes and masks
Set of instruments
Tourniquet
- Scalpel blades and handles
- Forceps
- Scissors
- Elevator
- Suture material: Needle-thread combination

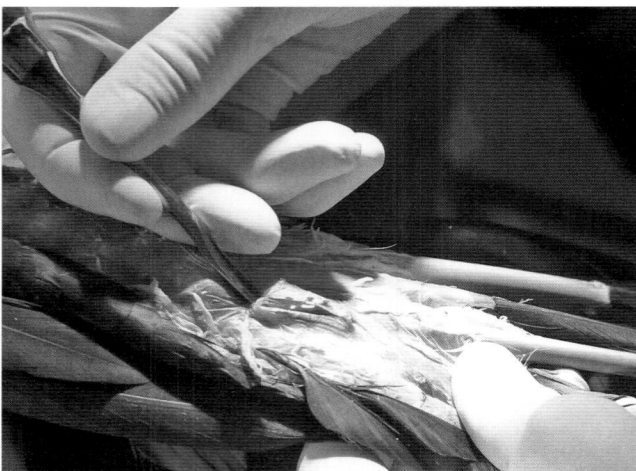

Figure 36-3

Large birds (e.g., marabou). The incision is made parallel on the feather shaft. The feather follicle is found at the end of the evaluator.

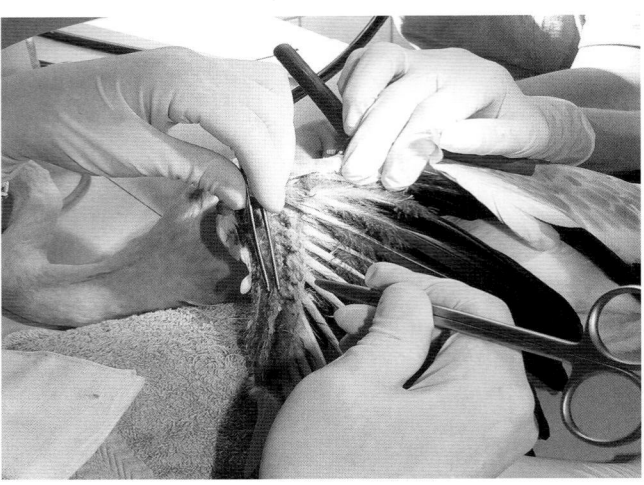

Figure 36-4

Small birds (e.g., flamingo). One incision is made parallel to the metacarpus.

First, in larger birds such as marabou and other storks and pelicans, the extirpation is done with single vertical incisions. This prevents the surgery field from becoming unnecessarily large. Each cut is placed parallel to the feather shaft. The skin may be bluntly separated with scissors or an elevator from the end of the shaft. This should be done very gently to avoid tearing the thin avian skin. Attention should be directed toward avoiding the larger blood vessels running parallel to the metacarpus. The follicles are then dissected and up to 1 cm of the tip will be removed on every flight feather. The remaining part of the feather remains in the skin.

The remaining feather, including the vane, is trimmed to facilitate placement of a bandage following surgery. This also reduces the weight of the wing in compensation for the weight of the bandage. The remaining feather will be released during the next molting period. Only then will the result of the surgery be evident Depending on the size of the incision, the skin will be closed with one or two sutures. A monofilament, resorbable, needle-thread combination with a tapered needle should be used to reduce traumatization of the tender skin. The suture will not need to be removed. The same is repeated with all flight feathers of the carpometacarpus; in total, 10 or 11 feather follicles have to be extirpated.

It is also necessary to extirpate approximately six body feathers in this area, especially in large and heavy birds. Experience has shown that storks or pelicans can get enough upwind to fly if only the flight feathers were removed.[5,9]

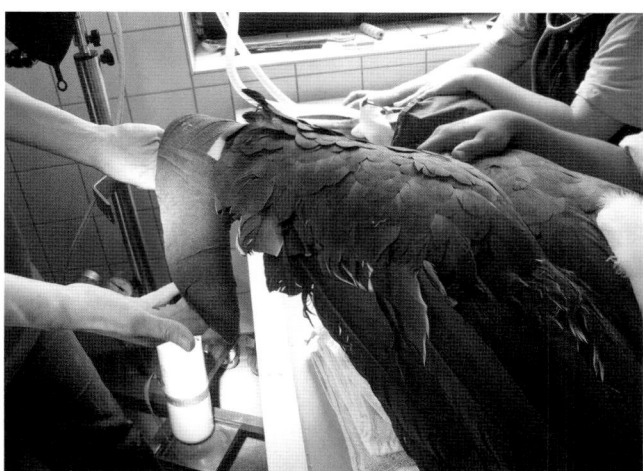

Figure 36-5

Marabou with bandage after follicle extirpation.

The other method involves only one incision with a scalpel parallel to the metacarpal bones, approximately 1 cm below the follicle. This can be used in small birds such as ducks. The skin is dissected along the incision to develop a flap, which will be lifted up cranially. Below the skin are the ends of the feather shafts, which have to be loosened and eventually cut with scissors, up to 6 to 8 mm, depending on the size of the bird. The incision may be closed with single stitches in smaller birds. Once the remains of the feathers below the wing are shortened, the wing will be covered with a bandage.[5,9]

Bandaging

The surgical field will be covered with a nonadhesive wound dressing after a wound gel or powder has been applied. To further protect the traumatized area, a thick layer of cotton gauze is then applied. in a figure-of-eight fashion so that the bird is able to rest the wing against the body. Finally, the wing is covered with a Vetrap bandage to protect the other bandage layers from dirt and moisture (Fig. 36-5). Water birds should not have access to bathing water. The tourniquet will be removed only after the bandage has been applied. A potential hemorrhage is prevented by the pressure bandage.

In any case, the bandage should be completely removed after 2 to 3 days to avoid ankylosis of the metacarpal joint. By then, the healing process is usually advanced enough so that no further wound protection is required. If needed, the wound may be treated with gel or powder.[5,9]

BOX 36-4	Risks and Advantages[9]

Risks and Problems

Risk of restraint and anesthesia

Invasive surgery that may result in complications:
- Large wound areas
- Tissue damage caused by trauma
- Excessive bleeding caused by insufficient tourniquet or careless dissection
- Risk of necrosis
- Risk of infections

Unwanted regrowth of flight feathers: Caused by insufficient removal of germinal tissue (particular risk in molting or young patients)

Advantages

Permanent flight restraint in adult birds

Bird caught only twice compared with regular clipping

Mating and other behavior not compromised when compared with complete pinioning (amputation)

No risk of injury at former surgical site compared with complete pinioning because no parts of the extremity become exposed

Recovery

Birds with long legs need to be supported by a person or hammock during recovery from anesthesia until they are able to stand by themselves (Box 36-4).[9]

REFERENCES

1. Bezzel E, Prinzinger R: Feder und Gefieder. Ornithologie, ed 2, Stuttgart, Germany, 1990, Ulmer Verlag, pp 71–94.
2. Cwiertna Z, Frak W: Über einige chirurgische Methoden zur Flugbeschränkung bei Zoovögeln. Proceedings 14. Visz, Hungary, 1972, pp 147.
3. D'Agostino JJ, Snider T, Hoover J, et al: Use of laser ablation and cryosurgery to prevent primary feather growth in a pigeon (Columba livia) model. J Avian Med Surg 20:219–224, 2006.
4. Engel H, Pagel TH: Flugunfähigmachen von Wasservögeln, Vortrag 62. Niedersachsen, Germany, 2005, Sitzung des Tierschutzbeirates des Landes.
5. Gauckler A, Baumgartner K: Die Exstirpation der Handschwingenpapillen bei Wasser- und Stelzvögeln. 21 Arbeitstagung der Zootierärzte im deutschsprachigen Raum, 2001.
6. Gylstorff I, Grimm F: Flugunfähigkeit—Operationsmöglichkeiten. Vogelkrankheiten. Stuttgart, Germany, 1987, Ulmer Verlag, pp 527–528.
7. Hatt JM: Anästhesie und Analgesie bei Ziervögeln. Schweizer Archiv für Tierheilkunde 144:606–613, 2002.
8. Korbel R: Schmerz und Analgesie beim Vogel. Erhardt W, Henke J, Haberstroh J: Anästhesie und Analgesie beim Klein- und Heimtier. Stuttgart, Germany, 2004, Schattauer Verlag, pp 745–747.
9. Krawinkel P, Weber H, Schauerte N, et al: Extirpation of feather follicles—a practical, acceptable and permanent method to prevent zoo birds from flying? Presented at the 7th Scientific Meeting of the European Association of Zoo and Wildlife Veterinarians (EAZWV), Leipzig, Germany, April 30-May 3, 2008.

10. O'Malley B: Klinische Anatomie und Physiologie bei kleinen Heimtieren, Vögeln, Reptilien und Amphibien. Munich, Germany, 2008, Urban & Fischer.

11. Paul-Murphy J, Fialkowski J: Injectable anesthesia and analgesia of birds. In Gleed RD, Ludders JW, editors: Recent advances in veterinary anesthesia and analgesia: Companion animals, 2001, (http://www.ivis.org/advances/Anesthesia_Gleed/toc.asp).

12. Rüedi D: Neue Coupiermethoden—Erfahrungen im Zoo Basel. 2nd Arbeitstagung der Zootierärzte im deutschsprachigen Raum, Dortmund, Germany, 1983.

13. Schaller K: Stelzvögel, Kraniche, Flamingos. In Gölthenboth R, Klös HG, editors: Krankheiten der Zoo- und Wildtiere, Berlin, 1995, Blackwell Wissenschaftsverlag.

14. West C, Jones D: Workshop on flight restraint in birds. Presented at the 62nd Annual Meeting of the World Association of Zoos and Aquariums, Budapest, August 26-30, 2007.

15. Williamson WM, Russell WC: Prevention of flight in older captive birds. J Am Vet Med Assoc 159:596–598, 1971.

16. Wissdorf H: Tenotomie als Möglichkeit zur Beseitigung der Flugfähigkeit bei Zoo- und Volierenvögeln. 2nd Arbeitstagung der Zootierärzte im deutschsprachigen Raum, Dortmund, Germany, 1983.

17. Wissdorf H, Heidenreich M, Brahm R, et al: Flugunfähigkeit-Durchgeführte Operationen bei Zoovögeln sowie Beschreibung einer neuen Tenotomiemethode. Internationalen Symposium über die Erkrankungen der Zootiere, Poznan, Poland, 1977.

CHAPTER 37

Squamous Cell Carcinoma in *Buceros* Hornbills

Kathryn C. Gamble

The rhinothecal ornamentation known as the casque is unique to the avian family Bucerotidae (hornbill).[9] The casque is an air-filled cavity with minimal cancellous bone caudally in all but one species, the greater helmeted hornbill *(Buceros [Rhinoplax] vigil)*.[7] This space is enclosed by a thin shell of bone and overlaid externally by keratin. The striking external casque contours and rhamphothecal coloration varies by species, gender, and sexual maturity.

Casque squamous cell carcinoma (CSCC) has been documented repeatedly in great hornbills *(Buceros bicornis)*, also called concave-casqued, great pied, giant, or great Indian hornbills, since the incident case was described in the literature in 1985.[7,9,12] Despite two other species in the genus and one species *(Buceros [Rhinoplax] vigil)* in a closely related genus, it is only the great hornbill that has presented this specific pathology. No such casque neoplasia has been presented in any other of the 50 extant hornbill species, although 27 others are found in Asia, and are even sympatric with *Buceros* in India, Thailand, Java, Sumatra, Vietnam, and southwestern China.

Great hornbills were exhibited in Association of Zoos and Aquariums (AZA) holding institutions without successful captive breeding until 1973.[13] Largely through importation, the managed population of great hornbills in the United States reached a maximum population of 79 in 1983. At the onset of active investigation of CSCC in 2006, only 52 birds were present in this group and, currently, the Species Survival Plan (SSP) reports only 43 individuals in 18 institutions. The great hornbill is slow to mature, requiring 5 to 6 years to reach phenotypic maturity, and unlikely to reproduce successfully before 10 years.[9] It is also long-lived, with more than 40 years not unexpected, although its median longevity is 10 to 13 years. The species has not been reported to breed successfully beyond 30 years of age,

when CSCC typically presents; however, six animals in the affected group were actively courting, mating, or nesting at the time of their diagnosis. Considering that the U.S.-managed population generally hovered between 40 and 50 individuals in the last 25 years, and that not all of these animals were adults, removal of 11 adults represents a loss of 20% of the population, which has not been counteracted by slow captive reproductive success.

Squamous cell carcinoma has been diagnosed previously in other avian species. It has been documented at the cere or in the oral cavity, but has not been reported previously with such a species-specific predilection.[12,14,15] Through 2010, 12 cases of CSCC in great hornbills have presented similarly in onset and progression, and consistently in location on the casque and rhinotheca. Until recently, only birds in AZA-holding institutions were reported, despite repeated inquiries to European Endangered Species Program–holding institutions.[8] However, in 2008, a single case was reported in the United Kingdom.[1]

Clustering of cases has occurred with five birds housed in two institutions, and the others spread among seven different facilities. An intriguing case clustering has been noted along two specific U.S. longitudinal measurements. All birds, except one AZA-held animal, were wild-caught animals and generally presented between the ages of 30 and 40 years; the single captive-born animal presented at 25 years. No gender predisposition is apparent.

CLINICAL PRESENTATION

The hornbill casque has a location vulnerable to trauma and environmental damage because of its protrusion from the rhinothecal contour. In the great hornbill, the square-ended rectangular casque interfaces with

281

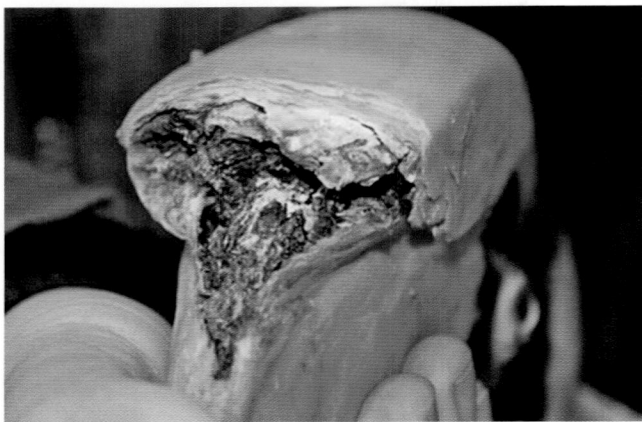

Figure 37-1

Head of an adult female great hornbill *(Buceros bicornis)* demonstrating gross appearance of squamous cell carcinoma of the rostral casque. *(Courtesy Dr. John Bainbridge.)*

the maxillary beak rostral to the external nares by approximately 50% of the casque length (see Fig. 37-2,A).[7] It is at this interface—the rostroventral casque and dorsocaudal maxillary rhampotheca—that CSCC consistently appears. In five of the CSCC-group, diagnoses of trauma, frostbite, bacterial sinusitis, or fungal infection of the casque were made prior to conclusive determination of neoplasia.

The external clinical presentation of CSCC is often limited to a focal softening, fissuring, or discoloration of the rostral casque or, occasionally, the maxillary rhinotheca near the casque, rather than the ulceration typically reported in other avian species.[14] Black, grey, or brown dry flaking tissue or actual necrosis with pink fleshy material is often found in the rostral casque once the bird is manually restrained and the abnormal keratin is debulked (Fig. 37-1). In warmer climates or seasons, myiasis has presented as a confounding problem. In several cases, before lesion identification, a pervasive yeast or necrotic odor was noted in the animal's enclosure or associated with the animal specifically. Although most of the birds had uneventful clinical histories prior to CSCC, three of them had notations of lost pieces of casque 1 to 4 years prior to CSCC diagnosis, and one had a notation of lost casque pieces and partial casque slough 11 years preceding neoplastic presentation.

DIAGNOSIS

The neoplasm is markedly aggressive locally. Softening, fissuring, and deep necrosis of the casque and its interface with the maxilla are observed. Abnormal

soft tissue, usually white or pink and fleshy, may be observed growing through the choanal slits on oral examination.

The full extent of CSCC is better appreciated by imaging. Simple radiography may detect soft tissue opacification of the affected areas, sinuses of the casque or maxillary beak, and potential bony invasion (see Fig. 37-2).[7] Multiple radiographic views may assist in staging debulking of the neoplasm but lateral images of the skull and casque will screen most rapidly for the presence of the neoplasm. These particular images are easily obtained under manual restraint, with the head and neck secured by tape or while the bird is fully anesthetized. Although advanced imaging has been performed in *Buceros* species, it is not considered necessary for conclusive CSCC diagnosis.[18]

Confirmatory diagnosis of CSCC may be challenging because of the overlying necrotic keratinous tissue. Multiple deep biopsies of the actual casque structure or the radiographically identified mass should be collected to maximize positive identification of the neoplasm. At this casque location in the giant hornbill, a CSCC-consistent lesion should be considered as neoplastic, even when negative biopsy results are obtained initially.

Culture of the affected tissue generally presents distracting organisms, which have misdirected treatment in many affected animals.[14] Mixed Gram-negative and Gram-positive bacteria may be cultured from biopsies of the affected casque, even when taken deeply. *Staphylococcus*, *Bacillus*, and coliforms—most commonly *Escherichia coli*, *Proteus*, and *Pseudomonas*—have been reported. Limited fungal organisms have been cultured, such as *Penicillium*, *Candida*, and *Chrysosporium*, and these organisms have similarly altered initial treatment protocols.

PATHOLOGY

Despite the marked local invasion of CSCC, metastasis has been observed only once in the 12 birds, which is consistent with reports in other avian species.[12,14,15,18,19] In the one case that received protracted (~4 years) treatment duration, splenic metastasis was identified.[2] Despite lack of metastasis, the local effects are sufficient to produce deteriorating effects on quality of life.

Marked epidermal necrosis and inflammatory cell infiltrates appear frequently on histopathology of CSCC samples. Bacterial or fungal organisms may be seen within the affected tissues. The neoplastic cells are polygonal, spindle, or stellate, with marked

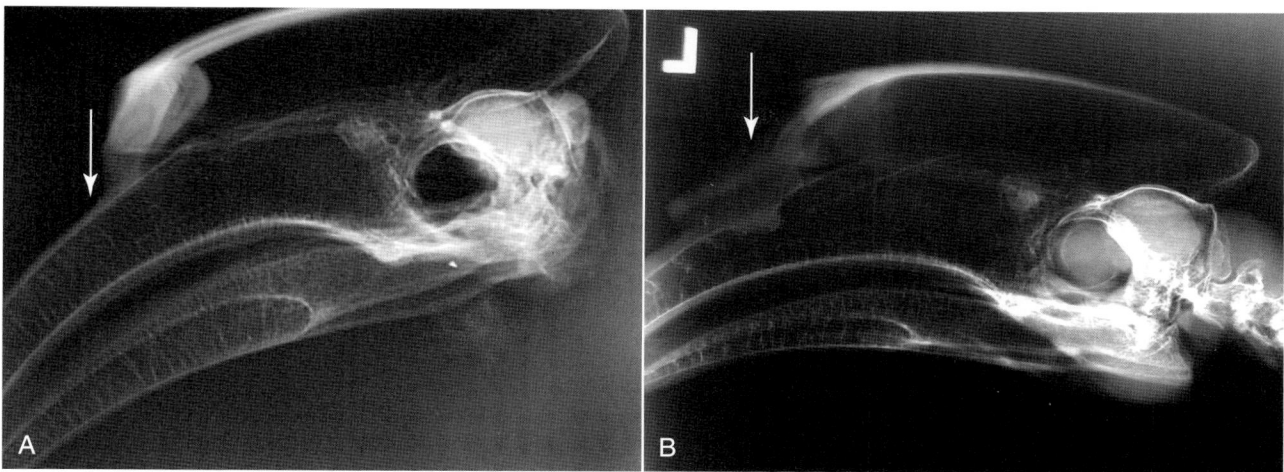

Figure 37-2

A, Lateral radiograph of normal skull and casque of an adult female great hornbill *(Buceros bicornis)*. Arrow indicates area of typical location of squamous cell carcinoma development. **B**, Lateral radiograph of skull and casque of an adult female great hornbill *(Buceros bicornis)* with squamous cell carcinoma *(arrow)* of the casque, invasion into the maxillary sinus with disruption of the maxillary bone, and thickened rhinotheca. *(B, Courtesy Dr. Eric Baitchman.)*

anisokaryosis in anastomosing cords.[14] In three cases, enhanced desmosomes were observed but, as the hallmark of SCC, keratin pearls were only reported in one case.[12,14,15,19] Mitotic figures may be present in limited to moderate numbers, or may not be evident. In four cases, cytoplasm of the neoplastic cells was specifically observed as eosinophilic.

TREATMENT

Radical surgical casque resection is disfiguring, but not technically challenging (Fig. 37-3). Casque and skull anatomy for surgical margins have been described in several hornbill species, including both *Buceros* species typically housed in zoos.[7] Debulking of neoplastic tissue is important in preparation for adjunctive treatment.[3,12,14,15,18] In three cases, standard radiation treatments at weekly intervals have been used, with only minor slowing of neoplastic growth.[17] Attempted photodynamic treatment with 2-(1-hexyloxyethyl)-2-devinyl pyropheophorbide-a (Photochlor) in one case demonstrated prompt tissue destruction and eschar formation at the treated casque site, but neoplastic growth persisted.

Antiangiogenic topical treatment (OLCAT-005a [off-label combinatorial antiangiogenic therapy—imiquimod 5%, tretinoin 0.1%, calcipotriene 0.005%, diclofenac 3%, and hydrocortisone valerate 0.2%) used in two cases has presented the most recent promise to address the debulked surgery site directly.[3,18] It has been

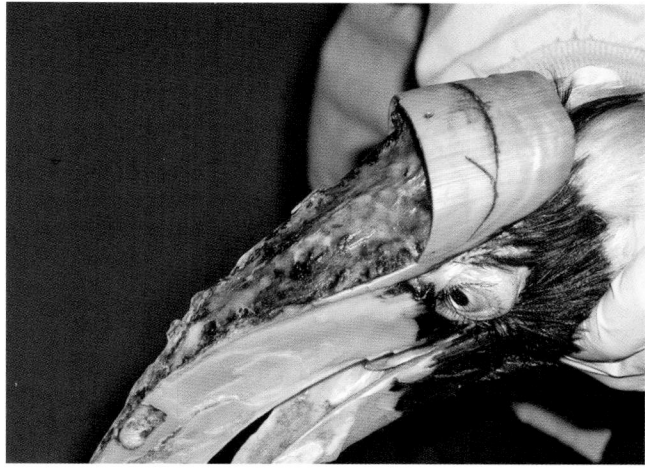

Figure 37-3

Head of an adult female great hornbill *(Buceros bicornis)* following radical casque resection to prepare site for application of antiangiogenic agents. *(Courtesy Dr. Eric Baitchman.)*

used once with and once without adjunctive radiation with similar results, extinguished neoplastic growth and negative repetitive biopsy results. Unfortunately, resumption of neoplastic growth recurs within weeks to months of discontinued treatment, so the repeated captures, long-term commitment, and significant financial impact cannot be alleviated.

Early detection of the neoplasm permits initiation of treatment promptly and remains a clear advantage for longer survival times. It has been reported that successful treatment of CSCC in giant hornbills has been accomplished.[4] Treatment has been uniformly unsuccessful to date to affect full neoplastic remission, although long-term survival possibilities have been enhanced for the individual. Newer technology, such as electronic brachytherapy (Xoft, Sunnyvale, Calif), may find successful application in future cases of CSCC in the great hornbill.[10]

PROGNOSIS

Repeated advocacy for early detection through annual casque radiographs for adult great hornbills older than 20 years has been made by the SSP Veterinary Advisor. Documented cases in the literature have reiterated this procedure as essential for early-onset detection and case management.[3,12,15,18]

Most cases of CSCC in great hornbills have presented without the opportunity for specific treatment. Before CSCC was known as a predisposing problem in this species with four or five cases, substantial time delay to actual diagnosis and misdirected treatment could occur, with 5 to 8 months typically reported. One bird with clinical presentation consistent with CSCC for 4 years rapidly deteriorated in 2.5 months once diagnosis was confirmed. Time delays were also presented in breeding season, when management was reluctant to disrupt the pair. With increased awareness of CSCC, cases that escaped early detection and presented with markedly advanced disease (four birds) were either immediately euthanized or within 2 weeks of presentation, which generally coincides with a positive histopathologic biopsy diagnosis. Overall prognosis for any bird with CSCC is guarded to grave, with steady progression to euthanasia for even aggressively treated birds. The longest survival time was almost 4 years with direct antiangiogenesis treatment.[3] However, surviving did not necessarily equate to thriving; the bird could not be paired successfully because of repeated captures required for treatment or marked neoplastic progression without treatment.[2]

ONGOING INVESTIGATIONS

An explanation for the species predilection for CSCC in great hornbills remains under active investigation by the SSP Veterinary Advisor. Rhinoceros hornbills *(Buceros rhinoceros)* that are often housed in zoos, and even in collections with great hornbills, have not been documented with any such neoplasms. These species are so closely related that they have been observed to hybridize in the wild, so it would seem that both species could be susceptible.[9]

A unique facet of the *Buceros* hornbills is that their casque pigmentation does not occur within the rhamphothecal keratin. Rather, the bright yellow (great hornbill) and deep orange (rhinoceros hornbill) coloration is applied cosmetically from preening oils produced in the uropygial gland.[9] Carotenoids (pigments of yellow and orange) have been reported with anti-inflammatory and immunomodulatory properties in other species, including birds, and have been specifically correlated as protective against ultraviolet light oxidative damage.[5,11,14]

To investigate this hypothesis, researchers in a project endorsed by the SSP gathered uropygial gland secreta from both species held in AZA-managed collections for semiquantitative carotenoid pigment profiling.[9] Four birds that were sampled ultimately presented with CSCC; three of these individuals had minimal gross yellow pigmentation of the uropygial gland oils evaluated. In one CSCC case prior to this study, clinical notes reported that the white bars on the rectrices were not pigmented yellow and the quantity of uropygial gland oils seemed markedly reduced from the quantity expected for this size of bird.[16]

To provide context for the analysis of carotenoid concentrations, housing, husbandry, and diet information was collected for not only the birds presenting with CSCC, but also unaffected great hornbills and rhinoceros hornbills as controls. Regression analysis has been performed to profile at-risk birds within the predisposed species, and may suggest species differences in carotenoids that presumably could protect the nontargeted species. Carotenoids could potentially be provided as a dietary source to enhance protection for the giant hornbill casque.

REFERENCES

1. Bainbridge J: Personal communication, 2008.
2. Baitchman E: Personal communication, 2010.
3. Baitchman E, Li VW, Li WW, et al: Treatment of squamous cell carcinoma in a great Indian hornbill *(Buceros bicornis)*. In Baer CK, editor: Proceedings of the Annual Meeting of the American Association of Zoo Veterinarians and Association of Reptilian and Amphibian Veterinarians, Los Angeles, 2008, pp 134–135.
4. Dutton DJ: Coraciiformes (kingfishers, motmots, bee-eaters, hoopoes, hornbills). In Fowler ME, Miller RE, editors: Zoo and wild animal medicine, ed 5, St. Louis, 2003, Elsevier, pp 254–260.
5. Ewen JG, Surai P, Stradi R, et al: Carotenoids, colour and conservation in an endangered passerine, the hihi or stitchbird *(Notiomystis cincta)*. Anim Conserv 9:229–235, 2006.
6. Gamble KC: Personal communication, 2010.

7. Gamble KC: Internal anatomy of the hornbill casque described by radiography, contrast radiography, and computed tomography. J Avian Med Surg 21:38–49, 2007.
8. Gamble KC, Kehl N: Risk factor analysis of squamous cell carcinoma in giant Indian hornbills *(Buceros bicornis)*. Vehr ber Erkrg Zootiere 42:222, single page 2005.
9. Kemp AC: Family Bucerotidae (hornbills). In del Hoyo J, Elliott A, Sargatal J, editors: Handbook of the birds of the world (mousebirds to hornbills), vol 6, Barcelona, Spain, 2001, Lynx, pp 430, 437, 440, 444, 446, 449, 503.
10. L.A. zoo announces successful cancer treatment of rhinoceros with electronic brachytherapy, 2009 (http://www.lazoo.org/about/press/1109/111609rhino.html).
11. McGraw KJ, Klasing KC: Carotenoids, immunity, and integumentary coloration in red junglefowl *(Gallus gallus)*, 2006 (http://www.public.asu.edu/~kjmcgraw/pubs/Auk2006.pdf).
12. Miller RE, Trampel DW, Boever WJ, et al: Carcinoma of a greater Indian hornbill *(Buceros bicornis)*. J Zoo Anim Med 16:131–136, 1985.
13. Myers MM, Schoen L, Lynch C, et al: Population analysis and breeding plan—great hornbill *(Buceros bicornis)*. Species Survival Plan. Chicago, 2009, Population Management Center Lincoln Park Zoo.
14. Reavill DR: Tumors of pet birds. Vet Clin North Am Exot Anim Pract 7:537–560, 2004.
15. Suedmeyer WK, McCaw D, Turnquist S: Attempted photodynamic therapy of squamous cell carcinoma in the casque of a great hornbill *(Buceros bicornis)*. J Avian Med Surg 15:44–49, 2001.
16. Wagner R: Personal communication, 1997.
17. Wagner W, Pirie G: Personal communication, 2003.
18. Wilson RW, Hammond EE, Gamble KC, et al: Squamous cell carcinoma in a great Indian hornbill *(Buceros bicornis)*. In Baer, CK, editor: Proceedings of the Annual Meeting of the American Association of Zoo Veterinarians, San Diego, 2004, pp 376–381.
19. Wüunschmann A, Weisman MJ, Rasmussen JM, et al: Squamous cell carcinoma in a greater Indian hornbill *(Buceros bicornis)*. Tieärztl Prax 30:214–218, 2002.

CHAPTER 38

The California Condor *(Gymnogyps californianus)* Veterinary Program: 1997-2010

The California condor recovery program has experienced tremendous growth in the decade since Ensley's report,[10] which included a thorough and comprehensive review of biologic data, captive management and husbandry, transportation, quarantine procedures, clinical techniques, annual examination, radiographic imaging, surgery, reproduction, medical conditions of chicks at hatch, gender determination, pathology, environmental contaminants affecting condor health, bacterial pathogens, fungal diseases, parasitology, clinical evaluation of a sick condor, and medical treatments for released condors through March of 1997. The aim of this chapter is not to reproduce this information, but to update it with new information. Also presented is an expanded section on free-ranging condors.

In March 1997, there were 132 birds, and captive breeders living in three facilities. The release program existed at three sites, two in California and one in Arizona, and included only 39 birds. Four institutions, in addition to the U.S. Fish and Wildlife Service (USFWS) Hopper Mountain staff, held captive or managed free-living California condors—the San Diego Wild Animal Park (captive birds only), Los Angeles Zoo (captive birds at the zoo and veterinary care for all released California birds), Peregrine Fund (captive birds at the World Center for Birds of Prey, and released birds at the Grand Canyon in Arizona), and Ventana Wilderness Society (released birds in this area). One veterinarian, the Veterinary Coordinator, oversaw the care of all wild birds and captive birds at the Los Angeles Zoo. Additionally, the Phoenix Zoo provided veterinary support for the Arizona release birds, and a private practice veterinarian provided emergency veterinary support for birds in central California.

In marked contrast, as of March of 2010, there were 347 birds, almost triple the total number of birds, and 184 birds in the wild, more than four times the original

number. Three additional institutions house captive birds; the Oregon Zoo joined the breeding program in 2003, and exhibit birds are now living at the Santa Barbara Zoo and Chapultepec Zoo in Mexico City. Two additional release sites were created: in 2003, Pinnacles National Monument (staffed by biologists from the National Park Service) and, in 2002, Sierra San Pedro de Martir National Park in Baja California. In Mexico, local biologists have worked with recovery team leader Mike Wallace in a release program run by the Zoological Society of San Diego. Southern California added another release site at Bitter Creek National Wildlife Refuge using biologists employed there as well. The Los Angeles Zoo continues veterinary support for all California field birds, now numbering 94, and the San Diego Zoo's Wild Animal Park provides veterinary support for the 17 birds in Baja California. Additional private practice veterinarians and the Santa Barbara Zoo have provided additional support for California's free-flying birds. The veterinary coordinator position remained, but to predominantly oversee care, rather than knowing each bird and providing individual care.

In addition to the growth in organizations and birds, released California condors began nesting in the wild, with the first wild hatch occurring in 2001. In 2003, the first fledging of a chick occurred in the wild. To date, 33 birds have been successfully fledged in the wild (of 49 hatches) in Arizona and California, and 25 wild-fledged birds are flying free. This aspect of the program has created a whole new field of veterinary care in the last decade.

The immense effort on the part of veterinarians, often on their own time for the wild population, to provide care is enormous. The knowledge base and communication, case load, questions that need answering, and looming disasters that need prevention often seem overwhelming as the program has grown.

However, providing care to the wild members of this species must be similar to being a physician on the front lines during war. We patch them up and ship them back out, sometimes to have them end up on a pathology table contributing to the knowledge and science needed to save them as a species, but not individually. I believe that the birds that gave their lives to hold a place in the wild for their descendants have not done so in vain, and all veterinarians who have helped a California condor should be recognized for their conservation efforts for this magnificent species. As long as these Pleistocene relics exist, there will be dedicated veterinarians in there fighting with them, hoping for a day when our intensive efforts are no longer needed.

CLINICAL CONSIDERATIONS

Normal hematologic values have been published.[9] California Condors at the Los Angeles Zoo are now restrained in a catch cage to allow for much improved capture, rather than attempting capture from large free-flight aviaries. This is highly recommended as a safer and less stressful way to capture birds.

Annual Examination, Bacterial Pathogens, and Parasitology

Captive adult or subadult birds may be examined annually, biannually, or opportunistically, depending on the facility. Recommended laboratory examinations include complete blood count (CBC) and complete chemistry panel, electrophoresis, and bile acid determination for captive birds that appear healthy. The volume of blood obtained is determined by the clinician at the institution based on laboratory needs. Two valuable female breeding birds with egg yolk peritonitis were radiographed and diagnosed solely because of abnormalities in electrophoretic patterns during routine examinations at the Los Angeles Zoo; both recovered well from surgery and resumed breeding with no further problems. It is recommended that valuable breeders be examined annually if this may be done safely. Routine fecal cultures are no longer considered to be necessary because no pathologic disease process has been seen in adult birds related to bacteria considered to be pathogenic to other species. Lead and zinc testing procedures are also unnecessary in captive birds with no history of metal exposure or ingestion. Additionally, *Aspergillus* testing is not necessary in normal adults and chicks (see fungal section). Serum banking is performed at

most institutions, and strongly recommended. The use of a Vacutainer butterfly (19- to 21-gauge needle, according to the size of vessel, largely dependent on the bird's temperature) is a fast and efficient way to obtain blood samples, because normal birds have a high enough blood pressure to fill large tubes easily. Annual fecal examinations for parasites are performed at some institutions and recommended. Strongyle nematode eggs have been seen and successfully treated at the Los Angeles Zoo. Coccidia has also been seen at more than one institution, without clinical signs.[30]

Clinical Techniques

Physical Restraint

Experienced handlers may hand-grab birds without using a net or, using condor techniques that relate to condors' intelligence, perceptive nature, and behavioral response to displays, restraint with a net may be accomplished with minimal stress. Operant conditioning and slow methodic methods have been very successful in decreasing stress and capture-related injury.[7] Also, if experienced, only one person may be needed for restraint (Fig. 38-1).

Care must be taken if the bird is held at the base of the skull not to press into the ventral neck. One case of postrestraint tracheal hemorrhage has been seen, likely because of improper restraint of the neck (the bird recovered without incident). An improved technique is to hold the bird by the beak only and push the head back toward the body. The bird cannot strike out this way, and does not struggle to do so (Fig. 38-2).

Restraint of very young chicks (younger than 1 month) should be done with caution for short periods and only with supplemental oxygen via mask provided, because young birds have lower red blood cell (RBC) parameters and are at higher risk of hypoxemia. Any ill bird should be supplemented with oxygen.

Capture myopathy has not been seen in California condors, even in field situations in which temperatures were high and laboratory findings indicated very high CPK (creatinine phosphokinase) levels. Regardless, care should be taken not to overexert or overheat birds, and spraying feet and wing webs with cool water is routine. Hot birds will take much longer to form a clot at a venipuncture site, especially when a larger gauge needle is used. Application of ice at the site appears to speed clot formation.

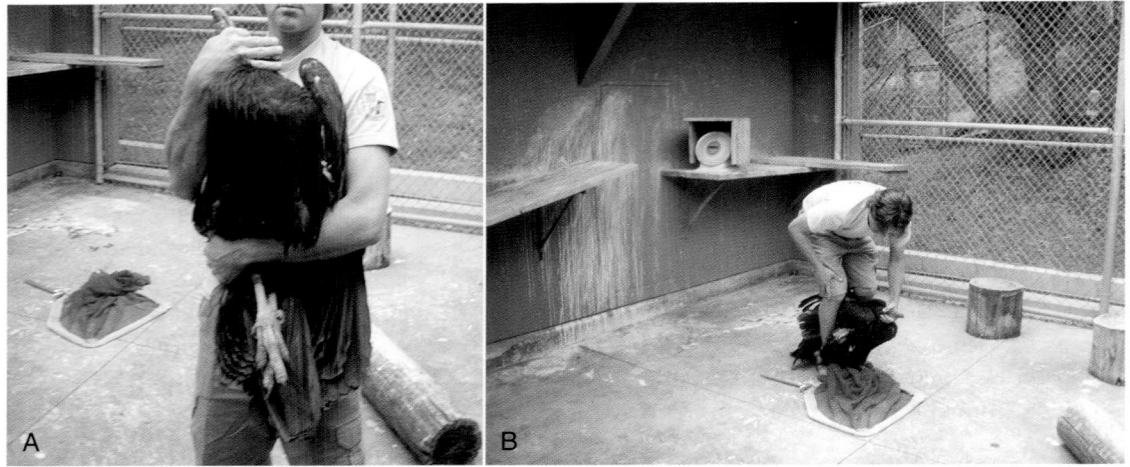

Figure 38-1

Restraint techniques. *(Courtesy J. Wynne.)*

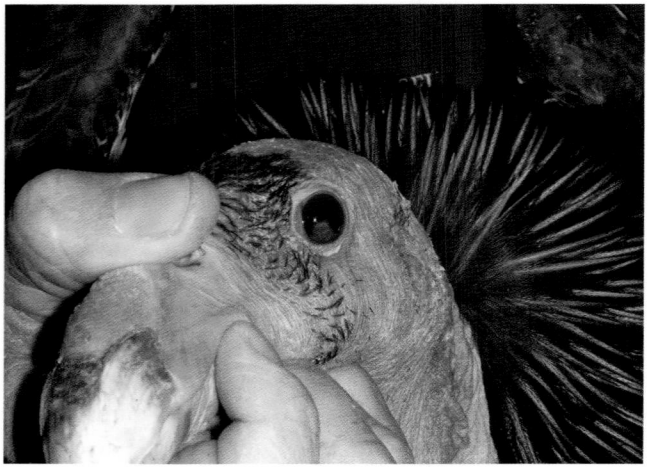

Figure 38-2

Proper beak restraint and finger placement. This bird has an iris mass seen in the left eye. *(Courtesy J. Wynne.)*

Oral Medication Administration and Oral Examination

Because of the strength of the beak, inserting fingers at the commissures of the beak allows an oral examination to be performed without risk of being bitten (see Fig. 38-2). Oral medication in chunks of meat may be force-fed in a similar manner by experienced handlers.[30]

Intravenous and Intraosseous Access

Although clinicians have used the jugular vein and ulnar vein for venipuncture, the medial metatarsal vein is the easiest IV access and location for maintaining an indwelling IV catheter. Intraosseous catheters are usually not needed because of the availability of this vein but, in one case, an intraosseous ulnar catheter was used for fluid administration and the bird suffered a fatal pulmonary edema. Further investigation showed the ulna to be pneumatized, with pneumatic foramina at the proximal and distal ends of the bones in this species (as well as in Andean condors and other species of storks and vultures examined).[23] One dissection has shown that the tibiotarsus may be a better location because it was the only marrow-filled long bone found,[30] but to date this has not been clinically attempted.

Anesthesia

Induction via mask and inhalation anesthesia is routinely performed using isoflurane gas. Once intubated, if positive pressure ventilation is initiated, the bird's neck will inflate because of cervical air sac anatomy that allows the bird to inflate the skin of the neck during displays. Bandaging material such as Vetwrap wrapped around the neck minimizes this inflation. Otherwise, anesthesia techniques and monitoring are as for other avian species.

Surgery

Numerous surgeries have been performed on this species, including orthopedic surgeries (Fig. 38-3) and ventriculotomies (see later). This species exhibits remarkable postsurgical healing and recovery abilities. Patagial tears caused by improper wing transmitter placement have been seen that required surgical repair, but severe tears that had torn completely through the patagium were not reparable.[30]

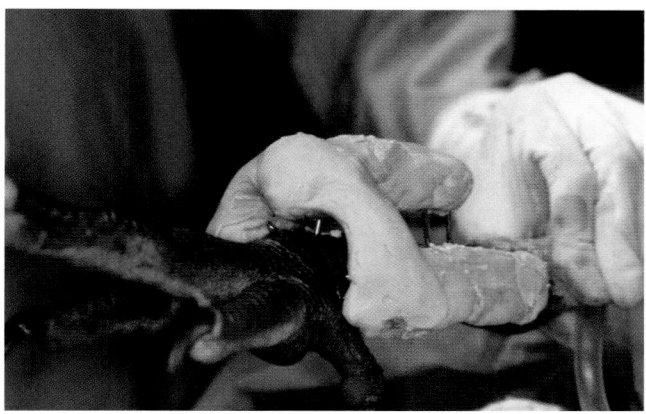

Figure 38-3

External fixator applied at the Los Angeles Zoo for treatment of open comminuted distal tarsometatarsal fracture secondary to gunshot. This severe fracture healed. *(Courtesy Charles Sedgwick.)*

Reproduction and Medical Conditions of Chicks at Hatch

Captive chick rearing methods have been detailed.[13] Intervention during hatching, if needed, has been detailed[10] and is routinely performed at most institutions. Egg yolk infections have been successfully treated by surgically removing the affected yolk, along with medical treatment. At the Los Angeles Zoo, a standard dose of ceftriaxone, 12.5 mg SC two to four times daily, is used for newly hatched chicks. The drug is applied to the shell membrane in chicks in the final days of development in an opened egg.

Clinical Examination of a Sick Condor

Although very resilient birds, any bird presenting as weak and debilitated should be stabilized before major procedures, especially if anesthesia and a prolonged procedure such as surgery is needed, because mortalities have occurred from shock in such cases. Sick condors, like birds in general, may not show the extent of their disease with clinical symptoms and may be difficult to assess for dehydration because of the normal appearance of the skin and mucous membranes. Careful critique by experienced staff, decreased size of the metatarsal vein, and decreased strength and struggling are good indicators of dehydration and a sick bird. Wild birds that are brought into captivity also produce hydrourate frequently, which could cause increased fluid loss, in addition to not eating immediately because of stress.

PATHOLOGY

Pathologic studies continue to be performed for the entire population by the Zoological Society of San Diego, with the exception of several birds that were suspected to have been killed in the wild, and necropsies were performed by the government for legal purposes. Mortality data for released birds from the beginning of the release program until 2002 have been published.[25] A complete review of released bird mortalities is in process.[22] After initial mortalities from electrocution and/or trauma from hitting power lines in California decreased because of experience and/or power pole aversion training, lead poisoning emerged as the most common single cause of mortality in free-flying released birds. Lead poisoning is the most frequent cause of death for free-flying wild birds in Arizona. Additional mortalities have been seen from trash ingestion (including zinc toxicity from pennies) in wild-hatched chicks, trauma and accidents (e.g., predators, conspecifics, rattlesnake bite, fire, accidental rope strangulation, drowning, fires), gunshot or arrow shot, ethylene glycol toxicity, and inanition and/or dehydration from failure to adapt. In captivity, causes of death for adults have included rattlesnake bite, trauma (primarily neck trauma caused by hitting fences; one case of head trauma likely caused by hitting the top of a crate), pulmonary edema secondary to an intraosseous catheter placed in the ulna, two deaths from unknown viral cause, and one death from West Nile virus. Poxvirus, likely from local wild birds, caused death in one chick, and various hatching malpositions and infections, West Nile virus, and parental trauma have been the causes of death in other chicks in captivity.

Fungal Diseases

Aspergillosis has been seen only in seriously ill debilitated condors. It has been associated with death in an adult with severe lead poisoning, leading to serious debilitation and long-term treatment, chicks with trash impaction (see later), and in two chicks that died with West Nile infection. Diagnosis in a live bird is based on auscultation and clinical signs, radiographic, endoscopic, surgical, and laboratory evidence. Laboratory tests include protein electrophoresis, white blood cell count, and *Aspergillus* antigen and antibody testing, although these may be difficult to interpret with changes in laboratories running specific *Aspergillus* tests. Debilitated condors should be monitored closely for this complication, and prevention with itraconazole therapy is used routinely.

Candida growth found on a cloacal culture from a debilitated bird with botulism who was on antibiotic therapy was treated successfully with itraconazole.[5]

Trauma

Several cases of a specific form of trauma have been seen in wild birds being held together in quarantine pens. A dominant bird will pick the tail and rear end of the subordinate bird raw, in some cases causing extreme trauma. Treatment has been as typically done for wound management and, even in severe cases, birds have recovered well, with two of three even regrowing tail feathers completely.

Beak tip injuries have occurred, some more severe than others, and healed well but are painful and cause inanition. Butorphenol, 1.5 to 4 mg/bird (given to effect) SID, SC or IM, has been efficacious in providing pain relief.[30] Wing tip injuries have also been seen caused by birds cling-flapping on chain link during capture attempts. Although one case involved osteomyelitis, necrotic bone, and lengthy wound care, this species' amazing healing abilities prevailed once again.

Cardiac Abnormalities

Cardiac murmurs have been auscultated in birds during routine examinations. Workups, including radiography and ultrasound examination, have not indicated abnormalities, and birds remained clinically normal. Some murmurs may be positional only in these large birds, and others appear to resolve as chicks mature. Further study, including genetic evaluation, may be warranted. An additional cardiac case is a geriatric founder bird diagnosed with congestive heart failure who is currently responding well to treatment.[32]

Ocular Abnormalities

An adult bird with a mass of the ciliary body being treated with photodynamic laser therapy has responded well to treatment (see Fig. 38-2).[30]

Infectious Diseases: West Nile Virus

West Nile virus (WNV) had caused significant morbidity and mortality in the eastern United States in native and exotic avian species since its emergence in New York City in 1999. Information about the species that appeared to be sensitive to the virus, in conjunction with information that two Andean condors at a zoo in New York had contracted the virus and become ill,[14] caused concern regarding exposure to the California condor. The only commercially available WNV vaccine at the time was Fort Dodge's killed West Nile equine product in the MetaStim adjuvant, which was not showing promising results in generating a protective titer in the initial studies of other species of birds receiving it. The Centers for Disease Control and Prevention (CDC) was testing new technology, a DNA vaccine, in American crows, with very encouraging results.[26]

In the fall of 2002, with WNV expected to reach the west in 2003, and through a tremendous cooperative effort, the CDC agreed to include the California condor in their research program; a private company, Aldevron (Fargo, ND), offered to make the DNA plasmid for the vaccine at no charge. After initial testing in Andean condors and then California condors of least genetic and breeding importance, staff and veterinarians at the Los Angeles Zoo, and then the San Diego Wild Animal Park, vaccinated two thirds of the captive condor population that winter—over 100 handlings of birds in a very short period of time before breeding season started (Fig. 38-4). Remaining captives in Boise and free-ranging birds were vaccinated the following spring, along with chicks that had hatched out.[7] A two-dose regimen (500 µg in aluminum hydroxide/1.0-mL dose, IM) was used 3 weeks apart in the leg in adults and chicks (at 3 months of age). However, many free-ranging condors were only able to be vaccinated once. Resulting titers were dramatic and deemed protective. In addition, surveillance at the Los Angeles Zoo showed WNV-positive mosquitos in the area in July 2004 and vaccinated condors that were exposed, based on titer changes, showed no symptoms of infection.[5] Importantly, chicks with maternal antibodies that were vaccinated also responded to the vaccine, showing no interference from those antibodies.[3]

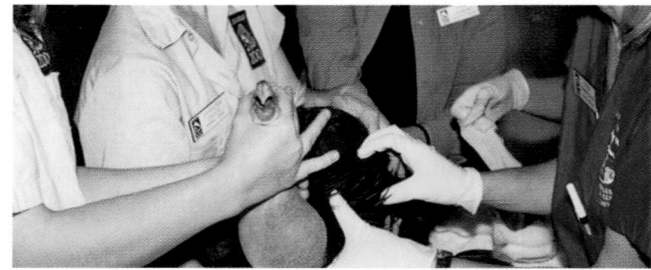

Figure 38-4

West Nile vaccination at the Los Angeles Zoo.

This vaccine continues to be used to date, but 2010 will be the last year of the study because the vaccine has been made available commercially as an equine vaccine but in a decreased concentration, and with the Meta-Stim adjuvant (Pfizer West Nile Innovator DNA, Pfizer Animal Health, New York). The experimental vaccine also appears not to be causing the same serologic responses it did in the initial study, but this has not been associated with WNV morbidity or mortality. Vaccine handling, storage, formulation differences, and other factors are being investigated. Discussions are in process to determine which currently available vaccine will be used and more research will continue. In adults, titers are monitored routinely for each individual in the population, and appear, overall, to be long-lived but not lifelong. Once natural exposure occurs, revaccination has not been deemed necessary.[4]

In the entire necropsied population of condors (all captives and all retrievable wild bodies, roughly 65%), there have been nine mortalities from WNV. In July 2006, after discontinuing the vaccination program, the Boise breeding facility experienced a mortality event over a 10-day period in four birds, one adult and three unvaccinated chicks ranging from $2\frac{1}{2}$ to 5 months of age. Despite emergency vaccinations in the face of the outbreak, two additional chicks in the same age range died in the next month—one developed symptoms 9 days after one vaccination and died 4 days later, and the other developed symptoms 20 days after one vaccination and died 11 days later. The adult who died had been vaccinated in 2003 but had not developed a titer response. Additionally, one unvaccinated 8-month-old who had just been transferred from Boise to Arizona also died that July from WNV. The remaining cases were a 3-month-old chick in a wild California nest in 2005 that was deemed too difficult to reach for vaccination, and a 19-month-old bird who had been in captivity and treated for lead toxicity the month before her death in December 2008. Both California cases also had severe Aspergillus pneumonias. Vaccine history and titers for the 19-month-old wild California bird are under review. Overall, clinically, the vaccine has appeared to be protective, with only one case of WNV in an appropriately vaccinated bird, and that bird had not mounted a serologic response to the vaccine.

RELEASE PROGRAM IN MEXICO: OUT OF COUNTRY CHALLENGES

The release program in Baja California, Mexico, began in 2003 and has been detailed.[17] Veterinary challenges have included exotic Newcastle disease, avian influenza and salmonella testing and paperwork, and communication in a foreign language, a short timeline required to ship condors from the United States to Mexico, quarantine requirements (at the release site) once they arrive, and biologic samples with limited ability to come back into the United States. Despite these challenges, veterinarians involved in this release program have been able to address them successfully.

ENVIRONMENTAL CONTAMINATION

Botulism

Botulism has been reported in a 15-month-old released condor being held in a holding pen that had not been cleaned for $2\frac{1}{2}$ weeks. This bird presented nonresponsive with flaccid paralysis but stable vital signs and responded well to supportive care and antitoxin administration.[19] Two possible additional cases have been seen, both from a field pen, that presented at the same time; there was one mortality and one clinical case that presented with flaccid paralysis and responded well to supportive care over time, however botulism was unable to be definitively proven as the cause.[30]

Lead

Lead poisoning in wild condors is the most serious threat to success of the wild recovery program. Without intensive management and treatment, mortalities would no doubt be much higher.[11] Diagnostic and treatment regimens have been published for Arizona[21] and are in process for California. Routine screening occurs during hunting season and when animals are reported or observed feeding on hunter-killed carcasses. This includes the use of a handheld portable tester (LeadCare portable field tester, ESA, Chelmsford, Mass) for immediate field screening, with samples being sent to a diagnostic laboratory for correlation.[1] Portable x-ray techniques have been attempted but are difficult because of field conditions, and birds that are at a high level on the LeadCare machine are usually transported to a medical facility for radiography (Fig. 38-5). Birds in a gray area (lead concentration, 30 to 60 µg/dL) may be held, treated, and/or radiographed depending on clinical history, signs, and resources. In clinically normal birds, standard treatments include subcutaneous fluids and calcium EDTA injected twice daily at standard avian doses. An alternative once-daily treatment using calcium EDTA and succimer[8] together (to minimize handling and stress) was successful in California for many cases, but appeared to be linked to acute gout deaths in several birds and was discontinued. California condors are extremely resistant to the acute effects of lead, and routinely fly around with levels that would cause mortality in other species. Birds with extremely high levels (1000 to 5000 µg/dL, or 1 to 5 ppm) have been treated successfully, showing little to no clinical symptoms. Conversely, there have been several cases of severe clinical signs, likely the result of more chronic exposure, that have required months of treatment (Fig. 38-6).[31] Some of these cases have pulled through with extensive support.[20]

Although no legislation will be possible in Arizona because of the legal status of release birds there, California represents a different scenario. After data analysis and testimony by the Veterinary Coordinator clearly stating morbidity and mortality rates in California from lead poisoning, and testimony regarding current isotope studies performed at University of California, Santa Cruz, linking poisoning to ammunition,[6] lead ammunition was banned in condor ranges in 2007[16] (see Fig. 38-6). Unfortunately, cases and mortalities continue as implementation and enforcement issues work their way to resolution.

In addition to acute and chronic poisoning in adults, two cases have now been seen in chicks in the nest, one with both parents being treated at the same time. Developmental effects and long-term effects from lead being deposited in bone and released chronically over time have been well documented in humans[2,18] and are cause for concern, although difficult to study in wild condors. Veterinarians new to the program may be alarmed at the levels that are not treated in this species, but the practicality of treating all low levels (below 30 µg/dL) in wild birds is daunting.

Captive held condors in Baja California have been inadvertently poisoned by food fed to them in the pen

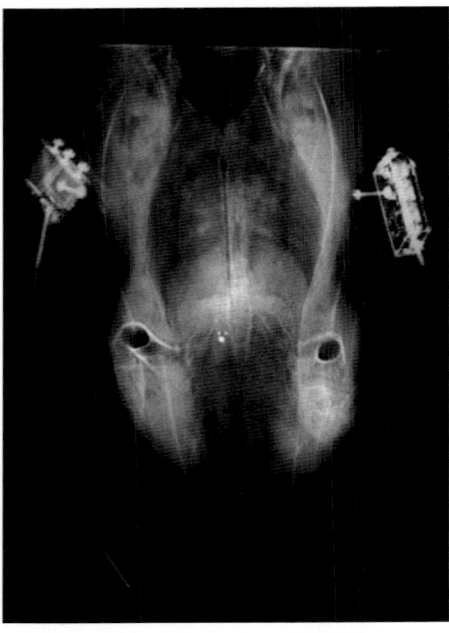

Figure 38-5

X-ray of California condor AC8, an original founder bird who immediately returned to captivity with lead poisoning after re-release. Note metal densities apparent in the ventriculus on this radiograph.

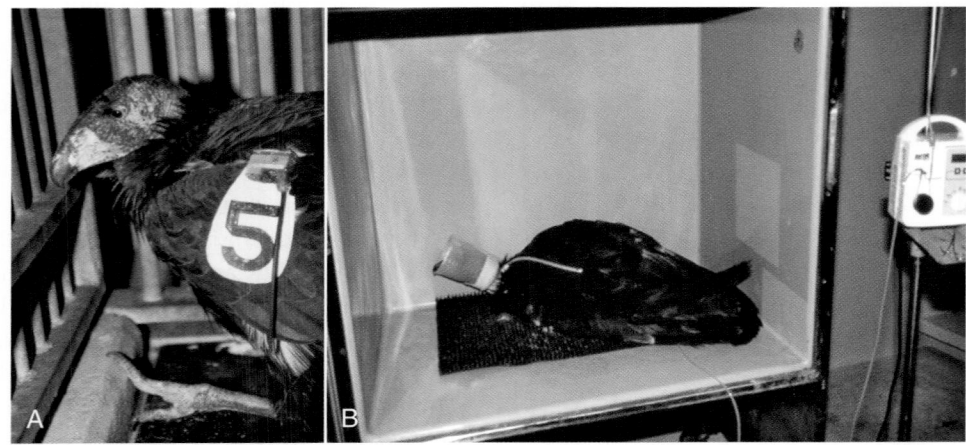

Figure 38-6

California condor W5 presented with limb paralysis and crop stasis from lead poisoning. Treatment included the use of an enteral feeding pump at the Los Angeles Zoo. (*Courtesy Charles Sedgwick.*)

that unknowingly contained lead shot, with transport of birds to the United States for treatment being required.[33] Screening of food has been changed to prevent this from occurring in the future.[27]

Copper

As ammunition changes to copper, investigation of normal copper levels and possible pathology is being investigated by the Zoological Society of San Diego Wildlife Disease Laboratories.[22] To date, there have been cases where copper levels may have been higher than seen routinely, but no pathology seen at necropsy has been attributed to copper. Increased copper levels in proferred calf carcasses have also been implicated as a possible cause.

DDT and DDE

DDT (dichlorodiphenyltrichloroethane) and DDE (dichlorodiphenyldichloroethylene) are currently under investigation regarding possible eggshell thinning in central California, where marine mammals are a staple food source.

WILD CHICKS: INTENSIVE NEST MANAGEMENT PROGRAM

Poor survival of chicks hatched in the wild in California without intervention has been well-described for the period from 2001 to 2005, primarily because of junk ingestion—trash brought to nest sites and fed to chicks by parents.[15] This problem, along with concerns about WNV and lead exposure, have led to an intensive nest management program in California. This program has become more intense every year and, in 2007, routine visits were initiated to each nest site (usually at 30, 60, 90, and 120 days of age) through the efforts of expert climbing biologists and helicopter use to reach previously inaccessible sites (Fig. 38-7). Nests are checked for trash, chicks are examined and blood taken for health evaluation, including lead levels, in addition to measurements taken for growth and evaluation of plumage development. Chicks are vaccinated for WNV at 1 month of age, serologic results are checked, and additional vaccination performed, if needed, at later visits. Many of these nest sites require extremely strenuous hiking and climbing skills by veterinarians involved, and more than one incidence of medical treatment has been needed for veterinarians postnest visit.

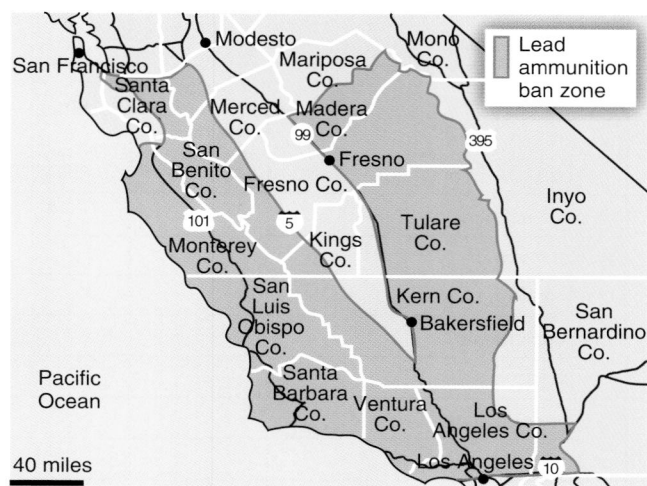

Lead ammo banned in condor range
The California Fish and Game Commission on Friday banned lead bullets in the current and historic range of the endangered California condor, shown here. The new regulations took effect July 1, 2008.

Figure 38-7

Map of California lead ban.

Additionally, field observations may be the cause of an unscheduled visit or a chick to be helicoptered out of the nest on an emergency basis.

Numerous ventriculotomies have been performed at the Los Angeles Zoo on ill chicks to remove trash (Figs. 38-8 and 38-9). Three of these cases were returned to the nest 36 hours postsurgery, and two of three successfully went on to fledge in the wild under parental care. An additional case in Arizona was similarly successful postventriculotomy for stick impaction. This intensive program—clean-up efforts, management techniques to attempt to limit parents from accessing trash during nesting season, and intensive nest monitoring by dedicated biologists and volunteers—has improved successful fledging in California. It appears that the ability of chicks to cast up trash starts at about 5 to 6 months of age (fledging age), providing a developmental time window during which intensive veterinary management may be successful in fledging chicks in the wild who otherwise would have died. This program requires extremely close cooperation and intensive communication between field biologists and veterinarians.

REVIEWS OF THE PROGRAM

Extensive reviews of the program, or aspects of it, have taken place using detailed veterinary data to make conclusions. Constant scrutiny by media and private groups

Southern California Nest Entry Schedule 2007 Breeding Season

Stage of development:	Egg stage (56-58 days)		Chick stage				
Entry #	1	1.5	2	2.5	3	3.5	4
	Fertility check, dummy replacement	Pipping egg replacement	WNV vaccination	Optional	Health/ developmental check	Critical response	Tagging
Time frame (days of stage)	12-16	50-60*	28-32	58-62	88-92	90-120	118-124
Additional activities:							
Physical exam			X	X	X	X	X
Sift substrate	X	X	X	X	X	X	X
Bone supplements	?	X	X	X	X	X	X
Chick weight			X	X	X		X
Tail feather measurements						X	X
Blood samples			X			X	
Personnel							
Vet	No	No	Yes	No	Yes	Yes	No
Number to Nest	2	2	3	3	3	3	3
Total	4	4	4	4	5	5	4
Helicopter	Yes	Depends on site	No	No	No	Yes	No
Breeding pairs 2007							
21+192	11-Feb	11, 15, 23-Mar	25-Apr	25-May	24-Jun	?	24-Jul
111+125	NA	7-May**	4-Jun	4-Jul	3-Aug	?	2-Sept
107+161	NA	8-May**	5-Jun	5-Jul	4-Aug	?	3-Sep
206+255***	24-Apr	30-May	est. 28-Jun	28-Jul	28-Aug	?	28-Sep
Big Sur 168+208 (laid Feb 14)	9-Mar	6-Apr	9-May	9-Jun	8-Jul		7-Aug
Big Sur 167+190 (laid Mar 13)	14-Apr	7-May*	7-Jun	7-Jul	6-Aug		5-Sep

(*To be determined by availability of captive eggs) (**Enter only if egg remains unhatched at day 60) (***Dates may change after fertility check)

Figure 38-8

Example of chick nest entry schedule in California. *(Courtesy Joseph Brandt, USFWS.)*

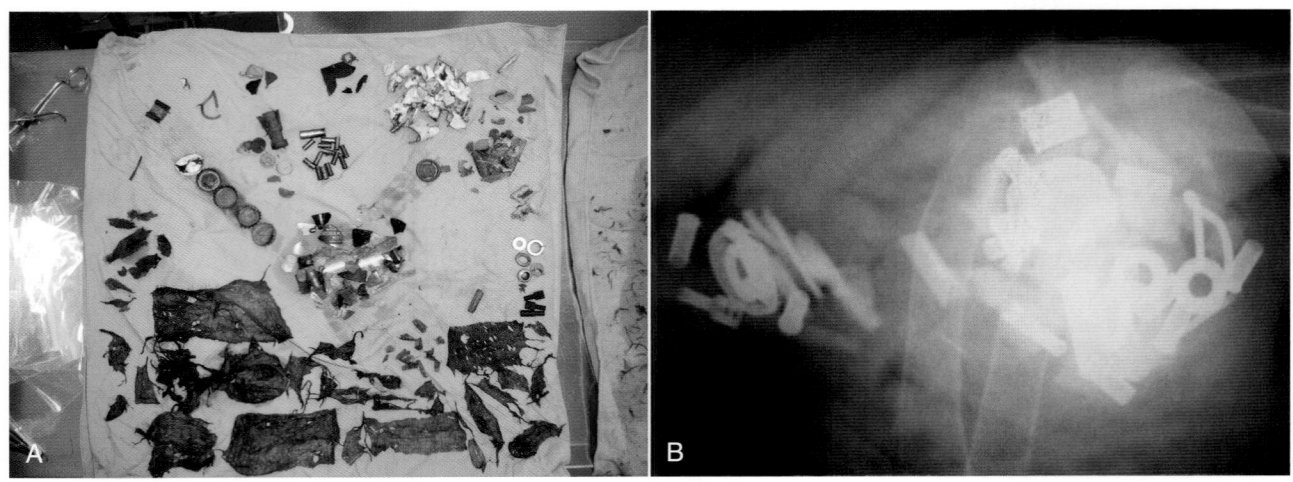

Figure 38-9

A, Example of junk removed during ventriculotomy from a wild California chick in 2005. **B,** Radiograph of wild California condor demonstrating junk ingestion.

continues unabated because of the controversial nature of the high-profile release program, and especially of the lead debate. This highlights the importance of providing accurate and consistent veterinary data for use by outside agencies and media, especially morbidity and mortality data.

University of California, Davis, Report

A private report was commissioned to University of California, Davis (UCD) by the California Department of Fish and Game and released in February of 2007.[12] Several inaccuracies were reported in this document because of unintentionally inaccurate data provided to the investigators. The most important of these was an inaccurate report of mortalities from copper.

American Ornithologists' Union Report

From 2007 to 2008, the American Ornithologists' Union (AOU) investigated the condor program and issued a 125-page report in August 2008.[29] A detailed analysis of the program with specific recommendations, including veterinary recommendations, may be found in this report.

CONCLUSIONS

It cannot be stated more emphatically that California condors are the toughest of patients. They are extremely strong birds that tolerate severe disease processes, toxicity, trauma, and invasive and prolonged treatment. From a veterinary standpoint, they are rewarding patients, often allowing us to push the envelope in avian care, with positive outcomes. Additionally, providing veterinary care to this species is an excellent example of the increasingly blurred line between zoo and wildlife medicine. Many techniques and learning what is normal, especially in regard to chick development, have been tried on birds in captivity and then applied to birds in the wild—often in extreme conditions. The intensive veterinary nest management program in the wild in California would no doubt be much less successful without veterinarians who did not have extensive experience and expertise with condor chicks in captivity. On an even larger scale, the AOU report has described condors as "the canaries in the coal mine" in their habitat in North America, referring specifically to lead. The huge strides in educating the public about the debilitating toxicity of lead poisoning in California condors has also indicated an increasing concern about the

effect of this metal in our own species. As harbingers of the One Health message, veterinarians in the condor program have also contributed much to the larger world picture.

Acknowledgment

Thank you to Janna Wynne for reviewing and adding much important information to this chapter, and to Kathy Orr, Don Janssen, and Jesse Grantham for their reviews and comments.

REFERENCES

1. Bedrosian B, Parish CN, Craighead D: Difference between blood lead level detection techniques: Analysis within and among three techniques and four avian species. In Watson RT, Fuller M, Pokras M, Hunt WG, editors: Ingestion of Lead from Spent Ammunition: Implications for Wildlife and Humans, 2009, pp 287 (http://www.peregrinefund.org/lead_conference/2008PbConf_Proceedings.htm).
2. Bunning M, Chang J: Personal communication, 2006.
3. Centers for Disease Control and Prevention (CDC) Advisory Committee on Childhood Lead Poisoning Prevention: Interpreting and managing blood lead levels <10 microg/dl in children and reducing childhood exposures to lead: Recommendations of CDC's Advisory Committee on Childhood Lead Poisoning Prevention. MMWR Recomm Rep 56(RR-8):1–16, 2007.
4. Chang J: Personal communication, 2005.
5. Chang GJ, Davis BS, Stringfield CE: Prospective immunization of the endangered California condors *(Gymnogyps californianus)* protects this species from lethal West Nile virus infection. Vaccine 25:2325–2330, 2007.
6. Church ME, Gwiazda R, Risebrough RW, et al: Ammunition is the principal source of lead accumulated by California condors reintroduced to the wild. Environ Sci Technol 40:6143–6150, 2006.
7. Clark M: Personal communication, 2010.
8. Denver MC, Tell LA, Galey FD, et al: Comparison of two heavy metal chelators for treatment of lead toxicosis in cockatiels. Am J Vet Res 61:935–940, 2000.
9. Dujowich M, Mazet JK, Zuba JR: Hematologic and biochemical reference ranges for captive California condors *(Gymnogyps californianus)*. J Zoo Wildl Med 36:590–597, 2005.
10. Ensley PK: Medical management of the California condor. In Fowler ME, Miller RE, editors: Zoo and Wild Animal Medicine: Current Therapy 4, Philadelphia, 1999, WB Saunders, pp 277–292.
11. Hunt WG, Parish CN, Orr K: Lead poisoning and the reintroduction of the California condor in northern Arizona. J Avian Med Surg 23:145–150, 2009.
12. Johnson CK, Vodovoz T, Boyce WM, et al: Lead exposure in California condors and sentinel species in California, 2007 (http://www.biologicaldiversity.org/species/birds/California_condor/pdfs/Johnson-et-al-2007-DFG-Report.pdf).
13. Kasielke S: Condors. In Gage LJ, Duerr RS, editors: Hand-Rearing Birds, Ames, Iowa, 2007, Blackwell, pp 171–186.
14. Mace M: Personal communication, 2001.
15. Mee A, Rideout BA, Hamber JA, et al: Junk ingestion and nestling mortality in a reintroduced population of California condors *Gymnogyps californianus*. Bird Conserv Int 17:119–130, 2007.
16. Meeting of CA Fish and Game Commission, October 27, 2007. http://www.cal-span.org/cgi-bin/media.pl?folder=CFG.

17. Mercado JA, Zuba JR, Fernandez FS, et al: California condor *(Gymnogyps californianus)* conservation in Baja California: Successes and challenges across the border. In Proceedings of the Annual Meeting of the American Association of Zoo Veterinarians, 2006, pp 36–39.
18. Needleman HL, McFarland C, Ness RB, et al: Bone lead levels in adjudicated delinquents. A case control study. Neurotoxicol Teratol 24:711–717, 2002.
19. Orr K: Botulism in a California condor *(Gymnogyps californianus)*. In Proceedings of the Annual Meeting of the American Association of Zoo Veterinarians, 2002, pp 101–103. Milwaukee, WI, Baer, ed.
20. Orr K, Wynne J: Personal communication, 2000–2010.
21. Parish CN, Heinrich WR, Hunt WG: Lead exposure, diagnosis, and treatment in California condors released in Arizona. In Mee A, Hall LS editors: California condors in the 21st century, Washington DC, 2007, American Ornithologists' Union, pp 97–108.
22. Rideout B: Personal communication, 2009.
23. Stacy B: Personal communication, 2004.
24. Stringfield CE, Davis BS, Chang GJ: Vaccination of Andean condors *(Vultur gryphus)* and California condors *(Gymnogyps californianus)* with a West Nile virus DNA vaccine. In Proceedings of the Annual Meeting of the American Association of Zoo Veterinarians, 2003, pp 193–194. Minneapolis, MN, Baer.
25. Stringfield CE, Wong A, Wallace M, et al: Causes of death in released California condors *(Gymnogyps californianus)* from 1992-2002. In Proceedings of the Annual Meeting of the American Association of Zoo Veterinarians, American Association of Wildlife Veterinarians, Wildlife Disease Association Joint Conference, 2004, pp 85–86. San Diego, CA, Baer, ed.
26. Turell MG, Bunning M, Ludwig GV, et al: DNA vaccine for West Nile virus infection in fish crows *(Corvus ossifragus)*. Emerg Infect Dis 9:1077–1081, 2003.
27. Wallace M: Personal communication, 2007.
28. Walters JR, Derrickson SR, Fry DM, et al: Status of the California condor and efforts to achieve its recovery, 2008 (http://www.aou.org/committees/conservation/docs/AOU_Condor_Report.pdf).
29. Wynne J: Personal communication, 2010.
30. Wynne JE, Stringfield CE: Treatment of lead toxicity and crop stasis in a California condor *(Gymnogyps californianus)*. J Zoo Wildl Med 38(4):588–590, 2007.
31. Zuba J: Personal communication, 2007.
32. Zuba J, Lamberski N: Personal communication, 2007.

CHAPTER 39

Avian Circovirus and Polyomavirus Diseases

Shane R. Raidal

Psittacine beak and feather disease (PBFD) and budgerigar fledgling disease are well-characterized causes of disease in captive psittacine birds. However, since beak and feather disease virus (BFDV) was first characterized, the *Circovirus* genus has grown to contain a growing number of viruses from a diverse range of bird species.

Although budgerigar fledgling disease polyomavirus is the name designated by the International Committee on Taxonomy of Viruses for the first avian member of the Polyomaviridae to be discovered, the term *avian polyomavirus* (APV) is more commonly used. This better reflects the range of passerine and non-passerine bird species that are now known to be susceptible to APV infection. The abbreviation APV also avoids confusion with BFDV and will be used herein.

PSITTACINE BEAK AND FEATHER DISEASE

PBFD, arguably the most recognizable disease of Psittaciformes, is a major problem of wild psittacine birds in Australasia and in captive birds worldwide. The disease was first recorded in wild Australian sulfur-crested cockatoos *(Cacatua galerita)* in 1903,[16,17] and a second report in 1907[2] described feather disease affecting red-rumped parrots *(Psephotus haematonotus)* in South Australia. Affected birds were described as "quite healthy, except being destitute of feathers." PBFD has since come to be recognized as the most common disease of wild and captive psittacine birds, with a worldwide distribution, and posing a threat to the conservation of endangered psittacine birds in Australia, South Africa, and New Zealand.

Cause

Measuring only about 20 nm in diameter, circoviruses are comparatively small, nonenveloped, icosahedral viruses that contain relatively simple, circular, single-stranded DNA genomes, making them among the smallest and simplest pathogens so far known. Their small genomes of approximately 2 kb encode for only two major proteins, the structural capsid (Cap) protein and a replicase (Rep) protein. Compared with budgerigar fledgling disease polyomavirus and other DNA viruses, they are genetically diverse, even within species. Despite this, little association has been demonstrated between genotypes and pathotypes of any of the members of the Circoviridae.

Clinical Signs

PBFD generally affects juvenile or young adult psittacine birds but all ages may succumb to the disease. Two syndromes are recognized, an acute form, which occurs in nestlings and African grey parrots *(Psittacus erithacus)*, and a chronic form, which occurs in many species of psittacine birds. In acute disease, there is rapid development of depression associated with leucopenia, green diarrhea, and death caused by hepatic necrosis. High titers of BFDV may be detected in the liver and bile of affected birds and some may die of liver failure without obvious feather lesions. African grey parrots often die within 1 week of the development of clinical signs and, depending on the age of the nestling, many diseased contour feathers may be shed all at once or only the primary flight feathers may be affected. Feather necrosis causing fractures of the developing calamus and accompanying intrapulp hemorrhage are the predominant clinical findings. Affected feathers fracture from the point of necrosis, usually before the feather has

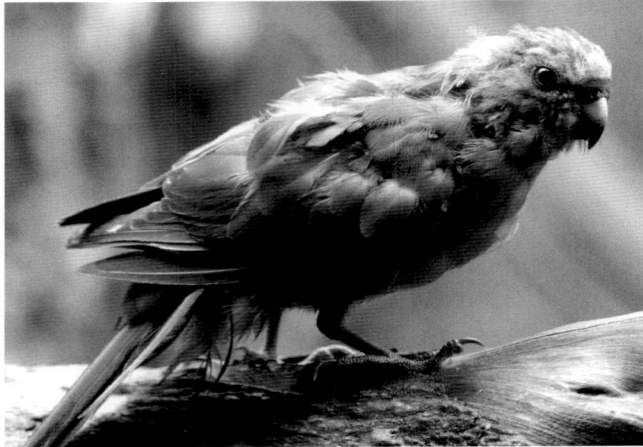

Figure 39-1

Chronic PBFD in a yellow crowned kakariki *(Cyanoramphus auriceps)* demonstrating generalized plumage deficits caused by bilaterally symmetrical feather dystrophy.

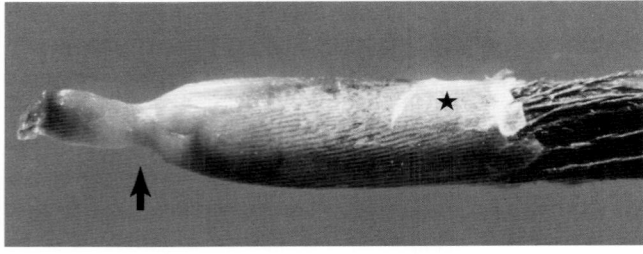

Figure 39-2

PBFD-affected feather demonstrating annular constriction of the developing calamus *(arrow)* and thickening of the feather sheath *(star)*.

unsheathed. Feather tracts may become acutely swollen and sensitive because of inflammation and edema, and the birds often become systemically ill, anorexic, and/or regurgitate food. Death may occur suddenly within 1 to 2 weeks of developing clinical signs.

More commonly, PBFD develops as a chronic disease that is insidious in its development and progression; dystrophic feathers replace normal ones as they are molted. In this manner, a PBFD-affected bird may gradually lose its plumage without other signs of illness (Fig. 39-1). The pattern of feather dystrophy is related to the stage of molt that the bird is in when the disease first begins; it is usually bilaterally symmetrical and slowly progressive. Dystrophic feathers are usually short and have one or more of the following characteristics: fault lines across the vanes; a thickened or retained feather sheath; blood within the calamus; an annular constriction of the calamus; and curling (Fig. 39-2).

In cockatoos, the powder-down feathers, or pulviplumes, are often the first feathers affected. PBFD-affected pulviplumes are fragile or develop an abnormally thickened outer sheath that fails to disintegrate. Pulviplume follicles may atrophy and thus create bare powder-down patches. Arrested production of powder down causes the plumage to become dull and the beak to become glossy. Claw abnormalities occur occasionally, and generally develop well after feather and beak lesions become apparent. Feather loss is symmetrical, usually affecting the powder-down feathers first in cockatoos, and then flight and tail feathers, before progressively involving the rest of the body until birds appear to be bald. The pattern of feather loss is dependent on the stage of molt that the bird is in when clinical signs commence. Affected developing feathers fracture at an annular constriction, typically near the calamus. The beak becomes progressively elongated, develops fracture lines, and may eventually fracture or slough off. Chronically affected birds are predisposed to secondary infections, presumably because of immunosuppression.

On the extremities, PBFD-induced hyperkeratosis may cause the skin to appear excessively scaly or it may be thickened and moist. Sunlight-exposed skin may become darkly pigmented. Chronic skin ulcers may occur at the elbows and wing tips. Beak, and less commonly, claw deformities occur in some PBFD-affected birds, particularly in cockatoos. The beak may become abnormally soft and brittle and the upper and lower tips elongated. Transverse or longitudinal fractures or delaminations often occur. In severe cases, necrosis of the oral epithelium and osteomyelitis may cause the beak to slough. Secondary disease problems commonly exist. These include cryptosporidiosis and bacterial, mycotic, and other viral infections. Most birds with chronic disease eventually have difficulty eating, lose weight, and die.

In smaller grass parrots such as *Psephotus* and *Neophema* spp., apparently normal feathers which fall out or are effortlessly plucked, may be the only clinical sign. The first clinical sign in birds with green plumage may be the development of yellow feathers, which may appear normal in other respects.

Diagnosis

PBFD has distinct pathologic features and, although in most circumstances a presumptive diagnosis may be achieved by clinical examination alone, further tests must be done to differentiate PBFD from similar diseases of the integument (e.g., acute avian polyomavirus infection, chronic hypothyroidism). Clinicopathologic derangements such as anemia and hypoproteinemia are nonspecific. Histologic examination of feather follicle or feather biopsies may confirm clinical disease but is not suitable for diagnosing incubating BFDV infection or detecting BFDV carriers. Necrosis of feather epidermal cells and the presence of relatively large intracytoplasmic inclusions in macrophages and keratinocytes is characteristic of the disease. Similar viral inclusions occur in the bursa of Fabricius. Lesions are usually absent in the apterial and interfollicular skin, although BFDV antigen may be found here by immunohistochemistry. This may also be used to detect antigen in the bursa of Fabricius, spleen, pharynx, crop, esophageal epithelium, and other tissues.

Unlike other members of the *Circovirus* genus, BFDV is a hemagglutinating virus and has been shown to agglutinate erythrocytes from guinea pigs, geese, and many species of psittacine birds. To date, no method has been described to cultivate BFDV in vitro successfully. Thus, research into the biologic characteristics, pathophysiology, and mode of replication has required the use of virus purified from the tissues of infected birds or recombinant proteins.

Virus detection by hemagglutination (HA) assay is a sensitive diagnostic test for detecting BFDV antigen emission in feather material. Chronically affected birds typically excrete very high titers (>1 : 40,960), often in the absence of detectable antibodies measurable by hemagglutination inhibition (HI) assay.[10] HA may be used to detect virus excretion in feathers, liver, bile, and feces and may be performed on actively growing feather pulp or dry keratinized feathers.

Virus DNA detection by polymerase chain reaction (PCR) assay is also available as a diagnostic test and may detect BFDV infection in circulating leucocytes or feather material. The results must be interpreted in relation to the clinical signs and results of other tests, because cross-contamination caused by unclean collection and laboratory technique is possible.[4,10,12]

Serology may be done by HI, enzyme-linked immunosorbent assay (ELISA), or blocking ELISA (bELISA) and is useful for detecting BFDV-infected flocks or seroconversion in individual birds.[8,10,24] A high plasma HI antibody titer (>1:320) in an adult bird is a good indicator that it does not have chronic PBFD. Nestlings with incubating infection or acute disease may have low and declining antibody titers. The HI test may be done on serum, plasma, or whole blood collected on filter paper.

Pathogenesis and Epidemiology

The incubation period of PBFD may be as short as 21 days but it is probably dependent on the dose of virus, age of the bird, stage of feather development, and absence of immunity. Primary virus replication probably occurs in the bursa of Fabricius and/or gastrointestinal tract lymphoid tissue. Secondary virus replication occurs in the liver and thymus, and probably in other tissues. The target organ is the epidermis and the manifestation of skin disease requires a molt. Consequently, birds that become infected after feather development has completed may not develop clinical signs until their next molt. This could take 6 months or longer. Most birds that succumb to PBFD are younger than 2 years. However, all age groups should be considered susceptible to circovirus infection. Long-term exposure and/or stress are probably required for infection and seroconversion in adult birds.

Very little is known about the steps involved in the replication of BFDV but it is possible that it uses a similar mechanism for cellular entry into macrophages as that discovered for porcine circovirus The capsid protein contains a nuclear localization signal that assists viral entry into the nucleus,[7] but the genome may also be able to enter the nucleus during mitosis by associating itself with cellular chromatin. Circoviruses are highly dependent on cellular enzymes for their replication via the synthesis of a complementary strand to form a double-stranded DNA (dsDNA) replicative form and then by rolling circle replication. How assembled virions are transported into the nucleus to form the characteristic paracrystalline arrays, which are readily seen histologically, is not precisely known, but BFDV Cap and Rep are known to interact,[7] which may facilitate transport of encapsidated virions into the cytoplasm.

BFDV is epitheliotrophic and primary sites of replication include the skin (including the epithelium of the beak and claws), liver, gastrointestinal tract, and bursa of Fabricius. The virus replicates to high titers in these tissues and also spreads to the spleen, thyroid, parathyroid, and bone marrow. Skin lesions are associated with apoptosis of keratinocytes.

The maximum incubation period of PBFD is unknown, because the appearance of clinical signs depends on the stage of molt of the bird; however, experimentally infected nestlings may show signs of acute disease from 21 to 28 days postinfection. BFDV is excreted via the feathers and the gastrointestinal tract. Consequently, high concentrations of BFDV antigen may be detected in liver tissue, bile, crop secretions, feces, and feather dander. Horizontal transmission by oral and/or intracloacal ingestion of virus excreted via feces, feather dander, and crop secretions is likely the primary mechanism of viral spread. Experimental infection may also be accomplished by intramuscular administration of the virus. Vertical transmission is suspected, because BFDV DNA has been amplified from embryonated eggs by PCR assay.[18]

All species of psittacine birds should be considered to be susceptible to BFDV. Depending on the species and age, not all birds infected with BFDV progress to develop clinical signs of disease. Spontaneous clinical recovery from acute PBFD may occur rarely in many species, including budgerigars *(Melopsittacus undulatus)*, lorikeets, and *Eclectus* and *Agapornis* spp. but these birds typically become carriers. However, most chronically affected birds do not recover from the disease. Individual lorikeets and eclectus parrots may develop protective HA antibody with intermittent cessation of virus excretion. In contrast, others, such as African grey parrots and black cockatoos *(Calyptorhynchus* and *Callocephalon* spp.), appear highly susceptible and may die before clinical signs of feather loss develop. In contrast, cockatiels seem to be resistant to BFDV infection and subsequent PBFD.[23] White cockatoos *(Cacatua* spp.) typically develop the chronic form of the disease, with high HA titers detectable in feathers and feces and no detectable HI titer. The reasons for the variations in clinical disease remain to be explained.

Compared with APV, BFDV is a relatively genetically diverse species, with BFDV nucleotide sequence similarities reported to range from 84% to 99%. Based on phylogenetic analyses and differences in pathogenicity, the existence of strains of BFDV has been proposed but this has yet to be confirmed experimentally. Individual serotypes were not found in the one cross-reactivity study[10] undertaken to date. However, studies on BFDV isolates from PBFD-affected cockatiels *(Nymphicus hollandicus)* have shown some degree of serologic and phylogenetic divergence, but this is insufficient to justify classifying these as distinct strains or species.[23]

In infected flocks viral DNA may be detected in up to 28.0% of birds[6] in wild flocks and up to 83% to 90% of birds in captive flocks.[10] Seroprevalences up to 62% in captive flocks and up to 94% in wild flocks have been reported. In wild birds, PBFD has been confirmed in most Australian psittacine bird species, as well as in parrots and cockatoos throughout Indonesia, Papua New Guinea, and New Zealand. In Australia, flocks of wild cockatoos may have a disease prevalence of 20% and a seroprevalence of 60% to 80% and infection is probably maintained in a population by diseased birds and contaminated nest hollows. Epidemics may occur in susceptible wild or aviary flocks. Virus transmission is probably predominantly by horizontal spread, but carrier birds may contribute by vertical transmission. Virus infectivity probably persists in contaminated nests for many months or years. Aviary flocks with a history of PBFD usually have a high seroprevalence. In these situations, PBFD-affected birds are often the progeny of hens with low or nondetectable serum antibody levels.

Prevention and Control

Aviary birds should be maintained as a closed flock and new birds only received from PBFD-free flocks. Extended quarantine, and/or repeated PCR testing within quarantine, is recommended because of the variable incubation period of the disease. The appropriate use of disinfectants such as glutaraldehyde, which are suitable for inactivating environmentally resistant viruses, should be recommended for disinfecting contaminated utensils, cages, and rooms.

Experimental inactivated vaccines have been used in nestlings as young as 10 days. However, immunity takes at least 10 days to develop and a booster is required at least 1 month after the first vaccination. Vaccination does not prevent infection, and transient viral replication in developing feathers and vaccination of already infected nestlings may exacerbate the progression of natural disease.[5]

CIRCOVIRUSES IN OTHER AVIAN SPECIES

Circovirus infections have been demonstrated in a diverse range of passerine hosts, including canary *(Serinus canaria)*, gouldian finches *(Erythrura gouldiae)*, common starling *(Sternus vulgaris)*, and raven *(Corvus coronoides)*. Nonpasserine birds such as anatids, lariids, and columbids are also well represented, with circovirus species found in various species of duck geese, swan, gull, and pigeons.[26,27] Pigeon, goose, and canary circovirus have all been officially classified as members of the genus *Circovirus* and they share similar genomic and structural characteristics with other circoviruses. Pigeon circovirus (PiCV), associated with lethargy, anorexia, runting, and poor racing performance as part of a multifactorial syndrome known as young pigeon disease syndrome,[21] is distributed worldwide, and a range of molecular diagnostic assays have been developed to detect PiCV DNA.[15] Goose circovirus (GoCV) is associated with a runting syndrome and is also expected to have a worldwide distribution. Dot blot and PCR assays have been developed for the detection of viral DNA[3] and an indirect immunofluorescence assay using a recombinant GoCV capsid protein has been developed for serologic screening.

AVIAN POLYOMAVIRUS DISEASE

Like circoviruses, avian polyomaviruses are also nonenveloped with a circular, but larger, dsDNA genome of approximately 5 kb in size. At least two species of polyomaviruses are currently recognized to infect birds; there is phylogenetic evidence to support their reclassification into an *Avipolyomavirus* genus[25] within the Polyomaviridae. Unlike their mammalian polyomavirus relatives, which cause low pathogenic and persistent infections, avian polyomaviruses have an acute replication strategy that is often associated with disease and mortality. Goose hemorrhagic polyomavirus, which causes fatal disease in geese aged from 3 to 12 weeks,[11] is closely related to but clearly distinct from APV.[13] The more commonly encountered APV, however, is a recognized cause of acute fatal disease of Psittaciformes and sporadically occurs in a wide range of passerine and nonpasserine birds.[1,16] Two more avian polyomaviruses have been characterized in the Eurasian bullfinch *(Pyrrhula pyrrhula griseiventris)* and Eurasian jackdaw *(Corvus monedula)*, tentatively designated as finch polyomavirus (FPyV) and crow polyomavirus (CPyV), respectively.[9,28]

Like BFDV, APV is probably capable of causing disease in all psittacine species. However, nestling and juvenile birds are most susceptible. Most birds that recover from the acute phase of APV disease make a complete clinical recovery. Chronic progressive skin disease is not always a feature of APV infection, but may occur in nestling birds, and persistent virus infection and excretion are common sequelae. Concurrent APV and BFDV infection occurs often and the latter has been implicated in exacerbating APV-induced disease, presumably because of immunosuppression.[20]

Clinical Signs

In budgerigars *(Melopsittacus undulatus)* and *Neophema* spp., APV infection may cause severe clinical signs and mortalities in susceptible nestlings between 10 and 25 days of age. APV replication occurs in all tissues, including the brain, and affected nestlings may be ataxic or have head tremors. There may be abdominal distension

caused by hepatomegaly and ascites; subcutaneous petechiae or ecchymosis or a generalized pallor. The mortality rate in this age group may be 100%, with death occurring rapidly following the development of clinical signs. Gross necropsy lesions may be absent but the crop is often distended with food. Older budgerigar nestlings may fail to develop normal contour feathers and affected contour feathers may lack normal barbs. The rectrices and secondary remiges may fail to develop. There may be a lack of down feathers on the back and abdomen and a lack of contour feathers on the head and neck. At necropsy, there may be cardiomegaly, hydropericardium, and hepatomegaly or focal hepatic necrosis.

In other species, APV may cause nonspecific signs of illness, including anorexia, crop stasis, depression, paresis, and ataxia. Sporadic sudden deaths may occur in juvenile or adult birds with or without the presence of feather abnormalities and may be accompanied by a membranous glomerulopathy.[14] All age groups should be considered to be susceptible to infection. Mortalities typically occur in conures younger than 6 weeks, in macaws and eclectus parrots younger than 14 weeks and, in *Agapornis* spp., deaths may occur in birds up to 1 year old. Cockatoo species appear to be very resistant to developing disease, despite being susceptible to infection.

Diagnosis

A presumptive diagnosis of APV infection may be made from the history, clinical, and pathologic features. However, histopathologic, bacteriologic, and serologic investigations should be used to rule out differential diagnoses, such as adenovirus or herpesvirus infection and acute hepatotoxicity. PCR assay is currently the main technique for confirming APV infection and may be performed on blood and or cloacal swabs.[15]

APV infections cause marked basophilic karyomegaly in many tissues, in particular the feather follicles, kidney, and liver. Basophilic intranuclear inclusions may be found in persistently infected kidneys but cannot be differentiated morphologically from other viral infections, particularly adenovirus infections. A definitive diagnosis of the cause of intranuclear inclusions requires the use of electron microscopy or in situ hybridization using APV-specific DNA probes.[20]

APV may be cultured in vitro in budgerigar embryo fibroblast, chicken embryo fibroblast, or chicken embryo kidney cell cultures. However, virus isolation is generally not available for routine diagnosis. Antibodies to APV have been detected by immunodiffusion, virus neutralization assay, and indirect immunofluorescence, but serology is not routinely available despite it being possibly more sensitive than cloacal PCR assay for detecting APV infection on a flock basis.

Epidemiology

Horizontal transmission is the major method of APV infection in an epidemic but vertical transmission probably also occurs. Virus is excreted in feather dander and droppings. Infection persists in the kidneys of carrier birds and virus is excreted intermittently in the droppings, probably during times of stress. Polyomaviruses are thermostable, may withstand freeze-thawing, and remain infective in contaminated environments. Aviary flocks with endemic APV infection may have a seroprevalence from 11% to 100%. APV carriers may be seropositive or seronegative and their serologic status may change over time. Up to 100% of birds in a flock may be persistently APV-infected, but not all will be excreting virus at the time of sampling. There have been few studies of the epidemiology of avian polyomaviruses in wild birds,[1,9] but a high seroprevalence has been demonstrated to APV in flocks of *Cacatua* spp. but not the galah *(Eolophus roseicapillus)* in Australia.[19]

Prevention and Control

APV-free bird collections should be encouraged to maintain a closed flock with strict hygiene and quarantine procedures. This includes eliminating exposure to free-flying wild birds and regulating all food, utensils, and humans with access to the birds. Polyomavirus particles probably remain infectious on utensils, clothing, and hands of well-meaning visitors for long periods. New stock should only be obtained from seronegative and APV-free aviary flocks and held in quarantine and confirmed as APV-free, preferably both by serology and PCR, before being incorporated into an existing flock.

An APV vaccine is available in some countries,[22] although the effectiveness of vaccination to protect the most susceptible groups such as nestling birds is somewhat controversial. Passive transfer of maternal immunity is probably insufficient to protect this group and vaccination of older nestlings is unlikely to protect them in an already contaminated environment.[14]

Nevertheless, vaccination is likely to protect fledglings leaving an APV-free aviary and should be considered a valuable tool, along with appropriate hygiene, for controlling the infection. In an endemic situation, an effort should be made to eradicate horizontal transmission between birds and between batches of young birds. Accurate record keeping and regular disease monitoring are most important. It may be desirable to identify APV carriers and isolate these birds in a separate facility.[14] Complete cessation of breeding activity for 6 months may eradicate infection from a flock provided that all utensils, incubators, and brooders are thoroughly cleaned and disinfected between clutches. Chlorine, synthetic phenol, stabilized chlorine dioxide, sodium hypochlorite, and 70% ethanol have been effective in reducing the infectivity of APV, and rooms should be fitted with air filtration systems that eliminate aerosolized virus.[14]

REFERENCES

1. Arroube AS, Halami MY, Johne R, et al: Mortality due to polyomavirus infection in two nightjars *(Caprimulgus europaeus)*. J Avian Med Surg 23:136–140, 2009.
2. Ashby E: Parakeets Moulting. Emu 193–194, 1907.
3. Ball NW, Smyth JA, Weston JH, et al: Diagnosis of goose circovirus infection in Hungarian geese samples using polymerase chain reaction and dot blot hybridisation tests. Avian Pathol 33:51–58, 2004.
4. Bonne N, Clark P, Shearer P, et al: Elimination of false-positive polymerase chain reaction results resulting from hole punch carryover contamination. J Vet Diagn Invest 20:60–63, 2008.
5. Bonne N, Shearer P, Sharp M, et al: Assessment of recombinant beak and feather disease virus (BFDV) capsid protein as a vaccine for psittacine beak and feather disease (PBFD). J Gen Virol 90:640–647, 2009.
6. Ha HJ, Anderson IL, Alley MR, et al: The prevalence of beak and feather disease virus infection in wild populations of parrots and cockatoos in New Zealand. New Zealand Vet J 55:235–238, 2007.
7. Heath L, Williamson A, Rybicki EP: The capsid protein of beak and feather disease virus binds to the viral DNA and is responsible for transporting the replication-associated protein into the nucleus. J Virol 80:7219–7225, 2006.
8. Johne R, Raue R, Grund C, et al: Recombinant expression of a truncated capsid protein of beak and feather disease virus and its application in serological tests. Avian Pathol 33:328–336, 2004.
9. Johne R, Wittig W, Fernandez-de-Luco D, et al: Characterization of two novel polyomaviruses of birds by using multiply primed rolling-circle amplification of their genomes. J Virol 80:3523–3531, 2006.
10. Khalesi B, Bonne N, Stewart M, et al: A comparison of haemagglutination, haemagglutination inhibition and PCR for the detection of psittacine beak and feather disease virus infection and a comparison of isolates obtained from loriids. J Gen Virol 86:3039–3046, 2005.
11. Lacroux C, Andreoletti O, Payre B, et al: Pathology of spontaneous and experimental infections by Goose haemorrhagic polyomavirus. Avian Pathol 33:351–358, 2004.
12. Olsen G, Speer B: Laboratory reporting accuracy of polymerase chain reaction testing for psittacine beak and feather disease virus. J Avian Med Surg 23:194–198, 2009.
13. Perez-Losada M, Christensen RG, McClellan DA, et al: Comparing phylogenetic codivergence between polyomaviruses and their hosts. J Virol 80:5663–5669, 2006.
14. Phalen DN, Wilson VG, Graham DL: Characterization of the avian polyomavirus-associated glomerulopathy of nestling parrots. Avian Dis 40:140–149, 1996.

15. Phalen DN, Wilson VG, Graham DL: Polymerase chain-reaction assay for avian polyomavirus. J Clin Microbiol 29:1030–1037, 1991.

16. Potti J, Blanco G, Lemus JA, et al: Infectious offspring: How birds acquire and transmit an avian polyomavirus in the wild. PLoS ONE 2:e1276, 2007.

17. Powell AM: Nude cockatoos. Emu 3:55–56, 1903.

18. Rahaus M, Desloges N, Probst S, et al: Detection of beak and feather disease virus DNA in embryonated eggs of psittacine birds. Vet Med 53:53–58, 2008.

19. Raidal SR, Cross GM, Tomaszewski E, et al: A serological survey for avian polyomavirus and Pacheco's disease virus in Australian cockatoos. Avian Pathol 27:263–268, 1998.

20. Ramis A, Latimer KS, Niagro FD, et al: Diagnosis of psittacine beak and feather disease (PBFD) viral infection, avian polyomavirus infection, adenovirus infection and herpesvirus infection in psittacine tissues using DNA in situ hybridization. Avian Pathol 23:643–657, 1994.

21. Raue R, Schmidt V, Freick M, et al: A comprehensive study on a disease complex associated with pigeon circovirus infection, young pigeon disease syndrome. Avian Pathol 34:418–425, 2005.

22. Ritchie BW, Latimer KS, Leonard J, et al: Safety, immunogenicity, and efficacy of an inactivated avian polyomavirus vaccine. Am J Vet Res 59:143–148, 1998.

23. Shearer P, Bonne N, Clark P, et al: Beak and feather disease virus infection in cockatiels (Nymphicus hollandicus). Avian Pathol 37:75–81, 2008.

24. Shearer PL, Sharp M, Bonne N, et al: A blocking ELISA for the detection of antibodies to psittacine beak and feather disease virus (BFDV). J Virol Methods 158:136–140, 2009.

25. Stoll R, Luo D, Kouwenhoven B, et al: Molecular and biological characteristics of avian polyomaviruses—isolates from different species of birds indicate that avian polyomaviruses form a distinct subgenus within the polyomavirus genus. J Gen Virol 74:229–237, 1993.

26. Todd D, Duchatel J-P, Bustin SA, et al: Detection of pigeon circovirus in cloacal swabs: Implications for diagnosis, epidemiology and control. Vet Rec 159:314–317, 2006.

27. Todd D, Fringuelli E, Scott ANJ, et al: Sequence comparison of pigeon circoviruses. Res Vet Sci 84:311–319, 2008.

28. Wittig W, Hoffmann K, Muller H, et al: Detection of DNA of the finch polyomavirus in diseased birds of the order Passeriformes. Berl Münch Tierärztl Wochenschr 120:113–119, 2007.

CHAPTER 40

Veterinary Care of Kakapo

Richard Jakob-Hoff and Brett Gartrell

The kakapo, *Strigops habroptilus* (family Strigopidae, subfamily Strigopinae) is a critically endangered endemic New Zealand parrot. Once common throughout New Zealand, the species was brought to the edge of extinction by a combination of habitat loss and predation by introduced rats and carnivores, especially stoats, *Mustela erminea*, and now survives only on predator-free offshore islands.[11,25] From a low of 51 in 1995, intensive management by the New Zealand Department of Conservation (DOC) has increased the number to 123 as of March 2010. The current rarity of this species has meant that few veterinarians have had the opportunity to work with kakapo. However, this is changing as the numbers continue to increase and DOC is placing greater emphasis on the display of the species for educational and advocacy purposes. Our objective in this chapter is to provide information for the guidance of clinicians faced with the opportunity to provide veterinary care for this unique species.

UNIQUE AND UNUSUAL FEATURES

The kakapo is flightless and nocturnal and has the biggest body mass and most extreme sexual dimorphism of any parrot. Males weigh 1.6 to 3.6 kg (mean, 2.11 kg) and females weigh 0.9 to 1.9 kg (mean, 1.45 kg).[13,25] Average seasonal weight gains can be as much as 23% to 25%, but individuals can fluctuate by 100% in the course of a year.[12] The ventral surface of the strong broad rhinotheca is equipped with transverse serrations used, with the tongue, to crush and extract nutrients from a wide range of leaves, fruits, seeds, grasses, fern fronds, and rhizomes that comprise its herbivorous diet.[8,30] The crop is unusually large and pendulous to accommodate this highly fibrous, low-nutrient diet. When full, it overlies the thorax ventrally, where the birds have the markedly reduced keel and

pectoral muscle mass associated with their inability to fly. The simple gut includes a relatively thin-walled gizzard and no caecum.

BEHAVIOR AND REPRODUCTION

Perhaps the most unusual aspect of this bird's biology is its lek mating system. This involves the construction, maintenance, and defense, by the male, of a display territory known as a track and bowl system. These are usually located on an elevated site and are comprised of one or more shallow excavations (bowls), linked by clearly defined tracks. The male stands within the bowl and, after massively inflating his cervicocephalic air sacs, emits a series of low-frequency booms that may be heard for a distance of up to 5 km.[25] This serves to proclaim territory and attract females for mating. Females subsequently lay a clutch of two to four eggs in natural holes or cavities at ground level within their own home range. The male takes no part in the incubation of eggs or rearing of the altricial chicks, which hatch after 30 days.[13]

There is some indirect evidence to suggest that kakapo are very long-lived. Clout[9] has speculated that some may survive for over a century. Breeding is irregular and occurs only every 2 to 7 years, stimulated by the fruiting of podocarp trees, especially the rimu, *Dacrydium cupressinum*, whose protein-rich seeds and fruit form the basis of the diet on which the chicks are reared.[10,25,30] Males reach sexual maturity at approximately 5 years of age and females by at least 6 years.[12]

HOSPITALIZATION

Only one adult kakapo, a human-imprinted male, has been publicly displayed in captivity to date. Although some individual adult birds have been hospitalized for extended periods of up to several months, it can take several weeks before they settle enough to self-feed. Consequently, daily supplementary feeding with a crop tube is required to ensure adequate nutrition. When this is necessary for prolonged periods, either a stainless steel crop tube or a soft flexible tube (26-Fr Foley catheter) inserted through an oral gag can be used to minimize trauma to the upper gastrointestinal mucosa. Harrison's neonate, juvenile, and recovery formulas (HBD International, Brentwood, Tenn) provide adequate nutrition for weight gain and maintenance of body condition but the thick consistency of this food requires the 26-gauge soft tube. Kaytee Exact hand-rearing formula for macaws (Kaytee Products, Chilton, Wisc), mixed at 28% solids, is equally effective and can be fed through a stainless steel crop tube. The capacious crop can accommodate up to 70 to 100 mL comfortably in most adult birds. Twice-daily feeds are given initially and the evening feed is gradually reduced to encourage normal nocturnal self-feeding on a variety of native browse supplemented with apples *(Malus domesticus)*, kumara (sweet potato, *Ipomoea batatas*), and carrots *(Daucus carota* subsp. *sativus)*. To minimize fecal contamination, food can be provided in hoppers placed at the bird's head height. These are used to supplement free-living birds who readily learn to lift the lid that excludes other wild birds. Similarly, young birds readily learn to drink from up-turned sipper bottles with metal tubes that provide controlled water flow.[29] For adults, water is supplied in a shallow dish or an up-turned water hopper, as used for poultry.[22] It is important for this solitary cryptic species that they be provided with a quiet environment that provides opportunities to hide under large, up-turned leafy branches of nontoxic native plants, which also provide the birds with climbing, roosting, and chewing opportunities (Fig. 40-1). Kakapo do not tolerate prolonged environmental temperatures above 25° C (77° F).

Because the aim of hospitalization is to rehabilitate sick or injured kakapo for return to the wild, strict hygiene and quarantine barrier techniques must be used to minimize risk of nosocomial infections being inadvertently transferred to the wild population. On admission, it is standard practice to run a full health screen comprised of a physical examination (including body weight and examination for ectoparasites), complete blood count, avian biochemistry panel, polymerase chain reaction (PCR) assay for psittacine circovirus (PBFD), immunoassay for *Chlamydophila*, fecal wet preparation and flotation for gastrointestinal parasites, and whole-body lateral and ventrodorsal radiographs.

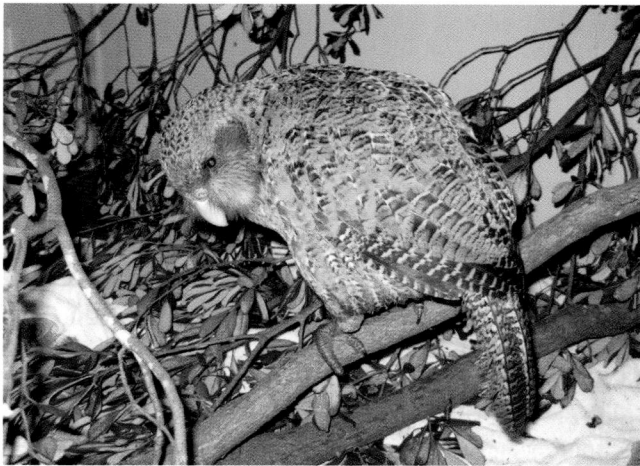

Figure 40-1

Hospitalized kakapo. *(Courtesy Auckland Zoo, Western Springs, New Zealand.)*

The PBFD test is repeated just prior to discharge. The captive care of juvenile birds has been described in detail by Eason and Moorhouse.[14]

RESTRAINT

Physical

Kakapo differ in their response to handling depending on whether they are hand-raised or parent-reared. However, all kakapo are subject to regular capture and examination. For some hand-raised birds only minimal physical restraint need be applied for handling and examination while others can struggle more than parent-reared kakapo. For the more resistant birds, standard practice for restraint of large parrots can be applied. The birds have a large, strong bill, sharp claws, and strong feet. Consequently the head is secured first in one hand by grasping around the back of the head and onto both mandibles which allows complete control of the head. The bird can then be allowed to stand for examination or with the legs supported. A light towel may be wrapped around the bird to aid in restraint. Generally, physical restraint is sufficiently well tolerated to enable physical examination, the collection of diagnostic samples such as blood, crop washes, cloacal swabs and feathers, and the administration of medications.

There are some peculiarities of the physical examination of kakapo compared to other parrots. The pectoral musculature cannot be used to reliably condition score the birds due to the very shallow keel, and use of the epaxial muscles of the spine and muscles over the pelvis and thighs is recommended instead. During the breeding season, the cervicocephalic air sacs of the male are inflated for booming and care must be taken to avoid damage to this area. The wings are functional but have little power.

Reference ranges for hematology and serum biochemical analysis have been published for wild kakapo.[6,18] For venous access, the medial metatarsal, brachial, and jugular veins have all been used successfully. Microscopic examination of crop washes and fecal smears also differs from other parrots in that kakapo have mixed gram-positive and gram-negative gastrointestinal flora, low numbers of budding yeasts *(Candida famata, C. guilleamondi)*, and flagellated protozoa, similar in morphology to *Trichomonas* spp,. are commonly seen in samples from healthy wild birds.

Chemical

We have only used inhalation of isoflurane in oxygen to induce and maintain anesthesia in kakapo. Butorphanol, 1 to 4 mg/kg slow IV, has been used intraoperatively, which appears to have an isoflurane-sparing effect. General anesthesia using isoflurane has been successfully carried out in the field with adults and in veterinary hospitals in both chicks and adults. As with other parrots, uncuffed endotracheal tubes are recommended to prevent mucosal irritation. Complications of anesthesia, including regurgitation, hypoventilation, hypothermia, hypotension, and cardiac arrhythmias, have been encountered and should be minimized with preoperative fasting, intraoperative fluid therapy, thermal support, and minimizing the concentration of anesthetic used. Standard anesthetic monitoring devices such as Doppler blood pressure monitors, capnography, pulse oximetry, and electrocardiography should be used. Pulse oximetry probes have been successfully used on the upper bill and ventral elbow of kakapo.[8]

Analgesics used in kakapo include butorphanol, 1 to 4 mg/kg IV or IM, and meloxicam, 0.2 mg/kg PO SID. No pharmacokinetic studies exist to support this use, although our clinical experience suggests that they are effective.

DIAGNOSTIC IMAGING

Diagnostic imaging modalities that have been applied to kakapo include radiography, ultrasonography, laparoscopy, and computed tomography (CT). Ultrasonography and echocardiography have been carried out with the kakapo conscious but all other modalities require general anesthesia to obtain images of acceptable diagnostic value. Standard techniques were used for these modalities and normal examples of radiographs and CT scans from healthy kakapo are illustrated in Figures 40-2 and 40-3. Imaging anatomy mirrors the anatomic peculiarity of the species with the large pendulous crop, minimal keel and pectoral muscles, and a strong appendicular skeleton (see Fig. 40-2). The lungs of kakapo

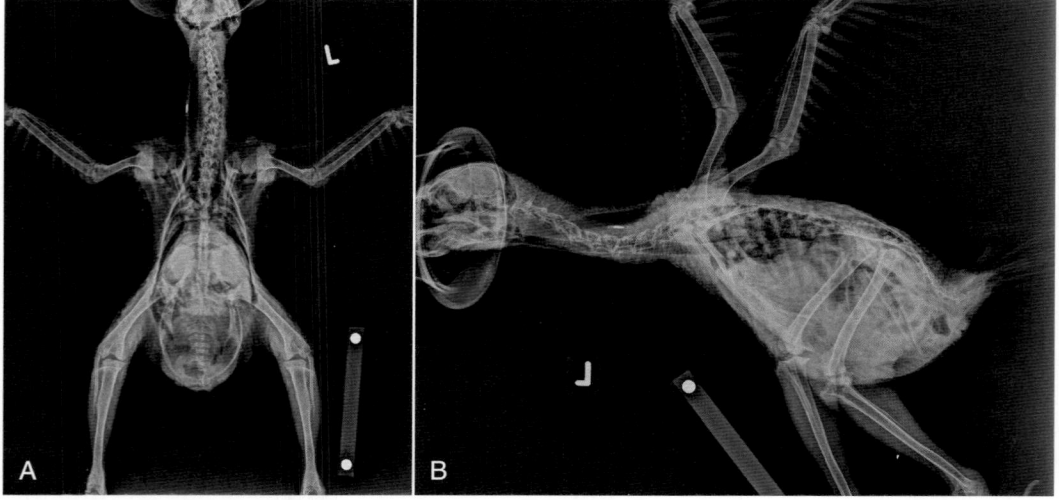

Figure 40-2

Radiographic anatomy of a juvenile male kakapo in lateral and ventrodorsal positioning. *(Courtesy Massey University, Palmerston North, New Zealand.)*

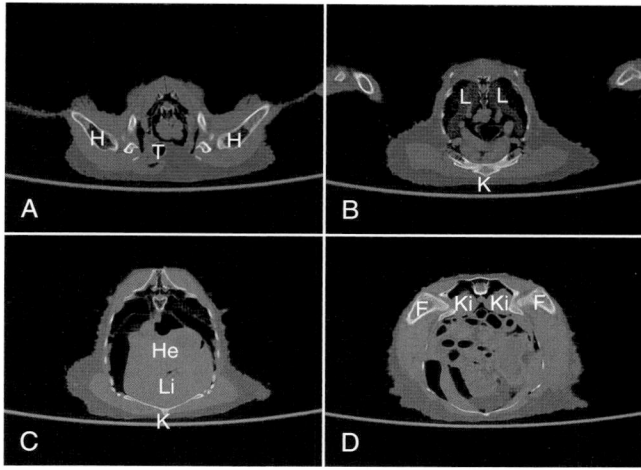

Figure 40-3

CT scans of a juvenile male kakapo showing cross-sectional anatomy of the thoracic inlet (**A**), lungs (**B**), heart and liver at the caudal extent of the lungs (**C**), and pelvis (**D**). *F,* Femurs; *H,* pneumatic humerus; *He,* heart; *K,* keel; *Ki,* kidneys; *L,* lungs; *Li,* liver; *T,* trachea. *(Courtesy Massey University, Palmerston North, New Zealand.)*

differ from those of other parrots on CT in that there appears to be a network of large parabronchi close to the ribs, but the significance of this finding is uncertain (see Fig. 40-3).

DISEASES

Diseases Associated With Incubation and Hand Rearing

Kakapo females are diligent and dedicated mothers but, because of the small size of the remaining population, slow natural breeding cycle, and frequency with which natural rimu fruit crops fail to ripen, all birds and nests are closely monitored to maximize chick survival. Closed-circuit cameras in each nesting burrow and daily examination and weighing of chicks enable rapid identification of problems and appropriate interventions. This hands-on management technique has played a critical role in the successful conservation management of this species to date; details of the methodology have been well described by Eason and Moorhouse.[14]

Incubation

The chilling of eggs that inadvertently rolled out of the nest during the late stages of incubation resulted in late embryonic death associated with acute bacterial egg yolk sacculitis in one chick, and malpositioning

requiring assisted hatching in another. The latter egg was removed for incubation, but the chick died 36 hours post-hatching with omphalitis and aspiration pneumonia.

Neonatal Period: 7 to 10 Days

Because kakapo chicks are only removed for hand rearing following evidence of injury or disease, the bird's health is compromised from the outset.[14] Given this, it is a tribute to the expertise and dedication of their carers that the vast majority are raised to fledging. The first chick hatched in captivity died at 4 days from aspiration pneumonia and enteritis associated with a pure growth of *Klebsiella ozaenae*.[4] Acute, necrotizing, umbilical infection with acute bacterial aspiration pneumonia and a septicemia resulting in peracute multifocal hepatitis were responsible for two other neonatal deaths; another chick died shortly after hatching because of a traumatic injury that ruptured its yolk sac. Three 2- to 4-day-old hand-reared chicks with suspected omphalitis and enteritis recovered following treatment with ciprofloxacin (Ciprofloxacin),10 mg/kg PO twice daily, fluconazole (Diflucan), 2.5 mg/kg PO twice daily, and lactulose (Lactulose), 0.3 mL/kg PO twice daily for 5 days.

Juvenile Prefledging Period

Hand-reared chicks have fledged at 90 to 110 days of age.[14,27] Signs of illness recorded in this age group include, in decreasing order of frequency, crop stasis, slow gut transit time, lethargy, anorexia, poor growth, regurgitation, dyspnea, diarrhea, straining to pass droppings and, rarely, traumatic wounds. Dyspnea, inappetance, and depression following episodes of food regurgitation have resulted in the deaths of some chicks caused by aspiration pneumonia.[24] Gastrointestinal signs have been attributed to the composition and consistency of the hand-rearing formula, the volume, frequency, and temperature of the formula feeds, mycotic (*Candida* spp.) and bacterial infections, and the effects of starvation, dehydration and/or chilling suffered prior to being removed from the nest. Although classic gastrointestinal signs and lesions of clostridial enteritis have not been observed to date, *Clostridium perfringens* is commonly isolated from the feces of hand-raised chicks but not from adults or parent-reared chicks.

In an epidemiologic analysis of illness in seven hand-reared chicks, Potter and McKenzie[24] concluded that a bacterial septicemia was the most likely cause, although no specific pathogen was identified. (In 2009,

Escherichia coli was cultured from the blood of one sick chick and *Enterococcus faecalis* from another; both survived with intensive treatment.[12]) One indicator of this condition was a heterophilic leucocytosis, in which total white blood cells exceeded 40×10^9/liter as compared with a mean of 20.7×10^9/liter for 17 healthy chicks raised in previous years. One chick in this study died following food aspiration in its weakened state but also had the histopathologic features of an interstitial pneumonia. The cause of this lesion was not established. The other six birds recovered within a 2-week period following combined antimicrobial (amoxicillin-clavulonic acid) and antifungal (itraconazole) treatment. Actions taken to prevent and/or mitigate these adverse events have included modification of the hand-rearing formula to resemble the high-fiber diet of wild-reared chicks more closely, use of prepathogen screened adult feces to inoculate chicks with the birds' natural gut flora, comprehensive documentation and charting of chick behavior, growth, and development, strict consistency in feeding practices, strict nursery hygiene, and the isolation of sick from healthy chicks.[14]

Infectious Diseases of Adult Kakapo

Erysipelas

Infection in animals with the bacteria *Erysipelothrix rhusiopathiae* is known as erysipelas.[7] Erysipelas in birds is characterized by acute fulminating infections or, more rarely, by chronic infections causing infertility in male birds and reduced egg production in females. Three juvenile kakapo from a group of 19 translocated birds died within 72 hours of transport between New Zealand off shore islands. Clinical findings, gross necropsy changes, cytology, histopathology, and bacterial culture confirmed systemic disease caused by *E. rhusiopathiae*. On the island from which the kakapo were sourced, positive cultures of *E. rhusiopathiae* were obtained from the medulla of the ulna from 10 of 15 seabird carcasses examined. These were found to be the same genotype as the bacteria isolated from the kakapo, confirming the seabirds as a reservoir of infection for the parrots. Immediately after the diagnosis, all 16 remaining translocated birds were recaptured and treated with antibiotics. Vaccination with a commercial killed bacterin for turkeys was initially instigated for all kakapo, with the exception of six adult males, followed by boosters at 1 and 12 to 16 months.[1,15]

An erysipelas antibody enzyme-linked immunosorbent assay (ELISA) was developed and serum was collected at the time of vaccination to detect naturally occurring exposure. Preliminary results have indicated that, at the time of sampling, serum antibodies were present in most adult birds.[22] Vaccination is currently used only with nestlings and hand-reared chicks. Despite the evidence of continued exposure of kakapo to the bacteria in the island environments, regular vaccination of adults was discontinued, partly because of a concern over a reported low incidence of endocarditis in vaccinated turkeys[7] and the development in approximately 50% of birds of a pea-sized granuloma at the injection site, which erupted from the skin after 2 years.

Parasites and Parasitic Diseases

Protozoal Cloacitis

Small motile protozoa have been found associated with firmly adherent caseous necrotic plaques in the cloacal proctodeum of two birds younger than 5 years. These were accompanied by hyperemia of the cloacal mucosa and ulcerative wounds at the mucocutaneous junction of the vent. Although both birds had lost weight, they were bright and active on presentation. One of us (RJH) has speculated that the ulcerative lesions were initiated by self-inflicted trauma in an attempt to relieve irritation from the parasitic infection, and these wounds became secondarily infected by gut flora. Both birds responded to treatment with metronidazole (Trichozole,), 20 mg/kg PO twice daily for 5 to 8 days, combined with supportive topical and antimicrobial treatment for secondary infection. Carnidazole (Spartrix), 20 mg/kg PO, repeated twice at 10-day intervals, was successful in treating a mild cases of cloacal trichomoniasis detected in an older male during semen collection.[4] These protozoal organisms have yet to be formally identified, but they have two paired flagellae and are motile and similar in appearance to *Trichomonas* spp. These protozoa have also been observed in low numbers in the feces of clinically healthy wild kakapo and may be part of normal gut flora.

Coccidia

No clinical cases of coccidiosis have been recorded to date, but coccidian oocysts are identified in feces occasionally, and some have recently been identified as an *Eimeria* spp.[20]

Hemoparasites

None were found by light microscopic examination of thin blood smears in 207 samples recorded in the National Wildlife Health database.

Helminths

The only gastrointestinal helminths recorded in kakapo to date are the species-specific cestode, *Stringopotaenia psittacea*,[21] and a *Capillaria* spp. nematode.[20] No clinical disease associated with endoparasitism has been recorded to date.

Ectoparasites

Feather lice are frequently seen in low numbers.[12] *Heteromenopon kea* was identified from one bird on Pearl Island. The feather mites *Megninia androgynes*, *Mesalges lyurus*, and *Protalges psittacinus* and the flea *Parapsyllus nestoris nestoris* have been recorded occasionally.[3] One juvenile bird on Codfish Island has been found on three occasions with a single immature tick attached to an eyelid, and tentatively identified as *Ixodes pterodromae*.[12]

Noninfectious Diseases

Aflatoxicosis

An adult male kakapo was found dead in the wild, with no prior signs of illness. Gross postmortem examination revealed a firm, massively enlarged, rounded liver, with multifocal to coalescing cream lesions throughout the parenchyma. Histopathologic examination showed a severe inflammation and necrosis, with an irregular multifocal to coalescing distribution. Mycotoxin analysis on the crop contents revealed an extremely high level of aflatoxins. Analysis of supplementary food offered to the kakapo at feed stations showed that high levels of aflatoxins were present in the walnuts offered and trace levels were found in almonds and old food from the hoppers in the bush. Based on these findings, regular screening of supplemented foods for aflatoxins was implemented and the hygiene of feed stations was improved.[2] Nuts, in combination with honey water, had been the only supplementary foods on which kakapo were able to rear their own chicks without ripe rimu fruit. However, in the 2009 breeding season, Harrison's high-potency coarse pellets were used by six birds to feed their young.[12]

Heavy Metal Toxicosis

In September 2008, a male kakapo, probably older than 30 years, was found to be weak and in emaciated body condition, having lost 41% of his body weight in the 4 months following translocation from Codfish Island to Anchor Island. Additional clinical findings following transfer to a veterinary hospital were mild depression (but no other neurologic abnormalities), moderate numbers of *Capillaria* spp. ova in feces, and a blood lead level of 0.62 mg/liter. No evidence of heavy metal ingestion was found on whole body radiographs, and hematology and biochemical parameters were within normal limits. A blood lead concentration higher than 0. 2 mg/liter is considered abnormal[26] and higher than 0.5 mg/liter is considered diagnostic of lead toxicity.[17] Consequently, chelation therapy with calcium disodium versenate (CaEDTA) at 50 mg/kg SC twice daily for 5 days was instituted in conjunction with nutritional and oral fluid support and preventive antimicrobial therapy (amoxicillin-clavulonate [Clavulox], 125 mg/kg PO twice daily for 5 days) and antifungal therapy (itraconazole [Sporanox], 5 mg/kg PO twice daily). Lead levels decreased to 0.021 mg/liter 2 weeks post-treatment and remained at this level 1 month after presentation. An elevation in the serum uric acid level from 63 mmol/liter on day 7 to 444 mmol/liter on day 14 raised concern about possible nephrotoxicity associated with the chelating agent, but this parameter returned to within normal limits 2 weeks later.[18] Although insufficient blood was collected initially to test for zinc exposure at the time of admission, testing following chelation therapy revealed a serum zinc level of 20.8 µmol/liter. A serum concentration above 30 µmol/liter is considered diagnostic of zinc toxicity by a number of authors,[17,26] although ranges of 7.65 to 84 µmol/liter have been recorded in psittacines.[19] The bird's initial concentration is likely to have been depressed by chelation therapy, because retesting 4 weeks later found a concentration of 50 µmol/liter. Although food had been provided in a galvanized dish, there was no evidence of chewing and no other source of zinc that could have contributed to this level in the hospital environment. A course of chelation therapy with dimercaptosuccinic acid (DMSA, Captomer), 30 mg/kg PO twice daily for 10 days, reduced the serum zinc level to 37.2 µmol/liter. After a 2-month period, the bird was vigorous and had regained 53% of his initial weight loss. Tragically, a crop rupture occurred on the day prior to his planned discharge and he died during surgery.

A survey by DOC staff to ascertain lead and zinc exposure of other kakapo resident on Codfish and Anchor islands ($N = 23$) found a mean blood lead concentration of 0.0426 mg/liter and a range of 0.0207 to 0.1500 mg/liter,[23] well within the acceptable range for other bird species.[28] The mean serum zinc level in free-ranging kakapo, however, was 34.8 µmol/liter, with a range of 20.6 to 59.2 µmol/liter. Extensive searching on both islands found the most likely source to be wire mesh used on pens, and this bird had been seen clinging to the mesh of a pen in which he had been temporarily accommodated. Testing of this mesh revealed that it contained 1.1 g/m³ lead and 3100 g/m³ zinc, making it the most likely candidate for the source of lead; the two other types of wire mesh on the islands used to cover boardwalks had similar zinc content, but contained just 0.42 and less than 0.0021 g/m³ lead, respectively.

TRAUMA

Traumatic Cloacitis

A mature female kakapo presented with necrotic ulcerative lesions of the cloacal proctodeum, covered in caseous exudate and associated with mucosal erythema and pain on palpation. No trichomonads were detected at the time of presentation (see earlier) but a heavy growth of *E. coli* and moderate growth of *Enterococcus* spp. were cultured from the lesions. A heterophilic leucocytosis (white blood cells, 38.6 × 10⁹/liter, 86% heterophils) with toxic heterophils were consistent with active infection. The lesions healed and the bird fully recovered over a 26-day period, during which she received systemic antimicrobial therapy—initially, cefaclor (Cefaclor), 25 mg/kg PO twice daily, followed by amoxicillin-clavulonic acid, 125 mg/kg PO twice daily, and prophylactic antifungal therapy (nystatin [Nilstat Oral Drops]), 120,000 IU/kg PO twice daily. Meloxicam (Metacam) at an initial dose of 0.35 mg/kg followed by 0.17 mg/kg PO SID, was provided for pain relief for the first 2 weeks.[16]

A 2-year-old female kakapo developed exudative dermatitis of the vent that was unresponsive to conservative treatment (Fig. 40-4). The vent was surgically débrided, but the dermatitis recurred multiple times over a 177-day period. Diagnostic testing including biopsies, culture of wounds and feces, hematology, and biochemistry, and psittacine circovirus PCR assay failed to detect any underlying cause of disease. Multiple attempts at surgical débridement and combination treatment with a range of topical and oral medications were eventually successful in resolving the dermatitis.

Both these birds fully recovered and laid fertile eggs in the subsequent breeding season.

Traumatic injuries have been observed in a number of other kakapo. Causes have included misadventure—although flightless, kakapo are nevertheless capable of moving at some speed and may crash down gullies and into thick shrubbery or fall out of trees, particularly fledging chicks, providing plenty of opportunities for self-harm—territorial fighting between males, and

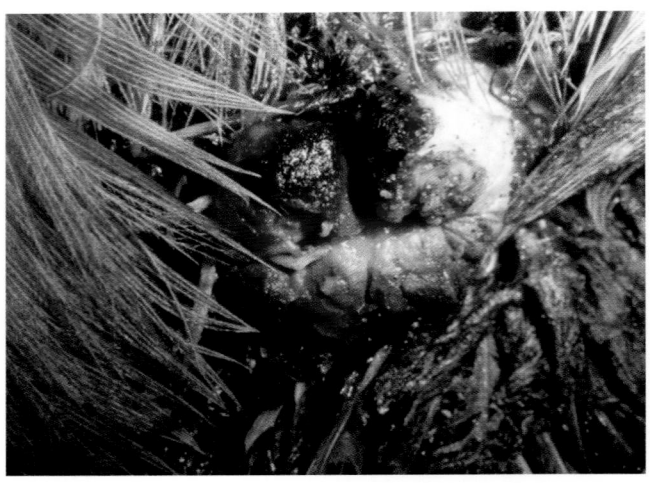

Figure 40-4

Severe exudative dermatitis and fissuring of the vent in a subadult female kakapo. (*Courtesy Massey University, Palmerston North, New Zealand.*)

injuries to chicks in the nest inflicted by resident subadult males.[22] Two birds have also suffered deep constriction wounds from transmitter harnesses that became overly tight.[5] One bird suffered a coxofemoral dislocation that was reduced while the bird was being positioned for radiography under general anesthesia. The dislocation did not recur.

Ocular Lesions

Bilateral cataracts have been observed in at least two male kakapo and, given the probable extreme age of the two birds, are likely to reflect a normal degenerative process. One of these birds also developed chronic keratitis, possibly of traumatic origin resulting from misadventure associated with decreased vision.

Acknowledgments

We are indebted to the many people who have documented their research on this unique bird over the years. In particular, we want to thank Daryl Eason and Ron Moorhouse of the Department of Conservation Kakapo Team, who have freely shared their knowledge and experience with us and, in many cases, made available unpublished information for inclusion in this chapter. They, along with John Potter, Kate McInnes, and Deidre Vercoe, have provided valuable comment on the manuscript. The following also provided assistance with specific topics: Maurice Alley (pathology), Meg Curnick (heavy metal toxicosis), Kerri Morgan (clinical expertise, aflatoxicosis), and Nicola Smith (anesthesia).

REFERENCES

1. Alley MR, Gartrell BD, Mack HJ, et al: *Erysipelothrix rhusiopathiae* septicaemia in translocated kakapo *(Strigops habroptilus)*. N Z Vet J 53(1):94, 2004.
2. Alley M, Gartrell B, Morgan K: Aflatoxicosis in a kakapo, *Strigops habroptilus*. Kokako 12:29, 2005.
3. Bishop DM, Heath, ACG: Checklist of ectoparasites of birds in New Zealand. Surveillance 25:13–31, 1998.
4. Blanco J: Personal communication, 2009.
5. Boardman WSJ: Auckland Zoo's veterinary involvement in the kakapo recovery program. Proc Am Assoc Zoo Vet 175–180, 1993.
6. Boardman WSJ, Boyd S, Smits B: Clinical pathology baseline normal data for the kakapo *(Strigops habroptilus)*. Kokako 2:12–13, 1995.
7. Bricker J, Saif Y: Erysipelas. In Calnek BW, editor: Diseases of poultry, Ames, Iowa, 1997, Mosby-Wolfe, pp 302–313.
8. Butler DJ: The habitat, food and feeding ecology of kakapo in Fiordland: A synopsis from the unpublished MSc thesis of Richard Gray. Notornis 53:5–9, 2006.
9. Clout MN: A celebration of kakapo: Progress in the conservation of an enigmatic parrot. Notornis 53:1–2, 2006.
10. Cottam Y, Merton DV, Hendricks W: Nutrient composition of the diet of parent-raised kakapo nestlings. Notornis 53:90–99, 2006.
11. Department of Conservation: Kakapo recovery programme 2006-2016, 2008 (http://www.riotinto.com/documents/Kakapo_Brochure_2_0_NZAS_.pdf).
12. Eason D: Personal communication, 2010.
13. Eason D, Elliot GP, Merton DV, et al: Breeding biology of kakapo *(Strigops habroptilus)* on offshore island sanctuaries, 1990-2002. Notornis 53:27–36, 2006.
14. Eason D, Moorhouse RJ: Hand-rearing kakapo *(Strigops habroptilus)*, 1997-2005. Notornis 53:116–125, 2006.
15. Gartrell BD, Alley MR, Mack H, et al: Erysipelas in the critically endangered Kakapo *(Strigops habroptilus)*. Avian Pathol 34:383–387, 2005.
16. Jakob-Hoff R, Potter JS, Shaw SD, et al: Traumatic cloacitis in a kakapo, *Strigops habroptilus*. Kokako 16:1–53, 2009.
17. LaBonde J: Toxic disorders. In Rosskopf WJ, Woerpel RW, editors: Diseases of cage and aviary birds, ed 3, Baltimore, 1996, Lea & Febiger, pp 514–519.
18. Lowe M, Eason D, McInnes K, Paul-Murphy J: Haematological and biochemical reference ranges for the kakapo *(Strigops habroptilus)*: generation and interpretation in a field-based wildlife recovery program. J Avian Med Surg 20:80–88, 2006.
19. McDonald D: Nutritional considerations. Section I: Nutrition and dietary supplementation. In Harrison GJ, Lightfoot TL, editors: Clinical avian medicine, vol 1, Palm Beach, Fla, 2006, Spix, pp 83–140.
20. McKenna P: Personal communication, 2010.
21. McKenna PB: Special issue: parasites of birds in New Zealand: checklist of helminth and protozoan parasites—Part II: Parasite list by parasite. Surveillance 25:10–12, 1998.
22. McInnes K: Personal communication, 2010.
23. Moorhouse RJ: Personal communication, 2010.
24. Potter J, McKenzie J: Report on kakapo chick illness in 2008. (Unpublished report to the New Zealand Department of Conservation, November 3, 2008.)
25. Powlesland RG, Merton DV, Cockrem JF: A parrot apart: The natural history of the kakapo *(Strigops habroptilus)*, and the context of its conservation management. Notornis 53:3–26, 2006.
26. Richardson JA: Implications of toxic substances in clinical disorders. In Harrison GJ, Lightfoot TL, editors: Clinical avian medicine, vol 2, Palm Beach, Fla, 2006, Spix, pp 711–719.
27. Sibley MD: First hand-rearing of kakapo *(Strigops habroptilus)* at the Auckland Zoological Park. Int Zoo Yb 33:181–194, 1994.
28. Sigurdson CJ, Franson JC: Avian toxicological diagnosis. In Fudge AM, editor: Laboratory medicine: Avian and exotic pets, Philadelphia, 2000, WB Saunders, pp 174–184.
29. Westera B: Personal communication, 2009.
30. Wilson DH, Grant AD, Parker N: Diet of kakapo in breeding and non-breeding years on Codfish island (Whenua Hau) and Stewart Island. Notornis 53:80–89, 2006.

CHAPTER 41

Avian Analgesia

Joanne Paul-Murphy and Michelle G. Hawkins

RECOGNIZING PAIN IN BIRDS

All vertebrate animals share similar neuroanatomic and neuropharmacologic components required for nociception—detection, transmission, and response to noxious stimuli. Pain is the sensory and emotional experience associated with actual or potential tissue damage. Pain affects the animal's physiology and behavior to reduce or avoid the injury and minimize the likelihood of recurrence. Assessment of pain must give consideration to species, gender, age, strain, environment, and concurrent disease as well as the type of pain, such as acute, chronic, somatic, visceral, clinical, or neuropathic. Species variability occurs because of differences in pain sensitivity, the conscious response to pain, and the physiologic response to analgesic therapy. Pain is subjective and, in humans, we accept that pain is what the patient says it is but, with birds, people's perceptions of the bird's behavior determine what is recognized as pain.

Behavioral changes may be very cryptic and subtle, but are often the earliest signs of pain detected by animal care staff or owners. Behavioral changes are often species-specific, and observers must be familiar with the full range of normal behaviors for the species as well as the individual. It is important to observe birds at appropriate times for each species, such as observing nocturnal species at night. Certain behaviors have evolved and have survival value; for example, immobility is a common behavior displayed by birds when being observed or examined, making pain evaluation challenging. In chickens, immobility has also been associated with prolonged pain, stress, and fear responses. Feather grooming is an avian behavior that may express the full spectrum of change associated with pain, both acute and chronic. Grooming activity may decrease when a bird is in pain or, conversely, overgrooming and feather destructive behaviors have been associated with chronic pain. In a social species housed with a group, a painful bird frequently isolates itself and may sleep apart from the rest of the flock, and mutual grooming is often decreased. In some species, a display of discomfort, illness, or weakness may gain support or protection from conspecifics, but similar behavior in another species may attract attention from predators or lower its status in the flock's social order. Increased grooming activities to themselves or other birds may also be an intentional distraction. Studies using chickens with experimental arthritis have demonstrated that shifting attention may reduce painful behaviors and potentially reduce peripheral inflammation.[9]

Treating avian pain is limited by the reliability of pain assessment, which remains highly subjective, and clinicians often need to rely on indirect measures of pain. Identifying a behavior or set of behaviors that correlate with pain provides a basis to monitor analgesia therapy. Pain scales and score sheets are tools that are increasingly being used to assess pain in animals, especially when specifically designed for a given species under well-defined conditions. Pain score sheets may help maximize the efficacy of pain scoring and score sheet descriptions of behavior must be refined, including clearly defined terms to reduce observer bias and interobserver variability. Once such a system is implemented, scoring may be performed by well-trained non–veterinary staff.

Pain occurs along a gradient and, in lieu of species-specific pain score sheets for birds, there is tremendous value in using a generic pain scale of 1 to 10 to evaluate a bird's pain and response to treatment. In one study, pigeons following orthopedic surgery were evaluated using a detailed numeric rating scale plus a simple 1 to 10 pain scale, and there was significant correlation between both methods.[23]

Effective analgesia is expected to show a marked, easily discernible change in posture or behaviors that will effect a reliable change in the subjective pain score. If no change in pain score occurs, then the drugs, dosage, or frequency of administration need to be reevaluated for that individual patient.

EVALUATION OF ANALGESICS

To determine the efficacy of an analgesic in any species, it is important to determine the pharmacokinetics (PK) and pharmacodynamics (PD) of the drug in that species. Integrating PK and PD data provides a basis for selecting clinically relevant dosing schedules. When the same dose produces different plasma concentrations in different species of birds, the variance is caused by PK. When the same plasma concentration produces different responses in different species, the variance is caused by PD. PK studies of analgesic drugs are insufficient to determine appropriate doses and dosing frequencies because plasma concentrations of opioids and nonsteroidal anti-inflammatory drugs (NSAIDs) do not always correlate with delivery of analgesia. Plasma concentrations provide guidance for dosing frequencies, but it has been shown that the duration of the analgesic effect of NSAIDs may be longer than that predicted from plasma levels. The PK of analgesics varies considerably across all species that have been studied, so extrapolating clinical doses and dosing intervals from one species to another species is not appropriate. To date, very few PK studies have been published for analgesics in birds (Tables 41-1 and 41-2).

Anesthetic-sparing studies provide an in vivo PD technique for objective evaluation by measuring the minimum anesthetic dose (MAD) necessary to provide anesthesia following administration of an analgesic. This type of testing has been used in many species to evaluate analgesic drug properties, particularly opioids. Although this approach provides meaningful information, there are limitations because the anesthetic itself may be a confounding variable and, when evaluating opioids, it is difficult to assess whether an observed effect is an analgesic or a sedative response to the drug.

Inflammatory models are used to create painful conditions with repeatable behaviors or weight bearing that may be quantified, such as acute synovitis-arthritis models in chickens and parrots.[12] In one model, the injection of urate microcrystals into the intertarsal joint caused acute inflammatory arthritis, leading to measurable changes in weight bearing and lameness. A study with Hispaniolan Amazon parrots *(Amazonia ventralis)* differentiated significant weight-bearing improvement when birds were given butorphanol versus less improvement in the same birds given carprofen.[26] Evaluating the response of a bird to a noxious stimulus with and without analgesics is used to determine efficacy when thresholds may be measured. The noxious stimuli used in avian analgesia studies are variable, but usually include withdrawal thresholds to thermal, electrical, or pressure stimuli. Experimental models have been developed in chickens and parrots, but these models may not extrapolate to pain behaviors relevant to clinical pain. Therefore, the doses and dosing frequencies recommended in the published reports should always be critically evaluated on a case by case basis.

Preemptive Analgesia

Recent evidence has suggested that surgical incisions and other painful procedures in humans may induce prolonged central nervous system (CNS) changes that later contribute to postoperative pain. This noxious stimulus–induced sensitization may be prevented or "preempted" by the administration of analgesic agents prior to tissue injury. Preemptive analgesia with opiates, NSAIDs, or local anesthetics may block sensory noxious stimuli from onward transmission to the CNS, thus reducing the overall potential for pain and inflammation and potentially improving the patient's short-term and long-term recovery.

Opioids

Opioids are used for moderate to severe pain, such as traumatic or surgical pain. Opioids reversibly bind to specific receptors in the central and peripheral nervous system. These drugs are categorized as agonists, partial agonists, mixed agonists-antagonists, or antagonists based on their ability to induce an analgesic response once bound to a specific receptor. The agonist drugs have a linear dose-response curve that may be titrated to reach the desired effect, whereas the agonist-antagonist drugs may reach a ceiling effect, after which increasing the dose does not appear to provide additional analgesia. During anesthesia, opioids are used to provide perioperative analgesia that may reduce the concentrations of volatile anesthetics (e.g., gas anesthesia–sparing effects). The most common adverse effects reported with opioids are cardiac and/or respiratory depression. In many cases, these drugs may be reversed with antagonists, which will also terminate analgesia. The application and dosages of several opioid

TABLE 41-1   Opioid Analgesics Evaluated in Avian Species by Pharmacokinetic (PK) or Pharmacodynamic (PD) Studies

Study (Year)	Drug	Dosage (mg/kg)	Route	Frequency (per hr)	Species	Comments	Type of Study
Riggs et al 2008[28]	Butorphanol	0.5	IM, IV (median ulnar vein; medial metatarsal vein)	Single injection	Red-tailed hawks; great horned owls	$t_{1/2}$ IV, IM very short (≈1-2 hr); significantly more rapid clearance and shorter $t_{1/2}$ when given IV medial metatarsal than IV median ulnar vein	PK
Paul-Murphy (2010)[23a]	Butorphanol	5	PO	Single dose	Hispaniolan Amazon parrots	Oral bioavailability <10%; do not recommend this route of administration	PK
Sladky et al (2006)[30]	Butorphanol	2-5	IM	Single injection	Hispaniolan Amazon parrots	PK: Low mean plasma concentrations at 2 hr after injection PD: Withdrawal thresholds to electrical stimuli reduced after 2 mg/kg IM	PK, PD
Curro et al (1994)[5,6]	Butorphanol	1	IM	Single injection	Cockatoos; African grey parrots, blue-fronted Amazon parrots	Isoflurane-sparing study showed significant reduction in isoflurane MAD in cockatoos and African greys, but not Amazon parrots	PD
Paul-Murphy et al (1999)[24]	Butorphanol	1-2	IM	Single injection	African grey parrots	Electrical stimuli to assess withdrawal thresholds: More significant reduction of withdrawal response at 2 mg/kg	PD
Klaphake et al (2006)[14]	Butorphanol	2	IM	Single injection	Hispaniolan Amazon parrots	Safe and effective preemptive analgesia with sevoflurane anesthesia for endoscopy	PD

TABLE 41-1	Opioid Analgesics Evaluated in Avian Species by Pharmacokinetic (PK) or Pharmacodynamic (PD) Studies—cont'd						
Study (Year)	Drug	Dosage (mg/kg)	Route	Frequency (per hr)	Species	Comments	Type of Study
Hoppes et al (2003)[13]	Fentanyl	0.02 0.2	IM SC	Single injection	Cockatoos	PK: Rapid absorption and elimination PD: Withdrawal thresholds to electrical and thermal stimuli; 0.02 mg/kg did not affect either threshold; 0.2 mg/kg affected both withdrawal thresholds but only some birds; hyperactivity in first 15-30 min	PK, PD
Hawkins (2010)[11]	Fentanyl	Targeted controlled infusions	IV	Constant rate infusion	Red-tailed hawks	Reduced isoflurane MAD 31% to 55% in dose-related manner, without significant effects on heart rate, blood pressure, $Paco_2$, or Pao_2	PD
Paul-Murphy et al (1999, 2004)[24,25]	Buprenorphine	0.1	IM	Single injection	African grey parrots	PK: May not achieve effective plasma concentrations at this dose PD: No change in withdrawal response to noxious stimuli	PK, PD
Gaggermeier et al (2003)[8]	Buprenorphine	0.25 0.5	IM	Single injection	Domestic pigeons	Increased latency period for withdrawal from a noxious electrical stimulus of 2 hr at 0.25 mg/kg and for 5 hr for 0.5 mg/kg	PD
Paul-Murphy (2010)[23b]	Nalbuphine	12.5, 25, 50	IM	Single injection	Hispaniolan Amazon parrots	PK: $t_{1/2}$ IM and IV less than 0.35 hr Excellent IM bioavailability PD: 12.5 mg/kg produced 3-hr analgesia; higher doses, no increase in analgesic duration	PD

$t_{1/2}$, Half-life.

TABLE 41-2 Nonsteroidal Anti-Inflammatory Drugs Evaluated in Avian Species by Pharmacokinetic (PK) or Pharmacodynamic (PD) Evaluations, or Toxicologic (TOX) or Clinical Studies

Study (Year)	Drug	Dosage (mg/kg)	Route	Frequency (per hr)	Species	Comments	Type of Study
Hocking et al (2005)[12]	Sodium salicylate	100-200	IM	Single injection	Chickens	Arthritis painful behaviors partially reduced 1 hr after acetylsalicylic acid treatment	PD
Baert and De Backer (2003)[1]	Sodium salicylate	25	IV	Single injection	Chickens, ostriches, ducks, turkeys, pigeons	Rapid clearance except long $t_{1/2}$ in pigeon	PK
Hocking et al (2005)[12]	Carprofen	30	IM	Single injection	Chickens	Arthritis painful behaviors reduced 1 hr after treatment	PD
Paul-Murphy et al (2009)[26]	Carprofen	3	IM	12	Hispaniolan Amazon parrots	Arthritis pain partially reduced, effect less than 12 hr	PD
McGeowen et al (1999)[18]	Carprofen	1	IM	Single injection	Chickens	Improved locomotion of lame birds 1 hr after treatment	PD
Machin et al (2001)[17]	Flunixin meglumide	5.0	IM	Single injection	Mallard ducks	12-hr activity but muscle necrosis at injection site	PD
Pereira and Werther (2007)[27]	Flunixin meglumide	5.5	IM	24 for 7 days	Budgerigars	Severe renal lesions	TOX
Baert and De Backer (2003)[1]	Flunixin meglumide	1.1	IV	Single injection	Chickens, ostriches, ducks, turkeys, pigeons	Chickens had long half-life but 10 min $t_{1/2}$ in ostriches	PK
Hocking et al (2005)[12]	Flunixin meglumide	3	IM	Single injection	Chickens	Arthritis painful behaviors reduced 1 hr after treatment	PD
Graham et al (2005)[10]	Ketoprofen	2.0	IV, IM, PO	Single injection	Quail	Low bioavailability IM, PO; short IV $t_{1/2}$	PK
Hocking et al (2005)[12]	Ketoprofen	12	IM	Single injection	Chickens	Arthritis painful behaviors reduced 1 hr after treatment	PD
Pereira and Werther (2007)[27]	Ketoprofen	2.5	IM	24 for 7 days	Budgerigars	Tubular necrosis	TOX
Machin et al (2001)[17]	Ketoprofen	5	IM	Single injection	Mallard ducks	12-hr activity	PD
Mulcahy et al (2003)[19]	Ketoprofen	2.0 5.0	PO IM, IV	12-24	Eiders	Mortality associated with male eiders	CS
Cole et al (2009)[3]	Meloxicam	1	IM	12	Hispaniolan Amazon parrots	Improved weight bearing on arthritic limb	PD
Pereira and Werther (2007)[27]	Meloxicam	0.1	IM	24 for 7 days	Budgerigars	Glomerular congestion	TOX
Baert and De Backer (2003)[1]	Meloxicam	0.5	IV	Single injection	Chickens, ostriches, ducks, turkeys, pigeons	Variable distribution, slow clearance except in ostriches	PK
Naidoo et al (2008)[21]	Meloxicam	2	IM, PO	Single treatment	Cape Griffon vultures	Short $t_{1/2}$, less than 45 min	PK
Paul-Murphy (2010)[23]	Piroxicam	0.5-0.8	PO	12	Whooping cranes	Used for acute myopathy and chronic arthritis	CS

CS, *Case series*; TOX, *toxicity*.

formulations have been scientifically evaluated and clinically applied in birds (see Table 41-1).

Most opioid analgesics are used parenterally because of poor oral bioavailability associated with the first-pass effect. Once absorbed, oral opioids first pass through the liver, where they are metabolized, releasing a significantly lower amount of active drug into the general circulation. For example, the bioavailability of 5 mg/kg orally administered butorphanol in Hispaniolan Amazon parrots was lower than 10%, making this route ineffective.[23a]

Opioids vary in their receptor specificity and efficacy in mammals, which results in a wide variety of clinical effects in different species. It is reasonable to presume that this opioid variability will also have a wide range of clinical effects in avian species. The distribution of opiate receptor types is well conserved across all mammalian species in the brainstem and spinal cord, but may vary markedly in the forebrain and midbrain. There is an overall lack of published data concerning differences in opioid receptor distribution, density, and functionality in birds. However, early work showed that the regional distribution of mu, kappa, and delta receptors in the forebrain and midbrain of pigeons were similar to mammals, but 76% of opiate receptors in the forebrain were of the kappa type. Kappa receptors have multiple physiologic functions in the bird and the analgesic function of these receptors still needs further investigation. It has been postulated that this difference in receptor distribution and density may partially explain why some avian species do not appear to respond to mu agonists in the same manner as mammals. However, in day-old chicks, marked dissimilarities to this distribution suggest either age- or species-related differences. It has been postulated that birds may not possess distinct mu and kappa receptors or that the receptors may have similar functions. This may explain in part why the isoflurane-sparing effects of mu and kappa agonists in chickens appear to be similar to those in mammals.[4]

Fentanyl

Fentanyl is a short-acting mu receptor agonist that has not been used commonly in avian medicine because historical investigations with morphine (the standard for mu opioids) administered to chickens were confusing and clinically inconclusive. Fentanyl, 0.02 mg/kg IM, did not affect the withdrawal thresholds to electrical or thermal stimuli of white cockatoos; a tenfold increase in the dosage (0.2 mg/kg SC) did produce an analgesic response, but many birds were hyperactive for the first 15 to 30 minutes after receiving the high dose.[13]

Fentanyl had rapid absorption and elimination in parrots, with mean residence times of less than 2 hours (see Table 41-1). Because of its short-acting properties, fentanyl delivered via constant rate infusion (CRI) is an excellent choice as an analgesic adjunct to inhalant anesthesia in mammals and, when used at low doses as a CRI, we have found fentanyl may also be effectively used in avian anesthetic protocols. Fentanyl administered as an IV CRI in red-tailed hawks (*Buteo jamaicensis*) to target plasma concentrations of 8 to 32 ng/mL reduced the MAD of isoflurane 31% to 55% in a dose-related manner, without statistically significant effects on heart rate, blood pressure, $PaCO_2$, or PaO_2.[11] Fentanyl may also be combined with ketamine as a CRI, thereby reducing the dosages of each that are needed.

Butorphanol

Butorphanol is a mixed agonist-antagonist with low intrinsic activity at the mu receptor and strong agonist activity at the kappa receptor. Adverse effects associated with butorphanol such as dysphoria have not been reported in birds. Preoperative butorphanol administration (2 mg/kg IM) did not show significant anesthetic (including time to intubation and extubation) or cardiopulmonary changes in Hispaniolan Amazon parrots anesthetized with sevoflurane, suggesting that it may be useful as part of a preemptive analgesic protocol (see Table 41-1).[14] Earlier isoflurane-sparing studies using 1 mg/kg IM butorphanol in cockatoos, African grey parrots (*Psittacus erithacus erithacus*), and blue-fronted Amazon parrots (*Amazona aestiva*) showed a significant MAD reduction in the cockatoos and African grey parrots, but not in the blue-fronted Amazon parrots.[5,6] In a study using withdrawal thresholds to electrical stimuli in conscious African grey parrots, butorphanol, 1 to 2 mg/kg showed a decreased withdrawal effect that was more significant at 2 mg/kg.[24] Butorphanol dosages of 3 to 6 mg/kg IM had similar analgesic effects on Hispaniolan Amazon parrots. Based on these studies, dosages of 1 to 4 mg/kg have been suggested in birds. A recent study evaluating the PK of 0.5 mg/kg butorphanol in red-tailed hawks (*Buteo jamaicensis*) and great-horned owls (*Bubo virginianus*) found half-lives of 0.93 and 1.78 hours, respectively, when given IV and 0.94 and 1.84 hours, respectively, when given IM.[28] Similarly, low serum butorphanol concentrations were evident in Hispaniolan Amazon parrots 2 hours after a single IM administration of a 5-mg/kg dose.[30]

These data suggest that frequent dosing of butorphanol may be necessary in birds. This frequency of dosing is, in some cases, impractical because of lack of personnel to provide frequent dosing and the stress of frequent handling on the patient. A liposome-encapsulated, long-acting form of butorphanol tartrate was shown to be safe and effective in Hispaniolan Amazon parrots for up to 5 days following SC administration,[30] and was also shown to be an effective analgesic in Hispaniolan Amazon parrots with induced arthritis (see Table 41-1).[26] The results from these studies are encouraging because a long-acting formulation of butorphanol would allow for both reduced frequency in butorphanol dosing and handling of avian patients for drug administration. Unfortunately, this formulation is not yet commercially available.

Buprenorphine

Buprenorphine is a slow-onset, long-acting opiate with a unique and complex pharmacological profile. Buprenorphine is thought to act as a partial mu agonist but its kappa receptor activities are less well defined. Several studies have suggested that buprenorphine demonstrates kappa receptor agonist effects but other evidence in mammals and pigeons has suggested that it also displays some kappa antagonistic activities. Buprenorphine has unusual receptor binding characteristics that appear to be the result of slow drug dissociation from opioid receptors. It may exhibit a plateau or ceiling analgesic effect in which increased doses may result in no additional analgesia or may have detrimental effects. Few studies have been published evaluating the use of buprenorphine in birds. Buprenorphine, 0.1 mg/kg IM, in African grey parrots did not have an analgesic effect when tested by PD analgesimetry, but PK analysis has suggested that this dose may not achieve effective plasma concentrations (see Table 41-1).[24,25] Pigeons given 0.25 and 0.5 mg/kg IM buprenorphine had an increased latency period for withdrawal from a noxious electrical stimulus of 2 and 5 hours, respectively.[8] Further work is required to determine whether clinical efficacy may be obtained using different buprenorphine doses in other avian species.

Nalbuphine Hydrochloride

Nalbuphine hydrochloride (HCl) exerts its agonist activity principally at the kappa receptor and is a partial antagonist at the mu receptor. It is used as an analgesic in the treatment of moderate to severe pain in humans and has a relatively lower incidence of respiratory depression that does not increase with additional dosing. Nalbuphine HCl was rapidly cleared after both IM and IV dosing of 12.5 mg/kg to Hispaniolan Amazon parrots and had excellent bioavailability following IM administration, with little sedation and no adverse effects.[23b] The same dosage increased thermal foot withdrawal threshold values in this species for up to 3 hours; higher dosages (25 and 50 mg/kg IM) did not significantly increase thermal foot withdrawal threshold values above those of the 12.5-mg/kg dosage. Because of its low abuse potential, this opioid is currently not a U.S. Drug Enforcement Administration (DEA)–scheduled substance. Based on the receptor activity of this drug, and its potential for minor to few side effects, nalbuphine HCl may show promise as an analgesic in pain management protocols in avian patients.

Nonsteroidal Anti-Inflammatory Drugs

NSAIDs are the most common class of analgesic drugs prescribed in small animal medicine. NSAIDs are used to relieve musculoskeletal and visceral pain, acute pain, and chronic pain, such as in osteoarthritis. The pharmacologic activity of NSAIDs has been reviewed in veterinary articles and textbooks and, although most reviews do not consider avian applications, it is assumed that the chemistry and mechanism of action are similar when administered to birds.[22] NSAIDs are characterized by their anti-inflammatory effects on cyclooxygenase (COX) enzymes expressed in peripheral tissues and also have centrally acting antinociceptive effects. A broad tissue distribution of COX receptors has been demonstrated in chickens. The relative expression of COX-1 and COX-2 enzymes varies between species and both enzymes are important in avian pain, but more information is needed to differentiate their physiologic effects in avian species.

The application and dosages of several NSAID formulations continues to be scientifically evaluated and clinically applied in birds (see Table 41-2). The intention of recently developed NSAIDs has been to spare COX-1 and emphasize COX-2 inhibition with the goal of providing analgesia and suppressing inflammation without inhibiting physiologically important prostaglandins. The common NSAIDs used in avian medicine at the time of this writing include meloxicam, carprofen, ketoprofen, celecoxib, and piroxicam, each with a distinct COX-1/COX-2 ratio and differing reports of effectiveness and toxicity in birds.

The selection of NSAID is determined by the ease of administration best suited to the situation—for example, giving an injectable formulation at the time of surgery, followed by oral formulation of the same or different NSAID postoperatively. There is little scientific support for a washout period when switching NSAIDs.[22] In cases of acute or chronic pain, there may be a benefit to changing the NSAID and a washout period could put the bird at risk of having untreated pain. Only one NSAID should be used at a time but, in cases of chronic pain, the response to therapy needs to be frequently reevaluated and the NSAID may need to be changed or augmented with other analgesics if the response is poor or diminishing.

Anti-inflammatory and analgesic effects of NSAIDs continue longer than predicted by plasma half-lives. One explanation for this long duration of effect is the high protein binding, such as the protein in an inflamed site, which may act as a reservoir for the drug after it has been eliminated from the plasma. There are tremendous species differences in drug elimination among the NSAIDs.

The best example of avian species variability is the PK study of meloxicam, flunixin, and sodium salicylate administered intravenously to chickens, ostriches (*Struthio camelus*), mallard ducks (*Anas platyrhynchos*), turkeys (*Meleagris gallopavo*), and pigeons (*Columba livia*).[1] All three NSAIDs were rapidly eliminated in these species, but the volume of distribution was highly variable, which may reflect species differences in protein binding. Although the distribution, half-life, and clearance have been characterized for some NSAIDs in a few species of birds, this information has not always been of use for predicting safe and effective dosage regimens.

NSAID PD studies have been published describing the effects of ketoprofen and flunixin on thromboxane B2 (TBX) concentrations in mallard ducks.[17] Because NSAIDs block the binding of arachidonic acid with COX enzyme, preventing conversion to TBX, plasma TBX is used to estimate the duration of NSAID action. In mallard ducks, flunixin (5 mg/kg) and ketoprofen (5 mg/kg) suppressed TBX levels for up to 12 hours, suggesting that their physiologic action may be that long.[17]

Several analgesimetry models have been used to evaluate the PD of NSAIDs in chickens. Dose responses for carprofen, flunixin, ketoprofen, and sodium salicylate for the treatment of inflammatory pain were determined in chickens using the articular pain model to measure the effect on specific behaviors.[11] Sodium salicylate was determined to be less effective than the other NSAIDs and large doses of carprofen were needed to return to nonarthritic behaviors; minimum effective doses determined in this study are listed in Table 41-2. A similar experimental arthritis model in parrots (*Amazona ventralis*) was used to evaluate NSAID treatment by measuring the return to normal weight

bearing.[3,26] Carprofen (2 mg/kg IM every 12 hours) was less effective than butorphanol. Alternatively, in a similar study, meloxicam (1 mg/kg IM every 12 hours) was effective at returning the parrots to normal weight bearing on the arthritic limb throughout the 36 hours of observation.[3]

Adverse Effects

The most common adverse actions of NSAIDs in mammals include effects on the gastrointestinal system, renal system, and coagulation. NSAIDs have been recently implicated in humans and mammals with regard to an increased risk of myocardial infarction and delays in bone healing, but these effects have not been substantiated in birds. However, it is prudent to be aware that these adverse effects are often dose-dependent and associated with chronic administration. The most common adverse effect of NSAIDs reported in avian species is the impact on renal tissue and function.

Prostaglandins in the kidney have an important role in regulating water and mineral balances and modulating intravascular tone. In chickens, COX-2 metabolites have been implicated in the maintenance of renal blood flow, mediation of renin release, and regulation of sodium excretion. Therefore, in conditions of relative intravascular volume, depletion and/or renal hypoperfusion, such as dehydration, hemorrhage, hemodynamic compromise, heart failure, and renal disease, interference with COX-2 activity may have significant deleterious effects on renal blood flow and glomerular filtration rate. When budgerigars were treated with 5.5 mg/kg flunixin meglumine, 2.5 mg/kg ketoprofen, or 0.1 mg/kg meloxicam for 3 or 7 days, plasma uric acid and protein levels did not change but a low frequency of glomerular congestion, degeneration, and dilation of tubules was seen.[27] Lesions were more severe in birds treated with flunixin meglumine for 3 or 7 days, with increased mesangial matrix synthesis.

The recent massive mortalities in three vulture species on the Asian subcontinent have led to the banning of the NSAID diclofenac (DF) on the Indian subcontinent (see Chapter 46). Common findings of diffuse visceral gout and proximal convoluted tubular damage indicated that the site of toxicity was the kidneys or the renal supportive vascular system. The association of DF with vulture mortalities led to several investigations to establish the mechanism of toxicity for DF and other NSAIDs in several avian species. Recent studies have determined that vulture susceptibility to DF results from a combination of an increased reactive oxygen species, interference with uric acid transport, and duration of exposure.[20] Both DF and meloxicam were found to be toxic to renal tubular epithelial cells following 12 hours of cell culture exposure because of an increase in production of reactive oxygen species although, when cultures were incubated with either drug for only 2 hours, meloxicam showed no toxicity in contrast to DF. DF also decreased the transport of uric acid by interfering with the *p*-aminohippuric acid channel. Additionally, the half-life of DF in vultures (14 hours) is much longer than chickens (2 hours), thus exposing vultures to the toxic effects of DF for prolonged periods.

Formulations

Ketoprofen

Ketoprofen is a potent nonselective COX-1 inhibitor that has been used extensively in small animal medicine. The excellent oral bioavailability of ketoprofen in mammals makes this drug attractive for oral dosing. However, ketoprofen is most commonly used parenterally in birds because of limited oral PK data and difficulty in accurately dosing the oral formulation in small species. PK studies evaluating a single dose of 2 mg/kg ketoprofen given PO, IM, and IV in Japanese quail *(Coturnix japonica)* have shown very low oral (24%) and IM (54%) bioavailability of the drug and the shortest half-life reported for this NSAID in any species.[10] Additional studies are needed to determine whether drug formulations or physiologic differences between species could account for these differences. PD studies of 5 mg/kg IM ketoprofen in mallard ducks *(Anas platyrhynchos)* found an overall decrease in the inflammatory mediator TBX for approximately 12 hours after administration.[17] This suggests that the duration of anti-inflammatory effect in the mallards may parallel that of some mammals studied, and further studies are needed to evaluate the duration of effect and bioavailability in additional avian species. When ketoprofen (2 to 5 mg/kg IM) was administered to free-ranging spectacled eiders *(Somateria fischeri)* and king eiders *(Somateria spectabilis)*, four of ten male spectacled eiders and five of six male king eiders died within 1 to 4 days after surgery,[19] with histologic findings that included renal tubular necrosis, acute rhabdomyolysis, and mild visceral gout. Strong consideration was given to the male behaviors during mating season that may have predisposed these birds to dehydration and the adverse effects of COX inhibition.

Carprofen

Carprofen (CAR) may be administered parenterally or orally and is well absorbed through the gastrointes-

tinal tract in mammals. The mechanism of action of CAR has not been fully elucidated. It is a weak inhibitor of COX at therapeutic doses, yet exhibits good anti-inflammatory activity. This weak inhibition of both COX isoforms may explain its wide margin of safety in comparison with other NSAIDs and it may achieve its therapeutic effects partially through other pathways. CAR given SC significantly improved the speed and walking ability of lame chickens in a dose-dependent manner.[18] An extremely high CAR dose of 30 mg/kg IM was needed for analgesia in chickens with experimental arthritis.[12] An analgesia study with Hispaniolan Amazon parrots with experimental arthritis noted that 2 hours following CAR administration, lameness was markedly improved, but the analgesic effect was very short term because carprofen, 3 mg/kg IM every 12 hours, did not significantly improve the weight-bearing load of the arthritic limb for the 30-hour study period.[26] More work is needed to determine appropriate dosages, dosing routes, and dosing frequency of carprofen in birds.

Meloxicam (MEL)

Meloxicam (MEL) is a COX-2 selective oxicam NSAID. In recent years, MEL has become the most widely used anti-inflammatory medication in exotic animal practice. A survey to determine NSAID toxicity in captive birds treated in zoos reported zero fatalities associated with MEL, which was administered to over 700 birds from 60 species.[7] MEL is currently available as an oral suspension and injectable form. A dose-response analgesia study with Hispaniolan Amazon parrots with experimental arthritis has determined that MEL, 1 mg/kg IM every 12 hours, was necessary to achieve significant return to baseline weight bearing.[3] Oral administration of MEL suspension, 1 mg/kg, to Amazon parrots had lower bioavailability than when administered parenterally, and the highest mean concentration expected to provide analgesia was 6 hours after administration.[23c] Ostriches given MEL IV exhibited the most rapid half-life (0.5 hours) when compared with ducks, turkeys, pigeons, and chickens, respectively.[1] Clinical recommendations for the treatment of parrots with high dosages of MEL need to await critical examination of its effect on renal parenchyma. Future studies to evaluate the PD and PK of MEL administered by different routes in different avian species are necessary to determine appropriate meloxicam analgesic dosages and dosing schedules in avian patients.

Piroxicam

Piroxicam (PIRO) is a nonselective NSAID used for its anti-inflammatory properties as well and for its value as a chemopreventive and antitumor agent. It has a much higher potency against COX-1 than COX-2. Piroxicam has good oral bioavailability and a long half-life in mammals, but PD and PK studies have not been carried out in any avian species. Despite the high incidence of negative side effects of piroxicam used in humans, there are no reports of its toxicity in birds. It has been used clinically for the long-term treatment of chronic arthritis in cranes.[23]

Regional Anesthesia and Analgesia

In all vertebrates, including birds, local anesthetics block sodium channels in the nerve axon, interfering with the generation and conduction of action potentials along the nerve. When local anesthetics are used preemptively, the number and frequency of impulses are reduced, thereby reducing nociceptor sensitization, which has the beneficial effect of minimizing central sensitization. Regional infiltration using a local line or splash block is the most common method. The subcutaneous space in most avian species is very thin so a small-gauge needle is recommended to make several SC injections into the operative area. Although lidocaine and bupivacaine have been used for brachial plexus blockade in a variety of avian species, a recent evaluation of bupivacaine (2 and 8 mg/kg) and lidocaine with epinephrine (15 mg/kg) found that neither effectively blocked nerve transmission in the brachial plexus of mallard ducks.[2]

Local anesthetics are absorbed by the vasculature in the region being blocked. Systemic uptake of local anesthetics may be rapid in birds and metabolism may be prolonged, increasing the potential for toxic reactions. The duration of action depends on the molecular properties and lipid solubility of the drug. Neither the time to effect nor duration of action has been determined in birds. Dosage recommendations are lower for birds than mammals because birds may be more sensitive to the effects of the drug. Chickens given intra-articular injections of high doses of bupivacaine (2.7 to 3.3 mg/kg) showed immediate signs of toxicity, such as drowsiness and recumbency. Other toxic effects reported in birds include fine tremors, ataxia, recumbency, seizures, stupor, cardiovascular effects, and death. Toxic effects may be acute if accidentally injected intravenously.

Lidocaine

Lidocaine is available as a commercial preparation of 2% (20 mg/mL) and the formulation without epinephrine is recommended. Based on empirical use, the recommended dosage is 2 to 3 mg/kg, although 15 mg/kg with epinephrine had no adverse effects when used for

brachial plexus block in mallard ducks.[2] For small birds, the commercial preparation may need to be diluted 1:10 to achieve an effective volume for the block. It is unknown whether this dilution allows appropriate tissue drug levels for analgesia to be reached or the expected duration of analgesia to occur.

Bupivacaine

Bupivacaine is the most clinically useful perioperative local anesthetic in mammals because it is long acting, but it has been used conservatively in birds because of concerns that toxic effects may also take longer to resolve. The commercial preparations of bupivacaine available are 0.25%, 0.5%, and 0.75% solutions (2.5, 5, and 7.5 mg/mL, respectively), and the lower concentration may not need dilution for birds. The recommended maximum dose of bupivacaine for mammals is 2 mg/kg. One study in which bupivacaine, 2 mg/kg SC, was administered to mallard ducks has suggested that it may be shorter acting in ducks than in mammals.[15] In this study, bupivacaine showed a faster absorption versus elimination rate and sequestration and redistribution of bupivacaine were suggested by increases in plasma concentrations at 6 and 12 hours after administration, making it possible for toxicity to be delayed. Higher doses of 8 mg/kg had no adverse effects when used for brachial plexus block in ducks.[2]

Other Analgesics

Tramadol

Tramadol hydrochloride is an analgesic that has become popular recently despite minimal evidence as to its efficacy. It is active at opiate, alpha-adrenergic, and serotonergic receptors. Tramadol is a weak mu agonist but the O-desmethyl metabolite (M1) is a much more potent agonist in mammals. The conversion to the M1 metabolite is variable among species but it is known that it is produced in bald eagles,[32] red-tailed hawks, and Hispaniolan Amazon parrots.[31] It is available in PO and injectable formulations and currently the drug is not a controlled substance. The oral (11 mg/kg) and IV (4 mg/kg) PK of single-dose tramadol have been evaluated in bald eagles,[32] but its analgesic efficacy at these plasma concentrations have not been established. The oral bioavailability of tramadol (mean ± SD = 97.94% ± 0.52%) was higher than that observed in humans and dogs, suggesting this as a useful route of administration in this species. Tramadol, 11 mg/kg PO, achieved concentrations in the human analgesic range for 10 hours in five of six bald eagles; M1 plasma concentrations reached the human analgesic range in only two eagles at much earlier time points.[32] Until specific analgesic plasma concentrations are known, it is difficult to predict how these differences may affect appropriate dosing frequency after repeated doses. Mild transient bradycardia was observed immediately after IV administration in three of six birds, but was not considered clinically significant. Although tramadol holds great promise for use in birds, studies are needed to evaluate the efficacy, safety, and appropriate dosing in different species.

Gabapentin

Gabapentin, a gamma-aminobutyric acid (GABA) analogue, has been used to treat neuropathic pain in humans for almost a decade. Its exact mechanism of action is unknown, but its therapeutic action on neuropathic pain is thought to involve voltage-gated N-type calcium ion channels. To date, there is only one published report on the clinical use of gabapentin as part of a multimodal therapeutic plan for suspected neuropathic pain in birds.[29]

Balanced or Multimodal Analgesia

Combinations of drugs acting at different points in the nociceptive system provide a greater effect and have potentially less toxicity than single drugs. For example, opioids generally act centrally to limit the input of nociceptive information into the CNS, whereas NSAIDs primarily act peripherally to decrease inflammation, thus limiting the nociceptive information that initially enters the CNS. Balanced analgesia with opiates, NSAIDs, and/or local anesthetics administered before a painful procedure may block sensory noxious stimuli from onward transmission to the CNS, thus reducing the overall potential for pain and inflammation. These synergies have been demonstrated in laboratory animals and are now being used in the clinical environment. Balanced analgesia should be considered in almost every avian patient because the use of multimodal therapy may maximize analgesic efficacy and minimize individual drug toxicity in these patients, for which few analgesic data are available.

CONCLUSION

Avian analgesia is finally recognized as a critical component of avian medicine and surgery. The need to recognize pain and provide pain relief is the first step, and many anecdotal therapeutic dosages extrapolated from other companion animals have been developed. Several published research investigations, using several species of birds, have begun to provide avian analgesia therapeutics with empirical information for clinical application. The challenge is to continue pushing this research forward, recognizing that there are approximately 10,000 known species of birds, perhaps 200 species commonly kept as pets, and that each species has a range of behaviors as varied as their species-specific PK and PD for each analgesic drug.

REFERENCES

1. Baert K, De Backer P: Comparative pharmacokinetics of three non-steroidal anti-inflammatory drugs in five bird species. Comp Biochem Physiol C Toxicol Pharmacol 134:25–33, 2003.
2. Brenner DJ, Larsen RS, Dickinson PJ, et al: Development of an avian brachial plexus nerve block technique for perioperative analgesia in mallard ducks (Anas platyrhynchos). J Avian Med Surg 24:24–34, 2010.
3. Cole GA, Paul-Murphy J, Krugner-Higby L, et al: Analgesic effects of intramuscular administration of meloxicam in Hispaniolan parrots (Amazona ventralis) with experimentally induced arthritis. Am J Vet Res 70:1471–1476, 2009.
4. Concannon KT, Dodam JR, Hellyer PW: Influence of a mu- and kappa-opioid agonist on isoflurane minimal anesthetic concentration in chickens. Am J Vet Res 56:806–811, 1995.
5. Curro TG: Evaluation of the isoflurane-sparing effects of butorphanol and flunixin in psittaciformes. Proc Assoc Avian Vet 17–19, 1994.
6. Curro TG, Brunson DB, Paul-Murphy J: Determination of the ED50 of isoflurane and evaluation of the isoflurane-sparing effect of butorphanol in cockatoos (Cacatua spp.). Vet Surg 23:429–433, 1994.
7. Cuthbert R, Parry-Jones J, Green RE, et al: NSAIDs and scavenging birds: Potential impacts beyond Asia's critically endangered vultures. Biol Lett 3:90–93, 2007.
8. Gaggermeier B, Henke J, Schatzmann U: Investigations on analgesia in domestic pigeons (C. livia, Gmel., 1789, var. dom.) using buprenorphine and butorphanol. Proc Eur Assoc Avian Vet 70–73, 2003.
9. Gentle MJ, Tilston VL: Reduction in peripheral inflammation by changes in attention. Physiol Behav 66:289–292, 1999.
10. Graham JE, Kollias-Baker C, Craigmill AL, et al: Pharmacokinetics of ketoprofen in Japanese quail (Coturnix japonica). J Vet Pharmacol Ther 28:399–402, 2005.
11. Pavez JC, Pascoe PJ, DiMaio Knych HK, Kass PH, Hawkins MG: Effect of fentanyl target-controlled infusions on isoflurane MAD for red-tailed hawks. Proceedings of the Association of Avian Veterinarians Annual Meeting 29, 2010.
12. Hocking PM, Robertson GW, Gentle MJ: Effects of non-steroidal anti-inflammatory drugs on pain-related behaviour in a model of articular pain in the domestic fowl. Res Vet Sci 78:69–75, 2005.
13. Hoppes S, Flammer K, Hoersch K, et al: Disposition and analgesic effects of fentanyl in white cockatoos (Cacatua alba). J Avian Med Surg 17:124–130, 2003.
14. Klaphake E, Schumacher J, Greenacre C, et al: Comparative anesthetic and cardiopulmonary effects of pre- versus postoperative butorphanol administration in hispaniolan amazon parrots (Amazona ventralis) anesthetized with sevoflurane. J Avian Med Surg 20:2–7, 2006.
15. Machin KL, Livingston A: Plasma bupivicaine levels in mallard ducks (Anas platyrhyncos) following a single subcutaneous dose. Proc Am Assoc Zoo Vet 159–163, 2001.

16. Machin KL, Livingston A: Assessment of the analgesic effects of ketoprofen in ducks anesthetized with isoflurane. Am J Vet Res 63:821–826, 2002.

17. Machin KL, Tellier LA, Lair S, et al: Pharmacodynamics of flunixin and ketoprofen in mallard ducks (*Anas platyrhynchos*). J Zoo Wildl Med 32:222–229, 2001.

18. McGeowen D, Danbury TC, Waterman-Pearson AE, et al: Effect of carprofen on lameness in broiler chickens. Vet Rec 144:668–671, 1999.

19. Mulcahy DM, Tuomi P, Larsen RS: Differential mortality of male spectacled eiders (*Somateria fischeri*) and king eiders (*Somateria spectabilis*) subsequent to anesthesia with propofol, bupivacaine and ketoprofen. J Avian Med Surg 17:117–123, 2003.

20. Naidoo V, Swan GE: Diclofenac toxicity in Gyps vulture is associated with decreased uric acid excretion and not renal portal vasoconstriction. Comp Biochem Physiol C Toxicol Pharmacol 149:269–274, 2008.

21. Naidoo V, Wolter K, Cromarty AD, et al: The pharmacokinetics of meloxicam in vultures. J Vet Pharmacol Ther 31:128–134, 2008.

22. Papich MG: An update on nonsteroidal anti-inflammatory drugs (NSAIDs) in small animals. Vet Clin North Am Small Anim Pract 38:1243–1266, vi, 2008.

23. Paul-Murphy J: Personal communication, 2010.

23a. Sanchez-Migallon Guzman D, Paul-Murphy JR, Barker SA, Tully TN: Plasma concentrations of butorphanol in Hispaniolan Amazon parrots (*Amazona ventralis*) after intravenous and oral administration. Proceedings of the Association of Avian Veterinarians 23–24, 2008.

23b. Sanchez-Migallon Guzman D, Keller D, Kukanich D, et al: Pharmacokinetics and antinociceptive effects of nalbuphine hydrochloride in Hispaniolan Amazon parrots (*Amazona ventralis*). Proceedings of the Association of Avian Veterinarians 27–28, 2010.

23c. Molter C, Court MN, Cole GA, Gagnon D, Klauer JM, Paul-Murphy J: Pharmacokinetics of pareneteral and oral meloxicam in Hispaniolan parrots (*Amazona ventralis*). Proceedings of the Association of Avian Veterinarians 317–318, 2009.

24. Paul-Murphy J, Brunson DB, Miletic V: Analgesic effects of butorphanol and buprenorphine in conscious African grey parrots (*Psittacus erithacus erithacus* and *Psittacus erithacus timneh*). Am J Vet Res 60:1218–1221, 1999.

25. Paul-Murphy J, Hess J, Fialkowski JP: Pharmokinetic properties of a single intramuscular dose of buprenorphine in African Grey Parrots (*Psittacus erithacus erithacus*). J Avian Med Surg 18:224–228, 2004.

26. Paul-Murphy JR, Sladky KK, Krugner-Higby LA, et al: Analgesic effects of carprofen and liposome-encapsulated butorphanol tartrate in Hispaniolan parrots (*Amazona ventralis*) with experimentally induced arthritis. Am J Vet Res 70:1201–1210, 2009.

27. Pereira ME, Werther K: Evaluation of the renal effects of flunixin meglumine, ketoprofen and meloxicam in budgerigars (*Melopsittacus undulatus*). Vet Rec 160:844–846, 2007.

28. Riggs SM, Hawkins MG, Craigmill AL, et al: Pharmacokinetics of butorphanol tartrate in red-tailed hawks (*Buteo jamaicensis*) and great horned owls (*Bubo virginianus*). Am J Vet Res 69:596–603, 2008.

29. Shaver SL, Robinson NG, Wright BD, et al: A multimodal approach to management of suspected neuropathic pain in a prairie falcon (*Falco mexicanus*). J Avian Med Surg 23:209–213, 2009.

30. Sladky KK, Krugner-Higby L, Meek-Walker E, et al: Serum concentrations and analgesic effects of liposome-encapsulated and standard butorphanol tartrate in parrots. Am J Vet Res 67:775–781, 2006.

31. Souza MJ, Sanchez-Migallon Guzman D, Paul-Murphy J, Cox S: Tramadol in Hispaniolan Amazon parrots (*Amazona ventralis*). Proceedings of the Association of Avian Veterinarians 293–294, 2010.

32. Souza MJ, Martin-Jimenez T, Jones MP, et al: Pharmacokinetics of intravenous and oral tramadol in the bald eagle (*Haliaeetus leucocephalus*). J Avian Med Surg 23:247–252, 2009.

CHAPTER 42

Prehatch Protocols to Improve Hatchability

Meg Sutherland-Smith and Pat Witman

Artificial incubation of avian eggs is a valuable tool that has facilitated breeding programs for numerous species. Removing eggs for artificial incubation frequently leads to double or triple clutching, thereby increasing the fecundity of a pair in any given season. Management of artificial incubation focuses on minimizing contamination and using best practice incubation conditions to maximize hatchability. This involves developing protocols for sanitation, incubation, egg management, record keeping, and egg necropsy. An overview of these topics will be covered in this chapter. An understanding of avian egg and embryo development is important when working with artificial incubation techniques. There are several comprehensive works on avian development.[6,7,19,20]

FACILITIES AND EQUIPMENT

Primary considerations for facilities related to hatchability involve environmental conditions and sanitation. It is ideal to have separate areas for incubation, hatching, and hand-rearing to facilitate one-way traffic flow from the incubation area. All surfaces should be amenable to disinfection. The ability to control temperature, humidity, and air flow within a facility is important. Practices that restrict access to personnel working with egg incubation, as well as work routines that allow incubation duties to be performed prior to working in other collection areas, may minimize the risk of contamination. Because eggs are a perfect medium for bacterial growth, the importance of strict hygiene to minimize contamination cannot be over-emphasized. Rigorous disinfection should be done once to twice weekly. Ultraviolet radiation in the incubator room as well as ozonation of empty incubators is performed weekly at our facility as part of disinfection protocols.

Temperature, humidity, and egg rotation are primary factors in avian incubation, so the ability to maintain, adjust, and monitor these parameters is important. The primary equipment needed for artificial incubation includes incubators, hatchers, candlers, and scales. Incubators are typically described as still air or forced air. Forced air machines are most commonly used and are designed with a fan to circulate the air within the unit. This facilitates a uniform temperature throughout the incubator as well as influx of oxygen and dissipation of carbon dioxide produced by eggs. Some machines come equipped with digital readouts for temperature and humidity, but we believe that best practice is also to place a separate mercury thermometer in the machine to use for daily monitoring. Digital thermohygrometers have been used, but limiting factors include variable life spans and, when they fail, the temperature readings may be off by only 1°. This change would go undetected unless a second thermometer is in use for comparison. A backup generator to maintain incubator function is essential in case of a power outage.

Humidity is provided by automatic humidifiers or through evaporation from one or more water pans placed in the bottom of an incubator. Humidity may be measured by a hair hygrometer, wet bulb hygrometer, or digital hygrometer. We prefer the wet bulb technique. It is simpler to have several incubators maintained at different humidity settings so that eggs may be moved to an appropriate humidity level as needed, based on egg weight loss, rather than changing humidity levels in an incubator during incubation.

Commonly used incubators have automated turning systems that rotate eggs every 1 to 2 hours. Embryonic development may be improved by hand turning three times a day to ensure that an egg has been turned completely, because some automatic turners do not roll an egg over completely. Studies have shown that some of

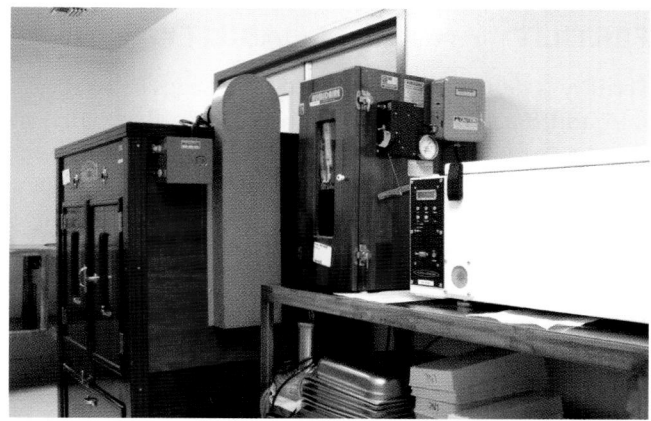

Figure 42-1

Several types of incubators are utilized at the author's facility.

the smaller eggs, such as most passerine species, may benefit from more turning than larger eggs, such as ratite eggs.[3] Fig. 42-1 shows several types of incubators within the incubation room at the author's facility.

Hatchers are similar to incubators, but without turners. Incubators may be used as hatchers, although it is not recommended to do so at the same time as the eggs are being incubated because of the increased risk of contamination. Hatchers are typically set at 0.5° F to 1° F (0.27° C to 0.55° C) lower than the temperature used for incubation. A candler is used for evaluating egg condition at the start of incubation and monitoring the development of the circulatory system throughout incubation. High-quality scales are necessary for accurate and precise monitoring of egg weights. Otherwise, errors may be introduced into calculations of egg weight loss. A more in-depth discussion of incubation equipment has been covered by others.[12]

EGG MANAGEMENT AND RECORD KEEPING

A first step in egg management is to decide which species are candidates for artificial incubation. If possible, take measures to ensure a clean nest environment. Personnel should ensure that their hands are washed or wear examination gloves when handling eggs. Egg collection may occur before or after incubation has started. Eggs may benefit from partial parental incubation. Once incubation has started, eggs may be transported in a small cooler containing clean warm (95° F [35° C]) millet deep enough to cover at least half of the egg. Millet is readily available, is clean, and functions as a

shock absorber when moving eggs from the nest to the incubator. Other systems for egg collection have also been used.[1] Anything that may absorb moisture also increases the risk of contamination.

When feasible, choose eggs for incubation that have no evidence of heavy contamination or trauma. Genetic importance of an egg or a poor parental history will sometimes necessitate incubating eggs in less than ideal conditions. Gross contamination may be removed by gently wiping away debris with a soft clean or sterile cloth. Fine sandpaper may be used to remove buildup of dried debris, but care must be taken to preserve the cuticle. Several methods for repairing damaged eggs have been described.[12] Candling eggs prior to being set for incubation allows documentation of conditions and developmental stage. Additionally, this may be done daily as long as safe techniques are used, such as not holding an egg up to a hot lamp for more than a few seconds at a time. If an embryo is determined to have died, it should be removed from the incubator as soon as possible to avoid contamination. Eggs may be weighed daily or biweekly to determine the percentage of egg weight loss. An example of how record keeping, egg weighing, and candling equipment are set-up in a clean environmental space at the author's facility is shown in Fig. 42-2.

It is a common practice in commercial poultry operations to use egg dips, washes, or fumigation to reduce external egg contamination. These processes need to be carefully monitored because the dip or wash solution needs to be warmer than the egg or the solution and surface bacteria will be drawn into the egg as it cools. Also, some solutions may damage the protective cuticle layer of the egg. One epidemiology study evaluating

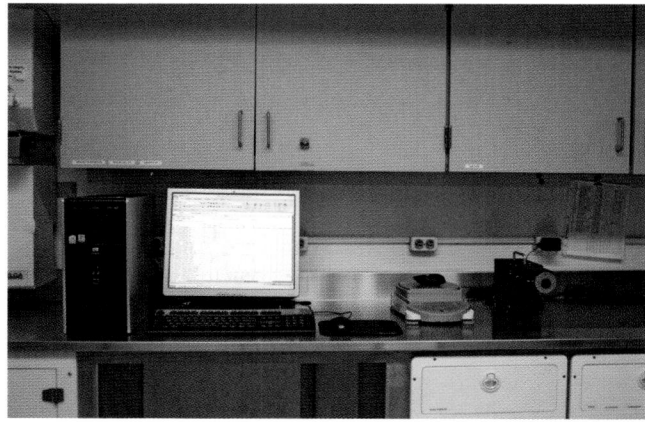

Figure 42-2

Examples of record keeping, egg weighing, and candling equipment at the author's facility.

hatchability in broiler breeder flocks in a number of poultry operations has found that those not using any egg disinfection had better results than those using dips, sprays, or formalin fumigation.[9]

Formaldehyde fumigation of freshly laid eggs is no longer used at our facility because of regulations and human health hazards. Dips and sprays are generally not recommended for most exotic eggs because of a lack of information regarding their safety. Spot-cleaning soiled eggs with liquids is not recommended. In situations in which infections have been documented, dips may be appropriate for thick-shelled eggs. A fine mist of a phenolic or quaternary ammonium disinfectant applied to moist or contaminated eggs is used in the ostrich industry.[23]

A new technique recently evaluated for the poultry industry uses electrolyzed oxidizing (EO) water spray on eggs to reduce microbial contamination.[5] The authors of this study concluded that the use of EO water reduces microbial contamination without affecting hatchability of the eggs. This could prove to be an option for nondomestic operations in the future.

Treating potentially infected eggs during incubation has been reported. Piperacillin has been injected into the air cell of psittacine eggs at days 14, 18, and 22 (4.0 mg for macaw eggs and 2.0 mg for cockatoos or smaller) to improve hatchability.[16] Tylosin (0.5 to 1.0 mg) injected into the air cell at the start of incubation has been used to treat *Mycoplasma* infections in eggs.[17] Others have studied the effects of gentamicin injection (0.2 mg) into the albumen of chicken eggs at 15 days of incubation.[2] There was no adverse effect on hatchability of treated eggs versus control eggs. Despite gentamicin levels being below the limit of detection in yolks and embryos, hatchability was significantly improved in the gentamicin-treated eggs. Dipping eggs into antibiotic solutions has also been used to treat infected eggs.

Tracking incubation parameters through detailed record keeping is essential for retrospective analyses evaluating egg outcomes. As noted, temperature and humidity readings for facility rooms and each individual incubator are recorded twice daily at our facility to confirm that proper parameters are being maintained. Egg records include date laid, date set, initial egg weight and measurements, condition of egg, incubator model, incubation parameters, egg turning, daily weights, candling results, internal and external pip, hatcher parameters, date hatched, and condition of chick and umbilicus. This information also helps establish incubation parameters for unfamiliar species.

FERTILITY AND HATCHABILITY

Fertility is defined as the ratio of fertile eggs to total eggs laid and hatchability is the ratio of eggs that hatch to the total number of fertile eggs. Factors affecting both should be considered when evaluating eggs that do not hatch and may be divided into three periods—prior to oviposition, preincubation, and incubation. Incompatible pairs or interference by enclosure mates may affect fertility. Some parameters such as the genetics of the parents or age of the hen are difficult to control. Abnormally sized and shaped eggs are not uncommon in very young or old hens. Eggshell thinning may occur as females reach reproductive senescence. Inadequate nutritional status of the parents will affect the quality of eggs produced. A review of maternal nutrition and hatchability is useful.[24] Low hatchability and poor chick survival in artificially incubated black stilt (*Himantopus novaezelandiae*) prompted an investigation that identified iodine-deficient diets as the problem.[21] Exposure to toxins is generally not a problem in captive settings, but could be a consideration where eggs are collected from nests in the wild.

Eggs produced from highly stressed hens are also likely to have reduced hatchability.[22] Certain diseases such as exotic Newcastle disease, avian influenza, or trematode infestation in the oviduct may affect shell quality. Infections acquired via vertical transmission of pathogens from the hen to the egg or from the external environment may result in embryo mortality. Others have summarized pathogens infecting avian embryos.[17]

How eggs are handled and stored prior to incubation also affects hatchability. The ideal conditions to store eggs are between 55°F to 60°F (12.8°C to 15.6°C), because embryo development does not start until the egg temperature is higher than 70°F (21°C). Because excessive water loss will occur in most ambient conditions, a relative humidity of 70% to 80% is recommended. Storing eggs facilitates synchronizing hatching and rearing of clutches. A general rule of thumb is to store eggs no longer than 7 days. Eggs in which incubation has commenced are not candidates for storage.

Aviculturists working with nondomestic species have used protocols established for domestic species as guidelines to refine incubation protocols for nondomestic species based on their experience.* In general, small eggs have shorter incubation times at higher

*References 1, 4, 10, 13, 15, and 23.

Temperature, °F (°C)*	Order or Species Artificially Incubated†
96.5 (35.83)	Ratites (3)
97.5 (36.38)	Kiwi (1), California condor
98.0 (36.66)	California condor, Andean condor, Harpy eagle
98.5 (36.94)	Psittaciformes (40), crested screamer
99.0 (37.22)	Elegant crested tinamou, Pelecaniformes (2), Ciconiiformes (11), Anseriformes (29), Falconiformes (5), Galliformes (20), Gruiformes (12), Charadriiformes (4), Psittaciformes (2), Cuculiformes (5), Strigiformes (3), Caprimulgiformes (1), Coraciiformes (5), Piciformes (1)
99.5 (37.50)	Galliformes (33), Gruiformes (2), Charadriiformes (5), Columbiformes (6), Psittaciformes (11), Cuculiformes (3), Coraciiformes (2), Passeriformes (6)
100.0 (37.77)	Cuculiformes (2), Coraciiformes (2)
100.5 (38.05)	Columbiformes (16), Cuculiformes (2), Piciformes (3), Passeriformes (37)

TABLE 42-1 Artificial Incubation Temperatures for Various Orders and Species of Birds

Dry bulb temperature.
†*Number of species successfully hand-reared from eggs artificially incubated at these temperatures in parentheses.*

temperatures, whereas larger eggs incubate for longer periods at lower temperatures. Table 42-1 lists incubation temperatures for a variety of species successfully used at our facility. Incubation temperature is sometimes determined by the temperature of available incubators, demonstrating that some species may tolerate a wider range of incubation temperatures. It is recommended to avoid temperature fluctuations greater than ±0.5°F (0.28°C) in an incubator. Incubation temperatures that are too high may result in chicks that are smaller than normal and have abnormal umbilical seals, and/or unretracted yolk sacs.[12,17] Scissor bill, curled toes, and twisted necks may also be the result of elevated incubation temperatures. Incubation temperatures below normal may result in late dead embryos as

well as chicks that are larger than normal and weak, and have abnormal umbilical seals or yolk sacs.

Weight loss is a normal process during egg development caused by evaporation through the pores of the eggshell. We have found that most eggs lose 12% to 18% of their weight (linear rate of loss) during incubation. Too high or too low incubator humidity will result in inadequate or excessive weight losses, respectively. Malpositioned chicks, edematous chicks, and unretracted yolk sacs may result from inadequate weight loss.[12] Excessive weight loss may impair calcium transport, resulting in poor bone mineralization, weakness, and dehydration.[14,17] Therefore, the humidity to which an egg is exposed should be adjusted accordingly to weight loss trends during incubation.

Inadequate turning of eggs may result in abnormal membrane development, malpositioned chicks, and/or poor nutrient assimilation and may cause the embryo to stick to the egg shell. Turning needs to occur in alternating opposite directions to prevent the chalazae from wrapping around the embryo and rupturing. Physical trauma, such as jarring or shaking when eggs are collected or handled during incubation, may damage the developing embryo. Excessive carbon dioxide and/or insufficient oxygen levels will adversely affect chick development. This is generally more of a problem with still air incubators or at high altitudes.

To evaluate and understand problems with hatchability, complete necropsies, including histopathologic evaluation, should be performed on all eggs that die during incubation or fail to hatch.[11,12] Necropsy techniques have been previously described.[18] Time of embryonic death during incubation may provide information regarding the cause of death. Also, chick mortality during the first 10 days may be linked to problems during incubation. As an example, the combination of necropsy information and review of incubation parameters has identified several problems contributing to low hatchability in trumpeter swan (*Cygnus buccinator*) eggs being incubated as part of a restoration program in Canada.[8]

Despite the circumstances that are out of an aviculturist's control, there are many factors that may be influenced to maximize successful artificial incubation. The two most important are to start with the cleanest egg possible and use sound incubation practices.

REFERENCES

1. Aourir M, Znari M, El Abbassi A, et al: Reproductive parameters in captive hand-reared black-bellied sandgrouse. Zoo Biol 27:269–281, 2008.

2. Calle PP, Janssen DL, Kuehler CM, et al: Gentamicin injection of incubating avian eggs. In Wharton, D, editor: Proceedings of the Annual Conference of the American Association of Zoo Veterinarians, 1989, pp 83–89.
3. Deeming DC: Patterns and significance of egg turning. In Deeming DC, editor: Avian incubation: Behavior, environment, and evolution, Oxford, 2002, Oxford University Press, pp 161–178.
4. Ellis DH, Gee GF, Mirande CM: Cranes: Their biology, management and conservation, Blaine, Wash, 1996, Hancock House (http://www.pwrc.usgs.gov/resshow/gee/cranbook/cranebook.htm).
5. Fasenko GM, O'Dea EE, McMullen LM: Spraying hatching eggs with electrolyzed oxidizing water reduces eggshell microbial load without compromising broiler production parameters. Poult Sci 88:1121–1127, 2009.
6. Freeman BM, Vince MA: Development of the avian embryo, London, 1974, Chapman and Hall.
7. Hamburger V, Hamilton HL: A series of normal stages in the development of the chick embryo. J Morphol 88:49–89, 1951.
8. Hamilton EC, Hunter DB, Smith DA, et al: Artificial incubation of trumpeter swan eggs. In Wharton, D, editor: Selected factors affecting hatchability. Zoo Biol 18:403–414, 1999.
9. Heier BT, Jarp J: An epidemiological study of the hatchability in broiler breeder flocks. Poult Sci 80:1132–1138, 2001.
10. Jordan R: Parrot incubation procedures, Ontario, 1989, Silvio Mattacchione.
11. Joyner KL, Abbott UK: Egg necropsy techniques. In Proceedings of the American Association of Avian Veterinarians, 1991, pp 146–152.
12. Kasielke S: Incubation of eggs. In Gage LJ, Duerr RS, editors: Hand-rearing birds, Ames, Iowa, 2007, Blackwell, pp 39–54.
13. Kuehler CM, Good J: Artificial incubation of bird eggs at the Zoological Society of San Diego. Int Zoo Yb 29:118–136, 1990.
14. Kuehler CM, Loomis MR: Artificial incubation of nondomestic bird eggs. In Kirk WR, Bonagura JD, editors: Current veterinary therapy XI, Philadelphia, 1992, WB Saunders, pp 1138–1141.
15. Kuehler CM, Lieberman A, McIlraith B, et al: Artificial incubation and hand-rearing of loggerhead shrikes. Wildl Soc Bull 21:165–171, 1993.
16. McDonald SE: Injecting eggs with antibiotics. J Assoc Avian Vet 1:9, 1989.
17. Olsen GH, Clubb SL: Embryology, incubation, and hatching. In Altman RB, Clubb SL, Dorrestein GM, et al editors: Avian medicine and surgery, Philadelphia, 1997, WB Saunders, pp 54–71.
18. Rideout BR, Kuehler CM: Pathology of the avian embryo: What veterinarians need to know about pathology as a disease surveillance tool for avian captive propagation programs. In Proceedings of the American Association of Avian Veterinarians, 2000, pp 329–334.
19. Romanoff AL, Romanoff AJ: The avian egg, New York, 1949, John Wiley & Sons.
20. Romanoff AL, Romanoff AJ: The avian embryo, New York, 1960, MacMillan.
21. Sancha E, van Heezik Y, Maloney R, et al: Iodine deficiency affects hatchability of endangered captive Kaki (black stilt, Himantopus novaezelandiae). Zoo Biol 23:1–13, 2004.
22. Schmidt JB, Satterlee DG, Treese SM: Maternal corticosterone reduces egg fertility and hatchability and increases the numbers of early dead embryos in eggs laid by quail hens selected for exaggerated adrenocortical stress responsiveness. Poult Sci 88:1352–1357, 2009.
23. Stewart J: Hatchery management in ostrich production. In Fowler ME, editor: Zoo and wildlife medicine: Current therapy 3, Philadelphia, 1993, WB Saunders, pp 206–211.
24. Wilson HR: Effects of maternal nutrition on hatchability. Poult Sci 76:134–143, 1997.

CHAPTER 43

West Nile Virus in Raptors

Nicole M. Nemeth

HISTORY AND BACKGROUND

West Nile virus (WNV; family Flaviviridae, genus *Flavivirus*) is a member of the Japanese encephalitis virus antigenic complex. Initial virus isolation and characterization occurred in Uganda in 1937, with subsequent detections in southern and northern Africa, the Middle East and, later, Europe. More recently, its range has expanded to the Western Hemisphere and now encompasses the contiguous United States, southern Canada, Mexico, and portions of Central and South America.

Increased WNV virulence in birds first became evident in migrating storks and domestic geese in the Middle East in the late 1990s. Since then, WNV has emerged as an important pathogen of wild and captive birds in the United States and Canada. There is a broad range of susceptibility to WNV disease across avian taxa, the reasons for which are not well understood. Although high rates of lethal WNV infection among numerous corvid species have led to conservation concerns, the risk posed by WNV to the health of both captive and free-ranging raptors also merits attention.

EPIDEMIOLOGY

Birds are the primary amplifying host of WNV and infections have been detected in more than 300 species of native and exotic birds in North America, including raptor species of five families.[15] Raptor species, including the American kestrel *(Falco sparverius)*, red-tailed hawk *(Buteo jamaicensis)*, Eastern screech owl *(Megascops asio)*, and great horned owl *(Bubo virginianus)*, have been deemed reservoir competent via laboratory-derived infections.[10,15,16] Additionally, raptors have presented with a variety of WNV-associated clinical syndromes at rehabilitation, education, propagation, and zoological centers in the United States and Canada.*

Transmission of WNV in nature is maintained between avian hosts and mosquito vectors (most notably *Culex* spp.) with occasional transmission to dead-end hosts (e.g., humans and horses). Natural infection of vertebrates occurs primarily through mosquito blood feeding, although additional transmission routes of lesser epidemiologic importance likely occur. For example, laboratory infections of birds resulted after ingestion of infectious prey or liquid as well as contact with infectious conspecifics.[10,15] The latter most likely occurs because of virus-laden oral secretions being ingested or virus entering microabrasions in oral mucosa or skin during allopreening, aggressive behavior, or parental feeding of offspring or mates. Nonmosquito arthropods such as swallow bugs *(Oeciacus vicarious)*, louse flies *(Icosta americana)*, and ticks *(Carios capensis)* have been assessed for WNV vector competence, and laboratory-controlled transmission to birds was demonstrated by the latter. However, whether these nontraditional vectors successfully transmit WNV under natural conditions is unknown.

Within tropical and subtropical climates, WNV transmission may occur year-round, whereas temperate regions experience seasonal transmission (from about June through October in the United States and Canada). However, annual and seasonal transmission rates vary, depending on environmental, host, and vector-related factors. Infection rates in birds as estimated by seroprevalence vary geographically and topographically, as well as taxonomically. WNV has been documented in raptors occupying multiple geographic regions throughout the contiguous United States and southern Canada, including owls, hawks, eagles, falcons, and osprey.†

*References 1, 2, 4, 6, 9, 18, 23, and 24.
†References 2-4, 8, 9, 12-14, 18, 19, and 23-27.

PATHOGENESIS, IMMUNITY, CLINICAL COURSE, AND OUTCOME

As the natural reservoir host of WNV, most birds are susceptible to infection, which often involves marked virus replication in blood and other tissues followed by a robust humoral immune response. Experimental WNV infection in raptors and other birds has led to a better understanding of timing and intensity of shedding, viremia, tissue tropism, seroconversion, and clinical outcomes. Notably, some if not most WNV-infected raptors experience viremia and shed virus soon after infection, usually prior to onset or in the absence of clinical signs. Shedding of infectious WNV via oral and cloacal secretions typically begins within 1 to 3 days after infection and may continue intermittently through 14 or more day(s) postinoculation (DPI), albeit at low titers after 7 DPI. Viremia is often detectable by 1 DPI and is cleared by 6 to 8 DPI in raptors that survive acute infection (i.e., approximately 10 DPI or later); peak viremia titers of some experimentally inoculated raptors were relatively high (i.e., >$10^{7.5}$ plaque-forming units/mL serum) between 2 and 4 DPI. WNV also infiltrates multiple organ systems soon after infection and, again, is usually cleared within approximately 1 to 2 weeks in survivors. However, WNV has been detected in tissues of clinically normal raptors for up to 27 DPI.[10,15,16] For raptors that succumb to WNV relatively early after infection (i.e., within 1 to 2 weeks), viral titers in tissues are relatively high at the time of death.

Although the specific roles of innate and adaptive immunity following WNV infection in birds are not known, evidence in mammals suggests that humoral immunity is critical to survival. In raptors, serum antibodies are detectable by approximately 5 to 7 DPI and antibody titers usually increase fourfold or more within the first month after infection; antibodies persist and protect against subsequent infections for 4 years or longer.[15-18]

Clinical responses to WNV infection among raptors range from subclinical (likely the most common) to fatal. Although many species are susceptible to WNV neurologic disease, neurologic syndromes appear to be more common in strigiforms, such as the great horned owl, whereas nonspecific syndromes (e.g., emaciation and dehydration) and feather abnormalities (e.g., pinched-off feathers at the calamus, stunted feather growth) may be more common in some falconiforms, such as the American kestrel, red-tailed hawk, and Swainson's hawk (Buteo swainsoni) and can also occur in owls and eagles[9,18,23] (Figs. 43-1 to 43-4). Consistent with the wide array of WNV clinical manifestations among raptors, death may be rapid and unexpected, whereas complete recovery may be prolonged.[18,24] The precise timeline between WNV infection and subsequent onset and duration of clinical signs has been difficult to determine in naturally infected birds; death occurred between 4 and 13 DPI in experimentally inoculated birds, including two screech owls at 8 to 9 DPI.[10,16]

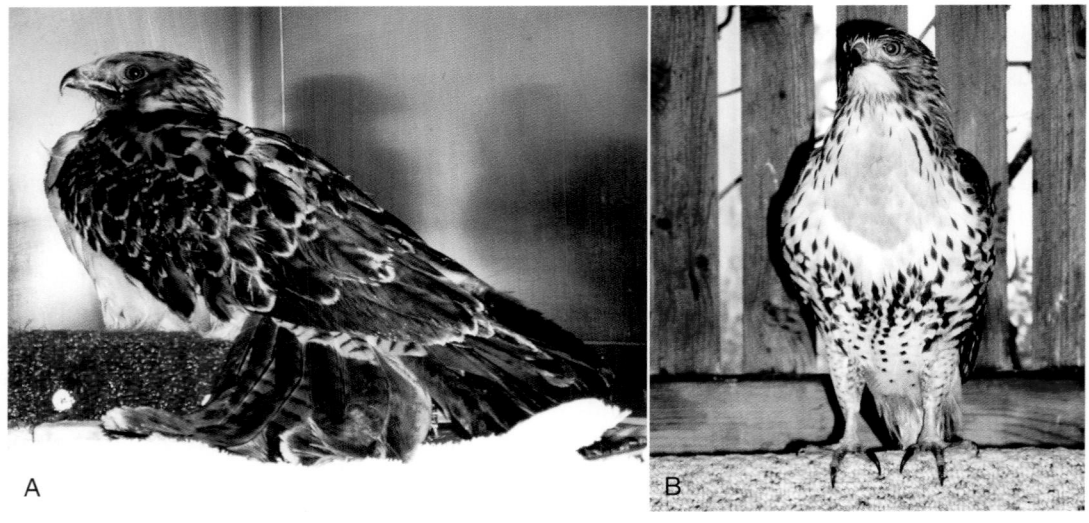

Figure 43-1

A, Red-tailed hawk with acute WNV infection, August 2005, with head tremors, dysphagia, and ataxia.
B, Marked improvement was seen after 10 weeks of supportive and homeopathic care.

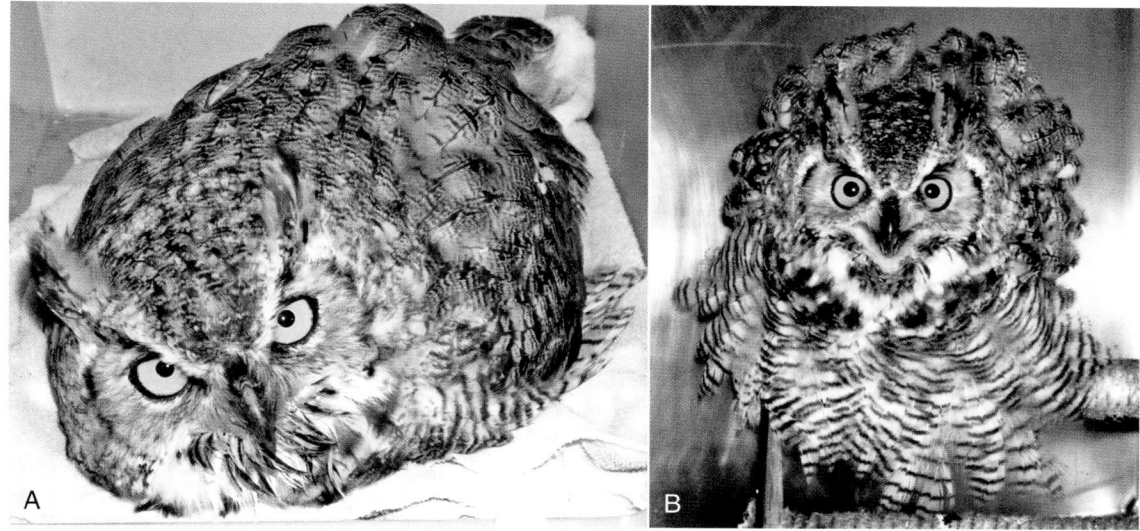

Figure 43-2

A, Great horned owl with acute WNV infection, August 2005, with hindlimb paresis, ataxia, depression, and dysphagia. **B,** Marked improvement was seen after 10 weeks of supportive and homeopathic care.

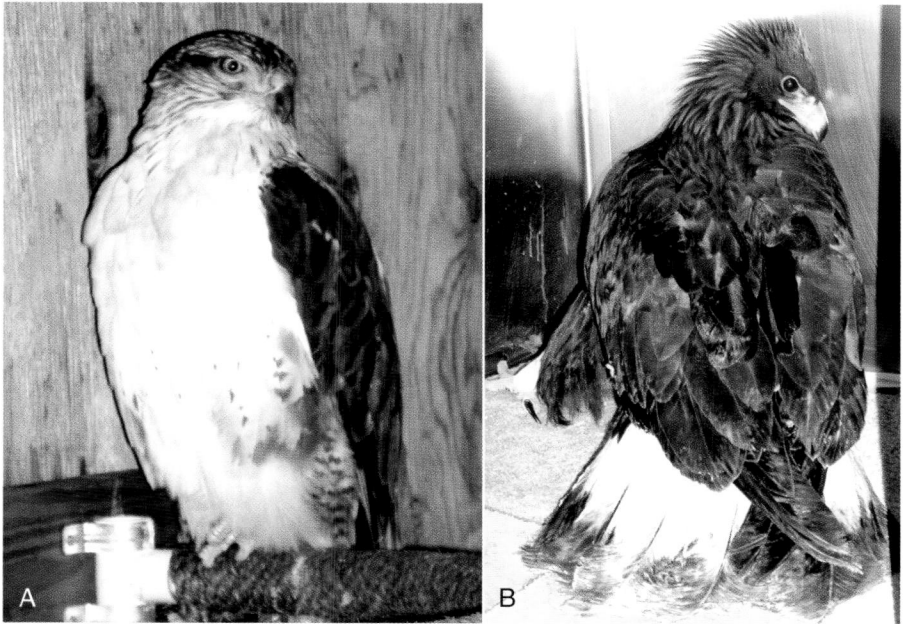

Figure 43-3

WNV-infected raptors. **A,** Recovering educational ferruginous hawk *(Buteo regalis)* that received supportive care early in the course of infection. Clinical signs included ataxia, dehydration, and lethargy of several weeks duration followed by full recovery in approximately 6 weeks. **B,** Golden eagle in rehabilitation that was emaciated and dehydrated and had head tremors and hindlimb rigidity (euthanized 10 weeks after admission).

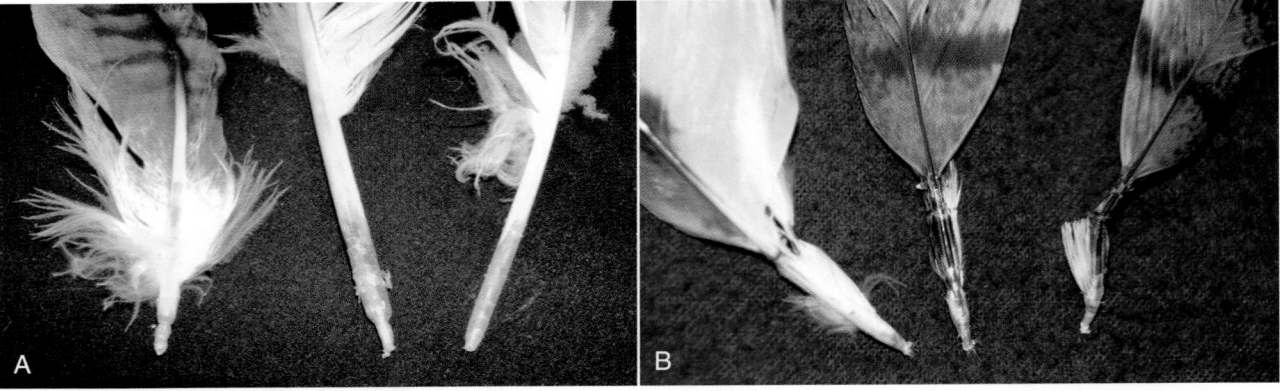

Figure 43-4

Feathers with abnormal morphology that molted prematurely from WNV-infected raptors. **A,** Red-tailed hawk. **B,** Barn owl.

The most commonly reported neurologic signs in WNV-infected raptors include ataxia, head tremors and tilt, and depression. Less commonly reported signs include torticollis; nystagmus and other abnormal pupillary responses; circling; abnormal positioning of tongue, wings, or tail; dysphagia; hind-limb rigidity or paresis; hypersensitivity; and seizures (see Figs. 43-1A, 43-2A, and 43-3B). Although additional causes of neurologic disease should be considered (e.g., trauma, bacterial, toxic, parasitic, metabolic), time of year and recent confirmed presence of WNV in the area are supportive of WNV diagnoses. Nonspecific signs, such as emaciation, dehydration, and lethargy, are also commonly reported and may be the sole indicator of disease or accompany neurologic signs. Less commonly, WNV-infected raptors experience vomiting, peripheral nerve damage, hyperthermia, and gastrointestinal stasis.[9,18,23] Ophthalmic lesions in WNV-infected raptors have included exudative chorioretinal lesions and scarring and anterior uveitis in red-tailed and Cooper's hawks *(Accipiter cooperii)*.[22] Visual impairment has led to blindness in red-tailed and Cooper's hawks and northern goshawks *(A. gentilis)*, and unilateral blindness in bald *(Haliaeetus leucocephalus)* and golden eagles *(Aquila chrysaetos)*.[18,26,27]

The prognosis of WNV-associated disease in raptors is likely affected by health status at the time of infection and timing of initiation of treatment. Raptors provided with appropriate and early supportive care following WNV infection may have an increased chance of surviving acute infection and in some cases appear to fully recover (see Figs. 43-1B, 43-2B, and 43-3A), but some may subsequently suffer from low-grade chronic disease. Little information is available on long-term WNV-

associated neurologic damage in birds, although fatigue, faulty memory, weakness, and motor skill abnormalities have occurred in humans more than 1 year after infection. Subclinical WNV pathology in experimentally inoculated raptors has suggested a potential risk of associated mortality in the wild.[15] In some captive raptors, subtle neurologic signs and feather abnormalities suggestive of WNV infection have been evident for years after initial infection.[18] The occurrence and effects of recrudescent or persistent WNV infection in birds are not well understood.

The outcomes and impacts of WNV infection among free-ranging raptors are difficult to assess. Trauma is not uncommon in WNV-infected raptors admitted to rehabilitation centers and likely occurs after infection as a result of debilitation, starvation, or neurologic deficits; in cases of subclinical WNV infection, trauma may occur independently of infection.[2,9,18,23] Long-lasting feather abnormalities have delayed the release of raptors in rehabilitation, although effects on survival of free-ranging raptors are unknown. Relatively high release rates have been achieved among WNV-infected raptors in rehabilitation, and WNV-associated neurologic disease did not alter the probability of release, although long-term survival outcomes were unknown.[18] Serosurveys among wild raptors have demonstrated that healthy, breeding, WNV-immune individuals were relatively common in regions of Florida, California, Pennsylvania, and Wisconsin.[8,12,14,25]

DIAGNOSIS

Reaching a definitive diagnosis of WNV may be challenging in birds, especially beyond the acute to subacute phases of infection. This is because of the relatively rapid clearance of virus from tissues and secretions of birds that survive these phases, and the variable timing of clinical disease onset. However, controlled infection studies and careful examination of naturally occurring WNV cases have led to a better understanding of the use of various ante mortem and post mortem diagnostic methods.*

Sample collection for ante mortem WNV testing in birds may include blood (i.e., serum or plasma), oral and cloacal swabs, and feathers. Serology is most useful when applied to paired (acute and convalescent) serum samples. Although the presence of anti-WNV antibodies in a single serum sample reveals past infection, little may be concluded about the timing of infection or clinical sequela, and other causes of disease cannot be excluded. On the other hand, a more than fourfold antibody titer increase between paired sera collected 2 to 4 weeks apart suggests recent WNV infection.[15,17-19] Plaque reduction neutralization test (PRNT) is the gold standard for anti-WNV antibody detection and titer determination, although an additional test may be necessary to rule out cross-reactive antibodies to other flaviviruses (e.g., St. Louis encephalitis virus). Alternatively, blocking enzyme-linked immunosorbent assay is useful for high-throughput screening and requires a lower biosafety level, but positive samples should be confirmed by PRNT.

Virus isolation by Vero cell plaque assay is the gold standard for the confirmation of acute WNV infection, and samples should be collected as early as possible to maximize detection probability. Infectious WNV may be detected in sera or swabs as early as 1 DPI and is usually undetectable after approximately 7 to 10 DPI. Reverse transcriptase polymerase chain reaction (RT-PCR) is commonly used as a diagnostic tool to demonstrate the presence of WNV RNA in swabs and tissues. Blood feathers and, to a lesser extent, mature feathers, may be homogenized and tested for WNV; the latter may be stored long term at room temperature prior to homogenization. However, sensitivity is lower than for other tissues.[16,20] VecTest WNV Antigen Assay (Medical Analysis Systems, Fremont, Calif) is a commercially available rapid test developed for mosquitoes that has been assessed for use in birds. Oral or cloacal swabs may be tested by VecTest, although sensitivity is variable and relatively low for some avian groups, including raptors.[5,13] Finally, hematologic abnormalities reported in WNV-infected raptors include anemia and heterophilic leukocytosis with or without monocytosis. However, these findings are inconsistent and likely transient.[1,9,22]

For postmortem diagnosis, virus isolation or RT-PCR of homogenized tissue may be useful. Kidney, spleen, heart, and brain are considered relatively sensitive tissues for WNV detection in birds that die of acute WNV infection, and may be pooled or analyzed singly. However, detection in tissues is rare more than 2 to 3 weeks after infection, making the diagnosis of chronic infection difficult, although feather and eye of several subclinically infected raptors and other birds tested positive relatively late (e.g., approximately 2 to 4 weeks after infection).[15,20] Samples intended for virus isolation or RT-PCR should be refrigerated or placed on wet ice as soon as possible and stored at $-80°$ C if testing is not done on the same day. Immunohistochemistry performed on frozen or formalin-preserved tissue sections may be used for WNV antigen detection.[2,3]

Diagnosis of WNV by gross and histologic examination is generally unreliable, although several lesion patterns may support the diagnosis. Gross lesions among WNV-infected birds have included splenomegaly, focal to multifocal myocardial pallor, cerebral congestion, subdural hematomas over the cerebellum, and intraosseous calvarial hemorrhage. Skeletal muscle wasting, meningeal hemorrhage, cerebral malacia, renal swelling, mottling, enlargement and/or congestion, intestinal and proventricular hemorrhage, and pulmonary congestion, edema, and hemorrhage have been less commonly reported. However, some WNV-infected birds may be in good body condition, with no gross lesions.*

The most common histologic lesions reported in naturally and experimentally WNV-infected raptors include myocarditis, skeletal myositis, encephalitis, meningitis, hepatitis, and interstitial nephritis. These inflammatory lesions are sometimes observed in conjunction with hemorrhage, congestion, necrosis, and/or fibrosis.† In addition, endophthalmitis was observed in great horned owls, goshawks, Cooper's hawks, and red-tailed hawks, with a combination of encephalitis, myocarditis, and endophthalmitis observed in the hawks.[26,27] Ocular lesions in WNV-infected red-tailed and Cooper's hawks included interruption of the retinal pigmented epithelium, retinal necrosis and atrophy, and uveitis. Retinal inflammation was often most pronounced adjacent to the optic disc, sometimes with bilateral or unilateral optic neuritis.[22]

---

*References 2, 5, 10, 15, 16, 19, and 24.

*References 2, 6, 15, 16, 24, and 26.
*References 2, 3, 6, 15, 16, 23, 24, 26, and 27.

TREATMENT, MANAGEMENT, AND PREVENTION

Because there is no specific treatment for WNV infection in raptors or other birds, minimizing mosquito contact to lessen the likelihood of infection is crucial. Environmental control may involve interrupting the mosquito life cycle through chemical, biologic, or mechanical methods such as drainage and irrigation systems, aerial insecticide spraying, and mosquito-eating predators. Smaller scale strategies include eliminating standing water, covering upright containers, and filling holes or depressions. For captive birds housed outdoors, mosquito nets or screens may be used to cover caging. Alternately, bird-safe mosquito repellents (e.g., geraniol, Fasst Products, Brooklyn, NY) aerosolized around caging have been shown to deter mosquitoes.[21]

Treatment of WNV infection in raptors consists of supportive care, such as fluid electrolyte therapy, supplemental heat or cold, antibiotic or antimycotic agents to treat or prevent secondary infections, assisted feeding or nutritional supplementation, and nonsteroidal anti-inflammatory drugs or corticosteroids. In addition, L-lysine and homeopathic remedies have been administered to help fight viral infection and counter specific clinical signs.[11]

Although no WNV vaccinations are currently approved for use in birds, several commercially available equine vaccines (e.g., killed and recombinant canarypox-vectored vaccines) and other vaccine candidates (e.g., plasmid-mediated DNA and recombinant virus chimera) have been tested in birds. Results thus far indicate that seroconversion rates are generally low following vaccination and may vary by species and vaccine construction. Furthermore, few data are available regarding vaccine-induced protection against virus challenge, especially in raptors. In addition, maternal antibodies may interfere with vaccine responses of young birds (e.g., younger than 8 weeks).[7]

Acknowledgments

Many dedicated raptor rehabilitators, educators, biologists, and volunteers have contributed to the understanding of WNV in raptors.

REFERENCES

1. D'Agostino JJ, Isaza R: Clinical signs and results of specific diagnostic testing among captive birds housed at zoological institutions and infected with West Nile virus. J Am Vet Med Assoc 224:1640–1643, 2004.
2. Ellis AE, Mead DG, Allison AB, et al: Pathology and epidemiology of natural West Nile viral infection of raptors in Georgia. J Wildl Dis 43:214–223, 2007.
3. Fitzgerald SD, Patterson JS, Kiupel M, et al: Clinical and pathological features of West Nile virus infection in native North American owls (family Strigidae). Avian Dis 47:602–610, 2003.
4. Gancz AY, Barker IK, Lindsay R, et al: West Nile virus outbreak in North American owls, Ontario, 2002. Emerg Infect Dis 10:2135–2142, 2004.
5. Gancz AY, Campbell DG, Barker IK, et al: Detecting West Nile virus in owls and raptors by an antigen-capture assay. Emerg Infect Dis 10:2204–2206, 2004.
6. Gancz AY, Smith D, Barker IK, et al: Pathology and tissue distribution of West Nile virus in North American owls (family: strigidae). Avian Pathol 35:17–29, 2006.
7. Hahn DC, Nemeth NM, Edwards E, et al: Passive West Nile virus antibody transfer from maternal Eastern screech-owls (Megascops asio) to progeny. Avian Dis 50:454–455, 2006.
8. Hull J, Hull A, Reisen W, et al: Variation of West Nile virus antibody prevalence in migrating and wintering hawks in central California. Condor 108:435–439, 2006.
9. Joyner PH, Kelly S, Shreve AA, et al: West Nile virus in raptors from Virginia during 2003: Clinical, diagnostic, and epidemiologic findings. J Wildl Dis 42:335–344, 2006.
10. Komar N, Langevin S, Hinten S, et al: Experimental infection of North American birds with the New York 1999 strain of West Nile virus, Emerg Infect Dis 9:311–322, 2003.
11. Kratz G: personal communication, 2008.
12. Medica DL, Clauser R, Bildstein K: Prevalence of West Nile virus antibodies in a breeding population of American kestrels (Falco sparverius) in Pennsylvania. J Wildl Dis 43:538–541, 2007.
13. Nemeth NM, Beckett S, Edwards E, et al: Avian mortality surveillance for West Nile virus in Colorado. Am J Trop Med Hyg 76:431–437, 2007.
14. Nemeth N, Dwyer J, Morrison J, Fraser J: Seroprevalence rates of West Nile virus and other arboviruses among crested caracaras (Caracara cheriway) in Florida. J Wildl Dis 45:817–822, 2009.
15. Nemeth N, Gould D, Bowen R, Komar N: Natural and experimental West Nile virus infection in five raptor species. J Wildl Dis 42:1–13, 2006.
16. Nemeth NM, Hahn DC, Gould DH, Bowen RA: Experimental West Nile virus infection in eastern screech owls (Megascops asio). Avian Dis 50:252–258, 2006.
17. Nemeth N, Kratz GE, Bates R, et al: Naturally induced humoral immunity to West Nile virus. EcoHealth 5:298–304, 2008.
18. Nemeth N, Kratz GE, Bates R, et al: Clinical evaluation and outcomes of naturally acquired West Nile virus infection in raptors. J Zoo Wildl Med 40:51–63, 2009.
19. Nemeth N, Kratz G, Edwards E, et al: Surveillance for West Nile virus in clinic-admitted raptors, Colorado. Emerg Infect Dis 13:305–307, 2007.
20. Nemeth NM, Young GR, Burkhalter KL, et al: West Nile virus detection in non-vascular feathers from avian carcasses. J Vet Diagn Invest 21:616–622, 2009.
21. Price A: personal communication, 2010.
22. Pauli AM, Cruz-Martinez LA, Ponder JB, et al: Ophthalmologic and oculopathologic findings in red-tailed hawks and Cooper's hawks with naturally acquired West Nile virus infection. J Am Vet Med Assoc 231:1240–1248, 2007.
23. Saito EK, Sileo L, Green DE, et al: Raptor mortality due to West Nile virus in the United States, 2002. J Wildl Dis 43:206–213, 2007.

24. Steele KE, Linn MJ, Schoepp RJ, et al: Pathology of fatal West Nile virus infections in native and exotic birds during the 1999 outbreak in New York City, New York. Vet Pathol 37:208–224, 2000.
25. Stout WE, Cassini AG, Meece JK, et al: Serologic evidence of West Nile virus infection in three wild raptor populations. Avian Dis 49:371–375, 2005.
26. Wünschmann A, Shivers J, Bender J, et al: Pathologic findings in red-tailed hawks *(Buteo jamaicensis)* and Cooper's hawks *(Accipiter cooperi)* naturally infected with West Nile virus. Avian Dis 48:570–580, 2004.
27. Wünschmann A, Shivers J, Bender J, et al: Pathologic and immunohistochemical findings in goshawks *(Accipiter gentilis)* and great horned owls *(Bubo virginianus)* naturally infected with West Nile virus. Avian Dis 49:252–259, 2005.

CHAPTER 44

Diagnosis of Aspergillosis in Avian Species

Carolyn Cray

Invasive aspergillosis presents a diagnostic dilemma in mammalian and avian species.[3,19,20,25,26] Traditional techniques such as routine hematology and plasma biochemistry may complement radiographic investigations but results rarely provide a definitive diagnosis. Endoscopy is often available but is invasive and may not be readily used on severely ill birds.[17] Serologic test panels have been recently implemented and described for use in avian species.* This chapter summarizes this information as well as these and other studies undertaking a multidimensional diagnostic approach to detecting this disease.

ANTIBODY DETECTION

In clinical veterinary medicine, the value of serodiagnostic testing to detect antibody levels has been described in horses, dogs, and birds.† Primary methodologies available at some veterinary laboratories include agarose immunodiffusion (AGID) and enzyme-linked immunosorbent assay (ELISA). For AGID, a positive reaction is displayed in the form of a precipitin line of antibody-antigen complexes in the agarose media. This test is qualitative or semiquantitative at best. The method offers no restrictions regarding the species from which the specimen is derived because no secondary reagents are needed. However, because the interpretation is visual, the sensitivity of the test is limited. In contrast, ELISA offers increased sensitivity and specificity although its use is restricted to specimens for which secondary reagents are available (e.g., anticanine immunoglobulin G [IgG]). In the United States, AGID remains the more commercially available method. In 1994, Brown and Redig[4] described the implementation and use of ELISA

in companion birds and raptors. This assay was commercially available for many years, as is the ELISA methodology currently offered by the University of Miami, which was described in a recent publication.[9]

Martinez-Quesada and coworkers have demonstrated antibody titers in pigeons that were immunized with *Aspergillus fumigatus* extracts.[24] In this study, IgG titers were demonstrable from 14 days postimmunization, with a peak at 63 days. Titers were demonstrable, albeit lower, through 210 days, but booster immunizations resulted in the production of high levels of antibody. A high seroprevalence of antibody has been described in captive and wild penguins by ELISA.[13,15,27] German and associates[13] have observed that 93% (of 61 penguins) were seropositive and serostatus could not be correlated with clinical disease. This was similar to another study of captive penguins, in which the high seroprevalence prompted the authors to suggest that most penguins are infected or colonized by *Aspergillus* spp.[27] In an experimental model of infection in two duck species, Graczyk and colleagues concluded that the applicability of the antibody ELISA is low.[14] These studies suggest that antibody levels may be high in many avian species with a normal clinical condition. These levels may be long-lived and perhaps subject to restimulation through continued environmental exposure to *Aspergillus* spp.

In a recent study that included a large serosurvey of different avian species ($N = 1314$), Cray et al.[9] reported that most avian species grouped as zoo species (mostly land and waterfowl species), raptors, and penguins were seropositive for antibody to *Aspergillus* spp. (Table 44-1). This was in contrast to the psittaciform group, which only had a 32% positive serostatus. Additional data was gathered on 303 of the submissions, which enabled them to be categorized as presumptive nonaspergillosis, probable (on the basis of clinical signs and response to

*References 1, 6, 7, 9, 21, and 22.
†References 2, 8, 12-14, 16, 21, 22, and 24.

TABLE 44-1	*Aspergillus* Panel Reactivity by Avian Groups Without Regard to Clinical Status*								
		ANTIBODY			GALACTOMANNAN			EPH	
Avian Group	No. in Study	Positive ≥1.4 (%)	Negative <1.4 (%)	Mean Index (SE)	Positive ≥0.5 (%)	Negative <0.5 (%)	Mean Index (SE)	Abnormal (%)	Normal (%)
1. Psittacine	886	32[†]	68	1.22 (0.01)[†]	44[¶]	56	0.85 (0.04)[†]	40[†]	60
2. Zoo	216	86[‡]	14	1.85 (0.03)[§]	20	80	0.39 (0.09)	61	39
3. Raptor	104	93	7	1.88 (0.04)[‖]	25	75	0.49 (0.12)	69	31
4. Penguin	108	98	2	2.01 (0.04)	23	77	0.43 (0.11)	64	36

*Percentage of positive and negative results and mean index (SE). EPH cases were assigned as abnormal based on an increase of at least 20% in any globulin fraction.[7,9]
[†]P < 0.001 versus groups 2-4.
[‡]P = 0.004 versus penguin group.
[§]P = 0.001 versus penguin group.
[‖]P = 0.023 versus penguin group.
[¶]P < 0.01 versus groups 2-4.

TABLE 44-2	Antibody, Polyclonal Antigen, and Galactomannan Assays by Clinical Group*				
Clinical Group	No. in Study	Antibody		Galactomannan	
Normal	70	1.26 ± 0.05	P[†]	0.64 ± 0.19	P
Probable	176	1.35 ± 0.03	0.131	1.13 ± 0.12	0.030
Confirmed	57	1.41 ± 0.06	0.059	1.68 ± 0.23	0.001

*Mean and standard error of index results.
[†]P values shown as analysis versus the normal group.[6,8]

treatment), or confirmed (on the basis of histology, culture, and/or polymerase chain reaction [PCR] assay on necropsy or biopsy tissues). Most of these cases represented psittaciform species. This data is presented in Table 44-2 and shows no significant differences between the clinical groups (P = 0.059). The results are consistent with a small study of seven psittaciform birds with confirmed aspergillosis.[17] Interestingly, when the data was examined as percentage positive cases (index ≥1.4), 69% of the presumptive normal birds were negative versus only 42% of the confirmed cases (P = 0.022).

Although the antibody ELISA may have limited value as a single serodiagnostic test for avian species, it may still have some applicability. Whereas antibody serostatus may be of small consequence in zoo species, raptors, and penguins, with most birds being seropositive, most psittaciform cases in this study were seronegative.[9] Therefore, the presence of antibody in this species would be considered unusual and perhaps clinically remarkable. In addition, positive antibody serostatus was more often observed in those birds with confirmed infection, although the actual antibody index

was not a strong indicator of infection. That is, the qualitative rather than the quantitative result may be helpful in some avian species.

It has been proposed that cell-mediated immunity, especially Th1 responses, are important in modulating macrophage responses in aspergillosis.[3] Given this premise, it would be expected that antibody responses, which are mediated via the Th2 pathway, would not be a primary effector mechanism in the proper response to *Aspergillus* spp., although it may provide help in the initial resistance to infection. Antibody titers may also vary with the health status of the patient. Low levels of antibody reactivity may be present because of the immunosuppressive properties of toxins secreted by *Aspergillus* spp.

The value of antibody detection in the diagnosis of avian aspergillosis should be revisited with modifications to existing ELISA methods and the use of other methods with greater sensitivity to specific antigens of *Aspergillus* spp. The current ELISA method uses a secondary reagent that is cross-reactive with many avian species, and this may limit assay sensitivity. It may also necessitate the definition of species-specific cutoff levels. That is, the use of the positive cutoff index of 1.4 may need adjustment for some species. Implementing an ELISA or Western blot test with select *Aspergillus* spp. antigens rather than a bulk unfractionated preparation may also improve assay sensitivity and specificity, as well as allow for the study of the relative importance of antigen specificity and particular humoral immune responses in the reaction to *Aspergillus* spp. infection. These types of assays may also provide better prognostic information.

ANTIGEN DETECTION: GALACTOMANNAN

Galactomannan is a major component of the fungal cell wall that is released during the growth of hyphae. With invasive infection, this antigen may be found in the blood circulation. A commercially available ELISA that is reactive to β-(1-5)-galactofuranose has been widely implemented in human clinical pathology laboratories for the detection of invasive aspergillosis in immuno-suppressed patients in whom fungal disease is opportunistic and often associated with high rates of morbidity and mortality.[26] This population, given the severe immunosuppression and presence of chronic disease, rarely produce antibody to *Aspergillus* spp., making an antigen detection test a potentially ideal method. The ELISA is based on the sandwich method and, because it is based on internal positive and negative controls, the result is reported as an index with no units. Because of changing guidelines for human use, many early studies (through 2006) often used an index of 1.5 or 1.0 as a positive cutoff value. To improve the sensitivity of the assay, the guidelines were later changed to 0.5. When reviewing the literature, especially with reference to sensitivity and specificity, it is important to reference the cutoff level that was used in the respective studies.

In addition to the validation of the galactomannan ELISA in human and animal models of invasive aspergillosis (including rodents, guinea pigs, and rabbits), the assay has been studied in horses, cows, dogs, and avian species.* In dogs with aspergillosis, Garcia and coworkers[12] reported a high frequency of antibody as measured by ELISA versus a variable presence of galactomannan. The latter was consistently observed only in a dog with systemic infection and a dog with a severe bronchopneumonia that progressed to death. In horses

*References 1, 6, 7, 18, 21, and 22.

that often demonstrated antibody reactivity to *Aspergillus* spp., galactomannan was detected in a case with systemic aspergillosis but not in those with guttural pouch infection, an important point to note.[16] In cows experimentally infected with *A. fumigatus* as well as in cows with naturally occurring systemic infection, galactomannan was detected.[18] Notably, this study also reported that the level of galactomannan likely is associated with the burden of infection, a finding that had also been suggested by reports of human cases and in laboratory animal models.[26]

In a study of experimental infection in ducks using an early bench top version of the galactomannan assay, Graczyk and colleagues[14] were the first to report the possible high predictive value for antigen detection in invasive aspergillosis. Le Loc'h and associates[21,22] reported a specificity of 86% and positive predictive value of 75% for the commercial galactomannan ELISA in a collection of specimens from psittaciform species with suspected infection. However, using a positive index cutoff of 1.0, they observed a low sensitivity of 30%. In those birds with the poorest general health, the galactomannan values were observed to be the highest (index >3.5). In addition, birds showing signs of invasive infection were twice as likely to be positive than those with only respiratory signs. The galactomannan ELISA was also evaluated in a large study of falcons.[1] Comparing confirmed cases and confirmed aspergillosis-negative cases, a sensitivity of 12% and specificity of 85% were reported. This study was also conducted with the higher 1.0 index cutoff level. Given this data analysis, it was concluded that the assay should not be used as a screening test for aspergillosis in falcon species.

Galactomannan was also examined in a large study by Cray and coworkers.[7] In a general serosurvey using a positive cutoff index of 0.5, 20% to 25% of zoo species, raptors, and penguins were found to be positive for circulating galactomannan (see Table 44-1). This was significantly lower than that observed in specimens from the psittaciform group. In the extended study of presumptive nonaspergillosis, probable, and confirmed cases (as described earlier), significantly higher levels of galactomannan were observed in the probable and confirmed groups (see Table 44-2). The sensitivity was 67% and the specificity was 73%. When the data were reanalyzed with a positive cutoff level of 1.0, the sensitivity decreased to 39% and the specificity increased to 83%. These results are consistent with those reported by Arca-Ruibal and colleagues[1] and Le Loc'h and associates.[21,22] Given the observation of the mean value of the presumptive nonaspergillosis group to be 0.64, the

University of Miami currently uses the value of 0.7 or higher as the positive cutoff index for avian samples.

The galactomannan ELISA is used in human patients with reservation. Some cross-reactivity has been reported with other microbial antigens, including *Penicillium* spp. and *Histoplasma capsulatum.*[26] In addition, positive indices may be observed in clinically normal individuals exposed to galactomannan in the environment via food, drink, intravenous hydration or nutrition fluids, use of piperacillin or other beta-lactam antibiotics, or environmental aerosols. Antigenemia is also considered to be variable under any infectious process. This has been observed in humans and in dogs in which periodic testing has been performed.[12] Biologic factors, including the site of infection and the microenvironment at the site, may help or hinder the presence of galactomannan in the blood circulation. In a report of several confirmed cases of aspergillosis, Cray and coworkers[6] found negative galactomannan levels in a cockatoo with infection limited to a tracheal granuloma. This is in contrast to two cases with lung and air sac involvement, in which indices ranged from 5.3 to 6.7. In addition, recent exposure to antifungal agents as well as the presence of anti-*Aspergillus* antibodies may affect the galactomannan levels. The latter may be especially problematic in use of the assay in avian species. As reported, zoo species, raptors, and penguins often have high circulating levels of antibody. The presence of antibody may effectively clear the circulating galactomannan such that it is not detected by the ELISA. This may account for the data in the current study. In psittaciform species, in which antibody reactivity is less frequently observed, higher levels of galactomannan were observed in the serosurvey versus zoo species, raptors, and penguins (see Table 44-1). I have frequently observed this dichotomy of antibody and galactomannan results in the laboratory. That is, very high-level antibody indices are often accompanied by negative galactomannan indices. Thus, although the predictive value of an individual antibody ELISA result is of questionable value, it is important to know the level of antibody when interpreting the galactomannan result.

PROTEIN ELECTROPHORESIS

Protein electrophoresis (EPH) has been implemented for use in veterinary medicine for many years with specimens from mammals and has been more recently recognized for its applicability in detecting acute phase and humoral immune responses in avian species.[6-8,10,23] Because inflammatory pathways may be common to many diseases, EPH may not be solely diagnostic of any one particular disease. It may be used in conjunction with serodiagnostic testing and routine clinical testing to determine the presence of underlying inflammatory or infectious processes.

Using species-specific reference intervals, the frequency of abnormal EPH results was studied as part of the general serosurvey described earlier.[7] A significantly lower percentage of specimens from psittaciform species were abnormal versus those specimens from zoo species, raptors, or penguins. (see Table 44-1). Results from specimens from presumptive nonaspergillosis cases were also compared with confirmed cases. Whereas only 30% of the presumptive group had abnormal EPH results, 72% of the confirmed group had abnormal EPH results. Increases in beta globulins were most common, followed by combined beta and gamma globulin increases and gamma globulin increases alone. The sensitivity of the test was 73% and the specificity was 70%. These results were supported by two smaller case studies of aspergillosis in psittaciform species.[6,17]

OTHER TESTS

Given variable test sensitivity and specificity, as well as the course of infection, a multidimensional approach to diagnosis is important.[19] Routine diagnostic test options include traditional hematology and plasma biochemistry. Hematologic changes have included a leukocytosis with a heterophilia, monocytosis, and lymphopenia, as well as possible nonregenerative anemia. Plasma biochemistry changes may include increases in aspartate aminotransferase (AST) and creatine kinase (CK) levels. In a recent review of aspergillosis cases in psittaciform species, we observed that less than 40% of cases demonstrated leukocytosis.[6] Mild heterophilia was observed in 27% of cases and no monocytosis or anemia was observed. Plasma biochemistry analyses were not consistently present as part of these evaluations although, of those available, both AST and CK levels were elevated. Other test options may become more readily available in the near future. These assays are summarized here.

Beta-Glucan

Beta-glucans are major components of the cell wall of most fungal species. A commercial assay is available to detect 1-3-beta-D-glucan and has been implemented in recent years for the detection of fungal infection, including aspergillosis, in human patients.[25] Some studies have suggested that beta-glucan detection may offer greater sensitivity than galactomannan for the diagnosis of invasive aspergillosis in humans, although its lack of specificity may limit its overall usefulness. The assay has been found to be reproducible except at levels near the positive cutoff, making low positive results problematic to interpret. It is also complicated by the high probability of false-positive results. In humans, false results have been observed in dialysis patients and those who have received commercial blood components, because beta-glucan is present in cellulose filters. Intraoperative gauze, many antibiotics, and bacteremia may also affect the test. Given its limitations of specificity, it has been suggested that a negative result may be more useful than a positive result.

Other than its use in laboratory animal models of invasive aspergillosis, studies of the application of beta-glucan to veterinary medicine remain unpublished. In a small study of confirmed cases of aspergillosis in duck species, I have observed positive beta-glucan results, although some control specimens also showed high beta-glucan levels. In a larger study of chickens with confirmed A. flavus infection, the value of beta-glucan also appeared limited, with very high levels observed in uninfected chickens.[28] In contrast, in a study of sea birds at a rehabilitation center, plasma beta-glucan levels were significantly higher in specimens from those birds with confirmed infection.[5]

Polymerase Chain Reaction

As with many other infectious diseases, the use of the PCR assay may offer increased sensitivity and specificity. Interestingly, when the PCR assay was used in cases of aspergillosis in human patients, sensitivity ranged from 36% to 98% and specificity ranged from 72% to 100%. These results reflect wide laboratory differences in this method, likely based on specimen type, extraction procedures, nucleic acid targets, and amplification platforms.[20] When a direct comparison was made between galactomannan and PCR tests, the PCR method was either no more sensitive or much less sensitive than galactomannan. The combined use of PCR and galactomannan ELISA appeared to provide higher sensitivity and specificity in many reports.

To date, a PCR method has not been validated for use with human specimens.[20] Several veterinary laboratories offer PCR for Aspergillus spp. Its best current use may be with the amplification of fungal DNA from granuloma biopsy or necropsy specimens or from a swab of the trachea, air sac, or air sac fluids. Testing of blood samples has been found to provide variable results. When positive, blood samples correlate well with clinical infection. However, negative blood PCR test results do not rule out active infection.[11]

SUMMARY OF AVIAN STUDIES

It is expected that additional studies on the test applications for the serodiagnosis of avian aspergillosis will be published in the near-future. This section summarizes published and unpublished data.

Antibody Detection

Birds immunized with A. fumigatus may mount significant humoral immune responses as measured by antibody detection methods, including ELISA. However, studies of both experimental and natural infection in avian species have suggested that the presence of antibody may have limited value for the diagnosis of aspergillosis.*

Antigen Detection

A commercially available test to detect galactomannan, which has been widely applied to human specimens with good results, has applicability for the diagnosis of aspergillosis in avian species. The presence of circulating galactomannan has been described to have a negative predictive value of 76% and a positive predictive value of 63% in a study of confirmed cases dominated by psittaciform species.[6,7] The sensitivity was 67% and the specificity was 73%. Using a higher positive cutoff level in other studies of psittaciform species and falcons, the specificity was very high but the sensitivity was greatly impaired.[1,21,22] Recently, a newly implemented assay for beta-glucan has been shown to have promise in human specimens but variable results were obtained in unpublished studies of avian specimens.

Protein Electrophoresis

Protein electrophoresis has been demonstrated to be a sensitive indicator of inflammation and infection in mammalian and avian species. Small studies of confirmed infection in psittaciform species have suggested that EPH abnormalities are the most consistent changes in plasma biochemistry.[6,17] Similar findings were observed in penguins with naturally acquired infection.[27] In a larger study of confirmed cases, Cray and

*References 2, 4, 9, 12-16, 21, 22, 24, and 27.

colleagues[7] examined specimens for a change in any globulin fraction. The presence of an abnormal EPH was reported to have a sensitivity of 73% and specificity of 70%. The negative predictive value was 76% and the positive predictive value was 66%.

Combination of Testing Options

Because no one test has 100% sensitivity and specificity, and infection may be acute or chronic, using a combination of testing options may be of benefit, at least in the initial testing phase. Interestingly, when galactomannan and EPH results were combined, the overall sensitivity increased to 89% but the specificity decreased to 48%, likely because of the wide ranges of conditions that may be reflected by EPH globulin abnormalities.[7] Overall, what is notable is that the value of the tests as a panel (antibody, galactomannan, EPH) may increase the sensitivity. I have noted that the more positives (or abnormals) that are recorded on the panel, the higher the predictive value.

Other Notable Unpublished Studies

Over a 2-month period, mortalities were observed in young chickens (18 to 32 days) caused by infection with *A. flavus*. The organism was observed not only in lungs and air sacs but, in many cases, infection was also invasive to other organs. Serum samples from these birds (*n* = 62) were analyzed by ELISA for *Aspergillus* galactomannan, *Aspergillus* antibody, and beta-glucan. Samples from a group of birds without *Aspergillus* lesions were used as a control (*n* = 10). Mean galactomannan values were 1.3 to 2.0 times higher in the infected chickens, although the mean value for galactomannan in the control birds was much higher than that reported in other species. Many antibody levels were two- to three-fold higher in the infected birds. Notably, there was no difference in beta-glucan levels between the groups.[28] The presence of high galactomannan levels in the control group may reflect a significant exposure to this organism in the environment in which they were housed. Similarly, the lack of a difference in beta-glucan levels may be attributed to environmental exposure to and/or colonization by other fungal or yeast species.

A small study was conducted on sea birds in a rehabilitation center in northern California. Plasma and tracheal lavage samples were collected from 13 confirmed aspergillosis-positive and 42 aspergillosis-negative birds based on the gold standard of culture and histopathology. Both tracheal lavage and plasma galactomannan

levels were significantly higher in the infected birds. Plasma beta-glucan levels were also significantly higher in this group. Consistent changes in protein electrophoresis results were observed, which included a decrease in albumin and elevation of gamma globulin levels.[5]

CURRENT RECOMMENDATIONS AND FUTURE DIRECTIONS

The current test panel of antibody ELISA, galactomannan ELISA, and protein electrophoresis is commercially available at the University of Miami Avian and Wildlife Laboratory. Specimens can be submitted directly to this laboratory or other reference laboratories. As noted, each test offers a different approach to the diagnosis of avian aspergillosis and the combined panel may offer more interpretive and predictive value rather being limited to the use of the individual test components. Once a diagnosis is reached, individual tests may be revisited for their prognostic value. Of note, most of the data collected thus far is based on specimens from psittacine species. Practitioners should seek updates, not only as the database of species is enlarged but also as new tests or new variations of current tests become readily available.

It is notable that the more recent methodologies for diagnosing invasive aspergillosis that have been pursued in avian medicine have been adapted from advancements made in human clinical pathology testing. These include galactomannan and beta-glucan detection and PCR technologies. Recently, the National Institute of Allergy and Infectious Diseases issued a request for applications entitled "Innovative Approaches to Target Identification and Assay Development for Fungal Diagnosis." These applications were reviewed in mid-2009 and work began in 2010. Several novel technologies and investigations have received funding that will likely benefit human and veterinary medicine in the future. Although there is always hope for a gold standard test in the diagnosis of this disease process to be developed, the variation in species, genetics, and course of disease will always necessitate a multidimensional approach to diagnosis.

REFERENCES

1. Arca-Ruibal B, Wernery U, Zachariah R, et al: Assessment of a commercial sandwich ELISA in the diagnosis of aspergillosis in falcons. Vet Rec 158:442–444, 2006.
2. Billen F, Peeters D, Peters IR, et al: Comparison of the value of measurement of serum galactomannan and *Aspergillus*-specific

antibodies in the diagnosis of canine sino-nasal aspergillosis. Vet Microbiol 133:358–365, 2009.

3. Blanco JL, Garcia ME: Immune response to fungal infections. Vet Immunol Immunopathol 125:47–70, 2008.

4. Brown PA, Redig PT: Aspergillus ELISA: a tool for detection and management. In Proceedings of the Annual Conference of the American Association of Zoo Veterinarians, 1994, pp 295–297.

5. Burco J: Personal communication, 2010.

6. Cray C, Reavill DR, Romagnano A, et al: Galactomannan assay and protein electrophoresis findings in psittacine birds with aspergillosis. J Avian Med Surg 23:125–135, 2009.

7. Cray C, Watson T, Rodriguez M, Arheart K: Application of galactomannan analysis and protein electrophoresis in the diagnosis of aspergillosis in avian species. J Zoo Wildl Med 40:64–70, 2009.

8. Cray C, Tatum L: Application of protein electrophoresis in avian diagnostic testing. J Avian Med Surg 12:4–10, 1998.

9. Cray C, Watson T, Arheart KL: Serosurvey and diagnostic application of antibody titers to Aspergillus in avian species. Avian Dis 53:491–494, 2009.

10. Cray C, Rodriguez M, Zaias J: Protein electrophoresis of psittacine plasma. Vet Clin Pathol 36:64–72, 2007.

11. Dahlhausen B: Personal communication, 2010.

12. Garcia ME, Caballero J, Cruzado M, et al: The value of the determination of anti-Aspergillus IgG in the serodiagnosis of canine aspergillosis: Comparison with galactomannan detection. J Vet Med B 48:743–750, 2001.

13. German AC, Shankland GS, Edwards J, et al: Development of an indirect ELISA for the detection of serum antibodies to Aspergillus fumigatus in captive penguins. Vet Rec 150:513–518, 2002.

14. Graczyk TK, Cranfield MR, Klein PN: Value of antigen and antibody detection, and blood evaluation parameters in diagnosis of avian invasive aspergillosis. Mycopathologia 140:121–127, 1998.

15. Graczyk TK, Cockrem JF: Aspergillus spp. seropositivity in New Zealand penguins. Mycopathologia 131:179–184, 1995.

16. Guillot J, Sarfati J, de Barros M, et al: Comparative study of serological tests for the diagnosis of equine aspergillosis. Vet Rec 145:348–349, 1999.

17. Ivey ES: Serologic and plasma protein electrophoretic findings in 7 psittacine birds with aspergillosis. J Avian Med Surg 14:103–106, 2000.

18. Jensen HE, Stynen D, Sarfati J, et al: Detection of galactomannan and the 18-kDa antigen from Aspergillus fumigatus in serum and urine from cattle with systemic aspergillosis. J Vet Med B 40:397–408, 1993.

19. Jones MR, Orosz SE: The diagnosis of aspergillosis in birds. Semin Avian Exotic Pet Med 9:52–58, 2000.

20. Klingspor L, Loeffler J: Aspergillus PCR: Formidable challenges and progress. Med Mycol 47(Suppl 1):S241–S247, 2009.

21. Le Loc'h G, Arne P, Bourgerol C, et al: Detection of circulating serum galactomannan for the diagnosis of avian aspergillosis. In Proceedings of the 16th International Congress for Human and Animal Mycology, 2006, Imedex, Atlanta, GA, P-0020.

22. Le Loc'h G, Deville M, Risi E, et al: Evaluation of the serological test Platelia Aspergillus for the diagnosis of aspergillosis. Proc Eur Assoc Avian Vet 260–266, 2005.

23. Lumeij JT: Avian clinical biochemistry. In Kaneko JJ, Harvey JW, Bruss ML, editors: Clinical biochemistry of domestic animals, ed 5, San Diego, Calif, 1997, Academic Press, pp 857–883.

24. Martinez-Quesada J, Nieto-Cadenazzi A, Torres-Rodriguez JM: Humoral immunoresponse of pigeons to Aspergillus fumigatus antigens. Mycopathologia 124:131–137, 1993.

25. Marty FM, Koo S: Role of (1->3)-beta-D-glucan in the diagnosis of invasive aspergillosis. Med Mycol 47(suppl 1):S233–S240, 2009.

26. Mennink-Kersten MA, Donnelly JP, Verweij PE: Detection of circulating galactomannan for the diagnosis and management of invasive aspergillosis. Lancet Infect Dis 4:349–357, 2004.

27. Reidardson TH, McBain JF: Diagnosis and treatment of aspergillosis in temperate penguins. Erkrank Zootiere 34:155–158, 1992.

28. Shivaprasad HL: Personal communication, 2010.

CHAPTER 45

Avian Influenza H5N1 Virus: Epidemiology in Wild Birds, Zoo Outbreaks, and Zoo Vaccination Policy

Martin Gilbert and Joost Philippa

Influenza A viruses are a genus of highly variable, negative-strand RNA viruses within the family Orthomyxoviridae. Influenza A viruses infect birds and a number of mammals, including humans, but exhibit greatest diversity among avian taxa, particularly Anseriformes (ducks, geese, swans, and allies) and Charadriiformes (waders, gulls, auks, and allies), which are widely believed to constitute the natural reservoir.[25] The genus is characterized using the antigenic characteristic of two surface glycoproteins, hemagglutinin (16 subtypes) and neuraminidase (9 subtypes). Some strains of the H5 and H7 subtypes are capable of causing high mortality in domestic poultry (up to 100%), and are termed *highly pathogenic avian influenza* (HPAI) viruses, with others causing low mortality to poultry being termed *low- pathogenic avian influenza* (LPAI) viruses.[26] HPAI virus strains are believed to arise through mutation and selection of an LPAI progenitor virus, following introduction into domestic birds.[2] In the last half-century, there have been 26 recorded epizootics of HPAI virus, the largest of which is the current epizootic of HPAI H5N1 virus that emerged in 1996.[2]

CURRENT HIGHLY PATHOGENIC AVIAN INFLUENZA H5N1 VIRUS EPIZOOTIC

In 1996, an HPAI virus of the H5N1 subtype was isolated from an outbreak affecting domestic geese in Guangdong Province, China. A year later, a related virus emerged in Hong Kong that affected poultry, and led to the first human clinical respiratory cases, with hospitalization of 18 patients, of whom 6 died. Subsequent isolates in neighboring territories from 1998 to 2002 suggested that the virus continued to circulate in China, undergoing a number of genetic reassortments.[23] In late 2003 and early 2004, eight countries in East and Southeast Asia reported outbreaks for the first time,[1] with the virus establishing itself in some areas, particularly those integrating rice cultivation with free grazing of domestic ducks.[13] By 2005, multiple sublineages of HPAI H5N1 virus had become established among domestic poultry in geographic subregions of Asia, indicating long-term endemicity and spatial isolation.[7] Phylogenetic classification of these viruses, using a unified nomenclature based on H5N1 hemagglutination (HA) sequences from the goose Guangdong lineage, identified 10 major clades (designated 0 to 9) and numerous subclades.[28] In spring 2005, an outbreak affecting wild migratory waterfowl in Qinghai Province, China,[6] marked the onset of a range expansion that saw outbreaks in wild and domestic birds recorded over an area extending progressively westward through Central Asia to Europe to the Middle East and Africa.

By the end of 2009, 62 countries or territories had recorded outbreaks of HPAI H5N1,[26] with 468 human cases and 282 deaths reported across 15 countries.[29] Cases have also been recorded in a number of mammalian species, including canids, felids, viverids, mustelids, lagomorphs, suids, and primates. Globally, the number of outbreaks or cases in poultry and humans peaked annually in the January through March period each year, but the size of these peaks has declined annually.[9] Although variation in the intensity of national surveillance and frequency of reporting inhibit firm conclusions, effective control measures appear to have led to a steady reduction in the numbers of countries affected, with the virus now largely confined to endemic regions in Northeast Africa and South and Southeast Asia.

The ongoing HPAI H5N1 epizootic has been unusual in the extent to which wild birds have been affected. Prior to this, the only records of HPAI in wild birds were the isolation of HPAI H5N3 virus following the death of 1300 common terns *(Sterna hirundo)* in South Africa in 1961 and a case of H7 infection in a saker falcon *(Falco cherrug)* in Italy at the time of an HPAI H7N1 virus outbreak affecting poultry. The first wild bird cases of HPAI caused by the H5N1 subtype were detected in Hong Kong in December 2002 in wild and ornamental birds at four sites. Initially, further (sporadic) cases in wild birds occurred in the vicinity of infected poultry and were likely the result of local spillover from poultry. The possibility that wild birds might be capable of long-distance transmission of virus arose with the mortality of over 6000 wild birds during the outbreak at Qinghai Lake in April 2005.[6] Although the 2005 mortalities at Qinghai remain the largest reported in wild birds, further outbreaks involving tens or hundreds of birds of more than 60 species occurred at sites in Europe and Central Asia in 2006 and 2007. The regularity of wild bird outbreaks of Qinghai-like HPAI H5N1virus (clade 2.2) has declined since 2007. However, evidence is emerging that another strain of HPAI H5N1 virus, clade 2.3.2, may have established itself in wild birds, with isolates from Hong Kong in 2007 and 2008, Japan in 2008, Russia in 2009 and Mongolia in 2009 and 2010.

CONSIDERATIONS IN WILD BIRDS

Ecology of Low and Highly Pathogenic Avian Influenza

The comparative lack of precedent for HPAI virus infections among wild birds prior to 2002 limits our ability to predict how HPAI H5N1 viruses will behave in wild populations. Although extrapolation based on the epidemiology of LPAI viruses may be helpful, inferences should not be overinterpreted, because differences in pathogenesis may significantly affect the dynamics of HPAI virus transmission in wild populations. Recognizing these shortcomings, a discussion of HPAI with reference to the ecology of LPAI may still be instructive in predicting the behavior of the virus.

Influenza A viruses are able to persist for a prolonged period in an aquatic environment, which together with ecologic factors, such as feeding behavior and sociality, may explain the prominence of water birds in the epidemiology of LPAI viruses in the wild.[17] LPAI viruses follow a fecal-oral transmission cycle, with viral replication and shedding occurring within the intestinal mucosa. By contrast, HPAI viruses have a wider tissue affinity, with greater respiratory involvement, although the significance of this on the ecology of the virus in wild birds is unknown.[22]

Infections with LPAI viruses are traditionally believed to incur minimal cost on wild bird hosts, in most cases remaining entirely subclinical. However, more recently, this view has been challenged, and LPAI infections may have more subtle affects on behavior and ecology, such as those on migration, feeding rate, and body weight.[24]

Immune status plays an important role in the cycling of LPAI virus in host populations, with prevalence rates highest among naïve juvenile birds, resulting in seasonal peaks of infection in the postbreeding period.[16] The role of prior exposure to influenza A viruses in the survival and viral shedding patterns of birds infected with HPAI viruses is poorly known, although experimental infection of mute swans has implied that naturally acquired avian influenza–specific antibodies protect swans from clinical HPAI H5N1 virus infection, although viral shedding still occurs.

Source of Highly Pathogenic Avian Influenza H5N1 Virus Infection

The vast majority of isolates of HPAI H5N1 virus from wild birds have been collected from incapacitated or dead birds,[2] but this is of limited value in understanding how the virus perpetuates in diverse avian communities. Of greater importance is the identity of species that may withstand, shed, and potentially disseminate the virus over moderate or longer distances. Species variation in survival and shedding of HPAI virus has been demonstrated experimentally, yet few isolates have been obtained from live, apparently healthy birds in the wild. The failure to identify wild asymptomatic carriers of HPAI viruses should not be taken as evidence that such birds do not exist, because the costs and logistics of obtaining statistically robust sample sizes are prohibitive. However, considering the many tens of thousands of wild, healthy birds that have been tested in endemic areas,[16] we may conclude that at most, asymptomatic carriers are extremely rare within the wild bird population. This should be contrasted with the observation that predominant strains of LPAI virus may be detected from multiple individuals within a migratory flyway in any year,[15] emphasizing the differences in the epidemiology of HPAI with respect to LPAI in wild birds.

There has been intense debate over the relative importance of wild birds and domestic fowl in the dissemination of HPAI H5N1 virus.[10,12] The situation is complicated by the presence of backyard or extensive husbandry systems employed in many areas, and the complexity of supply chains that serve the poultry industry. This extensive overlap of domestic and wildlife sectors, coupled with inherent difficulties in wild bird surveillance, make it impossible to draw firm conclusions about the source of outbreaks in most cases. However, the occurrence of outbreaks in remote areas such as Mongolia or the Tuva Republic, where poultry are effectively absent, suggests that wild birds are able to carry virus, at least over moderate distances, and seed new outbreaks. The frequency at which this occurs is unknown, and the continued absence of HPAI of the H5N1 subtype in some areas that receive large populations of migrants from endemic regions, notably Australasia, suggests that dissemination of virus by wild birds, at least in some taxonomic groups, is very rare indeed.

ZOO OUTBREAKS

Most zoological collections house their birds in enclosures that allow for contact with (excrement of) wild birds, thus potentially providing a route of introduction of HPAI viruses into the zoo. To date, 15 outbreaks of Asian lineage H5N1 HPAI virus have been documented in captive collections of nondomestic birds (Table 45-1). Although wild birds are often cited as one of the possible routes of introduction, the causative strain has not usually been compared with strains in poultry or wild birds in the area of the zoo outbreak, and these allegations remain unconfirmed. In contrast, in five zoo outbreaks, the source of these infections has been traced back to the feeding of infected chickens.

Confirmed outbreaks of the Asian lineage H5N1 HPAI virus in mammalian species in zoos have predominantly affected large felids (see Table 45-1), with clinical manifestations ranging from severe clinical signs with high mortality and tiger-tiger transmission in Thailand to unspecific clinical signs with no mortality in a variety of felids in Cambodia. Additionally, visitors and zoo staff at Ragunan Zoo, Indonesia, were confirmed with HPAI H5N1 infection during the outbreak, although all patients recovered.[27]

To curtail the HPAI H5N1 virus outbreaks in zoos, a combination of increased biosecurity measures (isolation and quarantine of infected animals, disinfection of the area), prohibition of feeding uncooked poultry, antiviral treatment of infected animals in quarantine areas, selective culling (of nonendangered or low value species), extensive monitoring, and vaccination have been used. In Europe, measures taken in response to an outbreak may vary between countries, but are based on current European Union (EU) legislation (Council Directive 2005/94/EC), which allows zoological collections to refrain from culling in case of a confirmed HPAI virus outbreak—thereby repealing Directive 92/94/EEC—provided that all birds may be confined and regularly tested according to the diagnostic manual decision 2006/437/EC.

ZOO VACCINATION
Policy

HPAI in birds and LPAI caused by the H5 and H7 subtypes in poultry are listed as notifiable diseases.[26] In most countries, routine preventive vaccination of poultry against avian influenza viruses is not practiced because of international trade agreements and eradication policies. However, the eradication measures normally used to manage HPAI virus outbreaks in poultry (e.g., confinement, large-scale culling) are considered detrimental to the welfare, conservation status, and breeding programs of unique, priceless, or endangered zoo birds,[8,20,21] so amendments to (local) laws and regulations have been made for zoos in some affected countries.

Recommendations by the World Organisation for Animal Health on whether to vaccinate poultry may vary by country based on factors such as the level of infection, circulating strains, structure of veterinary services, and characteristics of the poultry sector.[5] In several countries, previous bans on routine vaccination have been lifted because of endemicity of the HPAI H5N1 virus, which makes vaccination of poultry a useful tool in the control of the disease, whereas some other countries have lifted vaccination bans as a preventive measure without having experienced outbreaks or endemicity. These African and Asian countries, including Togo, Egypt, Mali, Mauritania, Ghana, Senegal, Mauritius, China, Vietnam, Indonesia, and Laos, therefore do not impose any regulations or policies specific to the vaccination of zoo birds. In several Asian zoos, vaccination has been used as a preventive measure[18] or to control outbreaks (Indonesia, Thailand, Cambodia, Kuwait). To our knowledge, zoos in Africa have not vaccinated their birds.

The European Union has experienced several outbreaks of HPAI H5N1 virus, but routine vaccination of poultry is not practiced (European Council Directive 92/40/EEC) although, more recently, Directive 2005/94/EC provides for preventive vaccination plans to be approved in certain circumstances in poultry and other captive birds. Without vaccination, confinement of the

TABLE 45-1 Documented Outbreaks of Highly Pathogenic Avian Influenza H5N1 Virus in Zoological Collections

Zoo	Year	Avian Taxonomic Orders Infected	Mammalian Species Infected	Reported Route of Introduction	Containment Measures
Suphanburi Zoo, Thailand	2003		Tiger, *Panthera tigris*	Feeding infected chickens	Isolation, quarantine, vaccination, antiviral treatment, disinfection
Sri Racha Tiger Zoo, Thailand	2004		Tiger	Feeding infected chickens	
Penfold Park, Hong Kong, People's Republic of China	2004	Anseriformes, Ciconiiformes		Wild bird introduction	Culling, disinfection, surveillance
Kowloon Park, Hong Kong, People's Republic of China	2004	Anseriformes, Phoenicopteriformes		Wild bird or poultry markets in close proximity	Vaccination, quarantine, isolation, disinfection, surveillance
Phnomh Tamao Wildlife Rescue Centre, Cambodia	2004	Ciconiiformes, Galliformes, Passeriformes, Gruiformes, Coraciiformes, Pelecaniformes	Lion, *Panthera leo*, tiger, Asiatic golden cat, *Catopuma temminckii*, leopard, *Panthera pardus*, clouded leopard, *Neofelis nebulosa*	Feeding of or contact with infected chickens, contact with wild birds	Zoo closure, isolation, disinfection
Ragunan Zoo, Jakarta, Indonesia	2005	Passeriformes, Anseriformes, Galliformes, Ciconiiformes, Accipitriformes	Humans	Feeding of or contact with infected chickens	Zoo closure, antiviral treatment, disinfection, surveillance
Owston's Civet Conservation Program, Cuc Phuong National Park, Vietnam	2005		Owston's palm civet, *Chrotogale owstoni*	Unknown	Unknown
Shanghai Zoo, People's Republic of China	2005		Tiger	Unknown	Unknown
Cairo Zoo, Egypt	2006	Anseriformes, Galliformes		Unknown	Culling, disinfection
Odessa Zoo, Ukraine	2006	Anseriformes, Columbiformes, Falconiformes, Pelecaniformes, Galliformes, Strigiformes		Contact with wild birds	Selective culling, quarantine, screening, zoning, disinfection
Tinjomoyo Zoo, Semarang, Indonesia	2006	Accipitriformes, Galliformes		Unknown	Zoo closure, quarantine, selective culling, vaccination, disinfection
Dresden Zoo, Germany	2006	Anseriformes		Contact with resident wild birds or from a recent acquisition	Isolation, quarantine
Islamabad Zoo, Pakistan	2007	Galliformes, Anseriformes		Contact with wild birds	Closure, culling, ring vaccination, disinfection
Kuwait Zoo, Kuwait	2007	Falconiformes, Galliformes		Unknown	Biosecurity measures, selective culling, surveillance, vaccination
Abbotsbury Swannery, United Kingdom	2007	Anseriformes		Introduced contamination by staff, wild birds	Unknown

whole bird collection is recommended, but this is likely to be unrealistic or unattainable in most zoos, and is associated with stress-related welfare problems and disease. To alleviate confinement measures, Decision 2005/744/EC, later replaced by the Commission of the European Communities (CEC) Decision 2006/474/EC, allowed vaccination against HPAI H5N1 virus in European zoos (as defined by 1999/22/EC), approved bodies, institutes, or centers. Zoo vaccination plans have to be submitted by the member state (MS) and approved by the commission. The vaccination plans should be carried out as quickly as possible (preferably within 1 week) and carried out under supervision from an official veterinarian of the competent authorities. Rigorous surveillance and control requirements include the following:

1. Birds should be marked Individually.
2. Wherever possible, blood has to be collected prior to and at least 30 days after vaccination.
3. Serologic test results should be kept for at least 10 years.
4. The inactivated vaccine used should be in accordance with the manufacturer and/or veterinary authorities.
5. Vaccinated birds should be kept out of the food chain.

Additionally, zoos should carry out appropriate and practicable measures preventing direct and indirect contact between wild birds and zoo birds to avoid the introduction of the H5N1 avian influenza virus.

Movement of vaccinated birds among zoos, approved bodies, institutes, and centers within or between an MS is permitted on a risk assessment basis and when the place of origin has no animal health restrictions in relation to HPAI in place. Birds must be accompanied by a health certificate that must state that "birds conform to Decision 2006/474/EC [and] were vaccinated against AI on (date) with vaccine (specify type, brand, batch number)." Authorities in the MS of origin must notify the authorities of the recipient MS. Regulations for movement of birds to countries outside the EU are not specified.

Currently, vaccination of zoo birds in Europe is strongly recommended by the European Association of Zoos and Aquaria (EAZA) and the European Food Safety Association (EFSA), and the CEC has approved vaccination plans for zoo birds in 16 member states.

Zoos on continents that have never experienced outbreaks of the HPAI H5N1 virus subtype (North America, South America, and Australia) have thus far refrained from large-scale vaccination campaigns because of movement restrictions imposed on vaccinated birds. However, vaccination in combination with sound biosecurity and surveillance programs are "to be considered when there is a substantial threat of an outbreak of HPAI in the region of a zoo."[3] In Australia, vaccination "will only be approved if HPAI virus is known or suspected (by the consultative committee) to be present or notifiable LPAI H5/H7 is recognized to be spreading in captive birds in Australia."

Practice and Experience

Vaccination against AI viruses of the H5 and H7 subtypes with most current commercially available, inactivated oil-adjuvanted poultry vaccines is safe and effective in terms of inducing hemagglutination inhibition (HI) serum antibody titers in most taxonomic orders of zoo birds.[4,11,18,20,21] Detailed information on vaccination against HPAI viruses in zoos has been presented by Philippa,[19] a scientific assessment of 2296 individual vaccinated birds in zoos in 16 European countries,[8] and other reviews.[14] These may be summarized as follows:

- Dose should be adapted to body weight.[21]
- Injection route (IM or SC), does not affect vaccine efficacy, except in birds with large subcutaneous air sacs (e.g., pelicans), in which the SC route appears to be less efficacious.[8]
- Mortality and adverse effects are low and mainly attributed to handling stress and trauma, and should thus be minimized by careful and professional handling of birds. Vaccination during breeding seasons should be avoided whenever possible to minimize breeding losses attributed to handling.[8]
- The immune response is broad, with documented antibody titers against prototype strains of four antigenic clades of Asiatic lineage HPAI H5N1 viruses.[20]
- Booster vaccinations seem to be required at 6- to 12-month intervals to maintain high titers. Antibody titers have decreased significantly in most taxonomic orders after 1 year. Only Phoenicopteriformes had a geometric mean antibody titer (GMT) considered to be protective, but high titers are seen after a single annual booster dose.
- The use of heterologous vaccines (using the same H subtype as the field virus, but a different N subtype), may differentiate between vaccinated and field-virus infected animals, although infection

with LPAI viruses through contact with wild birds may interfere with this theory.

• Inactivated adjuvanted vaccines have shown to protect cats and macaques from experimental infection, but currently there is no commercial vaccine available to protect mammals from HPAI H5N1 virus infection.

Vaccination of zoo birds should always be used as an additional preventive measure, because biosecurity measures remain the first line of protection of animals against the introduction of AI viruses.[8,20] These biosecurity measures should include strict hygiene and quarantine measures and exclude the introduction of AI viruses through feed animals (day-old chicks, chickens), other poultry, or their products. Continuous clinical monitoring of captive and wild birds in zoos should be practiced, and followed up by virologic monitoring in suspected cases for early detection. Strict biosecurity measures will also reduce the risk of subsequent infection of wild birds by zoo birds.

When biosecurity measures alone cannot sufficiently protect zoo birds from exposure to HPAI viruses—based on an overall risk assessment, which includes welfare aspects—vaccination should be used for protection because it allows for an alleviation of confinement measures—and is therefore beneficial to the health and welfare of these birds, and to the disease status of the zoo.

REFERENCES

1. Alexander DJ: Summary of avian influenza activity in Europe, Asia, Africa, and Australasia, 2002-2006. Avian Dis 51:161–166, 2007.
2. Alexander DJ, Brown IH: History of highly pathogenic avian influenza. Rev Sci Tech 28:119–138, 2009.
3. American Association of Zoos and Aquariums: Highly pathogenic avian influenza: Emergency guidelines for zoos. Yulee, Fla, 2006, American Association of Zoos and Aquariums.
4. Bertelsen MF, Klausen J, Holm E, et al: Serological response to vaccination against avian influenza in zoo-birds using an inactivated H5N9 vaccine. Vaccine 25:4345–4349, 2007.
5. Bruschke CJ, Pittman M, Laddomada A: International regulations and standards for avian influenza, including the vaccine standards of the World Organisation for Animal Health. Rev Sci Tech 28:379–389, 2009.
6. Chen H, Smith GJD, Zhang SY, et al: H5N1 virus outbreak in migratory waterfowl. Nature 436:191–192, 2005.
7. Chen H, Smith GJD, Li KS, et al: Establishment of multiple sublineages of H5N1 influenza virus in Asia: Implications for pandemic control. Proc Natl Acad Sci U S A 103:2845–2850, 2006.
8. European Food Safety Authority (EFSA): Opinion of the scientific panel on Animal Health and Welfare (AHAW) on a request from the commission related with the vaccination against avian influenza of H5 and H7 subtypes as a preventive measure carried out in Member States in birds kept in zoos under community approved programmes, 2007 (http://www.efsa.europa.eu/en/scdocs/scdoc/450.htm).
9. FAO (Food and Agriculture Organization)–GLEWS (Global Early Warning and Response System) Team: H5N1 highly pathogenic avian influenza—monthly global overview, 2009 (http://www.fao.org/avianflu/en/overview.htm).
10. Feare CJ, Yasué M: Asymptomatic infection with highly pathogenic avian influenza H5N1 in wild birds: How sound is the evidence? Virol J 3:96, 2006.
11. Furger M, Hoop R, Steinmetz H, et al: Humoral immune response to avian influenza vaccination over a six-month period in different species of captive wild birds. Avian Dis 52:222–228, 2008.
12. Gilbert M, Xiao XM, Domenach J, et al: Anatidae migration in the western palearctic and spread of highly pathogenic avian influenza H5N1 virus. Emerg Infect Dis 12:111650–111656, 2006.
13. Gilbert M, Xiao XM, Pfeiffer DU, et al: Mapping H5N1 highly pathogenic avian influenza risk in Southeast Asia. Proc Natl Acad Sci U S A 105:124769–124774, 2008.
14. Koch G, Steensels M, van den BT: Vaccination of birds other than chickens and turkeys against avian influenza. Rev Sci Tech 28:307–318, 2009.
15. Krauss S, Walker D, Pryor SP, et al: Influenza A viruses of migrating wild aquatic birds in North America. Vector Borne Zoonotic Dis 4:3177–3189, 2004.
16. Munster VJ, Baas C, Lexmond P, et al: Spatial, temporal, and species variation in prevalence of influenza A viruses in wild migratory birds. PLoS Pathogens 3:e61, 2007.
17. Munster VJ, Fouchier RAM: Avian influenza virus: Of virus and bird ecology. Vaccine 27:6340–6344, 2009.
18. Oh S, Martelli P, Hock OS, et al: Field study on the use of inactivated H5N2 vaccine in avian species. Vet Rec 157:299–300, 2005.
19. Philippa JD: Avian influenza. In Fowler ME, Miller RE, editors: Zoo and wild animal medicine: Current therapy, ed 6, Philadelphia, 2007, WB Saunders, pp 79–85.
20. Philippa J, Baas C, Beyer W, et al: Vaccination against highly pathogenic avian influenza H5N1 virus in zoos using an adjuvanted inactivated H5N2 vaccine. Vaccine 25:3800–3808, 2007.
21. Philippa JDW, Munster VJ, Bolhuis H, et al: Highly pathogenic avian influenza (H7N7): Vaccination of zoo birds and transmission to non-poultry species. Vaccine 23:5743–5750, 2005.
22. Sturm-Ramirez KM, Hulse-Post DJ, Govorkova EA, et al: Are ducks contributing to the endemicity of highly pathogenic H5N1 influenza virus in Asia? J Virol 79:11269–11279, 2005.
23. Tumpey TM, Suarez DL, Perkins LEL, et al: Characterization of a highly pathogenic H5N1 avian influenza a virus isolated from duck meat. J Virol 76:6344–6355, 2005.
24. van Gils JA, Munster VJ, Radersma R, et al: Hampered foraging and migratory performance in swans infected with low-pathogenic avian influenza A virus. PLoS ONE 2:e184, 2007.
25. Webster RG, Bean WJ, Gorman OT, et al: Evolution and ecology of influenza A viruses. Microbiol Rev 56:152–179, 1992.
26. World Health Organization/World Organisation for Animal Health/Food and Agriculture Organization H5N1 Evolution Working Group: Toward a unified nomenclature system for highly pathogenic avian influenza virus (H5N1) (conference summary), 2008 (http://www.cdc.gov/EID/content/14/7/e1.htm).
27. World Organisation for Animal Health (OIE): Update on highly pathogenic avian influenza in animals (type H5 and H7), 2010 (http://www.oie.int/downld/AVIAN%20INFLUENZA/A_AI-Asia.htm).
28. World Organisation for Animal Health (OIE): Avian influenza. In World Organisation for Animal Health: Terrestrial animal health code, ed 17, Paris, 2008, OIE, pp 430–446.
29. World Health Organization: Cumulative number of confirmed human cases of avian influenza A/(H5N1) Reported to WHO, 2009 (http://www.who.int/csr/disease/avian_influenza/country/cases_table_2010_02_17/en/index.html).

CHAPTER 46

Nonsteroidal Anti-inflammatory Drugs in Raptors

J. Lindsay Oaks and Carol Uphoff Meteyer

The use of analgesia has become standard, and appropriate, practice in avian medicine. As in mammals, pain control in avian patients is usually accomplished with opioids and nonsteroidal anti-inflammatory drugs (NSAIDs) used singly or in combination for a multimodal approach. Despite their usefulness, widespread use, and relative safety in clinical use, few controlled studies in birds have been conducted on efficacy, safety, and dosing. The guidelines for the use of NSAIDs in raptors and other birds have mainly been empirical. More recently, NSAIDs in free-living raptors have emerged as a major conservation issue with the discovery that diclofenac sodium was responsible for the population crash of three species of *Gyps* vultures in southern Asia. In this context, residues of veterinary NSAIDs in domestic animals are now considered environmental contaminants that can be significantly toxic to vultures and possibly other avian scavengers. Ironically, the disaster with Asian vultures has led to a considerable body of research on NSAIDs in raptors to the benefit of clinicians who now have scientific information available to help assess dosing, safety, toxicity, and pharmacokinetics of NSAIDs in their raptor patients.

CLASSIFICATION AND MECHANISM OF ACTION

NSAIDs inhibit one or both of the cyclooxygenase (COX) enzyme systems involved in prostaglandin synthesis. COX-1 enzymes are constitutively expressed and their primary function is homeostasis through the synthesis of physiologic prostaglandins, including those involved in the protection of the gastric mucosa, renal function, and platelet aggregation.[8] As such, COX-1 inhibition contributes primarily to the adverse effects of gastric bleeding, erosions, and ulcers. COX-2 enzymes

are inducible and involved with synthesis of prostaglandins that initiate inflammation, including pain, swelling, and stiffness. COX-2 enzymes are the primary therapeutic targets for NSAIDs, and selective inhibitors of COX-2 have the advantage of inhibiting inflammation while sparing the adverse effects associated with COX-1 inhibition.[8] Thus, attempts have been made to develop NSAIDs that are highly or preferentially selective for COX-2 enzymes. Most of the NSAIDs important to avian medicine are nonselective (e.g., diclofenac, flunixin meglumine, ketoprofen) or partially selective (e.g., carprofen, meloxicam) for COX-2 enzymes. However, the degree of selectivity can vary widely among species. Also, renal toxicity, the most significant adverse effect in birds, can occur with COX-2 preferential drugs.[2]

THERAPEUTIC USES IN CAPTIVE BIRDS OF PREY

Anecdotally, the NSAIDs commonly used in raptors are similar to those used in other birds. This has been substantiated by a recent survey of veterinarians, zoos, and wildlife rehabilitation facilities that found that in descending order of use, the most commonly used NSAIDs in various raptors are meloxicam, carprofen, ketoprofen, and flunixin meglumine.[2] Other NSAIDs used rarely include acetylsalicylic acid, ibuprofen, and phenylbutazone. The doses used in these studies were comparable to those previously published for avian use in general[19] (Table 46-1).

No studies have been conducted in raptors that demonstrate the efficacy of analgesia with NSAID therapy. However, studies with naturally lame chickens treated with carprofen[10] and with experimentally-induced arthritis in parrots (*Amazona ventralis*) treated with meloxicam[1] have demonstrated evidence of successful

TABLE 46-1	Doses of Commonly Used Nonsteroidal Anti-Inflammatory Drugs in Raptors and Other Birds*		
Drug	Route	Dosage in Birds (mg/kg)	Dosage in Raptors (mg/kg)
Carprofen	Oral	2.0-4.0	1.5-7.6
Flunixin	Intramuscular	1.0	0.5-12.0
Ketoprofen	Intramuscular	2.0	1.0-7.7
Meloxicam	Oral	0.1	0.1-0.75

*Dosages for birds are from Paul-Murphy and Ludders[19]; dosages for raptors are from Cuthbert and associates.[2] Dosages for raptors are those for which adverse events were not reported.

analgesia at doses comparable to the usual doses used in raptors. Therefore, it is reasonable to expect that some analgesia can be expected from NSAID use in raptors although, based on work in other birds, the actual level of analgesia achieved is likely to be dose-[1] and possibly species-[10,20] dependent.

NSAID therapy in mammals is well known to have a number of adverse effects, including ulceration of the gastrointestinal tract, decreased platelet function, and impairment of renal function. Much less is known about the adverse effects of NSAIDs in birds. There are some reports of possible gastrointestinal disturbance and bleeding associated with the use of flunixin meglumine in budgerigars (Melopsittacus undulatus) and a crane.[19] Flunixin meglumine has also been associated with localized muscle necrosis when used parenterally in mallard ducks (Anas platyrhynchos).[9] However, the most common adverse effect that appears to be associated with NSAID use in birds, including raptors, is renal impairment. Unfortunately, this can be severe and rapidly lead to renal failure, visceral gout, and death. In raptors, the NSAIDs with the most reports of renal toxicity were flunixin meglumine (7 of 24 birds treated) and carprofen (5 of 40 birds treated); there were no reports of renal toxicity with ketoprofen (20 birds treated) or meloxicam (739 birds treated).[2] Despite the apparent lack of problems with ketoprofen, published[12] and anecdotal[14] reports in other avian species have suggested that this drug may be toxic, which has been substantiated in more recent studies in Gyps vultures.[17] NSAID toxicity is generally dose-dependent, although this was not evident in the above raptor survey, in which toxicity was not well correlated with higher dose ranges. However, dose-dependent toxicity is consistently seen in controlled studies, including studies of Gyps vultures

treated with ketoprofen[17] or diclofenac,[14,24] and in other birds with ketoprofen.[21] Consequently, great caution should be exercised when treating raptors at the higher end of or beyond established dose ranges. Preexisting dehydration or renal disease are additional risk factors for NSAID-induced renal toxicity in humans, and dehydration is suspected as a complicating factor in the renal toxicity of ketoprofen in birds.[12,13]

Of more concern with the clinical use of NSAIDs in birds, however, is the marked difference in toxicity among different groups of birds, making adverse events potentially very unpredictable. In spectacled eiders (Somateria fischeri) and king eiders (S. spectabilis) treated with ketoprofen, even gender differences in renal toxicity have been noted.[12] Species differences in sensitivity to NSAIDs have been exemplified in the diclofenac-induced decline of Gyps vultures in Asia and in the subsequent research conducted to mitigate the problem.

DICLOFENAC AND VULTURES

Diclofenac is a relatively early NSAID that was, and still is, very commonly used in human medicine, primarily for rheumatoid and nonrheumatoid arthritis. After this drug was no longer covered by patent, generic forms became widely available in Asia and, in the early 1990s, found their way into veterinary medicine in India.[18] Diclofenac acts on both COX-1 and COX-2 enzymes and, in humans, although quite effective therapeutically, the drug is associated with substantial adverse effects on the gastrointestinal tract, platelet function, and renal function. In livestock, however, diclofenac appeared to be an ideal veterinary drug—it was cheap and perceived to be effective and safe for clinical use in mammals. Thus, diclofenac became widely available to and widely used by veterinarians in India.

Anecdotal and newspaper reports of disappearing vultures in India began to appear in the mid-1990s, and the decline was scientifically documented in 1997 when biologists from the Bombay Natural History Society (BNHS) documented the decline in Keoladeo National Park in northern India. At this site, the breeding population of Oriental white-backed vultures (Gyps bengalensis) had gone from about 250 breeding pairs in the mid-1980s to none in 1999. Subsequent and more geographically comprehensive studies found that between the early 1990s and 2000 there was a decline of at least 96% for white-backed vultures and 92% each for the long-billed vultures (G. indicus) and slender-billed vultures (G. tenuirostris).[18] Similar catastrophic declines were recorded in neighboring Pakistan and Nepal. In Pakistan, at the end of 2000, three breeding colonies being studied each had 420 to 760 active breeding pairs of white-backed vultures but, by 2003, two of these large nesting colonies were completely extirpated, followed by the third in 2007.[4] White-backed and long-billed vultures were once regarded as probably the most common large raptors in the world but, in about a decade, and with a total loss estimated at tens of millions of individuals, these birds were listed as critically endangered.

In 2003, the vulture decline in Pakistan was linked to the use of diclofenac in livestock.[14,23] Key findings from ecologic studies that initially focused attention on toxins indicated that the vulture population decline was being driven by abnormal mortality in the breeding adults, and that mortality was clustered temporally and spatially, suggesting a highly lethal point source—findings most compatible with a toxic cause.[4] Diagnostically, it was evident from the beginning that the abnormal mortality was associated with visceral gout (Fig. 46-1). Gross postmortem examinations done on 259 adult and subadult white-backed vultures found that 219 (85%) of these had visceral gout, indicative of renal failure. The investigation then focused on identifying the cause of renal pathology, which in wild birds would most likely be toxic or infectious. The histopathology in these affected birds was uniformly described as severe, acute, renal tubular necrosis and resultant uric acid crystal deposition in the kidneys and other tissues.[11] Importantly, there were no significant inflammatory

cellular infiltrates consistent with an infectious disease. Extensive testing was performed for the usual toxic causes of renal failure and/or acute death in wild birds, including the heavy metals cadmium, lead, and mercury, other metals, including arsenic, copper, iron, manganese, molybdenum, and zinc, and poisoning by organophosphate, carbamate, or organochlorine pesticides. The results of all this testing were negative.[14]

At this point, based on the observation that the primary food source for vultures in Pakistan was domestic livestock,[14] attention turned specifically to veterinary pharmaceuticals. Because toxins would most likely be ingested, it was logical to look at drugs that either went in, or on, livestock. This was assessed with a questionnaire that asked regional veterinarians and veterinary retail stores about the use of drugs in livestock. The survey identified 34 drugs that were commonly used. This list of drugs was then narrowed by applying the criteria of known nephrotoxicity in other birds or mammals via oral absorption, because the presumed route of exposure was ingestion of new and commonly used drugs, compatible with the epidemiology of the vulture decline. Strikingly, the results of this analysis left only a single drug, diclofenac. Assays for diclofenac were then performed on kidney samples from vultures with renal failure and control cases without renal failure; all the renal failure cases had residues of diclofenac, whereas none of the nonrenal failure cases were positive. The toxicity of diclofenac for white-backed vultures was then verified experimentally by orally dosing nonreleasable captive vultures with 2.5 mg/kg (the standard veterinary dose recommended for mammals) and 0.25 mg/kg of diclofenac. Both of the high-dose birds and one of the two lower dose vultures died with visceral gout within 58 hours postadministration. Similar experiments reproduced visceral gout and diclofenac residues in vultures that were fed meat from a buffalo treated with standard label doses of veterinary diclofenac. All the experimentally exposed vultures had renal lesions that were identical to those found in the field cases. These findings were soon replicated in India, documenting diclofenac toxicity across the geographic extent of the vulture decline and providing key evidence that diclofenac was responsible not just for vulture mortality, but for the actual population decline.

As expected, the experimental diclofenac exposures established that the toxicity of diclofenac was dose-dependent.[14] More notable was that the median lethal dose was only about 0.1 mg/kg, indicating that *Gyps* vultures were extremely sensitive to diclofenac.[24]

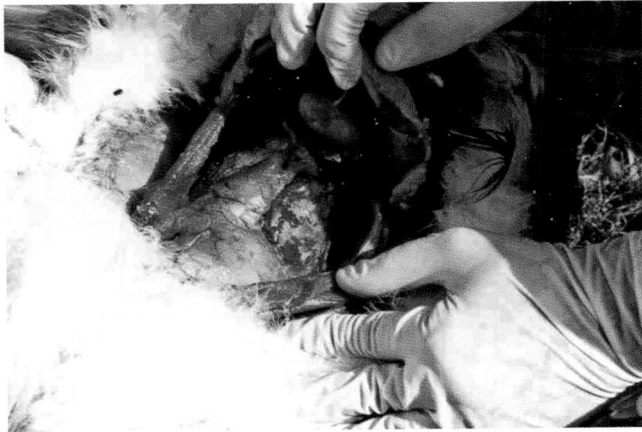

Figure 46-1

Gross appearance of visceral gout in an Oriental white-backed vulture in Pakistan. Visceral gout is evident as white deposits on the surface of the liver and other organs.

VULTURES AND OTHER NONSTEROIDAL ANTI-INFLAMMATORY DRUGS

Several questions arose from the finding that *Gyps* vultures were lethally sensitive to even residue levels of an NSAID. Was diclofenac uniformly very toxic to birds, or were *Gyps* vultures uniformly very sensitive to all NSAIDs? The answer to these questions had immediate conservation implications. One implication was that other NSAIDs were known to be used to treat livestock and could be found in livestock carcasses across India.[25] Thus, efforts to remove only diclofenac from the environment may not have solved the problem. Also, part of the strategy for facilitating a regulatory response banning the use of veterinary diclofenac was to identify a suitable, vulture-safe alternative for use in livestock.[2] This effort would not succeed if all NSAIDs were highly toxic to *Gyps* vultures.

Diclofenac is not uniformly toxic to birds. Turkey vultures *(Cathartes aura)*—in the family Cathartidae, and only distantly related to the *Gyps* vultures, which are in the family Accipitridae—dosed with up to 25 mg/kg of diclofenac had no ill effects.[22] A similar study using diclofenac doses of 0.25 to 20.0 mg/kg found variable sensitivities of chickens, pigeons *(Columba livia)*, Japanese quail *(Coturnix japonica)*, and common mynahs *(Acridotheres tristis)*. The minimum lethal doses for these birds occurred at 2.5, 0.25, 10.0, and 10.0 mg/kg of diclofenac, respectively.[6] Only pigeons had sensitivity comparable to *Gyps* vultures, whereas quail and mynahs were susceptible only to what would probably be considered supratherapeutic levels. Diclofenac has been found to be lethal to other *Gyps* vultures, including African white-backed vultures *(G. africanus)*, Eurasian Griffon vultures *(G. fulvus)*, and Cape Griffon vultures *(G. coprotheres)*, at similar median lethal doses as those found in Oriental white-backed vultures.[16,24] Thus, only some species of birds appear to be highly sensitive to diclofenac.

Fortunately, *Gyps* vultures are not uniformly sensitive to NSAIDs. After a survey that identified no reports of adverse effects with meloxicam in *Gyps* vultures and other raptors,[2] toxicologic studies were conducted to verify the safety of this drug using nonendangered African *Gyps* species, also shown to be extremely sensitive to diclofenac. The results indicated that meloxicam was safe in doses of 0.5 to 2.0 mg/kg.[24] The high dose in this study was about double the upper limit of standard therapeutic doses used in birds (see Table 46-1) and also exceeded the maximum likely residue exposure that *Gyps* vultures were likely to

encounter consuming the carcass of a treated animal. Although ketoprofen was initially thought likely to be safe for vultures, subsequent studies have found that doses approximating those typically used in avian therapeutics, and doses that could be consumed from the carcass of a treated animal, could cause renal failure in African white-backed and Cape Griffon vultures.[17]

Collectively, these studies illustrate the marked variation that can occur among different combinations of avian species and NSAIDs and the risk in extrapolation of data from one species to another. However, at least for *Gyps* vultures, meloxicam appears to be safe, both therapeutically and environmentally. Meloxicam has been heavily advocated as a potential replacement for diclofenac, and this research was important in achieving the ban on the sale and manufacture of veterinary diclofenac in India, Pakistan, and Nepal in 2006.[18]

PATHOLOGY AND PATHOGENESIS OF NONSTEROIDAL ANTI-INFLAMMATORY DRUG RENAL TOXICITY IN RAPTORS

NSAIDs have the potential to be extremely nephrotoxic in birds of prey. Necrosis of the proximal convoluted tubules is the hallmark of acute NSAID toxicity in susceptible raptors (Fig. 46-2). Because the proximal convoluted tubules are the primary site of NSAID and uric acid excretion, necrosis of these specialized cells can rapidly result in renal failure and visceral gout. Urate precipitation in visceral gout associated with NSAID toxicity has a predisposition for the kidney, quickly obscuring renal architecture and confounding the appearance of the inciting pathology in the renal cortex.[11] The lesions associated with NSAID toxicity in birds are similar to those induced by the pesticide Starlicide (Earth City Resources, Bridgeton, Mo; DRC 1339), which is the most likely cause of renal tubular necrosis and visceral gout in wild birds in the United States. However, Starlicide is unlikely to cause primary or secondary poisonings in raptors.

Spurred by the environmental problem of diclofenac and *Gyps* vultures, work is ongoing to determine the mechanism(s) whereby NSAIDs induce necrosis of proximal convoluted tubules in raptors. The proximal convoluted tubules are highly metabolic, with very steep energy and oxygen demands. These cells are also the primary route of uric acid excretion as well as

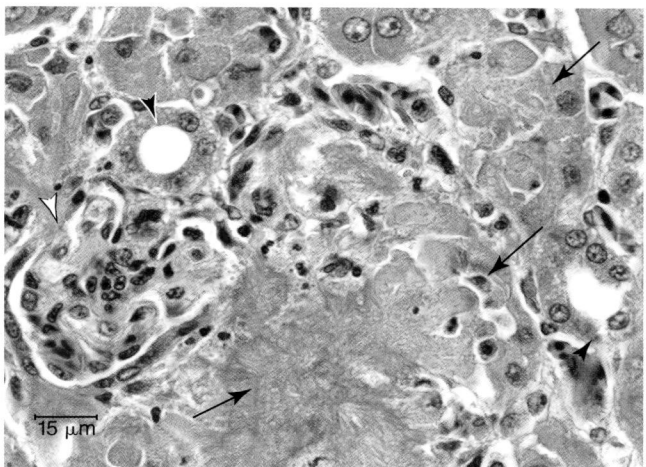

Figure 46-2

Photomicrograph showing acute necrosis of the renal proximal convoluted tubule in an Oriental white-backed vulture with visceral gout. Epithelial cells lining the proximal convoluted tubules are necrotic *(black arrow)*. Urate crystals are present *(white on black arrow)*. Adjacent distal convoluted tubules are unaffected *(black arrowhead)*, as is the glomerulus *(white on black arrowhead)*. A prominent inflammatory response is not present (hematoxylin and eosin stain, 60× magnification).

hydroxylation and clearance of NSAIDs. One route of NSAID toxicity on avian kidney may be through direct effects on the metabolism of the proximal convoluted tubules.[15] There is evidence that diclofenac has the potential to interfere with multiple proximal tubule cell functions. When explants of kidney tubule cells were treated with diclofenac, the cells showed inhibition of uric acid excretion, increase in reactive oxygen species (oxygen ions and free radicals), and subsequent damage to mitochondria, with cell death. If enzyme systems necessary for metabolizing NSAIDs are lacking in the proximal convoluted tubules of certain species of birds, this would decrease drug clearance, increasing the circulating parent compound and toxic effects of the drug.

Another hypothesis for NSAID toxicity is based on interference with the renal vascular supply and subsequent hypoxia, which is the most common mechanism of NSAID toxicity in mammals.[13] However, the vascular supply to the avian renal cortex is different from that in mammals. Blood to the avian renal cortex is supplied by the renal portal system, which differs anatomically among avian species.[7] Blood flow from the rear limbs to the renal cortex is controlled by the renal portal valve in the external iliac vein. When the renal portal valve is closed, blood is shunted through the renal cortex. When

the renal portal valve is open, blood is directed away from the kidney into the caudal vena cava. If there is a vascular component to the NSAID-mediated renal cortical necrosis, the renal portal system and functional response of the renal portal valve to NSAIDs would be logical to investigate.[11] Anatomic and physiologic variability in the functional response of the renal portal valve to COX-1 and COX-2 inhibitors may also contribute to the marked variability in species response to these drugs.

Whether death of renal cortical tubules is due to the result of hypoxia caused by NSAID-induced vascular shunting of blood away from the renal cortex, or by direct toxicity to cellular metabolism, the effect of proximal renal tubule cell necrosis is the same—decreased drug clearance, decreased uric acid excretion, acidosis, renal failure, and fatally elevated potassium levels with cardiac arrest.

The unpredictable toxicity of even the same NSAID to raptors, ranging from low to extreme toxicity,[14,22] presents a significant challenge to clinicians. Currently, testing to determine toxicity in avian species is limited to clinical trials in the species of interest with the drug of interest. If the link to understanding the selective toxicity of these drugs to certain species of birds does not involve the anatomy and function of the renal portal valve, but instead involves precise metabolic properties of the proximal renal tubule epithelium,[15] the potential to develop genetic markers of susceptibility for nonlethal prediction of species toxicity may be possible.

CONSERVATION IMPLICATIONS OF DICLOFENAC AND VULTURES

The effect of diclofenac on Asian vultures has exposed a new problem in environmental toxicology. The effect of human and veterinary pharmaceuticals on the environment has been a theoretical concern for some time, with the realization that massive quantities of inherently bioactive chemicals are entering the environment.[3] The vulture decline has made this concern no longer theoretical and has demonstrated that pharmaceuticals can be responsible for major ecologic damage. Several other findings from the vulture decline also make this situation unique, and alarming. The first, as noted, was the extreme sensitivity of an animal genus to a drug that would otherwise likely be regarded as safe at residue levels. This type of problem would not have been predicted or detected with current environmental assessments required for pharmaceuticals. Another was that this problem was not associated with environmental persistence and bioaccumulation of the chemical, but rather with a toxin that is present transiently and sporadically in the environment. Nonetheless, diclofenac effectively resulted in a continent-wide mass poisoning event, and this case illustrated the scope and scale of contemporary pharmaceutical use. And, finally, the vulture decline revealed the remarkable sensitivity that a population can have to a systematic disruption of their ecology. That diclofenac could cause renal failure and mortality in vultures was readily accepted by the scientists associated with the investigation. The ability of diclofenac poisoning to cause an actual population decline of the magnitude being observed—around 30%/year—was a different and more complicated question. Intuitively, it would seem that such a massive population effect would require some very large (and unlikely) proportion of the livestock population to be treated and then die. This issue was resolved by simulation modeling work that showed that for birds with the life history traits of *Gyps* vultures, an incidence of contaminated carcasses as low as 1/760 could have catastrophic population effects.[5] These startling results have shown that this relatively rare event is more than sufficient to have the observed population effect. This work also has shown that almost all the excess mortality driving the population decline could be attributed to diclofenac, and that the effect of other causes of vulture mortality is negligible.

These studies made it very clear that to save the Asian vultures from extinction, diclofenac use in livestock had to be stopped. In 2006, as a result of an extensive advocacy campaign by conservation groups, the manufacture of veterinary diclofenac was banned in India, Pakistan, and Nepal.[18] Unfortunately, 4 years after this regulatory success, diclofenac is still widely used in the region. Significant barriers remain in the areas of enforcement, prosecution, and awareness among farmers and veterinarians, and with inadequate incentives to use vulture-safe meloxicam. It remains to be seen whether NSAIDs will achieve the distinction of being the first pharmaceutical contaminant documented to cause extinction of a species.

REFERENCES

1. Cole GA, Paul-Murphy J, Krugner-Higby LA, et al: Analgesic effects of intramuscular administration of meloxicam in Hispaniolan parrots (*Amazona ventralis*) with experimentally induced arthritis. Am J Vet Res 70:1471–1476, 2009.

2. Cuthbert R, Parry-Jones J, Green RE, et al: NSAIDs and scavenging birds: Potential impacts beyond Asia's critically endangered vultures. Biol Lett 3:90–93, 2007.
3. Daughton CG, Ternes TA: Pharmaceuticals and personal care products in the environment: Agents of subtle change? Environ Health Perspect 107(Suppl 6):907–938, 1999.
4. Gilbert M, Watson RT, Virani MZ, et al: Rapid population declines and mortality clusters in three Oriental white-backed vulture *Gyps bengalensis* colonies due to diclofenac poisoning. Oryx 40:388–399, 2006.
5. Green RE, Newton I, Schultz S, et al: Diclofenac poisoning as a cause of vulture population declines across the Indian subcontinent. J Appl Ecol 41:793–800, 2004.
6. Hussain I, Khan MZ, Khan A, et al: Toxicological effects of diclofenac in four avian species. Avian Pathol 37:315–321, 2008.
7. Johnson OW: Urinary organs. In King AS, McLelland J, editors: Form and function in birds, London, 1979, Academic Press, pp 183–235.
8. Lees P, Landoni MF, Giraudel J, et al: Pharmacodynamics and pharmacokinetics of nonsteroidal anti-inflammatory drugs in species of veterinary interest. J Vet Pharmacol Therap 27:479–490, 2004.
9. Machin KL, Tellier LA, Lair S, et al: Pharmacodynamics of flunixin and ketoprofen in mallard ducks (*Anas platyrhynchos*). J Zoo Wildlife Med 32:222–229, 2001.
10. McGeown D, Danbury TC, Waterman-Pearson AE, et al: Effect of carprofen on lameness in broiler chickens. Vet Rec 144:668–671, 1999.
11. Meteyer CU, Rideout BA, Gilbert M, et al: Pathology and pathophysiology of diclofenac poisoning in free-living and experimentally exposed oriental white-backed vultures (*Gyps bengalensis*). J Wildl Dis 41:707–716, 2005.
12. Mulcahy DM, Tuomi P, Larsen RS: Differential mortality of male spectacled eiders (*Somateria fischeri*) and king eiders (*Somateria spectabilis*) subsequent to anesthesia with propofol, bupivacaine, and ketoprofen. J Avian Med Surg 17:117–123, 2003.
13. Murray MD, Brater DC: Renal toxicity of the nonsteroidal anti-inflammatory drugs. Ann Rev Pharmacol Toxicol 32:435–465, 1993.
14. Oaks JL, Gilbert M, Virani MZ, et al: Diclofenac residues as the cause of vulture population decline in Pakistan. Nature 427:630–633, 2004.
15. Naidoo V, Swan GE: Diclofenac toxicity in *Gyps* vultures is associated with decreased uric acid excretion and not renal portal vasoconstriction. Comp Biochem Physiol C Toxicol Pharmacol 149:269–274, 2009.
16. Naidoo V, Wolter K, Cuthbert R, et al: Veterinary diclofenac threatens Africa's endangered vultures. Regul Toxicol Pharmacol 53:205–208, 2009.
17. Naidoo V, Wolter K, Cromarty D, et al: Toxicity of non-steroidal anti-inflammatory drugs to Gyps vultures: A new threat from ketoprofen. Biol Lett 6:339–341, 2010.
18. Pain DJ, Bowden CGR, Cunningham AA, et al: The race to prevent the extinction of South Asian vultures. Bird Conserv Int 18:S30–S84, 2008.
19. Paul-Murphy J, Ludders JW: Avian analgesia. Vet Clin N Am Exotic Anim Prac 4:35–45, 2001.
20. Paul-Murphy J, Sladky KK, Krugner-Higby LA, et al: Analgesic effects of carprofen and liposome-encapsulated butorphanol tartrate in Hispaniolan parrots (*Amazona ventralis*) with experimentally induced arthritis. Am J Vet Res 70:1201–1210, 2009.
21. Pereira ME, Werther K: Evaluation of the renal effects of flunixin meglumine, ketoprofen and meloxicam in budgerigars (*Melopsittacus undulatus*). Vet Rec 160:844–846, 2007.

22. Rattner BA, Whitehead MA, Gasper G, et al: Apparent tolerance of turkey vultures *(Cathartes aura)* to the non-steroidal anti-inflammatory drug diclofenac. Environ Toxicol Chem 27:2341–2345, 2008.
23. Schultz S, Baral HS, Charman S, et al: Diclofenac poisoning is widespread in declining vulture populations across the Indian subcontinent. Proc Roy Soc Lond B 271(suppl 6):S458–S460, 2004.
24. Swan GE, Cuthbert R, Quevedo M, et al: Toxicity of diclofenac to *Gyps* vultures. Biol Lett 2:279–282, 2006.
25. Taggart MA, Senacha KR, Green RE, et al: Analysis of nine NSAIDs in ungulate tissues available to critically endangered vultures in India. Environ Sci Tech 43:4561–4566, 2009.

Haemosporidian Parasites: Impacts on Avian Hosts

Iris I. Levin and Patricia G. Parker

Haemosporidian parasites (order, Haemosporidia; phylum, Apicomplexa) are cosmopolitan intracellular protozoan parasites of birds, reptiles, and mammals.[25] Haemosporidian parasites develop in two types of hosts, vertebrates and invertebrate vectors (Insecta, Diptera, blood-sucking dipterans); the dipteran is considered the definitive host because it is the site of sexual reproduction. Avian haemosporidia include parasites from three genera—*Plasmodium*, which is typically vectored by mosquitoes (Culicidae); *Haemoproteus*, which is primarily transmitted by biting midges (Ceratopogonidae) and louse flies (Hippoboscidae), and *Leucocytozoon*, which is vectored by blackflies (Simuliidae). Historically, *Plasmodium* has been considered potentially very pathogenic and *Haemoproteus* relatively benign. In this chapter, we will summarize studies relevant to these common perceptions and present a detailed case study of an ongoing investigation of what is thought to be a recent arrival of *Plasmodium* in a naïve island population.

LIFE CYCLE OF HAEMOSPORIDIANS

The life cycle consists of several stages in tissue and circulating blood cells of infected hosts. An infected vector feeds on vertebrate host blood, inoculating the host with sporozoites and giving rise to agamic stages (referred to as exoerythrocytic meronts or schizonts), which undergo asexual reproduction in parenchymal tissue in the host. This asexual division, often called merogony or schizogony, results in uninuclear merozoites. Another cycle of merogony occurs in the host blood cells in *Plasmodium*, from which the parasite proceeds into the development of gametocytes; parasites in the genus *Haemoproteus* move quickly into the gametocyte stage in the blood. These cells produce macrogametocytes and microgametocytes, which are infective for the vectors. When an arthropod vector feeds on an infected bird, the change

in carbon dioxide and oxygen concentrations and temperature initiate gametogenesis in the midgut of the vector, resulting in a sexual process called oogamy. Macrogametocytes produce macrogametes, microgametocytes produce microgametes, and fertilization occurs extracellularly. The zygote forms an elongated mobile ookinete, which penetrates the epithelial layer of the vector's midgut, where it develops into an oocyst. Sporozoites, the stage that is infective for the vertebrate hosts, are formed in the oocyst and later move into the haemocoele of the vector, eventually penetrating the salivary glands. From there they may complete the infection cycle when the mosquito takes a second blood meal (Fig. 47-1).

PATHOGENICITY

Pathogenicity of haemosporidian parasites is complicated and varied. Infection in bird hosts follows four main periods:

1. Prepatent, in which parasite development occurs in parenchymal tissues outside the blood
2. Acute, characterized by the appearance of parasites in the host blood and an increase in parasitemia
3. Crisis, in which parasitemia reaches a peak
4. Chronic or latent, a period of sharp decrease in parasitemia caused by an immune response, following which parasitemia levels are then maintained at very low levels

Most research efforts aimed at understanding the effects of haemosporidia on host health have examined hosts during the crisis and chronic stages, in which the parasite in host erythrocytes can be detected by microscopy; parasite DNA can be amplified by a polymerase chain reaction (PCR) assay from DNA extracted from host blood. Once infected, birds usually maintain parasites for years, and relapses tend to occur during host reproduction or other times of physiologic stress.

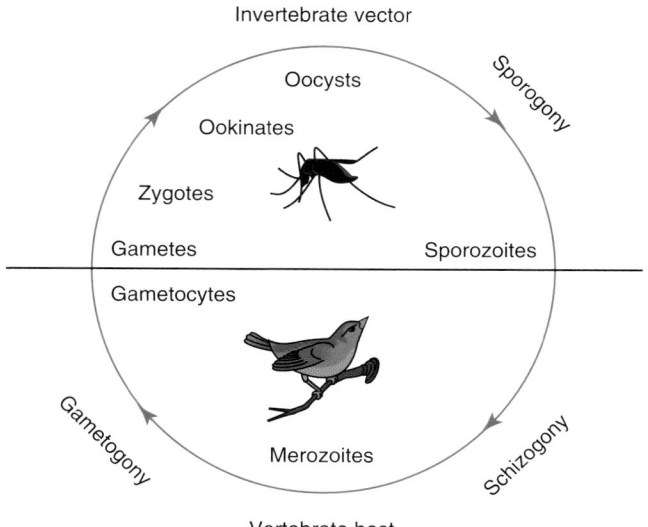

Invertebrate vector

Oocysts

Ookinates

Zygotes

Sporogony

Gametes

Sporozoites

Gametocytes

Gametogony

Merozoites

Schizogony

Vertebrate host

Figure 47-1

General schematic of the haemosporidian life cycle.

Much of our understanding of the pathogenicity of haemosporidian parasites is based on laboratory experiments on domesticated birds (canaries, chickens, ducks, pigeons, turkeys) or on accounts from infections in birds housed in zoos. In a review of pathogenicity of haemosporidian parasites in birds, Bennett and colleagues[4] found that 89% of published articles (5640 total) detailed mortality in domesticated birds, whereas 6% and 5% pertained to mortality in zoo and wildlife populations, respectively.

CAPTIVE POPULATIONS

Haemosporidian parasites (primarily *Plasmodium relictum* and *P. elongatum*) cause severe morbidity and mortality in penguin populations in zoos.[4] Most of the world's penguins are distributed near polar regions, where haemosporidia are scarce. Therefore, many of the penguin species found in zoos have not evolved in regions that support populations of suitable vectors, resulting in naïve hosts, which in turn contributes to the severity of the infections. Many of the examples of mortality in zoos caused by haemosporidia involve hosts challenged by parasites not found in their native distribution. One notable example is that of four Keas *(Nestor notabilis)* that were captured in New Zealand and moved to the Malaysian National Zoo in 1964. Native Kea habitat in New Zealand was free of haemosporidia but,

in captivity in Kuala Lumpur, where they were exposed to many blood-feeding vectors carrying local lineages of haemosporidia, all four died after 3 weeks in the new location because of infection by at least two *Plasmodium* species. *Leucocytozoon* spp. were found to be particularly pathogenic for birds in the orders Galliformes and Anseriformes (poultry and ducks, respectively).

We cannot easily extrapolate findings from zoo or domesticated birds to wild hosts, partly because of the shared evolutionary history between hosts and their haemosporidian parasites in their native geographic distributions. Although most haemosporidian parasites are not lethal in the wild, they may act as population modulators because they may reduce fitness or reduce the competitive ability of infected individuals.

HAEMOSPORIDIAN PARASITES IN HAWAII

We have learned a great deal about the impact of haemosporidian parasites on wild populations in Hawaii. This example has been so instructive because of the very short evolutionary history that Hawaiian birds have with *Plasmodium*. Like haemosporidia in zoos, this situation is not also entirely natural; however, globalization, tourism, and the pet trade have contributed to a world in which introduced diseases, such as *Plasmodium* in Hawaii, are no longer unusual. Prior to 1826, there was no competent vector for *Plasmodium* in Hawaii. When the southern house mosquito, *Culex quinquefaciatus,* was introduced to the islands, *P. relictum* was able to spread through native and introduced bird populations, contributing to substantial mortality (65% to 100%) in several species of Hawaiian honeycreepers (Drepanididae).

Intensive, long-term laboratory and field experiments have been conducted on Hawaiian avifauna, providing us with a complete understanding of the susceptibility of extant bird species to *Plasmodium*, the distribution (both across host species and in different habitats or elevation), and the prevalence (proportion of individuals infected) and intensity (proportion of cells infected within an individual) of infections in birds and in vectors. Native species were more susceptible to *Plasmodium* than were introduced species and more likely to have microscopically detectable infections during the nonbreeding season.[18] Many surviving species, particularly the susceptible and consequently endangered ones, persist only above 1500 m of elevation, where cooler temperatures prevent *Plasmodium* from effectively developing in mosquitoes. However, because of climate change and warmer temperatures, the prevalence of *Plasmodium* in Hawaiian forest birds sampled at 1900 m has more than doubled in over a decade.[8] Some Hawaiian bird species appear to be coping. The Amakihi *(Hemignathus virens)*, which exists in lowland areas in which mosquitoes and *Plasmodium* are prevalent, showed no significant reduction in reproductive success—as measured by clutch size, hatching success, fledging mass, number of nestlings fledged, daily survival, and minimum fledgling survival—while chronically infected with *P. relictum.*[11] These results are consistent with the hypothesis that offspring inherit genes for *Plasmodium* resistance from their infected parents that lead to increased survival, so it appears that the Amakihi is now a good reservoir for the parasite in the forest bird community. It remains unknown whether resistance will evolve in other species, because this requires both a growing population of resistant birds and heritable resistance to acute *Plasmodium* infection.

IMPACT ON LONG-TERM ASSOCIATIONS AND COMPARISON OF IMPACT ACROSS PARASITE GENERA

Haemosporidian parasites have been shown to affect hosts in situations in which the hosts have presumably evolved with both the vectors and parasites for far longer than in the case of the Amakihi in Hawaii. Much of the research on fitness consequences of haemosporidian has relied on correlative data in wild populations. Although these studies are important in adding to our understanding of the effects of these parasites, experimental manipulation may tease out the causal relationships involved. There are two main experimental approaches to understanding the impacts of haemosporidians on host fitness, brood size manipulation and medication experiments. By manipulating the reproductive effort or reducing natural parasite infection, experiments may reveal causal relationships. Some correlative and experimental studies that have demonstrated a potential fitness cost to haemosporidian parasites, and those that have shown no effect, are summarized in Table 47-1.[19]

Overall, it is clear that haemosporidian parasites may have a significant impact on their hosts, both in situations in which the parasite is recently introduced to naïve hosts and in situations in which hosts have evolved with local lineages for a long period. Parasites such as *Haemoproteus* that have historically been considered relatively benign often affect their hosts significantly.[13,14] Studying the pathogenicity of haemosporidian parasites in nature is challenging because of a low probability of capturing a severely ill bird; weaker individuals are usually not moving conspicuously or have been eliminated by predators. These moderately to highly pathogenic parasites may often be handled by the host's immune system, but may become even more dangerous or lethal when the host is coinfected with another pathogen, or a second haemosporidian lineage or species. Already infected hosts may have compromised immune systems and be more susceptible to coinfection. More studies, especially long-term studies, of the effects of haemosporidian parasites on host survival and reproduction are needed to add to this growing area of research.

PLASMODIUM INFECTIONS IN GALAPAGOS PENGUINS

We have recently detected a *Plasmodium* species infecting Galapagos penguins *(Spheniscus mediculus).*[12] Penguins tend to be very susceptible to *Plasmodium* in captive situations,[4] and Galapagos penguins are considered endangered because of small population size and restricted geographic range. Galapagos penguins exhibit low levels of genetic diversity and very low variation in major histocompatibility complex (MHC) genes,[5] both of which could contribute to the susceptibility of this population to infectious disease. The first task was to identify the parasite and place it in a phylogenetic context to begin to understand the potential for pathogenicity.

The two *Plasmodium* species that cause severe morbidity and mortality in captive penguin populations are *P. relictum* and *P. elongatum*, which belong to the subgenera *Haemamoeba* and *Huffia*, respectively. Using a PCR assay and subsequent DNA sequencing, we detected *Plasmodium* in 5% of 362 penguins tested.[12] Our phylogenetic analysis placed the parasite sequences within *Plasmodium* close to a *P. elongatum* sequence and other sequences belonging to the *Huffia* subgenus. The 19 positive penguins were widely distributed across nine sites of five islands in the Galapagos. Genetic analyses demonstrated that these penguins may move long distances and *Plasmodium* infections may be long-lasting, suggesting that the locations of infected penguins may tell us little about where (and when) the infections were contracted. Galapagos penguins

TABLE 47-1   Summary of Studies Measuring Impacts of Haemosporidian Parasites*

Study (Year)	Parasite	Host	Impact Measured	Result
Examples Showing Effects of Parasitism				
Zehtindjiev et al (2008)[29]	Plasmodium	Great reed warblers (Acrocephalus arundinaceus)	Primary (experimental) infection on previously uninfected juveniles versus chronic infections in adults	Naïve birds developed higher parasitemias; mortality rates in experimentally infected juveniles were high, although not all attributed just to haemosporidian infection (coinfection with Isospora).
Zehtindjiev et al (2008)[29]			Coinfection of naïve birds with two Plasmodium lineages	Strong positive correlation between parasitemias for both lineages
Norte et al (2009)[16]	Plasmodium, Haemoproteus, Leucocytozoon	Great tit (Parus major)	Body condition and plasma protein levels	Negatively affected by Leucocytozoon and Plasmodium
Norte et al (2009)[16]			Red blood cell glutathione peroxidase activity	Higher activity in birds infected with Leucocytozoon and Plasmodium
Norte et al (2009)[16]			Reproduction (egg weight)	Females that laid heavier eggs had higher probabilities of being infected by Plasmodium when feeding nestlings
Allander and Bennett (1995)[1]	Haemoproteus	Great tit	Egg laying, hatching	Delayed
Dawson and Bortolotti (2000)[6]	Haemoproteus	American kestrel (Falco sparverius)	Female condition	Poorer during incubation
Dawson and Bortolotti (2000)[6]			Female return rate	Lower for birds with higher intensity infections
Gilman et al (2007)[9]	Leucocytozoon, Plasmodium	White-crowned sparrow (Zonotrichia leucophrys oriantha)	Song behavior	Infected birds responded less to playback; song consistency affected
Weatherhead et al (1995)[27]	Haemoproteus	Red-winged blackbird (Agelaius phoeniceus)	Dominance	Uninfected individuals tended to be more dominant
Richner et al (1995)[17]	Plasmodium	Great tit	Brood size manipulation	Males attending enlarged broods had significantly higher prevalence
Fargallo and Merino (1999)[7]	Leucocytozoon, Haemoproteus, Hepatozoon	Blue tit (Parus caeruleus)	Brood size manipulation	Females caring for enlarged broods had higher intensity infections
Stjernaman et al (2008)[22]	Haemoproteus	Blue tit	Brood size manipulation	Poor nestling condition resulting from enlarged broods positively correlated with reduced long-term ability to control haemosporidian infections
Merino et al (2000)[14]	Haemoproteus	Blue tit	Medication experiment	Higher fledging success in broods of medicated females
Marzal et al (2005)[13]	Haemoproteus	House martin (Delichon urbica)	Medication experiment	Larger clutches in broods of medicated females, higher hatching and fledging success

Continued

TABLE 47-1	Summary of Studies Measuring Impacts of Haemosporidian Parasites—cont'd				
Study (Year)	Parasite	Host	Impact Measured	Result
Examples Showing No Effects of Parasitism				
Atkinson et al (2001)[2]	*Plasmodium*	Hawaiian thrushes (*Myadestes* spp.)	Serologic response, mortality, subsequent reinfection	Minor transient infections followed by immunity when rechallenged with the parasite
Tella et al (1996)[24]	*Haemoproteus*	Lesser kestrels (*Falco naumanni*)	Clutch size, adult survival	No effect
Shutler et al (1999)[21]	*Leucocytozoon*	Mallard (*Anas platyrhynchos*), American black duck (*A. rubripes*)	Duckling growth	No negative effect
Schrader et al (2003)[20]	*Haemoproteus*	Red-bellied woodpecker (*Melanerpes carolinus*)	Female condition, male and female survival	No effect; however, survival only measured by year to year survival over a 1-yr period
Hõrak et al (1998)[10]	*Haemoproteus*	Great tit	Brood size manipulation	No effect of enlarged broods on parasite intensity

Separated into those showing negative impacts of haemosporidian infection and those that do not demonstrate an effect.

are severely affected by El Niño; population sizes are reduced by as much as 50% during an El Niño year.[26] Penguins sampled (*N* = 94) before the most recent El Niño all tested negative for haemosporidian parasites,[15] suggesting that the population has not yet had to face the combined challenges of *Plasmodium* infection and the stressful environmental conditions of an El Niño year.

ONGOING WORK IN GALAPAGOS

Having identified what we believe is a recently arrived *Plasmodium* species infecting the Galapagos penguin, we have embarked on an extensive plan to determine the following: (1) whether it is infecting other species; (2) identifying the reservoir population; (3) identifying the arthropod vector; and (4) correlating infection with fitness and any morbidity in the population. Each will be discussed in turn.

Is It Infecting Other Species?

If the *Plasmodium* infecting the penguins is a recent arrival, we have grave concerns that a number of Galapagos endemic species may also be susceptible because of their long isolation without exposure. We have sampled a large number of passerine birds along the

coastlines where penguins congregate, knowing that infections must be originating where the parasite is completing its life cycle within a resident population and where the penguins are being bitten by the same arthropod vectors as the reservoir host.

We believe that the infections in penguins are not being sustained by a penguin-mosquito-penguin cycle, because this would require successful completion of the life cycle to the gametocyte stage in penguins. We have never seen the gametocyte stage in blood smears from Galapagos penguins, suggesting that the transmission cycle is through a reservoir species as yet unidentified and that when infected mosquitoes bite Galapagos penguins, the penguins become dead-end hosts. A good reservoir species would be one that is benign in both directions, with the parasite having little impact on the host and the host having little impact on the parasite, the type of relationship of mutual tolerance that permits both host and parasite to survive and reproduce in optimal fashion. This well-equilibrated relationship is more likely to have evolved in a host-parasite relationship of long duration. Because *Plasmodium* appears to be a recent arrival to Galapagos, this cannot characterize its relationship with any of the endemic lineages that have been there for hundreds of thousands or millions of years without exposure.

To date, we have found no evidence for *Plasmodium* infections in any other endemic birds of hundreds tested to date, including passerines of several finch species, yellow warblers, and mockingbirds, and including other nonpasserines such as the cormorants that share the penguins' range. We have not yet covered the entire coastal range of the penguins, however, and know that they are contracting infections somewhere that have successfully cycled through a bird host. Thus, we will continue our investigations; however, at this time, we have no evidence that the parasite has yet infected other endemic species.

Identifying the Reservoir Population

In our search for the reservoir species we focused initially on the only two introduced bird species currently residing on the islands, the smooth-billed ani *(Crotophaga ani)* and cattle egret *(Bubulcus ibis)*. Anis were first introduced by humans during the 1960s in the hope that they would reduce the tick burden on cattle and, although they are slated for eradication, they still occur in large numbers on several islands of the archipelago. In a sample of 60 anis collected from the island of Santa Cruz, where they are considered an invasive species, we found none that tested positive for haemosporidian blood parasites by PCR. It is still possible that the exotic ani is the reservoir species, or at least one of a number of competent reservoirs. We will also test the cattle egrets that were first documented in the 1960s and that are suspected to also have been introduced, although how they arrived is uncertain. In either case, both species occur in large numbers on the South American mainland, and cattle egrets throughout the world, where their ancestors have had long histories of exposure to haemosporidian parasites.

Identifying the Arthropod Vector

We are also working to identify the arthropod vector. Because *Plasmodium* is typically vectored by mosquitoes (Culicidae), we are trapping and testing mosquitoes of the three species occurring on the Galapagos Islands, the black salt-marsh mosquito *(Aedes taeniorhynchus)*, the southern house mosquito *(C. quinquefasciatus)*, and the yellow fever mosquito *(A. aegypti)*. The yellow fever mosquito is thought to be strongly specific to biting humans, and so is not considered a likely candidate, but we will test it because new host-parasite relationships may arise more commonly on islands where population densities of preferred hosts are sometimes

very low. The black saltwater mosquito arrived naturally to the archipelago some 200,000 years ago,[3] and is common throughout the archipelago on coastlines and other moist habitats and is capable of breeding in brackish water. The southern house mosquito is known to be the vector for *Plasmodium relictum* in Hawaii and has been established in Galapagos since the 1980s.[28] Unlike *A. taeniorhynchus*, *C. quinquefasciatus* requires fresh water to reproduce and so will be restricted in the Galapagos to the small number of areas with regular standing fresh water, which are also the sites inhabited by humans. For all three species, our tests will involve trapping blood meal–searching females, identifying the source of blood meals through molecular techniques, and then testing for the presence of *Plasmodium* by PCR assay for any species identified as feeding on birds. The final identification of vector status will require dissection of salivary glands for microscopic examination for the *Plasmodium* sporozoite stage.

Correlating Infection with Fitness and Morbidity in the Population

Finally, our ongoing monitoring work will continue to focus on identifying causes of morbidity or mortality in penguins. Because of the detection difficulty mentioned earlier, this requires regular and large-scale sampling to detect birds at the onset of acute or crisis stages before their behavior is drastically affected.

CAN IT BE ERADICATED?

We believe that there are circumstances under which this pathogen may be eradicated from the archipelago before any of the Galapagos endemic birds suffer the same sad fate as the Hawaiian honeycreepers. These conditions are the following:

1. The vector is identified as the southern house mosquito, *C. quinquefasciatus*. We believe that this is the most likely candidate because of its role as vector for *P. relictum* in Hawaii. Because of its requirement of fresh water, its distribution is severely restricted in Galapagos compared with that of *A. taeniorhynchus*.[3] With this level of localization, and with the historical success of malarial eradication through mosquito control, we are optimistic that this may be accomplished. Because *C. quinquefasciatus* is a recent arrival,[28] it is eligible for eradication, unlike any native species.

2. The reservoir species is identified as the smooth-billed ani *(C. ani)* or the cattle egret *(B. ibis)*, or both. Given their status as introduced species, either or both of these species is (are) eligible for eradication.

3. No endemic species has become a reservoir.

4. The Galapagos National Park, which oversees all management efforts on the islands, will undertake the eradication of the southern house mosquito, ani, cattle egret, or all three, in a historical attempt to divert a conservation crisis. The history of success in eradications in Galapagos of introduced birds (rock pigeons) and especially the destructive feral pigs, donkeys, and goats suggests to us that the willingness and commitment necessary for a program of this magnitude exists on the islands.

CONCLUSIONS

Studies of avian haemosporidian parasites have been increasing in number, partly because of the ease of testing for these parasites using molecular techniques. We have learned much from situations such as that in Hawaii and from the growing body of evidence that in many cases, haemosporidian parasites may have detrimental effects on reproduction and survival. Most of the research on the effects of haemosporidians is still correlative, and we need more experimental manipulation to investigate causal relationships between all the variables, particularly when correlations between some measure of haemosporidian infection and fitness may be explained in a number of ways. Additionally, relationships between fitness measures and parasitism may not be linear. A recent paper has shown that for blue tits *(Cyanistes caeruleus)* infected with *Haemoproteus*, maximum survival was found at intermediate levels of parasitism.[23] A significant negative quadratic effect was found between host survival and parasite intensity, suggesting that high parasite intensities are detrimental to the host, but that there are also disadvantages of controlling the parasites at low levels. Therefore, there may be a cost to being resistant, at least via actively mounting an immune response to suppress infection. More attention should be given to the possibility of nonlinear relationships between fitness costs of parasitism and haemosporidian infection. Additionally, we encourage more work in experimental infection and exploration of new frontiers in haemosporidian research involving multiple infections, with either of the two species of haemosporidia or haemosporidia(ns) and another parasite or pathogen.

REFERENCES

1. Allander K, Bennett GF: Retardation of breeding onset in great tits *(Parus major)* by blood parasites. Funct Ecol 9:677–682, 1995.
2. Atkinson CT, Lease JK, Drake BM, et al: Pathogenicity, serological responses, and diagnosis of experimental and natural malarial infections in native Hawaiian thrushes. Condor 103:209–218, 2001.
3. Bataille A, Cunningham AA, Cedeno V, et al: Evidence for regular ongoing introductions of mosquito disease vectors into the Galapagos Islands. Proc R Soc Lond B 276:3769–3775, 2009.
4. Bennett GF, Peirce MA, Ashford RW: Avian Haematozoa: Mortality and pathogenicity. J Nat Hist 27:993–1001, 1993.
5. Bollmer JL, Vargas FH, Parker PG: Low MHC variation in the endangered Galapagos penguin *(Spheniscus mendiculus)*. Immunogenetics 59:593–602, 2007.
6. Dawson RD, Bortolotti GR: Effects of hematozoan parasites on condition and return rates of American Kestrels. Auk 117:373–380, 2000.
7. Fargallo JA, Merino S: Brood size manipulation modifies the intensity of infection by haematozoa in female blue tits *Parus caeruleus*. Ardea 87:261–268, 1999.
8. Freed LA, Cann RL, Goff ML, et al: Increase in avian malaria at upper elevation in Hawaii. Condor 107:753–764, 2005.
9. Gilman S, Blumstein DT, Foufopoulos J: The effect of hemosporidian infections on white-crowned sparrow singing behavior. Ethology 113:437–445, 2007.
10. Hõrak P, Ots I, Murumägi A: Haematological health state indices of reproducing great tits: A response to brood size manipulation. Funct Ecol 12:750–756, 1998.
11. Kilpatrick AM, LaPointe DA, Atkinson CT, et al: Effects of chronic avian malaria *(Plasmodium relictum)* infection on reproductive success of Hawai Amakihi *(Hemignathus virens)*. Auk 123:764–774, 2006.
12. Levin II, Outlaw DC, Vargas FH, et al: Plasmodium blood parasite found in endangered Galapagos penguins *(Spheniscus mendiculus)*. Biol Conserv 142:3191–3195, 2009.
13. Marzal A, de Lope F, Navarro C, et al: Malarial parasites decrease reproductive success: An experimental study in a passerine bird. Oecologia 142:541–545, 2005.
14. Merino S, Moreno J, Sanz JJ, et al: Are avian blood parasites pathogenic in the wild? A medication experiment in blue tits *(Parus caeruleus)*. Proc Royal Soc Lond B 267:2507–2510, 2000.
15. Miller GD, Hofkin BV, Snell H, et al: Avian malaria and Marek's disease: Potential threats to Galapagos penguins *Spheniscus mendiculus*. Marine Ornithol 29:43–46, 2001.
16. Norte AC, Araújo PM, Sampaio HL, et al: Haematozoa infections in a great tit *Parus major* population in Central Portugal: Relationships with breeding effort and health. Ibis 151:677–688, 2009.
17. Richner H, Christe P, Opplinger A: Paternal investment affects prevalence of malaria. Proc Nat Acad Sci U S A 92:1192–1194, 1995.
18. van Riper C III, van Riper SG, Goff ML, Laird M: The epizooteology and ecological significance of malaria in Hawaiian land birds. Ecol Monogr 56:327–344, 1986.
19. Sanz JJ, Arriero E, Moreno J, et al: Female hematozoan infections reduces hatching success but not fledging success in pied flycatchers *Ficedula hypoleuca*. Auk 118:750–755, 2001.
20. Schrader MS, Walters EL, James FC, et al: Seasonal prevalence of a haematozoan parasite of red-bellied woodpeckers *(Melanerpes carolinus)* and its association with host condition and overwinter survival. Auk 120:130–137, 2003.
21. Shutler D, Ankney CD, Mullie A: Effects of the blood parasite *Leucocytozoon simondi* on growth rates of anatid ducklings. J Zool 77:1573–1578, 1999.

22. Stjernaman M, Råberg L, Nilsson JÅ: Long-term effects of nestling condition on blood parasite resistance in blue tits (*Cyanistes caeruleus*). J Zool 86:937–946, 2008.
23. Stjernaman M, Råberg L, Nilsson JÅ: Maximum host survival at intermediate parasite infection intensities. PloS One 3:e2463, 2008.
24. Tella JL, Forero MG, Gajón A, et al: Absence of blood-parasitism effects on lesser kestrel fitness. Auk 113:253–256, 1996.
25. Valki nas G: Avian malaria parasites and other haemosporidia, Boca Raton, Fla, 2005, CRC Press.
26. Vargas FH, Harrison S, Rea S, et al: Biological effects of El Niño on the Galapagos penguin. Biol Conserv 127:107–114, 2006.
27. Weatherhead PJ, Metz KJ, Shutler D, et al: Blood parasites and dominance in captive blackbirds. J Avian Biol 26:121–123, 1995.
28. Whiteman NK, Goodman SJ, Sinclair BJ, et al: Establishment of the avian disease vector *Culex quinquefasciatus* Say, 1823 (Diptera: Culicidae) on the Galápagos Islands, Ecuador. Ibis 147:844–847, 2005.
29. Zehtindjiev P, Ilieva M, Westerdahl H, et al: Dynamics of parasitemia of malaria parasites in a naturally and experimentally infected migratory songbird, the great reed warbler *Acrocephalus arundinaceus*. Exp Parasitol 119:99–110, 2008.

48 Rabies Management in Wild Carnivores

Dennis Slate and Charles E. Rupprecht

CHAPTER 48

Rabies Management in Wild Carnivores

Dennis Slate and Charles E. Rupprecht

Rabies is an acute progressive encephalitis caused by viruses in the family Rhabdoviridae, genus *Lyssavirus*. This zoonosis is global in distribution, maintained by bats and terrestrial mammalian carnivores. As one of the oldest infectious diseases, control of rabies in free-ranging wild carnivores has run the gamut from ignorance to population reduction prior to the 20th century. In contrast, animal vaccination (both trap, vaccinate, and release [TVR] and oral rabies vaccination [ORV]) has become a novel model for modern interventional wildlife management, using attenuated, modified live or recombinant rabies virus vaccines.[5-9,22,24] To put this effect in context, a review has generated an excellent historical perspective of rabies and its control in Europe.[10] Given that comprehensive contribution, other very recent literature on the topic, and space and citation limitations, this brief overview attempts to focus largely on timely progress in the field in North America since 2005.[16,21]

SHIFT FROM POPULATION REDUCTION TOWARD ORAL VACCINATION

Population reduction and vaccination are based on a similar tenet; that is, the number of susceptible animals is reduced by suppressed population density or by immunization to a threshold at which virus transmission rates are insufficient for rabies to be perpetuated. However, population reduction has proven to be a labor-intensive expensive approach, lacking social appeal as a sustainable control strategy for large land masses. Potential ecologic effects limiting population reduction as a stand-alone approach to rabies control include increased immigration of incubating or rabid animals from surrounding areas in which rabies is enzootic, and enhanced fecundity as a function of suppressed

target species densities, leading to relatively rapid (1 to 2 years) repopulation of treatment areas with susceptible animals.[13] Whereas successes that may be attributed to population reduction relate to the underlying goals of programs, there is no documentation of elimination of rabies in wild carnivores through population reduction in North America or Europe. Historically, the effect of suppression of fox populations in Europe over many years is reported to have produced only transient lulls in the prevalence of rabies.

Enhancement of population reduction was attempted through the integration of lethal gassing or toxicants delivered in eggs or other types of baits attractive to carnivores. For example, the effectiveness of controlling rabies—dampening broad outbreaks—in striped skunks in southern Alberta, Canada, from 1971 to 1986 was attributed in large part to the integration of strychnine delivered in tallow or egg baits, combined with trapping. Strychnine was also applied in tallow baits targeting rabies in foxes in the eastern United States in the 1960s, although the relative success of these efforts was never well documented. In Europe, gassing fox dens was reported as the single most effective rabies control method prior to the availability of vaccination. However, strychnine and other toxicants that were once widely used in rabies control are no longer legally available for that purpose in the United States (U.S. Environmental Protection Agency, 1996), in large part because of environmental concerns and low social acceptability.

More recently, population reduction (live trapping followed by euthanasia) has been integrated on a case by case basis into point infection control (PIC) campaigns conducted to prevent raccoon rabies from becoming established in Canada.[13] The PIC tactic calls for population reduction to be applied around detected cases as an initial phase of an integrated emergency rabies control strategy, followed by TVR and ORV, until the goal of disease elimination is achieved. This integrated strategy is credited with success in eliminating raccoon rabies from Ontario and New Brunswick. Quebec is nearing elimination of raccoon rabies using PIC, with only two cases remaining in skunks in the fall of 2009 from initial detection in June 2006 and a peak of 66 cases in 2007. The future role of population reduction in wildlife rabies control will likely be largely reserved for integration into contingency actions on a case-specific basis to enhance ORV or TVR, alone or in tandem, to address local emergencies. Continued objective study is warranted to evaluate the potential contribution of population reduction to other integrated rabies control strategies in specific local settings.

VACCINATION: CENTRAL TACTIC TO RABIES MANAGEMENT OF WILD CARNIVORES

The concept of ORV, conceived at the Centers for Disease Control and Prevention (CDC) by the late Dr. George Baer in the 1960s, has forever changed the approach to rabies control in wildlife. Initial laboratory proof of this concept, followed by field applications of ORV in red foxes *(Vulpes vulpes)* in Switzerland in 1978, demonstrated the potential to expand the capability to control rabies in specific wild carnivores. Through strategic spatiotemporal vaccination campaigns, the elimination of rabies in foxes from Switzerland by 1997 illustrated that ORV could be applied successfully on a landscape scale. The gradual evolution of ORV from original concept to field successes has led to a shift in emphasis, from population reduction as a conventional strategy for rabies control to an increasing use of ORV geographically and in diverse carnivore reservoirs.

Since its inaugural field use, ORV has been widely used in fox rabies control in western Europe, with expansion of control programs into eastern Europe.[7,10,12,19,22] In addition to foxes, ORV was expanded to a newly introduced wild carnivore, the raccoon dog *(Nyctereutes procyonides)* in Finland during 1988. Prior to the first use of a vaccinia-rabies glycoprotein (V-RG) vaccine in Belgium in 1988, all previous ORV programs were conducted with a variety of baits containing vaccine derivatives from a modified live SAD virus strain, including SAD-B19 and SAD-Berne or the newer generation of SAG1 and SAG2 vaccines, which were produced under monoclonal antibody selection that eliminated residual pathogenicity in rodents and other species. Canada followed with ORV in the mid-1980s using ERA vaccine,

and has almost achieved elimination of fox rabies virus, once widespread throughout the southern part of the province.[15] In 2007, Ontario began experimental field use of a human adenovirus–rabies glycoprotein vaccine (ONRAB) to address residual foci of fox rabies that had spilled over into striped skunks *(Mephitis mephitis)*, and that had also been used in raccoon *(Procyon lotor)* rabies control.[14] The United States was the first country to expand ORV to raccoons in the 1990s, and V-RG use expanded to coyotes *(Canis latrans)* and unique gray fox *(Urocyon cinereoargenteus)* variant rabies in Texas.[18]

The early promise of success with ORV led to an increase in rabies control programs that spanned state, provincial, and country boundaries, and that in turn require effective collaboration and coordination within and across those political boundaries for regional goals to be achieved. In the United States, for example, the broad scientific, regulatory, and management interface generated by wildlife rabies control involves collaboration among diverse disciplines and agencies, with specialized public trust niches, interests, and legislated mandates. State public health, agriculture, and wildlife agencies have authority and responsibility for specific aspects of control of rabies in wildlife. Also, federal agencies have mandated roles and responsibilities, such as the CDC, U.S. Department of Agriculture (USDA), Animal and Plant Health Inspection Service (APHIS), Wildlife Services, and the Center for Veterinary Biologics, and agencies such as the Bureau of Land Management, Forest Service, and Fish and Wildlife Service, whose responsibilities include management of federal lands. Planning, implementation, and coordination of surveillance and rabies control among states has been facilitated in part through a National Rabies Management Team from 1998 to the present. The ability to collaborate more effectively on rabies surveillance, control, and research with Canada and Mexico was recently enhanced by the signing of a North American Rabies Management Plan in 2008. This continental framework fosters interjurisdictional collaboration on rabies issues of mutual concern along international borders of North America and serves as a functional model for broader applications globally.

MEASURING ORAL RABIES VACCINATION SUCCESS

Typically, various ORV components are used as indirect markers of program evaluation, such as bait uptake, biomarker deposition, and seroconversion. Clearly,

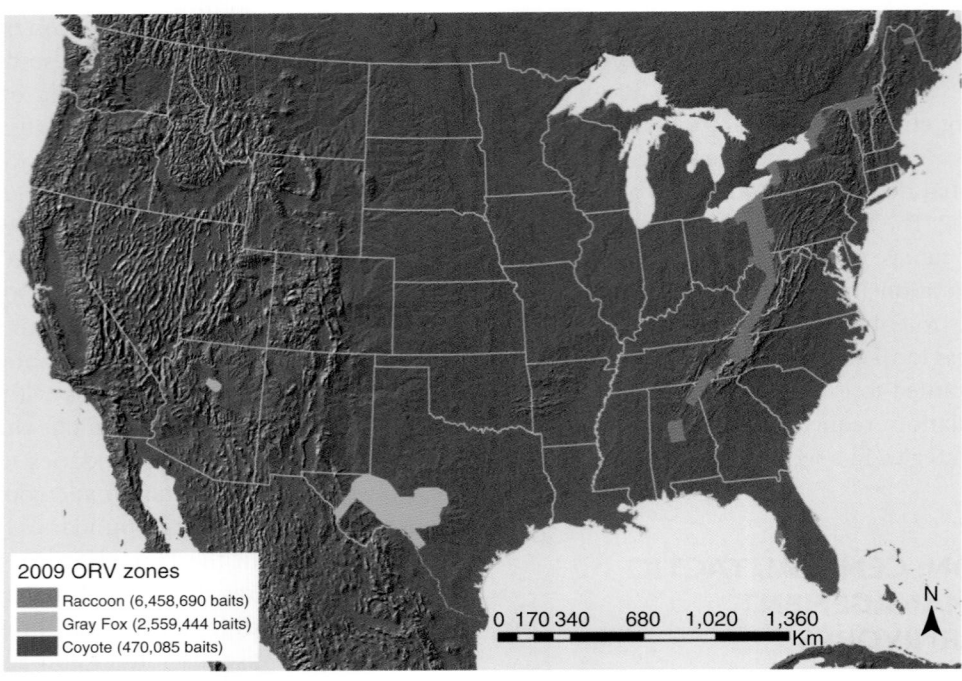

2009 ORV zones
Raccoon (6,458,690 baits)
Gray Fox (2,559,444 baits)
Coyote (470,085 baits)

0   170 340   680   1,020   1,360
Km

N

Figure 48-1

Oral wildlife rabies vaccination zones in the United States, 2009.

enhanced rabies surveillance is essential for measuring the most significant progress and success of ORV campaigns related to an actual decrease in disease occurrence.[21] The need is perhaps elevated even more when resources limit ORV application to smaller, strategically created vaccination zones near epizootic fronts to prevent spread (e.g., raccoon rabies in the eastern United States with an ORV zone less than 50 km wide). Inherent to enhanced surveillance is increased sampling intensity within and adjacent to ORV zones (Fig. 48-1) to complement information that may result from human and domestic animal exposure events brought to the attention of veterinarians and local public health officials.[1] Foci for enhanced surveillance range from road kills to strange-acting— extremely aggressive or docile behavior suggestive of rabies—animals where no human or domestic animal exposure has been reported. Enhanced rabies surveillance within a six-county area encompassing the suburban mosaic east of Cleveland, Ohio, from 2005 to 2007, where a raccoon rabies epizootic began in 2004, illustrates the premium value of testing strange-acting animals not involved in exposure events through enhanced rabies surveillance (Table 48-1). The fact that all rabid wild animal samples were derived

from enhanced surveillance sources in 2007 from this area, where exposures had been previously reported annually, provides an ideal example of the value of complementing public health surveillance to make the best informed rabies control decisions. Outreach, local coordination with state, county, and municipal public health officials, state wildlife officials, and veterinarians, and responsiveness in real time to pick up suspect animal samples are some key factors that drive effective enhanced surveillance.

Access to a direct rapid immunohistochemistry test (dRIT) developed at the CDC has facilitated enhanced local rabies surveillance.[1] Under the current paradigm, trained biologists with USDA and Wildlife Services perform the dRIT in several states, allowing for the real-time testing of high numbers of samples without overburdening state rabies laboratories that focus on investigating and diagnosing cases of public health significance as a priority. Since 2005, in excess of 36,000 samples have been tested using the dRIT in 19 states. All positives are confirmed and typed, and all data are entered into RabID, an interactive geographic information system (GIS)–based epidemiologic database with Internet mapping capability to assist in real-time ORV decision making.

TABLE 48-1 Raccoon Rabies Cases by Sampling Category in an Oral Vaccination Contingency Treatment Area for Ohio*

Reason for Testing	No. of Positives	No. Tested	Positive (%)
2005			
Odd behavior, sick, wounded	17	578	2.9
Found dead	2	142	1.4
Road kill	2	399	0.5
Surveillance trapped	1	738	0.1
Nuisance, otherwise healthy	0	1651	0.0
Pet, animal exposure	*13*	*154*	*8.4*
Human exposure	*3*	*202*	*1.5*
Unknown, no reason listed	0	3	0.0
Total	38	3867	10
2006			
Odd behavior, sick, wounded	5	263	1.9
Found dead	1	97	1.0
Road kill	0	159	0.0
Surveillance trapped	0	296	0.0
Nuisance, otherwise healthy	0	17	0.0
Pet, animal exposure	*3*	*136*	*2.2*
Human exposure	*2*	*136*	*1.5*
Unknown, no reason listed	0	6	0.0
Total	11[†]	1110	1.0
2007			
Odd behavior, sick, wounded	15	191	7.9
Found dead	3	106	2.8
Road kill	1	481	0.2
Surveillance trapped	0	90	0.0
Nuisance, otherwise healthy	0	12	0.0
Pet, animal exposure	*0*	*89*	*0.0*
Human exposure	*0*	*383*	*0.0*
Unknown, no reason listed	0	15	0.0
Total	19	1367	1.4

*Cuyahoga, Geauga, Lake, Medina, Portage, and Summit Counties during 2005-2007 (routine public health surveillance in italics).
[†]One opossum was not typed because of poor sample.

KEY ORAL RABIES VACCINATION PROGRAM CONSIDERATIONS

The underlying principle of ORV is that a sufficient proportion of a target population may be vaccinated to function as an immune buffer to disrupt the rabies transmission cycle (Fig. 48-2). As the percentage of the target population immunized increases, the risk of virus transmission decreases as a function of dwindling numbers of susceptible animals in the population. Unlike population reduction, in which removed individuals are ultimately replaced by susceptible animals, ORV may result in the survival of immune individuals for more than

1 year or for the life relatively short-lived (2 to 3 years) carnivores to meet rabies control goals. Oral rabies vaccine efficacy studies are expensive and often tailored to licensing requirements and, as such, often do not evaluate immune effects beyond 6-month study intervals. Retrospective studies of biomarker and virus-neutralizing antibody titers from field vaccinates may be an opportunistic means to evaluate this dynamic.

Vaccine-Bait Biomarker

An effective oral vaccine and bait attractive to the target species is the basic unit in ORV. Ideally, the vaccine and

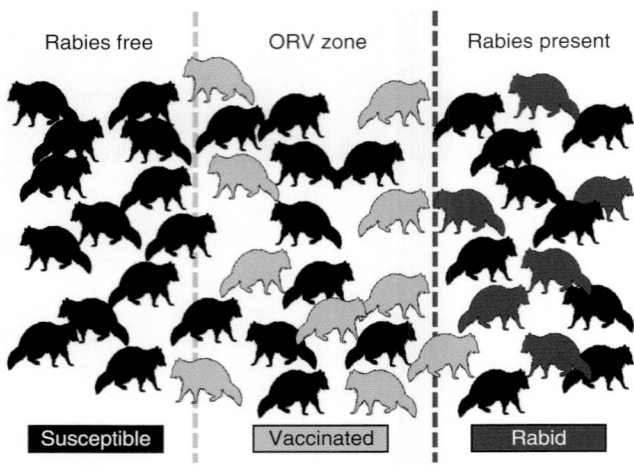

Rabies free   ORV zone   Rabies present

Susceptible   Vaccinated   Rabid

Figure 48-2

Conceptual model representing an oral wildlife rabies vaccination buffer zone.

a biomarker are incorporated into the bait matrix, without substantial aversive taste, to ensure consumption and ample vaccine contact in the oral cavity of the target species. Tetracycline remains a commonly used biomarker in oral baits and results in a long-term mark in bone and tooth. Concerns over antibiotic resistance could affect the use of tetracycline for this purpose in the future. A tetracycline biomarker in teeth provides an additional measure of bait uptake by gender and age cohort and is particularly useful if canine teeth are available from harvested animals for evaluation.[18] Sampling live-trapped animals for ORV evaluation requires a less intrusive extraction of the first or second premolar tooth, which are less than ideal tissues for consistent tetracycline deposition. The baits commonly used in North America contain the vaccine within a plastic sachet (V-RG) or blister pack (ONRAB) that is covered with the bait or attractants. Generally, bait innovations have not advanced with the pace of generational improvements in oral vaccines and, therefore, remains a critical area for research and development to improve vaccine delivery.

Bait Density

Baiting densities should be determined based on estimated population densities of the target species, which may vary spatially and temporarily because of a number of factors, including habitat, annual climatic effects, and management (e.g., harvest of furbearers. Projected

nontarget competition also is a factor in determining bait density. Opossums, for example, may represent strong competitors for baits distributed for raccoons, which may require increasing bait density in specific areas. A routine bait density for raccoons is 75 baits/km² but different bait densities are often warranted to optimize vaccination rates.[17] Commonly applied bait densities range from 19 to 27/baits/km² for coyotes and 27 to 39 baits/km² for gray foxes in Texas.[18] Given that baits are the single greatest cost driver in ORV, further refinements are needed in bait efficiency without sacrificing field performance, which may result in significant resource savings.

Bait Distribution

Large land masses are baited efficiently with fixed-wing aircraft equipped with global positioning system (GPS) capability for following planned flight lines and machinery to achieve prescribed ground bait densities. Fixed-wing machinery currently used to distribute baits in North America is by conveyor belt or hopper. Baiting in suburban and urban settings is typically conducted by helicopter or ground distribution to ensure proper bait densities and safety. Ground baiting may be accomplished by automobiles, four-wheelers, and walking, and has even included boats and bicycles for unique settings. Care is recommended in placing baits to minimize contacts by dogs, the most common source of human bait and vaccine exposures.[3] Bait stations also represent a potential option for baiting in suburban and urban settings, where concerns over human and dog bait contacts, and competition from nontarget species such as opossums, represent elevated concerns.[2]

Bait Distribution Patterns

Species targeted for ORV are typically clustered across the landscape according to spatiotemporal availability of food, water, and cover.[21] This ecologic phenomenon is not always in agreement with fixed aerial flight lines with even bait distribution, which may lead to adjustments in flight line spacing or omitting less than optimal habitats from baiting along fixed flight lines. Continued evaluation of these management effects on baiting efficiency and performance is warranted as sophistication is added to ORV operations.

Social behavior of a target species is a key consideration in bait distribution patterns. Flight line adjustments to intercept territories are required to ensure access to bait throughout the target population. Flight line spacing for nonterritorial species, such as raccoons and skunks, may need to be adjusted to account for relatively small overlapping home ranges, which could result in high population densities. Clustered high-density baiting patterns in suburban habitats may increase seroconversion rates. Aerial pulse baiting (groups of baits, pulsed along flight lines) may be useful if higher vaccination rates can be achieved as a result of carnivore family groups intercepting baits as they travel together prior to seasonal dispersal.

Timing of Baiting

Raccoon ORV operations have occurred predominantly in late summer in the northern United States and southern Canada or early fall in the southern United States, after juveniles have entered the foraging population.[21] This new cohort is susceptible to rabies and expected to have high dispersal rates, which are primary reasons for baiting during this period, along with the need to obtain post-ORV serum samples and biologic information to evaluate program effectiveness before winter, when raccoons are less active. The potential of opposing effects of baiting during summer to early fall, when other foods (e.g., corn crops) are abundant but when raccoons are actively feeding before the onset of winter, particularly at northerly latitudes, requires further study. High ambient daytime temperatures may affect vaccine titer stability and is a primary consideration for the January ORV baiting schedule for coyotes and gray foxes in the southwestern United States.

Frequency of Baiting

Logistics and costs typically limit planned ORV operations to a single baiting/year. An evaluation of twice-yearly baiting (spring and late summer) in Ohio detected no significant difference in seropositivity rates, but a significant difference was noted after the fifth cumulative campaign.[17] Spring and fall baiting, often at high bait densities, was carried out several years, beginning in May 1994 in southeast Massachusetts adjacent to the Cape Cod Canal, but this zone was compromised in 2004 when cases were detected on Cape Cod. Twice-yearly baiting is currently reserved for areas in which there is an imminent risk of rabies spreading, such as in the contingency action zone in northeast Ohio, where twice-yearly baiting at higher densities occurred from 2004 to the present.

FOCUSED RABIES CONTROL IN NORTH AMERICA

Raccoons, skunks (primarily the striped skunk), foxes (red, gray and arctic foxes), coyotes, and small Asian mongoose (*Herpestes javanicus*) represent a diverse carnivore reservoir complex for numerous distinct variants of rabies virus within the United States and its territories.[1] Two of these variants no longer occur in the conterminous United States as a result of successful ORV programs in Ontario, Canada, and Texas. An arctic fox (*V. lagopus*) rabies virus was once widespread in red foxes (*V. vulpes*) throughout southern Ontario, Canada, with cases extending into the northeastern United States, but has almost been eliminated, except for isolated foci in the southwestern part of Ontario.[15] This variant has not been reported in New York, New England, or elsewhere in the United States since 2001, a direct benefit of systematic ORV in Ontario. In Texas, ORV was implemented to control rabies in coyotes (*C. latrans*) as a result of spillover from a canine rabies virus.[18] Integration of ORV with parenteral vaccination in dogs has been credited with eliminating canine rabies and allowed the United States to declare a canine rabies-free status in 2007.[25]

The geographic area occupied by specific rabies viruses and the costs of vaccine-laden baits and delivery typically require the application of phased ORV strategies—first, to prevent spread, followed by methods aimed at elimination of specific viruses as determined by surveillance.[1] Clearly, ORV targeting coyote rabies in the United States and fox rabies in southern Ontario serve as examples of successful phased strategies. Since ORV became operational in the United States, there have been other noteworthy accomplishments in controlling rabies in gray foxes and raccoons.[18,20] Since 1995, ORV has resulted in a more than 50% reduction in the area occupied by a gray fox rabies in west Texas. Recent spillover of this virus variant into coyotes has necessitated contingency baiting in additional areas in west Texas, including a small area of southeast New Mexico, to prevent further spread. If this virus can be eliminated from United States, surveillance and control will be required along the Rio Grande in Texas until sufficient activity occurs in Mexico to determine its status south of the U.S. border. Similarly, raccoon rabies spread has been abated via ORV.[11]

Coordinated ORV among states along the leading western and northern edges of raccoon rabies is credited with preventing this virus from establishing a broader geographic footprint in the United States.[11,21] This accomplishment has not been achieved without the need for contingency actions that might integrate additional ORV baiting (e.g., high bait densities, multiple baitings/year, or targeting a special area representing higher risk for spread) with TVR. Population reduction has also been an integrated tactic along with ORV and TVR, particularly to address incursions of raccoon variant rabies into Canada.[13]

Although contingency actions are an integral part of rabies management in wild carnivores in North America, they are labor-intensive, cost at least 2.5 times more than ORV alone, and are not sustainable over larger tracts of land or for extended time periods.[21] These actions represent special management tactics to prevent rabies from spreading and becoming established in new areas. Often, these actions are to preserve or restore existing ORV zones or to prevent rabies from spreading where no ORV zone has been established. The high frequency of raccoon rabies spillover into striped skunks in the eastern United States often necessitates TVR in contingency actions because of the limitations of V-RG in skunks and the potential threat they pose to maintain the disease and confound local elimination efforts. For example, in the Ohio contingency action zone during 2009, there were only three cases of raccoon rabies virus detected, all in skunks, in an area that had been extensively treated with ORV and TVR since 2004. Access to an effective vaccine-bait to vaccinate skunks orally would ensure success better and allow resources to be shifted to other priority areas.

In 2009, an ORV zone was established around Flagstaff, Arizona, where the emergence of rabies in gray foxes and skunks has been attributed to a host shift of rabies virus variants from bats. This event represents the first real-time empirical evidence to support the hypothesis that bats are a primary source of rabies to mammalian carnivores. Intervention was considered prudent during 2009 in an attempt to prevent more widespread viral radiation and establishment in carnivores. The goal is to eliminate this focus, but lack of an effective vaccine-bait for skunks adds complexity to control measures that require periodic integration of TVR in an attempt to suppress disease.

KEY CHALLENGES FOR LONG-TERM ORAL RABIES VACCINATION SUCCESS

Rabies control in wild carnivores has established ORV as an integral adjunct to conventional prevention and control.[10,21] Conceptual, ecologic, technical, economic,

and environmental challenges must be addressed to ensure sustainability of cost-effective programs and achieve ultimate goals, such as true elimination of rabies in carnivores. The collective accomplishments of ORV throughout Europe and North America to date represent crucial building blocks for future successes. In turn, the hurdles encountered through these programs underscore many of the challenges that must be met to realize the promise of long-term success of ORV. Failure to demonstrate real-time progress toward meeting key challenges, such as shifting to more effective vaccine-baits and strategies, incorporating sensitive risk modeling for ORV decisions, and further reducing the threat of translocations, would likely lead to an erosion of public and resource support needed to continue such programs.

New Vaccine-Baits

Recent use of ONRAB vaccine in Canada represents a milestone in providing an alternative to ERA vaccine, a first-generation product previously used with success in fox rabies control.[1,13,14] Residual pathogenicity of ERA vaccine and lack of effectiveness in other species are among its limitations.[8] Prior to the availability of ONRAB, V-RG was used in integrated PIC strategies to target incursions of raccoon rabies into Canada. The recent shift to ONRAB for all Canadian rabies control, as a result of suggestive seroconversion in raccoons and skunks over V-RG, represents a key benchmark for measuring future success.

Challenges in the United States include improved bait development and access to alternative vaccines that perform better in raccoons, addressing rabies in skunks, and emerging host shifts from bat viruses in Flagstaff, Arizona. Serconversion as an index to vaccine-bait performance averages just above 30% in raccoons, with little indication of vaccine-induced antibody in wild skunks, and represents a contributing factor to the need for contingency actions in raccoon rabies control.[21] Field trials for prospective candidate vaccine-baits are in the early planning stages. Access to more effective vaccines and baits would set the stage for other meaningful applications, such as programs aimed at rabies elimination in the introduced small Asian mongoose in true insular settings in Puerto Rico and other Caribbean areas.

Species Challenges

As an ecologic generalist, the raccoon presents demanding rabies control challenges.[20] It occurs across a wide spectrum of habitats, including urban, suburban and rural environments. Local raccoon population densities vary widely, but often occur at higher densities (25 to 35/km^2) along rural-suburban interfaces, where anthropogenic food subsidies are often diverse and abundant, and represent competitive options against ORV baits. A high degree of spatiotemporal patchiness in habitats along this interface, as well as within urban-suburban habitats, adds logistic and environmental complexity to ORV campaigns. Home range overlap by raccoons is well documented but, in some suburban and urban settings, access points to food may concentrate raccoons at specific sites. Social networking studies have suggested a high degree of contact among such raccoons, which may enhance disease transmission. The juvenile cohort entering raccoon populations in an intensive contingency action zone, within the suburban sprawl east of Cleveland, Ohio, points to the potential value of contraception in local management actions. Currently, captive studies are underway to test the efficacy of parenteral delivery of such biologics, complemented with modeling to project the likely effect of fertility control on fecundity and site-specific disease control. Other species provide additional conundrums, which practical, safe, effective, and humane means of population control could help to address.

Translocation

Translocation represents a serious challenge and a continuing threat to rabies control efforts.[4] The commitment of millions of taxpayer dollars to establish ORV zones to contain rabies could be jeopardized by the movement of rabid individuals closer to naïve areas from enzootic sites. Raccoons and skunks are often among the top species involved as a result of nuisance wildlife control operations and rehabilitation, and untold numbers of these species may be trapped and moved by homeowners, who experience nuisance problems on their property. Unintentional movement of "hitchhiker" raccoons and skunks in trucks transporting garbage to regional landfills is another potential source of long distance translocation. The numbers of animals moved by this means is unknown, but likely pales in comparison to intentional translocation.

In the United States, the movement of raccoons from Florida to western Virginia and southern West Virginia in the late 1970s to supplement hunting opportunities illustrates the profound impact of translocation.

Prior to this event, raccoon rabies was confined to Florida and portions of Georgia, Alabama, and South Carolina.[1] Thereafter, raccoon rabies spread rapidly north and south, east of the Appalachian Mountains, forming a contiguous distribution from southwest Alabama to as far north as southern Ontario and Quebec, east to western New Brunswick, and west to northeastern Ohio. Another well-documented example involved the translocation of canine rabies in coyotes from South Texas to fenced fox pens in Florida in 1994, which resulted in rabies in hounds used for hunting in these pens. Timely detection prevented spread of this canine virus, which emerged in south Texas from Mexico.[25] A similar translocation event occurred in fox pens in Alabama. Since 2008, law enforcement officials have intervened in two major wild carnivore transportation cases in the southeastern United States, but these events suggest that translocation of carnivores (e.g., coyotes and foxes) to provide opportunities for hunting with dogs remains a threat of long distance movements of rabies.

Public health and agricultural officials and wildlife managers need to work together directly, as well as through their professional organizations, to promote effective outreach to educate citizens and encourage more effective legislation and policies, with strong enforcement, to prevent actions that pose a high rabies risk. Effective monitoring programs are necessary for better characterization of the movement of raccoons and other species to regional landfills in areas naïve to rabies, and are critical to determine practical management options to address such scenarios.

Dog-Wildlife Interactions

Spillover of canine rabies viruses into coyotes in south Texas serves to illustrate the active disease transmission interface between domestic animals and wildlife.[25] In turn, this example points to the dilemma posed by unvaccinated free-roaming dogs in regard to achieving rabies elimination. For example, in Mexico, mass parenteral rabies vaccination campaigns serve as a global model for effective dog rabies control. Recent field trials with SAG2 vaccine in free-roaming Mexican dogs represent an opportunity to vaccinate animals that are not readily accessible by parenteral means. Integration of trials with immunocontraceptive drugs is one requisite step toward the integration of fertility control in burgeoning animal populations that continue to tax vaccination campaigns.

ECONOMIC CONSIDERATIONS

Ultimately, rabies management directed at wild carnivore rabies reservoirs has to be viewed in the context of the overall economic benefits of such intervention.[23] In developing countries, where canine rabies is eliminated or controlled, primary considerations include improvements in public health (e.g., reduced human exposures) and agricultural benefits, as well as the potential to reduce the costs of living with rabies through targeting control in the reservoir. Extension in developing countries includes the obvious inclusion of ORV to free-ranging dogs in a similar capacity using a handout model of bait distribution. Moreover, protection of threatened and endangered species from rabies, such as the Florida panther *(Felis concolor)*, Ethiopian wolf *(C. simensis)* or African wild dog *(Lycaon pictus)* are relevant examples for which ecologic and other values associated with loss of a species are additive to human and agricultural benefits.

CONCLUSIONS

Great overall progress has occurred during the past 40 years in rabies management by the vaccination of wild carnivores. Disease elimination is possible through the strategic use of ORV.* However, setbacks are predictable, as evident from the frequent use of contingency actions.[20] As recently demonstrated with the reemergence of fox rabies in Italy, international coordination of surveillance and control among neighboring countries remains a challenge. Rabies viruses are highly adaptable, and host shifts are to be expected.[1] Reservoirs are extremely vagile, and population densities may exceed economic delivery of vaccine-laden baits. Translocation of infected animals adds additional complexity to control programs.[4] Adoption of new generational and recombinant rabies vaccines reemphasize the need for continued research and development and avid environmental stewardship.[6,9] Considerable costs of rabies control remain a central barometer against which benefits of success will be measured. Nevertheless, the contributions of modern technology applied to the age-old problem of this particular zoonosis demonstrates a model for extension to other emerging infectious diseases, and obviates the fact that chance does favor the prepared mind in a true One Health context.

*References 7, 10, 15, 16, 18, 21, 22, and 24.

REFERENCES

1. Blanton JD, Robertson K, Palmer D, et al: Rabies surveillance in the United States during 2008. J Am Vet Med Assoc 235:676–689, 2009.
2. Boulanger JR, Bigler LL, Curtis PD, et al: A polyvinyl chloride bait station for dispensing rabies vaccine to raccoons in suburban landscapes. Wildl Soc Bull 34:1206–1211, 2006.
3. Centers for Disease Control and Prevention: Human vaccinia infection after contact with a raccoon rabies vaccine bait—Pennsylvania, 2009. Morb Mortal Wkly Rep 58:1204–1207, 2009.
4. Chipman R, Slate D, Rupprecht C, et al: Downside risk of wildlife translocation. Dev Biol (Basel) 131:223–232, 2008.
5. Cliquet F, Combes B, Barrat J: Means used for terrestrial rabies elimination in France and policy for rabies surveillance in case of re-emergence. Dev Biol (Basel) 125:119–126, 2006.
6. Faber M, Dietzschold B, Li J: Immunogenicity and safety of recombinant rabies viruses used for oral vaccination of stray dogs and wildlife. Zoonoses Public Health 2009.
7. Freuling C, Müller T: Rabies bulletin Europe, 2010 (http://www.who-rabies-bulletin.org).
8. Geue L, Schares S, Schnick C, et al: Genetic characterisation of attenuated SAD rabies virus strains used for oral vaccination of wildlife. Vaccine 26:3227–3235, 2008.
9. Henderson H, Jackson F, Bean K, et al: Oral immunization of raccoons and skunks with a canine adenovirus recombinant rabies vaccine. Vaccine 27:7194–7197, 2009.
10. King AA, Fooks AR, Aubert A, Wandeler AI: World Organisation for Animal Health (OIE): Historical perspective of rabies in Europe and the Mediterranean basin, Paris, 2004, OIE.
11. Ma X, Blanton JD, Rathbun SL, et al: Time series analysis of the impact of oral vaccination on raccoon rabies in West Virginia, 1990-2007. Vector Borne Zoonotic Dis 2009 Dec 18.
12. Niin E, Barrat J, Kristian M, et al: First oral vaccination of wildlife against rabies in Estonia. Dev Biol (Basel) 125:145–147, 2006.
13. Rosatte RC, Donovan D, Allan M, et al: The control of raccoon rabies in Ontario Canada: Proactive and reactive tactics, 1994-2007. J Wild Dis 45:772–784, 2009.
14. Rosatte RC, Donovan D, Davies JC, et al: Aerial distribution of ONRAB baits as a tactic to control rabies in raccoons and striped skunks in Ontario, Canada. J Wildl Dis 45:363–374, 2009.
15. Rosatte RC, Power MJ, Donovan D, et al. Elimination of arctic fox variant rabies in red foxes, metropolitan Toronto. Emerg Infect Dis 13:25–27, 2007.
16. Rupprecht CE, Willoughby R, Slate D: Current and future trends in the prevention, treatment and control of rabies. Expert Rev Anti Infect Ther 4:1021–1038, 2006.
17. Sattler AC, Krogwold RA, Wittum TE, et al: Influence of oral rabies vaccine bait density on rabies seroprevalence in wild raccoons. Vaccine 27:7187–7193, 2009.
18. Sidwa TJ, Wilson PJ, Moore GM, et al: Evaluation of oral rabies vaccination programs for control of rabies epizootics in coyotes and gray foxes: 1995-2003. J Am Vet Med Assoc 227:785–792, 2005.
19. Singer A, Kauhala K, Holmala K, et al: Rabies in northeastern Europe—The threat from invasive raccoon dogs. J Wild Dis 45:1121–1137, 2009.
20. Slate D, Rupprecht CE, Donovan D, et al: Attaining raccoon rabies management goals: History and challenges. Dev Biol (Basel) 131:439–447, 2008.
21. Slate D, Algeo TP, Nelson KM, et al: Oral rabies vaccination in North America: Opportunities, complexities, and challenges. PLoS Negl Trop Dis 3:e549, 2009.

22. Smith GC, Thulke HH, Fooks AR, et al: What is the future of wildlife rabies control in Europe? Dev Biol (Basel) 131:283–289, 2008.

23. Sterner RT, Meltzer MI, Shwiff SA, Slate D: Tactics and economics of wildlife oral rabies vaccination, Canada and the United States. Emerg Infect Dis 15:1176–1184, 2009.

24. Thulke H-H, Eisinger D: The strength of 70%: Revision of a standard threshold of rabies control. Dev Biol (Basel) 131:291–298, 2008.

25. Velasco-Villa A, Reeder SA, Orciari LA, et al: Enzootic rabies elimination from dogs and reemergence in wild terrestrial carnivores, United States. Emerg Infect Dis 14:1849–1854, 2008.

Xenarthra

Section 6

CHAPTER 49

Feeding and Nutrition of Anteaters

Eduardo V. Valdes and Andrea Brenes Soto

The superorder Xenarthra (former Edentata) is grouped into two orders, Cingulata (armadillos) and Pilosa (anteaters and sloths). These are special mammals that show unique traits: (1) the existence of secondary articulations called xenarthrales located between the lumbar vertebrae and the spinal column; (2) the presence of fused pelvic bones; and (3) very low metabolic rate and variable body temperatures, which allow xenarthrans to conserve energy. They are also highly specialized, but diverse in terms of dietary needs. Xenarthrans include strict folivores such as the three-toed sloth (Bradypodidae), omnivore-generalists such as the two-toed sloth (*Choloepu*s spp.), specialized carnivores such as the giant anteater *(Mymecophaga tridactyla)*, and the tamanduas *(Tamandua tetradactyla, T. mexicana)*. Armadillos vary in their diet, with certain species feeding mainly on ants and termites but others, such as the common *Dasypus novemcinctus,* are omnivorous.

ANTEATERS

A few studies have been published on the dietary habits of anteaters that show the type and composition of prey selected by these animals in the wild. The natural diet of giant anteaters *(Mymecophaga tridactyla)* is composed 96% of ants and 4% of termites (*Camponotus* and *Solenopsis* spp.).[16,23] In Brazil, this species of anteater may consume approximately nine different ant species, but in June they switch to consume termites.[11] Some anteaters, such as the tamandua, are highly specialized predators, consuming mainly ants and termites, but preferring the reproductive and worker castes.[10,17] Occasionally, anteaters will consume other invertebrates but avoid prey with large jaws, strong chemical defenses, or spiny bodies. Anteater tongues may reach out 60 cm with an amazing mobility (150 times/min) and may consume up to 30,000 ants/day.[27] Silky anteaters *(Cyclopes*

didactylus), a nocturnal animal that lives mainly in the trees, will consume termites and beetles, but their main diet is ants. Medical issues (e.g., hair loss, conjunctivitis) has been observed when feeding silky anteaters captive diets in Peru consisting of a mixture of dog milk replacer, sunflower oil, barley, and yeast, with vitamin and mineral supplements.[26] Studies on the nutrient content of several species of termites have found that fat, ash, and nitrogen levels vary based on termite castes. Species that tended to be high in ash were low in fat and nitrogen. In the case of *Grigiotermes metoecus*, they are high in ash because of geophagy, with soldiers low in fat, but reproductive and alate forms were high in fat. Alate nymphs of *Procornitermes araujoi* had 24% fat; soldiers and workers of *Armitermes* had 42% ash and 3.64% nitrogen. In their natural environment, tamanduas feed almost exclusively (95% by volume) on termites (*Nasutitermes* spp.) and ants (*Crematogaster* and *Camponotus* spp.), with the rest of the diet consisting of stingless bees, heteropterans, unidentified insect pupae, and seeds.[2]

NUTRITIONAL CONSIDERATIONS

Nutritional Disorders

There have been a number of varied disorders seen in anteater species relating to nutrition. Rear limb paresis progressing to complete flaccid paralysis and extensive hyperostosis of the thoracic, lumbar, and coccygeal vertebrae has been reported in *T. mexicalis*.[3] The symptoms probably were related to vitamin A toxicosis or excess vitamin D and/or calcium.[21] Similar lesions have been reported in tamanduas in European zoos that had been consuming a diet with high levels of vitamin A (>20,000 IU/kg dry matter [DM]).[5] However, in one study of the natural diet of *T. tetradactyla*, the authors reported that the mean vitamin A value of *Nasutitermes* spp. was 24,773 IU/kg. Most of the invertebrates used in zoo diets will have much lower vitamin A levels, ranging from approximately 60 IU/kg (snails) to 2400 IU/kg (earthworms, crickets).[5,25] Requirements of vitamin A in domestic animals such as dogs and cats range from 5000 to 10,000 IU/kg DM.[20]

Other nutritional problems, including vitamin K deficiency, liquid feces probably caused by high levels of grain and lactose products in the diets, and constipation caused by lack of fiber and tongue problems, have been observed in anteaters kept in North American and European zoos.[18,19] Similar to domestic cats, low blood and plasma taurine concentrations have been associated with dilated cardiomyopathy in giant anteaters and used as early diagnostic indicators.[1,28] Taurine whole blood levels below 300 nmol/mL, (normal range = 300 to 600 nmol/mL) and plasma levels below 60 nmol/mL (normal range = 60 to 120 nmol/mL) might be associated with the presence of cardiomyopathies in giant anteaters. The use of dog chow as a food item has been given as the reason for the taurine-deficient dilated cardiomyopathy in giant anteaters.[1] Dogs, unlike cats, do not require taurine in their diet, provided there are sufficient sulfur amino acids for taurine synthesis. Similarly, symptoms of taurine deficiency have been reported in young tamandua when fed cat and dog milk replacers.[15] Vitamin K deficiencies in anteaters had been reported in the past. This suggested that ant and termite eaters have the tendency to have hemorrhagic problems unless supplemented, particularly when the animals had been treated with antibiotics.[12] In the last decade, diabetes has been reported in *T. tetradactyla* in zoological institutions.[24] In one case, the animal had been fed a mixture of primate and feline dry chows (see later). At the Cleveland Zoo, two tamanduas have been diagnosed with diabetes. Retrospective studies on the health and nutrition of tamandua in Association of Zoos and Aquariums (AZA) institutions are presently being conducted at Ohio State University–Cleveland Metro Parks Zoo.[4]

Anteater Diets in Zoos

It is difficult to mimic the natural anteater diet in zoos by providing specific ants and termites to consume, as in the free-ranging state, so alternative food choices available in the market are used to develop their diets. The selection of these foods becomes a challenge if we want to provide good nutrition and be able to satisfy behavioral needs. However, little is known of the exact

nutritional needs and nutrient requirements of insectivorous mammals, presenting another significant challenge for captive-kept animals. Because anteaters are specialized carnivores, the nutrient requirements established for domestic cats and dogs may be used as models when developing and evaluating the nutritional value of their diets in captivity. These data might be able to provide a range of nutrient values that can be used as general guidelines. Historically, in zoological institutions, anteaters are fed diets that consist of mixtures of different ingredients; these may include milk products, eggs, ground raw meat (horse or beef), dog chow, canned dog food, yogurt, commercial carnivore diets, multivitamins, trace mineral supplements, human protein supplements, and fruits (e.g., ripe bananas, oranges, limes, avocados, mangos). Normally, the ingredients were offered as a gruel mix, with additional vitamin K possibly added. Diets that include these ingredients have been previously described and were extensively used when zoos first added anteaters to their animal collections.[7-9,12-14] These diets, developed at Lincoln Park Zoo, led to some success in maintaining and reproducing anteaters. However, until the early 1990s, North American and South American zoos had a poor record of keeping and reproducing tamanduas.[3] Poor survival during the early years was probably related to their specialized dietary requirements. Several problems with the first diets used in zoos led to the development of new diets in the early 1990s.

One of the diets, developed in the early 1990s was based on a study of the nutrient composition of the natural diet of tamandua in the Llanos of Venezuela.[21] The goal of this study was to obtain baseline information through the collection and analysis of termites, one of the tamanduas' main prey items, as well as tamandua stomach contents. The summary of the results is given in Table 49-1. We found that the consumed diet of free-ranging tamandua contained 50.9% crude protein, 11.2% fat, 13.9% ash, 31.3% acid detergent fiber, 0.11% calcium, 0.41% phosphorus, 2.52 µg/g retinol, 44.35 µg/g α-tocopherol, and 4.58 kcal/g of gross energy on a dry matter basis. This information was used to help with the formulation of tamandua and anteater zoo diets in North American institutions and elsewhere. For example, after adjusting nutrient levels (e.g., calcium), the Toronto Zoo was able to replace or modify the traditional Lincoln Park Zoo diets (Table 49-2). This or similar diets are also used in other North American and Central and South American zoos.[22] With the development of commercial insectivore pellets (see Table 49-2), feeding anteaters has become easier, although

TABLE 49-1 Selected Chemical Analyses of Termites (*Nasutitermes* spp.) Consumed by Tamandua (*T. tetradactyla*) in Their Natural Environment: Comparison With Tamandua Stomach Contents

	TERMITES			
Analysis	Workers	Alates	Overall	Stomach Contents
DM (%)	24.7	41	29.4	17.8
CP (%)	66.7	48.8	58.2	50.8
Fat (%)	2.2	40.2	15	11.2
GE (kcal/g)	—	6.9	6	4.6
NDF (%)	—	23.4	30.8	32.2
ADF (%)	27	13	25	31.3
Lignin (%)	—	13	17.2	16.1
Ash (%)	4.6	3.7	4.1	13.8
Ca (%)	0.2	0.24	0.26	0.1
P (%)	0.4	0.36	0.38	0.4
Mg (%)	0.13	0.15	0.14	0.1
Fe (ppm)	—	394	246	652
Zn (ppm)	—	144	184	163
Retinol (μ/g)*	—	0.65	7.4	2.5
α-Tocopherol (μg/g)	—	40.4	92.5	44.3

ADF, Acid detergent fiber; CP, crude protein; DM, dry matter; GE, gross energy; NDF, neutral detergent fiber.
*Conversion factor: 0.3 μg retinol = 1 IU vitamin A; 1 mg α-tocopherol = 1.49 IU vitamin E.

not perfect. The gruel-type diets such as the one developed in Toronto, are better than previous anteater gruel diets because the nutrient profile is generally closer to the one found in the natural diet, avoiding excesses, like the ones previously reported.[3] However, this diet still lacks sufficient amount of daily fiber (acid detergent fiber [ADF]) if compared with the natural diet (see Table 49-1). The addition of artificial fiber (e.g., Solka-Floc, International Fiber, Tonawanda, NY) or commercial insectivore pellets to the gruel diets may improve their fiber content (see Table 49-2).

During the 1990s, a new diet was introduced aimed at simplifying the giant anteater diet through the elimination of milk products, including yogurt, and the elimination of raw meat, among other dietary ingredients. These changes also aimed to improve the nutrient concentrations, eliminate the presence of potentially harmful components, improve diet consistency, and improve stool consistency. This diet consisted of a finely ground mixture of equal proportions of a dry cat chow and a higher fiber primate chow.[6] The diet may be offered dry or wet (thin paste consistency with the addition of water). The composition of this diet mix is given in Table 49-2. Certainly, this diet has the advantage of being simple to prepare in contrast to the gruel-type mixes. However, simplicity does not mean that the diet

is better in terms of nutrients when compared with a more natural anteater diet (see Table 49-1). The main drawback of this mix is the very high level of starch (calculated value above 20%) and other soluble carbohydrates (above 20%). Starch content is extremely low in the natural diet of specialized carnivores, such as tamandua and giant anteaters. Because of the reported cases of diabetes in tamandua, the use of this mix of traditional high-starch commercial diets (primate and feline chow) is not recommended.

With the development of commercial insectivore pellets in the early 2000s (see Table 49-2), feeding anteaters has become easier. This relatively new commercial insectivore pellet, with less than 10% starch content, is a better alternative to the primate or feline chows. Some institutions will use a combination of the new gruels (Box 49-1) and the commercial insectivore pellet. Although the diets presented in Tables 49-2 and Box 49-1 represent an improvement from the original gruel diets from the 1970s, they are still highly digestible, unlike the natural anteater diets. A study of the metabolic rate and food digestibility in free-living southern tamandua has found that the dry matter digestibility is low, averaging 50%, mainly because of the presence in the digesta of large portions (51.5%) of matter with little metabolizable energy content, such as sand and

TABLE 49-2   Chemical Composition of Selected Tamandua Diets

Analysis	Tamandua Gruel*	Complete Tamandua[†]	Mazuri Insectivore pellets[‡]	DFPC 50:50 Diet[§]	NRC Reference[¶] Ranges
H_2O, %	79	74.4	4.1	6.51	—
DM, %	21	25.6	95.9	93.5	—
CP, %	52.2	31.6	31	30.9	25-50
ADF, %	3.32	10.7	20.1	—	—
NDF, %	4.74	23.7	30.8	—	—
Lignin	nr	nr	4.1	—	—
Starch, %	2.8	6.8	13.1	20[‖]	—
Sugar, %	24.6	19.3	2.7	—	—
C fat, %	15.6	13.5	14.6	14.7	13.8-22.5
Ash, %	5.96	7.53	9.31	6.3	—
Ca, %	0.9	1.25	1.26	1.07	0.72-1
P, %	0.69	0.85	0.97	0.84	0.64-0.75
Mg, %	0.08	0.13	0.17	—	100-150
K, %	0.85	0.85	0.82	—	1-1.3
Na, %	0.376	0.388	0.361	—	170-200
Fe, ppm	145	329	312	231	7.5-20
Zn, ppm	58	101	115	188	15-18.5
Cu, ppm	11	20	24	—	1.2-7.5
Mn, ppm	7	72	90	—	1.2
Mo, ppm	0.3	1.2	0.9	—	—
S, %	0.52	0.43	0.46	—	—
Cl, %	0.58	0.62	nr	—	—
Se, ppm	1.34	0.48	0.64	—	75-87
Co, ppm	0.16	0.62	1.49	—	—
Vitamin E (mg/kg)	541	82.43	84.8	196.3	7.5 -10
Vitamin A (IU/kg)	2964	4960	7576	18,137	250-379
Vitamin D (IU/g)	0.112	2.31	nd	—	1.4-1.75
Vitamin C (mg/kg)	0.48	24.32	nd	—	—
GE (cal/g)	5789	4766	4449	—	—
Sat FA g/100 g	5.99	1.24	4.27	—	—
PUFA g/100 g	3.43	0.87	3.75	—	—
Omega-3, g/100 g	1.53	0.06	0.34	—	—
Omega-6, g/100 g	1.8	0.77	3.2	—	—
Lysine, %	3.74	0.51	1.71	1.64	0.88

*Disney's Animal Kingdom gruel diet.
[†]Disney's Animal Kingdom Complete Tamandua diet (mix of gruel and commercial insectivore diet).
[‡]Mazuri Feeds.
[§]DFPC = 50:50 mix of Iams Cat Food, Dry, and Marion Zoological Leafeater Primate Diet, Dry.[6]
[‖]Calculated value.
[¶]NRC requirements: Protein, fat, Ca, P, g/1000 kcal metabolizable energy (ME); Mg, Na, Fe, Cu, Zn, mg/1000 kcal ME; vitamin A = μg RE/1000 kcal ME, vitamin E = mg/1000 kcal ME; vitamin D = cholecalciferol = μg/1000 kcal ME; daily ME for exotic cats = 55-260 × kg body weight $(BW)^{0.75}$; daily ME for dogs = 95-200 × kg $BW^{0.75}$; daily ME for T. tetradactyla = 107 kcal/day (5.1 kg BW).

BOX 49-1	Sample Anteater Diets

Ingredients	g/day
Disney's Animal Kingdom Gruel Diet	
Beef heart	213
Water	128
Banana	21
Chitin	0.3
Vitamin B complex with B_{12}*	0.6
Honey	5
Hardboiled egg	17
Nutrigro powder†	17
Flax	4
Vitamin E powder (40 IU/g)	1.5
Calcium carbonate	0.9
Vitamin C powder	0.6
Zoological Society of San Diego Giant Anteater Diet	
Mazuri Insectivore Diet 5MK8‡	750
Disney's Animal Kingdom Complete Tamandua Diet	
Mazuri Insectivore Diet 5MK8	293
DAK Tamandua Liquid Diet	161
Flax Oil	5
Jello, sugar-free	25
Waxworm	3.2
Superworm	14.6
Avocado	8.1
Banana	67
Mango	40
Zoological Society of San Diego Complete Tamandua Diet	
Banana	2.74
Water	710
Mazuri Insectivore Diet 5MK8	216
Mealworms§	0.17

*Goldline, 0.6 g = half-tablet.
†Grober.
‡Mazuri Feeds.
§Zoological Society of San Diego mealworms fed a high-calcium diet.

metabolic rate of tamandua was found to be approximately 42% lower than that expected for a nonherbivorous eutherian mammal of its size, with a mean energy expenditure of 449 kJ/kg/day or 107 kcal/day. Based on this information, it is important to adjust the present diets used in zoos to meet the lower energy requirements and lower digestibility coefficients found in the natural environment. The latter might be achieved by adding a source of indigestible fiber, such as chitin or cellulose, to the new gruels or insectivore pellets.

Acknowledgment

Katie Sullivan is greatly acknowledged for her assistance with the manuscript.

REFERENCES

1. Aguilar RF, Dunker F, Garner M: Dilated cardiomyopathy in two giant anteaters (Myrmecophaga tridactyla). In Kirk Baer C, editor: Proceedings American Association of Zoo Veterinarians, 2002, Milwaukee, October 5–10, 2002, Wisconsin, pp 169–172.
2. Bosque C, Hernandez M, Pannier E: Metabolic rate and food digestibility in free-living southern tamanduas (Mammallia:myrm ecophagidae). In Proceedings of the first comparative nutrition society symposium, Leesburg, Virginia, August 2-6, 1996, Published by Comparative Nutrition Society, pp 16–17.
3. Crawshaw GM, Oyarzun S: Vertebral hyperostosis in anteaters (Tamandua tetradactyla and Tamandua mexicana): Possible hypervitaminosis A and/or D. J Zoo Wildl Med 27:158–169, 1996.
4. Dennis P: Investigation of diabetes in tamandua in AZA institutions, 2010 (http://www.clemetzoo.com/whats_new/research.asp).
5. Dierenfeld ES, Barker D, McNamara TS, et al: Vitamin A and insectivore nutrition. Verh Ber Erkrg Zootiere 37:245–249, 1995.
6. Edwards MS, Lewandowski A: Preliminary observations of a new diet for giant anteaters (Myrmecophaga tetradactyla). Proc Am Assoc Zoo VetLeesburg, Virginia 496–499, 1996.
7. Divers BJ: Edentata: Diseases. In Fowler ME, editor: Zoo and wildlife animal medicine, ed 2, Philadelphia, 1986, W. B. Saunders, pp 621–630.
8. Gillespie D: Edentata: Diseases. In Fowler ME, editor: Zoo and wild animal medicine: current therapy, Philadelphia, 1993, W. B. Saunders, pp 304–309.
9. Gillespie D: Xenarthra: edentata (anteaters, armadillos, sloths). In Fowler ME, Miller RE, editors: Zoo and wild animal medicine: current therapy, Philadelphia, 2003, W. B. Saunders, pp 397–407.
10. Lubin YD, Montgomery GG: Defenses of Nasutitermes termites (Isoptera termitidae) against tamandua anteaters (Edentata, Myrmecophagidae). Biotropica 13:66–76, 1981.
11. Meri I, De Miranda G, Arada A: [Dieta de tamandua bandeira (Myrmecophaga tridactyla) no pantanal da Nhecolondia, Brasil.] Edentata 5:29–33, 2003.
12. Merritt DA: Edentate diets currently in use at Lincoln Park Zoo, Chicago. Int Zoo Yb 10:136–138, 1970.
13. Merritt DA: The lesser anteater (Tamndua tetradactyla) in captivity. Int Zoo Yb 15:41–45, 1975.
14. Merrit DA: The nutrition of edentates. Int Zoo Yb 16:38–46, 1976.
15. Miranda M, Loyola M, Cordeiro M, Cancado R: [Deficiencia de taurina en filote de tamandua-Mirim (Tamandua tetradactyla) Alimentado com substitutes de leite para caes e gatos.] Ciencia Anim Brasila 9:1004–1009, 2008.
16. Montgomery GG: Impact of vermilinguas (Cydopes, Tamandua: Xenarthra = Edentata) on arboreal ant populations. In Montgomery GG, editor: The evolution and ecology of armadillos, sloths, and vermilinguas, Washington DC, 1986, Smithsonian Institution Press, pp 351–363.
17. Montgomery GG: Movements, foraging and good habits of the four extant species of neotropical vermilinguas (Mammalia: Myrmecophagidae). In Montgomery GG, editor: The evolution and ecology of armadillos, sloths, and vermilinguas, Washington DC, 1986, Smithsonian Institution Press, pp 365–377.
18. Moford S, Meyers M: Giant anteater (Mymecopha tridactyla) diet survey. Edentata 5:5–20, 2003.

19. Moford S, Meyers M: Giant anteater *(Mymecopha tridactyla)* health care survey. Edentata 5:20–24, 2003.
20. National Research Council: Nutrient requirements of dogs and cats, Washington, DC, 2006, National Academies Press.
21. Oyarzun SE, Crawshaw GJ, Valdes EV: Nutrition of the tamandua: 1. Nutrient composition of termites (*Nasutitermes* spp.) and stomach contents from wild tamanduas *(Tamandua tetradactyla)*. Zoo Biol 15:509–524, 1996.
22. Perez JG, Gonzalez GG: [Evaluacion de una dieta para tamanduas (*Tamandua* spp) utilizada en el Jardin Zoologico de Rosario, Argentina y el Zoologico de la Aurora, Guatemala.] Edentata 6:43–50, 2006.
23. Redford KH: Feeding and food preference in captive and wild giant anteaters *(Mymecophaga tridactila)*. J Zool 205:559–572, 1985.
24. Stetter M: Personal communication, 2010.
25. Sullivan KE, Livingston S, Valdes EV: Vitamin A supplementation via cricket dusting: The effects of dusting fed and fasting crickets of three sizes using two different supplements on nutrient content. In Ward A, Treiber K, Schmidt D, Coslik A, Maslanka M, editors: Proceedings of the Eighth Conference of the Association of Zoos and Aquariums Nutrition Advisory Group on Zoo and Wildlife Nutrition, pp 160–162. 2009. Tulsa, OK, 24-28 October 2009, Published by Nutrition Advisory Group, pp 160–162.
26. Vargas A: [Formulacion de dietas en cautiverio de serafin del platanal *(Cyclopes didactylus)* en el parquet zoologico Huachipas.] Edentata 7:18–23, 2006.
27. Wainwright M: The natural history of Costa Rican mammals, Miami, 2003, Zona Tropical.
28. Wilson ED, Dunker F, Garner M, et al: Taurine deficiency associated dilated cardiomyopathy in giant anteaters *(Myrmecophaga tridactyla)*: Preliminary results and diagnostics. Proc Am Assoc Zoo Vet 155–159, 2003.

Marsupials

CHAPTER 50

Tasmanian Devil Facial Tumor Disease

Peter H. Holz

Tasmanian devil facial tumor disease (DFTD) was first recognized in Tasmanian devils *(Sarcophilus harrisii)* in northeastern Tasmania in 1996. Its origin remains unknown, but it appears to be a newly emerging disease because no devils trapped between 1964 and 1995 showed any evidence of DFTD.[2]

SIGNS AND SYMPTOMS

Affected devils develop tumors that present as large, solid, soft tissue masses that ulcerate, first appearing on the head and/or neck regions. Histologically, they form subepithelial expansile masses of round to spindloid cells with abundant eosinophilic cytoplasm encased within a pseudocapsule. Mitotic figures range from 0 to 12 and average 4/high-power field. The tumor is locally aggressive and metastasizes in 65% of cases, 57% of these to the local lymph nodes. Tumors similar to those on the face may occur later in other parts of the body.[6] Devils younger than 2 years are rarely affected, with males and females being equally represented. Once clinical, the course of DFTD is rapid, with tumors enlarging from small nodules to large friable masses over the course of 2 to 3 months, and death usually occurs within 6 months.[8] Mortality is 100%, mostly because of starvation, because the tumor destroys facial bones and dental arcades. In areas that have been affected for a long time, mature adults are scarce, with most animals being 2 years of age and younger. There is no treatment.

DIAGNOSIS

Early lesions need to be diagnosed histologically because devils commonly develop neoplasms, which could be confused with DFTD grossly (Figs. 50-1 and 50-2). Once the condition is advanced, the gross appearance alone is diagnostic (Fig. 50-3).

CAUSE

Initially, a viral cause was suspected, but transmission electron microscopic examination of tumor cells did not find a virus. Research based on immunohistochemical stains have indicated that the tumor appears to be an undifferentiated sarcoma of possible neuroendocrine origin.[7] However, a more recent study has shown that DFTD is a peripheral nerve sheath tumor that arose from a Schwann cell or Schwann cell precursor, because all tumors produce the Schwann cell–specific myelin protein, periaxin.[10]

Direct exposure to tumor cells is necessary for the development of DFTD but that alone is not sufficient for disease to occur. Damage to the skin or mucous membranes around the head and neck, as occurs with fighting, scratching, and biting, is also required before DFTD may develop. Most biting injuries occur between adult males and females during the 6-week mating season (February to March).[3,4] It is noteworthy that lesions are rarely observed on other parts of the body that are also subject to trauma. Aerosol transmission and vertical transmission both appear unlikely. Transmission via fomites on carcasses or by cannibalism of diseased devils has not been discounted.[4]

The incubation period is unknown but one animal developed DFTD after 10 months in captivity without apparent exposure to tumor cells during that time.[8]

Tasmanian devils have 14 chromosomes. However, the tumors only have 13 chromosomes, lacking both sex chromosomes, both chromosomes 2, and one chromosome 6. All tumors studied have the same chromosomal anomalies, indicating their origin as clones from a rogue cell line that are transferred between individuals as allografts.[11] Being different from the host cells, the tumor cells should be recognized as foreign and rejected. However, this is not the case, with lymphocyte

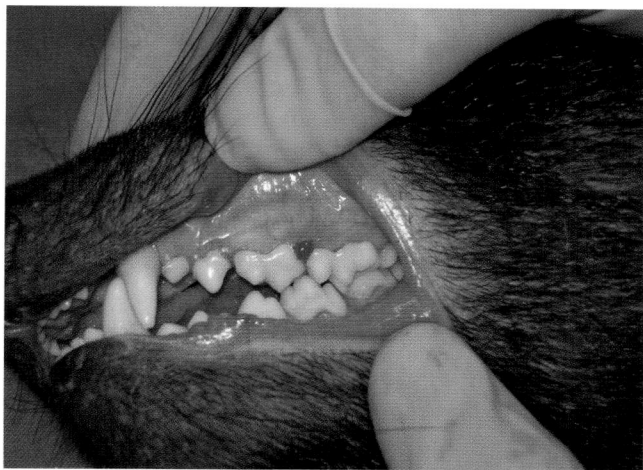

Figure 50-1

Small mass on the gingiva of a Tasmanian devil. Histologic examination identified the mass as a hemangioma.

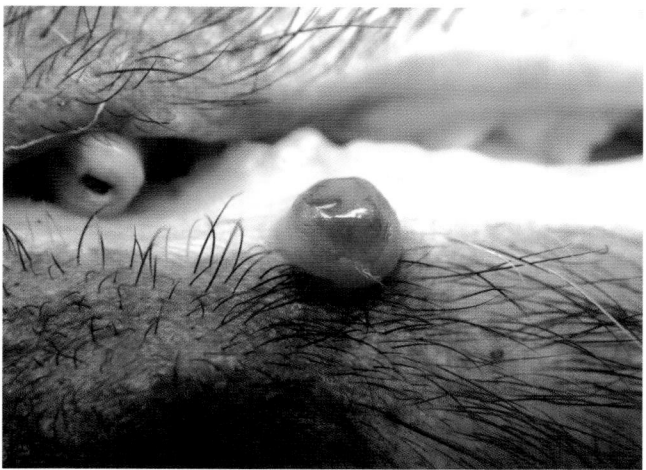

Figure 50-2

Small mass on the lip of a Tasmanian devil. Histologic examination identified the mass as DFTD.

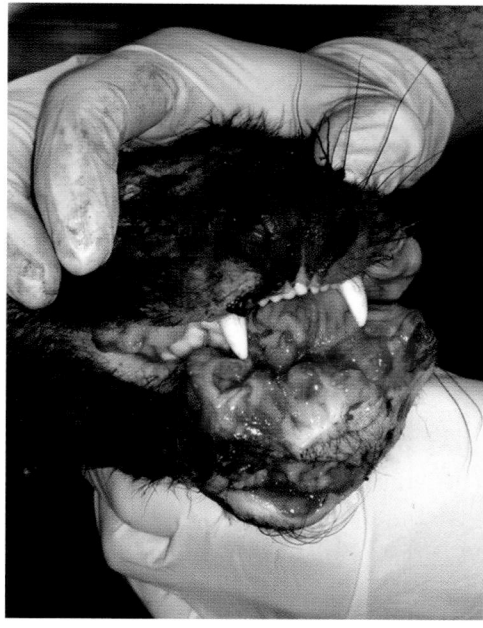

Figure 50-3

Advanced case of DFTD. *(Courtesy Alexandre Kreiss.)*

DEVIL FACIAL TUMOR DISEASE AND POPULATION

Before the arrival of DFTD, Tasmanian devils did not usually breed before their second year with, 0% to 12.5% of 1-year-old females breeding. Because the disease has now killed most mature age devils, precocial breeding has increased to 13.3% to 83.3% of 1-year-old females, depending on region. Whereas devils previously would produce a litter each year for 3 years until reproductive senescence set in after 5 years, devils in affected areas now only live long enough to produce one litter.[3]

Having first been observed in the northeast of the state, the distribution of DFTD has progressively spread south and west, with affected devils now being found over much of the eastern half of Tasmania. Devil numbers peaked at 130,000 to 150,000 in the mid-1990s. Total population decline since then has been in excess of 60%, with declines over 90% in the northeast. DFTD does not disappear at low population densities, meaning that it could cause the extinction of the Tasmanian devil in the wild.[3] At the current rate of spread and decline, it is estimated that this extinction could occur within the next 25 to 30 years.[8]

In the short term, the most likely scenario is one of local extinctions, with local persistence of diseased devil populations. Given the precipitous decline in devil

infiltration into DFTD tumors rarely observed. Research has shown that devils do have a competent immune system, similar to that of other mammals.[13] However, they have low genetic diversity, particularly at the major histocompatibility complex (MHC) locus. Therefore, tumor cells are not recognized as being foreign, so no immune response is mounted against them.[12] Given the genetic similarity of tumors, it is not surprising that no cases have been seen in any other species.

numbers, several ecosystem effects are beginning to emerge. Macropod prey densities are increasing and carrion is persisting longer in the landscape. Numbers of spotted-tail quolls *(Dasyurus maculatus)*, the second largest Tasmanian carnivore, are also increasing as are feral cats and foxes.[4]

The state's northwest still appears to be free of the disease. No cases of DFTD were seen in 705 devils trapped between 2004 and 2007[9] and the population was still considered to be DFTD-free as of February 2010.[1] Despite the devil's low genetic diversity, some of the northwestern animals are genetically distinct from the eastern animals. A lack of suitable habitat connecting the two areas has resulted in physical and genetic barriers between the two groups.[5] The different genetics of the western population and the lack of DFTD in this population has led to speculation that devils in this group may have some level of resistance to the disease. In a recent study, two western devils were injected with dead tumor cells. One devil mounted an immune response but the other did not. The devil that responded had MHC genes that were different to the tumor, thus recognizing it as foreign. The MHC genes of the other devil were similar to the tumor, hence the lack of response. When challenged with live tumor cells, the devil that responded remained clinically unaffected whereas the other devil developed signs of DFTD 12 weeks later. The disease does, however, appear to be evolving and several different strains have now appeared. When the clinically unaffected devil was injected with live cells of a different strain 1 year after the last immunization, tumors did appear 6 months postchallenge. Consequently, western devils seem to have some degree of resistance against some of the DFTD strains. This may open the way for the possible development of a vaccine, which is currently being investigated. Delivering that vaccine to the wild population will be challenging.

MOVING FORWARD

A number of other management options have been proposed and implemented. These have the goal of maintaining genetic diversity for 50 years to enable the reestablishment of reintroduced wild populations.[4] Insurance populations comprising disease-free subadult devils have been established both in Tasmania and on mainland Australia. In 2005, the first animals were shipped to a number of mainland institutions for housing and breeding. These animals have reproduced well and totaled 196 by the end of 2009. In 2008,

a 12-hectare (120,000 m^2) free-range enclosure was established in Tasmania and populated with six female and five male devils. There are plans for three more similar enclosures. Proposals have also been discussed to establish populations of disease-free devils on some of Tasmania's offshore islands. However, individually, these islands are too small to sustain a functioning Tasmanian devil population and maintain genetic diversity. This approach could be augmented by strategic exchanges of animals among several islands.[4]

Studies to control the disease through selective culling began in 2004. Infected devils on the Forestier peninsula were trapped and euthanized. After 12 months, fewer animals with large tumors were being found and population density remained at 1.6 devils/km^2 compared with a similar area with no culling, where devil density decreased from 0.9 to 0.6 devils/km^2 over this time period. However, 99% of affected devils would need to be removed to have a long-term effect on transmission, but hair and scat analysis have indicated that it has not been possible to trap up to 25% of the devils, so that a source of DFTD remains in the population.[4]

If the Tasmanian devil does become extinct, there will be significant consequences for the Tasmanian ecosystem. Preventing the loss of this iconic marsupial carnivore, the largest still alive today, will require careful planning and management and will need to use a variety of available options. Research into this unusual disease is ongoing with new information appearing frequently. To keep abreast of the latest developments, consult the following website: http://tassiedevil.com.au/disease.html.

Acknowledgment

The author would like to thank Alexandre Kreiss at the University of Tasmania for his valuable input and suggestions to improve the manuscript.

REFERENCES

1. Department of Primary Industries, Parks, Water and Environment: Science of devil facial tumor disease, 2010 (http://www.dpiw.tas.gov.au/inter.nsf/WebPages/JCOK-65X2Y6).
2. Hawkins CE, Baars C, Hesterman H, et al: Emerging disease and population decline of an island endemic, the Tasmanian devil *Sarcophilus harrisii*. Biol Conserv 131:307–324, 2006.
3. Jones ME, Cockburn A, Hamede R, et al: Life-history change in disease-ravaged Tasmanian devil populations. Proc Natl Acad Sci U S A 105:10023–10027, 2008.
4. Jones ME, Jarman PJ, Lees CM, et al: Conservation management of Tasmanian devils in the context of an emerging, extinction-threatening disease: Devil facial tumor disease. EcoHealth 4:326–337, 2007.

5. Jones ME, Paetkau D, Geffen E, et al: Genetic diversity and population structure of Tasmanian devils, the largest marsupial carnivore. Mol Ecol 13:2197–2209, 2004.

6. Loh R, Bergfeld J, Hayes D, et al: The pathology of devil facial tumor disease (DFTD) in Tasmanian devils *(Sarcophilus harrisii)*. Vet Pathol 43:890–895, 2006.

7. Loh R, Hayes D, Mahjoor A, et al: The immunohistochemical characterization of devil facial tumor disease (DFTD) in the Tasmanian devil *(Sarcophilus harrisii)*. Vet Pathol 43:896–903, 2006.

8. McCallum H, Jones M, Hawkins C, et al: Transmission dynamics of Tasmanian devil facial tumor disease may lead to disease-induced extinction. Ecology 90:3379–3392, 2009.

9. McCallum H, Tompkins DM, Jones M, et al: Distribution and impacts of Tasmanian devil facial tumor disease. EcoHealth 4:318–325, 2007.

10. Murchison EP, Tovar C, Hsu A, et al: The Tasmanian devil transcriptome reveals Schwann cell origins of a clonally transmissible cancer. Science 327:84–87, 2010.

11. Pearse AM, Swift K. Allograft theory: transmission of devil facial-tumour disease. Nature 439:549, 2006.

12. Siddle HV, Kreiss A, Eldridge MDB, et al: Transmission of a fatal clonal tumor by biting occurs due to depleted MHC diversity in a threatened carnivorous marsupial. Proc Natl Acad Sci U S A 104:16221–16226, 2007.

13. Woods GM, Kreiss A, Belov K, et al: The immune response of the Tasmanian devil *(Sarcophilus harrisii)* and devil facial tumour disease. EcoHealth 4:338–345, 2007.

CHAPTER 51

Viral Chorioretinitis of Kangaroos

Leslie Anne Reddacliff

A widespread outbreak of viral chorioretinitis in wild kangaroos received considerable media attention in Australia and worldwide in the 1990s. Many blind kangaroos were first observed along the Darling River in western New South Wales between April and July 1994. Between March and June 1995, the disease reappeared, with larger numbers of affected animals, and extended into northwestern Victoria and southeastern South Australia. The condition reappeared again the following year and, between December 1995 and April 1996, kangaroos in southern Western Australia were also affected. There had been anecdotal reports of similar outbreaks of blindness in kangaroos as early as 1905, and in the 1940s through the 1960s, but these were never investigated in any detail, so the cause remained uncertain. However, an outbreak of kangaroo blindness in northwestern Victoria in 1975 with similar histopathologic findings was retrospectively confirmed as viral chorioretinitis by polymerase chain reaction (PCR) testing of archived material. Durham and colleagues[2] have described the condition as seen in South Australia, and field observations and epidemiology were described by Curran and associates.[1] Comprehensive laboratory investigations (e.g., virus isolation, serology, histopathology, electron microscopy, molecular testing) of field cases indicating a viral cause were described by Hooper and coworkers.[3] A viral cause was confirmed when the disease was replicated by experimental inoculation of captive kangaroos, as described by Reddacliff and colleagues.[4]

NATURAL HOSTS

The disease was most common in western grey kangaroos (*Macropus fulginosis*), but was also detected in eastern grey kangaroos (*M. giganteus*), red kangaroos (*M. rufa*), and euros (*M. robustus*). Other macropods

within affected areas, including captive red-necked wallabies (*M. rufogriseus*) and swamp wallabies (*Wallabia bicolour*), had positive serologic results to two orbiviruses but no evidence for any ocular disease. There have been no surveys of other marsupials. Sheep from affected areas were shown to be seropositive, but had no signs of disease.

CAUSE

Serology and virus isolation from field cases consistently implicated two orbiviruses, Wallal and Warrego viruses. The Wallal virus isolated was a variant of reference strains. It was closely associated with active retinal lesions in immunohistochemical and molecular studies. The condition was reproduced experimentally by inoculating Eastern and Western grey kangaroos with Wallal virus. However, it was not possible to rule out involvement of the Warrego virus because the inocula also contained very low levels of Warrego virus and most inoculated animals, including all those that developed chorioretinitis, had seroconverted to both viruses.

EPIDEMIOLOGY

These orbiviruses are transmitted by biting midges (*Culicoides austropalpalis*, *C. dycei*, and *C. marksi*), whereas other insects, especially mosquitoes, appear not to be involved. Wallal and Warrego viruses circulate regularly between midges and macropods in northern Australia, apparently without clinical signs of disease. *C. austropalpalis* is known to prefer feeding on birds, but avian involvement in maintenance and transmission of the viruses in nature is unclear. A possible explanation for the occurrence of outbreaks may be the entry of the viruses, or at least a pathogenic strain, into southern vector populations and, in turn, the infection of susceptible groups of macropods. Infection is widespread during outbreaks, but often asymptomatic. Surveys at the peak of the outbreak in 1995 showed 50% to 85% of kangaroos in affected areas to be seropositive to both viruses, whereas estimates for prevalence of blindness ranged from less than 5% to approximately 50% in the worst affected areas. Only severely affected animals that become blind are noticed. Animals are viremic—thus capable of transmitting infection to biting midges—for less than 2 weeks, within several weeks of first infection, and weeks to months before clinical signs appear. There is no evidence for any direct transmission from kangaroo to kangaroo. In experimental transmission studies, control kangaroos kept in insect-proof enclosures with infected animals remained seronegative. There is no known risk of direct zoonotic infection.

CLINICAL SIGNS AND DIAGNOSIS
Signs
Severely affected kangaroos are blind, stumbling into bushes and other objects, especially when disturbed. The gait is affected, with shorter and higher hops, sometimes hopping in circles. The head may be elevated in a star-gazing posture when disturbed. These changes seem secondary to visual impairment, rather than caused by any neuromuscular problem. Otherwise, animals are apparently normal, being able to hear, move, and feed freely and, if feed is plentiful, may maintain body condition. Any deaths appear to be secondary to blindness, from malnutrition, dehydration, or misadventure.

Apart from blindness, there are few external signs of eye disease. Some animals have only small focal retinal lesions that have minimal or no clinical manifestations, but these may be observed ophthalmoscopically. Many apparently normal wild kangaroos from affected areas have lesions when examined pathologically. Changes in eye reflectivity when spotlighted at night may indicate early retinal changes. Occasional acutely affected animals that have accompanying anterior uveitis may show cloudy or watery eyes. In severely affected cases, acute and chronic, the pupils may be dilated and animals may not squint as is usual in bright sunlight. Cataracts were seen in some chronically affected kangaroos, but it is not clear whether these resulted from the chorioretinitis or from accidental eye damage. Increased rectal temperature is not a reliable indicator of viremia in this condition; in experimentally infected animals, this varied from 35.2°C to 38.9°C, depending on ambient conditions and excitement during capture.

Ophthalmoscopic Examination
The fundus of kangaroos is readily examined after pupillary dilation with 1% tropicamide drops using an indirect ophthalmoscope. (Chemical restraint should be considered to reduce stress on both animals and humans.) The normal fundus of the kangaroo has a paucity of fine, short retinal vessels emanating from the periphery of the optic disc and the background color is usually a bland reddish brown (representing choroidal vasculature), with no tapetum. Some animals have a pale area surrounding the optic disc that is a normal variation, in which there is an area of thin retina surrounding the optic disc that appears hyperreflective. Acute lesions of active retinal and/or choroidal inflammation appear as progressive focal to extensive pale areas in the retina. In addition to chorioretinitis, some acutely affected animals may also have anterior uveitis, which if moderate to severe may preclude meaningful fundic examination. Chronic retinal lesions are hyperreflective, pigmented, and nonprogressive.

Laboratory Investigations
Histopathology
For best results, eyes should be collected into Bouin's fixative within 15 minutes of death, one eye fixed whole and the other opened and fixed after samples are collected for virus isolation and electron microscopy. However, routine fixation in 10% neutral buffered formalin may give reasonable results. The brain and optic nerve should also be collected into formalin, and a wide range of other tissues should be collected for differential diagnosis. Typical findings are described.

Immunohistochemistry
Indirect immunofluorescence testing has been conducted on fixed eyes and brains. Strong positive fluorescence for only Wallal virus was seen in degenerate retinas of acute experimental cases. The reaction was confined to the retina and was absent in the inflamed choroid, degenerate optic nerve, and all other tissues.

Electron Microscopy
Ideally, 1-mm cubes of retina and underlying choroid should be collected within 15 minutes of death, fixed for 4 hours in 2.5% glutaraldehyde in phosphate-buffered saline, pH 7.5 (PBS), and then stored in PBS until further processed at the laboratory. However, routinely formalin-fixed material may also yield acceptable results. Icosahedral virus particles 65 nm in diameter are

associated with disrupted and degenerative photoreceptor cells and macrophages of affected retinas. Virus inclusion bodies and cytoplasmic virus–specific 30-nm diameter tubules may be seen in infected cultured cells. Such findings are characteristic of the genus *Orbivirus*, and may be confirmed with immunogold labeling.

Virus Isolation

Wallal and Warrego viruses have been isolated from acute, but not chronic, cases in BHK-21 cells, in primary retinal cell cultures, and in joey kidney and lung cells.

Polymerase Chain Reaction

A PCR test was developed for both the variant and reference Wallal and Warrego viruses, and could be used on fresh and fixed tissue. Variant Wallal virus was detected by PCR assay in both eyes and brain collected at necropsy from experimentally and naturally infected kangaroos with eye lesions. Warrego virus was also detected in some wild animals. The test may also be applied to insect samples, and was used during outbreaks to detect the viruses in three species of midges (see earlier).

Serology

Virus neutralization tests have been used in the investigation of outbreaks, for arboviral monitoring in sentinel animals, and in experimental infections. Seroconversion is widespread during outbreaks (see earlier).

Hematology and Serum Biochemistry

There appear to be no detectable changes in routine parameters attributable to this infection, consistent with the absence of clinical signs of significant systemic disease.

Further Diagnostic Considerations

In animals euthanized because of blindness during an outbreak in the endemic areas of Australia, the histopathologic lesions are pathognomonic. For isolated cases with similar pathology, PCR or immunoperoxidase testing should be used as confirmatory tests. Contact CSIRO, Australian Animal Health Laboratory, PO Bag 24, Geelong, Victoria 3220 regarding access to specific testing. In live animals with clinical signs, positive serologic results are not helpful because many unaffected animals have antibodies to both viruses. Negative serology, however, would suggest some other cause. Toxoplasmosis, head trauma, and toxicoses should be considered as differential diagnoses of clinical blindness in macropods.

PATHOLOGY AND PATHOGENESIS

The principal lesions are retinitis and/or retinal degeneration and uveitis. The retinal lesions vary in extent from small segmental lesions to cases in which the whole of the retina is involved. Acute cases show active retinal degeneration, with necrotic retinal cells, neutrophils, gitter cells, and often copious protein-rich exudates (Fig. 51-1), disrupting the normally ordered retinal structure (Fig. 51-2). Long-standing cases (>1-month duration) have segmental to extensive atrophic retinal remnants and few inflammatory cells (Fig. 51-3). The uveitis in acute and chronic cases is characterized by infiltration with mononuclear cells, including prominent plasma cells, and is most severe in the choroid overlying the affected retina. The lesion is spectacular in acute cases, with markedly thickened choroid. Wallerian degeneration, a secondary change that is the result of the loss of ganglion cells from the retina, is seen in optic nerves in acute cases, extending into the optic tracts in chronic cases. Mild multifocal nonsuppurative encephalitis occurs in some cases, possibly a direct result of viral infection, but has no clinical manifestations.

This disease is not a simple viral infection, and the eye lesions may be immunologically mediated. The eye is recognized as a privileged immunologic site, which normally contains no lymphocytes and no antigen-processing macrophages.[5] Activated lymphocytes are produced in the spleen in response to leakage of foreign antigen from the eye. These reach the eye approximately

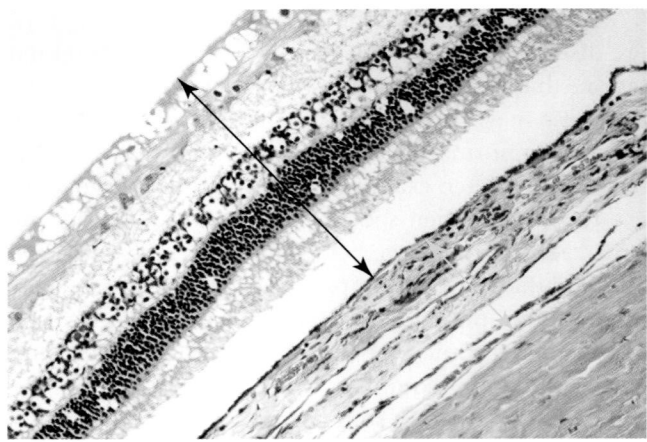

Figure 51-1

Section of normal eye from a Western grey kangaroo (*black arrow* spans the retina, *yellow arrow with solid arrowheads* spans the choroid). The space at the base of retina is a common artifact in paraffin-embedded histologic preparations (H & E stain, 400×).

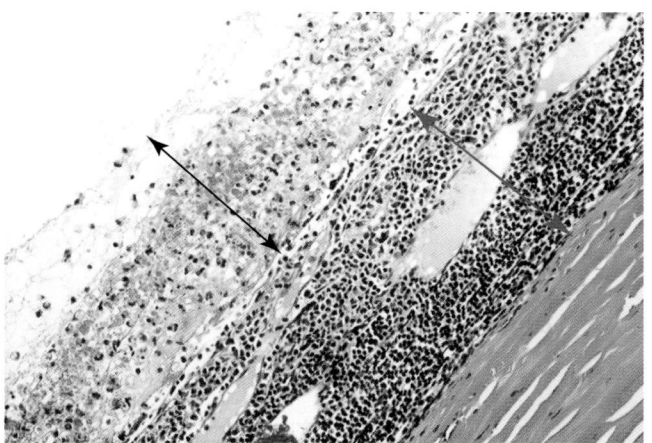

Figure 51-2

Section of eye from an acutely blind Western grey kangaroo. There is severe retinal degeneration, with abundant necrotic retinal cells, gitter cells, and some mixed inflammatory cells (*black arrow* spans the retina). The markedly thickened choroid has chronic lympoplasmacytic infiltration (*red arrow with solid arrowheads* spans the choroid; H & E stain, 400×).

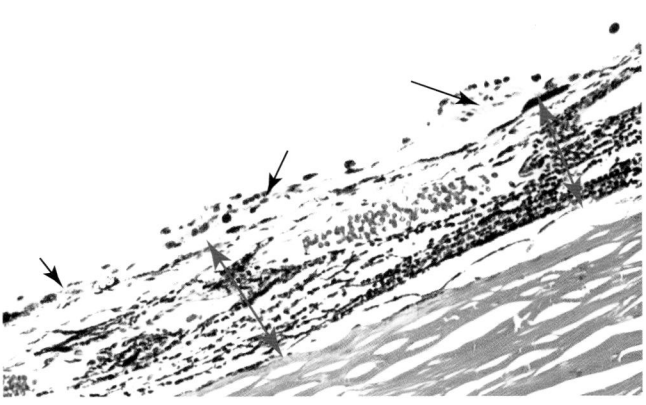

Figure 51-3

Section of eye from a long-standing case of viral chorioretinitis in a blind Western grey kangaroo. There is severe retinal atrophy *(black arrows)*, and a chronic nonsuppurative choroiditis (*red arrows with solid arrowheads* span the choroid; H & E stain, 400×).

1 week later and, once present, are capable of responding to a range of antigenic stimuli leading to the typical recurrent nature of uveitis in most domestic species. It is reasonable to assume that the initial infection of the eye in kangaroos occurs coincident with, or soon after, the detectable viremia. Stimulated lymphocytes reach the eye 1 week later, at about the same time as seroconversion. However, fundic changes are not seen for at least a further 2 weeks, suggesting an immunologic pathogenesis for the retinal damage. The pathology of acutely affected kangaroos supports this contention. Acute retinal degeneration coincident with a subacute to chronic lymphoplasmacytic choroiditis implies that choroidal changes may precede the retinal lesions. The anatomy of the macropod eye, with a paucity of retinal vessels such that the retina is more dependent on choroidal blood supply than in eutherian mammals, might predispose to retinal damage secondary to choroidal inflammation. Although Wallal virus seems to be the main virus involved, a dual infection may be necessary to precipitate the appearance of serious eye lesions. All experimental cases and almost all field cases of this disease had antibodies to both viruses, and the retina from an archival case had genetic material from an unknown but related orbivirus, as well as Wallal virus. The role of sequential or dual infections with closely related viruses, and the enhancement of infection and/or severity of clinical disease by antibody, have been investigated for other viral diseases, notably dengue fever and Murray Valley encephalitis. Further studies are necessary to clarify the pathogenesis of viral chorioretinitis in macropods.

TREATMENT, PREVENTION, AND CONTROL

Assuming an immunologic pathogenesis, local or systemic corticosteroid treatment might be helpful to reduce retinal damage in acute cases, but this is unproven. Currently, no treatment is practical, and retinal damage is permanent. However, animals with limited sight may adapt, especially in captivity, where their needs are well met; even blind wild animals in good seasons may maintain body condition. As an insect-borne disease, this condition is not directly contagious and highly unlikely to occur in zoological collections outside of the endemic areas in Australia. The period of viremia is brief and no carrier state is known, so the risk of transport of infected macropods, except from affected areas during an outbreak, is minimal. A national arbovirus monitoring program in Australia plots the extent of arboviral spread on an annual basis, allowing rational decisions to be made to avoid risk of moving potentially infected animals. A 1-month quarantine of animals imported in insect-proof enclosures from endemic areas would remove any risk of introduction.

REFERENCES

1. Curran G, Reddacliff LA, Menke L: Investigating the epidemiology of a new disease: Viral blindness in kangaroos. Presented at the VIII International Symposium on Veterinary Epidemiology and Economics, France, 1997 (http://www.sciquest.org.nz/elibrary/download/62111/Investigating_the_epidemiology_of_a_new_disease_%3A_viral_blindness_in_kangaroos?#search=%22Investigating%20the%20epidemiology%20of%20a%20new%20disease%20viral%20Viral%20%20blindness%20in%20kangaroos%22).
2. Durham PJ, Finnie JW, Lawrence DA, Alexander P: Blindness in South Australian kangaroos. Aust Vet J 73:111–112, 1996.
3. Hooper PT, Lunt RA, Gould AR, et al: Epidemic of blindness in kangaroos—Evidence of a viral aaetiology. Aust Vet J 77:529–536, 1999.
4. Reddacliff L, Kirkland P, Philbey A, et al: Experimental reproduction of viral chorioretinitis in kangaroos. Aust Vet J 77:522–528, 1999.
5. Wilcock BP: The eye. In Jubb KVF, Kennedy PC, Palmer N, editors: Pathology of domestic animals, San Diego, 1993, Academic Press, pp 441–521.

Primates

CHAPTER 52

Degenerative Skeletal Diseases of Primates

Michael J. Adkesson and David A. Rubin

Degenerative pathology affecting the skeletal system is well recognized in all classes of animals, with significant overlap among the conditions recognized in standard veterinary models (canine, feline, and equine) and humans. As a new One Health initiative philosophy emerges in the veterinary and medical fields, an obvious area of benefit is the veterinary care of nonhuman primates (NHPs). Through improvements in husbandry and care in recent decades, zoo clinicians are now routinely challenged with providing geriatric care to NHPs. Degenerative joint disease (DJD) is just one of many diseases more common in such geriatric populations.

Diagnosis and management of DJD in NHPs has traditionally followed veterinary impressions derived from our knowledge of traditional veterinary models. This approach, however, neglects a vast amount of knowledge existing in the human medical field. With osteoarthritis affecting an estimated 27 million Americans, veterinary care of NHP may benefit greatly by using the information on DJD derived from the human medical field. NHPs also bridge the divide between quadrupedal animals and bipedal humans. Thus, the veterinary approach to DJD in NHPs may at times be misguided if knowledge based only on animal models is applied, rather than considering the manifestations in bipedal humans. Furthermore, humans are able to describe clearly whether a condition is causing pain versus stiffness, joint locking, or joint instability. Humans are able to communicate whether a therapy is effective and are evaluated with diagnostic modalities not routinely available in the veterinary field. This type of information could greatly benefit the medical care of NHPs in zoological settings.

This chapter aims to discuss the most common DJDs in NHPs affecting the peripheral joints and spine, with incorporation of knowledge from the human medical field. Existing literature on DJD in NHPs focuses heavily on laboratory specimens and skeleton data from wild specimens. As veterinary care of zoo and wild primates continues to advance, the less described clinical diagnosis and treatment of DJD in NHPs will expand in importance.

Degenerative arthropathies in the peripheral synovial joints are best characterized as osteoarthritis (OA). Degenerative arthropathy in the spine, generically termed *spondylosis*, includes OA of the synovial joints (facet, uncovertebral, atlantoaxial, and sacroiliac joints), degenerative disc disease (DDD) of the fibrocartilaginous intervertebral discs, and senescent changes in the attachments of the fibrous supporting structures (degenerative enthesopathy).

OSTEOARTHRITIS

Osteoarthritis refers to the pathologic failure of synovial joints characterized by the mechanical destruction of articular cartilage, with secondary changes in the subchondral bone (osteophytes, sclerosis, and eburnation). Morphologically, it is well established that human OA resembles the disease in baboons and macaques, which are used as experimental models.[2,4,6] OA is distinct from erosive and infectious arthritis, in which cartilage dissolution and erosion of exposed bone surfaces are predominantly mediated by inflammatory changes in the synovial lining (pannus formation), without reactive bone proliferation (osteophytosis). No longer considered simply age-related or trauma-induced wear and tear, OA is the result of complex structural and biochemical changes in the synovial membrane and fluid, chondrocytes, collagen matrix and proteoglycans, and underlying cortical and cancellous bone.[13] Additionally, genetic predispositions strongly influence the development of OA in humans.[25] When no specific underlying condition is identified, the term *primary osteoarthritis* is used. *Secondary osteoarthritis* results when an underlying joint condition or systemic disease leads to premature joint degeneration.[17] Previous extremity trauma is the most common predisposition in humans.[8] Intra-articular fractures may result in incongruence of the articular surfaces, whereas extra-articular malunions may alter weight bearing, stance, gait, and joint loading. Ligament, tendon, meniscal, and muscle injuries will also affect biomechanics, especially if they result in joint instability. Similarly, osteomyelitis and septic arthritis, bleeding diatheses, crystal deposition diseases (e.g., gout), or osteonecrosis will change the physical characteristics of the articular surfaces of the bones, a risk factor for the development of OA.

Degenerative arthritis is recognized in free-ranging wild primates. Reported prevalence varies widely among studies, because data interpretation from wild specimens is often confounded by limited information on age, unknown history of injuries, and variation in observer interpretations. OA prevalence in wild great apes has been reported at 1% to 3%,[9] although much higher frequencies have also been reported.[5] Similar frequencies of OA were found in large studies of free-ranging prosimians (1.4%) and Old World (0.9%) and New World monkeys (1.5%).[21,22]

Assessing OA prevalence in wild populations is difficult because of the presumed impact of OA on survival. Selective pressures are likely to remove affected animals from the population rapidly. Captivity itself may play a role in the development of OA through alterations in environment, but this becomes difficult to evaluate because of the bias resulting from longer life expectancies in captive primates. Age is the most consistent risk factor for OA development in humans[26] and similar increases in prevalence and severity with age has been noted in baboons and macaques.[2,4,6] OA was found to be four and six times more common in captive Old World primates and prosimians, respectively.[21] Another study found OA in 12.5% of captive New World primates, compared with only 1.5% of wild specimens.[22] Housing may also play a role; captive macaques in a free-range setting had a higher prevalence and severity of OA than those in cages, possibly because of the protective trauma-free environment afforded by the cages.[6,10]

A higher incidence is seen in women and has been similarly reported in female rhesus macaques,[2] as well as an increased incidence in females with higher parity.[6] In humans, obesity is associated with earlier onset, increased prevalence, and more rapid progression of knee OA, but not necessarily hip OA.[16] Body weight was not found to be an influence in two studies of NHPs[2,4]; however, it is uncommon for NHPs in research settings to display significant obesity.

Clinical Signs

Signs of OA in NHPs may include alterations in gait, reluctance to walk and climb, appreciable lameness, and joint swelling.[6,10] Pain is difficult to assess accurately, but the clinician should err on the side of assuming that pain is present when OA is suspected. In humans, although joint pain is the most common clinical manifestation of OA, not all arthritic joints are symptomatic, and the severity of pain does not necessarily correlate with radiologic or histologic findings. When present, the pain of osteoarthritis increases with activity and improves with rest. Stiffness and decreased range of motion are also common. Mechanical symptoms—catching, locking, clicking—often indicate a complication of the disease, such as the development of loose bodies. Instability and malalignment caused by OA typically only occur in end-stage disease. Because of an often stoic nature and inability to describe pain verbally, NHPs with severe radiologic changes (Fig. 52-1) may show only mild clinical signs of discomfort (see later).

Joints Affected

In humans, primary OA in the upper extremity most commonly affects the basal joints of the thumbs, proximal and distal interphalangeal joints of the fingers, and glenohumeral and acromioclavicular joints in the shoulder.[17] Involvement of the elbows, metacarpophalangeal joints, and wrists is uncommon. In the lower extremities, hip, knee, and great toe metatarsophalangeal joint disease is most common. Spinal column OA occurs primarily in the facet joints of the lower cervical and lumbar spines, uncovertebral joints in the lower cervical spine, and the articulation between the anterior ring of C1 and the dens. Secondary osteoarthritis caused by trauma may afflict any joint, but most cases of OA in the ankles, hindfeet, midfeet, and elbows are post-traumatic. Atypical polyarticular distributions are often a clue to an underlying systemic condition.

In NHP, clear patterns of distribution are not as well defined, but several studies have noted similarities and differences from human patterns. As in humans, stifle, hip, interphalangeal, and spinal OA are common in NHP.[6,10,21,22] In contrast, primary elbow OA is uncommon in humans, but is seen frequently in

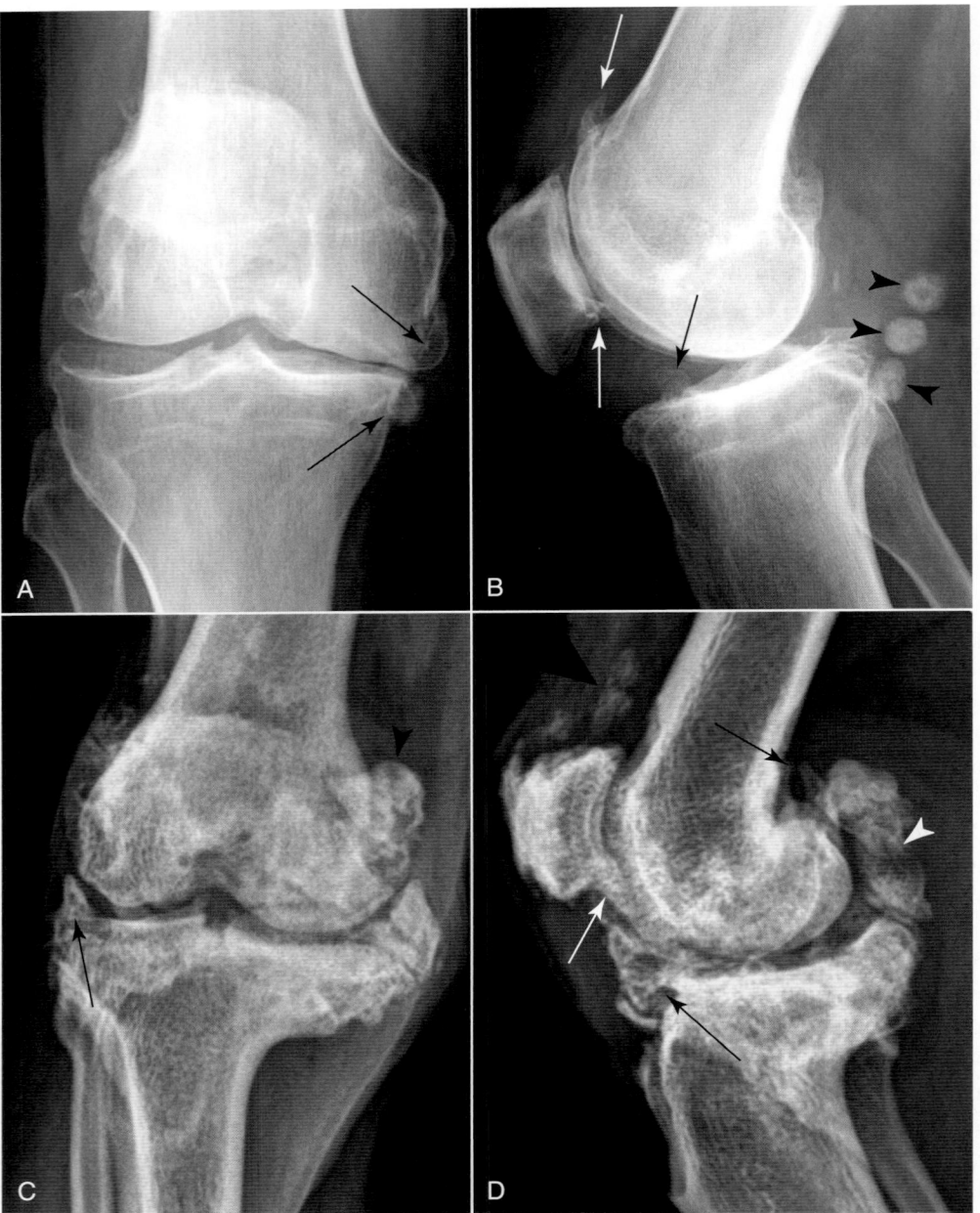

Figure 52-1

Osteoarthritis (OA). Shown are anteroposterior (AP) (**A**) and lateral (**B**) knee radiographs in a human who had intermittent knee locking and pain with walking. Note the severity of the medial and patellofemoral joint spaces compared with the lateral compartment. Peripheral osteophytes *(arrows)* emanate from the bones, while loose osteocartilaginous bodies *(arrowheads)* are present in the posterior joint space. Also shown are AP (**C**) and lateral (**D**) knee radiographs from a *Papio papio* with severe OA. This animal displayed no perceivable clinical signs, but pain and discomfort were presumed to be present. Large osteophytes *(arrows)* and loose bodies *(arrowheads)* are similar in distribution to those of the human.

geriatric quadrupedal and arboreal NHPs (Fig. 52-2). Interestingly, the relative risk of OA affecting the thumb base was almost eight times higher in humans than in a colony of macaques.[12] The more rudimentary NHP opposable thumb may be less prone to OA, because the evolutionary incongruence between joint design and altered functional demand in humans leads to increased OA. Studies in wild chimpanzees have shown OA to be more prevalent in the joints of the forelimbs than the hindlimbs.[5]

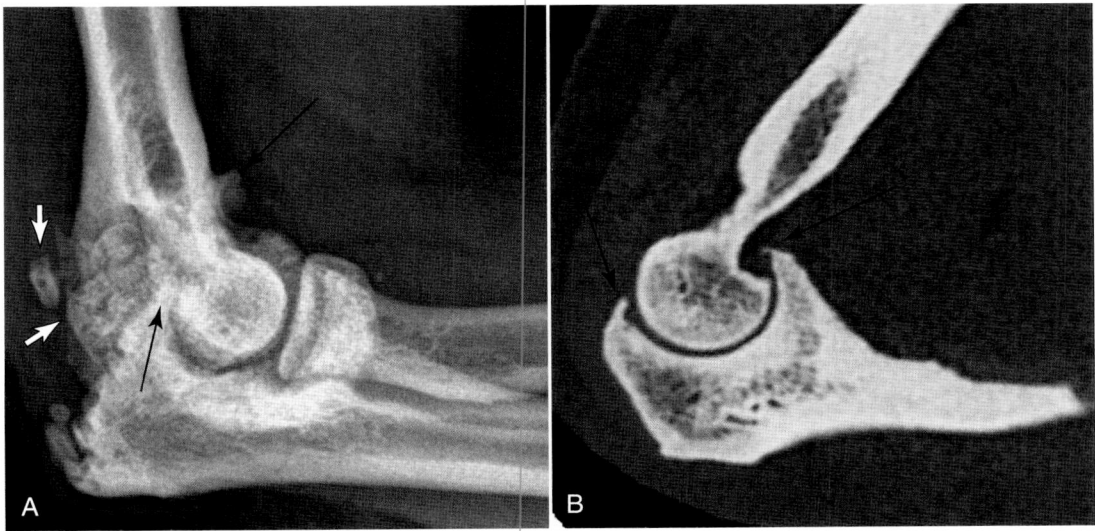

Figure 52-2

Elbow osteoarthritis. **A,** Lateral radiograph from a *Papio papio.* **B,** Sagittal reconstruction from a postmortem CT scan image of an orangutan showing narrowing of the humeroulnar joint and marginal osteophytes *(arrows).* Note the loose bodies *(white arrows)* in A, as well as the ossification attached to the olecranon, a manifestation of DISH. Primary elbow osteoarthritis is unusual in bipedal humans, but may occur in geriatric quadruped and arboreal primates.

Skeletal distribution of OA may also differ between captive and wild NHPs. Among Old World primates, the elbow was more commonly affected in captive specimens and the knee more so in wild specimens.[21] In captive New World monkeys, OA more commonly affected the shoulder, compared with the elbow and knee in free-ranging monkeys.[22]

SPONDYLOSIS

Spondylosis is a generic term that refers to degenerative arthropathy in the spine, including OA of the synovial joints (facet, uncovertebral, atlantoaxial, and sacroiliac joints), DDD of the fibrocartilaginous intervertebral discs, and senescent changes in the attachments of the fibrous supporting structures (degenerative enthesopathy).

Understanding the general anatomy of the primate spine is important for understanding degenerative changes. The spine consists of multiple motion segments, each composed of an adjacent pair of vertebrae and the connective tissues between the two.[18] Anteriorly, the vertebral body endplates are attached to the fibrocartilaginous disc through strong fibrous attachments called Sharpey's fibers. Each disc has a fibrous annulus surrounding a spongy nucleus. Strong longitudinal ligaments run the length of the spine craniocaudally, attached to the anterior and posterior margins of

the vertebral bodies and annulus fibrosus of the discs. Posteriorly, paired synovial facet joints are supported by the ligamentum flavum between the lamina and interspinous ligaments further dorsally. The orientation of the facet joints differs throughout the spine, so that the cervical spine motion segments demonstrate angular excursion (flexion-extension), rotation, and lateral bending, the lumbar spine shows angular excursion and lateral bending, and the thoracic spine is largely limited to a small amount of flexion-extension. The cervical spine also has specialized synovial joints in addition to the facets. These joints include the articulations between the lateral masses of C1 and C2 and the articulation between the anterior ring of the atlas and odontoid process, which allow for neck rotation.

Attachments of other elements of the axial skeleton also provide stability and protection of critical organs at the expense of decreased mobility. These structures include the ribs in the thoracic spine (each rib has three synovial joints linking it to each thoracic motion segment) and the sacroiliac joints, which have both synovial and ligamentous components, between the lower spine and pelvis.

The synovial joints in the spine are commonly affected by OA, analogous to the synovial joints in the extremities. In addition to pain and stiffness, facet and uncovertebral joint OA may result in radiculopathy in humans. The spinal nerves run adjacent to the joints, so osteophytes are an important cause of nerve compression.[7] Based on large numbers of wild ape specimens, spinal degenerative disease was found to be significantly more prevalent in humans than apes.[9] The human bipedal stance exerts greater compressive forces on the vertebral column than that seen in quadrupeds and may account for this disparity. Although quadrupedal for locomotion, many NHP still spend most of their time in an upright position.

Degenerative Disc Disease

Degeneration of the fibrocartilaginous interbody joints likely begins in the nucleus pulposus of the disc, which desiccates with age. As the process progresses, radially oriented tears occur within the annulus fibrosis. Herniated nucleus material may extend through these defects, protrude beyond the confines of the disc, or even extrude through the longitudinal ligaments. Gas clefts or calcification may develop in the degenerating discs. Collapse of the disc is a relatively late manifestation. These morphologic changes each affect the biomechanics of the motion segment. Specifically, loss of disc height and turgidity (often combined with facet joint osteoarthritis) increase the load in the vertebral endplates, and predispose to segmental hypermobility. The response of the endplates is marginal bone proliferation, similar to the formation of osteophytosis in synovial joint osteoarthritis.[1] Like osteophytes, this endplate remodeling increases the weight-bearing surface area of the bone, decreasing strain. Formation of primarily horizontally oriented vertebral endplate remodeling may also be in response to stress from chronic pulling of the Sharpey's fibers.

Baboons have been shown to be a natural model for human DDD, displaying similar disc space narrowing, endplate changes, and facet joint arthropathy.[11] Severe kyphosis may be present in NHPs, seen first as a loss of spinal flexibility on physical examination and later as an obvious structural abnormality. As in humans, the process is correlated with age.

Degenerative disc disease in humans produces symptoms in a variety of ways.[23] Provocative discography, in which a patient's typical pain is reproduced by injection into the disc, has shown that some degenerated discs may be pain generators, even without disc herniation. Neurologic symptoms may result from endplate remodeling or disc herniation. In the cervical and thoracic spine, stenosis of the central canal caused by bone overgrowth or disc protrusion may cause cord compression and upper motor neuron symptoms, whereas in the lumbar spine lower motor neurons are usually affected after they have exited the cord, but are still in the neural canal; in humans, the conus medullaris is typically located at the L1-L2 level. Throughout the spine, posterolateral disc herniation and endplate remodeling often produce foraminal stenosis, impinging on exiting nerve roots and resulting in radicular pain and weakness.

Diffuse Idiopathic Skeletal Hyperostosis

The fibrous soft tissues supporting the spine, primarily the ligaments and joint capsules, may also undergo degeneration. The primary manifestation is development of ossification that begins at the enthesis, the fibrocartilaginous junction between the bone and ligament, tendon, or capsule. When multifocal, the condition is termed *diffuse idiopathic skeletal hyperostosis* (DISH) or Forestier's disease. In the spine, ossification is most frequent in the anterior longitudinal ligament, iliolumbar ligaments, and sacroiliac joint capsules. In humans, DISH is often asymptomatic. When extensive, confluent ossification of the anterior longitudinal ligament will effectively fuse a portion of the spine and result in stiffness and decreased range of motion.[14] Long-segment spinal fusion also predisposes the patient to pathologic fractures with relatively low-force trauma.[15] Patients with bulky longitudinal ligament ossification in the cervical spine may also complain of difficulty swallowing because of the mass effect on the posterior esophagus. Much less commonly, DISH occurs in the posterior longitudinal ligament or ligamentum flavum; in the cervical spine, ossification of these ligaments causes spinal stenosis, cord compression, and myelopathy (see later, Fig. 52-5A).[3]

Although the findings of DISH are most common in the spine, the same process occurs in the extremities, frequently at tendinous attachments around the pelvis, calcanei, olecranon, and patellae (see Fig. 52-2A). Unless ossification is bulky enough to present as a palpable mass, DISH in the appendicular skeleton is typically asymptomatic in humans. Both in the spine and peripheral skeleton, the main risk factor for developing DISH is advanced age, and the disease is more common in men.[19]

DISH in NHP is poorly described, but likely occurs with high regularity. Veterinarians may fail to differentiate radiologic changes associated with DISH from those of DDD (see later, Fig. 52-5A). Isolated reports in geriatric primates exist,[24] but the prevalence is not well established. Veterinarians working with geriatric

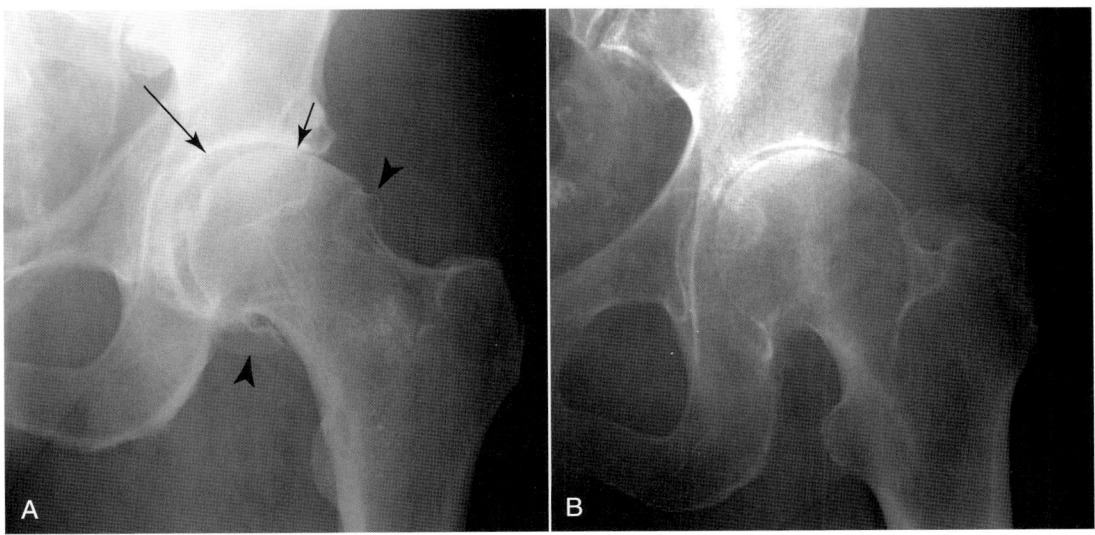

Figure 52-3

Hip arthritis in humans (AP radiographs). **A,** Osteoarthritis. Note the variability of the joint space loss, which is more severe superolaterally *(short arrow)* compared with medially *(long arrow);* also note the large osteophytes *(arrowheads).* **B,** Rheumatoid arthritis. In contrast, the joint space loss is relatively uniform and there are no osteophytes in this inflammatory arthritis. Both patients had hip and groin pain.

primates are likely to encounter the disorder frequently if they learn to recognize radiologic changes.

The bulky ligamentous ossification of DISH differs from the thin gracile syndesmophytes seen in inflammatory spondyloarthropathy, which primarily involve only the outer disc annulus and not the paraspinous ligaments. Similarly, fusion of the sacroiliac joints in spondyloarthropathy results from erosion and inflammation of the synovial part of the joint, separate from the fibrous joint capsule that is affected by DISH (see later, Fig. 52-5C). Spondyloarthropathy is a recognized disease process in NHPs, with prevalence as high as 20% in some populations of great apes, baboons, and rhesus macaques.[20] Numerous causes have been proposed for these erosive arthropathies; their discussion falls outside the scope of this chapter, but the link between infectious agent diarrhea (*Escherichia coli, Salmonella, Shigella, Campylobacter, Clostridium,* and *Giardia*) and spondyloarthropathy is worth noting briefly due to concerns with these infectious agents in zoo and wild animal populations.

DIAGNOSTIC IMAGING

Radiographs remain the cornerstone of diagnosis for degenerative skeletal diseases in both veterinary and human medicine. Digital radiography offers numerous benefits and is quickly becoming standard practice.

Radiologic features of OA are the same in humans, NHPs, and other mammals. The hallmarks are nonuniform joint space narrowing and reactive osteophyte formation[17] (Fig. 52-3; see Figs. 52-1 and 52-2). These findings are in contradistinction to inflammatory and infectious arthritides, in which synovial inflammation destroys the articular cartilage uniformly and the process does not incite bone production; these conditions are characterized by uniform joint space loss and lack of osteophytes (see Fig. 52-3B). Whereas subchondral cyst formation may occur in OA, cysts may be radiographically indistinguishable from erosions and their presence is not useful to distinguish degenerative from inflammatory arthritis. Late in the course of OA, the subchondral bone may develop sclerosis or eburnation in response to the overlying cartilage degeneration. Furthermore, damaged cartilage may break loose from the articular surface and migrate within the joint. If these microscopic fragments attach to synovium and establish a blood supply, they may grow, calcify, or ossify and thus be visible as joint mice radiographically (see Fig. 52-1). As more cartilage and underlying bone is destroyed, the ligaments and capsules supporting the joints become lax and joint subluxation may develop.

In both humans and NHPs, DDD has radiologic features that are complementary to those of OA.[11] Disc space narrowing and endplate remodeling in the degenerated spine are analogous to joint narrowing and

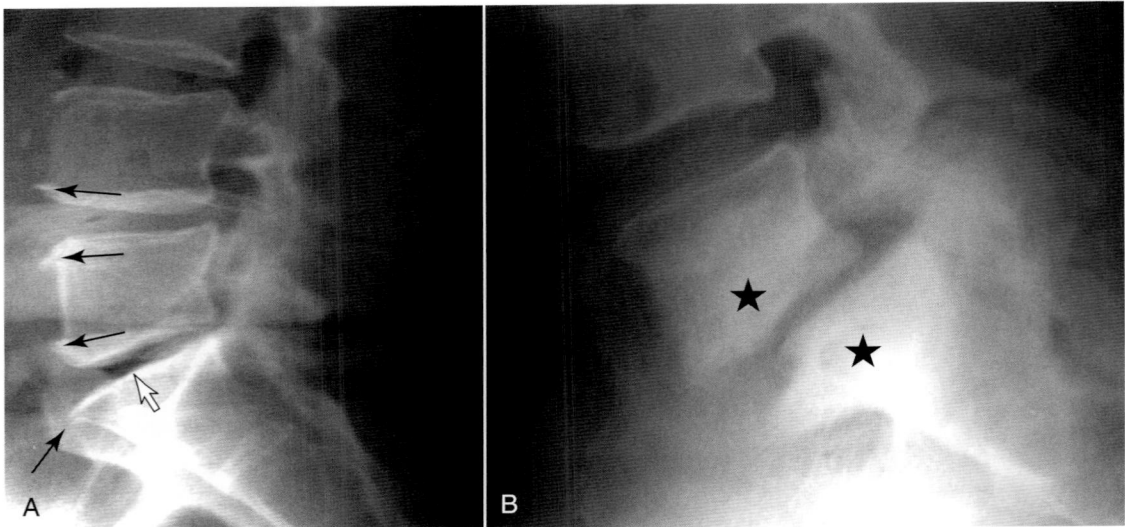

Figure 52-4
Degenerative disc disease (DDD) in humans (lateral lumbar spine radiographs). **A,** Moderate multilevel disease. Note the narrowing of the two most caudal disc spaces and the associated endplate remodeling *(solid arrows)*. A gas cleft in the L5-S1 disc *(white arrow)* represents a vacuum phenomenon. **B,** Severe single-segment disease. In a second patient, the most caudal disc space is almost obliterated and the adjacent vertebral bodies are sclerotic *(stars)*. Note the anterior subluxation (listhesis) of L5 on S1. Both patients complained of low back pain.

osteophytes in OA (Fig. 52-4). Desiccated discs may develop clefts that fill with gas because of internal negative pressure (vacuum phenomenon; see Fig. 52-4A), or may undergo dystrophic calcification (see later, Fig. 52-5B). In more advanced cases, sclerosis in the adjacent vertebra may occur. The combination of disc degeneration together with facet osteoarthritis often results in listhesis (subluxation) in the diseased segments (see Fig. 52-4B).

The main radiologic finding in DISH is solid, mature ligamentous ossification, most frequently in the anterior longitudinal ligament in the spine,[19] but also affecting other spine ligaments and capsules (Figs. 52-5 and 52-6). Ossification may flow from one spinal segment to the next, resulting in fusion. In humans and NHPs, DISH commonly coexists with degenerative spondylosis, likely because the main risk factor for both conditions is advanced age (see Figs. 52-5B and 52-6A).

Radiographs often provide all the information needed for diagnosis and treatment planning. In humans, CT is mainly used when the normal anatomy is severely distorted (e.g., because of prior trauma or surgery), for cross-sectional analysis (e.g., to assess the spinal canal or search for entrapped loose bodies), or for planning complex orthopedic procedures. Computed tomography (CT) use in veterinary medicine is becoming more common and will aid in the diagnosis

of more subtle degenerative lesions, but at present remains expensive and logistically more challenging because of the need for anesthesia with veterinary patients. Other imaging modalities such as ultrasound and magnetic resonance imaging (MRI) have a role in human medicine to visualize radiolucent soft tissues (e.g., articular cartilage, menisci, and intervertebral discs), and may be useful when the radiographic findings do not account for all the clinical symptomatology (Fig. 52-7). Contrast myelography may provide valuable information in NHPs with DDD when CT or MRI is not available.

Predicting the severity of discomfort in NHPs based on radiographic changes may be challenging. In humans, there is a weak correlation between radiographic severity and pain in both the peripheral joints and spine. Other symptoms, such as mechanical locking of a joint or radiculopathy in a limb, are more predictable based on specific radiologic features, allowing extrapolation to observed clinical signs in NHPs.

ANESTHESIA CONSIDERATIONS

Special consideration should be given to anesthesia of NHPs with moderate to severe degenerative skeletal diseases. The use of remote delivery systems (darts) and squeeze cages are standard practice with NHPs for

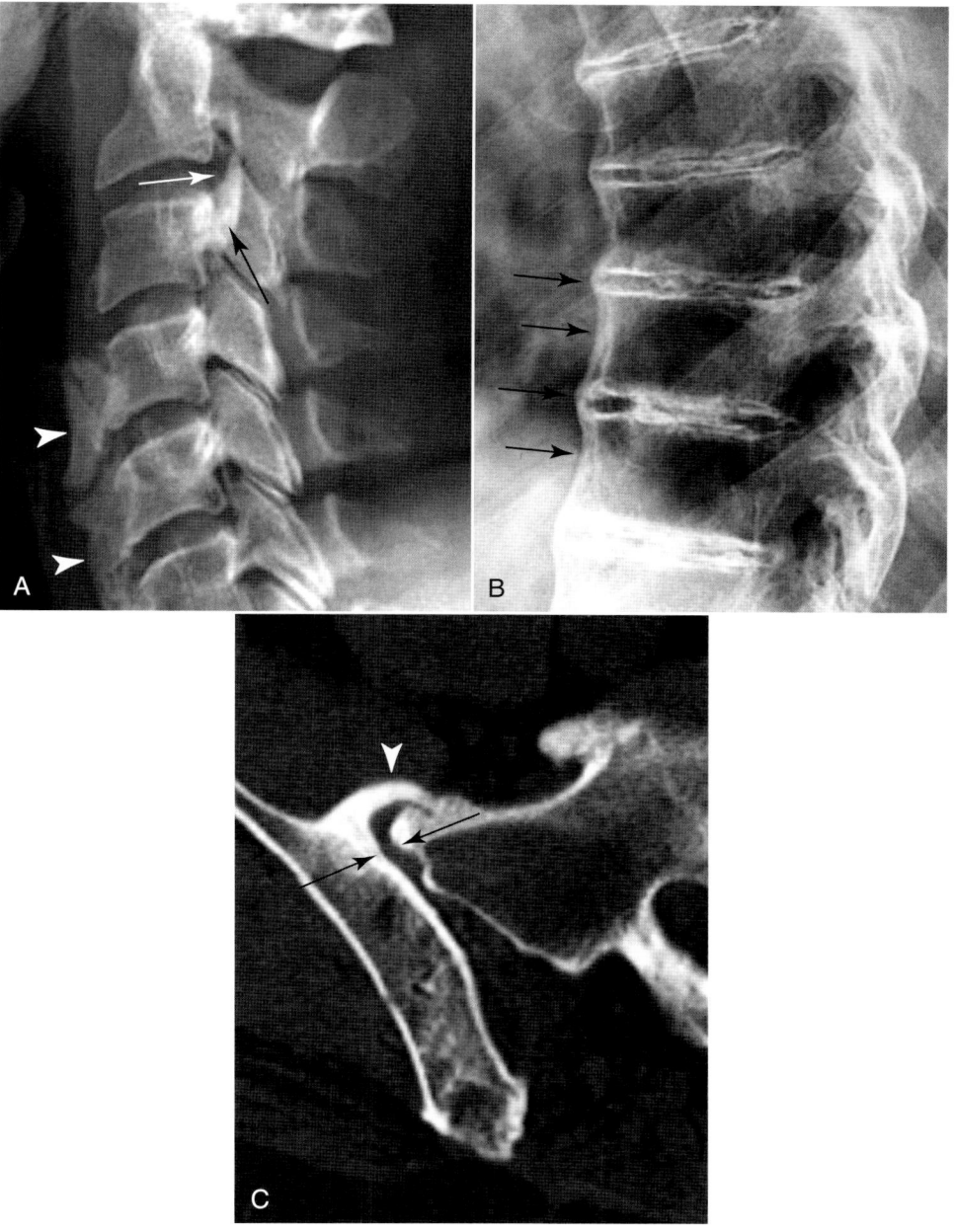

Figure 52-5

Diffuse idiopathic skeletal hyperostosis (DISH) in humans. **A,** Lateral radiograph, cervical spine. The bulky ossification in the anterior longitudinal ligament *(arrowheads)* may not be symptomatic, but the ossification in the posterior longitudinal ligament dorsal to C3 *(arrows)* results in spinal stenosis. **B,** Lateral radiograph, thoracic spine. Flowing ligament ossification *(arrows)* fuses adjacent segments. Note the concomitant disc narrowing and calcification, indicating coexistent DDD. **C,** CT scan image of the sacroiliac joint. Bridging ossification of the anterior joint capsule *(arrowhead)*, sparing the synovial part of the joint *(arrows)*, distinguishes the process from spondyloarthropathy.

human and animal safety. Careful dart selection and placement is necessary with geriatric NHPs, because muscle wasting associated with DJD increases the risk of a dart hitting bone. Special consideration should be given to animal location, because there is a greater risk of skeletal fracture from a fall during anesthetic induction in primates with DJD and/or vertebral fusion. Ideally, affected animals should be darted in enclosures with low vertical height and no climbing structures. Designing adequate spaces for anesthetic induction of

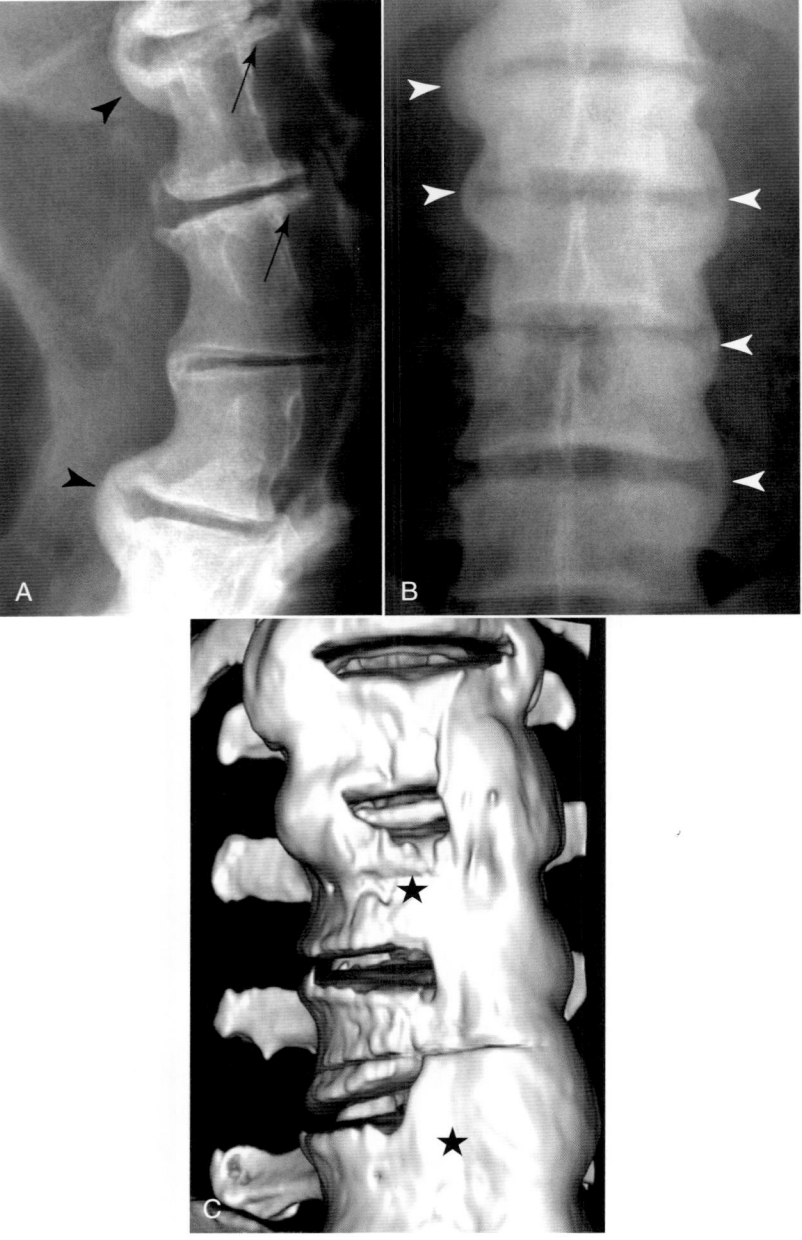

Figure 52-6

Lumbar spine DISH in nonhuman primates. **A,** Lateral radiograph, colobus monkey. Segmental bridging ossification of the anterior longitudinal ligament *(arrowheads)* likely contributes to stiffness. However, dorsal endplate remodeling *(arrows)* from coexistent DDD narrows the central canal, predisposing to neurologic symptoms. **B,** AP radiograph, orangutan. Paraspinal ossification is most apparent laterally *(arrowheads)*. **C,** Anterior three-dimensional CT reconstruction from the same orangutan as in **B** demonstrates that ossification also involves large portions of the anterior longitudinal ligament *(stars)*, which is difficult to appreciate on the AP radiograph in **B.** This animal had severely restricted motion.

geriatric NHPs should be part of new exhibit planning. Bedding the floor with straw, shavings, or blankets may decrease the risk of injury further. Squeeze cages present a reasonable alternative when available but care should be taken to avoid excessive pressure, because decreased joint motion and vertebral fusion may limit the appropriate degree of compression compared with a normal NHP. Similar care should be exercised with manual restraint of small NHPs to minimize pressure and torque exerted on the joints and spine.

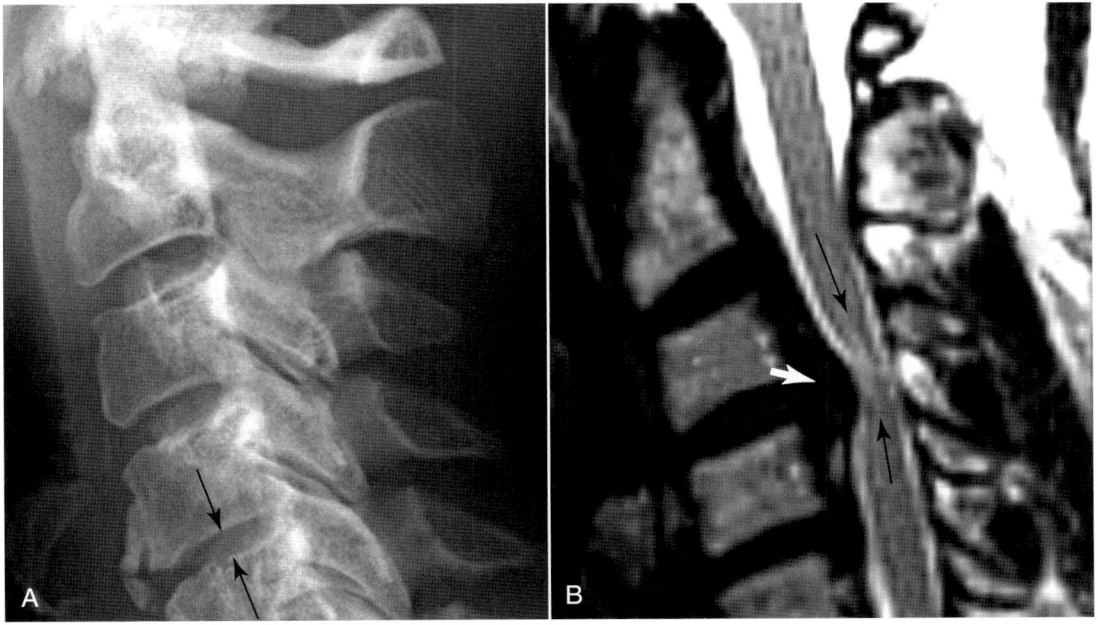

Figure 52-7

Advanced imaging of degenerative disease in a human. **A,** Lateral radiograph, cervical spine, shows mild DDD at C4-C5 *(arrows)*; C3-C4 appears normal. **B,** Sagittal T2-weighted MR image shows a large C3-C4 disc extrusion *(white arrow)* compressing the spinal cord, producing myelomalacia *(arrows)*. This patient had severe bilateral leg pain and hyperreflexia. Both the herniated disc material and the spinal cord compression are not visible on the radiographs in **A.**

Anesthetic recovery carries similar risks. Recovery in small enclosures without climbing structures will prevent the risk of fractures secondary to a fall while the animal regains coordination. NHPs, particularly larger apes, with severe OA or vertebral fusion may have difficulty sitting up if left in lateral recumbency. Placing such animals against enclosure mesh, a solid structure, or a rope may assist them in pulling themselves upright. With such animals, we routinely place fingers through the cage mesh when reversing anesthesia, since an NHP will often grasp the mesh to stabilize itself during recovery. Respiratory compromise and airway occlusion are concerns with large NHPs that roll into dorsal recumbency during recovery and are unable to move back into lateral recumbency.

TREATMENT

Determining when therapy is indicated for DJD is challenging, because many NHPs will hide signs of discomfort. The stoic nature of many NHPs adds a further challenge in determining when therapies are effective. NHPs that hide discomfort when a veterinarian is present may be more relaxed around routine caretaker staff and communication with these staff members is paramount. In some cases, however, even animal care staff may not observe clinical signs, despite significant radiologic changes of DJD being present (see Fig. 52-1). Decisions regarding treatment must therefore be guided not only by clinical signs, but also by interpretation of diagnostic imaging and physical examination findings. Decreases in passive range of joint motion, loss of spinal flexibility, joint crepitus, and other signs may indicate that some degree of discomfort is likely present. Serial monitoring of range of motion with a goniometer and radiologic changes may help determine when adjustments in therapy are indicated.

As with humans, significant individual variability exists with regard to which therapeutic modalities are effective. Through trial and error, veterinarians should work closely with animal care staff to determine which agents appear to be most effective in each case. Data on the efficacy and safety of many analgesics in the treatment of DJD in NHPs is lacking.

Nonsteroidal anti-inflammatory drugs (NSAIDs) are a primary treatment for DJD. Both human products (e.g., ibuprofen, naproxen) and veterinary products (e.g., carprofen, deracoxib) have been used in NHPs. Gastrointestinal and renal system side effects are most common and baseline blood and urine values should be monitored prior to and during treatment. NSAIDs such as meloxicam, which selectively inhibit cyclooxygenase (COX)-2 over COX-1 have a decreased potential for side effects. Newer drugs that specifically target COX-2, such as celecoxib and firocoxib, are presumed to be the safest option for long-term therapy. We have used celecoxib with success in several apes and monkeys with severe OA.

Tramadol acts as an agonist at mu opioid receptors and may be beneficial for the treatment of moderate to severe arthritic or spinal pain. The drug has fewer side effects than other opioids and is generally well tolerated.

Gabapentin and pregabalin have been shown to be beneficial in the treatment of neuropathic pain in humans. Their exact mechanism of action is unclear. Gabapentin has been used empirically in veterinary medicine for the treatment of spinal pain and may be beneficial in severe cases of DDD and DISH when nerve root compression is present. We have seen subjective improvement with the use of gabapentin in NHP with spinal pain refractory to NSAIDs and tramadol.

The effects of nutraceuticals, such as glucosamine and chondroitin sulfate, on DJD are not clear. A wide variety of these products is available for humans and companion animals. Solid scientific data on efficacy does not exist, but many people taking these products report improvement. The intra-articular administration of polysulfated glycosaminoglycan (Adequan) is routinely performed in horses and may be beneficial in NHPs, although no evidence has been reported. Intra-articular corticosteroid administration may also be considered.

The benefits of physical therapy, exercise, and a proper environment should not be overlooked. Treatment and even surgery for peripheral DJD and spine degeneration in humans is most effective when combined with an organized program of strength training and flexibility exercises. Providing stimulating environments and adequately sized enclosures to NHPs encourages normal activity and may help preserve range of motion and joint function. Soft substrates and nesting material may prevent excessive impact and joint strain. Similarly, providing stable, well-conceived climbing structures and ramps for older primates may prevent jumping and other high-impact activities that could exacerbate joint degeneration. Operant conditioning may be used to encourage exercise and activity further. We have observed improved flexibility and mobility in gorillas with DJD through operant conditioning. Specific stretches and simple exercises may be designed to exercise various joints by having the animal follow a target. Consultation with physical therapists may identify specific activities to improve comfort and mobility in NHPs with various DJD concerns.

With refractory OA pain in a single joint, advanced surgical procedures (e.g., joint replacement) may be an option. Similarly, disc herniation secondary to DDD may be surgically corrected. However, refractory pain is often caused by degeneration in multiple joints. In such cases, the ability to maintain a satisfactory quality of life in an NHP may become a concern. Euthanasia may be justified in such cases on the basis of refractory pain or discomfort, severely impaired mobility, and/or the inability to be maintained within a social group.

REFERENCES

1. Aoki J, Yamamoto I, Kitamura N, et al: End plate of the discovertebral joint: Degenerative change in the elderly adult. Radiology 164:411–414, 1987.
2. Black A, Lane MA: Nonhuman primate models of skeletal and reproductive aging. Gerontology 48:72–80, 2002.
3. Cammisa M, De Serio A, Guglielmi G: Diffuse idiopathic skeletal hyperostosis. Eur J Radiol 27(suppl 1):S7–S11, 1998.
4. Carlson CS, Loeser RF, Purser CB, et al: Osteoarthritis in cynomolgus macaques III: Effects of age, gender, and subchondral bone thickness on the severity of disease. J Bone Min Res 11:1209–1217, 1996.
5. Carter ML, Pontzer H, Wrangham RW, et al: Skeletal pathology in *Pan troglodytes schweinfurthii* in Kibale National Park, Uganda. Am J Phys Anthropol 135:389–403, 2008.
6. Châteauvert JMD, Grynpas MD, Kessler MJ, et al: Spontaneous osteoarthritis in rhesus macaques. II. Characterization of disease and morphometric studies. J Rheumatol 17:73–83, 1990.
7. Ebraheim NA, Lu J, Biyani A, et al: Anatomic considerations for uncovertebral involvement in cervical spondylosis. Clin Orthop 334:200–206, 1997.
8. Gelber AC, Hochberg MC, Mead LA, et al: Joint injury in young adults and risk for subsequent knee and hip osteoarthritis. Ann Intern Med 133:321–328, 2000.
9. Jurmain R: Degenerative joint disease in African great apes: an evolutionary perspective. J Hum Evol 39:185–203, 2000.
10. Kessler MJ, Turnquist JE, Pritzker KPH, et al: Reduction of passive extension and radiographic evidence of degenerative knee joint diseases in cage-raised and free-ranging aged rhesus monkeys *(Macaca mulatta)*. J Med Primatol 15:1–9, 1986.
11. Lauerman WC, Platenberg RC, Cain JE, et al: Age-related disk degeneration: Preliminary report of a naturally occurring baboon model. J Spinal Disorders 5:170–174, 1992.
12. Lim KT, Rogers J, Shepstone L, et al: The evolutionary origins of osteoarthritis: A comparative skeletal study of hand disease in 2 primates. J Rheumatol 22:2132–2134, 1995.
13. Loeser RF: Molecular mechanisms of cartilage destruction: Mechanics, inflammatory mediators, and aging collide. Arthritis Rheum 54:1357–1360, 2006.
14. Mata S, Fortin PR, Fitzcharles MA, et al: A controlled study of diffuse idiopathic skeletal hyperostosis. Clinical features and functional status. Medicine (Baltimore) 76:104–117, 1997.
15. Paley D, Schwartz M, Cooper P, et al: Fractures of the spine in diffuse idiopathic skeletal hyperostosis. Clin Orthop 267:22–32, 1991.

16. Reijman M, Pols HA, Bergink AP, et al: Body mass index associated with onset and progression of osteoarthritis of the knee but not of the hip: The Rotterdam Study. Ann Rheum Dis 66:158–162, 2007.

17. Resnick D: Degenerative disease of extraspinal locations. In Resnick D, editor: Diagnosis of bone and joint disorders, ed 4, Philadelphia, 2002, WB Saunders, pp 1271–1381.

18. Resnick D: Degenerative disease of the spine. In Resnick D, editor: Diagnosis of bone and joint disorders, ed 4, Philadelphia, 2002, WB Saunders, pp 1382–1475.

19. Resnick D, Niwayama G: Radiographic and pathologic features of spinal involvement in diffuse idiopathic skeletal hyperostosis (DISH). Radiology 119:559–568, 1976.

20. Rothschild BM: Primate spondyloarthropathy. Cur Rheumatol Rep 7:173–181, 2005.

21. Rothschild BM, Woods RJ: Osteoarthritis, calcium pyrophosphate deposition disease, and osseous infection in Old World primates. Am J Phys Anthropol 87:341–347, 1992.

22. Rothschild BM, Woods RJ: Arthritis in New World monkeys: Osteoarthritis, calcium pyrophosphate deposition disease, and spondyloarthropathy. Int J Primatol 14:61–78, 1993.

23. Russell EJ: Cervical disk disease. Radiology 177:313–325, 1990.

24. Swezey RL, Cox C, Gonzales B: Ankylosing spondylitis in nonhuman primates: The drill and the siamang. Semin Arthritis Rheuma 21:170–174, 1991.

25. Valdes AM, Spector TD: The contribution of genes to osteoarthritis. Med Clin North Am 93:45–66, 2009.

26. van Saase JL, van Romunde LK, Cats A, et al: Epidemiology of osteoarthritis: Zoetermeer survey. Comparison of radiological osteoarthritis in a Dutch population with that in 10 other populations. Ann Rheum Dis 48:271–280, 1989.

CHAPTER 53

Cardiovascular Disease in Great Apes

Rita McManamon and Linda Lowenstine

Cardiovascular disease (CVD, or heart disease) is a major cause of mortality in all four great ape taxa managed in captivity: gorillas (*Gorilla gorilla gorilla*), orangutans (*Pongo pygmaeus, P. abelli*, and *P. pygmaeus abelli* XP hybrids), chimpanzees (*Pan troglodytes*), and bonobos *(Pan paniscus)*. These primates are critically endangered in the wild and, in international zoological collections, they are among the most beloved and charismatic animals. In laboratory animal facilities, they contribute vital information and medical insights, which highlight their close phylogenetic relationship with human primates. Other apes are held, individually or in groups, in various sanctuaries, rehabilitation centers, private collections, or semicaptive situations. Thus, the impact of cardiovascular disease in apes crosses many phylogenetic, geographic, institutional, scientific, and conservation boundaries. Scientists and caretakers, across a wide swath of disciplines, must share knowledge, insights, and techniques so we can understand, address, and manage this devastating problem.

HISTORICAL PERSPECTIVE

Anecdotal press reports and published journal articles describing ape deaths caused by cardiac disease date back to the mid-20th century.[16] However, recognition of clinical signs of cardiac disease in apes, and scientific case reports detailing antemortem recognition of CVD, were scarce through the 1980s. Unfortunately, in both zoological and vivarial settings, clinical recognition of ape cardiac disease was rare, and heart disease was initially detected only in individual apes during postmortem examinations.[31] In 1990, a survey of diseases of great apes at the National Zoological Park drew attention to cardiovascular disease.[22] In 1994, a survey of gorilla mortality indicated that cardiovascular disease was the primary, or an important contributory, cause of death in 41% of adult gorilla necropsy reports in the Association of Zoos and Aquaria (AZA) North American Species Survival Plan (SSP).[18] A series of cases of aortic dissections and a seminal article reporting fibrosing cardiomyopathy in gorillas were published in 1994 and 1995, respectively.[12,27] Since then, systematic reviews of necropsy reports from captive zoo gorillas, orangutans, chimpanzees, and bonobos in their respective North American SSPs by a veterinary pathologist with expertise in primate pathology have revealed a similar pattern of myocardial fibrosis, in the absence of coronary atherosclerosis, in the other ape taxa.[14] In addition to the 41% incidence in gorillas, 20% of orangutans, 38% of adult zoo chimpanzees, and 45% of bonobos have been noted to have died of CVD.[2,5,15,18] Recent reviews have also confirmed the significant incidence of cardiac disease in chimpanzees in laboratory settings.[4,13,31] Although detailed analysis of trends and underlying factors is still in progress, CVD appears to be most frequent and severe in apes during mid- to late adulthood, with males affected more than females. Cardiovascular disease, including myocardial fibrosis, has also been recognized in wild mountain gorillas. In the wild, this is usually a contributory, not primary, cause of death, and occurs at a much lower incidence than that seen in captive apes. As of early 2010, neither anecdotal nor comprehensive cardiovascular postmortem reviews of apes in rehabilitation or sanctuary situations have been compiled.

Growing recognition of the importance of ape CVD has stimulated coordination of clinicopathologic, diagnostic, and therapeutic strategies in gorillas (see later, "Gorilla Health Project"), and has raised the index of suspicion for cardiac disease in all great apes. Increasing the availability and affordability of sophisticated cardiac ultrasound equipment and techniques for use in zoos, including occasional access to expensive transesophageal probes, which improve cardiac imaging capabilities, during the late 1980s and 1990s has resulted in improved cardiac monitoring during emergency and routine procedures. Improved access to appropriate equipment also coincided with the recruitment of voluntary clinical veterinary advisors within the AZA ape SSPs and taxon advisory group (TAG), enhanced promulgation of standardized AZA husbandry recommendations and veterinary examination protocol guidelines, and greater accessibility to inhalational anesthetic protocols. Such efforts led to more frequent routine physical examinations, including cardiac evaluations, in most SSP-managed captive apes, by 2000.

CURRENTLY IDENTIFIED TYPES

Several types of CVD are seen in apes, but the most common entity, based on published reports and analyses of SSP necropsy data, is characterized by an idiopathic scattered pattern of "myocardial replacement fibrosis with atrophy and hypertrophy of cardiac myocytes, absent or minimal inflammation, and no apparent etiology or associated disease."[27] This pattern has been termed *fibrosing cardiomyopathy* in gorillas, orangutans, chimpanzees, or bonobos or *idiopathic myocardial fibrosis* in chimpanzees.[11-15,27,31] Grossly, these lesions may be dramatic (Fig. 53-1), but often they are subtle. Histologically (Figs. 53-2 and 53-3), pathologists have noted that these patches of fibrosis arise most frequently near or around small-caliber intrinsic coronary arterioles, which are often thick-walled and hyalinized (arteriosclerosis). Larger coalescent areas of dissecting fibrosis may extend throughout the walls of all chambers, but not to the extent seen with myocardial infarction resulting from major coronary vessel occlusion. In many cases, the heart is enlarged with left ventricular hypertrophy, but in some cases the heart may be dilated and flabby. Myocardial fibrosis, per se, is an end-stage lesion, which does not imply a particular etiology or pathogenetic mechanism. It can develop as a consequence of several different types of injury to the myocardium (hypoxia, ischemia, necrosis, inflammation), and its cause(s), which are likely multifactorial, remain to be elucidated. However, the changes frequently seen in intrinsic arteries of the myocardium suggest that either transient (e.g., catecholamine-induced vasospasm) or systemic hypertension may be present. Many of the apes with myocardial fibrosis die suddenly and unexpectedly while on exhibit, in their night houses, or under anesthesia, presumably due to dysrhythmias, although in some cases more indolent

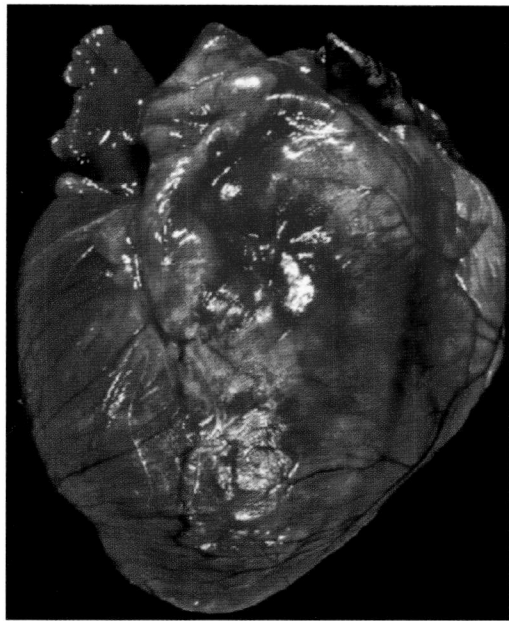

Figure 53-1

Heart of an adult male chimpanzee that died unexpectedly, with myocardial fibrosis. *(Photo credit: Linda J. Lowenstine.)*

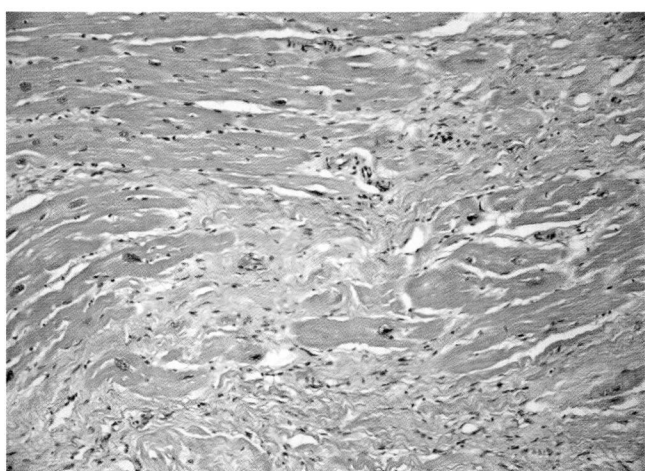

Figure 53-2

Histologic section of the myocardium of an adult male chimpanzee (H&E stain, ×20). *(Photo credit: Daniel C. Anderson.)*

congestive heart failure develops. Other types of ape cardiac and vascular disease that have been reported in the literature or gleaned from the SSP databases include aortic dissection, myxomatous valvular degeneration (endocardiosis, or nodular mucinosis), atherosclerosis, congenital heart defects, infectious myocarditis and

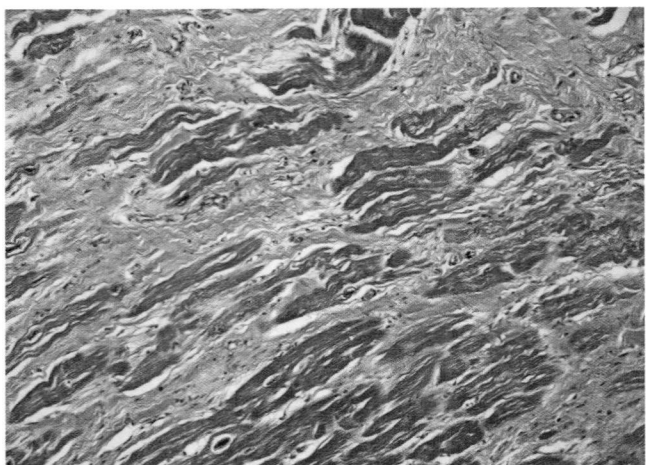

Figure 53-3

Histologic section of the myocardium of an adult male chimpanzee. Note extensive fibrosis *(blue)* separating and replacing cardiomyofibers *(red;* Masson's trichrome stain, ×20). *(Photo credit: Daniel C. Anderson.)*

valvular endocarditis, and hypertensive congestive heart failure.*

Aortic dissection and sudden death in gorillas was first described in 1970 and its importance was highlighted by the report of eight cases by Kenny and colleagues in 1994.[12,21] Since then, an additional four cases have been seen in gorillas[6] and three in bonobos.[2] In all cases, the tear was in the ascending aorta, not far from the valve, and was not associated with atherosclerosis. The causes of aortic dissection and rupture in apes are not fully understood, but hypertension has been implicated, as it is in more than half of the human cases. Left ventricular hypertrophy seen in these cases suggests either preexisting hypertension or increased workload resulting from the dissection, which is often chronic and forms a double-barreled aorta. Death ultimately is due to failure of the vessel wall, causing cardiac tamponade or intrathoracic hemorrhage. Occasional cases in which vessels other than the aorta (e.g., cerebral or pulmonary vessels) suffer from aneurysms, dissections, thrombosis, or rupture have been reported in the literature or identified in SSP databases. Although CVD in apes is generally not associated with atherosclerosis, occasionally atherosclerosis does occur in apes in the context of coronary arterial heart disease.[14] Most often, atherosclerosis is an incidental finding, which is occasionally severe, and usually confined to the descending abdominal aorta and internal iliac vessels. Reports are more common in the older literature than in the SSP databases, perhaps

*References 1, 8, 10-12, 14, 18, 19, and 29.

because in earlier times the diets of apes were often modeled on human diets.

Degenerative valvular disease characterized by nodular thickening and mucinosis of valve margins occurs with low frequency in the SSP databases, and has been seen in wild mountain gorillas as well. In apes, it is usually an incidental finding at necropsy of older individuals. This is in contrast to humans and domestic dogs, in which symptomatic valvular insufficiency occurs more frequently.

Congenital heart defects, including intra-atrial and intraventricular septal defects, have been identified in all ape taxa.[8] Often identified in very young animals, a few cases have been identified in apes that survived into adulthood, such as the case of coarctation of the aorta identified in a 7-year-old male gorilla.[30]

Causes of infective myocarditis reported to have resulted in death in apes include encephalomyocarditis viral (EMCV) infection in orangutans and bonobos, coxsackie B4 viral infection in an orangutan,[20] and Chagas disease (*Trypanosoma cruzi* infection) in a chimpanzee.[1] Vegetative endocarditis has been associated with alpha-hemolytic *Streptococcus* and *Gemella* spp. in gorillas.[6]

POSSIBLE ETIOLOGIES AND PATHOGENESIS

As noted, fibrosing cardiomyopathy is the most frequent form of CVD in apes and myocardial fibrosis is the result of insult to the myocardium. Its presence interferes with cardiac function through altered contractility or conduction. Factors that have been historically and anecdotally reported in great apes, which could logically be associated with some or all of the cardiac lesions seen in apes include the following: obesity or inactivity; dietary factors and chemical imbalances such as high lipids, iron overload, hypovitaminosis D and E, high salt content, and absence of plants eaten by wild apes that might be cardioprotective[17,25]; personality type and behavioral issues that might be associated with psychosocial stress and catecholamine release; endocrinopathies such as diabetes and hypothyroidism; primary or secondary hypertension; and intercurrent diseases, such as renal disease, dental disease, and osteoarthritis.

Many captive apes, whether born in the wild or in captivity, have had many different diets and social, environmental, and other experiences over their relatively long life spans. Similarly, current zoological exhibits often provide younger apes with larger social setting and enhanced exercise opportunities than were available in the past. Intercurrent diseases are often present in apes with CVD, and the interplay between cardiovascular disease and other diseases is under investigation. In orangutans, there is a statistically significant association between renal disease and fibrosing cardiomyopathy,[15] and concurrent renal and heart failure have been reported in a gorilla. It is not known which problem comes first, because chronic renal disease can cause secondary hypertension and primary hypertension can damage the renal vasculature and lead to renal failure. Further characterization of renal disease in apes is warranted to try to answer this question.

ANTEMORTEM CONSIDERATIONS

Clinical Documentation and Diagnosis

Timely antemortem detection of CVD in individual apes currently remains a challenge because of limited access to species-specific norms and standardized cardiac examination protocols. Significant progress toward developing these essential tools for gorillas has been made by the Gorilla Cardiac Database (GCD) group since 2000 and the Gorilla Heart Project (GHP) since 2006 (see later). Currently, population-wide, consensus-based normal values and protocol recommendations for orangutans, chimpanzees, and bonobos have not been established.

Clinicians anticipating an ape cardiac examination, as well as their collaborators, should familiarize themselves with the differences between human and ape CVD patterns (see earlier). Ideally, clinicians, consulting cardiologists, and/or ultrasonographers should also proactively seek out the assistance of the relevant ape SSP advisor and other experienced subject matter experts (SMEs) to anticipate and address technical and logistical concerns and establish an agreement on sample collection and data sharing for the benefit of the individual and the captive population. For three taxa (orangutans, chimpanzees, and bonobos), normal and abnormal, gender-specific, and age-specific comparative cardiac values are lacking, and it is difficult to draw definitive conclusions about where any one individual might fit on the spectrum of unaffected to severely affected. Clinical findings and data analyses conducted by the GCD and GHP have cast serious doubt on the validity of simply extrapolating human normal functional and anatomic measurements to apes. For all four taxa, antemortem clinical imaging and/or cardiac biomarker data have not been matched against the degree or pattern of myocardial fibrosis, nor with adequacy or impairment of cardiac function. It would be useful to know whether the amount or the pattern of fibrosis (i.e., how much, or where, the electrical conduction systems are disrupted) can assist in understanding disease severity, prognosis, and best treatment regimens. Electrical conductions systems have not been mapped in the four taxa (see later, "Future Directions"). Currently, taking endomyocardial biopsies for the diagnosis of myocarditis or cardiomyopathy, as is done in humans, is not performed in apes. Coronary angiography and placement of implantable monitors or defibrillation devices are rare in apes.[26,28]

Despite these current challenges, the approach taken by the GCD and GHP groups for gorillas represents an excellent model for conducting and analyzing cardiac examinations in any ape.

Gorilla Cardiac Database and Gorilla Health Project

A key model for standardized ape cardiac evaluation was created in 2000, when zoo veterinarian Dr. Hayley Murphy (Project Director) and physician cardiologist Dr. Ilana Kutinsky established the Gorilla Cardiac Database. When Kutinsky systematically reviewed over 170 cardiac imaging examinations from more than 100 gorillas, including serial examinations on some individuals, several key insights were revealed and disseminated through presentations and publications. Conclusions included the findings that in comparison to humans, normal gorilla heart rates are faster, blood pressures are higher, left ventricular muscle is thicker and hyperdynamic, and left ventricular ejection fraction is higher (about 60%).[23,24] Thus, some gorillas with apparently normal functional measurements, by human standards, were later proven to have significant myocardial fibrosis and profoundly impaired cardiac function. Preliminary gorilla specific-ranges have been published and are actively reevaluated and updated by the GCD group.[23,24] Initiation of treatment in some animals, which might not have needed intervention by human standards, is now considered by the GCD SMEs and zoo veterinarians in accordance with preliminary gorilla (not human) criteria.

In 2006, the Gorilla Health Project expanded on this effort, made specific recommendations for standardized cardiac examinations, medical history, and clinical data documentation and for sample submission of blood, serum, and plasma for current and future cardiac biomarker analysis. The group currently recommends a standardized cardiac examination when animals are anesthetized for physical examinations. Parasternal transthoracic (or transesophageal if available) ultrasound examination in specific positions is recommended. Measurements (in centimeters) are recorded (and reported to the centralized database) for aortic root diameter and left atrial and right atrial and ventricular chamber sizes. Measurements of the left ventricle, taken at or just below the tips of the mitral leaflets, in long- and short-axis views, are recorded for left ventricular internal diameter in systole (LVIDs), and diastole (LVIDd), diastolic interventricular septal thickness (IVS), and posterior wall thickness (LVPW). Fractional shortening and ejection fraction are calculated. Digital recording of black and white, and/or color flow Doppler examinations are encouraged, submitted, and reviewed by the GCD group, as needed. Additional data collected with the cardiac examination and analyzed by the GHP group are a 6- or (ideally) 12-lead electrocardiogram (ECG), if available, chest radiograph, heart rate, blood pressure, anesthetic regimen, and physical examination results. Blood, serum, and/or plasma are collected for complete blood count (CBC), chemistry panel, brain-type natriuretic peptide (BNP), and metabolic syndrome cardiac biomarkers such as insulin-to-glucose ratio and insulin, oxidized low-density lipoprotein (LDL), leptin, and cholesterol levels.[23,24,32] In humans, grouping of some metabolic issues such as obesity, hyperglycemia, hyperinsulinemia, dyslipidemia, and hypertension is termed *metabolic syndrome*, which has been associated with cardiovascular disease.[3] The GHP also encourages training the animals for nonanesthetized weight monitoring, blood pressure monitoring, blood collection, and awake cardiac ultrasound. The awake measurements cannot be taken in a parasternal position, and standardized techniques and measurements have not yet been developed. As of early 2010, discussions were underway with stakeholders working with the other ape taxa (see later discussion of the Great Ape Cardiac Disease Working Group) to replicate or adapt this general model to the other taxa.

Biomarkers

The rapidly expanding use of antemortem serologic biomarkers to help identify cardiac patients, direct ideal treatment regimens, and monitor therapeutic progress has been exciting in both human and veterinary medicine.[32] Determination of ideal biomarkers or biomarker panels for apes, identification or recruitment of laboratories that will accept nonhuman primate samples, and validation of those samples within and across ape taxa is in progress. Results with BNP appear promising and the usefulness of other biomarkers is being explored.[23] Comprehensive biomarker microarrays have been tested in chimpanzees in vivarial settings. Results indicate that BNP and cardiac troponin I (CTnI) show potential for distinguishing affected from nonaffected animals.[4] However, additional work is necessary to validate these tests in other species. An ideal biomarker for zoological, vivarial, sanctuary, and host country applications would be relatively adaptable to field applications, require minimal sample volume, be easy to obtain during voluntary blood draws with operantly trained cooperative animals, and remain stable during shipment and long-term banking to permit retrospective and population-wide studies to be conducted. The potential power of having access to minimally invasive, cooperative serial biomarker monitoring for animals at risk for developing heart disease, or for those being monitored under treatment for cardiac disease, is enormous. Blood samples from affected animals are precious and limited, especially historical banked samples. Effective foresight and coordination between collaborators and species veterinary advisors is critical, so that maximum benefit is gained from any analysis.

Treatment and Monitoring

Extrapolating potent cardiovascular therapeutic regimens to ape patients when the underlying disease process is not fully characterized or understood carries some risk. The risk is enhanced because few ape patients tolerate, or have access to, the routine monitoring techniques used in humans (e.g., regular body weight measurements, strict fluid and salt intake and output control, awake blood pressure measurements, electrocardiography, and/or serial cardiac ultrasound), which help fine-tune daily drug dosages and avoid hypotensive crises. However, skilled collaborating veterinary and physician SMEs, by assessing the available data and applying general principles, have successfully managed several gorillas and chimpanzees with chronic cardiac disease, with notable improvement in their quality of life.*

Such care must be highly individualized. Concurrent positive reinforcement training for noninvasive monitoring procedures is highly desirable and may increase treatment success. Most treatment regimens

*References 7, 13, 19, 23, 24, 29, and 31.

use angiotensin-converting enzyme (ACE) inhibitor therapy when significant left ventricular hypertrophy is diagnosed. Beta blocker therapy is considered if signs of cardiomyopathy (depressed ejection fraction [EF]) are also present. Diuretic therapy is used, as needed.[23,24] Digitalis-based cardioglycosides have been used in the past, but are not typically recommended for gorillas by the GCF. Careful patient monitoring of diet, exercise tolerance, potential fluid retention, and body weight are indicated, as for human cardiac patients.

FUTURE DIRECTIONS

The GHP has made significant progress toward collecting a tremendous amount of life history and medical history data on captive gorillas and toward analyzing the contributory factors that may initiate, or worsen, ape CVD. Similar early efforts are needed for orangutans, chimpanzees, and bonobos. Recently, a cross-disciplinary collaborative group of experienced veterinary and physician specialists—clinical generalists, pathologists, cardiologists, ultrasonographers, and medical instrumentation specialists—and caretakers with behavioral training and other expertise formed the Great Ape Cardiovascular Disease Working Group (GACDWG). This group is working to develop coordinated and standardized CVD diagnostic, treatment, and control strategies within and across taxa. Making sense of how this data relates to the pathophysiology of ape CVD, and establishing methods to control, reduce, and/or eliminate ape CVD, are the ultimate goals. Correlation and communication among all these stakeholders is critical if rapid progress is to be made. Here we present a noncomprehensive list of some issues being explored by the GACDWG.

Improved Clinicopathologic Characterization

To understand CVD characteristics within and across taxa better, and to correlate antemortem findings with lesions found on postmortem examination, veterinary and physician clinicians and anatomic and clinical pathologists must understand which data and resources each discipline needs, and must share data dynamically. The GACDWG is investigating how to optimize cross-disciplinary coordination before and after antemortem and postmortem examinations for asymptomatic as well as high-risk patients to improve sample collection and speed the analysis and dissemination of results. Proactive collaboration among clinicians, management

groups, and caretakers can use behavioral training to carry out noninvasive procedures such as chest auscultation, blood pressure measurement, and some ultrasound examinations and minimally invasive, cooperative blood collection. Such efforts will not eliminate the need for comprehensive examinations under anesthesia, but they may reduce their frequency and length and will provide essential complementary data.

The GACDWG is currently exploring ideal clinical pathology panels, which may provide insight across or within taxa. In addition to BNP and CTnI, other potential biomarker assays, such as metalloproteinase or micro-RNA assays, are being considered. Some of these might be applicable to antemortem situations and in tissue analysis of postmortem specimens, and might thus provide correlative insight. Taxa-specific multiplex arrays may also be applied or developed for diagnostic use.

The potential application of enhanced imaging modalities (computed tomography, magnetic resonance imaging, and positron emission tomography) to antemortem or postmortem examinations is being explored.[9] Animal size currently presents a challenge in some patients, such as adult male gorillas. In other taxa, this may be more practical.

Some implanted instrumentation devices are currently useful for CVD diagnostic, monitoring, or therapeutic purposes in humans and in some veterinary species. The use of instrumentation may prove to be practical and beneficial for apes in the future.[9] Using data from awake patients sent from such devices might allow therapeutic regimens to be adjusted and quality of life to be enhanced while reducing the frequency and risk of anesthetic episodes.

Through necropsy compilation and analysis across all ape taxa, anatomic pathology has provided critical historical insights into cross-taxa CVD manifestations. Recent improvements and standardization in antemortem imaging and clinical pathology characterization now provide an opportunity to match these findings through improved communication among physician and veterinary anatomic and clinical pathologists, clinicians, cardiologists, and ultrasonographers. The GACDWG hopes to work toward more precise standardization of terminology across taxa, mapping of the electrical conduction systems in all four taxa, and adaptation of the current AZA standardized necropsy cardiac examination protocol to correlate with antemortem ultrasound images and postmortem electromechanical analyses to improve clinicopathologic insights. Detailed epidemiologic studies are needed to assess the relative contributions of proposed causative factors (see earlier), correlate them with the antemortem information provided by individual examinations, and with the postmortem information provided by a comprehensive necropsy and standardized cardiac necropsy examination. Current ape SSP pathology protocol instructions for opening and examining the heart were originally developed for gorillas. Development of taxa-specific postmortem dissection protocols through collaboration between physician and veterinary pathologists, is planned. More advanced molecular or ultrastructural diagnostic analysis of postmortem specimens is also envisioned.

Finally, there is a need to recruit new collaborators from institutions that house great apes, as well as academic institutions in veterinary and human medicine, to provide expert consultation for diagnosing, treating, and monitoring current and future patients and provide research expertise to further our understanding of CVD in apes. Investigating and controlling CVD in apes is not merely an interesting academic exercise. It is imperative for improving management of all four ape taxa. The overriding aim must be to establish the pathophysiology of ape CVD and develop guidelines for diagnosis, treatment, and monitoring that will be effective and/or easily adaptable for all four taxa in whatever setting they are found—captive, rehabilitant, or wild. With such tools, heart disease in apes can be effectively understood, diagnosed, treated, reduced, and prevented, thus improving longevity and quality of life for these endangered and charismatic animals.

Acknowledgments

We gratefully acknowledge Dr. Hayley Murphy and innumerable other caretakers working with and for the benefit of apes for their contributions to the preparation of this manuscript. Part of this work was supported by National Institutes of Health grant to the Yerkes National Primate Research Center (RR000165).

REFERENCES

1. Bommineni YR, Dick EJ Jr, Estep JS, et al: Fatal acute Chagas disease in a chimpanzee. J Med Primatol 38:247–251, 2009.
2. Clyde V: Personal communication, 2010.
3. De la Sierra A, Ruilope LM: Management of cardiovascular risk factors in patients with metabolic syndrome. Cardiovasc Hematol Agents Med Chem 5:209–214, 2007.
4. Ely JJ, Bishop MA, Lammey ML, et al: Use of biomarkers of collagen types I and III fibrosis metabolism to detect cardiovascular and renal disease in chimpanzees (Pan troglodytes). Comp Med 60:1–5, 2010.
5. Gamble KC, North MCK, Backues K, Ross SR: Pathologic review of the chimpanzee (Pan troglodytes): 1990-2003. In Baer CK, editor: Proceedings of the American Association of Zoo Veterinarians/American Association of Wildlife Veterinarians, Annual Meeting, San Diego, California, 2004, pp 565–570.
6. Gorilla SSP: Unpublished data, 2010.
7. Harris DM, Kutinsky IB, Myers GE, Barrie MT: Treatment of hypertrophic cardiomyopathy in a western lowland gorilla (Gorilla gorilla gorilla). In Baer CK, editor: Proceedings of the American Association of Zoo Veterinarians/American Association of Wildlife Veterinarians, Annual Meeting, Tulsa, Oklahoma, 2009, pp 127.
8. Hendrickx AG, Binkerd PE: Congenital malformations. In Jones TC, Mohr U, Hunt RD, editors: Nonhuman primates I (ILSI monographs on pathology of laboratory animals). Berlin, 1993, Springer-Verlag, pp 170–180.
9. Hilton C: Personal communication, 2010.
10. Hruban Z, Meehan T, Wolff P, et al: Aortic dissection in a gorilla. J Med Primatol 15:287–293, 1986.
11. Jones P, Mahamba C, Rest J, et al: Fatal inflammatory heart disease in a bonobo (Pan paniscus). J Med Primatol 34:45–49, 2005.
12. Kenny DE, Cambre RC, Alvarado TP, et al: Aortic dissection: An important cardiovascular disease in captive gorillas (Gorilla gorilla gorilla). J Zoo Wildl Anim Med 25:561–568, 1994.
13. Lammey ML, Doane CJ, Gigliotti A, et al: Diagnosis and treatment of pulmonary arterial hypertension and atrial fibrillation in a chimpanzee (Pan troglodytes). J Am Assoc Lab Anim Sci 47:1–5, 2008.
14. Lowenstine LJ: A primer of primate pathology: Lesions and nonlesions. Toxicol Pathol 31(suppl):92–102, 2003.
15. Lowenstine LJ, McManamon R, Bonar C, et al: Preliminary results of a survey of United States and Canadian orangutan mortalities in the North American SSP population from 1980 to March 2008. In Baer CK, editor: Proceedings of the American Association of Zoo Veterinarians/American Association of Wildlife Veterinarians, Annual Meeting, Los Angeles, California, 2008, pp 40.
16. Manning GW: Coronary disease in the ape. Am Heart J 23:719–724, 1942.
17. McNamara T, Dolensek EP, Liu S, Dierenfeld ED: Cardiomyopathy associated with vitamin E deficiency in two mountain lowland gorillas. In Baer CK, editor: Proceedings of the First International Conference on Zoological and Avian Medicine, Oahu, Hawaii, 1987, pp 493.
18. Meehan TP, Lowenstine LJ: Causes of mortality in captive lowland gorillas: A survey of the SSP population. In Baer CK, editor: Proceedings of the American Association of Zoo Veterinarians/American Association of Wildlife Veterinarians, Annual Meeting, Pittsburgh, Pennsylvania, 1994, pp 216–218.
19. Miller CL, Schwartz AM, Barnhart JS, et al: Chronic hypertension with subsequent congestive heart failure in a western lowland gorilla (Gorilla gorilla gorilla). J Zoo Wildl Anim Med 30:262–267, 1999.
20. Miyagi J, Tsuhako K, Kinjo T, et al: Coxsackievirus B4 myocarditis in an orangutan. Vet Pathol 36:452–456, 1999.
21. Morgan DG: Dissecting aneurysm of the aorta in a gorilla. Vet Rec 86:502–505, 1970.
22. Munson L, Montali RJ: Pathology and disease of great apes at the National Zoological Park. Zoo Biol 9:99–105, 1990.
23. Murphy HW: Fibrosing cardiomyopathy in gorillas: Front-line diagnostics. In Burrows C, editor: North American Veterinary Conference Proceedings, 2010, pp 1853–1855.
24. Murphy HW, Dennis PM, Devlin W, et al: Echocardiographic parameters of captive western lowland gorillas (Gorilla gorilla gorilla). J Zoo Wildl Med (in review).

25. Popovich DG, Jenkins DJ, Kendall CW, et al: The western lowland gorilla diet has implications for the health of humans and other hominoids. J Nutr 127:2000–2005, 1997.

26. Rush EM, Hall J, Ogburn AL, et al: Implantation of a cardiac resynchronization therapy device (CRT) in a western lowland gorilla *(Gorilla gorilla gorilla)* with cardiac disease. In Baer CK, editor: Proceedings of the American Association of Zoo Veterinarians/American Association of Wildlife Veterinarians AZA/NAG Joint Conference, Omaha, Nebraska, 2005, pp 159–160.

27. Schulman FY, Farb A, Virmani R, et al: Fibrosing cardiomyopathy in captive western lowland gorillas *(Gorilla gorilla gorilla)* in the United States: A retrospective study. J Zoo Wildl Anim Med 26:43–51, 1995.

28. Scott NA, McManamon R, Strobert EL, et al: In vivo diagnosis of coronary artery disease in a western lowland gorilla *(Gorilla gorilla gorilla)*. J Zoo Wildl Anim Med 26:139–143, 1995.

29. Sleeper MM, Doane CJ, Langner PH, et al: Successful treatment of idiopathic dilated cardiomyopathy in an adult chimpanzee *(Pan troglodytes)*. Comp Med 55:80–84, 2005.

30. Trupkiewicz JG, McNamara TS, Weidenham KM, et al: Cerebral infarction associated with coarctation of the aorta in a lowland gorilla *(Gorilla gorilla gorilla)*. J Zoo Wildl Anim Med 26:123–131, 1995.

31. Varki N, Anderson D, Herndon JG, et al: Heart disease is common in humans and chimpanzees, but is caused by different pathological processes, 2008 (http://cmm.ucsd.edu/lab_pages/varki/varkilab/Publications/A173.pdf).

32. Vasan R: Biomarkers of cardiovascular disease: Molecular basis and practical considerations. Circulation 113:2335–2362, 2006.

CHAPTER 54

Ebola Hemorrhagic Fever

Kenneth N. Cameron and Patricia E. Reed

DEFINITION AND CAUSE

Ebola hemorrhagic fever (EHF) is a hemorrhagic disease of humans and nonhuman primates caused by the Ebola virus, a biosafety level (BSL) 4 biologic agent.[20] Ebola hemorrhagic fever (EHF) was first described in 1976 during hemorrhagic fever outbreaks in the Democratic Republic of Congo (DRC, former Zaïre) and Sudan.[17] Since then, its ecologic and epidemiologic characteristics largely remain a mystery.

EPIZOOTIOLOGY

Ebolavirus (EBOV) and *Margburgvirus* make up the family Filoviridae; enveloped, nonsegmented, negative-stranded RNA viruses. There are currently five recognized species of *Ebolavirus*: *Zaïre ebolavirus* (ZEBOV), *Sudan ebolavirus* (SEBOV), *Côte d'Ivoire ebolavirus* (CIEBOV), *Reston ebolavirus* (REBOV), and *Bundibugyo ebolavirus*.[4,17,23]

Viral Distribution

The geographic range of EBOV is associated with humid tropical forest ecosystems in sub-Saharan Africa and the Philippines.[10] Confirmed human and animal outbreaks have occurred in Côte d'Ivoire (CIEBOV), Democratic Republic of Congo, Republic of Congo, Gabon (ZEBOV), Sudan (SEBOV), and Uganda (SEBOV and *Bundibugyo ebolavirus*). REBOV outbreaks in American and European primate facilities have been traced back to the Philippines. Serologic surveys and ecologic niche modeling have suggested that the virus may also be endemic in Cameroon, Madagascar, Mozambique, and Tanzania.[14]

Reservoirs

Studies have suggested that EBOV circulates in the environment at levels difficult to detect and that viral titers may be very low in naturally infected reservoir species.[13,22] Tens of thousands of animals (bats, other vertebrates, and arthropods) have been tested from several central African countries since 1976, but live EBOV has not been isolated.[17] There is a growing body of evidence to support certain bat species as reservoirs of EBOV. In studies in which dozens of plant, vertebrate, and invertebrate species were inoculated with EBOV, viral amplification occurred only in bats. EBOV gene sequences were detected in 13 bats of three species—hammer-headed fruit bat (*Hypsignathus monstrosus*), Franquet's epauletted bat (*Epomops franqueti*), and little collared fruit bat (*Myonycteris torquata*). Recent detection of ZEBOV-specific IgG antibodies in 95 bats of six species (*E. franqueti*, *H. monstrosus*, *M. torquata*, *Micropteropus pusillus* [Peter's dwarf epauletted fruit bat], *Mops condylurus* [Angolan free-tailed bat], and *Rousettus aegyptiacus* [Egyptian fruit bat]), indicate prior exposure to EBOV and may support the assertion that they are reservoirs of ZEBOV.[12] Confirming bats as reservoir hosts will require additional evidence, including isolation of live virus from the animal, establishing persistence of infection, and confirming transmission to a target species.[10]

Epizootics

Captive Primates

On at least six different occasions since its discovery in 1989, REBOV was isolated from cynomolgus macaques (*Macaca fascicularis*) showing signs of viral hemorrhagic fever.[15] The macaques had been imported to America and Europe from a single breeding facility in the Philippines.[10] In one case, 82% of animals died and many were found to be coinfected with simian hemorrhagic fever virus. The significance of the coinfection is unknown. In almost all cases, affected macaques originated from a single breeding facility in Laguna Province, the Philippines. In 1996, an investigation at that facility reported a 14% mortality rate, with viral antigen detected in 32% of symptomatic and 4% of asymptomatic monkeys.[3] Three of 301 cynomolgus macaques were positive for IgG antibodies.[7] The source of infection for the macaques was not determined, but poor husbandry practices contributed to disease dissemination. Many macaques in both U.S. and Philippine centers were subsequently destroyed, and in 1997 the Laguna facility was closed. There have been no further REBOV cases reported in primates imported to the United States since that time.

Free-Ranging Primates

Chimpanzees *(Pan troglodytes)* and western lowland gorillas *(Gorilla gorilla gorilla)* appear to be dead-end hosts for ZEBOV infection. ZEBOV antigen was detected in 16 chimpanzee and gorilla carcasses discovered during epizootics associated with large great ape declines in central Africa.[19,25] Based on temporal and spatial links between large-scale great ape mortality and confirmed ZEBOV epidemics and epizootics, case-fatality rates in great apes have been estimated at roughly 90%.[24] The detection of *Ebolavirus*-specific IgG antibodies in 31 western lowland gorillas and chimpanzees suggests that they may survive infection or may be asymptomatically infected, or that assays are cross-reacting with an as yet unidentified, less virulent, strain of EBOV.[4,14]

Although the vastness and remoteness of the central African habitat makes precise great ape mortality impossible to determine, the impact of EHF on great ape populations appears dramatic.[17,24] Some field researchers have observed rapid and astonishingly high mortality in resident ape populations. Large-scale ecologic surveys carried out over the past decade have indicated dramatic declines (up to 95%) in great ape populations in some regions. In all cases, these declines were spatially and/or temporally linked with human or animal ZEBOV outbreaks, in which hunting and habitat loss were ruled out as contributing factors.[10] Given the context, it is reasonable to assume that the great ape declines were associated with EHF. The western lowland gorilla was reclassified as "critically endangered" by the International Union for the Conservation of Nature (IUCN), largely as a result of the threat of EHF.

Antibodies to ZEBOV were detected in eight wild-born monkeys of four species in Cameroon, Gabon, and the Republic of Congo, indicating virus circulation in nonhuman primates.[14] Monkey morbidity and mortality have been spatially or temporally linked with human ZEBOV, although tests were negative for ZEBOV.[10,25]

CIEBOV was associated with the deaths of 12 chimpanzees in the Taï forest of Côte d'Ivoire in 1994.[10] One chimpanzee was confirmed CIEBOV positive on immunohistochemistry (IHC) analysis, suggesting that chimpanzees are dead-end hosts.[26] Antibodies to CIEBOV were detected in a red colobus monkey *(Procolobus badius)* following the outbreak. All affected chimps were observed consuming the monkey 6 days prior to the outbreak, suggesting the monkey as the source of infection of the chimpanzees.

Wildlife morbidity and mortality associated with SEBOV and *Bundibugyo ebolavirus* have not been reported.

Other Potential Hosts

Relatively little is known about EBOV susceptibility of other species that may serve as reservoir, incidental or dead-end hosts. Positive serologic findings in central African domestic hunting dogs have suggested that canines may be naturally and asymptomatically infected.[3] Pigs *(Potamochoerus porcus)*, duikers (various species), porcupines *(Atherurus africanus)*, a civet *(Civettictis civetta)*, sitatungas *(Tragelaphus spekei)*, genets *(Genetta* spp.), an elephant *(Loxodonta. africana)*, pythons *(Python sebae)*, antelopes, rodents, a pangolin *(Manis* spp.), a mongoose (unspecified species), and a raptor have been reported dead in temporal or spatial coincidence with confirmed ZEBOV outbreaks in humans or nonhuman primates.[10] Of the species that were tested for ZEBOV by polymerase chain reaction (PCR) assay, only a blue duiker *(Cephalophus monticola)* tested positive.[19] A 50% decline in duiker populations was reported, coincident with ZEBOV outbreaks in humans and great apes in the Republic of Congo between 2000 and 2003, suggesting that duikers may be dead-end hosts for ZEBOV. Unconfirmed reports have also suggested the presence of EBOV in rodents *(Mastomys, Mus,* and *Praomys* spp.). In the Philippines, REBOV was recently isolated from domestic swine exhibiting a severe respiratory syndrome that were coinfected with porcine reproductive and respiratory syndrome virus.[3] Given this lack of strong evidence, additional studies on potential Ebola virus hosts are needed.

Transmission

EBOV is transmitted through direct contact with body fluids of infected animals or persons.[3,17] Increased risk of transmission occurs in the acute phase of infection, when patients are viremic. Once the virus is cleared, there is little risk of transmission. The exception may be with breast milk or semen, in which ZEBOV was detected in human patients at 15 and 91 days postinfection, respectively.

In a captive context, transmission is favored by poor husbandry conditions, poor compliance with infection control guidelines, and any other conditions that increase inter-animal contact.[15] However, there is evidence of ZEBOV transmission between monkeys separated by a distance of 3 m, perhaps involving conjunctival exposure occurring via aerosolization from urination or cage cleaning.[21]

Human ZEBOV outbreaks in central Africa have been linked to the handling of infected great ape carcasses and the consumption of bats.[12,17,18] Once in human communities, EHF spreads rapidly via person to person contact and in health care settings in which resources are limited or barrier nursing protocols are not implemented.[10] There is no evidence of aerosol transmission in humans. Accidental laboratory exposures have been reported, usually involving needle sticks or torn gloves. Evidence of previous exposure in animal handlers has been documented, however, sometimes in the absence of any illness or identifiable accident.[3]

The route of initial infection of wild great apes has not been confirmed, but the prevailing theory suggests direct or indirect (fruit consumption in the same tree) contact with reservoir species (largely believed to be bats) at common feeding sites.[10,16] Once EHF is initiated in the great ape population, viral transmission may be propagated by contact with an infected animal carcass and direct contact with other infected apes.[19]

ANIMALS AS DISEASE MODELS

Animal models have advanced our understanding of the pathogenesis of EHF and the development of vaccine platforms.[6,10] Laboratory models for ZEBOV include mice, guinea pigs, African green monkeys (*Chlorocebus aethiops*), cynomolgus macaques (*Macaca fascicularis*), rhesus macaques (*Macaca mulatta*), and hamadryas baboons (*Papio hamadryas*). Most laboratory experiments have involved REBOV and ZEBOV studies. Laboratory ZEBOV-infected macaques (*Macaca* spp.) show high mortality rates (≥90%) and some survivors exhibit neutralizing antibodies for 340 days. Given similar dose challenges, ZEBOV is less virulent to rhesus macaques than to cynomolgus macaques, making rhesus the preferred model for therapeutic studies and cynomolgus for vaccine studies. Of ZEBOV-infected hamadryas baboons, 60% to 75% develop a hemorrhagic syndrome. Case-fatality rates reached more than 80% in

macaques experimentally infected with REBOV, with clinical signs appearing late in the disease.[3] REBOV infections appear to be nonlethal in African green monkeys (*C. aethiops*). SEBOV is less virulent to rhesus macaques than is ZEBOV.

CLINICAL SIGNS

Clinical signs in experimentally infected animals are similar, but not identical, to those in humans. Primates experimentally infected with ZEBOV or SEBOV exhibit a wide variety of symptoms, typically within 3 days postinfection and include fever, lethargy, anorexia, maculopapular rash, diarrhea, melena, rectal bleeding, and hepatosplenomegaly.[3,10] Death generally occurs 5 to 8 days postinfection.

Clinical signs of EHF in humans are variable and include headache, fever, arthralgia, myalgia, maculopapular rash, hiccups, fever, convulsions, and muscle tonus.[10] Hemorrhagic manifestations are not always observed. Incubation periods are 4 to 16 days (ZEBOV) and 7 to 14 days (SEBOV). REBOV has not been reported to cause disease in humans.[17]

The sole indication of clinical signs in free-ranging nonhuman primates comes from a CIEBOV outbreak during which chimpanzees exhibited signs of abdominal pain, lethargy, and anorexia.[10]

PATHOLOGY AND POSTMORTEM FINDINGS

Information regarding postmortem lesions comes primarily from experimentally ZEBOV-infected primates, but is supplemented with observations associated with REBOV-infected macaques, a CIEBOV-infected chimpanzee, and a few human autopsies.[3,9,10,26] Gross lesions may include petechiae, ecchymoses, and frank hemorrhages involving a variety of organs, particularly the kidneys, liver, spleen, lung, and testes. Other potential findings include maculopapular rash, subcutaneous hemorrhages at venipuncture sites, hepatomegaly, splenomegaly, disseminated intravascular coagulopathy (DIC), and necrosis of the liver, lymphoid tissue, adrenal cortex, or pulmonary epithelium.[8]

ZOONOTIC POTENTIAL

The zoonotic potential of Ebola virus is well known. ZEBOV and SEBOV are the most pathogenic for humans, with case-fatality rates exceeding 80% and 50%, respectively.[10] To date, they have caused almost 1300 human deaths in the Democratic Republic of Congo, Republic of Congo, Gabon, Uganda, and Sudan.[17] Recent findings of ZEBOV seropositivity in rural people in Gabon have raised the question of its pathogenicity in humans.[1] *Bundibugyo ebolavirus*, the most recently discovered species, caused a human outbreak in Uganda in 2007, with a 34% case-fatality rate.[23] The sole confirmed human CIEBOV case, which was nonfatal, resulted from exposure during the necropsy of a CIEBOV-infected chimpanzee in Côte d'Ivoire in 1994. Although the recent discovery of REBOV in domestic swine in the Philippines raises public health concerns, it has not been shown to be pathogenic for humans.[3]

INFECTION CONTROL

Animal Trade

In response to the importation of REBOV-infected primates into American primate centers, the Centers for Disease Control and Prevention (CDC) have strengthened guidelines for the transportation, transit and quarantine of nonhuman primates in 1990. They include filovirus screening in the event of illness or death and a 31-day quarantine period for nonhuman primates; some scientists recommend 60 to 90 days quarantine.[21] In 1994, the Philippine Department of Agriculture implemented new measures, including a 45-day quarantine period prior to exportation and a ban on the export of wild-caught monkeys.[15]

Personal Protection

When working with animals in which EBOV exposure is a possibility (e.g., primate quarantine facilities or outbreak investigations), standard barrier nursing techniques are recommended to prevent infection.[10] Minimum protective clothing should include a proper fitting face mask, disposable gloves, gown or laboratory coat, long-sleeved shirts, and nonslip steel-toed boots.[21] In addition to these items, disposable protective suits with long sleeves, disposable boots, and three layers of latex gloves are used for wildlife necropsies in EBOV endemic regions (Fig. 54-1). However, once EBOV is identified as the cause of the mortality, positive-pressure hazmat suits and high-efficiency particulate air (HEPA) respirators are used. Face shields are useful when an aerosol potential exists. Special attention should be placed on protecting mucous membranes or skin lesions.[2] Guidelines have been developed

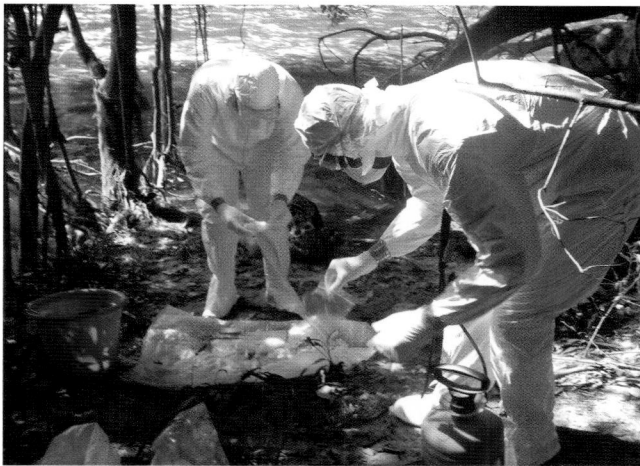

Figure 54-1

Minimum protective clothing used for initial outbreak investigations in Ebola virus endemic regions.

for dealing with an accidental exposure to EBOV-infected animals, blood, or tissue. They include cleaning with soap and disinfectant, irrigating mucous membranes, notifying health authorities, and possible isolation and surveillance of the affected person. BSL 4 facilities are required for manipulations involving known live EBOV virus.[9,20]

Disinfection

Nondisposable medical equipment and surfaces may be disinfected with a 1% to 5% sodium hypochlorite solution (5.0% chlorine concentration household bleach) for 30 minutes.[2] Delicate instruments, such as thermometers and stethoscopes, may be wrapped in a cloth soaked with rubbing alcohol (70% isopropyl) for 30 seconds and then air-dried. Inactivation of Ebola virus may be achieved with 1-hour exposure to formalin (1%), acetone, methanol, or diethyl ether. It has been reported that heating at 75°C for 30 minutes, 60°C for 60 minutes, exposure to ultraviolet light for 40 to 60 minutes, exposure to midday sun for 20 to 100 minutes, and irradiation will have the same effect.[3,10] Gamma radiation, 2% hypochlorite, 2% glutaraldehyde, 5% peracetic acid, 0.3% beta-propiolactone (37°C for 30 minutes), solutions containing sodium dodecyl sulfate (SDS) or polyethylene glycol *p*-phenylether, and standard hospital grade disinfectants have been recommended to neutralize Ebola virus.[21]

Outbreak Containment

Various approaches have been recommended for the management of an EHF outbreak in a nonhuman primate population. They include the following: obligatory use of personal protection equipment (including full face respirators) for all employees; cancellation of all animal shipments, suspension of activities other than once-daily feeding, observations, and cleaning; liberal use of 5% sodium hypochlorite as a disinfectant; and paraformaldehyde fumigation.[21] The efficacy of culling entire colonies to contain an outbreak is debated.

DIAGNOSIS

Diagnosis is based on the presence of antibody, antigen, or viral RNA. Key assays used today include reverse transcription PCR (RT-PCR) and antigen detection enzyme-linked immunosorbent assay (ELISA). However, virus isolation, quantitative real-time PCR assay, antibody capture ELISA, and antigen detection by IHC are also available.[3,4] The use of multiple diagnostic assays is recommended.[20]

Antigen capture ELISA is suitable for patients in the early stage of illness, when viral antigen may be detected in blood or tissues.[20] In fatal infections, humans and laboratory macaques often die before mounting an immune response. Viral RNA may be demonstrated in tissue using PCR and RT-PCR assays.[10] In the acute phase of human infections, EBOV has been detected in saliva, skin, breast milk, stool, tears, and semen.[3]

Serologic diagnosis (via ELISA or immunofluorescence antibody [IFA] analysis) is suitable for patients in the convalescent phase of illness, believed to appear 6 to 10 days after the onset of clinical signs.[3,10] Duration of immunity has not been determined, but in some human subjects IgG antibodies have been found up to 749 days postinfection. EBOV has been detected by RT-PCR assay in human breast milk and semen in the convalescent phase of infection.[3]

Histologic techniques, including antigen detection by IHC and IFA, are particularly useful for postmortem diagnosis. IFA may detect viral antigen in impression smears.[10] IHC analysis is a safe, sensitive, and specific method often used with skin biopsies, and may be performed on formalin-fixed tissue.[19]

Accurate diagnosis is particularly challenging in a tropical field setting, in which carcasses degrade quickly. Degraded tissue may be unsuitable for many diagnostic assays and more prone to false-negative results.[19] Antigen capture ELISA assays have detected EBOV in great ape tissue between 12 hours and 10 days old and PCR assay has detected viral RNA in 10-day-old degraded muscle tissue and 3-week-old bone marrow during epizootic investigations in central Africa. Attempts at viral isolation from decomposed carcasses are generally unrewarding. When cold chains are unavailable tissue may be preserved in RNAlater (Applied Biosystems/Ambion, Austin, Tex), excluding viral culture that requires fresh or frozen specimens.[11,20] Formalin-fixed tissues may undergo IHC analysis.[10]

Shipping of Samples for Diagnosis

In the United States, agencies regulating the shipping of biologic materials include the International Air Transport Association (IATA), U.S. Department of Transportation (DOT), U.S. Public Health Service (PHS), Occupational Health and Safety Administration (OSHA), and U.S. Postal Service (USPS). Those agencies regulating shipping of biologic samples originating from nonhuman species include the U.S. Fish and Wildlife Service (USFWS), which also regulates CITES (Convention on International Trade of Endangered Species) listed species, and the U.S. Department of Agriculture.

Differential Diagnosis

Acute signs of EHF in human and nonhuman primates may be somewhat nonspecific. Symptoms at any stage may vary in severity and hemorrhagic signs are not always present.[21] Differential diagnosis is dependent on the epidemiologic context and may include bacterial, viral, fungal, and parasitic causes.[10] Significant diseases to rule out include typhoid fever, shigellosis, rickettsial diseases, gram-negative bacterial septicemia, enterohemmorhagic *E. coli* enteritis, *P. falciparum* malaria, other viral hemorrhagic fevers, and platelet and vascular disorders.

TREATMENT

Treatment in humans consists of supportive therapy. No vaccines are licensed for human use, but at least one was reported to be effective in post-ZEBOV exposure treatment of rodents and nonhuman primates.[6]

REFERENCES

1. Becquart P, Wauquier N, Mahlakõiv T, et al: High prevalence of both humoral and cellular immunity to Zaire ebolavirus among rural populations in Gabon. PLoS One 5:e9126, 2002.

2. Centers for Disease Control and Prevention: Infection control for viral haemorrhagic fevers in the African health care setting, 2005 (http://www.cdc.gov/ncidod/dvrd/spb/mnpages/vhfmanual.htm).

3. Centers for Food Security and Public Health: Viral hemorrhagic fevers—Ebola and Marburg, 2009 (http://www.cfsph.iastate.edu/Factsheets/pdfs/viral_hemorrhagic_fever_filovirus.pdf).

4. Feldmann H: Personal communication, 2010.

5. Feldmann H, Geisbert, TW, Jahrling PB, et al: Family filoviridae. In Fauquet CM, Mayo MA, Maniloff J, et al, editors: Virus taxonomy. Eighth report of the International Committee on Taxonomy of Viruses, ed 2, San Diego, Calif, 2005, Elsevier/Academic Press, pp 645–653.

6. Feldmann H, Jones SM, Daddario-DiCaprio KM, et al: Effective post-exposure treatment of Ebola infection. PloS Path 3:54–61, 2007.

7. Geisbert TW, Hensley LE, Larsen T, et al: Pathogenesis of Ebola hemorrhagic fever in cynomolgus macaques: Evidence that dendritic cells are early and sustained targets of infection. Am J Pathol 163:2347–2370, 2003.

8. Jahrling PB, Geisbert TW, Jaax NK, et al: Experimental infection of cynomolgus macaques with Ebola-Reston filoviruses from the 1989-1990 U.S. epizootic. Arch Virol Suppl 11:115–134, 1996.

9. Kagan E: Ebola hemorrhagic fever: A paradigm of multiorgan dysfunction. J Organ Dysfunction 1:45–56, 2005.

10. Kuhn JH: Filoviruses, New York, 2008, Springer.

11. Leendertz FH, Pauli G, Maetz-Rensing K, et al: Pathogens as drivers of population declines: The importance of systematic monitoring in great apes and other threatened mammals. Biol Conserv 131:325–337, 2006.

12. Leroy EM, Epelboin A, Mondonge V, et al: Human Ebola outbreak resulting from direct exposure to fruit bats in Luebo, Democratic Republic of Congo, 2007. Vector Borne Zoonotic Dis 9:1557–7759, 2009.

13. Leroy EM, Kumulungui B, Pourrut X, et al: Fruit bats as reservoirs of Ebola virus. Nature 438:575–576, 2005.

14. Leroy EM, Telfer P, Kumulungui B, et al: A serological survey of Ebola virus infection in central African nonhuman primates. J Infect Dis 190:1895–1899, 2004.

15. Miranda ME, Ksiazek TG, Retuya TJ, et al: Epidemiology of Ebola (subtype Reston) virus in the Philippines, 1996. J Infect Dis 179:S115–S119, 1999.

16. Pourrut X, Delicat A, Rollin PE, et al: Spatial and temporal patterns of Zaire Ebola virus antibody prevalence in the possible reservoir bat species. J Infect Dis 196:S176–S183, 2007.

17. Pourrut X, Kumulungui B, Wittmann T, et al: The natural history of Ebola virus in Africa. Microb Infect 7:1005–1014, 2005.

18. Pourrut X, Souris M, Towner J, et al: Large serological survey showing cocirculation of Ebola and Marburg viruses in Gabonese bat populations, and a high seroprevalence of both viruses in Rousettus aegyptiacus. BMC Infect Dis 9:159, 2009.

19. Rouquet P, Froment JM, Bermejo M, et al: Wild animal mortality monitoring and human Ebola outbreaks, Gabon and Republic of Congo, 2001-2003. Emerg Infect Dis 11:283–289, 2005.

20. Saijo M, Niikura M, Ikegami T, et al: Laboratory diagnostic systems for Ebola and Marburg hemorrhagic fevers developed with recombinant proteins. Clin Vaccine Immunol 13:444–451, 2006.

21. Schou S, Hansen AK: Marburg and Ebola virus infections in laboratory non-human primates: A literature review. Comp Med 50:108–123, 2000.

22. Strong JE, Wong G, Jones SE, et al: Stimulation of Ebola virus production from persistent infection through activation of the Ras/MAPK pathway. Proc Natl Acad Sci U S A 105:17982–17987, 2008.

23. Wamala JF, Lukwago L, Malimbo M, et al: Ebola hemorrhagic fever associated with novel virus strain, Uganda, 2007-2008. Emerg Inf Dis 16:1087–1092, 2005.

24. Walsh PD, Abernethy KA, Bermejo M, et al: Catastrophic ape decline in western equatorial Africa. Nature 422:611–614, 2003.

25. Wittmann TJ, Biek R, Hassanin A, et al: Isolates of Zaire ebolavirus from wild apes reveal genetic lineage and recombinants. Proc Natl Acad Sci U S A 104:17123–17127, 2007.

26. Wyers M, Formenty P, Cherel Y, et al: Histopathological and immunohistochemical studies of lesions associated with Ebola virus in a naturally infected chimpanzee. J Infect Dis 179:S54–S59, 1999.

CHAPTER 55

Computed Tomography for the Diagnosis of Sinusitis and Air Sacculitis in Orangutans

Hanspeter W. Steinmetz and Nina Zimmermann

Captive orangutans *(Pongo pygmaeus, Pongo abelii)* have frequently been reported to suffer from upper respiratory tract disease, such as the common cold, sinusitis, and air sacculitis.[9,10,13,20] The exact reasons and pathogenesis are unknown until today, and the variety of microorganisms involved is broad. Predisposing factors that are discussed include increased microbacterial contamination of the environment, contact with humans, stress, and long-term antibiotic therapy. In humans, anatomic variations in the nose are the most important predisposing factors for sinusitis, leading to obstruction of the drainage pathways.[11,18,23]

Although air sacculitis is frequently diagnosed and recognized as a life-threatening disease, sinusitis in orangutans is probably underestimated or even unrecognized because diagnosis is difficult using common diagnostic methods. Also, the clinical signs are often vague. Most evident are chronic nasal discharge, halitosis, cough and, especially in air sacculitis, an enlarged air sac.[9,10,13] In recent years, the diagnosis of chronic sinusitis has received more attention, especially because an important correlation to the life-threatening air sacculitis has been suspected.[20,24]

Because of the inherent uncertainty associated with its diagnosis, more objective tools have been sought. In human medicine, computed tomography (CT) is the most important diagnostic aid to evaluate the upper respiratory tract and follow up on its response to treatment.[4,19] CT scanning of the head may represent an advanced imaging technique for the early diagnosis of upper airway diseases, especially of the sinuses, in orangutans.[20,24] This would allow the application of treatment modalities to prevent further serious infections of the upper respiratory tract. The increased speed of modern CT techniques and the increased availability of specialized institutions with CT equipment make this important diagnostic imaging technique more readily

available to zoological institutions. The purpose of the CT evaluation of the paranasal sinuses and related structures, including the air sacs, is to provide an accurate display of the regional anatomy, confirm the diagnosis, and characterize the extent and localization of disease.

NORMAL ANATOMY AND PHYSIOLOGY

The upper respiratory tract in primates includes the nose, larynx, and trachea. In addition to the wide range of size and external shapes of the nose, the internal anatomy and physiology vary considerably between humans and apes, and even between the different ape species.[3,14,16,17] A distinct feature of orangutans is the extent of the sinuses and laryngeal air sacs.

The primary function of the orangutan's nasal airway is breathing and, therefore, in contrast to olfactory-dependent mammals (e.g., carnivores), the anatomy is considerably simpler. A nasal septum in the midline divides the triangular-shaped nasal cavity into two separate passages. Each nasal cavity bears two well-developed scroll-like turbinates, or conchae, the maxilloturbinal inferior (inferior turbinates), and the ethmoturbinal posterosuperior (superior turbinates); the nasoturbinal anterosuperior (middle turbinates) is reduced to a small remnant rostral to the ethmoturbinal.[3] The turbinates divide the nasal airway into three groovelike air passages—upper, middle, and lower meatus—and are responsible for forcing inhaled air to flow in a steady regular pattern around the largest possible surface of cilia and climate-controlling tissue. In addition, the nasal passage may be divided into three regions on the basis of their functional significance. The main nasal airway extends from the floor of the nose upward to the middle and superior turbinates and from the tip of the nose backward to the posterior termination of the turbinates. Above the main nasal airway is the olfactory

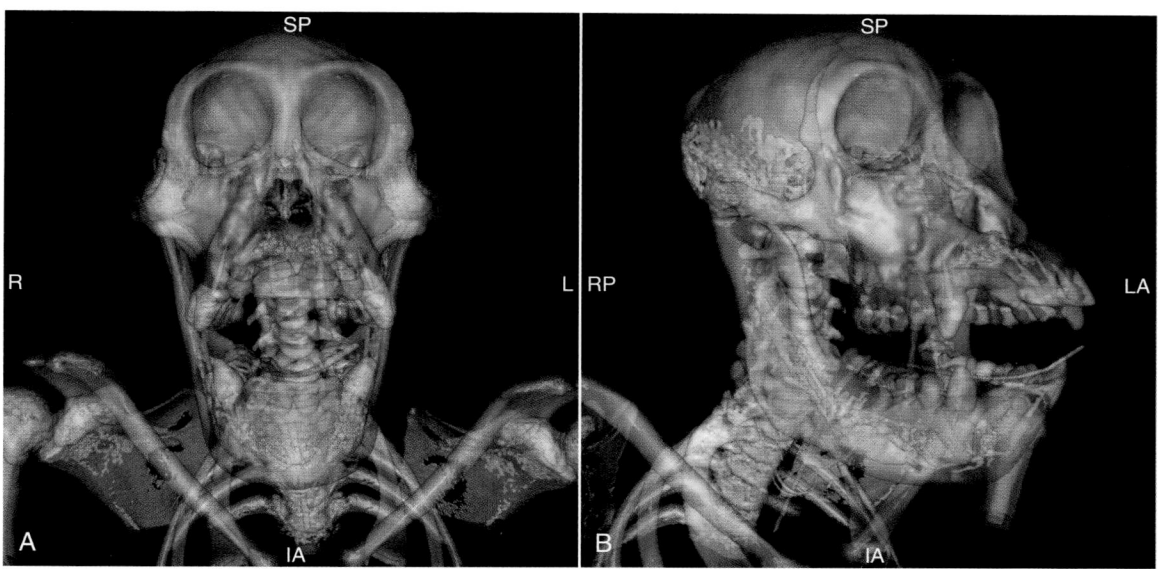

Figure 55-1

Three-dimensional reconstruction of the skull of an adult female orangutan *(Pongo abelii)* in frontal (A) and oblique (B) views. The sinuses are displayed in blue.

airway. The nasopharynx is the space posterior to the termination of the nasal septum and the turbinates and extends downward to the inferior termination of the soft palate. The nasal cavity is surrounded by two paranasal sinuses (Fig. 55-1), which develop as pneumatized expansions of the nasal cavity's mucosal recess.[8]

Orangutans differ from other apes in possessing a very narrow interorbital region. The paranasal sinuses include the maxillary and sphenoidal sinuses. Although the maxillary sinus is large, the sphenoidal sinus is significantly reduced in orangutans in contrast to other apes.[3] The maxillary sinus occupies the entire maxilla and extends into the lacrimal, frontal, ethmoid, zygomatic, palatine, and sphenoid bones. The sphenoidal extension is situated dorsal to the true sphenoidal sinus and invades both the pterygoid and zygomatic processes of the temporal bone. The nasolacrimal duct, infraorbital, and ethmoidal neurovascular structures pass the maxillary sinus, and the optic nerve and internal carotid artery encroach on its sphenoidal extension.[17] The sphenoidal sinuses are found in the most inferior part of the sphenoidal body and may be divided into right and left sinuses separated by an osseous septum. There is no frontal sinus but, in adult orangutans, a frontal recess of the maxillary sinus may extend superiorly to border much of the inferomedial corner of the orbit posterior to the lacrimal duct.[8] The extent of this frontal recess is variable, and may sometimes pneumatize the interorbital region of the frontal bone. Before the age of 8 to

12 years, the frontal recess is less developed and the nasal cavity is in direct contact with the medial orbital wall. The maxillary sinuses drain through ostia into the middle meatus, which lies superolaterally to the middle turbinate, whereas the sinus sphenoidalis opens into the upper meatus, which lies lateromedial at the posterior end. All the sinuses are normally in continuous communication with the nasal air.

The nasal cavity and paranasal sinuses are lined with respiratory ciliated epithelium containing serous and mucinous glands.[3] The cilia in the respiratory tract are in constant motion and act together to transport the mucus toward the external nasal cavity. In the maxillary sinus, the mucous flow originates along the floor and is centripetally directed toward the ostium, subsequently to the middle meatus, and ultimately to the nasopharynx.[5] The flow from the sphenoidal sinus enters the superior meatus and then the nasopharynx.

The larynx is situated in the anterior neck and connects the inferior part of the pharynx with the trachea. It provides a sphincter valve at the entrance to the trachea. The anatomy is similar to that of humans and the laryngeal skeleton consists of nine cartilages—three single (thyroid, cricoid, and epiglottic) and three paired (arytenoid, corniculate, and cuneiform). The hyoid bone is not part of the larynx, although it is connected to it. Slight differences in larynx anatomy have been a key factor in the evolution of human speech.[14] A remarkable feature of nonhuman primates is the laryngeal air

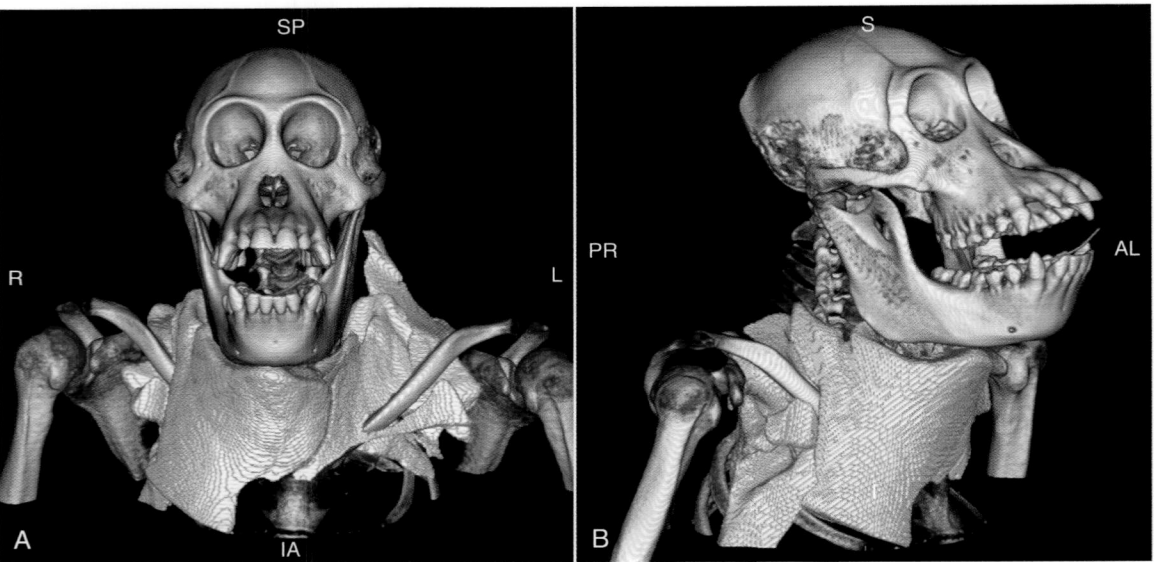

Figure 55-2

Three-dimensional reconstruction of the air sac system of an adult female orangutan *(Pongo abelii)* in frontal **(A)** and lateral **(B)** views. The air sacs are displayed in white and indicate an air-filled structure. Note that under anesthesia and in dorsal recumbency, the shape and extent of the air sac system might vary considerably among individuals because of different amount of air in the air sacs.

sac (Fig. 55-2), an accessory mucosal membrane pouch extending from a secondary valve formed by the inferior thyroarytenoid folds.[6] Its form and extent vary considerably among apes.[15]

Although there are slight differences in the sac configuration, all the great apes share a rapid expansion of the unilateral sac from the ventricles, which fuse with another sac inferiorly in the late juvenile period.[15] The fully developed extralaryngeal air sacs in orangutans extend inferiorly from the ventricles to the neck and axillary region, meet in the midline beneath the pectoral muscles, and are connected to the upper respiratory tract via two openings in the lateral larynx wall. When collapsed, the true capacity of these sacs is difficult to quantify. The air sac is lined with ciliated epithelium with a lamina propria consisting of a layer of loose elastic and collagenous fibers, with variable numbers of seromucinous glands.[6] The functions of the laryngeal air sac in primates are still a matter of debate. Suggested functions include storage of expired air to increase oxygen uptake, reduction of the hyperventilation caused by a long sequence of repetitive loud calls, generating another sound source in the laryngeal ventricles, resonating the laryngeal voice source to help produce loud and long calls, and buffering against the pressure induced by intensive expiratory air flow following air

trapping during three-dimensional arboreal locomotion. In humans, the saccule is probably the vestigial remains of the air sacs.

EQUIPMENT AND COMPUTED TOMOGRAPHY TECHNIQUE
Equipment

CT has been used in veterinary diagnostic imaging since the late 1970s. During a CT scan, a radiographic source rotates around the patient while x-ray detectors are positioned on the opposite side of the circle (gantry) from the x-ray source. Many data scans are progressively taken as the object is gradually passed through the gantry. They are combined together by mathematical procedures known as tomographic reconstruction. Although every slice was formerly taken step by step (sequence CT), newer technologies with faster computer systems and updated calculation software have allowed the production of continuously changing cross sections as the patient to be imaged slowly slides through the gantry within the x-ray circle (spiral CT). Adding multislice detectors to the scanner allows simultaneous scanning of multiple layers at the same time and improved image quality while scan time is reduced (multislice CT). The current newest technology combine two x-ray sources and detectors, which rotate around the patient at the same time and result in better image resolution, higher power, and reduced scan time while the x-ray dose is lowered even further (dual-source CT).[21] Reducing the energy dose is important in long-living animals to protect sensitive organs such as the thyroid gland, retina, lens, or gonads from the side effects of the radiation. Repeating a study results in a higher radiation exposure than an adequate energy setup that produces high-quality images.

The images generated are in the axial or transverse plane (slices) and the data of the moving individual slices may be used to generate a three-dimensional picture, viewable from different perspectives. The data obtained represent the varying radiographic intensity sensed at the detectors; through computer calculation, the radiographic density is displayed according to the mean attenuation of the tissue. The attenuation is expressed in Hounsfield units (HU) on a scale from +3071 (most attenuating) to −1024 (least attenuating) HU. Marker points are water, with an attenuation of 0 HU, and air, with −1000 HU; cancellous bone is typically +400 HU and more.[21] These Hounsfield units are displayed in terms of relative radiodensity as pixels in a two-dimensional and as voxels in a three-dimensional picture. Contrast medium (e.g., iodine) is sometimes used to highlight structures such as blood vessels to obtain functional information about tissues or to separate tissues of similar attenuation (e.g., mucous membranes and pus).

Positioning

Indications for the CT evaluation of the upper respiratory tract in orangutans include chronic nasal discharge, facial swellings, and suspected air sacculitis. Therefore, anesthesia should be regarded as a high-risk immobilization, especially because pulmonary aspiration of pathologic exudates from the sinuses or air sac must be expected. Anesthetized orangutans should be intubated immediately after induction for the entire procedure with an appropriate endotracheal tube to prevent aspiration of air sac or regurgitated stomach contents. Animals may be observed for cardiopulmonary stability (electrocardiography, noninvasive blood pressure determination, respiratory rate monitoring, capnography, pulse oximetry) with standard veterinary monitoring equipment. For CT scanning, orangutans should be positioned in ventral recumbency for best display of possible fluid levels, as recommended for humans.

Scanning Procedure

A high-resolution CT scanning technique for sinus evaluation in the orangutan is recommended. After positioning the animal, a scout image is obtained in dorsoventral and lateral projections. The scout image is used to select the anatomic region (scanning field) to be scanned and may later be used as a reference for location of individual slices. The dorsoventral projection is useful for evaluating bilateral symmetry and the lateral projection helps select the angle of the scan plane. The scanning field should start at the most frontal part of the head and reach down to the midthorax for assessment of the sinuses and air sacs. The field of view should be selected as small as possible to produce the best image quality. The setup of CT parameters follows the scout image. Slice thickness and slice interval (overlap) must be selected prior to scanning. Because fine details are required for sinus evaluation, a slice thickness less than 0.75 mm and slight overlap are recommended. The resolution, especially in small anatomic structures, is best with multislice CT. On single-slice spiral CT scanners, resolution is better with sequential protocols than with spiral protocols.[22] Because sinuses and the air sac are not moving anatomic structures, scanning time is not an important criterion. More important is the reduction of artifacts and best image quality. Therefore, a slight overscan with a pitch less than 1 is recommended for these structures. Many existing protocols for human sinus evaluation use high milliamperage (up to 200 mA) in the belief that this improves scan quality. However, studies in humans have shown excellent quality sinus scans with doses as low as 40 mA.[7] Although minimizing the radiation dose delivered to the patient is an important consideration, a dose of 120 mA is justifiable for orangutans because of their heavier skull anatomy. Recommended settings for sinus CT in orangutans are summarized in Table 55-1.

EVALUATION

The coronal plane perpendicular to the bony palate is the preferred plane for the sinus evaluation because it best displays the ostiomeatal unit and sinuses (Figs. 55-3 and 55-4), whereas the standard transverse plane is recommended for air sac assessment (Fig. 55-5). Nevertheless, all three planes should be assessed and a three-dimensional reconstruction is always recommended. A high-reconstruction algorithm is recommended, being aware to neglect the contrast, but

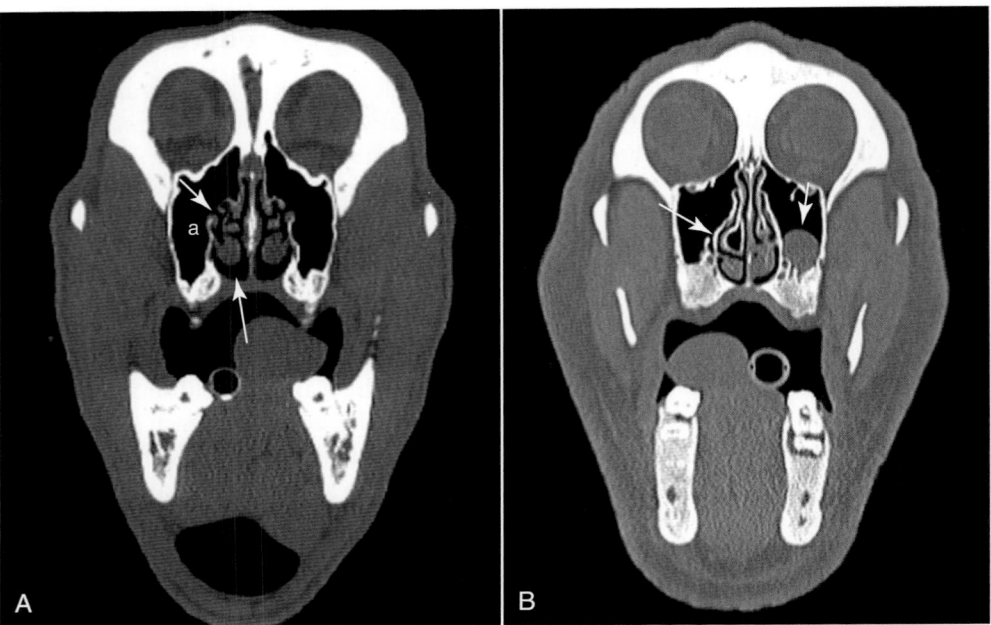

Figure 55-3

CT scans of an adult female orangutan *(Pongo abelii)*. **A,** Normal coronal CT scan of the paranasal sinuses. Shown are the normal maxillary sinus *(a)* and nasal cavity *(b)*; there are no signs of swollen membranes, fluid levels, or bone destruction. The ostium *(arrow)* is well displayed and connects the maxillary sinus with the nasal cavity. **B,** Anatomic variations of the paranasal sinuses shown in a coronal CT scan. A pneumatized superior turbinate *(long arrow)*, referred to as concha bullosa, can be seen in the right nasal cavity. A mucous retention cyst *(short arrow)* is displayed in the left maxillary sinus.

TABLE 55-1	Recommended Technique for CT Evaluation of Sinuses and Air Sacs in Orangutans *(Pongo* spp.)
Imaging Parameters	**Settings**
Position	Ventral recumbency
Extent of study	Top of head to midthorax
Section thickness	<0.75 mm
Pitch (table incrementation)	<1
Overlap	0.5
kVp	120
mA	120
Window width (HU)	1500
Window level (HU)	300

detailed reconstruction of anatomic structures within the sinuses and nasal cavity is most important. High-attenuation tissue (bone) next to low-attenuation tissue (air) allows the production of fine detail. The final image is converted in various shades of gray. Generally, 63 shades of gray are used to make the final image and each shade of gray represents a group of several

Hounsfield units. The HU window representing the gray scale may be adjusted to maximize the attenuation of the tissue of interest. The window width determines the HU range over which the available gray scale is spread. The window level is the median HU in the window. For sinus evaluation, a bone window is recommended, with the window width set at 1500 HU and window level set at 300 HU.

First, orientation in the various planes is achieved by the identification of anatomic structures. There are 12 anatomic structures that must be systematically evaluated. For ease and consistency of evaluation, these structures should be assessed anterior to posterior, in sequence. The sequence of evaluation is nasal cavity, the turbinates, lower, middle, and upper meatus, primary ostium, maxillary sinus, frontal recess, secondary ostium, sphenoidal sinus, larynx, and air sacs (Table 55-2). Special attention is given to any variation that is obstructing air passage, such as the presence of mucus or periosteal thickening, fluid-filled sinuses, or anatomic variations of the bony structures.

The normal sinus and nasal anatomy may differ considerably from animal to animal; certain anatomic variations are commonly observed in the whole

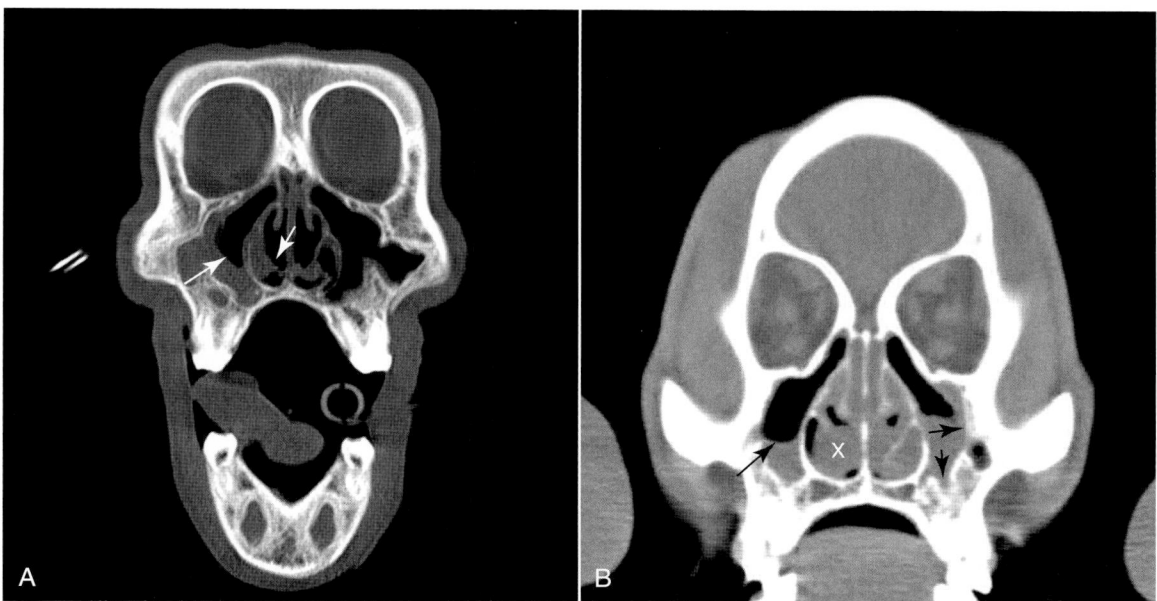

Figure 55-4

A, Coronal CT scan of the paranasal sinuses in a subadult male orangutan *(Pongo pygmaeus)* with mild sinusitis. Mildly swollen mucosal membranes in the nose *(short arrow)* and fluid levels *(long arrow)* in the right maxillary sinus can be seen. **B,** Coronal CT scan of the paranasal sinuses in an adult female orangutan *(Pongo pygmaeus)* with severe sinusitis. Severe swollen mucosal membranes in the congested nose *(X)* and horizontal fluid levels *(long arrow)* in both maxillary sinus can be seen. The primary ostium is completely blocked and bony alterations within the sinuses are present *(short arrows)*.

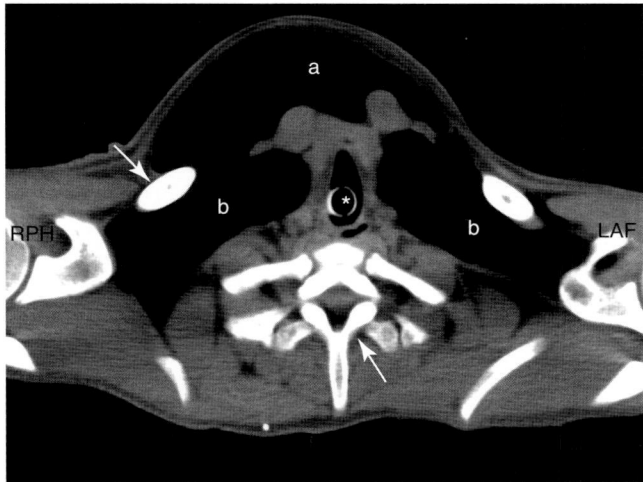

Figure 55-5

Transverse CT scan of the air sac system in an adult female orangutan *(Pongo abelii)*. Shown are the trachea, with endotracheal tube *(*)*, clavicle *(top arrow)*, spine *(bottom arrow)*, submandibular space *(a)*, and air-filled subclavicular and axillary spaces *(b)*.

population and others are seen more often in animals with chronic inflammatory disease (see Fig. 55-3). Thus, anatomic variations have to be assessed carefully and the significance of particular anatomic variants must be determined by their relationship with the ostiomeatal complex and nasal air passages. The ability of the variation to obstruct the air passages implies a role in the recurrence of sinusitis, and probably air sacculitis.[18,23]

All sinuses and the ostiomeatal complex must be evaluated for fluid content. The thickness of mucosal membranes should be judged carefully, although identification might be difficult. Magnetic resonance imaging (MRI) would display soft tissue better than CT. Repeated inflammation of the mucosa may lead to hypertrophy, polypoid thickening, areas of atrophy, and fibrosis. Because of mucosal swelling, two mucosal layers may become apposed, leading to stenosis and obstruction, which in turn reduce aeration and predispose for the accumulation of secretions in the sinus and make it prone to infection.[25] Similar cyclical changes in the mucosal lining of the sinuses, nasal cavity, and turbinates might occur and must be considered. Longstanding inflammation may cause reactive sclerosis of the adjacent bones; this sign may be used to suggest a diagnosis of chronic sinus disease. Therefore, osteal structures must be evaluated for reactive alterations, osteolysis, bone formations, and mass effects. Reactive bony sclerosis may be difficult to distinguish from osteomyelitis. Alterations may be caused by

TABLE 55-2   CT Staging System* for Sinusitis and Air Sacculitis in Orangutans *(Pongo pygmaeus, P. abelii)*

	LEFT				RIGHT			
Anatomic Structure	Anatomic Variation	Mucous Membranes	Bone	Fluid	Anatomic Variation	Mucous Membranes	Bone	Fluid
Nasal cavity								
Turbinates								
Lower meatus								
Middle meatus								
Upper meatus								
Primary ostium								
Maxillary sinus								
Frontal recessus								
Secondary ostium								
Spenoidal sinus								
Larynx								
Air sacs								

Each anatomic structure is scored according to the amount of the disease present. 0, No alteration or clear; 1, slight alteration or partial opacification; 2, severe alteration or total opacification.

anatomic variations, trauma, neoplasia, or inflammation. However, any narrowing in the ostiomeatal passages may lead secondarily to inflammation and further obstruction (see Fig. 55-4).

For evaluation of the air sac, the MRI would be preferable, but the clinical sign of a swollen air sac with palpable fluid accumulation may be confirmed in CT scans. Fluid levels within the air sac may be seen and, by attenuation measurement, may be distinguished from normal air (-1000 HU), fluid (0 HU), and identification of pus (≈ 20 HU). Mucosal thickening is more difficult to identify than in the ostiomeatal passages because high-attenuation differences between the skin and mucous membranes are missing (see Figure 55-5).

In an attempt to determine outcome indicators for the treatment of inflammatory sinus disease, several staging systems have been developed in human medicine.[12] Although results of the animal's medical history, laboratory findings, and possible rhinoscopic examinations should be included in the patient evaluation, CT findings have been proved to be the most useful and are accepted as the basis for a staging system. Because of the different anatomy and current lack of long-term experience in orangutans, it is difficult to determine a similar, significant, prognostic staging system; therefore, an adaptation in regard to treatment of the orangutan has been made. Each anatomic structure is scored according to the amount of disease present (see Table 55-2).

TABLE 55-3   Classification of Disease Severity in Orangutans *(Pongo* spp.) With Sinusitis and Air Sacculitis

Degree of Disease	Description
Healthy	Absent clinical signs, no score, except in anatomic variations; score not exceeding 1 (see Table 55-2)
Mild disease	Clinical signs, swollen mucosal membranes (up to score 2) and homogenous opacified sinus (up to maximum score 1) might be present; no bone lesions present and air sacs not affected.
Severe disease	Clinical signs, swollen mucosal membranes and homogenous opacified sinuses with bony lesions; if air sacs are affected, the degree of disease is always classified as severe.

TREATMENT

If any abnormalities are present on CT scans, they must be evaluated in the overall context of the animal's condition, as it provides important criteria for further treatment. Treatment options are chosen according to the CT scoring system (Table 55-3). Animals judged as healthy require no treatment, but anatomic variations might require future CT reexamination.

Medical Management

The goal of medical treatment is to reduce mucosal swelling and clear sinuses and air sacs from infection and fluid. Medical treatment may be attempted in animals with mild disease (see Table 55-3) that are asymptomatic or have only a homogenous opacified sinus without any signs of bony erosions and fluid accumulation in the air sacs. Broad-spectrum antibiotics according to sensitivity testing are given for 4 to 6 weeks, after which clinical signs are reassessed. Additionally, steroids and mucolytic agents are recommended. Antimycotic therapy might be indicated, depending on laboratory findings.

Surgical Management

Surgical treatment is indicated for any animal classified as having severe disease (see Table 55-3). Before surgical treatment is anticipated, medical treatment is recommended to reduce infection and swelling for 3 weeks. Treatments for air sacculitis are marsupialization of the air sac or even complete surgical resection of the air sac.[10,13] Surgical treatment of sinusitis is less well documented in orangutans. Although a craniotomy with maxillary sinus drainage has been described in one juvenile orangutan,[2] it appears that functional endoscopic sinus surgery (FESS) will be the future treatment of choice.[20] The FESS technique has shown good results in chronic sinusitis in humans[1] and has been described in a male orangutan with chronic severe sinusitis and air sacculitis. The purpose of FESS is to allow restoration of sinus drainage and ventilation by opening the natural ostium and preserving the mucosa.

CONCLUSION

CT is the modality of choice for imaging inflammatory disease of the ostiomeatal complex and sinuses. It should be considered for all orangutans with chronic nasal discharge, facial swelling, or a swollen air sac to confirm diagnosis. Furthermore, with the determination of the severity and localization of disease, treatment options, including a surgical approach, may be planned, and a better outcome might be attained.

Acknowledgments

We would like to acknowledge Jean-Michel Hatt and Mariano Makara for their time, expertise, and corrections. We thank the University of Zurich and Zurich Zoo for their financial support.

REFERENCES

1. Briner HR, Simmen D, Jones N: Endoscopic sinus surgery: Advantages of the bimanual technique. Am J Rhinol 19:269–273, 2005.
2. Cambre RC, Edwards JE, Wilson HL, et al: Maxillary and ethmoid sinusitis with orbital and intracranial extension in an infant orangutan *(Pongo pygmaeus)*. J Zoo Wildl Anim Med 26:144–151, 1995.
3. Cave AJ: The paranasal sinuses of the anthropoid apes. J Anat 74:493–523, 1940.
4. Danielsen A, Reitan E, Olofsson, J: The role of computed tomography in endoscopic sinus surgery: A review of 10 years' practice. Eur Arch Otorhinolaryngol 263:381–389, 2006.
5. Eggesbo HB: Radiological imaging of inflammatory lesions in the nasal cavity and paranasal sinuses. Eur Radiol 16:872–888, 2006.
6. Harrison DFN: The anatomy and physiology of the mammalian larynx, Cambridge, England, 1995, Cambridge University Press.
7. Kearney SE, Jones P, Meakin K. et al: CT scanning of the paranasal sinuses—The effect of reducing mAs. Br J Radiol 70:1071–1074, 1997.
8. Koppe T, Rae TC, Swindler DR: Influence of craniofacial morphology on primate paranasal pneumatization. Ann Anat 181:77–80, 1999.
9. Lawson B, Garriga R, Galdikas BM: Air sacculitis in fourteen juvenile southern Bornean orangutans *(Pongo pygmaeus wurmbii)*. J Med Primatol 35:149–154, 2006.
10. Loomis ME: Great apes. In Fowler ME, Miller RE, editors: Zoo and wild animal medicine, ed 5, St. Louis, 2003, WB Saunders, pp 381–397.
11. Lund VJ, Neijens HJ, Clement PA, et al: The treatment of chronic sinusitis: A controversial issue. Int J Pediatr Otorhinolaryngol 32(suppl):S21–S35, 1995.
12. Lund VJ, Kennedy DW: Staging for rhinosinusitis. Otolaryngol Head Neck Surg 117:S35–S40, 1997.
13. McManamon R, Swenson RB, Orkin JL, et al: Update on diagnostic and therapeutic approaches to air sacculitis in orangutans. Proc Conf Am Assoc Zoo Vet 1994:193–194.
14. Nishimura T: Comparative morphology of the hyo-laryngeal complex in anthropoids: Two steps in the evolution of the descent of the larynx. Primates 44:41–49, 2003.
15. Nishimura T, Mikami A, Suzuki J, et al: Development of the laryngeal air sac in chimpanzees. Int J Primatol 28:483–492, 2007.
16. Preuschoft H, Witte H, Witzel U: Pneumatized spaces, sinuses and spongy bones in the skulls of primates. Anthropol Anz 60:67–79, 2002.
17. Rossie JB: Anatomy of the nasal cavity and paranasal sinuses in Aegyptopithecus and early Miocene African catarrhines. Am J Phys Anthropol 126:250–267, 2005.
18. Scribano E, Ascenti G, Loria G, et al: The role of the ostiomeatal unit anatomic variations in inflammatory disease of the maxillary sinuses. Eur J Radiol 24:172–174, 1997.
19. Simmen D, Schuknecht B: Computerized tomography of paranasal sinuses—A preoperative check list. Laryngorhinootologie. 76:8–13, 1997.
20. Steinmetz HW, Briner HR, Vogt R, et al: Functional endoscopic sinus surgery in a Sumatran orangutan *(Pongo pygmaeus abeli)*. Verh Erkrg Zootiere 43:74–75, 2007.
21. Tidwell AS: Principles of computed tomography and magnetic resonance imaging. In Thrall DE, editor: Textbook of veterinary diagnostic radiology, ed 5, St. Louis, 2007, WB Saunders, pp 50–77.

22. Wallner CP, Roehrer-Ertl O, Schneider K: State-of-the-art com-
    puted tomography of primate skulls—Comparison of different
    scan-protocols. Ann Anat 186:521–524, 2004.
23. Zimmermann K, Heider C, Kosling S: Anatomy and normal varia-
    tions of paranasal sinuses in radiological imaging. Radiologe
    47:584–590, 2007.
24. Zimmermann N, Zingg R, Makara M, et al: Computer tomo-
    graphic evaluation of the upper respiratory tract in orangutans
    (Pongo pygmaeus, Pongo abelii), 2009 (https://www.zora.uzh.ch/
    18843/2/102_Zimmermann_N-1.pdf).
25. Zinreich SJ: Functional anatomy and computed tomography
    imaging of the paranasal sinuses. Am J Med Sci 316:2–12, 1998.

Chiroptera

CHAPTER 56

White-Nose Syndrome in Cave Bats of North America

Elizabeth L. Buckles and Anne E. Ballmann

White-nose syndrome (WNS), an emerging disease of hibernating insectivorous bats, is associated with unprecedented winter mortality at cave and mine hibernacula in the northeastern and mid-Atlantic regions of the United States.[2] The disease is named for the prominent white, powdery fungal growth around the muzzles of bats, although the fungus also appears on wings, ears, and tail membranes (Fig. 56-1). This fungus, which is consistently associated with WNS development and is the presumptive cause of the syndrome, is a newly discovered species named *Geomyces destructans*.[12]

The population effects of WNS have been profound and widespread. Several WNS-affected locations have reported 90% to 100% loss of the hibernating population after only two seasons of the disease.[23,30] Since its first detection in New York (February 2006), WNS has spread over 950 km, seemingly advancing 200 to 700 km/year. More than one million cave bats are estimated to have died.[8] The species most commonly observed to be affected is the little brown bat *(Myotis lucifugus)*, which had been the most abundant bat species in the region prior to the emergence of WNS.[11] Other hibernating species known to be susceptible to WNS include northern long-eared bats *(M. septentrionalis)*, tricolored bats *(Perimyotis subflavus)*, eastern small-footed bats *(M. leibii)*, big brown bats *(Eptesicus fuscus)*, and federally listed (endangered) Indiana bats *(M. sodalis)*. Within the WNS-affected region, Indiana bat winter counts decreased by 25,000 bats (30%) between 2007 and 2009.[29] Three additional *Myotis* spp. bats *(M. austrorparius, M. grisescens,* and *M. velifer)* may also be proven to be susceptible to WNS, however thus far only the genetic signature of *G. destructans* has been demonstrated in these species.[31]

The risk WNS poses to the rest of the North American bat population is unknown, but there is cause for concern. In all, 25 of 45 North American bat species hibernate in caves or mines[30] and therefore may be susceptible to WNS. Some of the country's largest and most species-rich bat hibernacula are located in the midwestern and southeastern United States,[29] just beyond the current leading edge of the disease. As WNS continues to spread further south and west, extensive hibernacula in Missouri, Tennessee, and Kentucky housing more than 100,000 bats, including endangered Virginia big-eared bats *(Corynorhinus townsendii virginianus)* and gray bats *(M. grisescens)*, are at risk.

EMERGENCE AND SPREAD

White-nose syndrome was first photodocumented in hibernating bats in a commercial cave near Albany, New York, in February 2006, although the disease went unrecognized until the following winter, when it was observed at four hibernacula within a 15-km radius near this presumptive index site. That same year (2007), the N.Y. State Department of Health received 10 times the 25-year average of bat submissions for rabies testing between January and April.[2]

Increased surveillance during the winter of 2007 to 2008 detected WNS at 33 sites in four states (New York, Connecticut, Massachusetts, and Vermont), with approximately 25% of all surveyed bat hibernacula affected within a 210-km radius from the presumptive New York epicenter. By the winter of 2008 to 2009, WNS expanded both within its original range and spread to another 27 sites in five additional states, including New Hampshire, New Jersey, Pennsylvania, Virginia, and West Virginia (Fig. 56-2). In winter 2009 to 2010, WNS reached eastern Tennessee and north into Quebec and Ontario although *G. destructans* DNA was recovered from bats as far west as Missouri and Oklahoma.[26] The pattern of expansion and the diversity of environmental variables among the growing number of affected sites

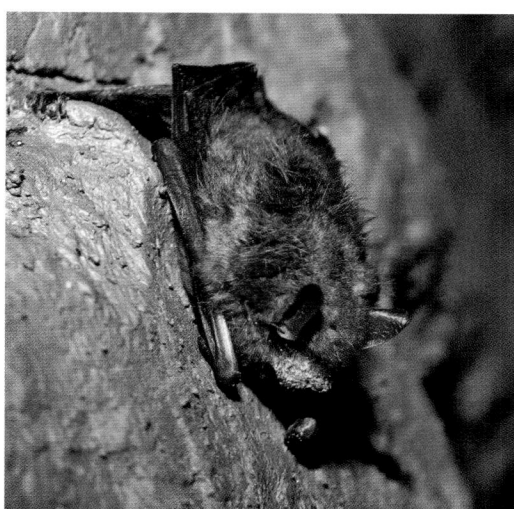

Figure 56-1

Tricolored bat *(Perimyotis subflavus)* in a Pennsylvania hibernaculum, March 2009. The white fungal plume of *Geomyces destructans* is evident on the muzzle. *(Courtesy Greg Turner, Pennsylvania Game Commission.)*

have supported WNS as an infectious disease rather than the result of contaminant exposure.[7,9]

EPIDEMIOLOGY

Visible evidence of cutaneous fungal growth on bats during the winter months is the hallmark of WNS; however, bats may have microscopic lesions on wing, muzzle, and ear caused by *G. destructans* without the visible manifestation of the fungus.[7,19] Even when visually present in the cave environment, the proliferative white fungal growth is easily disrupted and may disappear with handling.[7,19] Field observations have described pinpoint colonies of visible fungus around the nares of bats first developing in late November, although late September marks the earliest diagnosis of WNS skin infection in bats to date,[32] detected in a subclinical little brown bat collected from a hibernaculum confirmed as WNS-positive the previous winter. External signs of infection become more prominent on bats as hibernation continues.[7,19] Both adult and juvenile bats (~6 months old) are susceptible to WNS and associated winter mortality. *G. destructans* has been recovered from bats emerging from hibernacula with moderate to severe wing damage[19] and from postemergent females sampled at maternity colonies as late as May.[20] It has not yet been cultured from free-ranging bats collected between June and August within the affected region, nor has WNS been associated with summer bat mortality, including

that at maternity colonies,[31] although samples are limited.

In addition to the physical manifestation for which WNS is named, other characteristics accompanying the disease are often readily recognized in the field during the winter. Abnormal behavior such as bats observed outside in cold temperatures during daylight hours is often an early indicator of problems in the area. Large numbers of bats roosting near the entrances of hibernacula, particularly species not known to do so, and a delayed or lack of arousal response in the presence of human disturbance are other atypical behaviors commonly reported at affected sites. The gross appearance of *G. destructans* on torpid bats preceded behavioral changes and mass mortality in at least one affected site in Pennsylvania.[28] Most dead bats are often found at, or just outside, the hibernaculum entrance in poor body condition. Bats emerging in late winter and spring often have moderate to severe wing damage, including holes and tears, which may adversely affect their ability to forage.[23] The effects of this damage on survivorship and reproductive success of postemergent bats in maternity colonies are not yet well understood.[23]

PRESUMPTIVE CAUSE

The two most consistent findings from laboratory evaluations of dead bats with WNS are the presence of invasive fungi consistent with *G. destructans* on the glabrous skin and suboptimal body condition during late hibernation.[7,19] The presence of fungal hyphae on the WNS-affected bats is in clear contrast to the absence of invasive fungi on bats examined from areas not experiencing winter mortality or displaying signs of WNS. Furthermore, no consistent internal lesions have been identified in WNS-affected bats and ancillary tests failed to reveal any other consistent pathogen, mineral, or heavy metal–based toxicities.[3,9] Findings such as pneumonia and ectoparasitism and endoparasitism were interpreted as incidental because they were also found in bats from uninfected populations.[2,9]

G. destructans infections were prevalent on the wings where the fungal hyphae invaded into the dermis and, in severe cases, extended full thickness through the wing. On the face, fungal infections were not observed to infect mucosa beyond the anterior nares.[19] Although in vivo experiments demonstrating *G. destructans* as the causative agent of WNS mortality are ongoing, the strong correlation between the presence of this newly described fungus and WNS development make it the prime putative agent of the syndrome.[2]

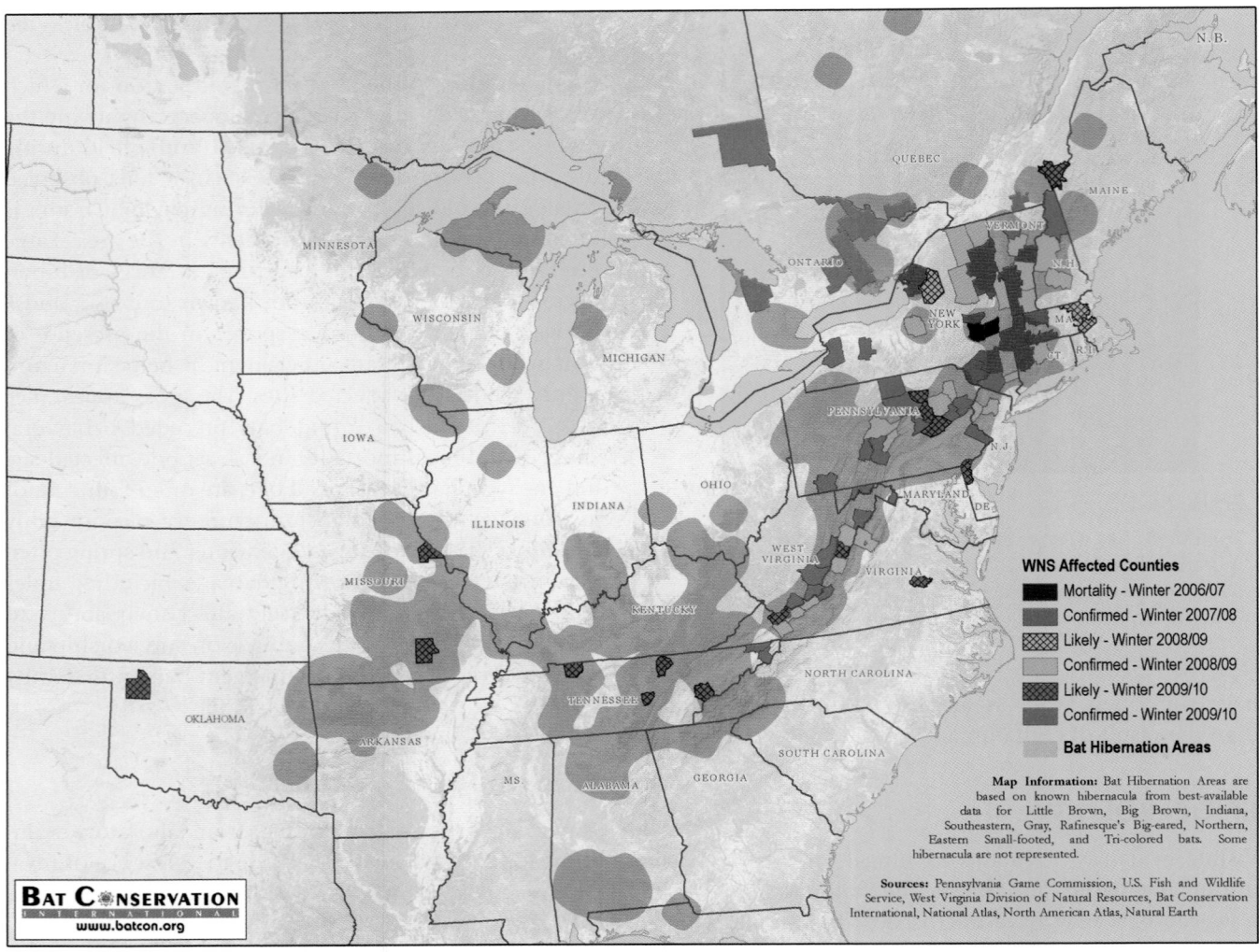

Figure 56-2

Map depicting the distribution of counties as of October 2010 where WNS (Confirmed) and *Geomyces destructans* DNA or field signs (Likely) have been detected in relation to existing bat hibernacula in North America occupied by at-risk species. *(Courtesy Bat Conservation International.)*

Classification of G. destructans

Phylogenetic analyses of two ribosomal RNA regions, the internal transcribed spacer (ITS) and small subunit (SSU), conducted on morphologically identical fungal isolates cultured from affected bats collected at different locations most closely resembled the anamorphic genus *Geomyces* (order Helotiales).[2,12] Morphologically however, the asymmetrically curved conidia appear to make this fungus unique among *Geomyces* spp., which are known to be psychrophilic (cold-loving) keratinophilic fungi (Fig. 56-3).[12] Other *Geomyces* spp. have been detected worldwide in soils and dust from cold climates as well as on the skin, hair, and feathers of animals from these areas.[15] Although rarely reported as a pathogen,

cutaneous infections by the closely related *G. pannorum* have been reported in humans.[13]

Culture Conditions

In the laboratory, optimum growing temperatures for *G. destructans* range from 4°C to 10°C (39.2°C to 50°F).[2] This is similar to the seasonal temperatures reported at WNS-affected hibernacula, where year-round growth may create reservoirs for infection.[2] Growth does not occur above 20°C (68°F). *G. destructans* grows well on antibiotic-infused Sabouraud dextrose agar[16] and other standard media[12,22] by placing wing or muzzle tissues directly onto culture plates.

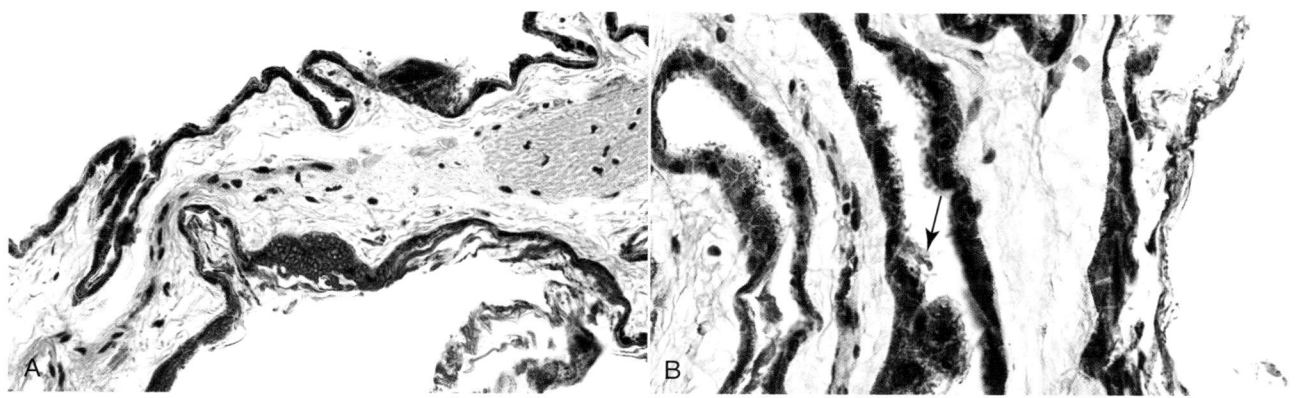

Figure 56-3

Photomicrographs showing morphologic *Geomyces destructans* infection on the wing of a little brown bat *(Myotis lucifigus)* from Vermont (2009). **A,** Fungal hyphae cover the surface of the skin, invade the keratin, and form a cuplike depression into the dermis (PAS, 60×). **B,** Sickle-shaped conidia *(arrow)* characteristic of *G. destructans* in tissue section. (PAS, 100×).

Colonies range from white to gray-green in appearance on the surface and are slow-growing, remaining small in diameter after 2 weeks of incubation.[12]

Other Diagnostic Criteria

In addition to isolation in fungal culture, the presence of *G. destructans* may be confirmed by examining fungal tape lifts from skin and fur of affected bats with light microscopy to observe the characteristic morphologic structure of conidia. Although the technique is not highly sensitive, fungal tape lifts collected from skin with grossly visible fungus (primarily the muzzle) have the advantage of being a nonlethal sampling technique. Swabbing flight membranes and muzzles of bats with a moistened sterile swab has also been used experimentally to collect *G. destructans* conidia for identification by light microscopy.[20] If further confirmation is warranted beyond that of conidial morphology, a polymerase chain reaction (PCR) assay targeting the ITS region of *G. destructans* rRNA gene has been used with variable success on tape or swab samples (USGS NWHC, unpublished data). PCR when applied to bat tissues has, however, demonstrated high levels of sensitivity and specificity that are comparable to those demonstrated by histologic evaluation.[16] PCR assay is a useful screening tool to detect the presence of *G. destructans* DNA on bat carcasses or wing biopsies collected from live animals. It does not, however, provide information about fungal viability as do fungal cultures or determine whether the fungus is associated with the cutaneous lesions that characterize WNS.

HISTOPATHOLOGY

Full details of the histologic appearance of *G. destructans* infection have been described elsewhere.[9,19] On hematoxylin and eosin preparations, *G. destructans* appears as masses of negatively stained hyphae on the surface of the skin and invading into the dermis and adnexa.[19] Fungal morphology is more easily visualized by the application of a periodic acid–Schiff stain (PAS) or a Gomori methenamine silver stain (GMS). Because fungal colonies may be regional or widely spaced, special stains to highlight fungi are suggested for all skin sections being evaluated for WNS (see Fig. 56-3). PAS is favored because it highlights fungal morphology without the background staining present in the GMS.

Distinctive conidia and patterns of colonization by *G. destructans* hyphae are the criteria for diagnosing WNS in tissue section.[19] The conidia are sickle-shaped, measuring 7.5 μm in length and 2.5 μm wide, with blunt apexes. The septate branching hyphae are more variable in appearance, ranging from 2 to 5 μm in diameter and may have parallel or irregular walls (see Fig. 56-3). When conidia are not readily apparent, the pattern of *G. destructans* growth and the appearance of fungal hyphae in tissue section may be used to distinguish it from incidental superficial fungal infections or postmortem invasion. In its mildest manifestation, *G. destructans* covers the surface of the skin and may fill adnexa. Large numbers of hyphae invade and fill the dermis in more severe infections and may breach the entire thickness of the wing membrane.[19] Postmortem fungi may also invade the dermis and subcutaneous tissues and stain PAS-positive, but these do not form the cupping epidermal erosions that are densely filled with G. *destructans* hyphae, as is seen in WNS.[19]

One striking feature of G. *destructans* infection is the lack of inflammatory response to the fungus among torpid animals. Although some inflammation may be detected, it is not severe during the winter months.[19] This lack of reaction is in contrast to the reactions noted in response to *Geomyces* spp. infections in other species.[13] Inflammation is seen most often in bats that have recently emerged from hibernation and consists of a mixture of neutrophils and smaller numbers of lymphocytes.[19] It is not clear whether this lack of a morphologically detectable inflammatory response is mediated by immune evasive features of G. *destructans*, or if this is a manifestation of immune suppression similar to that which has been documented in other hibernating animals.[21]

MODES OF TRANSMISSION

Preliminary results from infection trials in artificial hibernacula have demonstrated that direct bat to bat transmission of G. *destructans* occurs without requiring underlying skin damage or poor body condition to initiate infection.[25] Ongoing investigations to determine whether naive bats translocated to known WNS-positive hibernacula devoid of native bats develop the disease via environmental exposure have indicated that visible fungal infections, and possibly mortality, may develop in as little as 8 weeks postexposure.[14]

Although bat to bat transmission is likely the primary method of WNS spread, other proposed mechanisms for the rapid and extensive southern expansion of the disease are human or other nonbat movements. Anecdotal reports of newly identified WNS-affected sites occurring first in recreational sites, and large areas of seemingly unaffected hibernacula existing between affected sites in the 3 years since WNS emergence, suggest a pattern more consistent with selective visitation of hibernacula by humans as opposed to contiguous transmission resulting from local bat movements and interactions.[28] Such observations, however, may simply reflect surveillance biases and more systematic analysis is warranted. Finally, it is conceivable that animals other than bats could carry fungal spores on their body surfaces that could be transported to distant locations, as is known to occur with related *Geomyces* spp.[17] Evidence of avian and mammalian scavengers has been reported at the entrances of affected hibernacula.[14] Although characteristic signs of WNS have not been

reported in species other than bats, exhaustive surveillance has not been done at affected locations and the significance of nonbat movements to WNS spread is not known.

PATHOGENESIS

Relationship to Hibernation

Understanding WNS must be viewed in context of the natural history of the bats. All bats currently known to be affected by WNS survive winter by hibernating. Thus, WNS affects bats at a physiologically vulnerable time, a period when key metabolic processes such as temperature, respiration, cardiovascular output, and immune response are all downregulated.[15,21] Their ability to survive hinges on the measured metabolism of fat stores accumulated in the fall. Failure to acquire appropriate fat stores, improper metabolism during hibernation, or premature emergence from hibernation may all be fatal.[15,24]

Any infectious agent with the potential to alter these factors could pose a significant threat to the animals' survival.[24] The life histories of bats that hibernate are characterized by wide seasonal variations in activity, food availability, and population density. All are factors that may contribute to disease susceptibility. The life history of the little brown bat exemplifies these features. This small bat has a wide range in North America and, prior to the emergence of WNS, was the most abundant bat in the eastern United States. During the summer, little brown bats are very active and have low population density. They feed on a wide variety of insects and may form small roosting colonies during the day. Females form maternity colonies during pupping season. Males, however, remain more widely dispersed or roost on the periphery of the maternity colonies. Population densities increase in late fall, when bats from a wide geographic area congregate around hibernacula and feed extensively to accumulate white fat stores sufficient to sustain them during hibernation. Different species intermingle, and individuals come into contact with other bats that could carry a variety of pathogens.[11,15]

Population densities and bat to bat contact peak once animals enter the hibernacula. Here, bats downregulate their metabolism in a complex series of events that includes changes in hormonal secretions and intracellular signaling pathways.[15] During this time, little brown bats form dense clusters,[11] bat to bat intraspecies and interspecies contacts are frequent, and hibernating populations in a single cave or mine may exceed 10,000 bats. Activity during hibernation is markedly reduced compared with that in the summer and fall. Bats, however, periodically arouse from hibernation to drink and possibly to upregulate their immune systems temporarily to fight incidental pathogens.[15,21] These arousals typically occur every 10 to 14 days for little brown bats.[15] Although arousal is a natural part of the hibernation cycle, it is energetically costly and consumes large proportions of hibernation fat reserves.[4] Factors that alter natural arousal patterns may drastically influence the rate at which adipose tissue is metabolized and affect the ability of bats to survive the hibernation season.

Although the bat species affected by WNS share many life history characteristics with little brown bats, there are some differences. It is speculated that these differences may alter species' susceptibility to WNS. There are no clear data on how WNS differentially affects the various species; however, given that different species seek out different microhabitats within each hibernaculum, it is possible that different bat species may experience different temperatures, humidities, cluster sizes, and overall hibernation population densities in ways that could affect exposure to and the spread of pathogens, including G. destructans.[5]

Further research is needed to examine how species-specific microhabitat selection, hibernation population densities, and interspecies interactions affect susceptibility to WNS. This is particularly important because alterations in microhabitat selection by hibernating little brown bats is one characteristic of WNS. WNS-affected bats have been observed to congregate in areas of hibernacula colder than roost sites typically occupied by a particular species. Previous studies have demonstrated that thin bats or bats chemically rendered incapable of metabolizing fat select colder areas of hibernacula in which to hibernate.[3] A better understanding of the mechanism behind alterations in microhabitat selection by WNS-affected bats could provide clues about the pathogenesis of this disease, which may be key to implementing recovery and management strategies.

Another hallmark of WNS is early emergence from hibernation. Signals that regulate emergence from hibernation under normal circumstances are not well understood but are thought to include hormonal signaling or the sensing of the accumulation of metabolites that signal the need to arouse and leave the hibernaculum.[24] Because hibernating bats in temperate regions of the world are obligate insectivores, it is essential that emergence coincide with food availability. Furthermore,

it is essential that ambient temperatures be within a range that is suitable for these small, highly active animals. Emergence prior to either of these events may be devastating, as has been seen with WNS. It is possible that altered torpor patterns or fat metabolism in WNS-affected bats signal early emergence from hibernacula. Further research is needed to determine exactly how WNS alters bat physiology to result in the behavioral manifestations and mortalities associated with WNS.

Proposed Mechanism

Early observations in the emergence of WNS found that bats were markedly underweight, with depleted fat reserves at the time of their death, although it was not known if bats were entering torpor in poor body condition or if bats were consuming energy reserves at a faster rate because of changes in torpor behaviors secondary to, or as a direct result, of WNS.[4,30] Further investigation found that bats entered torpor with normal body mass at several locations in Pennsylvania that became positive for WNS during the winter of 2008 to 2009.[27] Postmortem studies have demonstrated that WNS-affected bats lack subcutaneous fat or have lower body mass compared with unaffected control bats by February and March.[7]

Studies have yet to demonstrate the causal relationship between infection with G. destructans and subsequent bat mortality. Infection trials did, however, produce histologic changes from G. destructans to wing membranes similar to those observed in naturally infected bats.[25] Preliminary findings from several studies have demonstrated that WNS-affected bats have shortened torpor cycles and maintain higher body temperatures during hibernation than control bats.[28] Mathematical models that increased the number of torpor cycles or increased the duration of arousal periods achieved similar patterns of winter mortality reported in bats from WNS-affected areas.[4] Research is focusing on finding the link between fungal infection and physiologic or behavioral changes in bats. Whether the link involves G. destructans stimulating the immune system of the bats, causing localized skin irritation, secretion of a mycotoxin, or some yet unidentified factor, is not known.

NEW PARADIGM OF BAT DISEASE

WNS is unique, not only because of its rapid emergence and spread, but also because it is one of the few mass mortality events ever documented among any of the over 1100 bat species that exist worldwide.[15] Despite the life history characteristics seemingly primed for disease spread—dispersal of individuals over large geographic areas, comingling of species during certain times of the year, and high population densities during hibernation when immune defenses and metabolism are depressed—reports of mass bat mortalities are limited. The most well-documented epizootic events have been related to bat rabies virus infections in massive colonies of free-tailed bats (*Tadarida brasiliensis*) in Texas and blue-green algae intoxication.[15]

Thus, WNS and *G. destructans* represents a new disease paradigm in the study of bat disease. *G. destructans* infects bats during the vulnerable time of hibernation and, unlike other bat pathogens in winter, is associated with death. This may have to do with the unique biology of *G. destructans*, in that it thrives at low temperatures. Other pathogens that have been detected in hibernating animals replicate best when animals are euthermic.[1] In hibernating ground squirrels, for example, hibernation has been shown to inhibit the replication of *Yersinia pestis* and allows squirrels to harbor the bacterium without disease until arousal.[1] Temperatures of bat hibernacula in the WNS-affected areas are within the optimal range for the growth of *G. destructans*, allowing for fungal proliferation and infection of the hibernating bats.[2]

An important question that remains to be answered is why WNS has occurred now. Is *G. destructans* a recently introduced pathogen to North America, or is it a ubiquitous organism that has recently acquired the ability to infect bats, either because of alteration in its biology or because bats have suddenly become susceptible? There is speculation that *G. destructans* may have originated from Europe and was inadvertently transported to North America by humans. Anecdotal reports from European bat biologists[10] have indicated that fungi on the muzzles of hibernating bats have been observed sporadically since 1983 in Germany. However, concurrent bat mortality similar to that which occurs in the United States has not been documented at affected European sites.[10,22,33]

Since the emergence of WNS in North America, extensive cave surveillance has been conducted across Europe to search for signs of the disease. *G. destructans*, has been identified using microscopy, fungal culture or DNA sequence analysis in five species of bats (*M. myotis, M. dasycneme, M. daubentonii, M. brandtii*, and *M. oxygnathus*) from France, Germany, Switzerland, and Hungary.[22,33] None of the early European fungi observed on bat muzzles (e.g., as noted by Feldmann[10]) exist in

culture for comparative studies with the more current isolates, so it is impossible to link early observations to the most recent European isolates conclusively.[22] Although it is possible that the *G. destructans* isolates observed in Europe may have only recently been carried there from the northeastern United States, the lack of associated mortality in European bat communities suggests that European bats coevolved with the *G. destructans* and developed a resistance to WNS, additional factors to *G. destructans* infection are required for mortality to occur, or there are differences between the European and North American strains. The recent complete genomic sequencing of a North American *G. destructans* isolate will facilitate these molecular epidemiology studies.[6]

TREATMENT

At the present time, there is no known treatment for WNS, but management strategies to slow the rate of disease spread or improve bat survival have been suggested. In March 2009, the U.S. Fish and Wildlife Service issued a recommendation for closure of caves in which bats are known to hibernate to recreational human traffic.[29] This was an effort to reduce the effects of disturbance on stressed populations and to prevent the inadvertent spread of the fungus from contaminated equipment. Stringent decontamination guidelines also exist in the hope of slowing any inadvertent advancement of WNS by humans. There is no evidence that WNS is a direct threat to human health, but increased numbers of dead or sick bats found in or near human dwellings may expose people to other zoonotic diseases harbored by bats, such as rabies.

Studies are underway to investigate the safety and efficacy of various antifungal agents on bats. The feasibility of implementing these treatments is unclear because treatment of free-ranging individuals is generally impractical, and the risks of introducing chemical agents into delicate subterranean ecosystems must be considered. It has been suggested that providing warm temperature refuges in hibernacula may increase bat survival by reducing the energy costs associated with shortened torpor cycles,[4] although its practicality remains doubtful. Medical treatment of bats may be most practical in a rehabilitation setting or in a captive propagation situation targeted at endangered bat species. Preliminary data have suggested that housing infected bats in warm temperatures and providing supplemental nutrition for several weeks may be enough to resolve cutaneous infections of *G. destructans*.[18]

CONCLUSIONS

WNS represents a novel and unique threat to vespertilionid bat populations, and management and mitigation of the disease will be dependent on a thorough understanding of the biology of the proposed causative agent, *G. destructans,* in concert with the biology and natural histories of bat species. Of major importance is that WNS affects bats during hibernation, a unique metabolic period of the life cycle when immunocompetence is low and population density is high. Thus, any future management strategies must account for the unique physiologic needs of bats in and around the time of hibernation.

The long-term implications of WNS have yet to be realized. Catastrophic population losses in bats associated with WNS will be slow to recover and the ecologic and economic consequences of these losses are difficult to predict. Bats are long-lived mammals, with typical life spans ranging from 10 to 30 years, and they produce only one pup annually.[30] Lower than expected reproductive rates have been reported at maternity colonies in WNS-affected areas.[23]

Bats are an important part of the ecosystem and likely play a significant role in controlling insect populations. It is estimated that a single little brown bat consumes approximately 4 to 8 g of insects every night when active.[4] Rough calculations estimate that one million bats could consume 694 tons of insects annually, many of which are considered forest and agricultural pest species, as well as disease vectors.[8] The loss of these insect predators could have profound effects on insect-induced crop damage and the prevalence of insect-vectored diseases. Furthermore, the sudden emergence of WNS and the resultant unprecedented bat mortality may mark a significant long-term shift in the dynamics of affected ecosystems.

There is much to learn about bats and WNS, and research into both is ongoing. Current research is focusing on the relationship between *G. destructans* and WNS and determining how fungal infection leads to the spectrum of behavioral and physiologic abnormalities observed in affected bats. Furthermore, research into how the immune status of bats during hibernation, microclimate selection within hibernacula, and species-specific life history differences may affect the outcome and susceptibility of bat populations are ongoing. More applied studies to determine the best method to curb the spread of WNS are also being conducted.

Although WNS is a devastating disease, it has opened the door for a better understanding of bats, hibernation physiology, and public education. It is hoped that the data generated will ultimately pave the way toward development of successful strategies to manage and control WNS and provide the basis for a better response to other emergent bat diseases.

Acknowledgments

We would like to thank state and federal biologists, especially A. Hicks, J. Okonewski, and G. Turner, for sharing field observations and Drs. D. Blehert, C. Meteyer, P. Curtis, J. Hermanson, D. Reeder, G. Kolias, and B. Akey for their review of this manuscript.

REFERENCES

1. Bizanov G, Dobrokhotova ND: Experimental infection of ground squirrels *(Citellus pygmaeus pallas)* with Yersinia pestis during hibernation. J Infect 54:198–203, 2007.
2. Blehert DS, Hicks AC, Behr M, et al: Bat white-nose syndrome: An emerging fungal pathogen? Science 323:227, 2009.
3. Boyles JG, Dunbar MB, Storm JJ, Brack V Jr: Energy availability influences microclimate selection of hibernating bats. J Exp Biol 210:4345–4350, 2007.
4. Boyles JG, Willis CK: Could localized warm areas inside cold caves reduce mortality in hibernating bats affected by white-nose syndrome? Front Ecol Environ 2:92–98, 2010.
5. Brack V Jr: Temperatures and locations used by hibernating bats, including *Myotis sodalis* (Indiana bat), in a limestone mine: Implications for conservation and management. Environ Manage 40:739–746, 2007.
6. Cuomo C. *Geomyces destructans* database. Broad Institute, 2010, (http://www.broadinstitute.org/annotation/genome/Geomyces_destructans/MultiHome.html).
7. Buckles EL, Behr M: White nose syndrome: A devastating emerging disease of bats. In American college of veterinary pathologists. Annual Meeting. 60th 2009, Red Hook, NY, 2010, Curran Associates, pp 103–105.
8. Consensus Statement: Second WNS Emergency Science Strategy Meeting, May 27-28, 2009, Austin, Texas (http://www.batcon.org/pdfs/whitenose/ConsensusStatement2009.pdf).
9. Courtin F, Stone WB, Risatti G, et al: Pathologic findings and liver elements in hibernating bats with white-nose syndrome. Vet Pathol 47:214–219, 2010.
10. Feldmann R: [Teichfledermaus-Myotis dasycneme (Boie, 1825).] In Schropfer R, Feldmann R, Vierhaus H, editors: Die Säugetiere Westfalens, 1984 (http://www.biostation-re.de/inhaltsseiten/Die%20Saeugetiere%20Westfalens.pdf), pp 107–111.
11. Fenton MB, Barclay MR: Myotis lucifugus. Mammalian Species 142:1–8, 1980.
12. Gargas A, Trest MT, Christensen M: *Geomyces destructans* sp. nov. associated with bat white-nose syndrome. Mycotaxon 108:147–154, 2009.
13. Gianni C, Caretta G, Romano C: Skin infection due to *Geomyces pannorum var. pannorum.* Mycoses 46:430–432, 2003.
14. Hicks A: Personal communication, 2010.
15. Kunz TH, Fenton MB: Bat ecology, Chicago, 2003, University of Chicago Press.
16. Lorch JM, Gargas A, Meteyer CU, et al: Rapid polymerase chain reaction diagnosis of white-nose syndrome in bats. J Vet Diagn Invest 22:224–230, 2010.

17. Marshall WA: Aerial transport of keratinaceous substrate and distribution of the fungus *Geomyces pannorum* in Antarctic soils. Microb Ecol 36:212–219, 1998.

18. Meteyer C: Personal communication, 2010.

19. Meteyer CU, Buckles EL, Blehert DS, et al: Histopathologic criteria to confirm white-nose syndrome in bats. J Vet Diagn Invest 21:411–414, 2009.

20. Okoniewski J: Personal communication, 2010.

21. Prendergast BJ, Freeman DA, Zucker I, Nelson RJ: Periodic arousal from hibernation is necessary for initiation of immune responses in ground squirrels. Am J Physiol Regul Integr Comp Physiol 282:R1054–R1062, 2002.

22. Puechmaille SJ, Verdeyroux P, Fuller H, et al: White-nose syndrome fungus *(Geomyces destructans)* in bat, France. Emerg Infect Dis 16:290–293, 2010.

23. Reichard JD, Kunz TH: White-nose syndrome inflicts lasting injuries to the wings of little brown myotis *(Myotis lucifugus)*. Acta Chiropterolog 11:457–464, 2009.

24. Ruf T, Arnold W: Effects of polyunsaturated fatty acids on hibernation and torpor: A review and hypothesis. Am J Physiol Regul Integr Comp Physiol 294:R1044–R1052, 2008.

25. Sleeman J: Update on white nose-syndrome. Wildlife Health Bulletin, vol 2. U.S. Geological Survey, National Wildlife Heath Center, 2009, (http://www.nwhc.usgs.gov/publications/wildlife_health_bulletins/WHB_2009-03.pdf).

26. Sleeman J: *Geomyces destructans* detected in Oklahoma Cave Myotis and listed Missouri gray bats. Wildlife Health Bulletin, #2010-04. U.S. Geological Survey, National Wildlife Heath Center, 2010, (http://www.nwhc.usgs.gov/publications/wildlife_health_bulletins/WHB_10_04.jsp).

27. Turner G: Personal communication, 2010.

28. Turner GG, Reeder DM: Update of white-nose syndrome in bats. Bat Res News 50:47–53, 2009.

29. U.S. Fish and Wildlife Service: White-nose syndrome in bats: Cave advisory, March 26, 2009 (http://www.fws.gov/WhiteNoseSyndrome/caveadvisory.html).

30. U.S. Geological Survey: White-nose syndrome threatens the survival of hibernating bats in North America, 2009 (http://www.fort.usgs.gov/WNS).

31. U.S. Geological Survey, National Wildlife Health Center: White-nose syndrome (WNS), 2010 (http://www.nwhc.usgs.gov/publications/quarterly_reports/2010_qtr_1.jsp).

32. USGS NWHC: unpublished data.

33. Wibbelt G, Kurth A, Hellmann D, et al: White-nose syndrome fungus *(Geomyces destructans)* in bats, Europe. Emerg Infect Dis 16:1237–1242, 2010.

Carnivores

CHAPTER 57

Updated Vaccination Recommendations for Carnivores

Nadine Lamberski

Protection against viral diseases is an important component of any preventive medicine or health care program for captive carnivores. Carnivores are susceptible to a variety of viral infections, the most significant of which also occur in domestic cats and dogs. For this reason, vaccination programs for wild carnivores are often modeled after recommendations for their domestic counterparts. The goal of this chapter is to assist the zoo veterinarian in developing a vaccination program that meets the needs of the individual animal, collection, and institution. Although carnivore vaccination programs are bound to be similar among institutions, they need not be identical to be effective. Factors to consider when developing these programs include the following: (1) the risk of exposure, including likelihood of exposure based on environmental factors and geographic location; (2) the severity of disease if exposed, which may vary with age, species, gender, and reproductive status; (3) the potential for adverse reactions to one or more vaccines; and (4) the availability of resources (e.g., time, finances, labor). Vaccination alone should not be relied on to prevent disease. Adjunct components to controlling infectious diseases are reducing exposure to these agents in the animal's environment through quarantine practices, cleaning and disinfection protocols, and pest and predator control programs, as well as minimizing factors such as stress, overcrowding, and inadequate nutrition that diminish resistance to disease.

Using the taxonomic classifications presented by Wilson and Reeder,[17] the order Carnivora is divided into two suborders, Feliformia and Caniformia (Table 57-1). Knowing which species are more catlike or more doglike may help predict disease susceptibility when published data are lacking. Commercial vaccines have been developed for use in domestic species, and using them in other carnivores constitutes extralabel use.

Although modified live and killed virus vaccines dominate the market, third-generation products are now complementing and in some cases replacing them.[4,8,11] This new technology should have a positive impact on current practices by improving the safety and efficacy of vaccines used in nondomestic carnivores.

Guidelines that have global application for the vaccination of cats and dogs have been compiled by the Vaccination Guidelines Group (VGG) of the World Small Animal Veterinary Association.[18] These guidelines were based on those provided by the American Animal Hospital Association (AAHA) Canine Vaccine Task Force and the Feline Vaccine Advisory Panel of the American Association of Feline Practitioners.[8,9] The guidelines are also consistent with those of the European Advisory Board on Cat Diseases and the South African Veterinary Council.[4,14] The information in this chapter is a condensed version taken directly from these guidelines, with special attention as to how they might be applied to nondomestic carnivores. This information is subject to change in light of developments in research, technology, and experience.

CORE VACCINES: UNIVERSALLY RECOMMENDED

The VGG recommends that all cats and dogs benefit from vaccination. Vaccination protects the individual and provides optimum herd immunity by reducing the number of susceptible animals in the regional population and decreasing disease prevalence. Specific recommendations are based on the concept of core vaccines. Core vaccines are those that every cat or dog, regardless of circumstances, should receive. Core vaccines protect animals from severe life-threatening diseases that have global distribution. Vaccination programs should

TABLE 57-1	Order Carnivora			
Suborder	Family	Subfamily	Genus	Common Name
Feliformia	Felidae	Felinae	*Acinonyx*	Cheetah
			Caracal	Caracal
			Catopuma	Bay cat, Asian golden cat
			Felis	Chinese mountain cat, domestic cat, jungle cat, Pallas' cat, sand cat, black-footed cat, wildcat
			Leopardus	Pantanal cat, colocolo, Geoffroy's cat, kodkod, Andean mountain cat, Pampas cat, ocelot, oncilla, margay
			Leptailurus	Serval
			Lynx	Canadian lynx, Eurasian lynx, Iberian lynx, bobcat
			Pardofelis	Marbled cat
			Prionailurus	Leopard cat, Iriomote cat, flat-headed cat, rusty-spotted cat, fishing cat
			Profelis	African golden cat
			Puma	Cougar, jaguarundi
		Pantherinae	*Neofelis*	Clouded leopard
			Panthera	Lion, jaguar, leopard, tiger
			Uncia	Snow leopard
	Viverridae	Paradoxurinae	*Arctictis*	Binturong
			Arctogalidia	Small-toothed palm civet
			Macrogalidia	Sulawesi palm civet
			Paguma	Masked palm civet
			Paradoxurus	Asian palm civet, Jerdon's palm civet, golden palm civet
		Hemigalinae	*Chrotogale*	Owston's palm civet
			Cynogale	Otter civet
			Diplogale	Hose's palm civet
			Hemigalus	Banded palm civet
		Prionodontinae	*Prionodon*	Banded linsang, spotted linsang
		Viverrinae	*Civettictis*	African civet
			Genetta	Abyssinian genet, Angolan genet, Bourlon's genet, crested servaline genet, common genet, Johnston's genet, rusty-spotted genet, Pardine genet, aquatic genet, king genet, servaline genet, Haussa genet, Cape genet, giant forest genet
			Poiana	Leighton's linsang, African linsang
			Viverra	Malabar large-spotted civet, large-spotted civet, Malayan civet, large Indian civet
			Viverricula	Small Indian civet
	Eupleridae	Euplerinae	*Cryptoprocta*	Fossa
			Eupleres	Falanouc
			Fossa	Malagasy civet
		Galidiinae	*Galidia*	Ring-tailed mongoose
			Galidictis	Broad-striped Malagasy mongoose, Grandidier's mongoose
			Mungotictis	Narrow-striped mongoose
			Salanoia	Brown-tailed mongoose
	Nandiniidae		*Nandinia*	African palm civet
	Herpestidae		*Atilax*	Marsh mongoose
			Bdeogale	Bushy-tailed mongoose, Jackson's mongoose, black-footed mongoose
			Crossarchus	Alexander's kusimanse, Angolan kusimanse, common kusimanse, flat-headed kusimanse

Continued

TABLE 57-1   Order Carnivora—cont'd

Suborder	Family	Subfamily	Genus	Common Name
			Cynictis	Yellow mongoose
			Dologale	Pousargues' mongoose
			Galerella	Angolan slender mongoose, Somalian slender mongoose, Cape gray mongoose, slender mongoose
			Helogale	Ethiopian dwarf mongoose, common dwarf mongoose
			Herpestes	Short-tailed mongoose, Indian gray mongoose, Indian brown mongoose, Egyptian mongoose, small Asian mongoose, long-nosed mongoose, collared mongoose, ruddy mongoose, crab-eating mongoose, striped-neck mongoose
			Ichneumia	White-tailed mongoose
			Liberiictis	Liberian mongoose
			Mungos	Gambian mongoose, banded mongoose
			Paracynictis	Selous' mongoose
			Rhynchogale	Meller's mongoose
			Suricata	Meerkat
	Hyaenidae		Crocuta	Spotted hyena
			Hyaena	Brown hyena, striped hyena
			Proteles	Aardwolf
Caniformia	Canidae		Atelocynus	Short-eared dog
			Canis	Side-striped jackal, golden jackal, coyote, wolf, black-backed jackal, Ethiopian wolf
			Cerdocyon	Crab-eating fox
			Chrysocyon	Maned wolf
			Cuon	Dhole
			Dusicyon	Falkland Islands wolf
			Lycalopex	Culpeo, Darwin's fox, South American gray fox, Pampas fox, Sechuran fox, Hoary fox
			Lycaon	African wild dog
			Nyctereutes	Raccoon dog
			Otocyon	Bat-eared fox
			Speothos	Bush dog
			Urocyon	Gray fox, island fox
			Vulpes	Bengal fox, Blanford's fox, Cape fox, Corsac fox, Tibetan sand fox, arctic fox, kit fox, pale fox, Ruppell's fox, swift fox, red fox, fennec fox
	Ursidae		Ailuropoda	Giant panda
			Helarctos	Sun bear
			Melursus	Sloth bear
			Tremarctos	Spectacled bear
			Ursus	American black bear, brown bear, polar bear, Asian black bear
	Otariidae		Arctocephalus	South American fur seal, Australasian fur seal, Galapagos fur seal, Antarctic fur seal, Juan Fernandez fur seal, brown fur seal, Guadalupe fur seal, subantarctic fur seal
			Callorhinus	Northern fur seal
			Eumetopias	Stellar sea lion
			Neophoca	Australian sea lion
			Otaria	South American sea lion

TABLE 57-1	Order Carnivora—cont'd			
Suborder	Family	Subfamily	Genus	Common Name
			Phocarctos	New Zealand sea lion
			Zalophus	California sea lion, Japanese sea lion, Galapagos sea lion
	Odobenidae			Walrus
	Phocidae		Cystophora	Hooded seal
			Erignathus	Bearded seal
			Halichoerus	Gray seal
			Histriophoca	Ribbon seal
			Hydrurga	Leopard seal
			Leptonychotes	Weddell seal
			Lobodon	Crabeater seal
			Mirounga	Northern elephant seal, southern elephant seal
			Monachus	Mediterranean monk seal, Hawaiian monk seal, Caribbean monk seal
			Ommatophoca	Ross seal
			Pagophilus	Harp seal
			Phoca	Spotted seal, harbor seal
			Pusa	Caspian seal, ringed seal, Baikal seal
	Mustelidae	Lutrinae	Aonyx	African clawless otter, Oriental small-clawed ottter
			Enhydra	Sea otter
			Hydrictis	Spotted-necked otter
			Lontra	North American river otter, marine otter, neotropical otter, southern river otter
			Lutra	European otter, Japanese otter, hairy-nosed otter
			Lutrogale	Smooth-coated otter
			Pteronura	Giant otter
		Mustelinae	Arctonyx	Hog badger
			Eira	Tayra
			Galictis	Lesser grison, greater grison
			Gulo	Wolverine
			Ictonyx	Saharan striped polecat, striped polecat
			Lyncodon	Patagonian weasel
			Martes	American marten, yellow-throated marten, Beech marten, Nilgiri marten, European pine marten, Japanese marten, fisher, sable
			Meles	Japanese badger, Asian badger, European badger
			Mellivora	Honey badger
			Melogale	Bornean ferret-badger, Chinese ferret-badger, Javan ferret-badger, Burmese ferret-badger
			Mustela	Amazon weasel, mountain weasel, ermine, Steppe polecat, Colombian weasel, long-tailed weasel, Japanese weasel, yellow-bellied weasel, European mink, Indonesian mountain weasel, black-footed ferret, least weasel, Malayan weasel, European polecat, Siberian weasel, back-striped weasel, Egyptian weasel
			Neovison	Sea mink, American mink
			Poecilogale	African striped weasel
			Taxidea	American badger
			Vormela	Marbled polecat
	Mephitidae		Conepatus	Molina's hog-nosed skunk, Humbolt's hog-nosed skunk, American hog-nosed skunk, striped hog-nosed skunk

Continued

Suborder	Family	Subfamily	Genus	Common Name
			Mephitis	Hooded skunk, striped skunk
			Mydaus	Sunda stink badger, Palawan stink badger
			Spilogale	Southern spotted skunk, western spotted skunk, eastern spotted skunk, pygmy spotted skunk
	Procyonidae		*Bassaricyon*	Allen's olingo, Beddard's olingo, olingo, Harris's olingo, Chiriqui olingo
			Bassariscus	Ringtail, cacomistle
			Nasua	White-nosed coati, South American coati
			Nasuella	Mountain coati
			Potos	Kinkajou
			Procyon	Crab-eating raccoon, raccoon, Cozumel racoon
	Ailuridae		*Ailurus*	Red panda

From Wilson DE, Reeder, DM (eds): Mammal species of the world. A taxonomic and geographic reference, ed 3. Baltimore, 2005, Johns Hopkins University Press.

include only those vaccines that the animal truly needs because all vaccines have the potential to cause adverse reactions.[18]

The core vaccines for felids are those that protect from feline parvovirus (panleukopenia) (FPV), feline calicivirus (FCV), and feline herpesvirus (FHV). Rabies virus is included in this core group in areas of the world in which rabies is endemic. With the exception of Australia, Great Britain, Japan, and some islands, rabies is present worldwide.[9] Parenteral killed FPV vaccine is usually preferred because vaccine-associated disease can occur if using a modified live (ML) product, although this has not been documented for ML FPV vaccine. Immunity takes 3 or more weeks to develop after a first dose of killed vaccine and at least 1 week after the second dose. This is in contrast to the ML FPV, which provides long-lasting immunity in approximately 3 days in cats older than 16 weeks. Products containing ML FPV also contain ML FCV and ML FHV. Similarly, products containing killed FPV contain killed FCV and FHV.[13]

Killed vaccines can be used in pregnant animals and should be used in disease-free collections. Using ML products (including the intranasal FPV-FCV-FHV vaccine) can introduce calicivirus and herpesvirus into collections that were previously free of these conditions and is not recommended for nondomestic carnivores. The protection afforded by the FCV and FHV vaccines (either killed or ML) will not provide the same efficacy of immunity as seen with the FPV vaccines. When vaccination does not prevent infection with FCV or

FHV, systemic and local cell-mediated and humoral immunity play important roles in preventing or reducing the severity of disease.[9] Although the FCV vaccines have been designed to produce cross-protective immunity against severe clinical disease, there are multiple strains of FCV. It is therefore possible for infection and mild disease to occur in the vaccinated animal.

Virulent systemic calicivirus (VSCV) has recently been described. Vaccination with current vaccines does not protect felids against field infections, but some protection has been shown experimentally.[13,18] There is no FHV vaccine (ML or killed) that can protect against infection with virulent strains of herpesvirus. Virulent strains of herpesvirus will become latent and may be reactivated during periods of severe stress for the life of the felid. The reactivated virus may cause clinical signs in the vaccinated animal or the virus can be shed to susceptible animals and cause disease. This is seen most frequently in captive cheetahs. Vaccination during pregnancy can help protect kittens by prolonging maternally derived antibody (MDA).[9] Cats may become infected with canine parvovirus and certain strains may cause signs of panleukopenia in cats.[7,15] Conventional FPV vaccines have been shown to protect against these canine parvoviruses, but there is a report of a cheetah vaccinated with a killed FPV vaccine that developed canine parvovirus infection (CPV-2b) and gastrointestinal disease.[3,6,16]

The core vaccines for canids are those that protect from canine distemper virus (CDV), canine adenovirus (CAV), and canine parvovirus (CPV). Rabies virus is included in this core group in areas of the world in which rabies is endemic. In areas or facilities in which CDV is not endemic in domestic or wild susceptible species, ML vaccines should not be used. The risk of introducing a virus into a host population is unacceptable.[11,18] Susceptible wild carnivore species do shed virus following ML CDV vaccine administration and may develop disease. This has been reported in the red panda, black-footed ferret, European mink, gray fox, kinkajou, South American bush dog, and maned wolf.[2] The ML CDV products available contain virulent strains and are for use in domestic dogs only. A poxvirus recombinant canine distemper vaccine (rCDV) is available in many countries and is considered the vaccine of choice for nondomestic carnivores to protect against vaccine-induced disease and natural infection. This recombinant vaccine has the added advantages of being safe in younger animals and more effective for immunizing carnivores with MDA. In the absence of MDA, rCDV vaccine provides immunity immediately after vaccination.[8,12] The rCDV vaccine is currently available as a monovalent product or combined with ML CPV and ML CAV, or with ML CPV, ML CAV, and canine parainfluenza virus (CPI). CPI is considered an optional vaccine (see later).

There are four genotypes of canine parvovirus that are recognized worldwide—CPV-2, CPV2a, CPV-2b, and CPV-c—and all genotypes are antigenically comparable. This means that vaccination with any one genotype provides protective immunity against all other genotypes.[9,18] CPV is hypothesized to be a natural genetic mutation of FPV that first emerged in dogs in 1978.[6,7] CPV strains can replicate in both canine and feline cells, but FPV has been shown to only replicate efficiently in feline cells. There are only a few killed CPV vaccines available and are less effective than the ML vaccines. In addition, they are often combined with a ML CDV vaccine. Although killed vaccines are preferable for use in wild or nondomestic species, this killed product may not be the best choice if it is part of a polyvalent vaccine that contains ML CDV for the reasons noted earlier. Canids are most susceptible to severe disease caused by CPV infection during the first year of life. Each institution should decide whether they could effectively isolate pups to prevent introduction of disease or whether the benefits of using a ML CPV product outweigh the risks. ML CPV vaccination will result in shedding of virus, and this virus could potentially revert to virulence, as well as infect other individuals or other species. Once in the environment, the virus can remain infectious for 1 year or longer.[8] Similar to ML FPV vaccines, ML CPV vaccines

provide immunity 3 days after vaccination. When CPV first appeared, FPV vaccines were used to provide some protection until a more specific vaccine was manufactured.[15] It is not known whether a killed FPV monovalent vaccine will protect against CPV in nondomestic carnivores but recent studies have suggested that it may offer some protection.[3] Alternatively, one could consider not revaccinating canids with a positive antibody titer to CPV postvaccination using a ML product, because life-long immunity should result.[12] Experimental canine DNA vaccines have been developed for CPV-2 and hold promise for the future. In contrast to ML CPV vaccines, ML CAV vaccine virus has not been shown to revert to virulence in back passage studies. ML CAV-2 containing vaccines are the most commonly available products. They will prevent infectious canine hepatitis (ICH) caused by CAV-1 and reduce the signs of respiratory disease caused by CAV-2. They also do not cause the adverse reaction commonly seen with CAV-1 vaccines, known as allergic uveitis, or blue eye.

MDA significantly interferes with the efficacy of most core vaccines currently available, with the exception of rCDV vaccine. Because the level of MDA varies among litters, young carnivores should receive three doses of vaccine. These repeated injections in the first year of life do not constitute boosters but rather are an attempt to induce a primary immune response. In general, passive immunity will have waned by 8 to 12 weeks to a level that allows for active immunization. The age at which to begin the vaccination series can vary, but vaccinations are typically begun between 6 and 9 weeks of age and then are readministered at 2- to 4-week intervals until the animal is 14 to 16 weeks of age; 16 weeks is usually preferable to ensure that the waning of maternal antibody is complete.[8,9,12,13,18] Starting the immunizations as early as 6 weeks may be appropriate in situations of high risk (e.g., FHV in cheetahs) and questionable MDA status. In situations in which only one vaccine can be administered, this should be done when the animal is immunologically capable of responding—that is, at the age of 16 weeks or older. After an initial series of three vaccines, the animal should receive a booster in 12 months. The initial series and this booster are referred to as the primary vaccination course. The booster at 12 months also ensures immunity for carnivores that did not adequately respond to the first series of vaccines. Core vaccines are given no more frequently than every 3 years thereafter. There are reports in the literature that suggest that the duration of immunity is at least 3 years when killed products are used.[4,8,10] A notable exception is that an annual booster is required for the recombinant virus, nonadjuvanted, canarypox-vectored rabies vaccine labeled for use in domestic cats. For this reason, the killed rabies vaccine is often chosen, despite concerns with the use of adjuvants. Primary rabies vaccination should occur at 12 to 16 weeks of age, with revaccination 1 year later. Annual or triennial vaccination should follow, depending on the type of vaccine used and applicable legal requirements. There is a push towards marketing vaccines with an extended duration of immunity (DOI). This will reduce the unnecessary administration of vaccines, thereby further improving vaccine safety.

NONCORE (OPTIONAL) AND NOT GENERALLY RECOMMENDED VACCINES

Noncore vaccines are those that are required only by those animals whose geographic location, local environment, or lifestyle places them at risk of contracting specific infections. There should be an assessment of the risks and benefits prior to choosing to use a noncore vaccine. This assessment includes an evaluation of the risk of infection, severity of disease, and efficacy of the products available.[8,9,18] Although feline leukemia virus (FELV) vaccine is recommended as a noncore vaccine in domestic cats that test negative for the virus, this vaccine is not recommended in nondomestic felids. Nondomestic felids should be tested for FELV and feline immunodeficiency virus (FIV), and negative and positive animals should be managed separately in lieu of vaccination. Antibodies produced following FIV vaccination interfere with all antibody-based FIV diagnostic tests and can be passed from queens to kittens in the colostrum. Additional noncore vaccines include *Chlamydophila felis* vaccine and *Bordetella bronchiseptica* vaccine. Although *Chlamydophila* and *Bordetella* can contribute to a feline respiratory disease complex, the value or need for these vaccines in the control of this complex disease is of questionable importance. Therefore, their use is of questionable importance in most cats. It should also be recognized that these two vaccines are associated with a variety of adverse reactions in a small percentage of animals.[13] rCDV vaccine would be a noncore vaccine that could be very valuable for use in nondomestic felids (e.g., genus *Panthera* or *Lynx*) or other susceptible catlike carnivores.[1,5] For species-specific recommendations, the reader is encouraged to refer to the guidelines provided by the Association of Zoo and Aquariums (AZA) Taxon Advisory Group (TAG) or Species Survival Plan (SSP) veterinary advisors. Similarly, the European Association of Zoos and Aquaria (EAZA) European Endangered Species Programmes (EEP) would also be a valuable resource.

The combination products with CPV-2, CDV, and CAV-2 currently often include CPI virus. New core-only products have been and are being developed that do not include CPI. However, the most effective route to vaccinate for CPI is intranasal, because local immunity is more important than systemic immunity.[8,12] Canine influenza virus (CIV) is antigenically unrelated to any other virus of dogs, but is related to equine influenza virus, which first infected greyhounds in Florida in 2004. The virus caused significant respiratory disease in that initial outbreak. At present, it is not known whether this virus will be an important cause of canine respiratory disease, nor if it will be an emerging disease of dogs. It is often acute, with mild to moderate clinical signs in most dogs. Mortality is very low. It does not readily spread to other dogs in the area; thus, it will remain relatively confined to the affected group. Many questions about the role of influenza virus, viruses other than CPI and CAV-2, bacteria other than *B. bronchiseptica*, various mycoplasmas, and other factors causing canine respiratory disease complex remain unanswered. *B. bronchiseptica* is an optional vaccine in nondomestic carnivores and is most likely not indicated for zoological collections. This organism can, however, be transmitted between canids and felids.[9] If used, it is important to realize that this vaccine needs to be given every 6 to 12 months.

Considering the low efficacy, adverse event rate, and minimal risk for leptospirosis in many regions of the United States, some practitioners are not using the current products. However, if an animal is in a high-risk environment for leptospirosis, the product to use should contain the four serovars (there is no significant cross protection), and the animal should be vaccinated starting no earlier than 12 weeks of age, revaccinated in 2 to 4 weeks, revaccinated at 6 months of age, revaccinated at 1 year of age, and may need to be revaccinated as often as every 6 to 9 months for optimal protection. Using this program, the animal should not develop clinical disease with *Leptospira*, but it may get infected and shed organisms in its urine.[12]

There are some vaccines that are classified as not recommended because of insufficient scientific evidence to justify their use. Currently, these include feline infectious peritonitis vaccine and feline *Giardia* vaccine.[9] The new FCV vaccine, a killed adjuvanted vaccine that is designed to aid in the prevention of VSCV, has not been in the field long enough to know whether it will be of any value in preventing or reducing the development of this extremely rare disease. VSCV was first recognized in cats approximately 10 years ago. It results when any one of the respiratory strains of calicivirus mutates to a variant that can cause an exceptionally virulent acute systemic disease. This acute disease can cause 50% to 75% or higher mortality. The use of this vaccine is not recommended at this time.[13]

The geographic distribution of Lyme disease suggests that vaccination would only be of benefit in certain U.S. regions. Thus, widespread use of this product is neither necessary nor desired. Tick control for prevention and antibiotics for treatment must be used in high-risk areas.[8,12] In the vaccination guidelines from the AAHA, neither *Giardia* nor *Coronavirus* vaccines are recommended unless they can be proven to be beneficial for a specific animal. There are also new vaccines for snake bite (*Crotalus* spp.) and for periodontal disease (*Porphyromonas* spp.) but no scientific research has been presented to support their use.

SEROLOGIC TESTING TO MONITOR IMMUNITY TO VACCINES AND DURATION OF IMMUNITY

Antibody tests are useful for monitoring immunity to the core vaccines FPV, CDV, CAV (CAV-1), and CPV (CPV-2). A negative test result indicates that the animal has little or no antibody and revaccination is recommended. Once a juvenile carnivore has completed the vaccine series at 14 to 16 weeks of age, the animal should test positive for antibodies. The serum sample should be collected 2 or more weeks after the last vaccination. Seronegative animals should be revaccinated and retested. There may have been interference from MDA (unlikely after 12 weeks of age) or the vaccine used was poorly immunogenic. If the animal again tests negative, it should be considered a nonresponder that is possibly incapable of developing protective immunity, or the immune system failed to recognize the antigenic determinants of the specific vaccine.[8]

Most vaccinated carnivores will have persistence of serum antibody (against core vaccine antigens) for many years. For core vaccines, there is excellent correlation between presence of antibody and protective immunity, and there is long DOI for these products. When antibody is absent, the animal should be revaccinated unless there is a medical or logistical basis for not doing so. Antibody determination to vaccine components other than those listed earlier are of limited

value because of the short time period for which these antibodies persist or the lack of correlation between serum antibody and protection (e.g., canine parainfluenza).[8] For FHV, the absence of detectable serum antibody levels in vaccinated felids does not necessarily indicate that cats are susceptible to disease because cell-mediated immunity plays an important role in protection. However, FHV seroconversion does correlate with protection against virulent FHV. Important considerations in performing antibody tests are cost and the time to obtain results.[9]

RECORD KEEPING AND ADVERSE EFFECTS

The VGG recommends that the following information be recorded in the animal's medical record[18]:
- Date of vaccine administration
- Identity (name, initials, or code) of the person administering the vaccine
- Vaccine name, lot or serial number, expiration date, and manufacturer
- Site and route of vaccine administration

Veterinarians are encouraged to report all possible adverse events to the manufacturer and/or regulatory authority to expand the knowledge base that drives development of improved vaccine safety. Adverse events are defined as any side effects or unintended consequences (including lack of protection) associated with vaccination, whether or not the event can be directly attributed to the vaccine.[18] Local (injection site) reactions following vaccinations include pain, pruritis, swelling, alopecia, abscess formation, granuloma formation, and neoplasia. Systemic reactions are events that involve the entire body or a defined location and/ or region other than the injection site, such as angio-edema, anaphylaxis, vomiting, diarrhea, respiratory distress, fever, lethargy, neurologic or behavioral changes, or immune-mediated disease.[8] Injectable adjuvanted vaccines have been associated with local inflammatory reactions at injection sites, with the degree of inflammation varying among products. The potential role of local inflammatory reactions in the genesis of vaccine-associated sarcomas remains controversial. All vaccines have the potential to cause adverse reactions and that reaction is dependent not only on the product but also on the individual animal. Often, there is a genetic predisposition that leads to adverse immune reactions and cancer. Current vaccine recommendations stress that veterinarians should administer only those vaccines that an animal truly needs. In addition, these vaccines should be given only as required, because all vaccines have the potential to cause adverse reactions.[13]

Acknowledgments

I gratefully acknowledge the contributions of Dr. Ron Schultz and Dr. PK Robbins and extend thanks to Valerie Stoddard, Linda Coates, and Andre Modin for technical assistance.

REFERENCES

1. Daoust PY, McBurney SR, Godson DL, et al: Canine distemper virus-associated encephalitis in free-living lynx *(Lynx Canadensis)* and bobcats *(Lynx rufus)* of eastern Canada. J Wildl Dis 45:611–624, 2009.
2. Deem SL, Spelman LH, Yates RA, et al: Canine distemper in terrestrial carnivores: A review. Zoo Wildl Med 31:441–451, 2000.
3. Gamoh K, Senda M, Inoue Y, et al: Efficacy of an inactivated feline panleucopenia virus vaccine against a canine parvovirus isolated from a domestic cat. Vet Rec 157:285–287, 2005.
4. Horzinek MC, Thiry E: Vaccines and vaccination: The principles and the polemics. J Fel Med Surg 11:530–537, 2009.
5. Kennedy-Stoskopf S: Emerging viral infections in large cats. In Fowler ME, Miller RE, editors: Zoo and wild animal medicine: Current therapy, ed 4, Philadelphia, 1999, WB Saunders, pp 401–410.
6. Nakamura K, Ikeda Y, Miyazawa T, et al: Characterisation of cross-reactivity of virus neutralizing antibodies induced by feline panleukopenia virus and canine parvoviruses. Res Vet Sci 71:219–222, 2001.
7. Nakamura K, Sakamoto M, Ikeda Y, et al: Pathogenic potential of canine parvovirus types 2a and 2c in domestic cats. Clin Diagn Lab Immunol 8:663–668, 2001.
8. Paul MA, Carmichael LE, Childers H, et al: 2006 AAHA canine vaccine guidelines. J Am Anim Hosp Assoc 42:80–89, 2006.
9. Richards JR, Elston TH, Ford RB, et al: The 2006 American Association of Feline Practitioners Feline Vaccine Advisory Panel report. J Am Vet Med Assoc 229:1405–1441, 2006.
10. Schultz RD: Duration of immunity for canine and feline vaccines: A review. Vet Microbiol 117:75–79, 2006.
11. Schultz RD: The immune response to traditional and recombinant vaccines (V189), 2008 (http://wvc.omnibooksonline.com/data/papers/2008_V189.pdf).
12. Schultz RD: What every veterinarian needs to know about canine vaccines and vaccination programs I & II (V190, V191), 2008 (http://wvc.omnibooksonline.com/data/papers/2008_V190_V191.pdf).
13. Schultz RD: What every veterinarian needs to know about feline vaccines and vaccination programs Western Veterinary Conference, Las Vegas, (V192), 2008.
14. South African Veterinary Council: www.savc.co.za.
15. Squires RA: An update on aspects of viral gastrointestinal diseases of dogs and cats. N Z Vet 51:252–261, 2003.
16. Steinel A, Munson L, van Vuuren M, et al: Genetic characterization of feline parvovirus sequences from various carnivores. J Gen Virol 81:345–350, 2000.
17. Wilson DE, Reeder DM, editors: Mammal species of the world. A taxonomic and geographic reference, ed 3, Baltimore, 2005, Johns Hopkins University Press.
18. World Small Animal Veterinary Association: Guidelines for the vaccination of dogs and cats, 2010 (http://www.wsava.org/PDF/Misc/VaccinationGuidelines2010.pdf).

CHAPTER 58

Medical Management of Maned Wolves (Chrysocyon brachyurus)

Elizabeth E. Hammond

BIOLOGY

The maned wolf (Chrysocyon brachyurus) is the largest canid in South America, with an average weight of 25 kg.[25] It is a member of the family Canidae in the order Carnivora, belongs to its own genus, and has a unique morphology. Its legs are long and stiltlike, an adaptation allowing it to maneuver easily in its native grasslands habitat, which it does with a pacing gait. The long hair coat is a rusty red color, with black or dark brown muzzle and legs (Fig. 58-1). A patch of black or dark brown hair runs along its withers and neck. This hair is often raised during encounters—thus the name "maned" wolf. The throat, inside of the large ears, and the tail tip are white. The maned wolf has a distinct odor that resembles that of a skunk. Its dental formula is I3/3, C1/1, PM4/4, M2/3 = 42.

The maned wolf is crepuscular or nocturnal and found in northeastern Brazil, northern Argentina, Paraguay, Uruguay, eastern Bolivia, and small regions of Peru.[25] In its native countries, it is known by several names: lobo de crin, aguará guazú, borochi, and lobo guará. The maned wolf prefers grassland, cerrado, and scrub forest habitat. The number of maned wolves in the wild is difficult to assess because of their secretive nature. A 2005 Population Viability and Health Assessment study in Brazil estimated the wild population at 23,000, with approximately 85% found in Brazil.[7] The maned wolf is classified as a Convention on International Trade in Endangered Species of Wild Fauna and Flora (CITES) Appendix II species, vulnerable by the International Union for Conservation of Nature (IUCN), endangered by the U.S. Department of the Interior (USDI), and endangered by the Brazilian government. The maned wolf's conservation status has been most affected by habitat loss because of agricultural development, but road kills and its reputation as a predator of domestic poultry in its native countries have also negatively affected its numbers in the wild.

HUSBANDRY

The maned wolf has been kept in captivity in the United States since the 1970s. Its secretive nature dictates special housing, especially for successful reproduction. Captive enclosures should be large (minimum, 930 m^2) and contain tall grass to provide the animals with cover.[15] In addition, captive maned wolves will forage natural prey items, such as insects, birds, and small mammals, which may have implications for pest control and internal parasites. Shade and hiding places should be available to allow the maned wolves to hide from public view and conspecifics.

Perimeter fencing should be a minimum of 2.3-m tall fencing, preferably with an inward overhang. The fence or a footer should be buried 46 cm in the ground to prevent wolves from digging out. Adequate shelter should be provided to protect maned wolves from the elements. Maned wolves should have access to a heated area if the temperature drops below 7° C (45° F).[15]

Maned wolves are often housed in male-female pairs, but same-sex sibling pairs or trios have also been successfully housed together. Attempts to introduce same-sex adults have not been successful. In addition, there are several reports of successful mixed species exhibits with maned wolves, including capybara (Hydrochoerus hydrochaeris), giant anteaters (Myrmecophaga tridactyla), and tapirs (Tapirus spp.).[15]

NUTRITION

Maned wolf nutrition is another unique aspect of this species and an area of intense ongoing research. As an omnivore, the maned wolf ingests approximately 51%

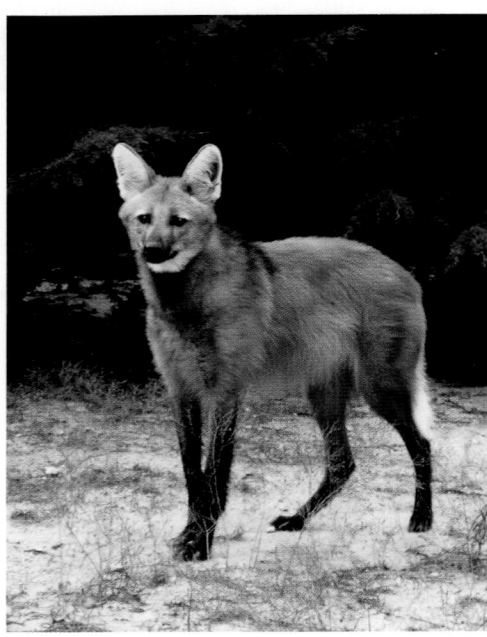

Figure 58-1

The maned wolf *(Chrysocyon brachyurus)* has a long, rusty red haircoat with black or dark brown muzzle, withers and legs. *(Courtesy Fossil Rim Wildlife Center, Glen Rose, Tex.)*

plant material and 49% animal protein, including mammals, birds, reptiles, and invertebrates, in the wild, and its diet varies seasonally.[8,21,25] In Brazil, a large proportion of the plant matter ingested by the maned wolf is *Solanum lycocarpum* (*lobeira*, or "fruit of the wolf"), a relative of the tomato.

The unique diet of wild maned wolves presents challenges in captivity. Historically, captive North American maned wolves were fed carnivorous diets. Problems such as urolithiasis, loose stool, and unthriftiness arose. These issues have been mitigated by feeding a more omnivorous diet, but the captive population continues to have some of these problems. Currently, zoological institutions strive to feed their maned wolves a varied diet that includes fruits, vegetables, and whole prey items, although commercial canine kibble still constitutes a large proportion (average, 71%) of the diet.[23] It is this discrepancy between the diets of zoo-housed and free-ranging maned wolves that is hypothesized to be a contributing factor to the morbidity of captive maned wolves.

A survey was conducted by the Maned Wolf Species Survival Plan in November 2006 to determine diets fed to captive North American maned wolves and correlate their health status. The survey identified approximately 26 different diets fed to maned wolves in 26 North American zoological facilities.[23] The survey also asked keepers to score fecal consistency in maned wolves. It was found that in one 24-hour period, many individual animals have a variety of fecal consistencies, from very loose to firm, that may vary according to what was ingested, activity, hydration status, among other factors.

Preliminary results from a study of nutritional blood parameters in captive North American maned wolves have demonstrated taurine and other amino acid deficiencies in several individuals. In addition, fatty acids vary greatly among individuals. I have noted that these variations may reflect the disparate diet of maned wolves in zoological facilities. Additional studies are needed to evaluate nutritional requirements in this species, including evaluating the nutritional blood parameters of wild maned wolves for comparison.

REPRODUCTION

Maned wolves are facultatively monogamous, with pairs uniting during the breeding season. Wild maned wolves are thought to be monestrous, with a 5-day estrous cycle. Gestation lasts 63 to 67 days. In the wild, maned wolves give birth during the dry season, from June to September.[25] In captivity in North America, pups are usually born from January to early March. The maned wolf litter size ranges from two to five pups, and captive male maned wolves have been observed assisting in pup rearing by regurgitating food and grooming pups.

Pregnancy may be determined by conventional methods such as radiography and ultrasound, but these usually require anesthesia. A recent study attempted to develop noninvasive pregnancy monitoring by measuring urinary relaxin.[26] Although the study showed a trend that urinary relaxin increased in some pregnant females, further investigations are required to establish a relaxin antibody that is specific to the maned wolf.

Contraception may be required in certain captive situations. Separating pairs is reversible and noninvasive, but problems may arise when reintroducing pairs, and space in zoological facilities may be a limiting factor. Spaying or neutering may be used to prevent pregnancies, but this is not reversible. The vasectomized male will continue to exhibit intact male behaviors, and there is a risk of pseudopregnancy in the female. Therefore, vasectomy is not recommended for maned wolves.

Historically, synthetic progestin implants, such as melengestrol acetate (MGA), have been used in female

TABLE 58-1	Selected Chemical Restraint Agents Used in Maned Wolves *(Chrysocyon Brachyurus)*		
Drug Combination	Dosage (mg/kg)	Reversal Agent (mg/kg)	Comments
Tiletamine/zolazepam (Telazol)[10]	2.77 IM	Flumazenil 0.1 IV, IM*	Free-ranging maned wolves; relaxed plane of anesthesia noted but recoveries may be prolonged; partial reversal with flumazenil may shorten recovery, but residual tiletamine may cause adverse effects.
Xylazine/ketamine[15]	1.1/6.0-8.0 IM	Yohimbine 0.1-0.2 IV, IM	Use alpha-2 adrenergic agonists with caution in debilitated animals.
Medetomidine butorphanol/midazolam	0.03/0.2/0.1 IM	Atipamezole 0.2/naltrexone 1.0/flumazenil 0.1 IM	Excellent muscle relaxation, option to reverse all or some of drugs, quick recovery

IM, Intramuscularly
*If using dexdetomidine, halve the dosage.

carnivores, including maned wolves. However, this form of chemical contraception has been associated with uterine pathology in zoo canids.[20] Because these side effects may cause irreversible damage to the reproductive tract, MGA implants are no longer recommended for contraception for maned wolves.

Gonadotropin-releasing hormone (GnRH) agonists are currently the recommended form of contraception for maned wolves. These agents suppress pituitary (luteinizing hormone [LH] and follicle-stimulating hormone [FSH]) and gonadal (estradiol and progesterone in females and testosterone in males) hormones. This form of contraception is reversible and may be used in males and females. Deslorelin implants and leuprolide acetate injections are the two most commonly used forms of GnRH agonists. Because they are relatively new, close monitoring of individuals treated with GnRH agonists is recommended, and results should be reported to the Association of Zoos and Aquariums Wildlife Contraception group.

RESTRAINT AND HANDLING

Care should be taken when handling maned wolves because they are wild animals, with large canine teeth and powerful jaws. However, their relatively timid nature allows some individuals to be restrained without anesthesia. Capture poles and squeeze cages may be used for minor procedures, such as phlebotomy. This may be stressful on the animal and on those involved in the procedure, so the benefits must be weighed against the risks. Using operant conditioning with food rewards,

the maned wolf may be trained for phlebotomy, hand injection of drugs, and other minor procedures.

ANESTHESIA

For refractory animals and long and/or painful procedures, general anesthesia should be used on maned wolves. Remote darting equipment may be used to administer the drugs. However, care should be taken when darting maned wolves because there have been several reports of fractured long bones secondary to capture darts. Many anesthetic protocols used for other canid species may be extrapolated to maned wolves, and drug choice depends on the clinician's preference. Several injectable protocols are listed in Table 58-1. Inhalant anesthesia is similar to that which is done for other canids, and isoflurane and sevoflurane are preferred. Monitoring during anesthesia and recovery is essential.

CLINICAL PATHOLOGY

Blood collection in maned wolves may be performed in a manner similar to techniques used for other canids. The jugular, cephalic, and saphenous veins are commonly used sites for venipuncture. Table 58-2 shows normal hematologic reference ranges for captive adult maned wolves. Serum chemistry reference ranges for captive adult maned wolves are shown in Table 58-3. Reference values for wild maned wolves in Brazil have been published recently by May-Junior and colleagues.[16]

TABLE 58-2 Hematologic Values for Adult Maned Wolves		
Parameter	Mean*	SD
White blood cell count ($\times10^3$/µL)	9.133	3.371
Red blood cell count ($\times10^6$/µL)	5.76	0.88
Hemoglobin (g/dL)	14.3	1.8
Hematocrit (%)	42.9	5.6
MCV (fL)	74.8	7.4
MCH (pg/cell)	25.4	2.3
MCHC (g/dL)	33.4	2.1
Platelet count ($\times10^3$/µL)	205	74
Segmented neutrophils ($\times10^3$/µL)	6.475	2.822
Neutrophilic bands ($\times10^3$/µL)	0.520	0.931
Lymphocytes ($\times10^3$/µL)	1.751	0.789
Monocytes ($\times10^3$/µL)	0.278	0.252
Eosinophils ($\times10^3$/µL)	0.609	0.447
Basophils ($\times10^3$/µL)	0.114	0.132

*Values are from Teare, ISIS.

TABLE 58-3 Serum Chemistry Values for Adult Maned Wolves		
Parameter	Mean*	SD
Calcium (mg/dL)	9.4	0.6
Phosphorus (mg/dL)	4.3	0.8
Sodium (mEq/liter)	145	3
Potassium (mEq/liter)	4.6	0.4
Chloride (mEq/liter)	115	3
Bicarbonate (mEq/liter)	19.2	4.0
Carbon dioxide (mEq/liter)	18.6	2.6
Iron (µg/dL)	107	36
Magnesium (mg/dL)	3.80	4.06
Blood urea nitrogen (mg/dL)	26	8
Creatinine (mg/dL)	1.5	0.3
Uric acid (mg/dL)	0.3	0.3
Total bilirubin (mg/dL)	0.3	0.2
Direct bilirubin (mg/dL)	0.1	0.1
Indirect bilirubin (mg/dL)	0.2	0.2
Glucose (mg/dL)	107	25
Cholesterol (mg/dL)	273	74
Triglyceride (mg/dL)	27	13
Creatine phosphokinase (IU/liter)	149	96
Lactate dehydrogenase (IU/liter)	157	147
Alkaline phosphatase (IU/liter)	41	43
Alanine aminotransferase (IU/liter)	95	83
Aspartate aminotransferase (IU/liter)	44	31
Gamma glutamyltrasferase (IU/liter)	4	3
Amylase (IU/liter)	490	379
Lipase (IU/liter)	174	78
Total protein (colorimetry) (g/dL)	6.6	0.6
Globulin (colorimetry) (g/dL)	3.5	0.5
Albumin (colorimetery) (g/dL)	3.1	0.3
Fibrinogen (mg/dL)	97	118
Progesterone (ng/dL)	1.680	0.000
Total triiodothyronine (ng/mL)	46.9	65.3
Total thyroxine (µg/dL)	1.7	0.5

*Values are from Teare, ISIS.

DISEASES

Wild Maned Wolves

Wild maned wolves are known to become infected with the giant kidney worm (*Dioctophyme renale*) by eating the paratenic (aquatic oligochaetes) or intermediate hosts (fish or frogs).[6,18] The parasite migrates to the right kidney, where it causes irreversible damage. However, maned wolves have been known to survive with one functioning kidney.

Nematodes (*Trichuris*, *Ancylostoma*, and *Toxocara* spp.) and cestodes have also been found in wild maned wolves, although their impact on morbidity and mortality is unknown. Ticks and screwworm larvae are ectoparasites that afflict wild maned wolves.

Cystinuria is another disease that has been reported in wild maned wolves. Field studies in Bolivia and Brazil have documented cystinuria, although its impact on the wild population is unknown.[5,8,27]

Maned wolves are susceptible to diseases afflicting domestic dogs, and recent studies have suggested that infectious diseases threaten wild maned wolf populations.[4,6] Domestic animals in rural areas are rarely vaccinated for common diseases. Human encroachment on maned wolf habitat provides the opportunity for domestic animal–wildlife interaction and increased exposure to domestic carnivore diseases, such as parvovirus, leptospirosis, and toxoplasmosis, is a significant concern.

Captive Maned Wolves

Canine distemper virus (CDV) is a morbillivirus causing significant morbidity and mortality in maned wolves.[14] Clinical signs of CDV are similar to those in dogs and include neurologic signs such as seizures and respiratory problems such as nasal discharge and sneezing. Treatment is rarely successful, and prevention by vaccination is the best way to control this disease. However, some commercially available canine modified live vaccines have been known to cause disease in naïve animals.[28]

Thus, the current recommendation is to use a recombinant canarypox-vectored or killed canine distemper vaccine annually.

Parvovirus is another disease that has been documented in maned wolves and may cause debilitating diarrhea and even death.[19] As with CDV, some modified live canine vaccines may cause disease in this species.[1] Thus, it is recommended to vaccinate young or naïve maned wolves with a killed parvovirus vaccine until serologic titers indicate an appropriate immune response (>1:80) and then to switch to a modified live vaccine, which may induce longer lasting, more effective protection against the disease.

Adenovirus is another viral disease of concern in maned wolves and is suspected to have caused hepatitis in a captive maned wolf.[11] The use of commercially available canine vaccines may be warranted, but they should be used with caution.

Maned wolves should also be vaccinated against rabies virus using a killed vaccine. Immunizations against other diseases may be warranted depending on which diseases are endemic. The risk of an adverse vaccine reaction may be reduced by avoiding multivalent vaccines in naïve animals.

The pancreatic fluke *Eurytrema procyonis* has recently been identified in captive maned wolves.[30] The normal host is the raccoon, and it is suspected to have an arthropod intermediate host.[29] Clinical signs may be subtle in maned wolves and may include thin body condition, with partial anorexia and loose stool. Fecal examination (sedimentation or float) may afford an antemortem diagnosis, but false-negative results are possible. Pancreatic biopsies may identify inflammation and possibly the trematodes in the pancreatic ducts. Treatment may be successful with praziquantel, and a pancreatic enzyme supplement may be warranted.

Preventive medicine for maned wolves should include treatment for endoparasites and ectoparasites. Routine fecal examinations and deworming based on results should be performed. Heartworm has been documented in maned wolves,[9] and heartworm prevention using commercially available canine formulations may be used monthly. Ectoparasites such as fleas and ticks may be problematic for maned wolves during warm weather. Monthly topical treatment with canine products has been used safely. In addition, it is recommended to treat the environment and shelters and to use oral products to sterilize adult fleas to break the life cycle. Tickborne diseases (including babesiosis) have been diagnosed in maned wolves, and tick prevention should be considered.[2]

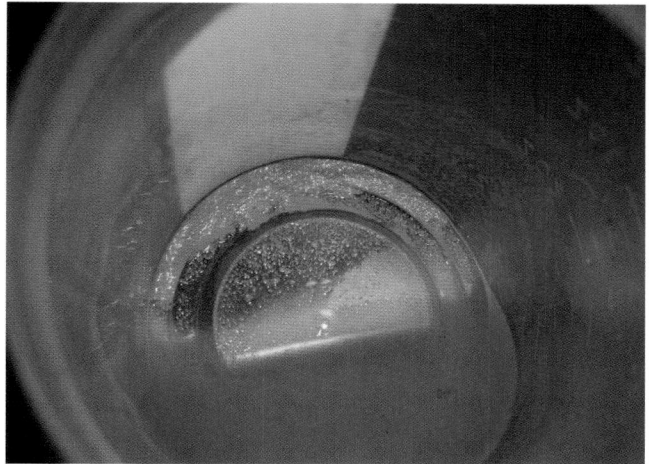

Figure 58-2

The maned wolf has a genetic predisposition to excrete cystine in the urine. Evaluation of the urine may show the characteristic yellow cystine "sludge."

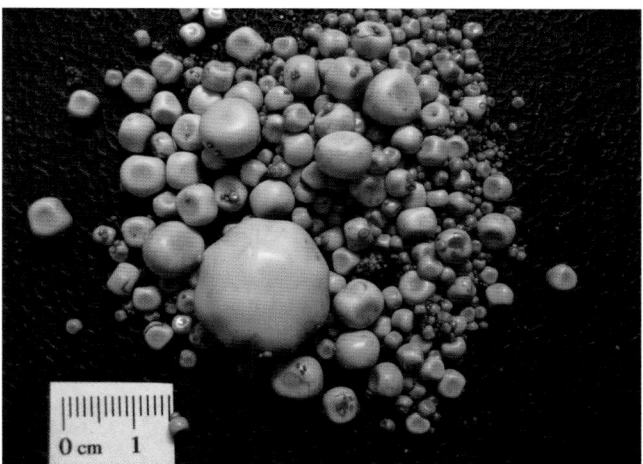

Figure 58-3

The cystine calculi shown in this picture were removed from the bladder of a maned wolf postmortem. Calculi may form when an imbalance is present. *(Courtesy Dr. Luis Padilla.)*

Cystinuria is commonly reported in captive maned wolves.[3,12,15] This may be caused by a genetic predisposition to excrete cystine in the urine, as evidenced by the presence of cystinuria in both wild and captive maned wolves. The cystinuria is often subclinical, but yellow cystine sludge may be seen in the urine (Fig. 58-2). Calculi may form when an imbalance is present. High-protein diets, diets containing high levels of methionine and cystine, and acidic urine may contribute to the formation of cystine calculi. These calculi may form in the urethra, bladder (Fig. 58-3), or kidney and pose a

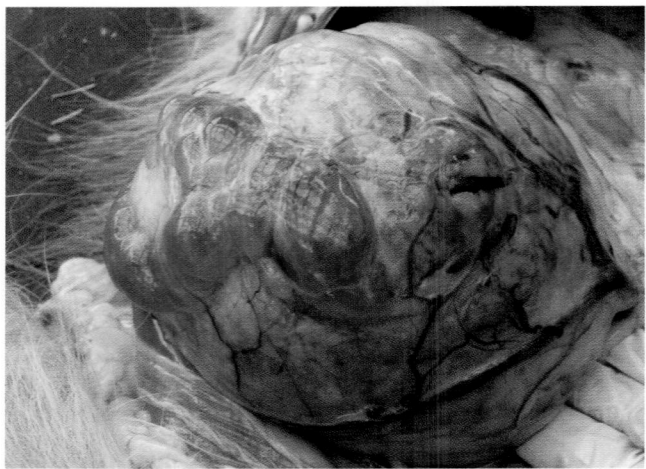

Figure 58-4

Ovarian dysgerminomas, as shown here, are frequently found in older female maned wolves at necropsy. *(Courtesy Dr. Holly Haefele.)*

significant health risk to the individual. Maned wolves with cystine calculi may present with stranguria; males are most often affected. Radiographs may reveal radiopaque stones. Urethral obstruction is a life-threatening emergency and should be treated as for domestic cats and dogs. If left untreated, bladder rupture and/or death may occur. Reducing animal-based protein in the diet and alkalinizing the urine by feeding potassium citrate or tiopronin may help prevent the formation of stones in the urinary tract, as seen in domestic dogs.[13] Research on this topic is ongoing.

Dermatitis is commonly reported in captive maned wolves. Interdigital dermatitis may have a mixed bacterial, fungal, and allergic cause. Lick granulomas, atopy, hot spots, allergic dermatitis, and other signs have been observed. Treating these conditions based on the principles used in domestic canine medicine has been successful.

Inflammatory bowel disease (IBD) has been documented in multiple captive maned wolves. Clinical signs include loose stool, weight loss, and unthriftiness. Definitive diagnosis requires biopsy of the affected gastrointestinal tract, which may show a lymphoplasmacytic and/or eosinophilic inflammation. Treatment is directed at removing the inciting cause and reducing the inflammation with steroids, antibiotics, and soluble fiber. Changing the kibble to a hypoallergenic formulation may also help assuage clinical signs.

Periodontal disease may afflict captive maned wolves. Dental prophylaxis under anesthesia should be performed annually, or when practical.

Neoplasia, such as fibrosarcomas and osteosarcoma, has been documented in captive maned wolves and is usually seen in older animals.[17,24] Ovarian dysgerminomas have frequently been seen in intact females (Fig. 58-4).[22]

Acknowledgments

I gratefully acknowledge the following people who have greatly contributed to the knowledge of maned wolves: Melissa Rodden, Dr. Mitchell Bush, Dr. Robyn Barbiers, Dr. Scott Citino, and Dr. Nucharin Songsasen. I extend thanks to Dr. Holly Haefele, Melissa Rodden, and Dr. Songsasen for reviewing this manuscript. This chapter is dedicated to the memory of Dr. Roy McClements, who was dedicated to researching maned wolf nutrition.

REFERENCES

1. Backues KA: Problems with maned wolf puppies and parvovirus immunization. Zoo Vet News 10:6, 1994.
2. Baeyens M: Personal communication, 2009.
3. Bovee KC, Bush M, Dietz J, et al: Cystinuria in the maned wolf of South America. Science 212:919–921, 1981.
4. Bronson E, Emmons LH, Murray S, et al: Serosurvey of pathogens in domestic dogs on the border of Noël Kempff Mercado National Park, Bolivia. J Zoo Wildl Med 39:28–36, 2008.
5. Deem SL: Personal communication, 2006.
6. Deem SL, Emmons LH: Exposure of free-ranging maned wolves to infectious and parasitic disease agents in Noel Kempff Mercado National Park, Bolivia. J Zoo Wildl Med 36:192–197, 2005.
7. De Paula RC, Medici P, Morato RG: [Plano de ação para conservação do Lobo-Guará: análise de viabilidade populacional e de habitat.] Brasilia, Brazil, 2008, IBAMA.
8. Dietz JM: Ecology and social organization of the maned wolf (*Chrysocyon brachyurus*), 1984 (http://si-pddr.si.edu/dspace/bitstream/10088/5348/2/SCtZ-0392-Lo_res.pdf).
9. Estrada AH, Gerlach TJ, Schmidt MK, et al: Cardiac evaluation of clinically healthy captive maned wolves (*Chrysocyon brachyurus*). J Zoo Wildl Med 40:478–486, 2009.
10. Furtado MM, Kashivakura CK, Ferro C, et al: Immobilization of free-ranging maned wolf (*Chrysocyon brachyurus*) with tiletamine and zolazepam in central Brazil. J Zoo Wildl Med 37:68–70, 2006.
11. Haefele H: Personal communication, 2009.
12. Hammond EE, Bush M, Citino SB, et al: Maned wolf (*Chrysocyon brachyurus*) species survival plan medical update. In Proceedings of the American Association of Zoo Veterinarians Annual Meeting, 2008, pp 192–193.
13. Hoppe A, Denneberg T: Cystinuria in the dog: Clinical studies during 14 years of medical management. J Vet Intern Med 15:361–367, 2001.
14. Maia OB, Gouveia AM: Serologic response of maned wolves (*Chrysocyon brachyurus*) to canine distemper virus and canine parvovirus vaccination. J Zoo Wildl Med 31:78–80, 2001.
15. Maned Wolf Species Survival Plan: Maned wolf husbandry manual. Silver Spring, Md, 2007, Association of Zoos and Aquariums.
16. May-Junior JA, Songsasen N, Azebedo FC, et al: Hematology and blood chemistry parameters differ in free-ranging maned wolves (*Chrysocyon brachyurus*) living in the Serra Da Canastra National

Park versus adjacent farmlands, Brazil. J Wildl Dis 45:81–90, 2009.

17. McNulty EE, Gilson SD, Houser BS, et al: Treatment of fibrosarcoma in a maned wolf *(Chrysocyon brachyurus)* by rostral maxillectomy. J Zoo Wildl Med 31:394–399, 2000.

18. Measures LN: Dioctophymatosis. In Samuel WM, Pybus MJ, Kocan AA, editors: Parasitic diseases of wild mammals, ed 2. Ames, Iowa, 2001, Iowa State University Press, pp 357–364.

19. Montali RJ, Kelly K: Pathologic survey and review of diseases of captive maned wolves *(Chrysocyon brachyurus)* and bush dogs *(Speothos venaticus)*. In Proceedings of the 31st International Symposium of Diseases of Zoological Animals, Berlin, 1989, Akademie-Verlag, pp 35–43.

20. Moresco A, Munson L, Gardner IA: Naturally occurring and melengestrol acetate-associated reproductive tract lesions in zoo canids. Vet Pathol 46:1117–1128, 2009.

21. Motta-Junior JC, Talamoni SA, Lombardi JA, et al: Diet of the maned wolf, *Chrysocyon brachyurus*, in central Brazil. J Zool London 240:277–284, 1996.

22. Munson L, Montali RJ: High prevalence of ovarian tumors in maned wolves *(Chrysocyon brachyurus)* at the National Zoological Park. J Zoo Wildl Med 22:125–129, 1991.

23. Phipps AM, Edwards MS: Diets offered to maned wolves *(Chrysocyon brachyurus)* in North American zoos: A review and analysis.

In Proceedings of the 8th Annual Conference of the AZA Nutritional Advisory Group on Zoo and Wildl Nutrition, 2009, pp 51–73.

24. Reid HL, Deem SL, Citino SB: Extraosseous osteosarcoma in a maned wolf *(Chrysocyon brachyurus)*. J Zoo Wildl Med 36:523–526, 2005.

25. Rodden M, Rodrigues F, Bestelmeyer S: Maned wolf *(Chrysocyon brachyurus)*. In Sillero-Zubiri C, Hoffmann M, Macdonald DW, editors: Canids: Foxes, wolves, jackals and dogs, Gland, Switzerland/Cambridge, England, 2004, IUCN/SSC Canid Specialist Group, pp 38–44.

26. Santymire RC, Steinetz B, Santymire RM, et al: Potential of urinary relaxin as a useful indicator of pregnancy in the maned wolf. Reprod Fertil Dev 21:182, 2009.

27. Songsasen N: Personal communication, 2010.

28. Thomas-Baker B: Vaccination-induced distemper in maned wolves, vaccination-induced corneal opacity in a maned wolf. In Silberman MS, Silberman SD, editors: Proceedings of the American Association of Zoo Veterinarians, Scottsdale, Ariz, 1985, American Association of Zoo Veterinarians, p 53.

29. Vyhnal KK, Barr SC, Hornbuckle WE, et al: *Eurytrema procyonis* and pancreatitis in a cat. J Feline Med Surg 10:384–387, 2008.

30. Weber M: Personal communication, 2010.

CHAPTER 59

Primer on Tick-Borne Diseases in Exotic Carnivores

Mark W. Cunningham and Michael J. Yabsley

Tick-borne diseases include bacterial, viral, protozoal, and even toxic diseases transmitted or caused by ticks. Ticks, especially *Amblyomma* spp., also may cause anemia and direct trauma leading to secondary infections and myiasis.[1] Tick-borne diseases of microbial origin are infectious but not contagious. For some organisms, such as *Ehrlichia canis* and *Cytauxzoon felis,* carnivores are the definitive host and serve as the reservoir for infection in other species, whereas for *Hepatozoon* spp., carnivores serve as the intermediate host. For other diseases, such as borreliosis, they are a dead-end or incidental host and do not play an important role in the epizootiology of the disease. These hosts, however, may be important in maintaining tick populations. Many infectious diseases, such as tularemia and yersiniosis, are more frequently transmitted by other mechanisms or vectors, but also may be transmitted by ticks. Recent advances in molecular analyses have improved sensitivity and, in many cases, have demonstrated that a much larger percentage of a given population is infected. These advances also have led to the identification of additional organisms and have changed the taxonomic classification of the causative agent for some diseases. Depending on geographic region and climate, there may be seasonal variation to disease occurrence because activity patterns of ticks, intermediate hosts, and definitive hosts vary through the year. The geographic distribution of tick-borne diseases generally is going to follow the distribution of competent vectors and hosts.

Coinfections with tick-borne organisms should be considered the rule rather than the exception. Individual ticks have been shown to be infected with multiple pathogens and carnivores are often infected with multiple tick species. Furthermore, infection with one pathogen may impair the immune response and increase susceptibility to other tick-borne pathogens. For example, coinfections of *Babesia* spp., possibly other

tick-borne diseases, and canine distemper virus may have resulted in a die-off of African lions *(Panthera leo)* in Ngorongoro Crater in 2001.[20]

Often, knowledge of clinical disease resulting from tick-borne infections in wildlife is lacking. Mortality studies using primarily adult animals (e.g., telemetry studies) may overlook morbidity and mortality in younger age groups, a demographic group particularly susceptible to many tick-borne pathogens. Also, clinical signs and hematologic changes resulting from tick-borne infections in exotic carnivores may be transient, only occurring during the acute stages. Captive adult animals also may be fully susceptible if never exposed at a young age. This could affect translocation projects because captive-bred animals, which were not exposed to tick-borne pathogens at a young age, may be susceptible when released into the wild.[23] Additionally, extreme stress, immunosuppressive coinfections, splenectomy, and other factors may precipitate clinical disease in infected carnivores.[5,20,31]

Diagnosis of infectious tick-borne diseases is based on clinical signs and history, direct visualization of organisms on histology or stained blood smears, serology, polymerase chain reaction (PCR) assay, and response to treatment. Most tick-borne bacteria are either obligate intracellular parasites or are otherwise difficult to grow, and some organisms such as *Rickettsia rickettsii* require enhanced biocontainment and select agent registration.[22] Therefore, culture is not routinely used as a diagnostic tool. Diagnostics should include tests for all potential tick-borne pathogens.

The control and prevention of tick-borne diseases are directed at control of ticks and management of their intermediate and/or definitive hosts. Topical acaricides may be used to control ticks on some host species and have been shown to reduce the transmission of some rickettsial diseases.[22]

458

Many tick-borne organisms infecting carnivores are zoonotic, including *Borrelia* spp., *Ehrlichia canis*, *E. chaffeensis*, *E. ewingii*, *Anaplasma phagocytophilum*, *Rickettsia rickettsii*, *Coxiella burnetii*, *Bartonella* spp., and Powassan virus, and thus carnivores may serve as sentinels for zoonotic tick-borne diseases. Ectoparasites in zoo settings have been found to carry zoonotic pathogens[21] and zoo animals, personnel, and visitors potentially are at risk if bitten by ticks. Appropriate personal protection equipment should be worn when handling blood or conducting necropsies on animals possibly infected with tick-borne diseases. Finally, the diagnosis, occurrence, and distribution of tick-borne diseases are increasing. This is likely the result of improved diagnostics, increased awareness, and changes in the environment and climate, resulting in an increase and expansion of tick populations and reservoir hosts.[20,22] Additionally, alterations in land management (e.g., prevention of natural wildfires) may lead to increased tick numbers and tick-borne diseases.

BACTERIA

Borreliosis

Lyme borreliosis is caused by a gram-negative spirochete belonging to the genus *Borrelia*. In the United States, *Borrelia burgdorferi sensu lato* is the primary cause of Lyme disease. This species complex shows considerable genetic diversity and includes the genotypes *B. burgdorferi sensu scricto*, *B. andersoni*, *B. bissettii*, and *B. carolinensis*. Transmission is primarily by *Ixodes* ticks, which usually parasitize different hosts as a larva, nymph, or adult. *Borrelia* is maintained in the vector by transstadial transmission and rodents are the principal reservoirs. For some *Borrelia* species, certain mammals are not important reservoirs but contribute to disease persistence by serving as a host for adult ticks (e.g., role of white-tailed deer *[Odocoileus virginianus]* in the ecology of Lyme disease).[6] Transplacental transmission has been demonstrated in several species, including the coyote *(Canis latrans)*. Among carnivores, infection with or antibodies reactive to *Borrelia burgdorferi s.l.* have been detected in captive and/or free-ranging canids, felids, ursids, mustelids, procyonids, and pinnipeds.[29]

In domestic dogs, clinical signs following experimental infection with *B. burgdorferi sensu stricto* occur months after exposure and include fever, inappetence, lethargy, lymphadenopathy, and polyarthritis.[13] An experimentally infected wolf *(Canis lupus)* developed a transient lymphadenopathy following intravenous inoculation of *B. burgdorferi*. Otherwise, clinical disease has not been described in naturally infected carnivores. The diagnosis of borreliosis may be difficult and is based on clinical signs, diagnostic tests (culture, PCR assay or, more commonly, serology), history of exposure, and elimination of other differential diagnoses.[6] Treatment is most beneficial early in the infection, and doxycycline is the antibiotic of choice. Other effective antibiotics include ampicillin or amoxicillin, some third-generation cephalosporins, and erythromycin. The development of an effective vaccine for borreliosis has been difficult because of the number of strains and species responsible for the disease; however, killed whole bacterin and recombinant vaccines labeled for use in dogs are available.

Rickettsial Diseases

Ehrlichiosis and Anaplasmosis

Ehrlichia and *Anaplasma* spp. are gram-negative obligate intracellular cocci in the family Anaplasmataceae that primarily infect leukocytes, although some species infect platelets. Several species have been described and each has a somewhat unique epizootiology, but all are transmitted by ticks. *Ehrlichia canis*, the cause of canine ehrlichiosis, is transmitted by the brown dog tick *(Rhipicephalus sanguineus)*, although *Dermacentor variabilis* also has been shown to be a competent vector. The reservoir hosts are domestic dogs and wild canids.[22] Antibodies to or infection with *E. canis* have been demonstrated in free-ranging and captive canids, felids, and procyonids.

In domestic dogs, the disease is characterized initially by depression and anorexia and may include weight loss, lymphadenopathy, nasal and ocular discharge, dyspnea, and edema. These transient signs may be followed by thrombocytopenia and leukopenia. Chronic infections may be mild or severe and may include bleeding tendencies, severe weight loss, debilitation, and neurologic signs. Putative *E. canis* infection and clinical signs have been reported in a captive gray wolf and in experimentally infected wild dogs *(Lycaon pictus)*. Wild dogs exhibited anorexia, depression, anemia, leukopenia, and mild thrombocytopenia. Experimentally infected jackals *(Canis mesomelas)* and foxes *(Vulpes* and *Urocyon)* did not show disease, although a mild thrombocytopenia, leukopenia, and anemia were seen in the acute stages of infection in foxes. Clinical disease has not been reported in other free-ranging carnivores.

Ehrlichia chaffeensis infects monocytes and is the cause of human monocytic ehrlichiosis. *E. chaffeensis* is transmitted by *Amblyomma americanum* and the white-tailed deer serves as its principal reservoir. This agent is zoonotic and also may infect domestic dogs. Antibodies reactive to *E. chaffeensis* have been reported from raccoons *(Procyon lotor)* throughout the southeastern United States.[32] Experimental inoculations of raccoons have resulted in short-term rickettsemias, but infected raccoons failed to transmit infections to ticks. Natural *E. chaffeensis* infections have been identified in free-ranging coyotes. Following experimental inoculation with *E. chaffeensis*, red foxes *(Vulpes vulpes)* became bacteremic, but gray foxes *(Urocyon cinereoargenteus)* were refractory. Clinical signs of *E. chaffeensis* infection in dogs may be similar to those of *E. canis* infections but typically are milder,[4] and clinical disease has not been reported in naturally or experimentally infected exotic carnivores.

Anaplasma phagocytophilum (formerly *Ehrlichia equi* and *Ehrlichia phagocytophila*) infects neutrophils, causing granulocytic anaplasmosis in humans, equids, and sheep. Rodents and some ruminants may serve as reservoirs for *A. phagocytophilum*, and transmission occurs via *Ixodes* spp. The epizootiology is similar to that of *Borrelia burgdorferi* and thus the two organisms have a similar distribution in North America.[22] Antibodies reactive with and/or DNA of *A. phagocytophilum* have been reported in canids, felids, ursids, procyonids, and mustelids.[7]

In domestic dogs, fever, lethargy, lameness, myalgia, and a reluctance to move are the most common physical examination findings. Significant hematologic findings may include lymphopenia, thrombocytopenia, and hypoalbuminemia, and long-term illness in dogs has been reported.[4] Natural infection in domestic cats does occur and may result in clinical disease.[18] Clinical disease has not been reported in infected exotic carnivores.

Anaplasma platys (formerly *Ehrlichia platys*) is the cause of canine infectious cyclic thrombocytopenia in dogs. *A. platys* is thought to be transmitted by the brown dog tick, although this has yet to be confirmed experimentally. *A. platys* infects platelets, but infection is not usually associated with significant clinical disease in domestic dogs. A mild normocytic, normochromic, nonregenerative anemia, leukopenia, hypoalbuminemia, and hyperglobulinemia have been observed in experimentally infected dogs.[4] Infections in wild canids have not been reported.

Other Anaplasmaceae infections have been detected in exotic carnivores. "*Candidatus* Neoehrlicia lotoris," an ehrlichial organism related to "*Candidatus* Neoehrlichia mikurensis," is common in raccoons in the southeastern United States.[34] A low percentage of coyotes from California were seropositive and PCR-positive for *Ehrlichia risticii*.[24] Clinical disease was not associated with infection in either host species.

Other Rickettsial Diseases

Rickettsia rickettsii is the cause of Rocky Mountain spotted fever (RMSF) in dogs and humans. The organism primarily is transmitted by *Dermacentor* ticks, although *Amblyomma cajennense* and *Rickettsia sanguineus* have been shown to transmit the organism in some areas.[22] *R. rickettsii* is maintained by a natural cycle between these ticks and small rodents, humans, and dogs. Carnivores are incidental hosts. Serologic evidence of exposure to *R. rickettsii* has been detected in canids, ursids, mustelids, and procyonids. The bacteria infects endothelial cells, resulting in vasculitis. The organism may cause severe disease in domestic dogs; however, infection is generally self-limiting and of short duration; it is characterized by fever, lethargy, vomiting, and occasional rash. In more severe disease, clinical signs include petechiae and ecchymotic hemorrhages, ocular lesions, neurologic abnormalities, and edema in the extremities.[4] There are no reports of overt disease in free-ranging carnivores, and experimentally infected domestic ferrets and coyotes have not exhibited clinical disease.

Diagnosis and Treatment of Rickettsial Infections

Early and definitive diagnosis of rickettsial infections is made by direct visualization of morulae in leukocytes (or platelets in the case of *A. platys*) using Romanowsky-type stains or by histology in the case of RMSF. Rickettsemia is often transient and smears collected after the initial stages of infection may result in false-negative diagnoses.[22] PCR assays currently are the primary diagnostic tool but may be of limited usefulness outside the clinical stages of the disease. Resolution of clinical signs of rickettsial disease following appropriate antimicrobial treatment and paired acute and convalescent serology with seroconversion also support the diagnosis.

Doxycycline is the mainstay of treatment for rickettsial diseases in humans and domestic animals. Fluoroquinolones also are effective for RMSF but not ehrlichiosis.[4] Often, treatment is based on clinical signs and a definitive diagnosis is never made. In many cases, early treatment is necessary to prevent debilitating infections.

Haemobartonellosis

Haemobartonellosis of felids and canids is caused by hemotrophic mycoplasmas (haemoplasmas), formerly known as *Hemobartonella* and *Eperythropozoon*. At least five species have been recognized, including *Mycoplasma haemofelis* (formerly *H. felis*). This larger and more pathogenic form causes feline hemotrophic mycoplasmosis (feline infectious anemia) in domestic cats. "*Candidatus* Mycoplasma haemominitum" is a smaller and less pathogenic hemoplasma of felids and a third species, "*Candidatus* Mycoplasma turicensis," recently has been discovered.[31] Canids may be infected with either *M. haemocanis* (formerly *H. canis*) or "*Candidatus* Mycoplasma haemoparvum."[30] Hemoplasmas are believed to be transmitted mechanically by blood-sucking ectoparasites, including ticks. Although the cat flea *(Ctenocephalides felis)* is a primary vector for *M. haemofelis*, hemoplasmas have been found in the brown dog tick in Africa and *Ixodes ovatus* in Japan. The brown dog tick has been shown to be a competent vector for *M. canis.*

Hemoplasma infections are common in free-ranging and captive exotic felid species worldwide.[30] The prevalence of infection with "*Candidatus* M. haemominutum" and/or *M. haemofelis* in free-ranging pumas (*Puma concolor* subspp.) in Florida has approached 90%, with dual infections common. Serial sampling of these pumas revealed conversion to negative status was routine for those infected with *M. haemofelis* whereas clearance of "*Candidatus* M. haemominutum" infections occurred only occasionally.

Following experimental infection, an incubation period of 2 to 34 days precedes extravascular hemolysis and acute anemia.[30] The parasitemia may be cyclic and infected animals generally remain carriers. Domestic dogs generally do not show clinical signs unless splenectomized or immunocompromised. Clinical signs and mortality only have been reported rarely in captive *Felis* spp. Hemoplasma infection in young and adult European wildcats *(Felis silvestris silvestris)* was associated with feline leukemia virus (FeLV) provirus-positive status.[31]

Diagnosis is based on the demonstration of organisms on the surface of infected erythrocytes; however, this lacks sensitivity and specificity, and PCR assay is used for definitive diagnosis.[30] Treatment of hemobartonellosis with doxycycline or enrofloxacin has been successful, although antibiotics do not completely clear the infection. Glucocorticoids also may be considered to prevent immune-mediated hemolytic anemia.

Bartonellosis

Bartonella spp. are gram-negative bacilli or coccobacilli that infect erythrocytes in mammals, leading to persistent bacteremia. Various *Bartonella* spp. have been identified in an increasing number of reservoir hosts.[5] The domestic cat and wild felids are the reservoir for *Bartonella heneslae* whereas the coyote may be the reservoir for *Bartonella vinsonii* subsp. *berkhoferfii*. Transmission of *B. henselae* primarily is via the cat flea, although ticks increasingly are being implicated as possible vectors for *Bartonella* spp. Nevertheless, currently there is no evidence that *Bartonella* spp.is able to replicate in ticks and transmission from ticks to vertebrate hosts has not been demonstrated.[2] *B. henselae*, has been detected by serology, PCR assay, and/or culture in a wide range of free-ranging and captive felids, and evidence of *Bartonella rochalimae* infection has been detected in canids and procyonids. Undescribed *Bartonella* spp. have been detected in free-ranging African lions *(Panthera leo)*, cheetahs *(Acinonyx jubatus)*, and North American river otters *(Lontra canadensis)*.[8,19]

Clinical disease most often occurs in nonreservoir hosts (hosts not adapted to the infecting *Bartonella* spp.) and vary by infecting species. Clinical signs of bartonellosis reported in domestic dogs include endocarditis, granulomatous lymphadenitis and hepatitis, polyarthritis, meningoencephalitis, ocular lesions, and peliosis hepatis.[5] Cats are usually asymptomatic, but fever, mild anemia, lymphadenopathy, uveitis, endocarditis, cholangitis, renal and urinary tract abnormalities, neurologic signs, and reproductive disorders have been reported. Concurrent immunoincompetence (e.g., coinfection with feline immunodeficiency virus) may exacerbate clinical signs. Clinical disease reported in exotic carnivores is limited to the finding of endocarditis in free-ranging sea otters *(Enhydra lutris)* infected with *Bartonella volans*–like sp. As with other tick-borne diseases, diagnosis may be challenging and is based on clinical signs, history, serology, PCR assay, and response to treatment. Detection of subclinical infection by *Bartonella* spp. in a reservoir host is commonly achieved by PCR assay; however, diagnosis in a nonreservoir host may be difficult. Treatment recommendations are based on extrapolation from infections in humans and options include azithromycin, fluoroquinolones (alone or in combination with amoxicillin), or doxycycline at high doses.

VIRUSES

Powassan Virus

Powassan virus (POWV) constitutes a genetically diverse group of flaviviruses that are transmitted among mustelids and some rodents by *Ixodes* ticks.[11] The virus is zoonotic and is a rare cause of encephalitis in humans. Virus has been isolated and/or antibodies to POWV have been detected in canids, mustelids, and procyonids. Deer tick virus, a POWV strain, caused a fatal encephalitis in a gray fox *(Urocyon cinereoargenteus)*. Experimental infection of striped skunks *(Mephitis mephitis)* and red and gray foxes, however, resulted in viremia but not clinical disease. Serology, virus isolation, and PCR may be used to diagnose infection. There is no vaccine approved for use in humans or animals.

PROTOZOA

Babesiosis

Numerous species of *Babesia* have been identified worldwide and are distinguished morphologically into small and large *Babesia* spp. However, these morphologic differences do not follow molecular phylogeny and demarcation of species now relies heavily on sequence analysis of various genetic targets.[23] For example, molecular techniques have shown that morphologically similar parasites in numerous hosts are distinct species, some of which, like piroplasms from humans, dogs, and some wildlife in the western United States, possibly are a new genus because they do not reliably group with either *Babesia* or *Theiliera*.[16] *Babesia* spp. are transmitted by *Ixodes, Haemaphysalis,* and *Rhipicephalus* ticks. Vertical transmission also may occur. Numerous *Babesia* spp. have been identified in a wide variety of carnivore hosts, including canids, felids, hyaenids, viverrids, mustelids, herpestids, and procyonids.

Clinical signs in infected mammals result from lysis of infected erythrocytes and subsequent hemolytic anemia. In domestic dogs infected with *Babesia* spp., the severity of disease depends on the infecting species or subspecies, coinfection with other tick-borne and viral diseases, and host immune status.[15,20] Chronic and subclinical infections may occur. In acute and peracute disease, domestic dogs infected with *Babesia* spp. develop hemolytic anemia, fever, pallor, depression, anorexia, and weakness. Clinical disease resulting from *Babesia* infection appears to be less severe or nonexistent in free-ranging carnivores unless exacerbated or predisposed by immunosuppression and/or stress. Approximately 95% of Florida panthers *(Puma concolor coryi)* examined by PCR assay were positive for *Babesia* spp., with none showing obvious signs of babesiosis, and Rotstein and colleagues[26] have found similar hematologic values in panthers with evidence of piroplasm infection on blood smears versus those without. Similarly, one field study found that 82% of river otters were infected with a *Babesia* sp.,[3] but recently a young otter from a rehabilitation center in Georgia died of fulminate babesiosis caused by the same *Babesia* sp.[27] Experimental coinfection of coyote pups with *Ehrlichia* spp. and *Babesia canis* resulted in severe clinical signs in less than 2 weeks postinfection, and fatal babesiosis in a captive juvenile wild dog was reported in a review by Penzhorn.[23] A splenectomized coyote experimentally infected with *Babesia gibsoni* died from severe anemia whereas intact coyotes had mild clinical signs characterized by regenerative hemolytic anemia.

A presumptive diagnosis of *Babesia* in domestic dogs may be made based on history, clinical signs, and serology. Definitive diagnosis in any species is based on observation of organisms in erythrocytes on blood smears using Romanowsky stains or PCR assay. Treatment of babesiosis in domestic dogs includes imidocarb dipropionate and supportive care for anemia. Diminizene aceturate also is effective but is not available in the United States.[15]

Cytauxzoonosis

Cytauxzoon spp. is among the few Theileridae known to infect carnivores. *Cytauxzoon felis* is transmitted by *Dermacentor variabilis* and *Amblyomma americanum*.[25] The definitive host is the bobcat *(Lynx rufus)* and prevalence rates vary by geographic locations but may be as high as 80% in highly endemic regions of the midwestern United States.[28] Infections also have been reported in pumas. In Florida panthers, the prevalence of infection based on PCR assay was 12%,[33] whereas only 3% of pumas from North Dakota were infected. *Cytauxzoon* spp. also have been reported from other felids in South America, Europe, and Asia.

Infections in bobcats and pumas are usually mild or subclinical. However, mild hemolytic anemia and probable liver injury following acute infection with *C. felis* have been reported in pumas,[14] and disease ranging from mild hematologic changes to mortality has been reported in experimentally and naturally infected bobcats. In other felids, *C. felis* often results in fatal disease, and domestic cats are particularly susceptible. Clinical signs are the result of severe intravascular hemolysis and include pallor, icterus, hepatomegaly, and splenomegaly. Mortality rates approach 100% within 2 weeks of infection although, rarely, individuals appear to recover and some free-ranging or feral cats may become subclinical carriers.[12] Fatal cytauxzoonosis caused by *Cytauxzoon* spp. has been reported in captive *Panthera* spp.

Definitive diagnosis of cytauxzoonosis is based on observation of organisms in erythrocytes on blood smears using Romanowsky stains, although the examination of blood smears was shown by Yabsley and associates[33] not to be sensitive enough to detect most subclinical infections. PCR assay may be used to diagnose clinical and subclinical infections. Treatment in susceptible species is largely unrewarding.

Hepatozoonosis

Hepatozoon spp. infect all classes of terrestrial vertebrates. Among carnivores, *Hepatozoon* infections have been reported from canids, felids, hyaenids, viverrids, mustelids, and procyonids.[9] Infection of the vertebrate intermediate host occurs by ingestion of an infected tick (definitive host) or by vertical transmission. In spotted hyenas *(Crocuta crocuta)*, juveniles often groom members of their social group to remove ticks, a behavior that would facilitate transmission of *Hepatozoon* infection.[10]

Clinical disease in domestic dogs results from pyogranulomatous inflammation, and chronic inflammation and immune complex disease may lead to glomerulonephritis and amyloidosis. Clinical signs are most severe with *H. americanum* infection and include depression, anorexia, fever, weight loss, hyperesthesia, and pallor.[15] A neutrophilic leukocytosis and a nonregenerative anemia are the most common clinicopathologic findings. *Hepatozoon* infections in exotic carnivores are generally subclinical, although granulomatous inflammation and myositis have been reported in infected raccoons, black-backed jackals, and martens (*Martes* spp.). Younger age groups may be more susceptible to infection, suggesting that the effect of *Hepatozoon* infection on wild carnivore populations may be underestimated. Clinical signs and mortality, similar to those reported for *Hepatozoon* infections in domestic dogs, have been reported in young spotted hyenas[10] and experimentally infected coyote pups.[17] Even in the absence of clinical signs, however, *Hepatozoon* infection may compromise immune status, thus predisposing the carnivore to infection with other pathogens. Similarly, immunocompromised individuals, such as those with concurrent immunosuppressive viral infections, may be more susceptible to severe *Hepatozoon* infection.

PCR assay may be used to diagnose *Hepatozoon* infections. Observation of gamonts in leukocytes on blood smears is unreliable; however, demonstration of cysts in muscle biopsies may provide a definitive diagnosis.[15] Treatment regimens, including trimethoprim-sulfadiazine, pyrimethamine, and clindamycin and toltrazuril, have provided short-term benefits but relapses were common.

TICK PARALYSIS

Ticks also may cause disease directly by toxicosis. Tick paralysis results from injection of a salivary neurotoxin by the tick during feeding, inhibiting the release of acetylcholine at the neuromuscular junction. In North America, tick paralysis is most commonly caused by *Dermacentor* spp.; however, numerous other species have been reported to cause paralysis in humans, domestic animals, and wildlife. *Ixodes holocyolus* is an important cause of tick paralysis in Australia. Clinical signs of an ascending flaccid paralysis occur 2 to 9 days after tick attachment. Paralysis eventually may affect the diaphragm, resulting in respiratory failure and death. Among exotic carnivores, tick paralysis has been reported in canids, mustelids, and ursids.[1] Diagnosis is based on history of exposure to ticks, clinical signs, and resolution of clinical signs following removal of ticks. Treatment is primarily supportive and recovery occurs within 1 to 2 days of tick removal.

CONCLUSION

Ticks cause disease in exotic carnivores by the transmission of infectious diseases, tick paralysis, and direct effects. Although reports of clinical disease in exotic carnivores are uncommon, infections may contribute to a reduction in fitness. Coinfections and/or infection in immunocompromised individuals also may result in clinical disease. Many tick-borne diseases are zoonotic and exotic carnivores may serve as sentinels for infection in humans and domestic animals. Tick control is the primary means to prevent tick-borne diseases. Climate change, natural or artificial range expansion of ticks and intermediate hosts, and possibly wildfire suppression will likely continue to result in an increasing incidence of tick-borne diseases.

REFERENCES

1. Allen SA: In Samuel WM, Pybus MJ, Kocan AA, editors: Parasitic diseases of wild mammals, Ames, Iowa, 2001, Iowa State University Press, pp 72–106.
2. Angelakis E, Billeter SA, Breitschwerdt EB, et al: Potential for tick-borne bartonelloses. Emerg Infect Dis 16:385–391, 2010.
3. Birkenheuer AJ, Harms CA, Neel J, et al: The identification of a genetically unique piroplasma in North American river otters (*Lontra canadensis*). Parasitol 134:631–635, 2001.
4. Breitschwerdt EB: Obligate intracellular bacterial pathogens. In Ettinger SJ, Feldman EC, editors: Textbook of veterinary internal medicine, St. Louis, 2005, Elsevier Saunders, pp 631–636.
5. Breitschwerdt EB, Maggi RG, Chomel BB, et al: Bartonellosis: An emerging infectious disease of zoonotic importance to animals and human beings. J Vet Emerg Crit Care 20:8–30, 2010.
6. Brown RN, Burgess EC: Lyme borreliosis. In Williams ES, Barker IK, editors: Infectious diseases of wild mammals, Ames, Iowa, 2001, Iowa State University Press, pp 435–454.
7. Brown RN, Gabriel MW, Wengert GM, et al: Pathogens associated with fishers. In US Fish and Wildlife Service Final Report: Pathogens associated with fishers (*Martes pennanti*) and sympatric mesocarnivores in California, Yreka, California, 2008, US Fish and Wildlife Service, pp 2–48.
8. Chinnadurai SK, Birkenheuer AJ, Blanton HL, et al: Prevalence of selected vector-borne organisms and identification of *Bartonella* species DNA in North American river otters (*Lontra Canadensis*). J Wildl Dis 46:947–950, 2010.
9. Craig TM: Hepatozoon spp. and hepatozoonosis. In Samuel WM, Pybus MJ, Kocan AA, editors: Parasitic diseases of wild mammals, Ames, Iowa, 2001, Iowa State University Press, pp 462–468.
10. East ML, Wibbelt G, Lieckfeldt D, et al: A *Hepatozoon* species genetically distinct from H. canis infecting spotted hyenas in the Serengeti ecosystem, Tanzania. J Wildl Dis 44:45–52, 2008.
11. Ebel GD: Update on Powassan virus: Emergence of a North American tick-borne flavivirus. Ann Rev Entomol 55:95–110, 2010.
12. Haber MD, Tucker MD, Marr HS, et al: The detection of *Cytauxzoon felis* in apparently healthy free-roaming cats in the USA. Vet Parasitol 146:316–320, 2007.
13. Hartmann K, Greene CE: Diseases caused by systemic bacterial infections. In Ettinger SJ, Feldman EC, editors: Textbook of veterinary internal medicine, St. Louis, 2005, Elsevier Saunders, pp 616–631.
14. Harvey JW, Dunbar MR, Norton TM, et al: Laboratory findings in acute *Cytauxzoon felis* infection in cougars (*Puma concolor couguar*) in Florida. J Zoo Wildl Med 38:285–291, 2007.
15. Holman PJ, Snowden KF: Canine hepatozoonosis and babesiosis, and feline cytauxzoonosis. Vet Clin Small Anim 39:1035–1053, 2009.
16. Kjemtrup AM, Thomford J, Robinson T, et al: Phylogenetic relationships of human and wildlife piroplasm isolates in the western United States inferred from the 18S nuclear small subunit RNA gene. ParasitolOGY 120:487–493, 2000.
17. Kocan AA, Cummings CA, Panciera RJ, et al: Naturally occurring and experimentally transmitted *Hepatozoon americanum* in coyotes from Oklahoma. J Wildl Dis 36:149–153, 2000.
18. Lappin MR, Breitschwerdt EB, Jensen WA, et al: Molecular and serologic evidence of *Anaplasma phagocytophilum* infection in cats in North America. J Am Vet Med Assoc 225:893–896, 2004.
19. Molia S, Chomel BB, Kasten RW, et al: Prevalence of Bartonella infection in wild African lions (*Panthera leo*) and cheetahs (*Acinonyx jubatus*). Vet Microbiol 100:31–41, 2004.
20. Munson L, Terio KA, Kock R, et al: Climate extremes promote fatal co-infections during canine distemper epidemics in African lions. PLoS One 3:e2545, 2008.
21. Nelder MP, Reeves WK, Adler PH, et al: Ectoparasites and associated pathogens of free-roaming and captive animals in zoos of South Carolina. Vector Borne Zoonotic Dis 9:469–477, 2009.
22. Nicholson WL, Allen KE, McQuiston JH, et al: The increasing recognition of rickettsial pathogens in dogs and people. Trends Parasitol 26:205–212, 2010.
23. Penzhorn BL: Babesiosis of wild carnivores and ungulates. Vet Parasitol 138:11–21, 2006.
24. Pusterla N, Chang CC, Chomel BB, et al: Serologic and molecular evidence of *Ehrlichia* spp. in coyotes in California. J Wildl Dis 36:494–499, 2000.
25. Reichard MV, Meinkoth JH, Edwards AC, et al: Transmission of Cytauxzoon felis to a domestic cat by *Amblyomma americanum*. Vet Parasitol 161:110–115, 2009.
26. Rotstein DS, Taylor SK, Harvey JW, et al: Hematologic effects of cytauxzoonosis in Florida panthers and Texas cougars in Florida. J Wildl Dis 35:613–617, 1999.
27. Ruder M: Personal communication. 2010.
28. Shock BC, Murphy SM, Patton LL, et al: Distribution and prevalence of Cytauxzoon felis in bobcats (*Lynx rufus*), the natural reservoir, and other wild felids in thirteen states. Vet Parasitol, in press.
29. Stoebel K, Schoenberg A, Streich WJ: The seroepidemiology of Lyme borreliosis in zoo animals in Germany. Epidemiol Infect 131:975–983, 2003.
30. Sykes JE: Feline hemotropic mycoplasmas. J Vet Emerg Crit Care 20:62–69, 2010.
31. Willi B, Boretti FS, Baumgartner C, et al: Prevalence, risk factor analysis, and follow-up of infections caused by three feline hemoplasma species in cats in Switzerland. J Clin Microbiol 44:961–969, 2006.
32. Yabsley MJ: Natural history of *Ehrlichia chaffeensis*: Vertebrate hosts and tick vectors from the United States and evidence for endemic transmission in other countries. Vet Parasitol 167:136–148, 2010.
33. Yabsley MJ, Murphy SM, Cunningham MW: Molecular detection and characterization of *Cytauxzoon felis* and *Babesia* species in cougars from Florida. J Wildl Dis 42:366–374, 2006.
34. Yabsley MJ, Murphy SM, Luttrell MP, et al: Characterization of "*Candidatus Neoehrlichia lotoris*" (family Anaplasmataceae) from raccoons (*Procyon lotor*). Int J Syst Evol Microbiol 58:2794–2798, 2008.

CHAPTER 60

Aging in Large Felids

Lesa Longley

Aging is not a disease, but its effects may influence how an animal responds to its environment and any interventions undertaken. Published data pertaining specifically to large felids are sparse. Veterinary clinicians are frequently required to apply small (domestic) cat veterinary knowledge to treatment of their larger relatives. This chapter will endeavor to cover current specific knowledge relating to aging large felids as well as outlining common conditions affecting older domestic cats.

AGING

Many theories attempt to explain how organisms age—evolution, genetics, metabolic damage, cellular senescence, and toxin accumulation—and the outcome is likely to be a result of a combination of several of these. Factors such as genetics and environment appear to be involved in how individual animals age.

Phenotypic changes may be seen with aging—for example in pelage, skin, or body condition. Internal physiologic changes will be less obvious. In free-ranging animals, these alterations frequently result in the individual succumbing to disease, predation, or starvation. Captive animals are protected from these, but as our captive population of large felids ages, we see more degenerative age-related alterations. One study on morbidity in jaguars has shown an increase in both incidence and variability of disease processes with aging.[11]

HEALTH CARE IN CAPTIVE AGING FELIDS

Older animals are predisposed to many health problems, and close monitoring of their physical and mental condition is advised. Physical signs of illness may be specific, but vague signs such as reduced appetite or weight loss should not be ignored. For several conditions, such as dental disease, osteoarthritis, and chronic renal failure, early detection and treatment will significantly improve (and may prolong) quality of life for the animal.[26]

Guidelines have been published by the American Animal Hospital Association for senior domestic cats, and the general principles may be well applied to large felids.[2] Routine physical examinations should form part of preventive medicine protocols for geriatric patients. These may permit samples to be collected and noninvasive imaging techniques to be performed (Fig. 60-1). This baseline profile of the individual's health will identify problems and be useful when assessing pharmacologic safety.

Anesthesia is not without risk in any age of animal, but aged individuals are more likely to have underlying chronic disease or degenerative organ dysfunction that may increase the risk. Before administering anesthesia, consideration should be given to some factors, including health status, attitude, and body weight, that may affect how the individual will cope with the drugs and procedure (Table 60-1). Ideally, animals should be trained for conscious phlebotomy so that blood parameters may be assessed before anesthesia. Blood pressure should be monitored directly or indirectly during anesthesia, and deviations (usually hypotension) should be corrected with appropriate fluid administration.

COMMON DISEASES

Renal System and Urinary Tract Disease

Chronic renal disease is commonly reported as a significant reason for morbidity and mortality in nondomestic geriatric cats. Causes of chronic renal failure (CRF)

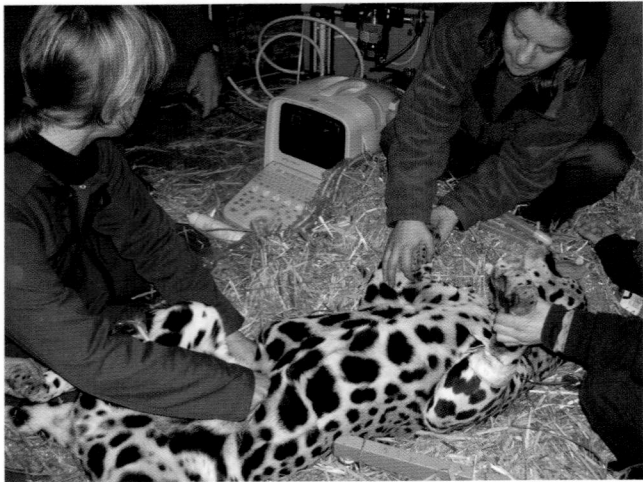

Figure 60-1

Ultrasonography is a useful diagnostic aid in health checks, such as in this 15-year-old jaguar *(Panthera onca)*.

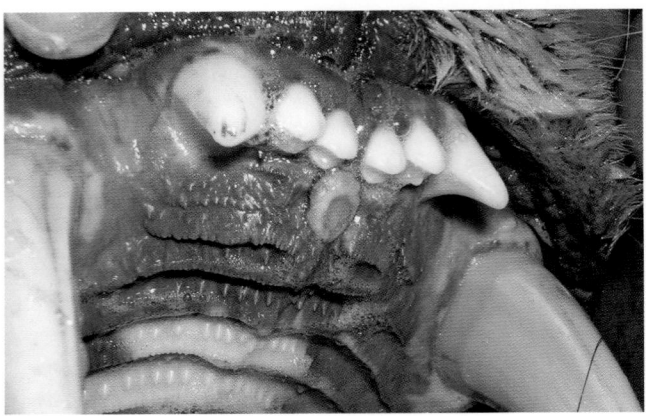

Figure 60-2

Differentials for oral lesions in aging large felids such as this lion *(Panthera leo)* include ulceration in renal failure and eosinophilic granulomas.

TABLE 60-1   Effects of Anesthetic Agents on Aged Felids

Drug or Combination	Comments
Atipamezole	Stimulates the central nervous system, so should be used cautiously in neurologic patients
Ketamine-midazolam	Good choice for debilitated animals, with wide safety margin; cardioprotective
Ketamine-midazolam-butorphanol	Recommended for debilitated or geriatric large felids
Medetomidine	Caution with preexisting cardiac conditions.
Medetomidine-butorphanol-midazolam	Fully reversible; useful for animals with renal or hepatic disease
Phenothiazines (e.g., acepromazine)	Depress physiologic functions (e.g., blood pressure and cardiovascular responses); should be avoided in animals with preexisting cardiovascular compromise
Propofol	May be useful alternative to isoflurane or ketamine for animals with renal or hepatic disease
Tiletamine-zolazepam	High safety margin and few cardiopulmonary side effects; not advised for tigers

Modified from Gunkel C, Lafortune M: Felids. In West G, Heard D, Caulkett N (eds): Zoo animal and wildlife immobilisation and anesthesia. Ames, Iowa, 2007, Blackwell, pp 443-457; and Lewis JCM: Veterinary considerations. Management guidelines for exotic cats. Bristol, England, 1991, Association of British Wild Animal Keepers, pp 118-145.

frequently include chronic pyelonephritis, glomerulo-sclerosis, or amyloidosis. Clinical signs include polyuria or polydipsia, reduced appetite, poor coat condition, salivation, oral ulceration (Fig. 60-2), weight loss, and vomiting. Wack[27] has outlined the diagnosis of CRF in detail; the mainstays of clinical pathology are blood and urine analysis. Renal changes are usually irreversible, with an extremely poor long-term prognosis.[16] Treatment is targeted to slow progression and alleviate clinical signs, and should combat the primary cause and common complications (Table 60-2).

Musculoskeletal Disease

One radiographic study has detected degenerative joint disease in 90% of domestic cats older than 12 years, with elbow joints most commonly (17%) affected.[8] Neurologic disease was associated with lumbosacral lesions. Osteoarthritis has been noted in *Panthera* species.[23] Lesions in large felids frequently affect vertebrae and elbow (Fig. 60-3) and stifle joints.[17] Animals housed on concrete appear to be more susceptible to the development of osteoarthritis.[26]

TABLE 60-2	Common Complications in Chronic Renal Failure[1,25]
Complication	Treatment
Anemia	Iron supplementation, erythropoietin and antacids (against gastric ulceration)
Bacterial urinary tract infection	Antibiotic therapy based on culture and sensitivity testing
Dehydration	Fluid therapy
Hyperphosphatemia	Correction of dehydration, low phosphate diets, and/or oral phosphate binders
Hypokalemia	Renal diets* and potassium supplementation
Metabolic acidosis	Correction of dehydration, renal diets, and in severe cases bicarbonate therapy
Nausea and vomiting	Antacids, with H2 blockers such as famotidine
Proteinuria	Angiotensin-converting enzyme (ACE) inhibitor therapy, such as benazepril
Systemic hypertension	Amlodipine and/or benazepril

*Large felids will not consume 100% commercial renal diet, but addition of such food as part of the diet is beneficial.

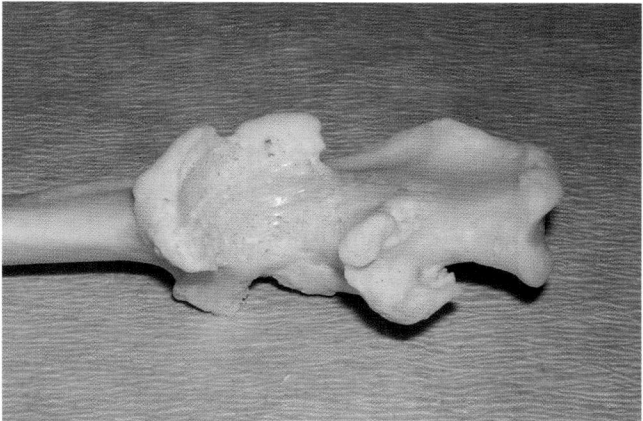

Figure 60-3

Osteoarthritis in a 15-year-old clouded leopard *(Neofelis nebulosa)*, with osteophytes, eburnation, and grooving of the proximal ulna.

Degenerative spinal disease in captive large felids is frequently associated with clinical signs, such as reduced activity, chronic intermittent hind limb paresis, and ataxia, becoming apparent at 10 to 19 years of age.[14] Antemortem diagnosis is possible using radiography. Lesions may include intervertebral disc mineralization or herniation, spondylosis, and spinal cord damage.

The aim of treatment for chronic age-related skeletal conditions is to optimize the individual's quality of life. Owston and colleagues[20] have recommended meloxicam and tramadol for the long-term treatment of chronic pain in nondomestic felids. Contraindications for the use of nonsteroidal anti-inflammatory drugs (NSAIDs) in aged animals include renal or hepatic insufficiency, dehydration, hypotension, conditions affecting circulatory volume (such as congestive heart failure or ascites), moderate or severe pulmonary disease, and gastric ulceration. Side effects include gastrointestinal ulcerations, nephropathies, and impaired coagulation.[6] Adverse effects may be minimized if the lowest effective dose is ascertained and by using lower doses with drug combinations with different pharmacologic action.[21] Weight reduction, nutritional supplements, and environmental manipulation may also alleviate discomfort.[8,24]

Reproductive

Most free-ranging nondomestic species die before the cessation of reproduction. Captive animals are more likely to survive beyond this point, and many pathologic conditions develop beyond the age of normal reproductivity. Older captive felids have a high prevalence of leiomyomas and leiomyosarcomas.[15]

Progestogen contraceptives, such as melengestrol acetate(MGA)–impregnated Silastic implants, are associated with progressive uterine growth in captive nondomestic felids, and are a risk factor for endometrial hyperplasia, uterine carcinomas or mammary neoplasia, pyometra, or ovarian cysts (see Chapter 2). Repeated sterile matings and pseudopregnancies result in the same uterine changes. Mammary carcinomata in felids rapidly metastasize to lymph nodes, lung, and liver.[9] These animals have a poor prognosis. Ovariectomy appears to protect against mammary carcinomas, but not benign mammary tumors. Because of the high risk of uterine and mammary neoplasia in felids with regular progestogen administration, these individuals should be regularly assessed clinically.

Cardiovascular and Respiratory Disorders

Cardiorespiratory disorders are particularly important if an older animal is to be anesthetized. Airway disorders such as chronic bronchial disease or pulmonary neoplasia may be significant problems in older animals. A variety of cardiac problems are reported in older domestic cats, including myocardial and degenerative valvular disease. Systemic diseases frequently show cardiopulmonary manifestations; feline hypertension is commonly seen associated with hyperthyroidism and chronic renal disease in domestic cats.

Neurologic Disorders

Senescent animals are physiologically and behaviorally susceptible to environmental stressors.[12] Animal behavior, in particular personality, has been shown to change with age in large felids—for example, as in snow leopards.[4] Behavioral abnormalities have been described in older jaguars.[11] Cognitive dysfunction associated with aging is well documented in domestic cats, with more than 50% older than 15 years of age having behavioral changes.[7,19] Beta-amyloid and abnormalities in tau phosphorylation have been demonstrated in brains from aged large felids.

Leukoencephalopathy in cheetahs is a slowly progressing condition, with degeneration and necrosis of the cerebral cortical white matter.[26] Most animals affected are older than 10 years.[22] This condition appears to be irreversible and treatment is supportive only.

Advanced imaging techniques, such as magnetic resonance imaging (MRI), may be useful to diagnose neurologic conditions antemortem, but often the diagnosis is made histologically postmortem.

Neoplasia

Neoplasia is frequently associated with aging animals.[20] Some benign conditions may progress to malignancy—for example, viral papillomatosis and squamous cell carcinoma in snow leopards.

Nutritional Disorders

Factors that predispose obesity in captive animals include genetics, lack of physical activity, diet, and female contraception.[5,16,26] Obesity exacerbates pressure on joints and degenerative musculoskeletal disease in aging individuals, and also predisposes to neoplasia and metabolic derangements (e.g., the development of

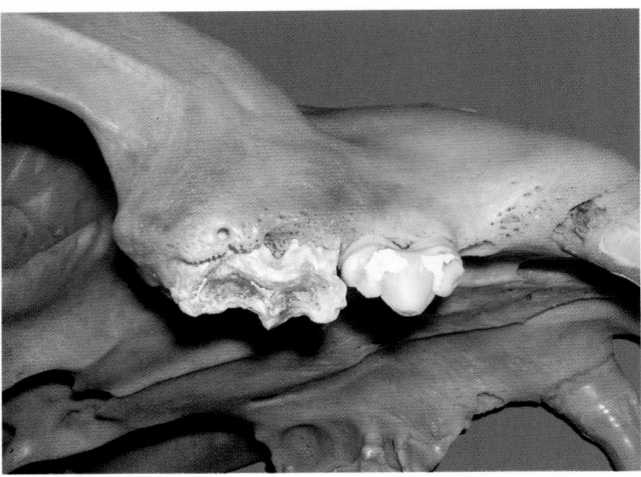

Figure 60-4

Dental fracture and calculus in a prepared skull from a 22-year-old captive lion *(Panthera leo)*.

diabetes or hepatic lipidosis). Some conditions may be avoided or reduced with appropriate nutrition. Food restriction will result in a lower incidence of osteoarthritis by reducing body weight and thus wear and tear of joints. Protein and phosphate restrictions increase the median survival time of cats with chronic renal disease.

Dental Disease

Dental disease is a significant cause of morbidity in older cats. Aged captive large felids are more likely to develop dental calculus and abscesses (Fig. 60-4) compared with their free-ranging counterparts, which frequently have dental attrition and fractures.[18]

Other Conditions

One may expect to see multiple organ system disease, as in domestic cats, in large felids. Thyroid adenocarcinomas have been detected in large felids postmortem, but to date there are no published reports of diagnosed hyperthyroidism in these species.

The gastrointestinal tract in older domestic cats has been shown to undergo various changes, with common disorders predominantly inflammatory in nature.[13] Several conditions result in chronic hepatic disease in nondomestic felids, such as neoplasia, cirrhosis, and toxic degeneration.[16] Treatment is supportive and the prognosis is often poor.

Ocular disease is frequent in aging patients—often due to chronic disease, neoplasia, degeneration, or age-related systemic diseases.[3] Hypertension often results in retinal detachment or hemorrhage.[10] Insular amyloidosis, which may be associated with type II diabetes, has been reported in several species of older nondomestic felids (older than 10 years). Oral eosinophilic granulomas have been reported in older tigers (8 to 16 years).[25]

In general, infectious disease is more commonly seen in younger, less immunocompetent animals. A few exceptions exist, with disease affecting adult animals more severely than younger individuals. Some diseases develop over several years and pathology and clinical signs are not present until animals are older—for example, feline spongiform encephalopathy.[22]

CONCLUSION

An increase in expected longevity of nondomestic felids in captivity heralds the onset of a new era of degenerative conditions. Care of these animals should be tailored to identify and treat these disorders to reduce morbidity and mortality.

REFERENCES

1. Caney S: Optimal care in dealing with feline chronic kidney disease. Vet Times 40:14–15, 2010.
2. Epstein M, Kuehn NF, Landsberg G, et al: Senior Care Guidelines Task Force, AAHA: AAHA senior care guidelines for dogs and cats. J Am Anim Hosp Assoc 41:1–11, 2005.
3. Fischer CA: Geriatric ophthalmology. Vet Clin North Am Small Anim Pract 19:103–123, 1989.
4. Gartner MC, Powell D: Personal communication, 2010.
5. German AJ: The growing problem of obesity in dogs and cats. J Nutr 136(Suppl 7):1940S-1946S, 2006.
6. Gunkel C, Lafortune M: Felids. In West G, Heard D, Caulkett N, editors: Zoo animal and wildlife immobilisation and anesthesia, Ames, Iowa, 2007, Blackwell, pp 443–457.
7. Gunn-Moore D, Moffat K, Christie LA, Head E: Cognitive dysfunction and the neurobiology of aging in cats. J Small Anim Pract 48:546–553, 2007.
8. Hardie EM, S. C. Roe SC, Martin FR: Radiographic evidence of degenerative joint disease in geriatric cats: 100 cases (1994–1997). J Am Vet Med Assoc 220:628–632, 2002.
9. Harrenstein LM, Munson L, Seal US, et al: Mammary cancer in captive wild felids and risk factors for its development: A retrospective study of the clinical behavior of 31 cases. J Zoo WildL Med 27:468–476, 1996.
10. Henik RA: Systemic hypertension and its management. Vet Clin North Am Small Anim Pract 27:1355–1372, 1997.
11. Hope K, Deem SL: A retrospective study of morbidity and mortality of captive North American jaguars: 1982–2002. (http://si-pddr.si.edu/dspace/bitstream/10088/900/1/Hope2006.pdf).
12. Hosey G, Melfi V, Pankhurst S: Housing and husbandry. In Hosey G, Melfi V, Pankhurst S, editors: Zoo animals: Behaviour, management, and welfare, Oxford, 2009, Oxford University Press, pp 168–218.
13. Jergens AE: Gastrointestinal disease and its management. Vet Clin North Am Small Anim Pract 27:1373–1402, 1997.
14. Kolmstetter C, Munson L, Ramsay EC: Degenerative spinal disease in large felids. J Zoo Wildl Med 31:15–19, 2000.
15. Langan JN, Dahill EM: Oncology in non-domestic species, 2002 (http://www.vin.com/proceedings/Proceedings.plx?CID=WSAVA 2002&Category=683&PID=4091&O=Generic).
16. Lewis JCM: Veterinary considerations. Management guidelines for exotic cats, Bristol, England, 1991, Association of British Wild Animal Keepers, pp 118–145.
17. Longley L: Assessment of skeletal aging in captive large felids. In Proceedings of the American Association of Zoo Veterinarians, 2006, Tampa, Florida, 2006, American Association of Zoo Veterinarians, pp 133.
18. Longley L, Kitchener A, et al: Gross dental pathology in free-ranging and captive lions (Panthera leo). In Proceedings of the 43rd International Symposium, Leibniz Institute for Zoo and Wildlife Research (IZW), Berlin. Edinburgh, 2007, p 213.
19. Deleted in proofs.
20. Owston MA, Ramsay EC, Rotstein DS: Incidence of neoplasia in a colony of captive felids at the Knoxville Zoological Gardens, 1979 to 2003. J Zoo Wildl Med 39:608–613, 2008.
21. Ramsay EC: Use of analgesics in exotic felids. In Fowler ME, Miller RE, editors: Zoo and wild animal medicine: Current therapy, ed 6, St Louis, 2008, WB Saunders, pp 289–293.
22. Robert N: Neurologic disorders in cheetahs and snow leopards. In Fowler ME, Miller RE, editors: Zoo and wild animal medicine: Current therapy, ed 6, St Louis, 2008, WB Saunders, pp 265–271.
23. Rothschild BM, Rothschild C, Woods RJ: Inflammatory arthritis in large cats: An expanded spectrum of spondyloarthropathy. J Zoo Wildl Med 29:279–284, 1998.
24. Stringfield CE, Wynne JE: Nutraceutical chondroprotectives and their use in osteoarthritis in zoo animals. In Proceedings of the American Association of Zoo Veterinarians, 1999.
25. Sykes JM, Garner MM, Greer LL, et al: Oral eosinophilic granulomas in tigers (Panthera tigris): A collection of four cases. In Proceedings of the AAZV, AAWV, WDA Joint Conference, 2004.
26. Wack RF: Felidae. In Fowler ME, Miller RE, editors: Zoo and wild animal medicine, ed 5, St. Louis, 2003, Elsevier Science, pp 491–501.
27. Wack RF: Treatment of chronic renal failure in nondomestic felids. In Fowler ME, Miller RE, editors: Zoo and wild animal medicine: Current therapy, ed 6, St Louis, 2008, WB Saunders, pp 462–465.

CHAPTER 61

Stargazing in Lions

Christian J. Wenker and Nadia Robert

Stargazing and related neurologic signs in lions is a well-known syndrome. The name of the disease relates to the characteristic attitude with the lion's head pulled backward, giving the impression that the animal is staring at the sky. It is understood that the proliferation of cranial bones with resulting compression of brain tissue, cause this clinical presentation. Recent reports have been limited to young and adolescent captive African lions (Panthera leo) and hypovitaminosis A has been proposed as the cause. There is no gender predilection. Interestingly, there are no reports in Asian lions and there are only rare historical reports of the condition in a 10-month-old tiger (Panthera tigris)[6] and in leopards.[8] It has to be clarified that stargazing is only one of a variety of neurologic signs of a vestibular disorder. The description is misleading and is not diagnostic for the syndrome. In most cases, stargazing was not even reported. It may also be discrete, absent, or hidden by other neurologic symptoms. Different terms are used for the same condition, such as Chiari I–like malformation or cerebellar herniation.* Arnold-Chiari malformation in humans and calves is almost always associated with spina bifida and/or a protruding meningomyelocele. These features were not found in affected lions and therefore we suggest to use the term with caution or to describe it as an Arnold-Chiari–like disorder when discussing the stargazing syndrome of lions.[4]

This chapter summarizes the current state of knowledge regarding pathogenesis, diagnosis, treatment, and prevention of the disease. Clinical observations and pathology are based on a recent case that we diagnosed, which is compared with relevant literature reports.

*References 1, 3, 10, 12, 15, and 19.

CLINICAL SIGNS

In recent cases, clinical signs were first observed in subadult lions at the age of 9 to 14 months. However, in rare cases, signs were already detected at the age of 2 months. Early detection of clinical signs is important because prognosis seems to be better at the beginning of the growing phase, when bone formation is more dynamic and may respond to therapy. Various occurrence histories have been reported in the literature, such as littermates of affected individuals that grew up normally, or whole litters affected to a higher or lesser extent, or with varying ages at the beginning. In the case that we diagnosed, the female (lion no. 1) of a litter of two was affected, with the first signs observed at the age of 12 months, whereas the male littermate (lion no. 2) grew up normally. A variety of neurologic signs, in most cases a combination of two to five signs, were reported. The signs may be summarized as the neuroanatomic expression of a peripheral or central vestibular disorder. Slow progression of the signs over weeks is a consistent feature. It is recommended to perform repeated video recording of the affected animal to allow for follow-up. This may also serve as a basis for discussion for the neurologist and helps locate the origin of the signs within the central or peripheral nervous system.

Initial signs include ataxia, lack of coordination, and difficulties in negotiating obstacles. Our first observation of signs in the affected lion was the sudden difficulty in jumping through a gate that had a 50-cm step, which connects the indoor and the outdoor enclosure. The animal fell back and it took a second attempt to cross this barrier finally. During the course of the disease, the affected animal eats and drinks normally, but takes smaller quantities, and therefore often appears smaller than other nonaffected members of the litter. Later, progressive ataxia, mild head tilt and cycling behavior (both often reported as left-sided), stargazing, nystagmus, fine head tremor, staring glare, and nonresponsiveness to new objects (neither playing nor defense behavior) are observed. At this stage, the affected lion often becomes lethargic and depressed. We observed that the ataxic signs worsened when the animal was excited, such as when the animal was separated from the group or when blow-darted. In single cases, abnormal vocalization, hypersalivation, and tongue protrusion were reported. We were able to test pupillary light reflexes, using a pocket lamp at a few centimeters' distance through the cage bars, and obtained a normal response. Late signs of the disease include blindness, convulsions, inability to stand, rolling over, recumbency, and death.*

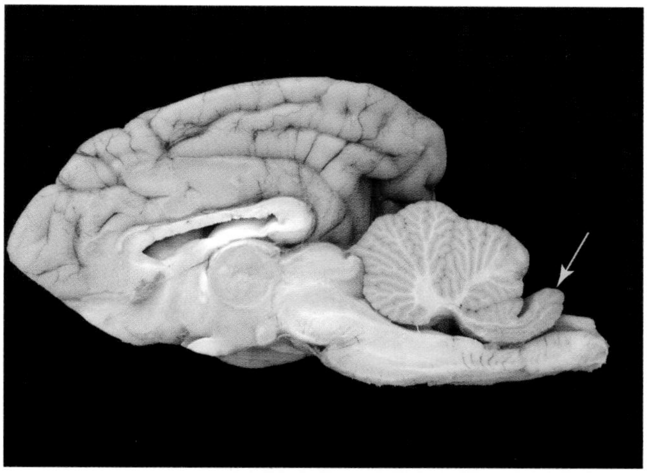

Figure 61-1

CT scan, sagittal view, showing the thickened tentorium cerebelli and occipital bones *(arrow)*. *(Courtesy Institute for Forensic Medicine, University of Bern, Switzerland.)*

DIAGNOSIS AND DIFFERENTIAL DIAGNOSES

After careful evaluation of the clinical symptoms, the neuroanatomic localization should be investigated. It is important to plan the diagnostic procedures carefully that will be performed during general anesthesia. A complete physical and neurologic examination, including blood and cerebrospinal fluid sampling, should be performed, taking samples for virology, microbiology, and parasitology, carrying out an examination with an otoscope, and having imaging techniques prepared (radiography, ultrasound) or organized (e.g., computed tomography [CT], magnetic resonance imaging [MRI]). Several differential diagnoses have to be considered and a rule-out protocol should be determined for trauma, infection (e.g., feline coronavirus, feline immunodeficiency virus, canine distemper), otitis media and/or interna, or a space-occupying process that compromises the central nervous system (e.g., hematoma, abscess, neoplasia, pathologic bone proliferation, congenital anomaly).

A complete feline hematology and serum chemistry panel, determination of serum vitamin A concentration, feline leukemia virus and feline coronavirus serology, and feline immunodeficiency virus (FIV) Western blot test should be carried out. Serology for *Toxoplasma gondii*, *Ehrlichia canis*, Lyme disease, and Rocky Mountain spotted fever antibodies may be added. Cerebrospinal fluid examination includes cell count and differentiation, protein determination, and polymerase chain reaction (PCR) assay for canine distemper. Ultrasound-guided liver biopsy may be used to measure

hepatic vitamin A concentration. Although reference ranges for serum or hepatic vitamin A concentrations have not been established for lions, they may be compared with values of most carnivores, including those of domestic cats. A detailed discussion on serum vitamin A concentrations in lions is presented in the next section of this chapter. Postmortem hepatic vitamin A concentration of the case that we observed was 0.34 µg/g. This is far lower than the hepatic vitamin A concentration of a single wild lion of 6075 µg/g, or references from two earlier postmortem samples from our zoo, 4060 µg/g and 907 µg/g, respectively.

For the detection of pathologic cranial bone thickening, specifically of the os tentorium cerebelli (Fig. 61-1), CT investigation is necessary. Both plain and contrast medium scans are useful. Alterations of brain tissue, such as the compression of the cerebellum, including herniation of the caudal folia through the foramen magnum occipitalis, is diagnostic for the syndrome and best visualized using sagittal MRI scans (Fig. 61-2). An objective interpretation of osseous cranial structures may be achieved by measuring the maximum diameter of the vitreous body of the eye and relating it to the thickest part of the occipital bone and os tentorium cerebelli.[7] Hyperintensity of sagittal images in the spinal cord consistent with syringohydromyelia and secondary enlargement of the lateral ventricles caused by stasis of cerebrospinal fluid were additional MRI findings in recent reports.[10,20]

*References 1-3, 7, 9-11, 15, 16, 19, and 20.

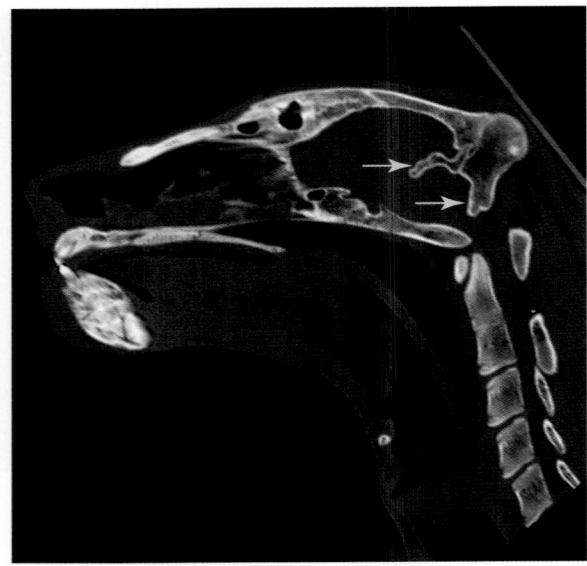

Figure 61-2

Sagittal MRI scan showing compression of the cerebellum, with herniation of the caudal cerebellar folia through the foramen magnum occipitalis *(top arrow).* The hyperintense area in the cervical spinal cord indicates syringomyelia *(bottom arrow). (Courtesy Institute for Forensic Medicine, University of Bern, Switzerland.)*

SERUM VITAMIN A CONCENTRATIONS IN LIONS

The accuracy of serum vitamin A (retinol) concentration certainly is lower than the value of the concentration in the liver, which is the reservoir organ for vitamin A. However, tissue analysis is impractical for routine clinical application in zoo animals and therefore serum values may serve as controls for vitamin A status or support a diagnosis of vitamin A deficiency. Table 61-1 shows the serum retinol concentrations of an affected lion cub (lion no. 1) before and after the appearance of the first clinical signs and before and after therapeutic supplementation. The results are compared with the concentrations from nonaffected pack mates and littermates, as well as individual concentrations from subadult free-ranging lions at capture and later as adults in captivity. Finally, serum samples from subadult and adult captive lions from the same zoo and from four other institutions referenced in the literature have been summarized as mean values.[5] Lion no. 1, which developed clinical signs of stargazing at the age of 12 months, showed the lowest serum retinol concentration at that time (37.4 μg/liter). This finding was confirmed by extremely low liver vitamin A values at necropsy (0.34 μg/g). Its littermate, lion no. 2, raised under

identical conditions, had a serum retinol concentration (122 μg/liter) that was approximately three times higher. Therefore, an individual problem, such as a congenital deficiency of specific lipoproteins, which are needed for endogenous vitamin A transport, may be theorized. After repeated parenteral vitamin A supplementation, lion no. 1 showed only a slightly increased retinol concentration (60.1 μg/liter), which indicates that the influence of parenteral vitamin A supplementation is limited in the short term. When compared with the reference values from the same institution before 1998, all concentrations measured in the current lion pack (nos. 1 to 4, 6, and 7) were low. Concentrations of free-ranging subadult lions at capture (nos. 3 to 5), which reflected true reference values from the natural availability of whole-prey diets, were also low when compared with those concentrations at the same zoo and four other zoos. They may reflect long-term vitamin A supplementation in a captive situation. We have concluded that serum retinol concentrations below 60 μg/liter are critical for the development of stargazing in growing lions, and values higher than 90 μg/liter are adequate and should be achieved by dietary measures in captivity.

CAUSE AND PATHOGENESIS

Although the stargazing syndrome in lions has been known for a long time, with the first cases described in two young lions with paraplegia, head tilts, and tremor,[17] the exact cause is still uncertain. The disease was first ascribed to vitamin B deficiency.[14] Later, the hypothesis of a lack of vitamin A was proposed, based on the empirical and experimental data obtained from puppies, calves, and pigs, although the effects of vitamin A on bone metabolism is incompletely understood. It has been suggested that the bony changes result from low vitamin A stores during growth and may not be seen when hypovitaminosis A occurs later in life. A dam with deficient vitamin A will have vitamin A–deficient milk, which may predispose her young to this syndrome. Vitamin A is reported to stimulate the activity of osteoclasts via an unknown mechanism, causing them to increase their acid phosphatase content and resorb bone. The underlying skeletal abnormality involves defective remodeling of membranous bone— development of bone tissue within connective tissue, as in the skull—presumably caused by the stimulatory effect of vitamin A on osteoclastic activity. In the cranium of vitamin A–deficient animals, there is inadequate resorption of endosteal bone, and consequently

TABLE 61-1	Serum Vitamin A Levels of Free-Ranging and Captive Lions at the Basel Zoo*		
Lion	Age	Vitamin A (μg/liter)	Remarks
No. 1, female, captive-born, Basel Zoo	6 mo	57.6	Radiographic lameness
	6.5 mo	40.4	Radiographic lameness
Developed ataxia within 12 mo	12 mo	37.4	Stargazing MRI scan
	13 mo	60.1	Euthanasia after 1 mo of parenteral vitamin A supplementation; liver vitamin A level at necropsy = 0.34 μg/g
No. 2, male (littermate of no. 1), captive-born, Basel Zoo	14 mo	122.0	Checkup
No. 3, female (mother of no. 1 and 2)			
Free-ranging†	10 mo‡	96.2	Sample taken at capture
Captive-born, Basel Zoo	5.5 yr‡	122.4	Implant for contraception
No. 4, female			
Free-ranging†	14 mo‡	109.0	Sample taken at capture
Captive-born, Basel Zoo	6 yr‡	54.2	Implant for contraception
No. 5, male, free-ranging	11 mo‡	93.5	Sample taken at capture
No. 6, male, captive-born, Basel Zoo	18 mo	61.6	Crating for transfer
No. 7, female, captive-born, Basel Zoo	18 mo	62.6	Crating for transfer
Values from 15 subadult and adult captive lions, Basel Zoo, 1987-1998 (mean ± SD)		163.8 ± 31.75	Miscellaneous immobilizations
Values from 14 lions, 1-17 yr old, from four U.S. zoos (mean ± SD)[5]		130.0 ± 33.0	

*Compared with reference levels from the Basel Zoo and four other zoos.
†National Park, South Africa.
‡Age estimated.

there is an asynchrony between the developing central nervous system (CNS) and the bones of the skull and spinal column, causing secondary changes in the CNS, with a variety of nervous signs. In the cranium, the defect is particularly severe in the bones of the caudal fossa and the cerebellum may herniate into the foramen magnum. In puppies with vitamin A deficiency, deafness is a prominent sign because of changes in the internal auditory meatus, whereas affected calves and pigs develop blindness caused by narrowing of the optic foramina and compression of the optic nerves. However, deafness has never been reported in affected lions and blindness only rarely. The basis for these variations among species is unclear, but the lesions are modified according to the severity of the deficiency and the stage of skeletal growth. Membranous bones in other locations, including the periosteal surface of the long bones, may also be affected and develop a coarse profile, but endochondral bone, as in the growth of the length of long bones, with gradual replacement of cartilage by bone tissue, does not appear to be directly influenced by vitamin A deficiency. Another proposed

mechanism causing clinical nervous signs might be related to hydrocephalus mainly caused by impaired absorption of cerebrospinal fluid into the blood, a process that occurs in the arachnoid villi. The villi are located in the tentorium cerebelli, which is affected by the thickening that occurs in the dura mater in vitamin A deficiency. Hypersecretion of cerebrospinal fluid also contributes to the development of hydrocephalus.[18] This hypothesis, based on vitamin A deficiency, has been reinforced by the fact that improvement and resolution of signs were achieved in young cubs through parenteral vitamin A supplementation.[7]

This vitamin A assumption was, however, refuted in a study done on 149 cases of affected lions and leopards in France.[8] The clinical signs appeared between day 1 and 2 years after birth, with a maximum peak between 3 and 10 months. In all cases, herniation of the cerebellar vermis through the foramen magnum was observed, but thickening of the occipital bone was present in only 50% of cases, contrary to the theory of a primary osseous lesion. Furthermore, similar cerebellar herniation was also observed in fetuses and in healthy adult lions. A pedigree analysis has failed to show a primary genetic problem, but an infectious viral cause has been proposed based on epidemiologic considerations and the observation of cytopathogenic effect on cell cultures from affected animals.

TREATMENT

Therapeutic measures include conservative and surgical treatment or a combination of both. Glucocorticoids are used to reduce the swelling or edema of brain tissue and neurologic signs may improve because of decompression and pain relief. The typical initial dose of dexamethasone is 2 to 3 mg/kg/day, which may later be reduced to 0.2 mg/kg/day. Alternatively, prednisone was used at a dosage of 1 mg/kg/day for 3 weeks, which was later reduced by 50%.[16] In addition, vitamin A should be administered. Reported dosages vary from 2000 IU/kg/wk IM for 4 weeks and then every 2 weeks for four more doses,[7] up to 5000 IU/kg/daily PO, until full adult size is reached.[10] It is recommended to start with a parenteral application because a disorder of enteral absorption of vitamin A may be present. Hartley and colleagues[7] have reported that all of the seven mildly affected cubs showed some improvement within 2 weeks and all clinical signs had disappeared after 3 months, using only vitamin A supplementation. The beneficial effect of conservative treatment was also initially reported in other cases. However, in most reports, there was consistent recurrence of neurologic signs and further deterioration. It is assumed that younger and/or mildly affected animals at an age when the cranial bones start to grow fast may respond better to a conservative approach. Recently, successful suboccipital craniectomy and laminectomy were performed in two cases to achieve surgical decompression of the caudal fossa, and the clinical signs disappeared quickly.[10,16] Surgical decompression, together with adequate preoperative and postoperative medical care, may be the only way to cure this condition. Individuals in an advanced state of disease should be euthanized immediately for animal-welfare reasons and submitted for postmortem examination.

NECROPSY AND HISTOPATHOLOGY

The most obvious lesion reported in all cases of lions with similar signs is the severe thickening of the osseum tentorium cerebelli and of the occipital bone, leading to crowding of the caudal fossa and subsequent herniation of caudal cerebellar folia through the foramen magnum occipitalis (Fig. 61-3). Closer

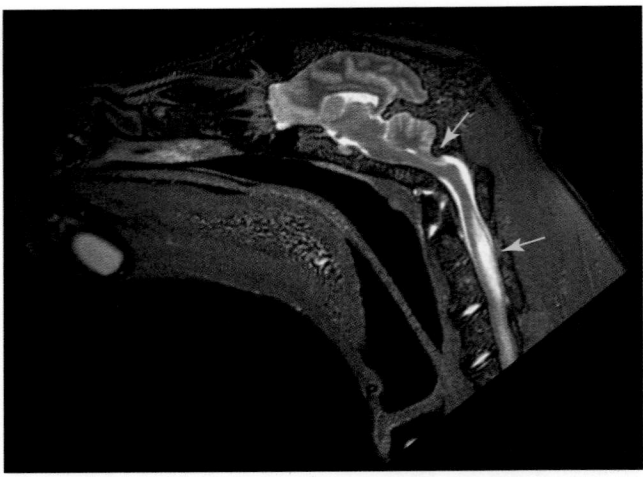

Figure 61-3

Sagittal midline section of the brain showing the herniated caudal cerebellar folia *(arrows)*.

inspection of the skull reveals increased thickness of all bones composing the brain case as well as thickened mandibular bones. Dilation of the lateral ventricles, as well as syringomyelia of the cervical spinal cord have also been observed. A few reports have also described fragile teeth, with thin enamel.*

Histopathologic lesions of the bones are characterized by thickened, poorly remodeled bone tissue caused by a shift from compact to cancellous bone. Examination of the tentorium cerebelli reveals thickening, mostly caused by the growth of new periosteal woven bone containing retained cartilaginous cores. Histologic lesions of the nervous tissue are mostly confined to the herniated cerebellar folia, compressed brainstem, and cervical spinal cord. Cerebellar lesions include thinning and rarefaction of the molecular layer, loss of Purkinje cells, granular cells associated with proliferation of Bergmann's glia, and disseminated punctate hemorrhages. Varying degrees of malacia and wallerian degeneration characterized by dilated myelin sheaths, axonal swelling (spheroids), and digesting chambers associated with astrogliosis may be observed in the white matter of the compressed cerebellar folia, medulla oblongata, and different tracts of the cervical spinal cord. Edema and the formation of syringomyelia are mostly observed in the dorsal tract of the cervical spinal cord. Meningeal lymphoplasmacytic infiltration, fibroplasia, and hemorrhages may also be observed focally in these compressed regions.

*References 1-3, 7, 11-13, 15, 19, and 20.

PREVENTION

Hypovitaminosis A is assumed to cause the skull bones to become thicker, which is responsible for the cerebellar compression of stargazing lions. Therefore, the diets of captive African lions, especially of growing cubs, need careful veterinary evaluation and supervision of the diet for adequate vitamin A content. Several case reports of stargazing lions have mentioned a history of meat or beef on the bone diets without supplementation. However, other reports have noted daily or weekly multivitamin supplements without indicating exact quantities.

Meat on the bone feeding is the most frequent diet given to the lions in our institution. Every ration includes a mineral and vitamin supplement in powder form containing 91,000 IU/kg of vitamin A. This supplement is added at a dosage of 5% to the total food ration. The keepers were made aware of the need to supplement minerals and vitamins, and were trained to provide sufficient supplementation—for example, by weighing samples, such as 50 g of supplement/kg of food, which is equivalent to 4550 IU vitamin A/kg of food. The powder supplement is applied to deep cuts in the meat, so that it cannot easily fall off. African wild dogs, wolves, snow leopards, cheetahs, and lions, including a healthy littermate of an affected lion, were raised in the zoo in the last decade without any problems and, to the best of our knowledge, there was no change in feeding regimen, technique, or staff. Usually, there are two irregular fasting days per week in the feeding management of the lion group. Additionally, freshly killed whole prey, such as rats, chicken, and hoofstock from the zoo, including their livers, which are rich in vitamin A, are fed at weekly or monthly intervals. Despite all these precautions, a fatal case of a stargazing lion occurred. We therefore find it difficult to believe that a lack of vitamin A intake is the sole cause in this case and other factors must be considered. Pathologic alterations in vitamin A absorption or metabolism have to be considered in individual cases. As opposed to the digestion of herbivores, vitamin A metabolism from carotene is not important because the enzyme carotenase is absent in felids. However, no morphologic signs of endogenous alterations have so far been found in necropsies. Further studies of vitamin A digestion, absorption, and metabolism in lions are required and need to be compared with those made in other felid species.

Practical feeding techniques, such as group feeding and their associated feeding-related social interactions, may be important because, under such conditions, the exact individual intake of supplemented food cannot be determined. Additional preventive measures in addition to supplementation include an increased quantity of whole-prey food or bovine liver on a weekly basis. Daily liver feeding is not recommended because it could result in diarrhea or hypervitaminosis A.

REFERENCES

1. Baker JR, Lyon DG: Skull malformation and cerebellar herniation in captive African lions. Vet Rec 100:154–156, 1977.
2. Bartsch RC, Imes GD, Smit JPJ: Vitamin a deficiency in the captive African lion cub *Panthera leo*. Onderstepoort J Vet Res 42:43–54, 1975.
3. Chandra SAM, Papendick RE, Schumacher J, et al: Cerebellar herniation in captive lions *(Panthera leo)*. J Vet Diagn Invest 11:465–468, 1999.
4. Chandra S: Letter to the editor concerning Arnold-Chiari malformation in a captive African lion cub. J Wildl Dis 36:190–191, 2000.
5. Crissey SD, Ange KD, Jacobson KL, et al: Serum concentrations of lipids, vitamin D metabolites, retinol, retinyl esters, tocopherols and selected carotenoids in twelve captive wild felid species at four zoos. J Nutr 133:160–166, 2003.
6. Demmel U: [Über Veränderungen am Schädel eines Tigers *(Panthera tigris* L.) bei therapieresistenten Paresen der Hintergliedmassen.] Zool Gart 31:327–336, 1965.
7. Hartley MP, Kirberger RM, Haagenson M, et al: Diagnosis of suspected hypovitaminosis a using magnetic resonance imaging in "African lions" *(Panthera leo)*. J South Afr Vet Assoc 76:132–137, 2005.
8. Leclerc-Cassan M: [La maladie des étoiles. Etude clinique et recherche étiologique.] Thèse de l'Université Paris, VII, 1982.
9. Maratea KA, Hooser SB, Ramos-Vara JA: Degenerative myelopathy and vitamin a deficiency in a young black-maned lion *(Panthera leo)*. J Vet Diagn Invest 18:608–611, 2006.
10. McCain S, Souza M, Ramsay E, et al: Diagnosis and surgical treatment of a Chiari I–like malformation in an African lion *(Panthera leo)*. J Zoo Wildl Med 39:421–427, 2008.
11. O'Sullivan BM, Mayo FD, Hartley WJ: Neurologic lesions in young captive lions associated with vitamin A deficiency. Austral Vet J 53:187–189, 1977.
12. Papendick R, Schumacher J, Wollenmann P: Arnold-Chiari-like malformation in a litter of lion cubs *(Panthera leo)*. Vet Pathol 32:578, 1995.
13. Perrin-Raybaud F, Guillon JC, Wyers M: [Contribution à l'étude de la "Maladie des Etoiles" du lion à propos de 4 observations.] Rec Med Vet 149:739–752, 1973.
14. Scheunert A: [Die Sternguckerkrankheit junger Löwen—eine Vitamin-B$_1$-Avitaminose.] Zool Gart 6:182–187, 1933.
15. Shamir MH, Horowitz IH, Yakobson B, et al: Arnold-Chiari malformation in a captive African lion cub. J Wildl Dis 34:661–666, 1998.
16. Shamir MH, Shilo Y, Fridman A, et al: Sub-occipital craniectomy in a lion *(Panthera leo)* with occipital bone malformation and hypovitaminosis A. J Zoo Wildl Med 39:455–459, 2008.
17. Sutton J: On some specimens of diseases from mammals in the society's gardens. Proc Zool Soc London 364–368, 1887.

18. Thompson K: Bones and joints. In Maxie GM, editor: Pathology of domestic animals, vol 1, ed 5, Philadelphia, 2007, Saunders Elsevier, pp 1–184.

19. Tuch K, Pohlenz J: Partielle cerebellarhernie beim löwen (*Panther leo* L.). Vet Pathol 10:299–306, 1973.

20. Wenker C, Völlm J, Steffen F, et al: [Hypovitaminose A bedingte Ataxie bei einem Junglöwen im Zoo Basel—eine vergessene Erkrankung? Tagungsbericht der 28.] Arbeitstagung der Zootierärzte im deutschsprachigen Raum 2008, pp 116–121.

CHAPTER 62

Pyometra in Large Felids

Stephanie McCain and Edward C. Ramsay

Pyometra is well described in domestic cats, but is relatively uncommon. However, pyometra appears to occur more often in large exotic felids.[9] It has been diagnosed in leopards, lions, tigers, and a liger, with lions being at an increased risk.[1,2,9] Most large felids that develop pyometra are older than 10 years, although it has been seen in a 5-year-old lion.[9]

Pyometra in domestic carnivores is associated with cystic endometrial hyperplasia,[3,6] which also appears to be the case in large felids.[9,10] In the development of pyometra, cystic endometrial hyperplasia is followed by secondary bacterial overgrowth of normal vaginal flora that enters the uterus during proestrus and estrus. The incidence of cystic endometrial hyperplasia in exotic felids increases with age.[10] Unlike with domestic felids, it is uncommon to spay large exotic felids in zoo collections for the prevention of pregnancy, but more common to contracept them. Historically, melengesterol acetate implants were commonly used for this purpose, although they are used less frequently now because of associated side effects. Cystic endometrial hyperplasia has been reported in felids both with and without a history of melengesterol acetate contraception.[10]

Pyometra is less common in the domestic cat than in the dog,[6] presumably because of cats being induced ovulators. In induced ovulators, uterine tissue is exposed to progesterone only after copulation or artificial stimulation. The uterus is not, therefore, exposed to progesterone in every estrous cycle, which reduces the risk for the development of cystic endometrial hyperplasia.

An early work suggested that lions are spontaneous ovulators,[12] but a more recent study has suggested that most lions are induced ovulators.[13] Like in the domestic cat,[5,8] spontaneous ovulation may occur with varying frequency in lions housed singly or with other females.[2,13] The same appears to be true for the tiger.[4] In contrast, the leopard has been shown to ovulate in the presence of other females, but not when housed singly. This suggests that they do not require intromission but do require stimulation for ovulation to occur.[2,11]

Histopathology of the reproductive tracts of large felids with pyometra has demonstrated at least one corpus luteum in most cases, indicating that ovulation had taken place within a few weeks prior to surgery.[9] One lion was housed only with other females, which confirms the previous findings that intromission is not required for ovulation in the lion. Additionally, one of two tigers and a liger were housed alone and also had multiple corpora lutea, supporting the occurrence of spontaneous ovulation in at least some large exotic felids.

CLINICAL SIGNS

The most common clinical signs are vulvar discharge, anorexia, and lethargy. The most consistent sign is 1 to 3 days of vulvar discharge. The discharge is typically purulent and white, tan, or green in color, although bloody discharges have also been observed. The appetite may be normal or decreased for a few days, or animals may be completely anorexic for several days. Similarly, the amount of lethargy cats demonstrate varies widely. Vomiting is also occasionally seen. Polydipsia and polyuria, commonly seen in domestic dogs with pyometra, are not routinely reported in domestic cats,[3] nor in large felids with pyometra. However, when cats are housed outdoors, evaluation of urination is a challenge. Cystitis is the most common differential diagnosis for pyometra in large felids.

DIAGNOSTIC FINDINGS

Leukocytosis caused by neutrophilia, with or without a left shift, is a common finding in large felids with

477

pyometra, although some affected animals have white blood cell counts within reference intervals. Normal or even decreased white blood cells are occasionally seen in domestic animals with pyometra, and may be related to septicemia or sequestration of white blood cells into the uterine lumen.[3,6] Common biochemical findings include hyperproteinemia and hyperglobulinemia, presumably caused by chronic antigenic stimulation. Azotemia may also be seen and is usually prerenal in origin, although concurrent primary renal dysfunction should be ruled out because both conditions are correlated with age.

Although radiographs are occasionally helpful in the diagnosis of pyometra in large felids, ultrasound is a superior modality for diagnosis. Radiographic findings are often nonspecific but may include a tubular soft tissue opacity dorsal to the urinary bladder, displaced intestinal loops, or poor serosal detail. In cases with an open pyometra, enough uterine drainage may have occurred to make visualization of the uterus difficult.

Abdominal ultrasonography is more sensitive and, in our experience, has been diagnostic in every case. The most common finding is a distended fluid-filled uterus. Thickened uterine walls may also be seen. Ultrasonography also allows for the evaluation of the presence of peritoneal effusion, which may indicate a ruptured uterus in some cases.

TREATMENT

Ovariohysterectomy is the treatment of choice for pyometra in domestic carnivores and is recommended for large felids as well. In valuable breeding animals that are not critically ill, medical treatment using prostaglandins and antibiotics could be considered. A technique for uterine lavage in large cats has also been described and used to treat a tiger with aseptic pyometra; however, that cat subsequently underwent an ovariohysterectomy.[7] The long-term effectiveness of this technique as a treatment for pyometra in large felids has not been evaluated.

If substantial vaginal discharge exists, one may assume that the cervix is open. In this case, if ovariohysterectomy cannot be performed immediately, and the patient is stable, broad-spectrum oral or injectable antibiotics should be initiated until surgery may be done. Animals with closed pyometra or critically ill animals should be treated as surgical emergencies.

At the time of surgery, perioperative broad-spectrum antibiotics should be administered. Clinicians may perform a lumbosacral epidural block for additional analgesia. Although more difficult because of the large size of these cats, the technique is the same as that for domestic carnivores. Typically, 0.06 to 0.12 mg/kg morphine sulfate, without preservative, is given epidurally to an adult lion or tiger. Intraoperative or immediately postoperative injectable nonsteroidal anti-inflammatory drugs (NSAIDs) are also used routinely.

The abdominal incision needs to be long and extend cranially to the umbilicus to gain adequate access to the ovaries. There are often two to three large vessels supplying the ovary, and these may be ligated individually or in groups. A modified Miller knot is useful if these vessels are ligated as a group. The uterus is often not as friable as that of domestic carnivores, but caution should still be used when exteriorizing the uterus. Several extra large Carmalt forceps are typically needed to cross-clamp the uterine body. A modified Miller knot may be useful to ligate the large uterine body, and clinicians may also consider oversewing the cut edge. After the uterus is removed, the abdomen should be lavaged with sterile fluid. Extensive lavage should be used in cases with uterine rupture or if the abdomen is contaminated during uterine ligation. Large-gauge suture (0 to 2) in an interrupted simple, mattress, or cruciate pattern should be used to close the linea alba to minimize the risk of dehiscence. Often, a four-layer closure is used rather than the traditional three-layer closure.

Postoperatively, broad-spectrum antibiotics should be administered pending culture and sensitivity results of uterine contents. *Escherichia coli* is the most common bacteria isolated; however, *Pseudomonas aeruginosa* and other bacteria have also been cultured.[9] Postoperative analgesia may be accomplished with oral or injectable NSAIDs and an oral opiate agonist, such as tramadol.

Prognosis is good if uterine rupture has not occurred and the ovariohysterectomy is performed in a timely manner. In the case of uterine rupture, the prognosis is fair to guarded. To date, we have diagnosed and treated 23 cases of pyometra in large felids, with only two major complications. One lion was euthanized postoperatively because of not recovering from anesthesia. This animal had a severe leukocytosis, ruptured uterus, and subacute peritonitis. A second lion had complete dehiscence of the abdominal wall. This cat underwent a second surgery for repair and subsequently recovered completely.

Pyometra is a potentially life-threatening condition that occurs during diestrus. An abdominal ultrasound is recommended for any intact, large, female felid with vulvar discharge, especially lions. Ovariohysterectomy is curative.

REFERENCES

1. Baker R, Henderson R: Pyometra in an African lioness. J Am Vet Med Assoc 183:1314, 1983.
2. Brown JL, Graham LH, Wielebnowski N, et al: Understanding the basic reproductive biology of wild felids by monitoring of faecal steroids. J Reprod Fertil Suppl 57:71–82, 2001.
3. Feldman EC: The cystic endometrial hyperplasia/pyometra complex and infertility in female dogs. In Ettinger SJ, Feldman EC, editors: Textbook of veterinary internal medicine: Diseases of the dog and cat. Philadelphia, 2000, WB Saunders, pp 1549–1555.
4. Graham LH, Byers AP, Armstrong DL, et al: Natural and gonadotropin-induced ovarian activity in tigers *(Panthera tigris)* assessed by fecal steroid analysis. Gen Comp Endocrinol 147:362–370, 2006.
5. Gudermuth DF, Newton L, Daels P, et al: Incidence of spontaneous ovulation in young, group-housed cats based on serum and faecal concentrations of progesterone. J Reprod Fertil Suppl 51:177–184, 1997.
6. Hedlund CS: Surgery of the reproductive and genital systems. In Fossum TW, editor: Small animal surgery, ed 2, St. Louis, 2002, Mosby, pp 639–644,
7. Hildebrandt TB, Göritz F, Boardman W, et al: A non-surgical uterine lavage technique in large cats intended for treatment of uterine infection–induced infertility. Theriogenology 66:1783–1786, 2006.
8. Lawler DF, Johnston SD, Hegstad RL, et al: Ovulation without cervical stimulation in domestic cats. J Reprod Fertil Suppl 47:57–61, 1993.
9. McCain S, Ramsay E, Allender M, et al: Pyometra in captive large felids: A review of 11 cases. J Zoo Wildl Med 40:147–151, 2009.
10. Munson L, Gardner IA, Mason RJ, et al: Endometrial hyperplasia and mineralization in zoo felids treated with melengestrol acetate contraceptives. Vet Pathol 39:419–427, 2002.
11. Schmidt AM, Hess DL, Schmidt MJ, et al: Serum concentrations of oestradiol and progesterone, and sexual behaviour during the normal oestrous cycle in the leopard *(Panthera pardus)*. J Reprod Fertil 82:43–49, 1988.
12. Schmidt AM, Nadal LA, Schmidt MJ, et al: Serum concentrations of oestradiol and progesterone during the normal oestrous cycle and early pregnancy in the lion *(Panthera leo)*. J Reprod Fertil 57:267–272, 1979.
13. Schramm RD, Briggs MB, Reeves JJ: Spontaneous and induced ovulation in the lion *(Panthera leo)*. Zoo Biol 13:301–307, 1994.

Marine Mammals

Section 11

CHAPTER 63

Longitudinal Monitoring of Immune System Parameters of Cetaceans and Application to Their Health Management

Jeffrey L. Stott and James F. McBain

Infectious disease, trauma, and stress are all important contributors to morbidity and mortality in zoo and free-ranging mammals. Routine health assessment at the individual level largely relies on observation of abnormal (condition), appetite and/or behavior and population stability. Clinical evaluation of individual animals is based on laboratory analyses of accessible samples, including blood, urine, and feces. Ancillary diagnostic aids applied to such samples include hematology, serum biochemistry, microbe isolation, and serology; these all include relatively solid baseline data from which to draw tentative conclusions. From a hematologic perspective, the complete blood count (CBC) associated with varied chemical analyses continues to serve as the gold standard for diagnostic testing. Accurate identification of the causative insult may be difficult, especially in the early stages of clinical disease. This is significant in view of the fact that successful treatment and prevention of disease progression and/or development of chronic debilitating sequelae relies on the early accurate identification of the likely insult and specific disease processes. The administration of broad-spectrum antimicrobial agents, with its associated risks, is common in affected individuals in the absence of a specific diagnosis.

ESTABLISHING BASELINE VALUES

Development of programs to train zoo and marine mammals to present themselves voluntarily for blood collection has provided a much desired alternative to physical or chemical animal restraint techniques that often place the animals at risk for injury or death. Blood collection via voluntary presentation of extremities has permitted the initiation of routine hematologic analyses in valued terrestrial and aquatic mammalian species. Such programs have accelerated the establishment of baseline values for a given species and for individual animals. The ability to identify abnormal values, based on an animal's own predetermined baseline, increases relative diagnostic sensitivity.

TOOLS FOR FLOW CYTOMETRY–BASED LEUKOCYTE PHENOTYPING

Establishment of routine bleeding programs in many marine parks has provided a window for advancing the science of clinical immunology in cetacean species. Successes enjoyed in human medicine, which have used analytic flow cytometry to identify perturbations in blood leukocytes, formulate prognoses, and evaluate the efficacy of treatment modalities, has logically inspired the initiation of similar approaches in veterinary medicine. Application of flow cytometry to zoo and free-ranging nondomestic species is limited in part by the paucity of monoclonal antibodies specific for leukocyte differentiation antigens; the great majority of antibodies developed for human, murine, and domestic mammals are species-specific and thus of limited use in comparative medicine. On a positive note, reagents developed for canine, feline, equine, and bovine species often cross-react with members in their greater families.

Toothed whales (suborder Odontoceti, order Cetacea), which are the primary focus of this chapter, have no close relatives in the world of domestic mammals, and thus limited immunologic reagents are available to assess perturbations in leukocyte phenotype. Given their monetary value, high visibility, and ongoing training programs directed at establishing voluntary fluke presentation for blood collection, efforts were successfully initiated to develop monoclonal antibodies specific for dolphin (*Tursiops truncatus*) and killer

TABLE 63-1 Monoclonal Antibodies With Specificities for Cetacean Leukocyte Differentiation Antigens

| CD Designation | Antibody Designation[1,3,5,11] | TARGET | | Cell Specificity (*Tursiops, Orcinus*) |
		Genus and Species	Common Name	
CD2	F21.I and F21.C	*Tursiops truncatus*	Bottlenose dolphin	T cell
CD19	F21.B	*Tursiops truncatus*	Bottlenose dolphin	B cell
CD21	F21.F	*Tursiops truncatus*	Bottlenose dolphin	B cell
CD45R	F21.H	*Tursiops truncatus*	Bottlenose dolphin	B cell, T cell subset
MHCII	F21.K	*Tursiops truncatus*	Bottlenose dolphin	Monocytes, lymphocytes
None	F21.D (CAM-D)	*Tursiops truncatus*	Bottlenose dolphin	Adhesion molecule*
MHCII	171.D3	*Bos taurus*	Bovine	Monocytes, lymphocytes
None	ILA.24	*Bos taurus*	Bovine	Myeloid
None	F6B	*Equus caballus*	Horse	Pan leukocyte

Putative leukocyte adhesion molecule.

whale *(Orcinus orca)* leukocyte differentiation antigens,[1-3] referred to in the literature as CD antigens; select monoclonal antibodies previously developed for equine[8] and bovine[5,11] species were also tested for cross-reactivity. A summary of these antibodies and their leukocyte differentiation antigen specificities, if known, are given in Table 63-1.

MARKERS

For T and B Lymphocytes

The antibodies shown in Table 63-1 have been applied to four killer whale populations over a period of 12 years. The antibody set was able to distinguish neutrophils (F6B+/ILA-24+, major histocompatibility complex [MHC] II−), monocytes (F6B+/ILA-24+/MHC II+), and lymphocytes (F6B+, MHC II+/ILA-24−). Lymphocytes could be divided into B cells (CD19+, CD21+) and T cells (CD2+), with T cells being subdivided further by differential density expression of CD2 and CD45R into naïve and memory T cell populations (CD2+/CD45R+/Hi and CD2+/CD45R+/Lo, respectively). The usefulness of using a longitudinal approach for identifying immunologic perturbations in killer whales was quickly revealed. As expected, all markers listed in Table 63-1 were determined to be susceptible to perturbation. Outliers could be identified through comparison to the baseline established for the total population. Sensitivity in identification of immunologic perturbations was increased for select animals—low variation in immune parameter values over time—when using their own individual baselines. Absolute numbers of T and B lymphocyte

subpopulations, representing a subset of the data collected over a 3-year period from 25 animals, are illustrated in Figure 63-1. Such data may only be developed for the individual through longitudinal sampling. Figure 63-1 illustrates the obvious variability in T and B lymphocyte subpopulations among animals. Those animals with dramatic fluctuations may be experiencing multiple and/or recurring insults, some outwardly visible and others subclinical. On inspection of all leukocyte subpopulation data, total numbers of memory T, naïve T, and B lymphocyte numbers were sometimes abnormally elevated and sometimes depressed; this often occurred differentially, resulting in altered ratios of total T versus B lymphocytes and naïve versus memory T lymphocytes. The clinical significance of the various patterns is currently a matter of investigation. Diagnostically speaking, point in time perturbations and trends toward becoming abnormal may be more readily identified with comparative analyses using a combination of the species' baseline and an animal's own individual baseline. However, age-associated changes in leukocyte subpopulation numbers must be taken into account when establishing baseline values for a species.

For Neutrophils

As noted, the cell surface density of select immune parameter markers has provided a sensitive measure of immunologic perturbation. From a diagnostic perspective, the relative density of the putative cell adhesion molecule, CAM-D, appeared to be telling. As determined by flow cytometry, decreased fluorescence intensity on a variable percentage of polymorphonuclear

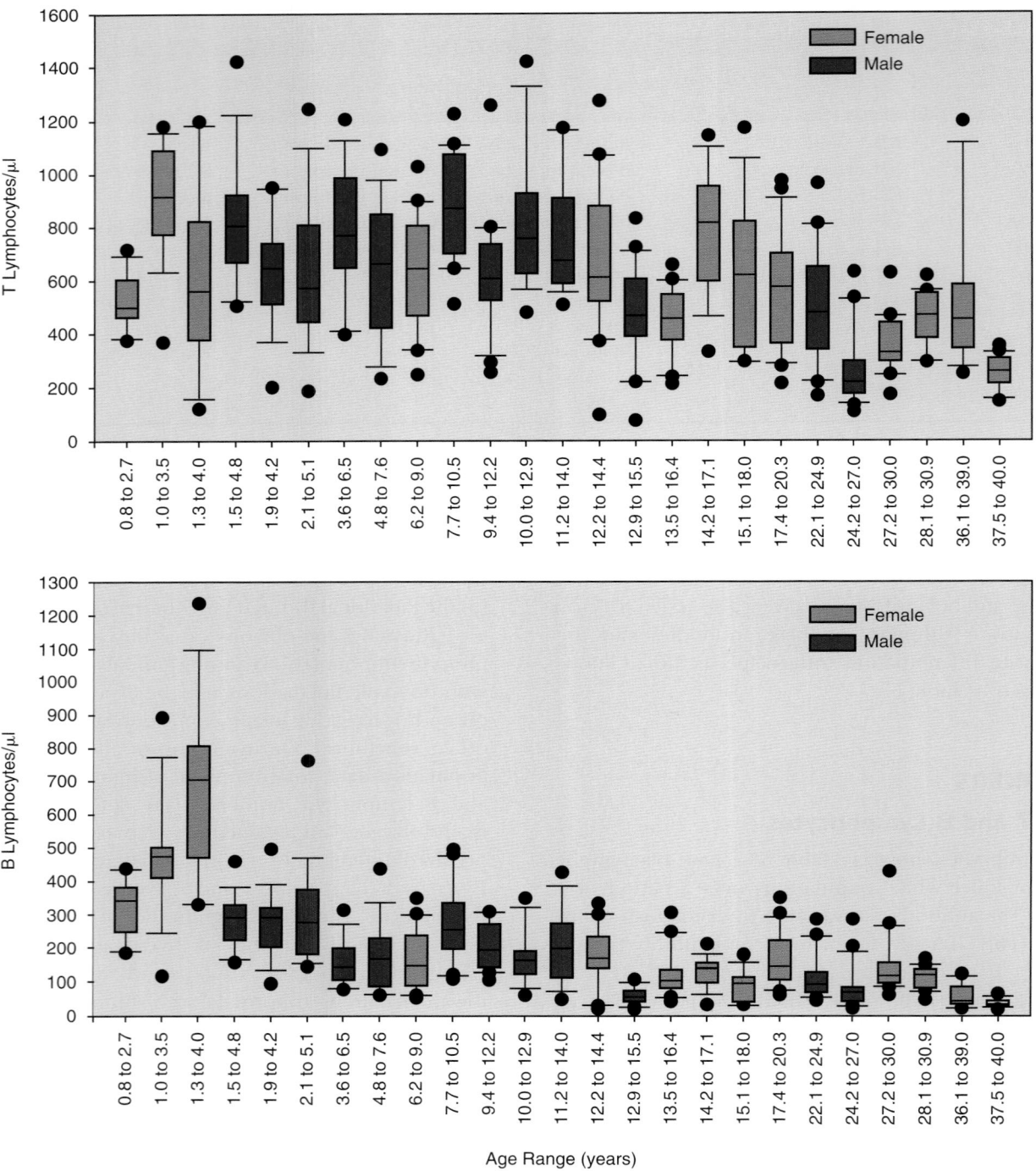

Figure 63-1

Absolute numbers of T and B lymphocytes in peripheral blood samples derived from 25 killer whales over a period of 3 years. The means, associated percentiles (10th, 25th, 75th, and 90th), and outliers for each animal (male and female) are illustrated. Sample size and animal numbers ranged from 12 to 22.

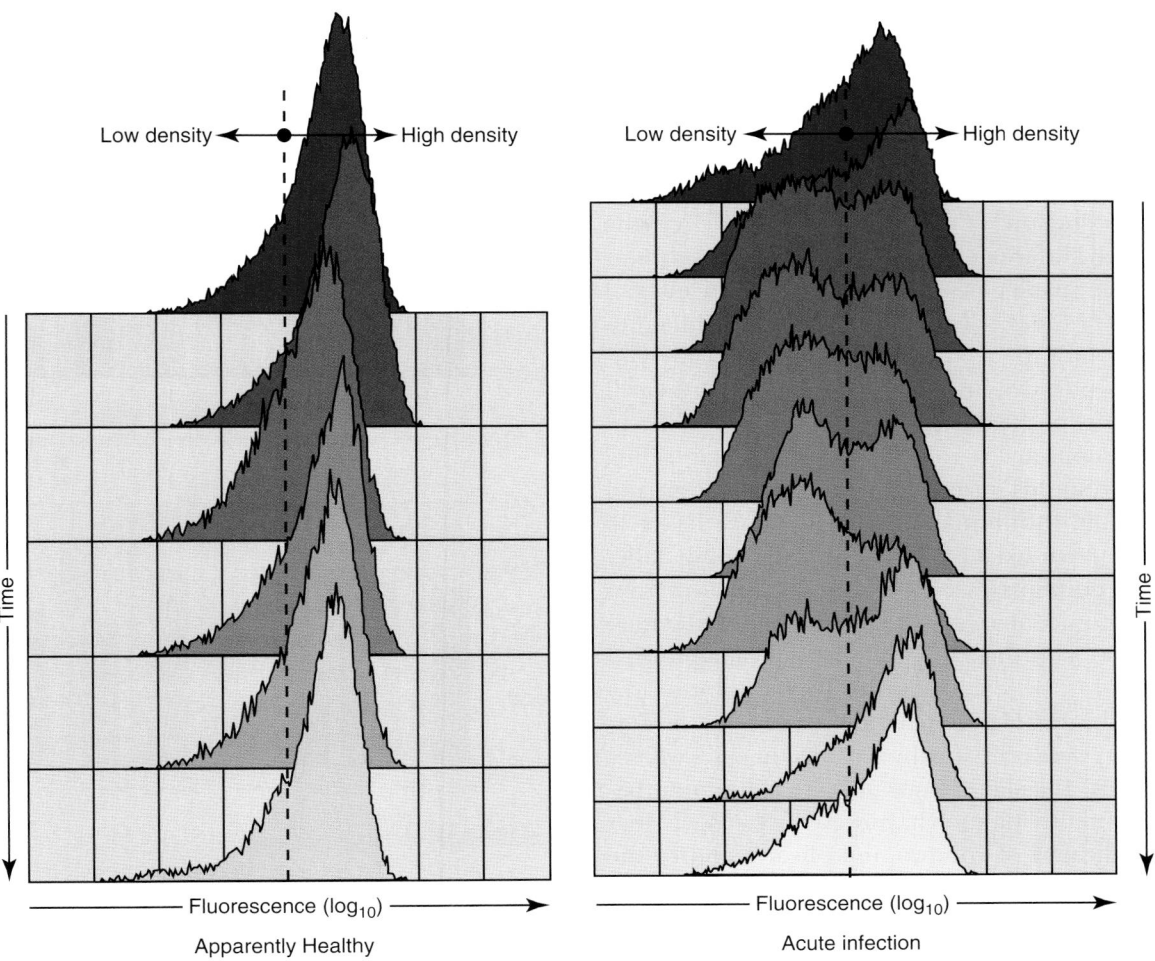

Figure 63-2

Alteration in the cell surface density of a putative cell adhesion molecule, CAM-D, on PMNs as a function of health. The clinical case is represented on the right and a time-matched healthy control on the left. Time points of blood collection for both animals are color-coded. Blood samples obtained from both the principal and control on the same date are illustrated in the same color. The first blood sample collected (at the time of clinical presentation) is at the top of the figure and subsequent samples are illustrated in a descending fashion. The unusual profile of high percentages of PMNs carrying a relative low density of CAM-D resolves with time.

leukocytes (PMNs) stained with fluorescein isothiocyanate (FITC)-labeled α–CAM-D was occasionally recorded. We have speculated that this could be the result of either a conformational change in the adhesion protein, resulting in reduced binding of the monoclonal antibody, or reduced cell surface density of the protein. Regardless, the appearance of a subpopulation of PMNs with low-density fluorescence was associated with clinical disease. Figure 63-2 illustrates a clinically ill animal with a subpopulation of PMNs expressing a low fluorescence as compared with those expressing a relatively high fluorescence following staining with α–CAM-D. Parallel samples obtained from a healthy companion

are illustrated for comparative purposes. The first time point was obtained at the initiation of acute illness (top of the figure); the PMN profile slowly returned to a pattern similar to that of the control following treatment.

For Mononuclear Leukocyte Activity

Determination of the cell surface density of MHC class II proteins on monocytes and lymphocytes, and CD19 on B lymphocytes, has allowed for assessment of the relative activation status of these leukocytes. Both monocytes and B lymphocytes are professional antigen-presenting cells (APCs) and play a pivotal role in displaying processed antigen in physical context with their MHC class II proteins, so that T lymphocytes may be induced to activate, differentiate, and proliferate in a pathogen-specific manner. These APCs respond to insult-induced proinflammatory mediators by increasing the production of MHC class II proteins; the increased cell surface density of these proteins serves as a phenotypic marker of activation. CD19, an integral component of the B cell coreceptor, has contributed to the evaluation of the relative activation status of B lymphocytes (hypoactive or hyperactive) based on the cell surface density of the differentiation antigen. Studies in mice have supported a role for CD19 in establishing signaling thresholds for regulating B cell activation and differentiation.[7] Abnormally low cell surface levels of CD19 were recorded in stressed animals (both killer whales and dolphins), whereas animals suffering from apparent chronic infections often had abnormally high levels of CD19 on their B lymphocytes. The abnormal expression of CD19 on a subset of T lymphocytes (low density) and variable percentages of PMNs (low and/or high density) were occasionally recorded in killer whales and dolphins. The significance of these latter perturbations (is) currently unknown; however, we suspect that they are indicative of compromised health and/or the result of an unusual immunologic response to a unique insult. Animals presenting with these unusual features often do so for weeks to months before returning to a normal profile.

LYMPHOCYTE FUNCTION

Flow cytometry–based leukocyte phenotype analysis was augmented by the functional analysis of lymphocytes using mitogen-induced (concanavalin A [ConA], phytohemagglutinin [PHA], and pokeweed mitogen [PWM]) mononuclear leukocyte proliferation; mitogens induce the proliferation of lymphocytes in a non–antigen-specific manner and serve as the gold standard in human and veterinary medicine when assessing lymphocyte function. Two concentrations of each mitogen were used, one being considered an optimal concentration and the other being suboptimal, in which the lowest concentration that induced a near-maximum response was used. Generally, we did not identify any substantial lymphocyte dysfunction that could not be attributed to daily variation. However, when responses to both concentrations (optimal and suboptimal) of mitogen were compared, periods of reduced lymphocyte responsiveness were identified. Figure 63-3

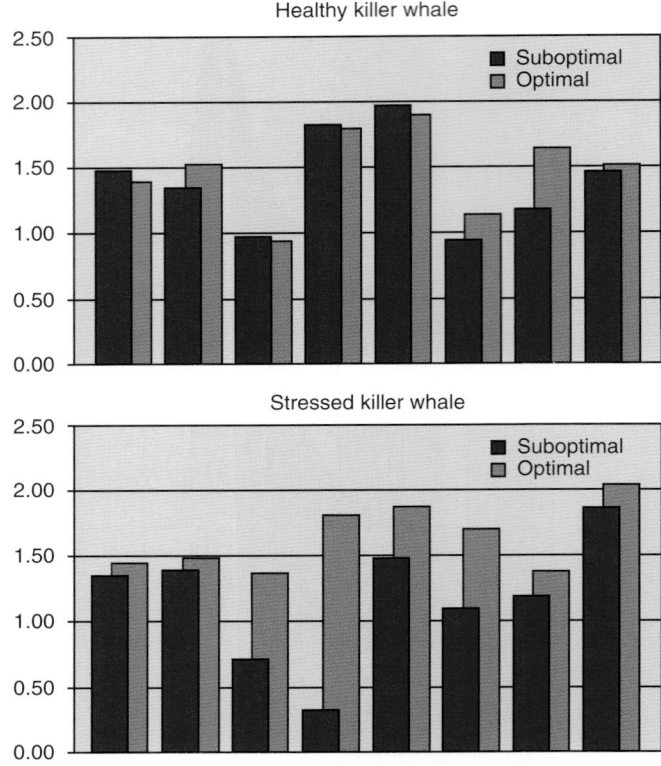

Figure 63-3

ConA-induced proliferation of mononuclear leukocytes using optimal (1.0 μg/mL) and suboptimal (0.1 μg/mL) concentrations of mitogen. The lower graph depicts data from a pregnant killer whale, with apparent stressors associated with birth (third time point), followed by negative behavioral changes (fourth time point). The upper graph represents an apparently healthy animal sampled over the same time period from the same park.

illustrates a longitudinal set of data on a killer whale that experienced an extended period of reduced lymphocyte function; an apparently healthy cohort is included for comparative purposes. A decreased response of lymphocytes to the suboptimal concentration of ConA developed when the principal female gave birth (third time point) and became further exacerbated as aggression toward her calf was expressed (fourth time point).

Applications In Clinical Research

The killer whale immune monitoring program is seen as a long-term commitment toward developing immunologic signatures that may assist with diagnostic procedures, design of treatment modalities, and prognosis. Many of the leukocyte phenotypic and functional perturbations statistically correlated with established

TABLE 63-2 Leukocyte Gene Transcripts Targeted by Quantitative Real-Time Reverse Transcriptase Polymerase Chain Reaction Assay

| Gene Transcript | TARGET | | Function* |
	Tursiops Truncatus	*Orcinus Orca*	
Interleukin-4 (IL-4)	X	X	Th2[†] activity
IL-10	X	X	Anti-inflammatory
IL-17	X	X	Proinflammatory
TNF-α	X	X	Proinflammatory
CD69	X	X	Leukocyte activation
IL-2Rα	X		Lymphocyte activation
IFN-α	X		Antiviral
Cyclooxygenase-2 (COX-2)	X	X	Oxidative burst
Myxovirus resistance 1 (MX-1)	X	X	Antiviral
IFN-γ	X	X	CMI[‡] activity
Fas-associated death domain (FADD)	X	X	Leukocyte apoptosis
S9	X	X	Housekeeping gene (control)

*A primary function for each leukocyte gene product is listed. However, all gene products can elicit a wide variety of immunologic responses.
†Th2 activity: T helper type 2 lymphocyte activity is associated with immune responses to helminthic pathogens and immediate-type (type 1) hypersensitivities. IL-4 is one of several cytokines that Th2 cells produce on activation.
‡CMI (cell-mediated immunity) activity is associated with immune responses to intracellular pathogens. Th1 (T helper type 1) lymphocytes, NK (natural killer) cells, and CTLs (cytotoxic T lymphocytes) all contribute to this activity by producing IFN-γ (classically referred to as macrophage activation factor).

hematologic markers of disease, but others fell short of significance. The latter does not necessarily bode poorly for the potential usefulness of those markers, but rather may prove to identify conditions that would otherwise have gone undetected and could benefit from treatment. Approaches and assays to assess immunologic health of cetaceans continue to be developed and applied. As an example, a robust kinetics-based neutrophil phagocytosis assay was applied in conjunction with leukocyte phenotyping to assess the potential efficacy of a purported immunoenhancing supplement in killer whales. No immunologic changes occurred after 1 month of treatment, suggesting that the product was not gaining systemic circulation.

PROFILING LEUKOCYTE GENE TRANSCRIPTIONAL ACTIVITY

More recently, a quantitative approach to measure leukocyte gene transcription was initiated to complement leukocyte phenotyping and function, and preliminary data are encouraging. Again, the longitudinal approach was taken in killer whales and dolphins in a wide variety of collections. Such an approach has been made possible with the advent of quantitative polymerase chain reaction (Q-PCR) assays and techniques for the immediate stabilization of mRNA in clinical blood samples. Validation of techniques required for the clinical application of Q-PCR has been established and successful application(s) have been described in human medicine.[4,10] A modest but select group of genes were chosen for development using a real-time reverse transcriptase PCR approach. The gene transcripts represented a cross section of activities (Table 63-2), including those encoding products with proinflammatory, anti-inflammatory, regulatory, and antiviral activities, respiratory burst, apoptosis, enhancement of cellular immunity, and enhancement of helminthic immunity and immediate-type hypersensitivities. At some point in time, perturbations in one or more gene transcripts were noted in both species, with all markers proving useful. Increased levels of select mRNA transcripts are readily interpretable as increased activity of select leukocytes, apoptosis, or antiviral genes. At the opposite extreme, several animals presented with abnormally low levels of select cytokine transcripts on multiple occasions, and such data are perplexing. This may best be interpreted as indicative of abnormally low levels of leukocyte activity; such suppressed activity has been described for T helper lymphocytes derived from humans with chronic viral infections.[6] Figure 63-4 selectively illustrates peripheral

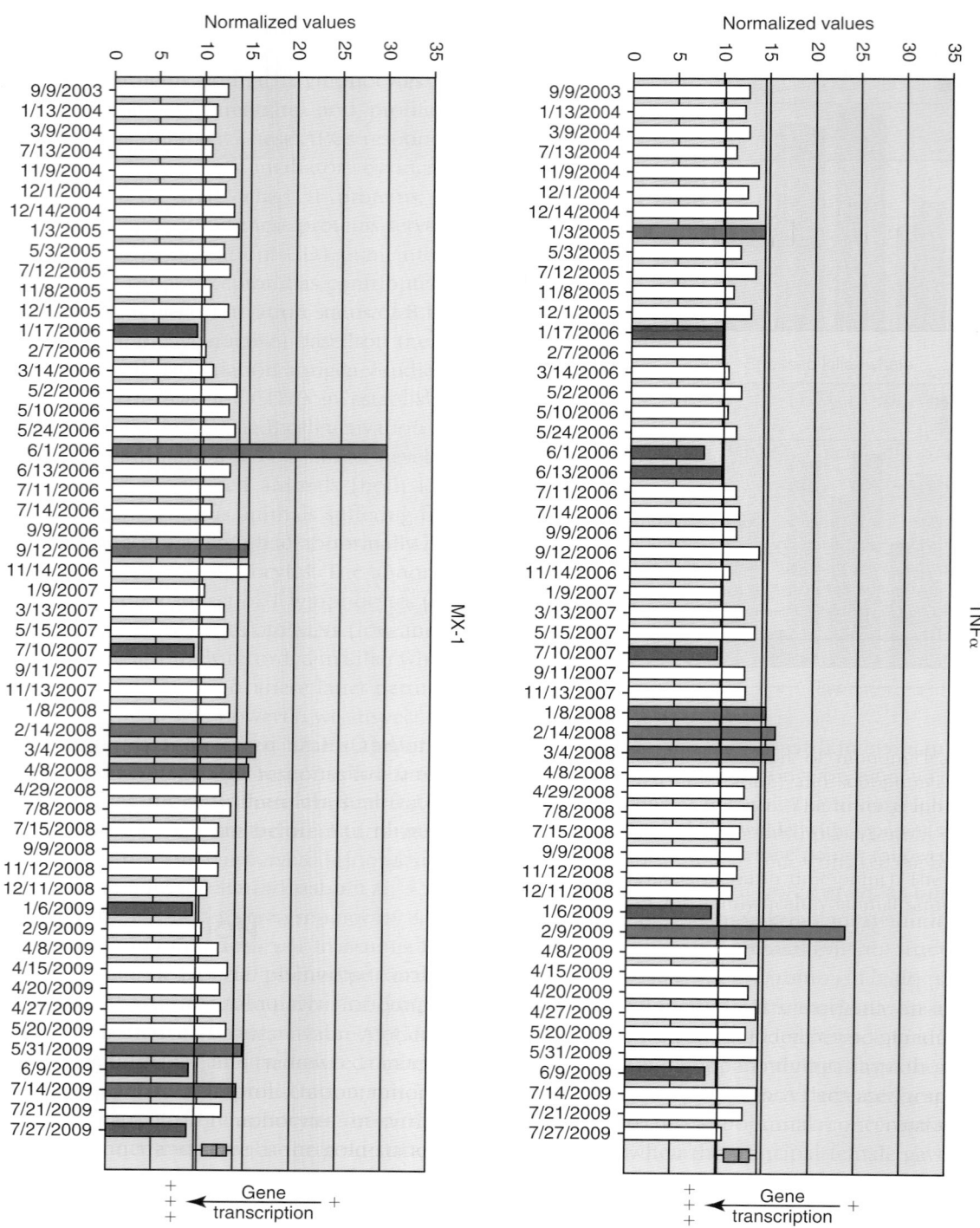

Figure 63-4

Leukocyte cytokine transcript profile of a killer whale over a 6-year period. Two select genes are illustrated, TNF-α, a gene encoding a proinflammatory mediator, and MX-1, a gene encoding a product with antiviral activity induced by myxovirus infection. Data are presented as normalized values (number of PCR cycles required to identify the DNA product minus the number of PCR cycles required to identify the housekeeping gene, 7S ribosomal gene). The graph is counterintuitive; abnormally high levels of cytokine transcript are detected at lower PCR cycle numbers *(red bars)* whereas abnormally low levels of transcript are detected at higher cycle numbers *(blue bars)*. Solid lines mark the 10th and 90th percentiles established using 158 data points derived from apparently healthy killer whales.

blood-derived cytokine gene transcript levels from a killer whale over a 6-year period. Five obvious episodes of elevated tumor necrosis factor-α (TNF-α) and four of MX-1 (antiviral; induced by myxovirus infection) levels were recorded. Interestingly, all four increases in MX-1 were mirrored by increases in TNF-α level. The exception occurred on June 1, 2006, in which TNF-α was elevated whereas levels of MX-1 were abnormally suppressed; this would not appear to be a coincidence given the magnitude of the MX-1 suppression.

Applications in Clinical Research

In addition to the routine longitudinal monitoring approaches described, a clinical approach was recently initiated with dolphins from multiple facilities. Dolphins were enrolled in the project when they presented with signs of distress and before initiation of treatment. Blood samples were collected for analysis on a longitudinal basis throughout the entire treatment regimen and again 30 days following termination of medications. Although these latter data are only now being analyzed, the long-term goal is to identify transcriptional signatures that may enable early identification of a general type of causative insult and/or prognosis, thereby facilitating application of timely and appropriate prophylactic measures.

As with many projects, techniques and data established for the immunology program have fostered new and unique approaches to address marine mammal health. The ability to assess the induction of T lymphocyte cytokines quantitatively has served as the basis of assessing the efficacy of a swine erysipelas vaccine in domestic cetaceans. Identification of vaccine-induced *Erysipelothrix rhusiopathiae*–specific memory T lymphocytes was realized using an in vitro blastogenesis assay in conjunction with quantitative PCR-based determination of interferon gamma (IFN-γ) mRNA transcripts.[9]

The application of health-based laboratory assays in zoo or marine park environments ultimately results in establishment of baseline values for a given species. The development of such data facilitates their application in establishing the health of free-ranging wild populations. Such is currently the case with the studies described earlier. Techniques initially established for killer whales have driven the application of leukocyte phenotyping, lymphocyte function, and leukocyte gene transcript analyses to a long-term collaborative health assessment of a free-ranging dolphin (*Tursiops truncates*) population in Sarasota Bay, Florida. Data obtained over a 5-year period are currently being compared with a recently

established apparently normal baseline using captive *T. truncatus*. Similar approaches are being successfully applied to associate environmental conditions with the immunologic health of captive and free-ranging populations of fur seals, monk seals, California sea lions, Steller sea lions, and sea otters.

CONCLUSION

The establishment and application of techniques for the routine immunologic evaluation of zoo and marine mammals is justified. This approach was endorsed at a 2007 National Oceanic and Atmospheric Administration (NOAA)–sponsored workshop entitled "Managing Cetaceans for Optimal Health." The group concluded that research directed at better defining environmental influences on the health of captive and free-ranging cetaceans was a priority and would result in improved management decisions; defining animal health was one of seven action plans developed at the workshop.

REFERENCES

1. De Guise S, Erickson K, Blanchard M, et al: Characterization of a monoclonal antibody that recognizes a lymphocyte surface antigen for the cetacean homologue to CD45R. Immunology 94:207–212, 1998.
2. De Guise S, Erickson K, Blanchard M, et al: Characterization of F21.A, a monoclonal antibody that recognizes a leukocyte surface antigen for killer whale homologue to beta-2 integrin. Vet Immunol Immunopathol 97:195–206, 2004.
3. De Guise S, Erickson K, Blanchard M, et al: Monoclonal antibodies to lymphocyte surface antigens for cetacean homologues to CD2, CD19 and CD21. Vet Immunol Immunopathol 84:209–221, 2002.
4. Deirmengian C, Lonner JL, Booth RE: White blood cell gene expression: A new approach toward the study and diagnosis of infection. Clin Orthop Relat Res 440:38–44, 2005.
5. Ellis JA, Davis WC, MacHugh ND, et al: Differentiation antigens on bovine mononuclear phagocytes identified by monoclonal antibodies. Vet Immunol Immunopathol 19:325–340, 1988.
6. Elsaesser H, Sauer K, Brooks DG: IL-21 is required to control chronic viral infection. Science 324:1569–1572, 2009.
7. Engel P, Zhou LJ, Ord DC, et al: Abnormal B lymphocyte development, activation, and differentiation in mice that lack or overexpress the CD19 signal transduction molecule. Immunity 3:39–50, 1995.
8. Lunn DP, Holmes MA, Antczak DF, et al: Report of the Second Equine Leukocyte Antigen Workshop, Squaw Valley, California, July 1995. Vet Immunol Immunopathol 62:101–143, 1998.
9. Sitt T, Lizabeth Bowen L, Blanchard MT, et al: Cellular immune responses in cetaceans immunized with a porcine erysipelas vaccine. Vet Immunol Immunopathol 137:181–189, 2010.
10. Stordeur P, Zhou L, Byl B, et al: Immune monitoring in whole blood using real-time PCR. J Immunol Methods 276:69–77, 2003.
11. Taylor BC, Choi KY, Scibienski RJ, et al: Differential expression of bovine MHC class II antigens identified by monoclonal antibodies. J Leuk Biol 53:479–489, 1993.

CHAPTER 64

Ocular Disease and Suspected Causes in Captive Pinnipeds

Laurie J. Gage

Ocular disease is one of the most common medical problems observed in captive pinnipeds, with a disproportionally higher prevalence when compared with similar eye problems in their wild counterparts or other captive mammalian species. Possible causes, both studied and anecdotal, are one or a combination of factors, including trauma, infection, periodic or persistent exposure to excessive chemical, oxidant, or noxious byproduct levels in the water, osmolality of the water, viral or bacterial pathogens, excessive ultraviolet (UV) light exposure, nutritional imbalances, and genetic predisposition.[5-7] When single or multiple pinnipeds develop recurrent eye problems, a comprehensive review of possible causative factors is advised. In addition to an ophthalmic examination, a thorough evaluation of oxidant levels in the pool, coliform counts, environmental conditions, including pool color and availability of shade, salinity, nutritional supplements, exposure to pathogens, and prevalence of trauma is warranted.

OCULAR DISEASE

Corneal disease is a painful and frequently recurrent problem in captive pinnipeds. Many have experienced mild to moderate ulcerative corneal disease and may become visually impaired by the time they reach their teenage years. Common corneal problems seen in pinnipeds are edema, opacities, and chronic keratitis. In one 6-year study conducted on 113 captive otariids in North America and the Bahamas, keratitis was identified in one or both eyes of more than 45% of the animals evaluated.[1] Flare-ups occurred in the most affected animals two to four times/year, primarily during seasons when the sunlight exposure increased or, in tropical climates, became more intense. In winter, flare-ups were seen when there were bright sunny days, with snow continuously on the ground. In two study facilities

in which animals lived primarily indoors, the resident pinnipeds had less severe corneal disease for their age and fewer annual flare-ups of keratitis. This study defined three stages of keratitis in otariids and identified this common syndrome as otariid keratitis (Fig. 64-1).[1] Repeated insults to the cornea could lead to secondary bacterial or fungal infections. When trauma and primary infectious processes are ruled out, frequent oxidant or noxious byproduct spikes in the water and excessive exposure to UV light are two of the more likely causes. An ongoing large-scale epidemiologic survey involving 20 facilities worldwide will help determine whether sun exposure is truly a risk factor for this disease.[1]

Another study has described cataracts or lens luxations in pinnipeds older than 5 years, which became increasingly more common in older animals. In a study group of 111 pinnipeds, the prevalence of cataracts, with or without lens luxation, was 21% in those aged between 6 and 10 years 58% in those between 11 and 15 years, 66% in those in the 16- to 20-year-old age group, 87% in animals between 21 and 25 years old; all 9 study animals older than 26 years had cataracts, and 5 of them also had lens luxations.[2] The risk factors for developing cataracts, lens luxations, or both that were identified in this study included increasing age, history of ocular disease, history of fighting, and lack of shade. Animals in this study without access to shade were 10 times more likely to develop cataracts or lens luxations.[2]

Other factors that may contribute significantly to ocular disease in pinnipeds are trauma, nutritional deficiencies, and genetic predisposition.

ENVIRONMENTAL ISSUES

The environment provided for captive animals must meet their physical and social needs, provide safe and secure living quarters, and not contribute to medical

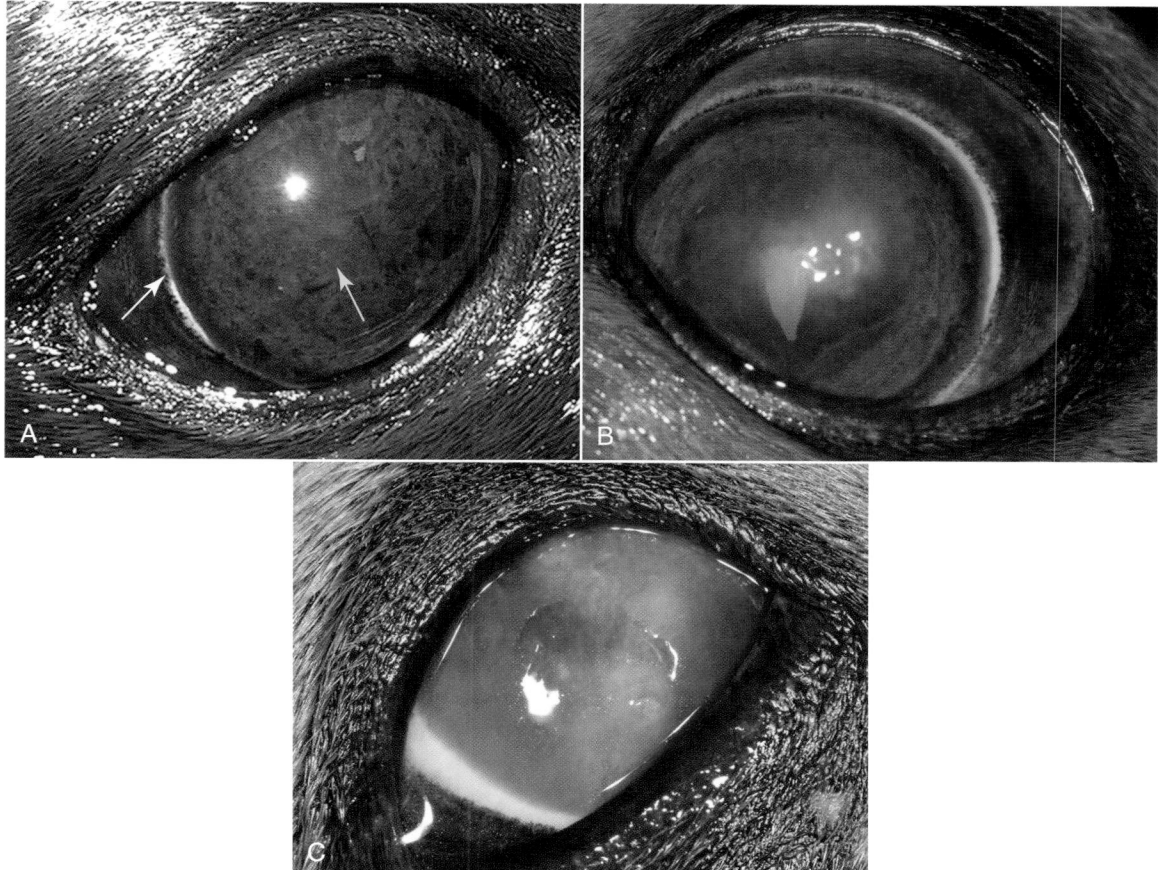

Figure 64-1

A, Stage 1 otariid keratitis. A faint gray-white corneal opacity is located dorsotemporal to the axial cornea *(yellow arrow)*. There is also perilimbal corneal edema *(white arrow)* seen as a gray line located just inside the limbus. There will often be small, superficial, corneal ulcers and there is clinical blepharospasm and epiphora when ulcers are present. **B,** Stage 2 otariid keratitis. A larger gray-white corneal opacity is located dorsotemporal to the axial cornea. The corneal surface in this area is variably irregular and often has recurrent ulcerations, with secondary opportunistic bacterial infections. The ulcers begin as superficial ulcers that have easily sloughed epithelium. The perilimbal corneal edema is also present and the limbal region may have mild corneal vascularization and pigmentation crossing the limbus. The clinical signs of pain (blepharospasm and epiphora) are more severe and chronic in this stage. These signs abate when ulcers, infection, and inflammation are controlled and disease is quiescent. **C,** Stage 3 otariid keratitis. This is the most severe manifestation of this disease. It encompasses most of the cornea with diffuse corneal edema, cellular infilatrate, and superficial to stromal ulceration. Perilimbal edema is present but less obvious because of diffuse edema throughout the cornea. Blepharospasm and epiphora are severe, and the eye may not open for many days without medications to control pain, inflammation, and infected ulcers.

problems. Although most of these criteria are met for captive pinnipeds, the alarming prevalence of painful and debilitating ocular disease must be addressed. Advances in technology to provide optimal water quality, combined with recent and ongoing studies identifying causative factors for keratitis, cataracts, and lens luxations, should help institutions make appropriate decisions for creating and maintaining an environment that will help prevent eye disease in pinnipeds.

Pool Color and Ultraviolet Light

Historically, many pinniped exhibit pools were painted a light blue color, and many exhibit pool and holding area walls are a light color or natural concrete. Most animals included in the cataract study were housed in these conditions for most of their lives. Efforts to create more naturalistic exhibits and paint pool surfaces tan or other less reflective colors have been more recent.

Although pool or exhibit color was not directly identified in the cataract study as a risk factor for developing lens luxations or cataracts, the lack of shade was significant.[2] This suggests that chronic excessive exposure to UV light is likely a factor in the early development of cataracts and/or lens luxations in pinnipeds. It might be argued that pinnipeds have evolved in a bright ocean environment, but wild pinnipeds are not exposed to the same amount of UVA and UVB light as many of their captive counterparts.

Comparing captive pinniped housing and behavior, which may contribute to the amount of UV light exposure that they experience over time, with that of wild pinnipeds may be revealing. Captive animals may be held in bright reflective pools, many of which are painted a light blue color. Although these bright pools may exhibit the animals nicely, they reflect a considerable amount of UV light back into the animals' eyes. Wild pinnipeds swim and feed in a nonreflective environment, looking downward into deeper darker water as they hunt for food. The ocean floor has a relatively nonreflective surface. Captive pinnipeds are more inclined to look up frequently toward the sky than their wild counterparts. Captive animals are usually fed by trainers holding fish for the animal to eat or by keepers who broadcast-feed the animals by throwing quantities of fish into the pool. Some facilities allow the public to feed the animals by having them throw or drop fish into the exhibit pool. In all these cases, the captive animals orient their eyes skyward to locate or receive their fish reward. In some cases, keepers or trainers feed the animals from one location in the exhibit throughout the day. Care should be taken to ensure that the animal never has to look directly into the sun when being fed. Wild animals may haul out on bright reflective beaches, but they typically rest or sleep with their eyes closed. They may occasionally look about their surroundings or at one another but rarely gaze skyward. Captive animals are frequently surrounded by natural concrete or light-colored walls in their exhibit or holding area. The combination of the light-colored reflective pools and the fish being fed from above ("sky fish") causes them to receive considerably more UV light exposure than their wild counterparts. Studies in humans and other animals have suggested that progressive eye damage may be the result of excessive UV light exposure.[3,4,9] A recent study has found that pinnipeds with lack of shade are 10 times more likely to develop cataracts and/or lens luxations.[2] This may explain why I have observed that captive pinnipeds held in U.S. facilities at latitudes below 33 degrees N with a preponderance of bright sunnydays, housed in light blue salt water pools, with no access to shade, appear to have a greater prevalence of clinically apparent eye disease than animals held indoors or in northern latitudes, especially considering that some of these sunny facilities have few, if any, water quality issues.

Water Quality

Clean pathogen-free water is desirable, but the use of excessive oxidants to keep the water pristine may, in turn, lead to oxidative damage to the eyes. If corneal problems are seen either repeatedly in a single pinniped or in multiple pinnipeds, reviewing the water quality records for chemical spikes or imbalances over the course of a year may help identify the problem.

Excessive Chemicals, Oxidants, or Noxious Byproducts in the Water

Chlorine, ozone and, to a lesser extent, bromine, are the most common oxidizing agents used to reduce pathogen levels in marine mammal life support systems. These compounds may cause damage to the corneal tissue by themselves when found in concentrations that are too high. They also combine with dissolved organic material, such as organic carbon and nitrogenous waste, to produce byproducts of disinfection, some of which may cause oxidative damage to ocular tissue. These compounds are rarely measured, and measurement may require different techniques for different compounds. Therefore, their presence and concentration are usually unknown. Compounds of interest include halogenated methanes; these include chloroform, bromoform, bromodichloromethane, and dibromochloromethane.[8] The presence of bromine in source water or its use as a disinfectant may contribute to the formation of many of these noxious byproducts.[8]

Chlorine is used at many facilities to maintain water quality. Total chlorine levels may spike on occasion; however, if these spikes occur repeatedly, the chlorine or its byproducts could cause damage to the cornea. Optimally total chlorine levels should not exceed 1 ppm. Consider that a spike of 0.5 ppm in a 24-hour period could cause corneal damage, even if the total chlorine levels remain under 1 ppm. Chlorine tablet dispensers seem more likely to cause frequent spikes in chlorine levels than gas or liquid chlorine dispensers. When municipal water is used as source water for the pools, chlorine levels should be measured before adding the water to the animal pools. Many municipalities maintain chlorine levels in city water at 2 to 4 ppm. Animals exposed to chlorine levels this high may suffer corneal damage. Repeated exposure to excessive chlorine in the pool may lead to irreparable damage to the eye.

Ozone systems must have an efficient method to degas the water. Occasionally, residual ozone may enter the animal pools, causing a number of animals to have clinical eye discomfort (e.g., blepharospasm, epiphora). Ozone is a powerful oxidant and there should be no measureable residual ozone in the animal pools. Ozone test kits are inexpensive and available commercially. Although these tests are not quantitative, they will accurately determine the presence of ozone in the water. If the test result is positive, measures must be taken to eliminate residual ozone from entering water in which animals are present.

Salinity

In a survey conducted in 1995, animals housed in freshwater systems appeared to have a higher prevalence of corneal edema than those housed in salt water systems.[4] Although most pinnipeds are now housed in salt water, there are some that continue to be housed in freshwater. At one northern latitude institution, there is a constant influx of fresh clean water into the pinniped pool and no chemical additives are necessary to maintain the water quality. Additionally, the pool color is almost black and nonreflective. Pinnipeds housed in that system exhibit few eye problems, suggesting that the osmolality of the water alone may be less of a factor in causing pinniped eye disease than previously thought.

Trauma

Injury to the eyes could occur from a punctate lesion to the cornea from a vibrissa or from a negative social interaction. Eye trauma may also occur from excessive debris in the water, such as pine needles or other plant materials. Fragments of fiberglass material have been found in pools in which residual ozone was causing the lining of some of the filtration system components to disintegrate, distributing them into the animal pools. Keepers and trainers should be aware of these issues and

vigilant in keeping animal pools free of all harmful debris. Animals should be housed in compatible groups to prevent fighting.

MINIMIZING EYE PROBLEMS IN FUTURE PINNIPED GENERATIONS

Captive pinnipeds tend to outlive their wild counterparts by as much as a decade. Age-related eye problems such as cataracts would be expected to occur in animals living into their 20s and 30s. However, progressive ocular disease is frequently seen in animals younger than 10 years. With some changes in the way pinnipeds are housed and cared for, these problems may be prevented. Addressing and controlling numerous factors would help eliminate the most common eye problems. These measures include eliminating or minimizing excessive oxidants or noxious byproducts in the water, with more checks and balances, providing shade and/or nonreflective pools and surrounding areas, never forcing animals to look directly toward the sun while feeding them, and placing them in compatible groups to avoid fighting. Early identification and aggressive treatment of existing eye problems by ophthalmologists familiar with pinniped eye disease would help slow the progression of existing eye problems.

Once keratitis is identified in pinnipeds, there is no known therapeutic or management regimen that will resolve this disease permanently.[1] Shade may help make animals with active disease more comfortable, and appears to slow the progression of ocular disease.[1] All superficial ulcers should have samples for culture and sensitivity submitted, because bacterial and fungal infections must be identified and treated aggressively, the prophylactic use of cyclosporine or tacrolimus topical medications may help minimize flare-ups of otariid keratitis.[1] Offering a wide variety of daily antioxidants in the diet may have a positive effect and help prevent or minimize damage to ocular tissues. Antioxidants that have been shown to protect the lens, such as the carotenoids lutein and zeaxanthin, protect ocular tissues against photo-oxidative stress and may be helpful.[2]

Acknowledgment

I thank Carmen Colitz for her assistance with this chapter.

REFERENCES

1. Colitz CMH, Renner MS, Manire CA, et al: Characterization of progressive keratitis in Otariids. Vet Ophthalmol 13(suppl):47–53, 2010.
2. Colitz CMH, Saville WJA, Renner MS, et al: Risk factors associated with cataracts and lens luxations in captive pinnipeds in the United States and the Bahamas. J Am Vet Med Assoc 237:429–436, 2010.
3. Cullen AP: Photokeratitis and other phototoxic effects on the cornea and conjunctiva. Int J Toxicol 21:455–464, 2002.
4. Delcourt C, Carriere I, Ponton-Sanchez A, et al: Light exposure and the risk of cortical, nuclear, and posterior subcapsular cataracts. Arch Ophthalmol 118:385–392, 2000.
5. Dunn JL, Overstrom NA, St. Aubin DJ: An epidemiologic survey to determine factors associated with corneal and lenticular lesions in captive harbor seals and California sea lions. In Proceedings of the 27th Annual Meeting of the International Association of Aquatic Animal Medicine, 1996, pp 108–109.
6. Gage LJ: Known and suspected factors contributing to chronic corneal lesions in captive pinnipeds. Presented at the 49th Annual Meeting of the American Association of Zoo Veterinarians, Tulsa, Oklahoma, October 2009.
7. Greenwood AG: Prevalence of ocular anterior segment disease in captive pinnipeds, 1985 (http://aquaticmammalsjournal.org/share/AquaticMammalsIssueArchives/1985/Aquatic_Mammals_11_1/Greenwood.pdf).
8. Latson E: Byproducts of disinfection of water and potential mechanisms of ocular injury in marine mammls. What you can't see might hurt them. In Proceedings of the 40th Annual Meeting of the International Association of Aquatic Animal Medicine, 2009, pp 186–188.
9. Newkirk KM, Chandler HL, Parent AE, et al: Ultraviolet radiation-induced corneal degeneration in 129 mice. Toxicol Pathol 35:819–826, 2007.

Elephants

CHAPTER 65

Elephant Herpesviruses

Laura K. Richman and Gary S. Hayward

A newly recognized, often fatal hemorrhagic disease attributed to elephant endotheliotropic herpesvirus (EEHV) has been found in North America, Europe, the Middle East, and Asia. Out of 156 Asian elephants born in captivity in North America during the modern era (between 1962 to 2007), about 25% were stillborn and 78 are still alive. However, of 35 deaths from all causes between the ages of 4 months and 15 years, 20 have been confirmed to be associated with EEHV disease. Overall, the disease has affected approximately 20% of all captive-born Asian elephant calves in North American and European zoos, and has been responsible for two thirds of all deaths of juvenile Asian elephants in captivity in North America. EEHV was first identified in 1995 in association with the index case of lethal acute sudden-onset hemorrhagic disease in a young Asian zoo elephant.[15] At least 60 cases with an 85% fatality rate have subsequently been identified by histopathologic examination and polymerase chain reaction (PCR) assay in elephant populations across North America and Europe.[4,5,11,14,16] Most of these cases have occurred since 1995 and the rest were detected retrospectively from archival pathologic samples dating back to 1978. Most cases (>80%) have occurred in captive-born juvenile Asian elephant (Elephas maximus) calves younger than 8 years old, with a peak in cases between the ages of 1 and 3 years. Several examples of systemic EEHV have also been confirmed in European stillborn fetuses,[18] as well as in older and wild-born animals, and there have been several cases in African elephants (Loxodonta africana). The systemic disease attributed to EEHV has a sudden onset and is characterized by subcutaneous edema of the head and proboscis, cyanosis of the tongue, possibly limb stiffness or lameness, decreased white blood cell and platelet counts, and internal hemorrhages. Histologic abnormalities are predominantly localized to the heart, liver, spleen, tongue,

and intestinal tract and other major organs and include the appearance of basophilic intranuclear viral inclusion bodies in the microvasculature of these organs.[13,17] By electron microscopy, the inclusion bodies have been found to contain viral capsids morphologically consistent with herpes virions. The virus has a predilection for endothelial cells (endotheliotropism), which is unusual for any of the previously characterized herpesviruses. The high fatality rate is attributed to acute myocardial failure and capillary injury and leakage resulting from endothelial cell damage caused by the presence of the herpesvirus. Nine calves have survived after early aggressive antiherpesvirus treatment with famciclovir or ganciclovir, but these agents were not uniformly successful in preventing deaths. Furthermore, as many as 18 recent deaths of orphan and wild Asian elephant calves in four different countries in Asia have also been attributed to EEHV.[12,23]

CAUSE

Current knowledge and all data generated to date have suggested that EEHVs are host-specific to elephants. In general, all mammalian species examined have been found to carry ubiquitous and well-adapted herpesviruses that have evolved colinearly along with their natural hosts. Many host species are infected with a number of different virus species from the alpha-, beta-, and gammaherpesvirus subfamilies. Herpesviruses in general usually cause only mild asymptomatic systemic primary infections at a very early age, then persist long term in a quiescent latent form (usually within neurons, lymphocytes, or monocytes), and occasionally reactivate as localized skin or mucosal epithelial lesions with active lytic infection. These lesions shed infectious virions that may be transmitted by cell to cell contact as well as in aerosols and in body fluids. In the occasional situations in which serious disease is encountered, it is usually presumed to involve a virus that has either become rare or was selected for unusual pathogenicity within its own natural hosts, or more likely has recently crossed species or subspecies boundaries. Alternatively, or in addition, it is also possible the host is immuno-suppressed or suffering from concurrent infections.

There are at least seven distinct species or subspecies of EEHV that have been identified and are now collectively classified as members of the *Proboscivirus* genus within the Betaherpesvirinae: EEHV1A, EEHV1B, EEHV2, EEHV3, EEHV4, EEHV5, and EEHV6.[6,9,25] Among the most recent 25 North American cases of systemic infection by EEHVs that have been confirmed, only two (the EEHV5 case and one example of EEHV1B) have not been associated with the typical signs and/or pathologic changes associated with acute hemorrhagic disease. None of the EEHVs have yet been grown in cell culture, but partial genomic DNA sequence analysis after PCR assay directly from necropsy tissue has revealed that they are a highly diverged group that evidently evolved separately from all other herpesvirus genera, beginning about 100 million years ago and corresponding to when the ancestors of modern elephants branched off from all other placental mammals. Three of these viruses (EEHV1A, EEHV2, and EEHV3) have also been found as typical localized reactivated infections in epithelial cells of skin, genital lesions, or pulmonary nodules in healthy African elephants, but EEHV has not been found in peripheral blood from healthy carrier elephants.

Preliminary PCR evidence in early studies has suggested that EEHV1, the virus found most commonly in Asian elephant disease cases, may in fact be endemic in healthy African elephants, because it was detected in an outbreak of skin nodules in several young African elephants from among a large group that was imported to Florida from Zimbabwe in the mid-1980s.[8,13,14,16] However, that conclusion has yet to be rigorously or unambiguously confirmed by extensive gene subtyping or in additional samples from wild elephants in Africa. It is plausible that an Asian elephant present at the same location could have transmitted EEHV1 virus to the Florida juveniles after arriving in Florida. On the other hand, EEHV2 was similarly implicated as being present in small nodules found in the lungs of healthy wild African elephants that were culled at Kruger National Park in South Africa in the late 1990s.[17] These pulmonary nodules were reported to occur in more than 50% of healthy adult free-ranging animals.[10] Furthermore, the presence of EEHV3 and EEHV6 in African elephant

lung nodules in high abundance has also recently been confirmed. The original hypothesis was that most cases of this disease in juvenile Asian elephants represent primary infection with a virus (EEHV1A) that has evolved naturally in African elephants, but not in Asian elephants. Over the past decade, this result has led to a significant awareness of and changes in the housing and management of the two species in facilities that keep mixed Asian and African herds, but some cases have occurred at facilities that appear never to have housed African elephants. Current serologic evidence implies that at least 8% of the wild-born adult captive Asian elephants in North America are also carriers of EEHV1 who must themselves have survived primary infection (possibly as infants in the wild), but little is known as yet about the EEHV1 serologic status of captive African elephants or of wild elephants in Asia or Africa. Over the last 2 years, necropsy samples from more than 10 cases of sudden death in both orphaned and wild Asian elephant calves in India were tested for the presence of EEHV by PCR assay. We were able to confirm the presence of EEHV1 DNA in frozen samples from eight of those cases. There have also been reports of at least eight other similarly suspected but unconfirmed cases in other parts of India, Thailand, and Sumatra, plus one PCR-confirmed EEHV1 case each in both Thailand and Cambodia.[12,23]

Despite over 15 years of research, EEHVs have not yet been successfully grown in cell culture, even in primary Asian or African elephant fibroblasts and placental umbilical cord endothelial cells, nor have stable lymphoid cell lines carrying the virus been established. Therefore, all DNA sequence analyses so far have had to be carried out directly from diseased necropsy tissue or from whole-blood DNA samples obtained from animals with acute EEHV-associated disease. Accurate sequence data have been obtained on both DNA strands for between 22 and 38 kb of EEHV DNA from necropsy tissue from each of five different EEHV1A, EEHV1B, and EEHV2 cases using a combination of lambda phage libraries and PCR approaches with redundant homologous primers.[17] Initial viral clones in the libraries were detected by hybridization with EEHV POL or TER probes; genome-walking techniques by direct and PCR-based sequencing were then applied. However, both libraries were incomplete because of the size and amount limitations for DNA recovered from necropsy tissue. Analyses of several additional segments of each virus not available from the libraries and of a few small loci in the four most recently discovered EEHV species were accomplished by direct PCR sequencing approaches based on known homologous motifs as data have been accumulated for more EEHV1 and EEHV2 genes. However, of necessity, all the data available are restricted to within the central core herpesvirus gene block covering about 80 kb out of an expected total genome size range of close to 200 kb for each EEHV species.

EPIDEMIOLOGY

All herpesviruses may persist in their host in the form of an episome within the nucleus of various cell types. Generally, the natural host range of herpesviruses is restricted to one species, although there are exceptions. During acute systemic disease, EEHV has been found at very high levels in whole-blood samples from all known cases, and this provides the only definitive test available. At necropsy, viral DNA is also found in all major organs tested in which focal hemorrhaging was evident, including heart, liver, spleen, kidney, colon, intestine, tongue, and brain. With the exception of the localized skin and lung nodules in African elephants and one older Asian elephant, EEHV DNA has never been found in the blood of healthy animals nor in any unrelated autopsy tissue samples. Even in the two cases in which no EEHV1 or EEHV2 was initially found, they eventually both proved instead to contain high levels of two other related viruses of this type, EEHV3 and EEHV4.[6,9]

EEHV DNA has been detected by PCR assay in necropsies or biopsies of two types of localized nodules found on the skin or in the lungs of otherwise asymptomatic African elephants.[17] However, in contrast to the acute disease, both EEHV1 in the skin nodules and EEHV2, EEHV3 and EEHV6 in pulmonary nodules were evidently undergoing productive lytic replication in dermal or alveolar epithelial cells, respectively, as judged by the presence of typical nuclear inclusion bodies. EEHV1 infection was also tentatively identified in vestibular lymphoid patches in some female African elephants, but very few such nodules or patches are known to have been observed in Asian elephants. Both the skin and lung nodules could presumably be considered the EEHV equivalents of reactivated herpes simplex lesions.

Most significantly, among 18 EEHV1A and five EEHV1B genomes for which up to 10 kb of DNA sequencing has been carried out, each by multilocus PCR gene subtyping, multiple minor subtype variants have been recognized.[25] In essence, modern EEHV1 genomes are made up of different scrambled combinations of pieces of two genomes that diverged 10 to 20 million years ago, plus residual pieces of three to five

distinct genome variants that diverged approximately 1 million years ago. This is superimposed on a common ancestral background from which all currently known individual isolates within both the EEHV1A and EEHV1B subgroups probably diverged within the past 100,000 years. Therefore, there is no doubt that one or the other elephant species has been the natural host of EEHV1 for at least that length of time, and each subtype cluster pattern is probably representative of the various distinctive herds or subpopulations of elephants—whether Asian or African—from which the individual donor wild-born elephant hosts were imported.

In addition to the novel EEHVs, five very distinct species of highly diverged gammaherpesviruses (or EGHVs) have now also been identified in captive Asian and African elephants.[22,25] Unlike the elephant EGHVs, which are periodically shed in oral, eye, and genital secretions, with or without visible lesions, in many captive Asian and African elephants, latent state infections have never been detected with any of the EEHVs by standard diagnostic DNA PCR assay in swabs or blood or autopsy tissues from healthy animals that were not already showing clinical signs of acute hemorrhagic disease. The only exceptions, in which EEHV DNA has been detected in blood of seemingly healthy animals, evidently represent either a transient reactivation event, as in the single case of EEHV5 in an older Asian adult, or a very early-stage primary infection in a herdmate of a parallel symptomatic case involving the identical EEHV1B strain. Unlike the pathogenic *Proboscivirus*, none of the EGHVs have been associated with any specific disease syndromes.

PATHOGENESIS

Two different but related EEHV species were implicated in our earliest studies, with that in two African elephant cases (EEHV2) being significantly different genetically (20% at the primary amino acid level in their encoded proteins) from Asian cases (EEHV1). Furthermore, two chimeric variants of EEHV1, EEHV1A and EEHV1B, were found in the Asian elephant cases.[1-3] Later, in 2007, we identified two more highly diverged species of *Proboscivirus*, EEHV3 and EEHV4, that have high GC content compared with the more AT-rich content of EEHV1 and EEHV2.[6,9] EEHV3 and EEHV4 differ by an average of 30% at the protein level from the other EEHVs and by 8% from each other. Subsequently, two single examples each of a fifth species (EEHV5), which is most closely related to EEHV2 (15% diverged), as well as a sixth species (EEHV6), which is most closely related to EEHV1

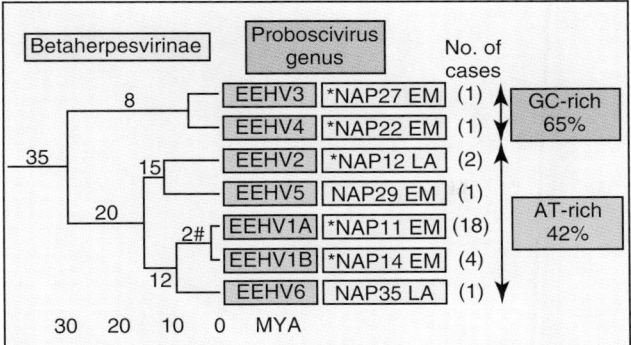

```
              Proboscivirus                 No. of
              genus                         cases
  Betaherpesvirinae
        8         ┌─ EEHV3 │*NAP27 EM│ (1)  ▲  GC-rich
                  └─ EEHV4 │*NAP22 EM│ (1)  │  65%
   35     15    ── EEHV2 │*NAP12 LA│ (2)  ▼
          20    ── EEHV5 │ NAP29 EM│ (1)  ▲
              2#┌─ EEHV1A │*NAP11 EM│ (18) │  AT-rich
                └─ EEHV1B │*NAP14 EM│ (4)  │  42%
          12    ── EEHV6 │ NAP35 LA│ (1)  ▼
   30   20   10    0  MYA
```

* = Lethal acute disease
EM = Elephas maximus (Asian)
LA = Loxodonta africana (African)
# = Plus chimeric segments
MYA = Million years ago

Figure 65-1

Summary of the average percentage of nucleotide differences, branching patterns, estimated evolutionary divergence dates, and number of cases detected of the seven distinctive EEHV species or subspecies.

(12% diverged), have also been identified (Fig. 65-1). The EEHV5 virus spiked briefly and at low levels in just two successive blood samples from a healthy older Asian elephant that was bled routinely every 2 weeks over a 2-year period. In comparison, EEHV6 was found at moderately high levels transiently in the blood of a 1-year-old African calf that had mild symptoms, but was treated with famciclovir (FCV) and recovered. The vast majority of cases that we have examined in detail were caused by EEHV1A (18 cases), but EEHV1B (four cases), plus EEHV2, EEHV3, EEHV4, and EEHV6 (one case each), have also been associated with acute systemic or disseminated disease, whereas EEHV5 was evidently observed just as a transient low-level reactivation from latency on one occasion so far. Recently, EEHV1B was detected transiently at a low level in the blood of a seemingly healthy calf 2 days after a herdmate with EEHV1B disease was diagnosed.

For EEHV1 gene subtype analysis, we selected seven representative EEHV1 PCR loci that display more extensive DNA sequence polymorphisms for detailed analysis of clustering patterns among the 25 most recent North American cases of EEHV1 disease.[25] Two zoo facilities have had six cases each in calves that were bred there, although several of these were afflicted after transfer to other facilities. Five cases each have also occurred among the progeny of two separate breeding bulls, and three each from two separate breeding cows, including some calves that had the same parents. However, in all such situations studied, multiple EEHV species and different

EEHV1 strains were involved, and all but two of the total of 25 EEHV1A plus EEHV1B cases analyzed proved to represent separate viral strains. Therefore, none of the cases at different facilities or even those among multiple cases that occurred at different times at the same facility, nor those that afflicted multiple offspring from one or both of the same parents, were directly or even closely linked epidemiologically.

The single case of two identical genomes occurred in a pair of 2-year-old calves that were evidently infected at the same time with the same EEHV1B strain at the same facility in 2009. In this case, the second calf had low levels of virus in the blood and was diagnosed only during preemptive screening of herdmates of the first symptomatic case. Both calves survived after ganciclovir (GCV) or FCV treatment, but the second calf never showed any clinical symptoms, presumably because prophylactic drug treatment was begun just after the first calf was diagnosed with typical symptoms. Curiously, an exactly analogous situation occurred with the same two calves about 6 months later, but in this case involving low levels of EEHV1A. Five elephant facilities are now known to have had elephants suffer from infections with both EEHV1A and EEHV1B, three in the United States and two in Europe.

Consequently, almost all known EEHV disease cases must have been derived from different source animals. Therefore, this is a sporadic (not epidemic or epizootic) disease; there was no linear chain of transmission involved. The most plausible interpretation is that these are uncontrolled primary infections that arise directly or indirectly through occasional cross-species infection from African elephants into Asian calves—but that must also include a number of asymptomatic Asian carriers as sources—leading to fulminant systemic infection in juvenile Asian elephants lacking any immune protection.

DIAGNOSIS

Clinical Pathology

Asian elephants with disseminated EEHV may become lymphopenic, thrombocytopenic, anemic, and dehydrated.[14] In the index case of EEHV in an Asian elephant, aerobic and anaerobic bacterial cultures of heart blood, pericardial and peritoneal fluid, cerebrospinal fluid, axillary lymph node, and liver were negative, and bacterial cultures of multiple segments of the gastrointestinal tract yielded no enteric pathogens. Cocultivation of the liver and heart were negative for any of the known herpesviruses or any other virus known to infect elephants.

Antemortem Diagnosis

Antemortem diagnosis of disseminated EEHV may be performed by PCR assay on a sample of whole blood, using both pan and specific primers directed toward the elephant herpesviruses.[15] Sensitive second-generation PCR-based DNA blood tests that are specific for EEHV have proven positive in all diseased animals, but almost never in any healthy animals.[9]

Differential Diagnosis

Where appropriate, encephalomyocarditis virus (EMCV) should be ruled out. Other diseases to consider include leptospirosis, other bacterial septicemias, toxicities, and nutritional deficiencies. There have been reports of blister beetles causing oral ulcers in elephants.

Postmortem Findings

Gross findings of elephants that have died with EEHV include pericardial effusion with extensive petechial to ecchymotic hemorrhages involving the epicardial and endocardial heart surfaces and throughout the myocardium, diffusely scattered petechiae within all the visceral and parietal peritoneal serous membranes, cyanosis and petechial hemorrhages on the tongue, hepatomegaly and, variably oral, laryngeal, and large intestinal ulcers. The microscopic findings consist of extensive microhemorrhages throughout the heart and tongue associated with edema and mild infiltrates of lymphocytes, monocytes, and neutrophils between myofibers. Multifocally, there is hepatic sinusoidal expansion with mild subacute inflammation and mild hepatocellular vacuolar degenerative changes. The capillary endothelial cells in the myocardium, tongue muscle, and within the hepatic sinusoids of the liver contain amphophilic to basophilic intranuclear viral inclusion bodies that are closely associated with the microhemorrhages (Fig. 65-2). Ultrastructural studies of the endothelial inclusion bodies reveal 80- to 92-nm diameter nucleocapsids morphologically consistent with the herpesvirus group.[14-16] The herpesvirus particles are most often present within the nucleus and rarely the cytoplasm, but have not been seen intercellularly.

TREATMENT

Prompt treatment with the human antiherpes drugs FCV and, more recently, GCV, appears to have been successful in saving nine confirmed PCR-positive afflicted

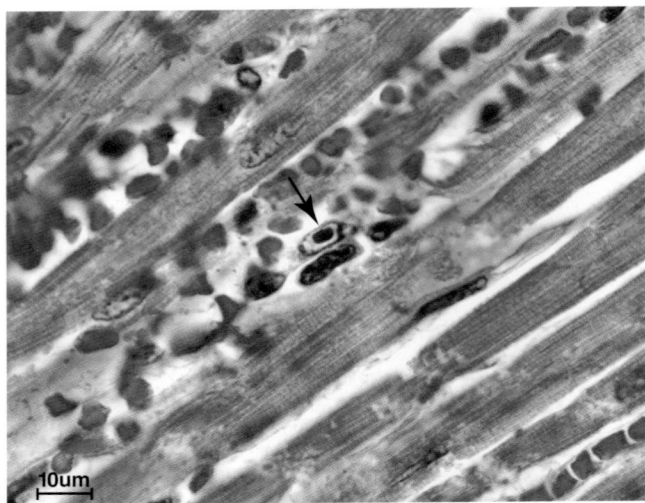

Figure 65-2

Photomicrograph of heart from an Asian elephant that died with elephant endotheliotropic herpesvirus (EEHV). The arrow indicates an intranuclear inclusion body within a capillary endothelial cell in the heart (hematoxylin and eosin stain).

calves, including two in Europe. These are the only known survivors of the disease, but similar medication was not effective in more than 12 other cases, in which it was likely started too late. High viral DNA loads were present in the blood of all acute disease cases, but this becomes undetectable several weeks after drug treatment in the survivors.[7,19,20] In the absence of drug treatment, there were also high levels of cell-free virus DNA found in the serum of several lethal cases, implying active lytic infection, but this has not been the case in the drug-treated survivors, in which the bulk of the viral DNA was present intracellularly in peripheral blood mononuclear cell (PBMC) fractions rather than in serum or plasma.

GLOBAL IMPLICATIONS

All seven species and subspecies of EEHV that we have identified have been found in captive elephants in North America, with five of them being associated with cases of fatal hemorrhagic disease. In addition, within the past few years, as many as 16 pathologically diagnosed cases of EEHV disease have now been recognized in captive and wild elephant calves in four Asian range countries. Zachariah and colleagues[23] have collected postmortem tissue samples from more than 10 lethal hemorrhagic disease cases in Kerala, India, over the past several years and have documented typical systemic hemorrhagic pathologic features, including microscopic detection of histochemically typical beta herpesvirus–like nuclear inclusion bodies in vascular endothelial cells in several of them. Diagnostic PCR tests carried out using PAN EEHV and specific EEHV1 primers have confirmed that necropsy tissue samples from eight of the cases examined contained high levels of EEHV1A DNA (for several of them in multiple tissues), whereas unrelated negative control tissue samples did not. However, we have not as yet been able to carry out any DNA sequencing for genotype analysis of such samples. Strain subtyping is critical to learn whether they involve EEHV1 strains similar to those seen in the United States and Europe or something novel, as well as whether the Indian and other Asian cases all involve the same strain or multiple different strains. The viral DNA sequence data here should provide immediate answers to major questions about whether this is a natural infection and an old disease in Asian elephants in India, or whether it was just introduced very recently from African elephants—perhaps, for example, via those that were housed at zoos there or possibly introduced instead during the Greek and Persian empires, whose armies travelled extensively with elephants of one or more species.

This question seems to be the most urgent and critical issue for understanding and combating the disease in captivity, at least by being able to assess intelligently whether having a seropositive mother portends well or ill for her calf. Whether there are just one or many different EEHV1 strains in the Indian cases will also have major implications about the origins and distribution of the virus within Asia. Our original concept, that EEHV1 is an endogenous virus of African elephants that must cross species barriers to kill Asian elephant calves in zoos, would certainly provide a logical explanation for the unexpectedly severe pathology of primary infection in naïve calves. However, this scenario also predicts that it should presumably occur only in captivity in zoos. Therefore, the discovery of EEHV1-like viruses causing exactly the same type of lethal hemorrhagic disease pathology in calves in Asian countries has disturbing implications. Not only does it negate any idea of this being just a disease of zoos or captivity, but it also seriously questions our notions about the origin of this virus. Either EEHV1 is an endogenous virus of Asian elephants, which means that some other explanation is needed to understand why it causes such a devastating disease, or the African virus has also somehow entered into the Asian elephant population in the wild. It now

becomes of critical importance to carry out specific serology assays to evaluate the extent of silent infections by the various EEHV species in all wild Asian and African elephant populations.

Recently, a real-time quantitative PCR assay was developed that has been used to detect the presence of pathogenic EEHVs in trunk wash samples obtained from healthy Asian elephants.[21] Within individual elephants, detection of EEHV1 DNA in trunk wash samples was variable over the course of the screening period, with the overall frequency of detection in the one herd examined being 31%. Two of the three positive healthy animals involved proved to be shedding an identical EEHV1A strain to that which killed a calf at the same facility 2 years earlier, whereas the third positive animal was shedding an EEHV1B strain and two other herdmates were negative over this period. The specific factors that result in a lethal infection in one elephant, but an asymptomatic infection in another, remain undetermined.

Overall, these data provide evidence supporting the hypothesis that trunk secretions may be a mode of transmission of pathogenic EEHV. Whatever the origins of the individual EEHV species, it is highly plausible that African and Asian elephants in the wild are normally infected universally and asymptomatically by multiple EEHV (and EGHV) species. Therefore, many of the adult wild-born animals in zoos have likely been carrying them from before they were originally captured and transported. The problem may be that unlike the EGHVs, the EEHVs are rather difficult to transmit and that unlike in the wild, the next generation of animals in captivity rarely encounter other infants and therefore do not acquire asymptomatic infections with multiple viruses at a very young age, when they are still protected by maternal antibodies. Instead, they may first become exposed to a relatively exotic nonadapted EEHV species at a much later age than normal and lack the immune protection that might normally be provided by antibodies developed against their own natural virus species. Determining which EEHV species a calf (and its mother) have been exposed to previously may well turn out to be the key for understanding the severity of EEHV-associated disease and assessing the risks involved in specific breeding and housing interactions between individual animals in captivity.

REFERENCES

1. Ehlers B, Burkhardt S, Goltz M, et al: Genetic and ultrastructural characterization of a European isolate of the fatal endotheliotropic elephant herpesvirus. J Gen Virol 82:475–482, 2001.

2. Ehlers B, Dural G, Marschall M, et al: Endotheliotropic elephant herpesvirus, the first betaherpesvirus with a thymidine kinase gene. J Gen Virol 87:2781–2789, 2006.

3. Fickel J, Lieckfeldt D, Richman LK, et al: Comparison of glycoprotein B (gB) variants of the elephant endotheliotropic herpesvirus (EEHV) isolated from Asian elephants *(Elephas maximus)*. Vet Microbiol 91:11–21, 2003.

4. Fickel J, Richman LK, Montali R, et al: A variant of the endotheliotropic herpesvirus in Asian elephants *(Elephas maximus)* in European zoos. Vet Microbiol 82:103–109, 2001.

5. Fickel J, Richman LK, Reinsch A, et al: Survey on the occurrence of the endotheliotropic elephant herpesvirus (EEHV) in Asian *(Elephas maximus)* and African *(Loxodonta africana)* elephants in European zoos, 2000 (http://library.vetmed.fu-berlin.de/resources/global/contents/VET164623/EAZWV/Parijs%20PDF/Microsoft%20Word%20-%20Fickel.pdf).

6. Garner MM, Helmick K, Ochsenreiter J, et al: Clinico-pathologic features of fatal disease attributed to new variants of endotheliotropic herpesviruses in two Asian elephants *(Elephas maximus)*. Vet Pathol 46:97–104, 2009.

7. Isaza R, Hunter RP, Richman LK: Famciclovir pharmacokinetics in young Asian elephants *(Elephas maximus)*. In Proceedings of the AAZV Annual Conference, Minneapolis, 2003, pp 82–83.

8. Jacobson E, Sundberg J, Gaskin J, et al: Cutaneous papillomas associated with a herpesvirus-like infection in a herd of captive African elephants. J Am Vet Med Assoc 189:1075–1078, 1986.

9. Latimer E, Zong J-C, Heaggans S, et al: Detection and evaluation of novel herpesviruses in routine and pathological samples from Asian and African elephants: Identification of two more proboscíciviruses (EEHV5 and EEHV6) and two more gammaherpesviruses (EGHV3B and EGHV5). Vet Microbiol 2010 (in press).

10. McCully RM, Basson PA, Pienaar JG, et al: Herpes nodules in the lung of the African elephant *(Loxodonta africana* [Blumebach, 1792]). Onderstepoort J Vet Res 38:225–235, 1971.

11. Ossent P, Guscetti F, Metzler AE, et al: Acute and fatal herpesvirus infection in a young Asian elephant *(Elephas maximus)*. Vet Pathol 27:131–133, 1990.

12. Reid C, Hildebrandt T, Marx N, et al: Endotheliotropic elephant herpes virus (EEHV) infection. The first PCR-confirmed fatal case in Asia. Vet Q 28:61–64, 2006.

13. Richman L: Pathological and molecular aspects of fatal endotheliotropic herpesviruses of elephants. Ph.D thesis. Baltimore, 2003, Johns Hopkins University.

14. Richman L, Montali R, Cambre R, et al: Clinical and pathological findings of a newly recognized disease of elephants caused by endotheliotropic herpesviruses. J Wildl Dis 36:1–12, 2000.

15. Richman LK, Montali RJ, Garber RL, et al: Novel endotheliotropic herpesviruses fatal for Asian and African elephants. Science 283:1171–1176, 1999.

16. Richman L, Montali RJ, Hayward GS: Review of a newly recognized disease of elephants caused by endotheliotropic herpesviruses. Zoo Biol 19:383–392, 2000.

17. Richman LK, Zong J-C, Latimer E, et al: The genomes of seven distinct elephant betaherpesviruses associated with endotheliolytic disease are highly diverged from both cytomegaloviruses and roseoloviruses and form a new proboscivirus genus (in preparation).

18. Schaftenaar W: Personal communication, 2004.

19. Schaftenaar W, Mensink JM, De Boer AM, et al: Successful treatment of a subadult Asian elephant bull *(Elephas maximus)* infected with elephant herpesvirus. In Hofer H, editor: Proceedings of the Institute for Zoo and Wildlife Research, ed 4, Rotterdam, The Netherlands, 2001, Institute for Zoo and Wildlife Research, pp 141–146.

20. Schmitt D, Hardy D, Montali R, et al: Use of famciclovir for the treatment of endotheliotrophic herpesvirus infections in Asian elephants *(Elephas maximus)*. J Zoo Wildl Med 31:518–522, 2000.

21. Stanton JJ, Zong J-C, Latimer E, et al: Detection of pathogenic elephant endotheliotropic herpesvirus in routine trunk washes from healthy adult Asian elephants *(Elephas maximus)* using a novel quantitative real-time polymerase chain reaction assay. Am J Vet Res 71:925–933, 2010.

22. Wellehan JF, Johnson AJ, Childress AL, et al: Six novel gammaherpesviruses of Afrotheria provide insight into the early divergence of the Gammaherpesvirinae. Vet Microbiol 127:249–257, 2008.

23. Zachariah A, Richman L, Latimer E, et al: Fatal endotheliotropic elephant herpesvirus infection in captive and free-ranging Asian elephants in South India. Presented at the International Elephant Conservation and Research Symposium, Bangkok, Thailand, November 2008.

24. Zong J-C, Latimer E, Heaggans SY, et al: Pathogenesis and molecular epidemiology of fatal elephant endotheliotropic disease associated with the expanding *Proboscivirus* genus of the Betaherpesvirinae. Presented at the International Elephant Conservation and Research Symposium, Pattaya, Thailand, 2008.

25. Zong J-C, Latimer E, Heaggans SY, et al: Viral gene subtyping of eighteen North American cases of EEHV hemorrhagic disease. Presented at the International Elephant Conservation and Research Symposium, Bangkok, Thailand, November 2008.

CHAPTER 66

Female Elephant Reproduction

Imke Lueders and Thomas Bernd Hildebrandt

Among our living terrestrial vertebrates, the three elephant species *(Elephas maximus, Loxodonta africana, Loxodonta cyclotis)* hold a unique position and differ in many ways from the general mammalian model. A fact that is most striking is in regard to their reproductive physiology. Many special reproductive features make the Asian and both African elephants subjects of great scientific interest. However, because of low numbers of available study animals, limited accessibility, their enormous size, and their endangered status, elephants are extremely challenging to study.

Through a combination of different approaches, such as postmortem structure analysis, biochemical investigations, application of imaging techniques, and behavioral observations, considerable advances have been made over the last 4 decades. This has assisted with the markedly improved breeding success of captive Asian and African elephants, as well as the management of their wild populations. The most recent accomplishments include successful manual semen collection, sorting, and freezing, as well as artificial insemination with fresh, chilled, or frozen semen.[9]

Nevertheless, several aspects of the female reproductive process remain unknown. Ongoing research efforts and the enhanced understanding of elephant reproductive physiology represent key factors for in situ and ex situ conservation of these magnificent creatures in the future.

FEMALE REPRODUCTIVE TRACT

The special anatomy of the elephant's reproductive organs is regarded as an adaptation to the previous aquatic life of their former ancestors.[10] In addition to the size of the entire female urogenital tract (Fig. 66-1), with a total length of about 3 m,[14] the most obvious difference compared with other ungulate species is the

extremely long vestibule (urogenital canal), which measures about 1.0 to 1.4 m and opens between the hind legs.[1,15,26] During urination and relaxation, the large clitoris becomes evident, protruding from the vestibule opening. The tubelike vestibule runs vertically and bends horizontally over the caudal pelvis (see Fig. 66-1L). At its cranial end, a hymen-like structure is found in nulliparous females, leaving only a small opening of approximately 0.4×0.2 cm into the vagina. For successful artificial insemination, this tiny vaginal os has to be penetrated with the insemination catheter to deposit the semen into the vagina. This true opening is flanked by two blind pouches. The whole hymenal structure will rupture during the first delivery, but not during mating, because the male elephant delivers his semen into the cranial part of the vestibule. After the first birth, the opening to the vagina is approximately 2 to 3 cm in diameter. The vagina is characterized by longitudinal folds and extends 30 to 50 cm cranially (see Fig. 66-1J, K). The cervix also shows longitudinal folds and is only approximately 15 cm long (see Fig. 66-1H, I). The portio cervices, as the caudal part of the cervix, prominently protrudes into the vagina. The uterus bicornis (see Fig. 66-1G) measures 0.8 to 1.5 m, including a short uterine body of only 5 to 10 cm. The endometrial thickness of the uterine body is different from the horns. The uterine body has a thinner endometrial lining, which may explain why implantation never occurs in this part. However, both body and horns have a similar uterine lining, which shows longitudinal rugae and a ciliated mucous membrane. Each pregnancy damages the endometrium where the placenta has been attached, leaving permanent scars. The comparably small ovaries measure $7.0 \times 5.5 \times 2.5$ cm and weigh approximately 60 g. They have a typical brainlike structured surface and are completely enveloped in a double-pouch formation. The inner serosal pouch forms the

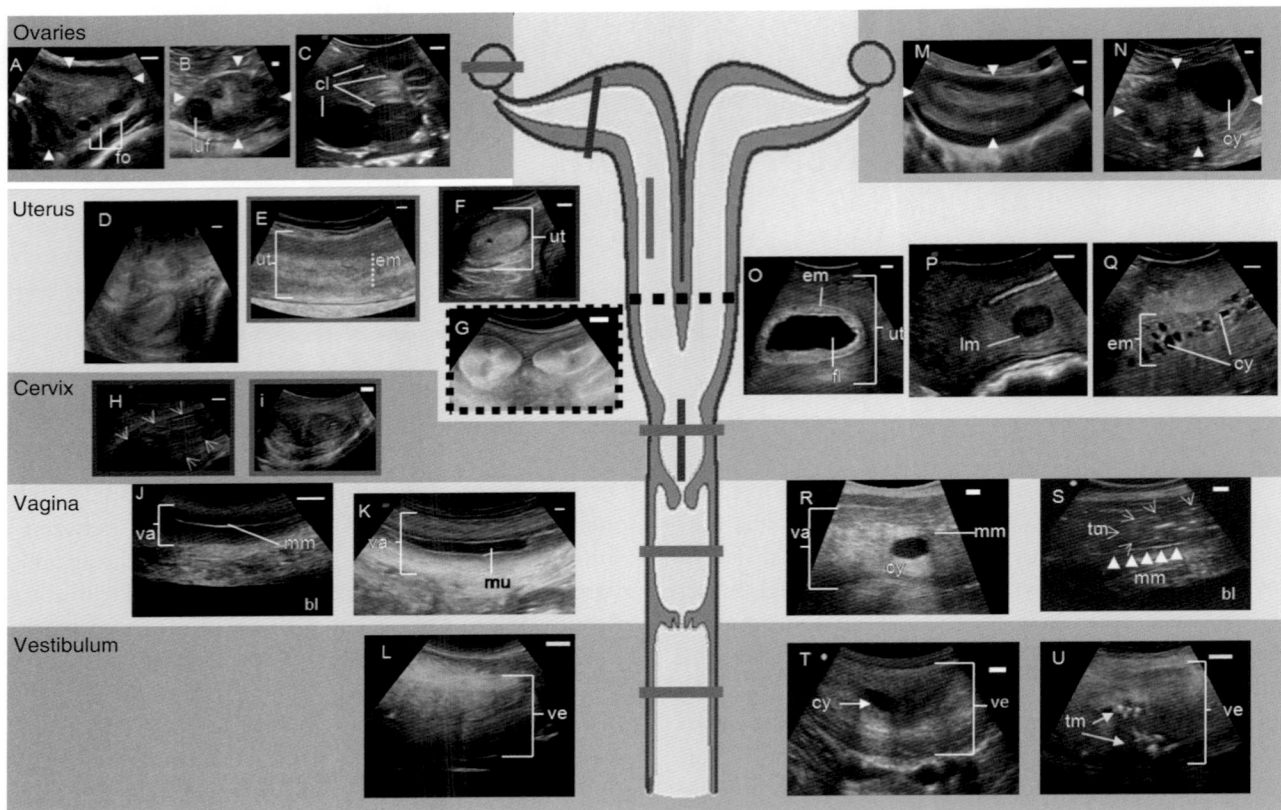

Figure 66-1

Physiologic *(left)* and pathologic *(right)* ultrasonographic appearance of the female elephant reproductive tract (bar = 10 mm). Normal: **A,** Ovary *(arrow heads),* follicular phase. **B,** Ovary *(arrowheads)* late follicular phase. **C,** Ovary, midluteal phase or pregnancy. **D,** Convoluted uterine horns shortly before ovulation. **E,** Flat uterine horn, longitudinal section, indistinct endometrium, late luteal phase. **F,** Uterine horn, cross section, bright distinct endometrium and small amount of intraluminal fluid, around ovulation. **G,** Uterine horns, cross-sectioned at bifurcation. **H,** Cervix *(arrows),* longitudinal section. **I,** Cervix, cross section. **J,** Vagina *(cross section)* around ovulation, prominent mucous membrane. **K,** Vagina *(cross section)* filled with mucus, typical for luteal phase or pregnancy. **L,** Vestibulum *(cross section).* Abnormal: **M,** Ovary *(arrowheads)* without any functional structures *(flatliner).* **N,** Ovary *(arrowheads),* showing large cyst. **O,** Uterine horn, filled with large amount of fluid. **P,** Leiomyoma. **Q,** Cystic endometrium. **R,** Vaginal cyst. **S,** Vaginal tumor. **T,** Vestibular cyst. **U,** Vestibular tumor. *bl,* Bladder; *cl,* corpus luteum; *cy,* cyst; *em,* endometrium; *fl,* fluid; *fo,* follicle; *lm,* leiomyoma; *luf,* luteinizing follicle; *mm,* mucous membrane; *tm,* tumor; *ut,* uterus, *va,* vagina; *ve,* vestibulum.

oviductal infundibulum. The outer pouch also encapsulates the ovary and their fat inclusions explain difficulties in imaging ovarian structures via ultrasound. In mature healthy females, the ovaries always contain functional structures (see Fig. 66-1A-C), except during late lactational anestrus. Most interesting is the occurrence of multiple corpora lutea (CLs) (up to 42; average, 4 to 6) of sizes between 10 and 50 mm, which protrude from the ovarian cortex in cycling as well as in pregnant cows.

ESTROUS CYCLE

In the wild, female elephants reach maturity at about 10 to 12 years. However, in captivity, puberty may be reached as early as 3.5 to 5 years.[16,25] The spontaneous ovulating, polyestric female is usually considered nonseasonal, with births occurring throughout the year, but peaks in the rainy season have been observed in their range countries. In captive herds, natural estrous synchronization has been observed,[29] but may rather be

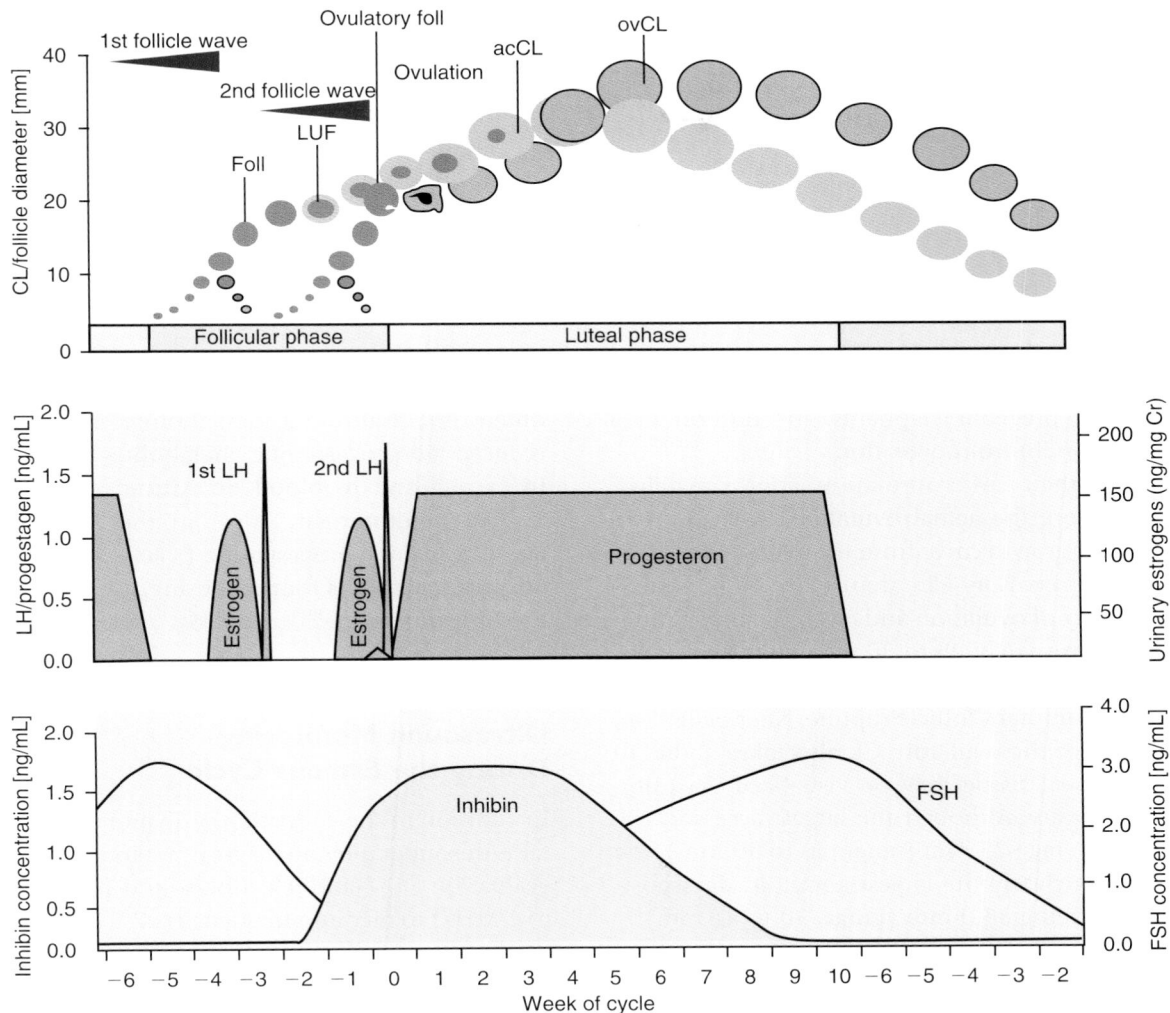

Figure 66-2

Schematic of events during the estrous cycle showing ovarian activity, development of follicles *(foll)*, luteinizing follicles *(LUF)*, accessory CLs *(acCL)*, and ovulatory CL *(ovCL)* in relationship to steroid hormones (progestagens, estrogen), inhibin and gonadotropin (luteinizing hormone *[LH]*, and follicle-stimulating hormone *[FSH]*) secretion.

an artificial condition because free-ranging elephant females spend most of their reproductive lifespan either pregnant or in lactational anestrus.

With a duration of 13 to 18 weeks, elephants exhibit the longest spontaneous estrous cycle of any mammal studied to date.[3,4] Seasonal differences in the length of the follicular and luteal phases may occur in Asian elephants in their natural environment.[27] Estrous cycle activity may be assessed by weekly progestagen determination from serum, urine, or feces. The typical cycle pattern shows a biphasic profile of interchanging periods of elevated (luteal phase, 6 to 12 weeks) and baseline (interluteal or follicular phase, 4 to 6 weeks) progestagen concentrations (Fig. 66-2).[3]

The most striking difference compared with other mammals is the occurrence of two distinct luteinizing hormone (LH) peaks, during the follicular phase of which only the second induces ovulation (see Fig. 66-2). These two peaks are 19 to 22 days apart and each one is preceded by an estrogen surge.[3,5] Each LH peak terminates a follicular wave , but only the second (ovulatory) LH peak will cause a dominant follicle of about 20.0 mm (range, 15.0 to 23.0 mm) to rupture 12 to 24 hours later.[11,15,21] The first (anovulatory) LH peak, however, has been shown to induce luteinization of larger follicles of the first follicle wave.[21] Luteinized follicles (LUFs) become ultrasonographically apparent about 10 days after the first LH peak. This is coincident with a sharp rise in the inhibin level. Luteal cells of the elephant's CLs appear to produce inhibin and might be a source of this hormone in addition to the dominant follicle.[19,22] Inhibin is known to be an important factor for the selection of the dominant follicle. Therefore, the first LH peak may be to induce luteinization of granulosa cells in larger follicles from the first wave and subsequently secrete inhibins, which in turn promotes deviation of a single dominant follicle at the end of the second follicular wave.[22] At the same time, the LUFs are the source of accessory corpora lutea.[11,21] There are approximately 2 to 10 of these accessory luteal structures on each ovary of cycling and pregnant elephants, in addition to a corpus luteum (CL) from ovulation.

Because of their earlier formation, approximately 8 to 10 days before the actual ovulation, accessory CLs have a different growth curve from the ovulatory CL (see Fig. 66-2). The accessory CLs are usually more numerous on the ovary of ovulation and reach their maximum diameter approximately 25 to 30 days after the second LH surge, about 10 days earlier than the single CL derived from dominant follicle rupture. After ovulation, the formation of the ovulatory CL also takes about 10 days before luteal tissue may be visualized via ultrasound in the ovary. Although the largest accessory CL measures on average 25 mm (range, 10 to 30 mm), the ovulatory CL is clearly the largest about 40 days postovulation, averaging 33.0 mm (range, 30 to 41 mm).[21]

Even though LUFs become distinct well before ovulation, progestagen levels only rise to luteal phase concentrations within 1 to 3 days after the second LH peak, but a preovulatory small progestagen rise has sometimes been seen (see Fig. 66-2). This occurs 1 to 3 days prior to the second LH peak and could be derived from the LUF to support ovulation. Regression of accessory CLs occurs approximately 1 week earlier than that of the ovulatory CL, without noticeable changes in progestagen levels. A decline in progestagen concentrations is soon followed by structural luteolysis of the ovulatory CL. Regression of all luteal structures is a slow process and functionally inactive CLs remain visible throughout the next follicular phase and even after the following ovulation, up to 3 weeks into the new luteal phase.[21]

Concentrations of follicle-stimulating hormone (FSH) rise during the luteal phase and peak at the beginning of the follicular phase, leading to the formation of fresh follicles as soon as progestagen levels are at baseline (see Fig. 66-2). Because inhibin and FSH are negatively correlated, the latter's concentration declines during the follicular phase and reaches baseline just before ovulation. The inhibin level remains elevated up to 5 weeks into the luteal phase, supporting the theory of luteal origin.[19,22]

In addition to the very unique formation of the CLs, their secretory capacity is also different from all mammals studied to date. There are only minute quantities of progesterone found, which is the main progestagen in other species. Instead, elephant CLs secrete predominately the reduced 5α-progesterone metabolites 5α-pregnane-3,20-dione (5α-DHP) and 3α-hydroxy-5α-pregnane-20-one (5α-P-3α-OH).[17] Correspondent receptors are demonstrated in the endometrium, confirming their biologic significance. The reduced 5α-progesterone metabolites are measurable in excreta and in blood. In African elephants, 5α-P-3α-OH predominates. Also, in the Asian elephants, the 17α-hydroxyprogesterone (17α-OH) metabolite of 5α-pregnanetriol is found in urine and feces, but not in the African species.[23]

Ultrasound Monitoring During the Estrous Cycle

In addition to the endocrine cycle monitoring, transrectal ultrasonography offers great potential for cycle stage evaluation.[11,15] Handheld ultrasound probes of low (4 to 2 MHz) to medium frequency (<7.5 MHz) are useful, but for the visualization of the cranial uterine parts and the ovaries, an extension (handle) for the scanner head might be necessary.[15]

During the luteal phase, many females develop an anechoic mucous plug within the vagina to protect the uterus from contamination (see Fig. 66-1K). Although the mucus is excreted in a nonconceptive cycle during the follicular phase (usually around the first LH peak, Fig. 66-3A), it is maintained during pregnancy. In the luteal phase, the uterus is relaxed and therefore is usually not totally accessible if the female is standing. The endometrium and myometrium appear less distinct (see Fig. 66-1E). The endometrial layer is thin, with a cross-sectional diameter of only 23.7 ± 0.21 mm as opposed to the 35.4-mm average in the follicular phase (see Fig. 66-1D, F). The ovaries show multiple large CLs (see Fig. 66-1C), of which the accessory CLs typically maintain a fluid-filled central cavity during the first 3 weeks after ovulation (see Fig. 66-1B). Antral follicles never occur during the luteal phase and therefore, in turn, the presence of multiple follicles is a good indicator that a female is in the follicular phase (see Fig. 66-1A).[11,21] Furthermore, a higher fluid content in the endometrium

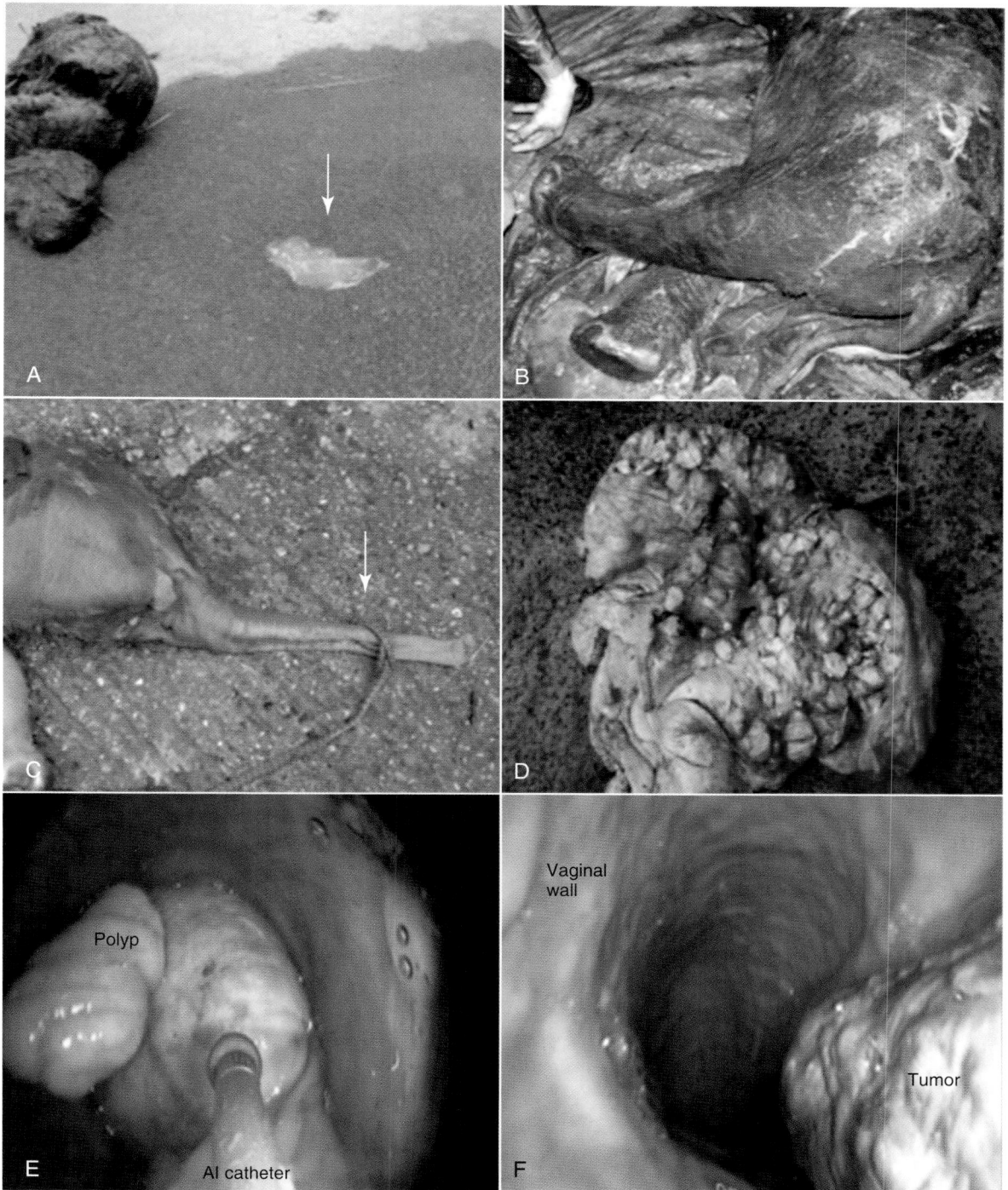

Figure 66-3

A, Typical mucous plug *(arrow)* from the vagina excreted during urination after the first LH peak. **B,** Mal-formed fetus (stiffening of the hind legs), leading to dystocia and uterine rupture in the dam. **C,** Use of the trunk rope *(arrow)* to extract a dead fetus during episiotomy. **D,** Uterus (opened) showing excessive uterine leiomyomas in a 40-year-old nulliparous Asian elephant female. **E,** Endoscopic image of a typical vestibular polyp. **F,** Endoscopic image of a vaginal tumor. *(A, Courtesy Guillaume Rebis; B, courtesy Belfast Zoological Gardens.)*

caused by low progestagen and increasing estrogen concentrations is noticeable during the follicular phase. Small amounts of free fluid might even accumulate within the uterine lumen 1 to 2 weeks before ovulation. The uterus becomes more toned toward the LH peaks; the horns appear convoluted and are now more easily accessible for the investigator because of retraction and elevation toward the pelvis (see Fig. 66-1G). Because of the more contracted myometrium, the tissues are denser and therefore the uterus appears increasingly bright in the ultrasound image. The endometrium becomes more distinct from the surrounding myometrium and shows a typical echogenicity of interchanging darker and brighter signals shortly before ovulation. After ovulation, the endometrial diameter decreases progressively and reaches the smallest measured thickness of 17 ± 1.5 mm in the early follicular phase of the next cycle.[11]

HORMONE CYCLE INDUCTION

Because of the significant differences during the elephant's estrous cycle (see earlier), endocrine treatments cannot be directly transferred from protocols for domestic animals. However, it is sometimes desirable to control the cycle and induce ovulation, especially for the application of artificial insemination. Information about possible hormonal manipulation is scarce and trials with commercially used drugs have not always produced the expected effects.[16]

Prostaglandin

Prostaglandin $F_{2\alpha}$ ($PGF_{2\alpha}$) is commonly used in domestic ruminants and horses to induce luteolysis and initiate a new estrous cycle. In a study on two cycling African elephants, $PGF_{2\alpha}$ was injected once IM at a dose of 80 to 125 mg/elephant on several different days during the luteal phase without any effect on serum progestagen secretion. Only in one female did progestagen levels decline 4 days after the injection, on day 60 postestrus. However, at this time, natural CL regression and termination of the luteal phase occurs (compare summary[16]).

In another case, $PGF_{2\alpha}$ was administered on three consecutive days to a young pregnant female to induce abortion at month 5 of gestation. Although urinary progesterone metabolite concentrations dropped to baseline during treatment, they returned to normal pregnancy concentrations 10 days after the last injection. A healthy calf was delivered by this dam.[24]

Therefore, functional luteolysis may be achieved; for structural luteolysis, however, a longer period of $PGF_{2\alpha}$ injection seems to be necessary.

Human Choriogonadotropin

To ensure ovulation at the time of artificial insemination (AI), human choriogonadotropin (hCG) has been used at a dosage of 5000 IU, injected at the time of the last AI. Subsequent ovulation was seen in six cases. However, coincidental occurrence of the natural second LH peak cannot be excluded because AI is usually timed 19 to 21 days after the first LH peak. Also, this treatment seems not to be completely reliable because in one case, injection of hCG 19 days after the measured first LH peak failed to induce ovulation. However, dominant follicle rupture then occurred on day 23 (following a natural second LH peak at day 22) after the first LH peak. This case indicates that the follicle needs to reach a certain size, or stage of maturation, to be receptive for ovulation induction. In another personal observation on an African elephant female, hCG led to the hyperstimulation of follicular development 5 days postinjection.[16]

Gonadotropin-Releasing Hormone

Several studies have suggested that the administration of gonadotropin-releasing hormone (GnRH) may induce the release of LH at levels lower than normal LH surges.[3] Thitaram and associates[28] have developed a method to induce the second LH peak by using a GnRH agonist (buserelin acetate) around the time of the first LH peak. Buserelin acetate given IV13 to 43 days after progesterone had reached baseline concentrations (but not earlier), at a dose of 80 µg resulted in an immediate anovulatory LH surge. This was followed by the second ovulatory LH surge 15 to 22 days later. One female conceived following this protocol. It was suggested in this study that the induction of the first LH peak in proximity to the time it would naturally occur would facilitate determination of the right time for breeding or AI. However, the range of 7 days for the occurrence of the second LH peak is still too imprecise. Another drawback is that the GnRH agonist needs to be administered in a restricted period of time during the long reproductive cycle (up to 4 months) to be effective. To determine this window, close monitoring of progestagen levels is necessary. Backing up the data with ovarian events during such hormone treatments will be very helpful.

PREGNANCY

Gestation length in both African and Asian species is 620 to 640 ± 14 days.[26] Progesterone levels during the first 6 weeks postconception are no different than those of a normal luteal phase. There is even a transient progestagen level decrease measurable at approximately 8 weeks postconception, when concentration nears baseline values. In case of pregnancy, these levels gradually increase again and reach concentrations above a nonconceptive luteal phase at 10 to 12 weeks of gestation.[3,26] Especially during the first half of gestation, the progestagen concentration may exceed that of the luteal phase by two to three times. However, the levels of progestagens are variable during the 22 months pregnancy and absolute values may not always exceed those observed during luteal phase.[3]

There are currently various possibilities to diagnose pregnancy in elephants[25]:

1. Progestagen
   - Elevation of progestagen levels beyond normal luteal phase length, more than 10 weeks above baseline level (from weekly samples)
   - For Asian elephants, the ratio of immunoreactive progesterone to 17α-hydroxyprogesterone (17α-OH) is significantly lower during the first 3 to 8 weeks of conception compared with a nonconceptive cycle.[23]
2. Prolactin
   - A single sample after 6 months for determination of prolactin is sufficient because this hormone rises 200 to 600 times higher than nonpregnant values.[3,4]
3. Ultrasonography
   - From day 50 postovulation, an embryonic vesicle may be detected in the uterine horn by transrectal ultrasound.[6,13]
   - From day 250, transabdominal sonography may be successful to visualize a fetus.

The origin of additional progestagen during pregnancy has been discussed at length. Conception initially prevents CL regression (luteal rescue) and thus prolongs progesterone metabolite secretion.

As described for the estrous cycle, a set of multiple CLs is present in elephants throughout the entire pregnancy.[1] Evaluation of their steroidogenic activity has suggested that they are mainly active between months 3 to 15 of gestation. In most species, there is a shift from luteal to placental progestagen secretion at a certain point of gestation. In elephants, immunocytochemical staining, gonadotropin extraction, and assays on placentas failed to detect any progestagen or gonadotropin activity, suggesting that elephant placental tissue has no endocrinologic competence.[1] Fetal gonads, in both genders, show an unusual enlargement during the second half of gestation. Furthermore, gonadal tissues incubated with progestin precursors exhibited copious production of progestins.[1] Therefore, their contribution to pregnancy progestagen concentration was considered.

A recently performed ultrasound study found CL diameters declining in weeks 6 to 8, reflecting the transient progestagen level decrease, as noted, after which a second growth phase occurred. This resulted in CL diameters significantly larger than during the estrous cycle. We noted that all CLs were maintained in size and number throughout the pregnancy and no additional follicles or CLs were observed to form. The factors that prolong luteal lifespan and initiate additional growth are not yet known. One study has suggested a choriogonadotropin with an LH-like action, measurable in elephant serum between weeks 8 and 13 of pregnancy, which could trigger luteal rescue.[18]

Another potential luteotropic factor could be prolactin. The secretion of prolactin increases between months 4 to 6 of gestation and concentrations up to 600 times above the normal estrous cycle levels may be measured.[3] The timing of increased prolactin secretion is too late to account for the initial extension of luteal lifespan. Nevertheless, it is likely to be associated with a continuous luteal output of progestagens.

The concentrations for LH and FSH during gestation were no different from those during the cycle. Relaxin was found to increase by week 20 of gestation and remained elevated most of the pregnancy, but declined toward the last weeks of gestation.[23] The exact endocrine events that trigger parturition have not yet been clarified.

Embryonic and Fetal Development

Data on embryonic and fetal development have been obtained from postmortem examination on culled African elephants as well as more recent in situ ultrasound observations. The latter allowed measurement of embryonic-fetal parameters such as crown-rump length (CRL; Fig. 66-4A), biparietal dimension (BPD; see Fig. 66-4B), thorax diameter (TH; see Fig. 66-4C), and femur length (FL; see Fig. 66-4D) and the development of a growth curve during the first 200 days of pregnancy.

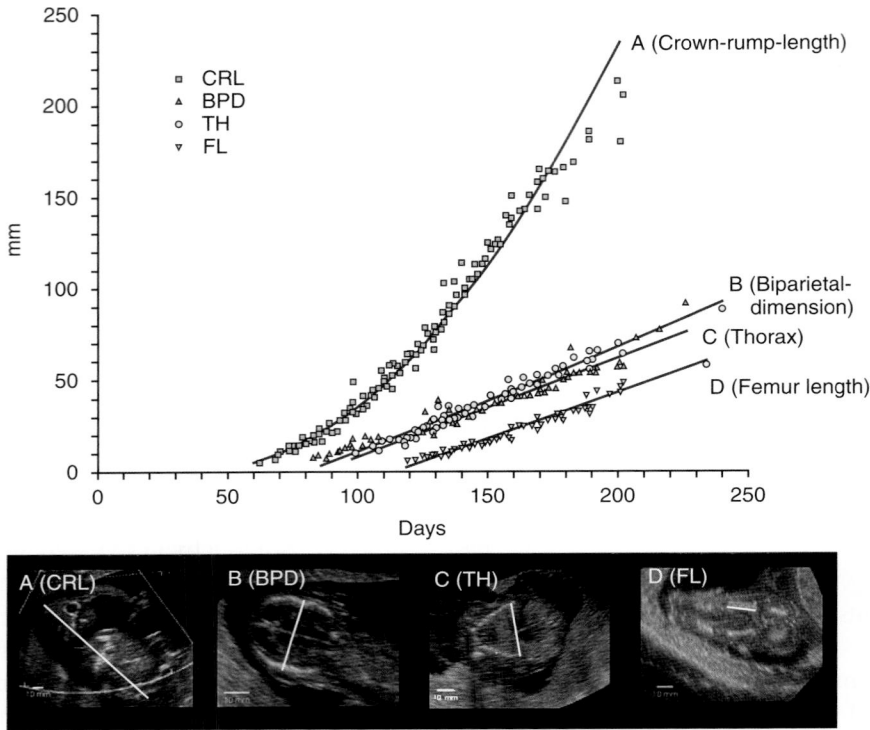

Figure 66-4

Growth curve for embryonic-fetal parameters assessed via ultrasound (bar = 10 mm). **A,** Crown-rump length (*CRL*). **B,** Biparietal dimension (*BPD*). **C,** Thorax width (*TH*). **D,** Femur length (*FL*).

Implantation seems to be delayed.[6] Based on serial sonography, the first constrained fluid accumulation within the uterine lumen was visualized between days 42 and 46 postconception, followed by a clear, round, embryonic vesicle (EV) near the uterine body on day 50 measuring approximately 8.0 to 10.0 mm.[13,14,20] The blastocyst (formed after fertilization of the oocyte) attaches itself in one of the four lateral clefts in the base of the ipsilateral uterine horn of ovulation by equatorial replacement of endometrium and derivation of an endotheliochorial zonary (girdle) placenta.[1,6,14]

The embryo becomes visible within the EV at 62 to 65 days. Initially roundish, the embryo becomes oblong and the attached prominent yolk sac becomes distinct by day 74. At this time, the placental band starts forming, visible as an echodense protrusion into the EV. During days 85 to 95 postconception, the allantois may be visualized with the embryo and the yolk sac. Between days 70 and 80, the heartbeat becomes visible and, by days 83 to 85, head and rump differentiation is observed, along with trunk formation. From day, 95 until day 120, a physiologic midgut herniation (dilation of the umbilical cord caused by prolapse of intestine) is present

because of the fast-growing embryonic liver occupying the abdomen. During days 100 to 120, forelimb and hindlimb formation in conjunction with straightening of the cervical flexure, formation of brain structures with surrounding ventricles, and organization and lining of lung, liver, kidneys and gastric vesicle, may be visualized. Beyond day 200 of gestation, transrectal visualization of the conceptus becomes difficult because the uterus disappears deep into the abdominal cavity. Transcutaneous scans might now be performed from behind, paramedian to the vestibule, or from the flank and inguinal regions with running water from a garden hose to increase coupling. This allows viability checks by detection of movements, evaluation of the fetal fluids, and even heartbeat visualization if the fetus is positioned conveniently.[6,13]

Parturition

There is currently no definite way to determine the day of delivery. However, several indicators help confine the due date, which also include close monitoring of behavioral changes. From day 620 on, daily samples for progestagen measurement are recommended. Usually, 1 to 5 days prior to parturition, progestagen levels reach nadir concentrations (less than 0.1 to 0.15 ng/mL). However, levels have been observed to be at baseline for as long as 2 weeks and even to bounce back up.[12,25] Also, a significant rise in relaxin as well as cortisol levels is measurable in the peripartum and immediate postpartum period.[23] Our preliminary work on serum and urine $PGF_{2\alpha}$ metabolites (PGF-M) has found an increase prior to birth and a subsequent fall of progestagen concentration, suggesting that $PGF_{2\alpha}$ is involved in luteolysis.

Other indicators that parturition is soon to begin are behavioral changes, including frequent passing of small fecal balls and increased nervousness, discomfort, and reduced feeding. The emission of milk from the mammary glands and passing the sticky mucus, which had served as a uterine seal within the vagina, are additional signs that parturition will occur within the next 24 to 48 hours. Approximately 12 hours prior to birth, the chorioallantoic sac pushes toward the pelvis and appears immediately when the investigator's hand is entering the rectum and is recognizable via palpation or ultrasonography. Also, the degree of cervical opening may be assessed by transrectal ultrasound. If the fetus has already progressed into the pelvis, its presentation and viability may be diagnosed.[12]

First-stage labor might remain unnoticed and little abdominal discomfort is obvious (stage 1). During this period, the fetus will be positioned correctly within the uterus in preparation for birth. Pregnant females have been observed to force the abdomen against structures such as rocks or logs within the enclosure to assist with proper repositioning. Active labor commences stage 2 of delivery, when the cervix dilates and the calf enters into the birth canal. Elephant calves are in usually born hind legs first. This posterior position serves to open up the birth canal and facilitate the passage of the large and rigid skull. As labor progresses, the chorioallantoic sac may rupture, leading to the discharge of a large volume of liquid, which is often difficult to distinguish from maternal urine. A large bulge will now occur under the tail, which becomes more prominent with every contraction; it first consists of the allantoic sac and then (front or hind) legs still enclosed in the amnion. The birthing process may remain in this stage for an extended period in primiparous females because the hymenal structure needs still to rupture. At this point, females may get very agitated, stretching or laying down and swiftly rising up again, kicking with the hind legs and sitting up. They may also press the head forcefully against solid objects. As soon as the calf passes the caudal rim of the pelvis, legs covered by remains of the amnion membranes appear in the opening of the vestibule and now the actual expulsion occurs rapidly. The calf, very often still enclosed in the amniotic sac, slides down the vestibule and drops between the dam's rear legs. Stage 3 of parturition involves expulsion of the placenta (usually within 10 hours after birth) and uterine involution, which may last several months. Neonatal care was described earlier.[25]

Pregnancy Loss

Abortion and embryonic resorption occur in captive breeding programs and also in wild elephants.[20] It is usually difficult to identify reasons for pregnancy failure, but common noninfectious causes such as severe stress, long duration of transport, or massive trauma have been reported anecdotally. Furthermore, intrauterine pathology, such as cystic endometriosis or leiomyoma, not only prevent implantation but also may compromise embryonic development and therefore are likely to lead to resorption.[20] As an infectious cause, salmonellosis has been identified in several cases.[7] Additionally, poxvirus and elephant endotheliotropic herpesvirus (EEHV) have been associated with cases of stillbirth.[20] Aborted materials or stillborn calves should be tested for these infectious diseases. Pregnancy wastage in very early embryonic or fetal stages (up to 150 to 200 days) might remain unnoticed if neither endocrine nor ultrasonographic monitoring is in place. Progesterone levels may decline several days or weeks after death of the conceptus and expulsion of the fetus may be delayed several months.

Dystocia Management

Generally, the risk of complication during birth increases with age in nulliparous females and first breeding is recommended 2 years after onset of puberty. To avoid a possible fatal outcome for the dam, the first parturition should take place no later than the age of 25 years. The main reasons for dystocia include the following[12]:

1. Weak uterine contractions or maternal expulsion forces caused by muscle exhaustion, lack of fitness, hypocalcemia, or labor cessation under stress.
2. Passage problems associated with viability, positioning, malformation (see Fig. 66-3B), size, or presentation of the fetus
3. Obstructed passage ways caused by pathologies, intact fibrotic hymen, edema, obesity of the cow, insufficient dilation, or lubrication if fetal sacs rupture too early

Options for the veterinarian to intervene include conservative and surgical methods. In any case, decisions should be made carefully and, because birthing in elephants may be a lengthy process, it is sometimes better to err on the side of caution. For several months prior to the presumed birth, the female should be frequently exercised to ensure good body condition and food should be rationed carefully to avoid obesity. Serum ionized calcium levels should be analyzed and, if necessary, the diet supplemented with vitamin D and calcium. A total calcium concentration of 2.5 to 2.9 mmol/mL serum is recommended.[13]

If there is uterine inertia after the fetus has entered the cervix, ultrasonographic observation is helpful to assess progress. However, as long as all membranes are still intact, there is no immediate intervention necessary and the cow may simply need a rest before entering the next delivery stage. Massage of the vaginal and cervical regions via the rectum may help make the female more comfortable and open up the passage. This transrectal stimulation activates the so-called Ferguson reflex, which is believed to induce vaginocervical receptors and trigger the release of oxytocin from both the posterior hypophysis and uterus.

A different approach to dilate the cervix further and help deliver the fetus into the birth canal is the application of estrogen and prostaglandin E gel or cream. Transrectal or transcutaneous application of estradiol, 600 to 800 mg, in the perineal region has had good success. Repeated application of half of the estradiol dose (300 to 400 mg) is possible 3 to 4 hours later. Prostaglandin E_2 (dinoprostone, 1.5 to 2.5 mg) administered transrectally over the cervical region also helps mature the cervix.[12]

To enhance labor contraction, the use of oxytocin remains controversial. A hyperreaction followed by exhaustion and total irresponsiveness, premature rupture of fetal membranes caused by enhanced contractions, decreased umbilical blood flow caused by myometrial spasm, and even uterine rupture have been reported in elephant cows. The uterine wall measures only approximately 10 mm in late pregnancy. In any case, it has to be confirmed that the cervix has sufficiently relaxed and the fetus is present in the birth canal. If it is a multiparous female, the birth passage is free and open and labor has stopped for at least 1 hour, an oxytocin injection of 25 to 60 IU IM may be considered and, according to the situation increased to 100 IU. The onset of contraction may take up to 20 minutes and last for approximately 40 minutes.[12]

If these measures fail to deliver the calf, further intervention depends on whether the allantoic sac is broken. If the membranes are still intact, but the calf is dead, it might be the best decision to leave it as a retained fetus. This has been shown to have the best prognosis for the cow and, in some cases, the fetus has even been delivered up to 1.5 years later without complications.[12]

Surgical intervention becomes mandatory in cases when the dead fetus is stuck in the birth canal, with a ruptured allantois and first signs of an ascending infection. Attempts at cesarean section have always ended fatally for both mother and calf. The only chance is to access the dead calf via episiotomy, which is only an option if fetal parts are present in the birth canal. If the fetus is in anterior position, it is essential for any extraction attempts to use ropes or chains, not only around the front legs but also through the trunk (see Fig. 66-3C). If the dead calf cannot be extracted via episiotomy, fetotomy is required, but has very often resulted in the death of the dam. Common complications after successful epsiotomy-fetotomy are infections as well as a permanent vestibular fistula.[12]

REPRODUCTIVE PATHOLOGIES

Up to 14% of Asian and 29% of African elephants in North America show no ovarian activity, exhibited by constant baseline serum progestagen concentrations, the so-called flatliner syndrome, with similar trends having been noted in Europe.[3] This acyclicity has been reported as temporary or permanent and is more often found in aged Asian elephant females (<30 years), but occurs in all age classes in African elephants.

There are various reasons for irregular or total absence of cycle activity. Seasonal changes (e.g., time spent indoors), distress-activated high cortisol levels (e.g., cycle cessation derived because of translocation), social factors such as hierarchy status (e.g., dominant African elephant females are reported more likely to be acyclic), or reproductive tract pathologies (ovarian and uterine cysts) are such factors.

Hyperprolactinemia often seems to be associated with acyclicity.[4] Average prolactin concentrations were reported to be significantly higher in one third of the noncycling African elephant females and in one case of an Asian elephant. Chronic elevated prolactin levels are known to cause infertility in women. In elephants, in addition to flatlining, development of the mammary gland, milk secretion, and mastitis have been observed in association with hyperprolactinemia.[4] The causes for chronic elevated prolactin concentrations are unknown, but may be induced by stress-related increases in adrenocorticotropin hormone and cortisol secretion. An effective treatment may be the dopamine agonist cabergoline.[3,4]

Another factor is so-called asymmetric reproductive aging in captive elephants. Long stretches of nonreproductive periods and the variation in exposure to endogenous sex steroids have been established to be problematic. The consequences are reduced fertility, shortened reproductive lifespan and, eventually, irreversible acyclicity.[10] Continuous frustrated cycles lead to a fast burnout of the ovarian resource and induce premature reproductive senescence. Extreme cases have demonstrated reproductive lifespans ending 15 years earlier compared with successfully reproducing females.[15]

Furthermore, repetitive bathing in reproductive hormones may lead to progressive development of genital pathology because estrogen and progesterone have been shown to promote steroid hormone–dependent tumor development and tumor growth.[15] Fibromas of the reproductive tract and/or cystic hyperplasia represent 80% of the most common lesions found in nonreproducing female elephants. Leimyomas, benign uterine smooth muscle tumors, are the most frequently seen genital abnormalities associated with age in Asian elephants, but have never been observed in African elephants.[10,14,15] An increased occurrence of leiomyomas (see Figs. 66-1P and 66-3D) and cystic endometriosis (see Fig. 66-1Q) reduce adequate endometrial surface for implantation.

In postreproductive females, a complete shutdown of ovarian activity may be considered to reduce steroid hormone–induced growth further of leiomyoma as well as the occurrence of tumor rupture and endometrial bleeding. This was previously attempted in an aged Asian elephant cow. However, the natural lavage effect (discharge) during the follicular phase was disabled and, in conjunction with a chronic endometritis, led to a fatal pyometra.[2]

In addition to intramural and submucous leiomyoma of the uterus, further genital abnormalities include the following (compare Figs. 66-1N with 66-1U).[14]

1. Cyst formation, commonly located in the vestibule, vagina, endometrium, oviduct, or ovary (see Fig. 66-1N, Q, R, T)
2. Nodular and pendulous fibroids of the vagina or vestibule (vestibular polyps only in African elephants; see Figs. 66-1S, U and 66-3E, F)

3. Fungal or bacterial infection and lesions of the vestibule and vagina, as well as in the uterus (see Fig. 66-1O)

Also, these pathologies are not fatal for the female and do not necessarily exclude a successful pregnancy; depending on location and severity, they may adversely affect fertility. Lesions and tumors of the vestibule or vagina may be diagnosed via endoscopy (see Fig. 66-3E, F). In the vestibule, they cause pain during mating, which leads to reluctance of the female for further breeding attempts by the bull. The female will typically cross her legs to avoid vestibular penetration. Larger cysts or fibroids within the vagina (see Fig. 66-1R, S) and in the upper vestibule (see Fig. 66-1T, U) may obstruct the passage of sperm. In both cases, artificial insemination is a potential method to fertilize these females.

Intraovarian cysts (see Fig. 66-1N) may induce acyclicity but, in many cases, do not affect the estrous cycle. Paraovarian cysts are usually unproblematic but, if they are located close to or at the oviduct, obstruction may occur.

Treatment for the described formation of reproductive tract pathologies is not existent. Their likelihood of occurrence may only be reduced by early breeding of these long-lived animals. All our efforts should be aimed toward this goal.

CONCLUSION

Research has brought great advances in our understanding of the elephant's reproductive physiology. The resulting increased successes in captive natural and artificial breeding are encouraging. Endocrine monitoring and ultrasonography have played a key role in this progress and their routine use to assess breeding herds is recommended.

However, we have not reached our goal, which is to establish self-sustaining populations in African and Asian elephants in our care. A number of problems have yet to be addressed, and gaps still remain. Endocrine treatments for acyclicity on the one hand, and controlling the estrous cycle on the other hand, especially need to be investigated in the future. Further hurdles such as high neonatal mortality and a skewed offspring-to-gender ratio need to be overcome.

REFERENCES

1. Allen WR: Ovulation, pregnancy, placentation and husbandry in the African elephant *(Loxodonta africana)*. Phil Trans R Soc B 361:821–834, 2006.

2. Aupperle H, Reinschauer A, Bach F, et al: Chronic endometritis in an Asian elephant *(Elephas maximus)*. J Zoo Wildl Med 39:107–110, 2008.

3. Brown JL: Reproductive endocrine monitoring of elephants: An essential tool for assisting captive management. Zoo Biol 19:347–367, 2000.

4. Brown JL, Walker SL, Moeller T: Comparative endocrinology of cycling and non-cycling Asian *(Elephas maximus)* and African *(Loxodonta africana)* elephants. Gen Comp Endocrinol 136:360–370, 2004.

5. Czekala NM, MacDonald EA, Steinman K, et al: Estrogen and LH dynamics during the follicular phase of the estrous cycle in the Asian elephant. Zoo Biol 22:443–454, 2003.

6. Drews B, Hermes R, Goeritz F, et al: Early embryo development in the elephant assessed by serial ultrasound examinations. Theriogenology 69:1120–1128, 2008.

7. Emanuelson KA, Kinzley CE: Salmonellosis and subsequent abortion in two African elephants *(Loxodonta africanus)*. Proc Am Assoc Zoo Vet 269–274, 2000.

8. Gaeth AP, Short RV, Renfree MB: The developing renal, reproductive, and respiratory systems of the African elephant suggest an aquatic ancestry. Proc Nat Acad Sci U S A 96:5555–5558, 1999.

9. Hermes R, Goeritz F, Streich WJ, Hildebrandt TB: Assisted reproduction in female rhinoceros and elephants—current status and future perspective. Reprod Domest Anim 42:33–44, 2007.

10. Hermes R, Hildebrandt TB, Goeritz F, et al: Reproductive problems directly attributable to long-term captivity-asymmetric reproductive aging. Anim Reprod Sci 82/83:49–60, 2004.

11. Hermes R, Olson D, Göritz F, et al: Ultrasonography of the estrous cycle in female African elephants *(Loxodonta africana)*. Zoo Biol 19:369–382, 2000.

12. Hermes R, Saragusty J, Schaftenaar W, et al: Obstetrics in elephants. Theriogenology 70:131–144, 2008.

13. Hildebrandt TB, Drews B, Gaeth AP, et al: Foetal age determination and development in elephants. Proc Royal Soc B 274:323–331, 2007.

14. Hildebrandt TB, Goeritz F, Hermes R: Aspects of the reproductive biology and breeding management of Asian and African elephants *Elephas maximus* and *Loxodonta africana*. Int Zoo Yb 40:20–40, 2006.

15. Hildebrandt TB, Goeritz F, Pratt NC, et al: Ultrasonography of the urogenital tract in elephants *(Loxodonta africana* and *Elephas maximus)*: An important tool for assessing female reproductive function. Zoo Biol 19:321–332, 2000.

16. Hildebrandt TB, Lueders I, Hermes R, et al: Reproductive cycle of the elephant. Anim Reprod Sci 2010 (in press). doi:10.1016/j.anireprosci.2010.08.027.

17. Hodges JK, Heistermann M, Beard A, et al: Concentrations of progesterone and the 5α-reduced progestins, 5α-pregnane-3,20-dione and 3α-hydroxy-5α-pregnan-20-one, in luteal tissue and circulating blood and their relationship to luteal function in the African elephant, *Loxodonta africana*. Biol Reprod 56:640–646, 1997.

18. Jayaram J: Potential gonadotropin activity during early pregnancy in elephants. Master's thesis, William H. Darr School of Agriculture, Missouri State University, May 2008.

19. Kaewmanee S, Watanabe G, Zhu Jin W, et al: Corpora lutea as a major source of inhibin secretion during luteal phase in the female Asian elephant *(Elephas maximus)*. Biol Reprod 81:211, 2009.

20. Lueders I, Drews B, Niemuller C, et al: Ultrasonographically documented early pregnancy loss in an Asian elephant *(Elephas maximus)*. Reprod Fertil Dev 22:1159–1165, 2010.

21. Lueders I, Niemuller C, Gray C, et al: Luteogenesis during the estrous cycle in Asian elephants *(Elephas maximus)*. Luteogenesis during the estrous cycle in Asian elephants *(Elephas maximus)*. Reproduction 140:777–786, 2010.

22. Lueders I, Taya K, Watanabe G, et al: Unique role of the double LH peak during the estrous cycle in Asian elephants *(Elephas maximus)*, submitted manuscript (Proc R Soc B).

23. Niemuller C, Brown JL, Hodges JK: Reproduction in elephants. In Knobil E, Neill J, editors: Encyclopedia of reproduction, vol 1, New York, 1998, Academic Press, pp 1018–1029.

24. Stephanie Sanderson S: Personal communication, 2008.

25. Schmitt DL: Proboscidea (elephants). In Fowler ME, Miller ME, editors: Zoo and wild animal medicine, ed 5, Philadelphia, 2003, WB Saunders, pp 541–550.

26. Schmitt DL: Reproductive system. In Fowler M, Mikota S, editors: Biology, medicine and surgery of elephants, Ames, Iowa, 2006, Blackwell, pp 347–355.

27. Thitaram C, Brown JL, Pongsopawijit P, et al: Seasonal effects on the endocrine pattern of semi-captive female Asian elephants *(Elephas maximus)*: Timing of the anovulatory luteinizing hormone surge determines the length of the estrous cycle. Theriogenology 69:237–244, 2008.

28. Thitaram C, Pongsopawijit P, Chansitthiwet S: Induction of the ovulatory LH surge in Asian elephants *(Elephas maximus)*: A novel aid in captive breeding management of an endangered species. Reprod Fertil Dev 21:672–678, 2009.

29. Weissenböck NM, Schwammer HM, Ruf T: Estrous synchrony in a group of African elephants *(Loxodonta africana)* under human care. Anim Reprod Sci 113:322–327, 2009.

CHAPTER 67

Digital Radiography of the Elephant Foot

Jessica L. Siegal-Willott, Amy Alexander, and Ramiro Isaza

Foot disease is a major cause of captive elephant morbidity and mortality.[4,6,10] Common foot problems encountered at the nail, skin, sole, or pad include penetrating injuries, trauma, cracks in the sole, nail, or cuticle, overgrown nail, sole, or cuticle, laminitis, ingrown nails, pododermatitis, osteomyelitis, arthritis, fractures, dislocations, abscesses, and degenerative joint disease.[2,5,12,13] Chronic foot disease that is unresponsive to medical and/or surgical management ultimately results in euthanasia.[9,17] Annual examination of captive elephants are recommended by the North American Species Survival Plan (SSP), including foot radiography in elephants with chronic foot disease.[14]

To date, elephant foot radiography reports have focused on conventional analog radiography (AR) techniques.[7,8,14] Recent advances in diagnostic medical imaging include the use of digital radiography (DR) for the clinical assessment of foot pathology in the captive elephant.

Digital Radiography Overview

Conventional radiography produces images using film coated with a light-sensitive, silver halide–containing emulsion. After exposure to x-rays or light, the silver halide crystals precipitate and remain on the film during processing. The amount of precipitation is directly related to processed film blackness. Film speed corresponds to the size or amount of silver halide crystals. High-speed films have crystals that are larger or more numerous. X-rays are more likely to precipitate these crystals, which will cause a greater area of exposure than with a slower speed film, resulting in less image detail with high-speed films. Intensifying screens in the form of film cassettes are used to convert x-rays to visible light to expose the film, because the film emulsion is more sensitive to light.[16] Using conventional analog techniques, standard portable radiographic units with 80 to100 kVp and 15 mA have produced reliable, diagnostic elephant foot radiographs.[7,14]

Digital radiography imaging systems include two basic types, computed radiography (CR) and direct digital radiography (DDR). Both systems use conventional x-ray equipment (e.g., machine, table, grids), but eliminate the need for film, processing chemicals, and light boxes. Instead, images may be adjusted and displayed on computer monitors. CR and DDR mainly differ in the method of image acquisition.

CR uses a detector, or image plate (IP), for image acquisition, an IP reader, an analog-to-digital converter (ADC), and a computer and software programs to process the digital image.[1,18] The IP is similar in appearance to conventional cassettes and is not directly attached to a computer. The IP functions similarly to conventional film-screen combinations, but uses photosensitive phosphors for image capture rather than crystals. The phosphors allow for latent image capture following x-ray exposure, similar to latent image capture with analog systems. In contrast to conventional radiography, CR latent images decay rapidly (minutes to days) and must be processed rapidly. The CR reader processes the latent image by converting stored energy into visible light and then into analog electrical signals, which are passed through an ADC to create a digital image for display on a computer monitor. Finally, the IP is erased using high-intensity white light to release residual energy, making the IP available for immediate reuse. The IP may be reused multiple times, with the actual number varying with protective plate quality and care during processing.

Computer software is used to process the digital image. Image contrast enhancement is possible with all digital imaging software using look-up tables (LUTs). LUTs enhance contrast by increasing the difference

515

among anatomic structures using preset pixel values specific for different body systems (e.g., thorax, abdomen, musculoskeletal). Default software settings also determine edge enhancement (sharpness), contrast resolution, and brightness.[18] Manual manipulations to adjust factors such as contrast, brightness, sharpness, and size can also be carried out.

In contrast to CR, DDR uses an integrated readout mechanism within the IP, producing a digital image following x-ray exposure that is sent directly to a computer via an attached cable.[1,18] Image acquisition is faster with DDR, because the need for an image-plate reader is eliminated. The IPs used in DDR include flat panel detectors (FPDs) and charge-coupled devices (CCDs). Both direct-converting and indirect-converting FPDs are available to transform x-rays into electrical signals. The specifics of direct and indirect FPDs are beyond the scope of this chapter, but are available in the literature. Image capture involves transforming x-rays to visible light, then to electrical charges, and finally from analog-to-digital format during the readout process.[16] The image minification process for visible light transformation into electrical signals with CCDs may result in greater image noise compared with FPDs. CCD systems also require more housing space than FPDs because of the optical system of the CCD and are nonportable, but tend to be less expensive than FPDs. Because of their nonportability, CCD systems are not currently applicable to large animal imaging outside the hospital setting. Comparisons among commercially available flat panel detectors are available. Digital data are processed on the computer as described for CR systems (see earlier).

Compared with DDR, CR's main disadvantage is the lack of direct readout. This becomes significant for the evaluation of elephants and other large mammals in which health examinations are conducted on site and not in the hospital setting. Using DDR, diagnostic digital images are obtained, processed, and evaluated patient side, eliminating the need to transport plates to the hospital for processing and evaluation. In addition, DR uses a single IP multiple times during a radiographic assessment, whereas CR uses multiple IPs that must be erased by the reader before reuse. Despite these limitations, CR is a more mature technology that has benefited from improvements and advancements over the years, whereas DDR is a relatively young imaging system.[18] In addition, with CR systems, the plate is not connected to a computer by a wire, an advantage when working with large animals. Both digital imaging systems enable users to send image data to a picture archiving communications system (PACS) for analysis

and storage. We expect to see continued advancement for both technologies in the future as digital radiography becomes more available to zoological and wildlife veterinarians.

ANALOG VERSUS DIGITAL

Using collimated, labeled, and correctly positioned equipment and animals, conventional and digital radiography systems produce diagnostic images of elephant digits. The advantages and disadvantages of each should be carefully considered in deciding which system is most appropriate for a given institution and situation.

Image format is the largest difference between the two systems. With AR, once the radiograph is printed, image adjustment is not possible. For digital radiographs, many factors may be manipulated following image acquisition that affect image appearance; these include contrast, brightness, magnification, monitor luminance, monitor size, and display resolution.[16,18,19] In addition to image format, digital systems allow for more rapid results given the ability to reuse cassettes without a need for replacing film (CR) or direct read-out ability (DDR). In this respect, DDR is especially beneficial because radiographs are available in seconds patient side, with fewer retakes necessary, allowing for rapid technique adjustments, modification of patient positioning, and radiographic assessments to obtain diagnostic images. The decreased time delay with digital systems becomes increasingly important when radiographing all digits on the four limbs at annual or baseline elephant foot examinations. Although digital systems lack the degree of spatial resolution possible with film-screen combinations, both digital radiography systems have diagnostic image quality equal to or better than that of analog radiology. This is largely because of superior contrast resolution and processing functions available with digital systems.[1]

Conventional radiography is further limited by the narrow exposure range, need for darkroom quality control, processor and chemical maintenance, cost of upkeep and purchase of chemicals and film, and hard copy image storage.[18] In contrast, digital radiography eliminates the need for film and chemicals, decreases the number of exposures for diagnostic images, decreases technician workload, and allows for rapid image acquisition.[1] Digital images are stored electronically—although some practices still prefer to maintain both hard and soft copies of patient records—and allow for easy remote consultation with specialists via the electronic exchange of digital images. Image capture, display, storage, adjustment, and communication are available for digital systems using PACSs.[1] In addition, digital imaging communications in medicine (DICOM) image file formats may be used for manipulation and storage of digital images from various medical imaging devices such as DR systems, as well as others such as computed tomography, magnetic resonance imaging, and ultrasound. DICOM allows for connectivity with PACS regardless of imaging modality or specific product used. Upkeep of digital systems may involve PACS software maintenance and general equipment and software upgrades, as well as monitor calibrations to minimize electronic image fading.[19]

Both CR and DDR offer improved exposure latitude, image contrast, and postimage capture processing ability compared with conventional radiography.[3,7] However, all three modalities require similar power techniques.[1] Because DR systems have a linear response to x-ray exposure (compared with a sigmoid response with conventional radiography), there is a wider exposure operating range, allowing for viewing of soft tissues and bony structures on the same image using the same exposure and technique. This becomes important in elephant foot radiography when assessing disease states of the soft tissues of the foot (e.g., cuticle, nail) and how they relate to the underlying bony structures (phalanges). Figure 67-1 displays D3 P3 from the same elephant using AR, CR, and DDR radiographic techniques.

Both CR and AR system equipment (e.g., cassettes, film, x-ray machine) are easily transported to the patient, whereas DDR systems are slightly more labor-intensive. In addition, DDR requires close proximity of a computer and cables to the elephant under study. Initial purchasing costs for conventional radiography are low compared with digital imaging systems, although costs incurred over the lifetime of digital systems compared with analog have yet to be evaluated.[18] Conventional systems may last an average of 7 to 10 years; the lifespan of digital systems is currently unknown. Considering the higher costs associated with digital system equipment purchase, repair, and replacement, all appropriate equipment safety measures should be used when evaluating elephants and other large mammals.

ELEPHANT FOOT RADIOGRAPHY

Anatomy

Elephants are ungulates with a modified digitigrade stance on the forefoot and semiplantigrade on the hind foot.[10] The number and location of toenails relative to each digit, and general anatomy of the elephant foot, are important when collimating radiographs to a specific digit, especially when nails are lacking. In both species, each foot has five digits, regardless of the number of toenails present. In the Asian elephant *(Elephas maximus)* forefoot, each of the five digits (D1

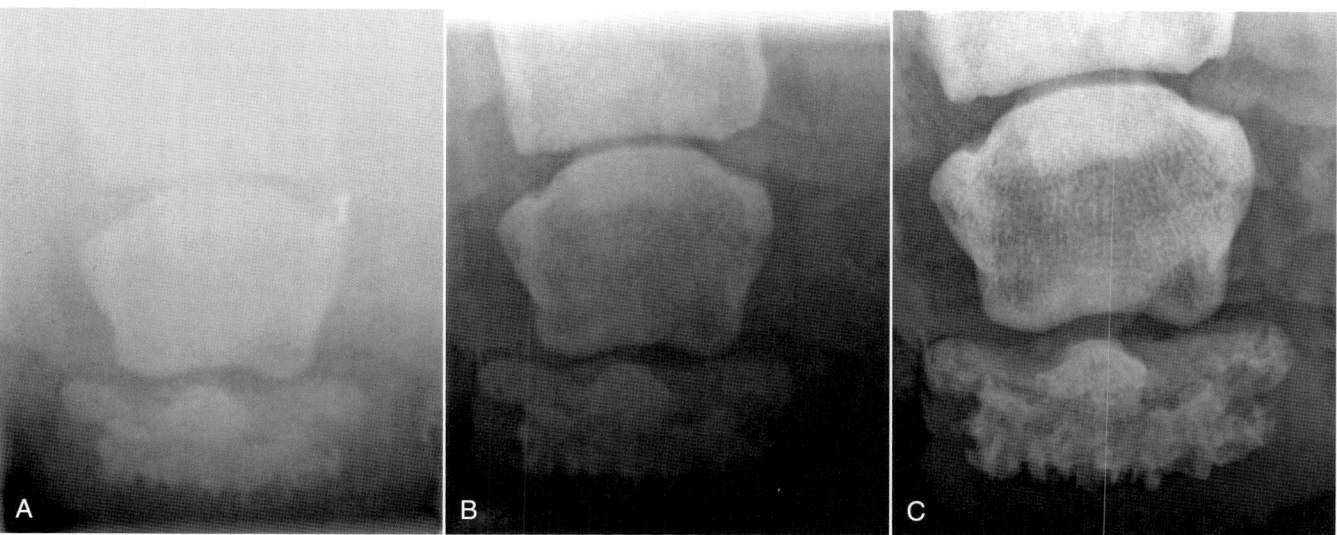

Figure 67-1

Conventional analog radiograph **(A)**, computed radiography image **(B)**, and direct digital radiograph **(C)** of an Asian elephant *(Elephas maximus)* foot, collimated on the distal phalanx (P3) of digit three (D3).

to D5) has an associated nail, whereas the hind foot typically has only four toenails (D2 to D5), although the number of nails may vary with the individual.[11] In the Asian elephant forelimb, the nails are intimately connected to the distal phalanx (P3) of D2 to D5 and underlying soft tissue structures.[2,14] Only two phalanges (P1 and P2) are present in D1, according to the literature, and a single phalanx without sesamoids is present on D1 of the Asian elephant hindlimb.

African elephants *(Loxodonta africana)* have four toenails on the forefoot and three on the hind, but the actual number may vary with subspecies and individual.[17] In the African elephant forelimb, D1 contains one phalanx and sesamoid, D5 has one phalanx and paired sesamoids, and D2 to D4 contain three phalanges each, with paired sesamoids.[11] African elephant hindlimb

digits differ in that D1 is represented by a sesamoid, D2 and D5 each have two phalanges, and D3 and D4 each have three phalanges.[2,15] Pathology in the nail, sole, and/or pad may lead to pathologic changes in the bones of the digits, most commonly in P3 of the weight-bearing digits, D2 to D5.

Patient Preparation

Optimal elephant foot radiographs require proper patient preparation. Training goals should incorporate foot handling, washing, and gentle placement on the radiographic tunnel in a free contact (FC) or protected contact (PC) setting. Elephant restraint devices (ERDs) should include accessible working areas for foot radiography (Fig. 67-2A, B). This may entail windows for foot

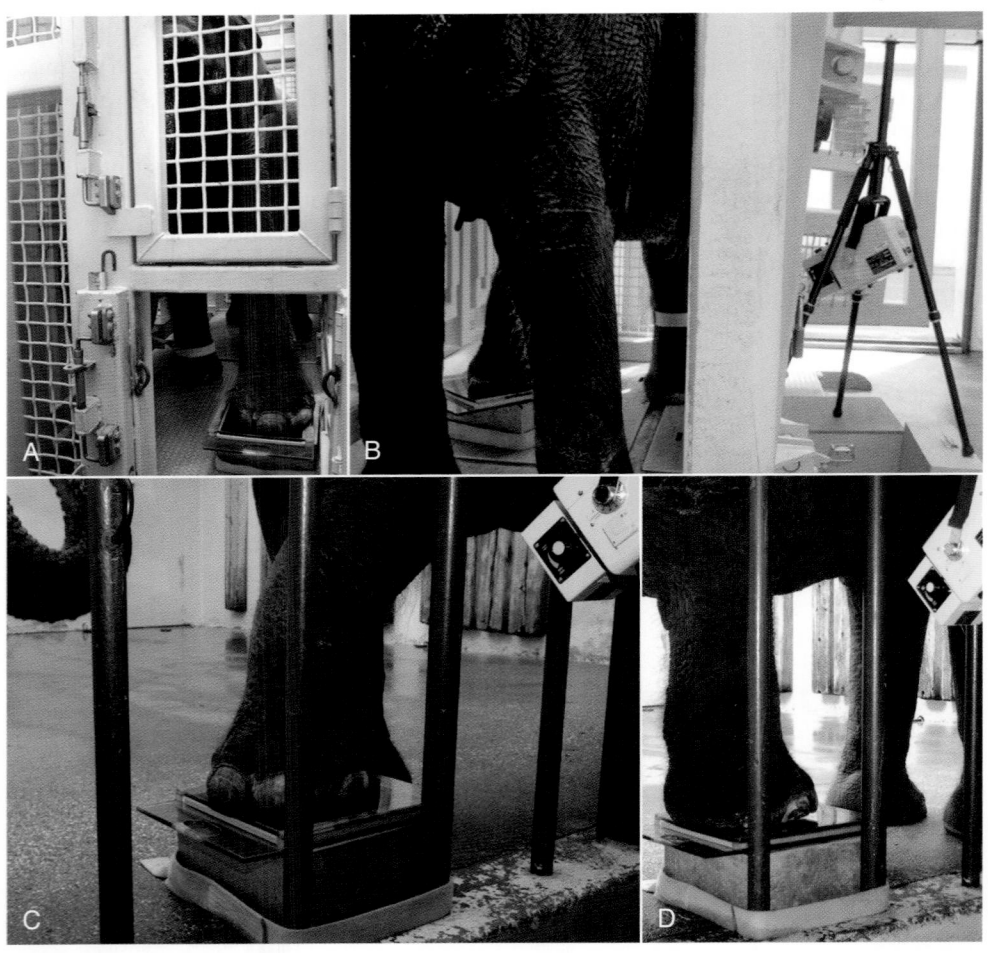

Figure 67-2

Asian elephant *(Elephas maximus)* positioning for digital foot radiography in a protected contact setting. **A,** Front foot using an ERD. **B,** Hind foot using an ERD. **C,** Front foot using an elephant enclosure. **D,** Hind foot using an elephant enclosure.

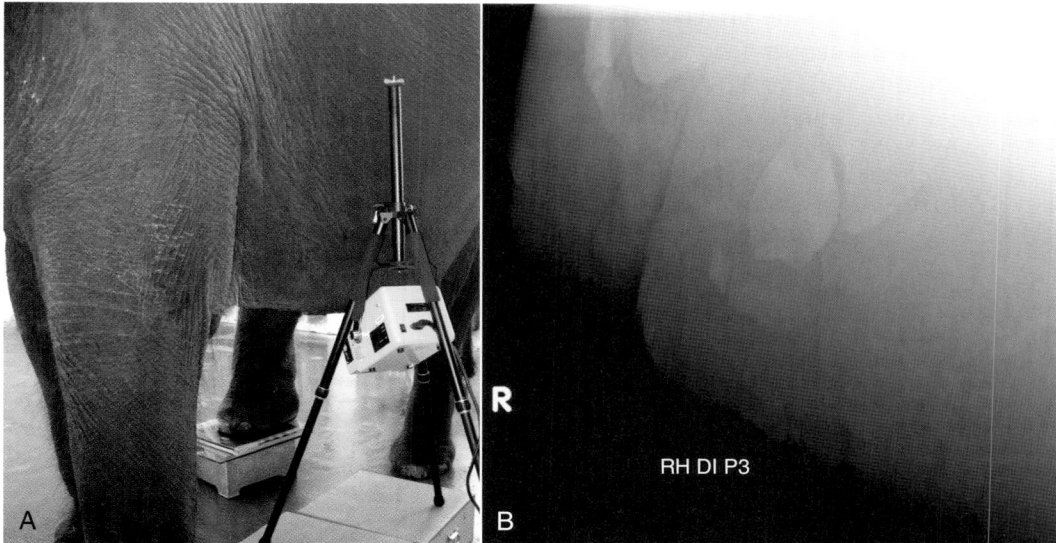

Figure 67-3

Asian elephant *(Elephas maximus)* positioning for hind foot digital radiographs in an FC setting. **A,** Radiograph of right hind foot (RH) distal phalanx (P3) of digit one (D1) obtained in an FC setting using MinXray HF 100/30, 100 kVp, and 14 mAs in a 45-degree dorsoproximal-palmarodistal oblique projection **(B).**

placement, or the ability to place secured platforms within the ERD, and windows for the x-ray machine. Alternatively, enclosure perimeters may be modified to allow for radiography in a PC environment (see Fig. 67-2C, D). Care should be taken to secure any loose items (e.g., foot stand, radiograph tunnel) to avoid manipulations by the elephant. Human and animal safety are the highest priorities for all elephant handling and radiographic situations; all necessary training should be in place prior to attempts at foot radiography.

All aspects of the foot must be thoroughly cleaned of debris and particulate matter to minimize radiograph artifact(s). This is accomplished using cleaning solutions, scrub brushes, and possibly picks or putty material to remove debris from within the sulci of the pad. Material remaining on the foot may appear on the radiographic image and be mistaken for foreign bodies, bony changes, or abnormalities within the soft tissues of the foot. If a tunnel is used to protect the radiographic plate, the foot need not be dried, but the tunnel should also be cleared of debris. Extreme caution is recommended if a protective tunnel is not used for the plate, because water, particulate matter (e.g., sand), and the mere weight of the elephant foot are likely to damage or destroy the image plate.[1,14]

The foot is positioned on the tunnel directly over the center of the IP, with only minimal weight bearing on the limb to be radiographed. Foot positioning often requires a degree of training, and low weight bearing on a particular limb is assisted by use of an elevated platform. Creative patient and equipment placement may be necessary in FC and PC settings, in particular for examination of the medial aspects of the hind feet (Fig. 67-3; see Fig. 67-2). Foot stands and radiographic tunnels may be secured in place using straps, welding, chains, or other means.

Equipment Setup

The elephant foot is positioned on a platform of hexcelite (0.5-inch or 1.3-cm thickness) within a wooden frame (tunnel), with dimensions large enough for a large radiographic image plate. The IP is placed within the tunnel under the hexcelite, protected from the weight of the elephant limb. A marker is essential to denote the foot and digit, as well as the medial and lateral aspects of the foot; lead shields (2-mm thick) are placed behind the plate within the tunnel to minimize artifact caused by scatter radiation (Fig. 67-4). For consistent standardized examinations, radiographs are collimated to evaluate each digit individually, and centered on the toe at a 45-degree angle to provide a dorsoproximal-palmarodistal oblique projection. Panoramic "foot-o-grams" are not recommended, because they lead to image distortion and inability to compare individual digit images over time (Fig. 67-5).[14] Bony changes associated with foot pathology may be missed in panoramic views, but are readily identified in collimated single-digit radiographs, as noted by the lucencies visible in D4 P3 in Figure 67-5. The diagnostic value of orthogonal views of the elephant digits are often limited because of the shape of the foot, and we do not generally recommend them as part of the routine foot examination.

The x-ray beam is centered at the cuticle for images of P3, and approximately 6 to 7.5 cm above the cuticle for images of P1-P2.[14] When using DR techniques, one of us (AA) has found that centering the x-ray beam higher on the foot may provide images of structures such as the metacarpals, metatarsals, carpus, and elbow.[7] Development of a technique chart detailing digit and phalanx examined, focal distance, location of x-ray beam relative to the cuticle, angle of the x-ray beam, kilovolt peak (kVp), and milliampere-seconds (mAs) is recommended for each institution, specific to the radiographic equipment used for each study (Table 67-1).

Use of a tripod is recommended to minimize human radiation exposure (see Fig. 67-4). Personal protective equipment, including lead body shields, thyroid protectors, and hand shields, are essential for handlers and veterinarians in proximity to the elephant and radiographic equipment. To ensure human safety, manual restraint of radiographic plates is not recommended.

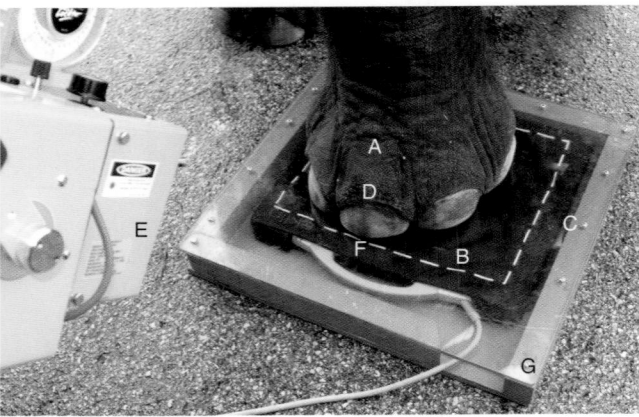

Figure 67-4

Equipment setup for digital radiography of the elephant foot. Note location of the foot *(A)*, image plate *(B)* with lead shield *(C)*, x-ray beam location on foot *(D)*, and positioning of portable radiography machine *(E)*. *F,* The position of a radiographic marker to denote the digit radiographed, as well as medial and lateral aspects of foot is indicated. *G,* The image plate and lead shield are housed within a hexcelite wooden tunnel for protection.

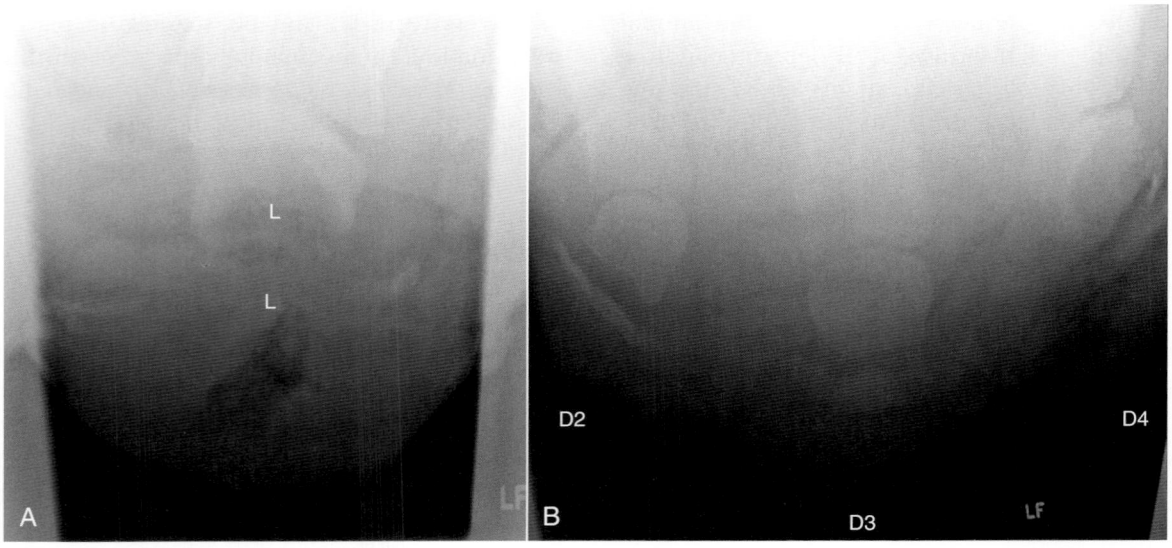

Figure 67-5

Digital radiographs of an Asian elephant *(Elephas maximus)* front foot using noncollimated, panoramic technique **(A)** and collimated, individual toe technique **(B)**. Digits two *(D2)*, three *(D3)*, and four *(D4)* are displayed in the panoramic technique **(A)** and D4 only in the collimated technique. Radiolucencies *(L)* in the distal phalanges of D4 are visible only in the collimated view.

Digit (D) and Phalanx (P) Radiographed	Location of Beam	Angle of Beam (Degrees)	kVp	mA	Seconds	mAs	Focal Distance (cm)
TABLE 67-1 Technique Charts for Asian Elephant *(Elephas maximus)* Foot Radiographs							
Analog Radiography							
D3P3	Cuticle	45	70	15	0.06	0.9	71
D3P1P2	6.35 cm above cuticle	45	75	15	0.1	1.5	71
Computed Radiography							
D3P3	Cuticle	45	80	15	0.16	2.4	71
D3P1P2	6.35 cm above cuticle	45	80	15	0.34	5.1	71
Direct Digital Radiography							
D3P3	Cuticle	45	80	25	0.14	3.5	71
D3P1P2	6.35 cm above cuticle	45	80	25	0.18	4.5	71

RADIOGRAPHIC ASSESSMENT

Positioning

The optimal elephant digit radiograph is collimated, labeled, obtained at a dorsal 45-degree proximal-palmarodistal oblique projection, using an appropriate technique to allow the bones, joints, and outline of the nail associated with the digit to be visible. Collimated views are strongly recommended to prevent unintentional oblique views of digits medial and lateral to the center of the x-ray beam. This projection angle and technique allow for visualization of the phalanges of interest, as well as the interphalangeal joints, without bony overlap.[14] Deviation from this angle produces nondiagnostic films, in which phalanges often overlap, joint spaces are obscured, and phalanx shape becomes distorted as it is viewed from a different angle. Most weight bearing occurs in digits two, three, and four, and correlates with where foot disease is most commonly recognized. All digits may be affected, however; obtaining repeatable, standardized, collimated radiographs of each digit is an essential component to the evaluation of elephant foot health.

Exposure

Proper exposure assessment and guidelines for the ideal elephant foot radiograph include the following: ability to visualize the phalanx, surrounding soft tissues, and cuticle of interest; minimal interference by artifacts; minimal pixilation of the image; proper positioning and use of markers; and proper degree of contrast.

Underexposure of digital images results in graininess or pixilation of the image. This results from statistical uncertainty in adjacent pixel, and worsens as the display size of the image is increased.[3] Similar to film-screen combinations using high-detail systems, DR requires the use of higher radiation exposure for increased anatomic detail. Thus, for an ideal image of the elephant foot, an appropriate exposure is needed to allow visualization of the bony and soft tissue structures of the foot, including the relationship of the distal phalanx to the cuticle. Underexposure may result in poor anatomic detail, crippling the radiographic assessment and interfering with diagnoses of elephant foot pathology. In general, slight overexposure is preferred to underexposure when radiographing elephant feet using digital equipment. However, overexposure of digital systems may result in saturation of the detector, with each pixel at its maximum value in the overexposed area. Margins of structures are no longer visible and, with some DR systems, planking or linear structures may appear in the background. Repeated radiographs using lower exposures will correct the image.

Given the greater exposure range of DR, more proximal aspects of the elephant limb (e.g., metacarpals, foreleg, elbow) are more readily obtained than with conventional radiography. This becomes important in older animals, commonly affected with degenerative joint disease and arthritic conditions.[6,17] Further evaluation of elephant proximal limb radiography techniques are necessary as DR becomes more commonly used across zoological institutions.

Artifacts

Artifacts are possible with both AR and DR systems, and may be caused by improper patient preparation, improper equipment setup or use, inappropriate technique, or processing errors. Classic artifacts such as patient motion, malpositioning, fog caused by scatter radiation, failure to label, debris on the foot (see earlier), and double exposures occur with conventional and digital systems.[1,3] Processing of analog films may result in artifacts caused by the following: improper storage of film and subsequent exposure to light; expired film; poor film handling (scratches, bends in film); poor quality control of processing chemicals or developer; and technical malfunctions of the processing machine. Additional artifacts are possible with DR systems, including LUT errors, image processing errors, exposure artifacts (see earlier), calibration errors, ghost images, excessive smoothing of an image, poor collimation, and image plate and plate reader artifacts (CR only).

During the application of LUTs in image processing in some systems, if the range of pixel values determined or area of the range of recorded exposures to apply a particular pixel range is incorrect, the LUT process will result in clipping. This results in information loss, and that part of the image is no longer available.[3] Digital display systems use window or contrast programs to adjust the range of pixel values, and level or brightness programs to adjust where the pixel range is centered. These programs, however, may not correct for any clipping that occurs in the processing phase; thus, radiographic artifacts may be created by LUTs in DR systems. Clipping errors may be corrected by reprocessing the film or repeating the radiographs if necessary.

In addition to changes in shape appearance when noncollimated radiographs are obtained (see Fig. 67-5), lack of collimation in CR systems results in improper processing of the image at the reader plate level and selection of an improper pixel histogram. The resulting image may be too light, or may be dark and grainy. With collimation, the reader detects the edges of the collimated view and creates a histogram within the appropriate area.[1,3] Finally, scatter radiation in the noncollimated portion of the radiograph interferes with detection of the collimated edge, and may result in improper histogram production, as well as fogging. For these reasons, collimated views of the elephant foot are strongly recommended, along with the use of a lead shield within the IP tunnel (see Fig. 67-4).

CR image plates become worn over time and may crack along the edge, resulting in linear artifacts on the image. Proper handling and storage of CR image plates are strongly recommended. CR image plate artifacts may also occur if the plate is incompletely erased prior to the next study, or if the plate reader is not cleaned regularly.

Additional artifacts possible with the use of CR and DDR systems are discussed elsewhere.[1,3]

CONCLUSIONS

Digital radiography offers the advantage of consistent, rapid, and easily obtainable diagnostic foot radiographs in FC and PC settings. Conventional techniques also allow for diagnostic images, and should not be abandoned by institutions without digital imaging capabilities. The decision to use conventional versus digital radiography systems depends on the needs, intended uses, and financial resources of each institution. Regardless of radiographic system used, elephant care staff and veterinarians are strongly encouraged to obtain labeled, collimated, 45-degree dorsoproximal-palmarodistal oblique projections centered at the region of interest during assessment of the elephant foot. It is essential to use the techniques outlined in this chapter consistently to allow for intraelephant and interelephant comparisons at the time of assessment and also over the lifespan of the individual. Use of a consistent technique across institutions will facilitate case consultation with radiography and zoological medicine specialists.[14] This will become increasingly important as digital image capture and electronic transfer of images for consultation becomes more common.

Acknowledgments

We would like to thank the following for their asssistance with this chapter: Marie Galloway and the elephant care staff and David Olsen and the veterinary technician staff at the Smithsonian Institution's National Zoological Park (SI NZP); elephant care and veterinary technician staff at Feld Entertainment; photographer Mehgan Murphy (SI NZP); and the Radiology Department Staff at the University of Florida's Veterinary Medical Teaching Hospital.

REFERENCES

1. Armburst LJ: Digital images and digital radiographic image capture. In Thrall DE, editor: Textbook of veterinary diagnostic radiology, ed 5, St. Louis, 2007, Saunders Elsevier, pp 22–37.
2. Benz A: The elephant's hoof: Macroscopic and microscopic morphology of defined locations under consideration of pathological changes, Ph.D. thesis, Zurich, 2005, Vetsuisse-Fakultat Universitat Zurich.
3. Drost WT, Reese DJ, Hornof WJ: Digital radiography artifacts. Vet Radiol Ultrasound 49:S48–S56, 2008.
4. Fowler ME: An overview of foot conditions in Asian and African elephants. In Csuti B, Sargent EL, Bechert US, editors: The elephant's foot: Prevention and care of foot conditions in captive

Asian and African elephants, Ames, Iowa, 2001, Iowa State University Press, pp 3–9.

5. Fowler ME: Foot care in elephants. In Fowler ME, editor: Zoo and wild animal medicine, ed 3, Philadelphia, 1993, WB Saunders, pp 448–453.

6. Fowler ME: Foot disorders. In Fowler ME, Mikota SK, editors: Biology, medicine, and surgery of elephants, Ames, Iowa, 2006, Blackwell, pp 271–290.

7. Gage LJ: Antemortem diagnostics: Section II: Radiology. In Fowler ME, Mikota SK, editors: Biology, medicine, and surgery of elephants, Ames, Iowa, 2006, Blackwell, pp 192–197.

8. Gage LJ: Radiographic techniques for the elephant foot and carpus. In Fowler ME, Miller RE, editors: Zoo and wild animal medicine, ed 4, Philadelphia, 1999, WB Saunders, pp 517–520.

9. Luikart KA, Stover SM: Chronic sole ulcerations associated with degenerative bone disease in two Asian elephants *(Elephas maximus)*. J Zoo Wildl Med 36:684–688, 2005.

10. Mikota SK, Sargent EL, Ranglack GS: The musculoskeletal system. In Mikota SK, Sargent EL, Ranglack GS, editors: Medical management of the elephant, West Bloomfield, Mich, 1994, Indira Publishing, pp 137–150.

11. Ramsay EC, Henry RW: Anatomy of the elephant foot. In Csuti B, Sargent EL, Bechert US, editors: The elephant's foot: Prevention and care of foot conditions in captive Asian and African elephants, Ames, Iowa, 2001, Iowa State University Press, pp 9–12.

12. Schmidt DL: Proboscidea (elephants). In Fowler ME, Miller RE, editors: Zoo and wild animal medicine, ed 5, Philadelphia, 2003, WB Saunders, pp 541–549.

13. Schmidt M: Elephants (proboscidea). In Fowler ME, editor: Zoo and wild animal medicine, ed 2, Philadelphia, 1986, WB Saunders, pp 884–923.

14. Siegal-Willott J, Isaza R, Johnson R, Blaik M: Distal limb radiography, ossification, and growth plate closure in the juvenile Asian elephant *(Elephas maximus)*. J Zoo Wildl Med 39:320–374, 2008.

15. Smuts MM, Bezuidenhout AJ: Osteology of the thoracic limb of the African elephant *(Loxodonta africana)*. J Vet Res 60:1–14, 1993.

16. Thrall DE, Widmer WR: Physics of diagnostic radiology, radiation protection, and darkroom theory. In Thrall DE, editor: Textbook of veterinary diagnostic radiology, St. Louis, 2007, Saunders Elsevier, pp 2–21.

17. West G: Musculoskeletal system. In Fowler ME, Mikota SK, editors: Biology, medicine, and surgery of elephants, Ames, Iowa, 2006, Blackwell, pp 263–270.

18. Widmer WR: Acquisition hardware for digital imaging. Vet Radiol Ultrasound 49:S2–S8, 2008.

19. Wright MA, Balance D, Robertson ID, Poteet B: Introduction to DICOM for the practicing veterinarian. Vet Radiol Ultrasound 49:S14–S18, 2008.

CHAPTER 68

Laparoscopic Surgery in the Elephant and Rhinoceros

Mark Stetter and Dean A. Hendrickson

Traditional abdominal surgery in the elephant and rhinoceros has rarely been performed and, in those cases in which it has, success has been limited.[1,4] Emergency cesarean sections in elephants have been attempted and have proved fatal for both the calf and mother. Successful castration of bull elephants has been described.[2,3,12] In these reports, young animals were castrated in a single procedure, whereas adults required multiple procedures. These elephant castration procedures were difficult and it was not uncommon for incisions to break down and heal by second intention. An abdominal exploratory and ovariectomy has been reported in an Indian one-horned rhinoceros, but the animal died 48 hours after the surgery.[11]

Abdominal surgery in the elephant and rhinoceros is difficult for several reasons, the first being the animal's overall size and how it affects the surgeon's ability to reach and manipulate organs. Second, there is considerable thickness to the skin and body wall, which requires larger incisions and an inordinate amount of time for closure. Surgical sites may also be predisposed to dehisce and break down.[2,12] An additional complicating anatomic variation in elephants is their peritoneum. Unlike most other mammal species, the peritoneum is covered by a fibroelastic layer and is itself redundant and only loosely attached to the body wall.[5] For this reason, entering the peritoneal cavity of elephants, even after making an incision through the dermis and associated muscle layers, may be very challenging. Finding a route to and through the peritoneum is much more of an issue when animals are in lateral recumbency (versus standing), when there is less tension on the peritoneum. Rigid laparoscopy, or minimally invasive surgery (MIS), offers a variety of advantages over traditional surgical procedures. In humans and animals, MIS has been shown to be less painful, requires

less healing time, allows faster return to normal function, and has less chance for infection.[19] For the elephant and rhinoceros, MIS has these advantages and thus makes abdominal surgery a realistic and much less risky procedure. Laparoscopic abdominal surgeries have been successfully performed in the African elephant, white rhinoceros, and black rhinoceros.[6,13,15-17] Procedures have included abdominal exploration with diagnostic sampling and a variety of reproductive surgical techniques.

LAPAROSCOPY IN THE ELEPHANT

Animal Positioning

Abdominal laparoscopic surgery in elephants is best accomplished in a standing position, either with the animal sedated and in a restraint device or under general anesthesia, with the animal in a standing position while being suspended from a crane truck.[6,15-17] Using MIS and maintaining the elephant in a standing position allows for small incisions, rapid access to the abdominal cavity, and excellent overall surgical success.[7] In captive situations, in which sedation may be used along with some degree of manual restraint, abdominal laparoscopic surgery may be readily accomplished. We have successfully used butorphenol and detomidine in conjunction with local analgesic nerve blocks with the elephant in a restraint chute (Fig. 68-1). The patient is sedated to the level at which it cannot lift its trunk and maintains a wide stance on all four legs, but is not likely to lie down. Once sedated, a regional analgesic block is accomplished using a 5-inch, 18-gauge spinal needle. In elephants, an elevated platform is used to place the surgeons at the level of the paralumbar fossa. This standing sedation approach has been used for abdominal exploratory

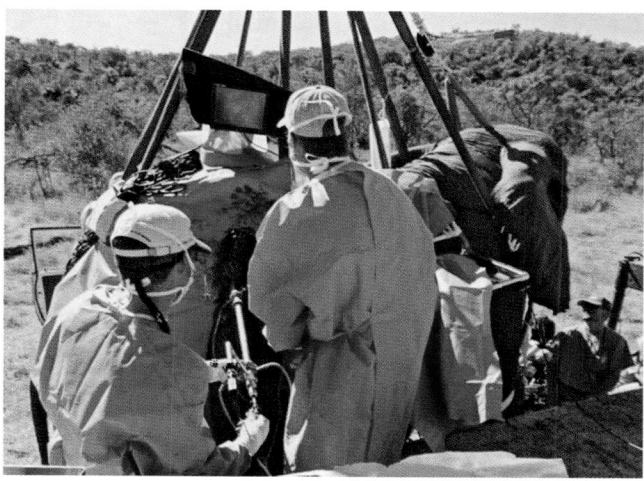

Figure 68-1

Standing sedation being used in an elephant chute for laparoscopic abdominal exploratory in a female African elephant. The surgeons' and associated equipment are on an elevated platform that provides access to the paralumbar fossa. The rigid laparoscope has been placed inside the elephant's abdomen. The surgeons are wearing video goggles, which are attached to the laparoscope camera unit and provide direct image viewing. These goggles significantly reduce glare issues when working outside in sunlight and allow both surgeons the same view without limitations of head position or monitor placement.

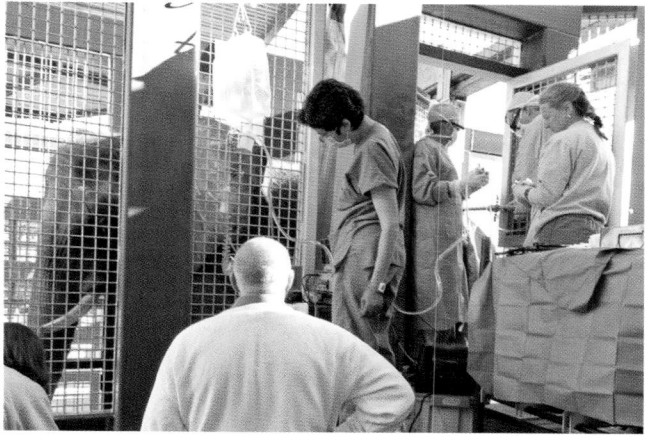

Figure 68-2

An anesthetized free-ranging bull elephant in South Africa undergoing laparoscopic surgery. Five-ton capacity ropes are used to suspend the animal from a crane truck in an upright standing position. The elephant has been intubated and is being provided with assisted ventilation. A rigid operating laparoscope has been placed into the abdominal cavity. The laparoscopic viewing monitor has been placed on the animal's dorsum so that the sun is behind it and the unit has been modified with the addition of black side panels to reduce glare.

and reproductive procedures in both adult elephants and rhinoceroses.

In free-ranging elephants, for which restraint facilities do not exist and the location of the patient is difficult to predict, the animals are placed under general anesthesia via a remote injection system. Once the patient is laterally recumbent, large padded straps or ropes (5-ton capacity with foam or wool padding) are placed around the proximal base of each leg and connected to the hook of a crane truck. These ropes are looped around the axilla or inguinal areas, ensuring limited pressure on the thoracic or abdominal cavities (Fig. 68-2). Limited pressure on the thorax greatly improves respiration and limited pressure on the abdominal cavity assists in insufflation and laparoscopic visibility. Once the ropes have been placed around each leg and secured to the crane, the elephant is lifted into a standing position. An additional rope is placed around the base of the tusks and attached with the other ropes so that the head is held in a normal upright position. In most cases, these animals are intubated to facilitate assisted ventilation when insufflation is applied.

Surgical Equipment

The nonlaparoscopic surgical instruments used for creating and closing the abdominal incisions are commonly available through veterinary surgical catalogues. In most cases, the large versions are used. The procedure benefits from two to four no. 8 surgical scalpel handles with no. 60 scalpel blades, and two to four long no. 4 scalpel handles with no. 22 scalpel blades. Elephant and rhinoceros skin is tough, dense, and thick, so many blades are generally used for a single incision. It is always better to have too many blades than not enough. Other instruments include penetrating towel clamps, large Mayo scissors, long needle holders, long thumb forceps, vulsellum forceps, wire needle holders, and wire cutters. Modified Finocetto rib spreaders are also used to distract the skin while making the primary incision (Fig. 68-3).

Laparoscopic Surgical Instruments

Laparoscopic surgical equipment for minimally invasive surgery in the megavertebrate species must be longer and stronger than traditional equipment. The telescope—a rigid laparoscope— should have at least an 80-cm working length for bull elephants younger than 20 years and for cow elephants. In larger bull

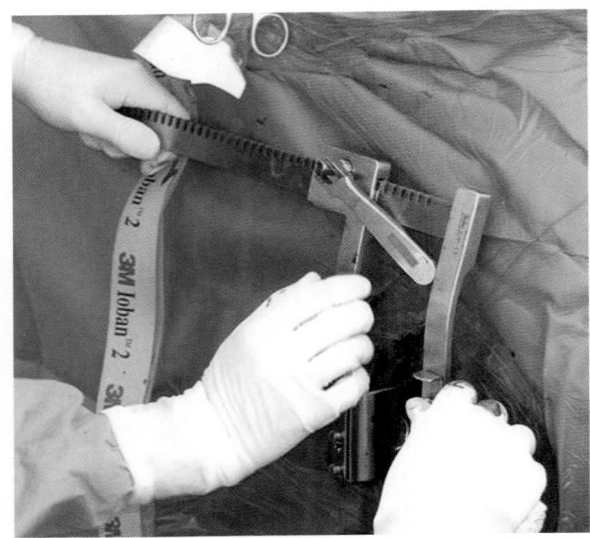

Figure 68-3

Skin incision made in the paralumbar fossa of an African elephant. Note the use of Finocetto rib spreaders to retract the skin margins and provide access and visibility to the underlying muscle layers. In larger animals, the blades of the rib spreaders will need to be lengthened to retract the entire body wall of the elephant. Once the laparoscope is placed into the abdomen and insufflation has begun, the rib spreaders are removed.

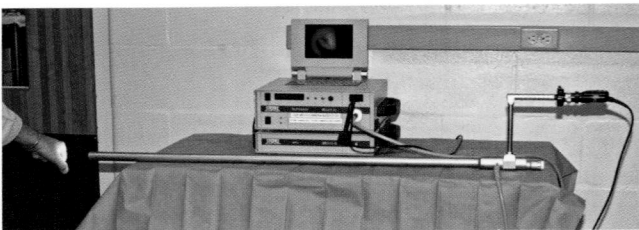

Figure 68-4

This 112-cm megavertebrate telescope (Karl Storz Endoscopy) has been developed for minimally invasive surgery in elephants and rhinoceros. This is an operating laparoscope, which has a 10-mm working channel for placement of laparoscopic instruments. The Techno Pack (Karl Storz Endoscopy) system is a self-contained, battery-operated light source, monitor, and camera. This system is easily transported in field situations. This is a halogen light system and a xenon light source may be required for optimum viewing in elephants.

elephants, a working length of 100 to 112 cm is helpful (Fig. 68-4). A traditional telescope may be used but, to reduce the number of portals necessary, an operating laparoscope is more useful. Specialty telescopes (Karl Storz Endoscopy, Tutlingen, Germany) with two light source input posts will improve the amount of light that

may be delivered into a potentially large peritoneal space. Visibility may be difficult because of the size of the abdominal cavity and the amount of fat and bowel distension that may occur. Having an appropriate amount of light is important. In the rhinoceros, depending on the size of the animal and procedure being attempted, an equine telescope (Hopkins Telescope, Karl Storz Endoscopy, 10 mm × 57 cm, 30-degree angle) may be used.[13]

Cannulas and Obturators

Laparoscopic cannulas are designed to allow exchange of instrumentation with minimal loss of intra-abdominal pressure, thereby maintaining an operating space within the abdominal cavity. Traditional diameter cannulas with their associated instruments and telescopes may be used. However, they should be 50 cm long and have thicker walls than traditional cannulas. If a larger diameter telescope is used, a larger diameter cannula is helpful. At least one of the cannulas should have two high-volume, stopcocks installed to allow larger volumes of insufflation gas to be instilled into the abdomen. The second stopcock may be used to measure intra-abdominal pressure. When using a longer large-diameter cannula as described earlier, the cannula should be at least 75 cm long but may be 50 cm long if the shorter telescope is used. In general, a large- diameter (30 mm for introduction of an operating telescope) and a traditional diameter (11 mm for introduction of instruments) cannula are used. This combination allows two instruments for diagnostics and surgical procedures. A third cannula would be necessary if a nonoperating telescope is used.

Obturators (trochars) for megavertebrate laparoscopy are similar to those used in traditional surgery. Because the primary cannula is placed using an open technique, no obturator is needed for the telescope. When placing the accessory instrument portal, a conical obturator is the best choice. This portal is placed blindly, after the abdomen has been insufflated, but the surgeon must be careful to avoid trauma to the bowel or other structures when placing the sharp obturator. The cannula-obturator unit is advanced until it may be seen laparoscopically tenting the peritoneum. The obturator is then removed and a hooked scissors is used to cut through and penetrate the peritoneum under direct visualization.

Hand Instruments

Hand laparoscopic instruments based on traditional instruments have been adapted for megavertebrate surgery. In general, these instruments have been designed with a 95- to 130-cm working length (Karl Storz Endoscopy and Surgical Direct, Deland, Fla). The most commonly used instruments are acute claw (Senn) graspers with lengthened jaws, atraumatic (Babcock) graspers, and scissors. Small-hook scissors tend to work best for entering through the peritoneum while placing the accessory portal and larger serrated scissors work best for transecting tissue such as the ductus deferens. Neither bipolar nor unipolar electrosurgery appears to be useful when using longer instruments and cannot be recommended at this time. Other instruments, including vessel-sealing devices and stapling equipment are being considered, but have not been tested at the time of this writing.

Instrument Sterilization

Instruments may be sterilized using ethylene oxide or glutaraldehyde solution. In general, the telescope and laparoscopic instruments are stored and sterilized inside a padded gun case. The case is left open for the sterilization process and then closed for transport after degassing. A challenge of ethylene oxide sterilization in outdoor environments may be low ambient temperatures that are often experienced when working in the field. A heated area would be ideal, but is rarely available. Specially designed portable tubs are used for glutaraldehyde sterilization because of the unique size and shape of the laparoscopic instruments. These lightweight plastic tubs allow cold sterilization between animals, when multiple procedures are occurring in a single day.

Light Source

As in all minimally invasive surgery, the light source is a critical piece of equipment. The anatomic and environmental considerations with the megavertebrate species require the best visualization possible to limit further complications. In our experience, a 300-W xenon light source may be effective in bulls that are 4500 kg or smaller. However, if the animal is larger, two light sources are helpful. The largest diameter light cords available should be used because they allow more light transmission into the abdominal cavity. When working outdoors, it is important that light sources are well built and sturdy enough to withstand the jostling that occurs with surgery in the bush. Having replacement light cords and light bulbs are a necessity when working in the field.

Camera and Monitors

The best-quality camera available should be used; the higher the quality of the camera, the better the image on the monitor. High-quality cameras will also provide better light-collecting capacity, reducing the amount of light required in the abdominal cavity. Positioning the monitor screen is one of the most challenging aspects of performing minimally invasive surgery in an outside environment. In general, the best monitor position is one in which the telescope may point at the monitor. Because of the size of the animal and limited positioning options, this generally means that the monitor must be placed on the animal's dorsum. When working outside, the direction of the sun is also important. Usually, having the sun behind the monitor is best. A better alternative to a single monitor is the use of video goggles. There are several commercially available sources for goggles that may be fed a video signal from the endoscopy camera unit. We have used goggles manufactured by MyVu (Wellesley, Mass; http://www.myvu.com) with good success. The main benefit to the use of video goggles is that the surgeon and assistant may be looking in the direction of the telescope at all times. The presence of bright sunshine is also less of a problem. The main detractor is that only those wearing goggles have access to the video image. This may be remedied by placing a small monitor (often a video recording device) in a position where staff and observers may watch.

Insufflation

As in all minimally invasive surgery, space must be created to maneuver the instruments in the peritoneal space. Traditionally, in domestic animals, CO_2 is used for insufflation and to create pneumoperitoneum. Access to compressed CO_2 in the field is limited. Consequently, other sources of compressed gas have been used. When working with free-ranging elephants, compressed air was selected because of the ease of access.[6,15-17] Compressed air is supplied via a commercially available 30-gallon tire inflation unit. The unit is plugged into a power generator for power and the air is filtered in line prior to entering the abdomen. In humans, a few studies have been performed comparing CO_2 with room air pneumoperitoneum. In one large study,[8] patients undergoing room air pneumoperitoneum were more likely to have wound infection and abdominal discomfort. However, it was concluded that room air pneumoperitoneum is safe, cheap, and available and can be used in low-resource settings. A more recent study comparing CO_2 and room air in both laparoscopy and natural orifice transluminal endoscopic surgery found it to be acceptable.[18]

In humans and animals, the recommended intra-abdominal pressure during laparoscopy is 10 to 15 mm Hg.[9] Pressures greater than 20 mm Hg for prolonged periods may produce negative cardiovascular and respiratory effects. However, when working with elephants and rhinoceros, traditional insufflators (0 to 20 mm Hg) do not provide enough intra-abdominal pressure to move the bowel out of the way and allow adequate visualization. An intra-abdominal pressure of between 0.5 and 3 psi (25 to 150 mm Hg) is necessary for most surgical procedures.[6,17] Although we recognize that this pressure is above what is used in other species, there have been no identifiable long-term consequences seen in 26 elephants that have undergone laparoscopic surgery. In general, intra-abdominal pressure is kept between 0.5 and 1 psi (25 to 50 mm Hg), except for short periods during which increased visualization is necessary. A specially designed insufflator that allows rapid air flow from the air compressor and continuous monitoring of the higher intra-abdominal pressures has also been used successfully (Fig. 68-5). Because of the potential respiratory complications associated with laparoscopy during general anesthesia, intubation and assisted ventilation are recommended in humans and veterinary species. It is important to have positive-pressure ventilation available when using any insufflator, especially when using higher pressures.

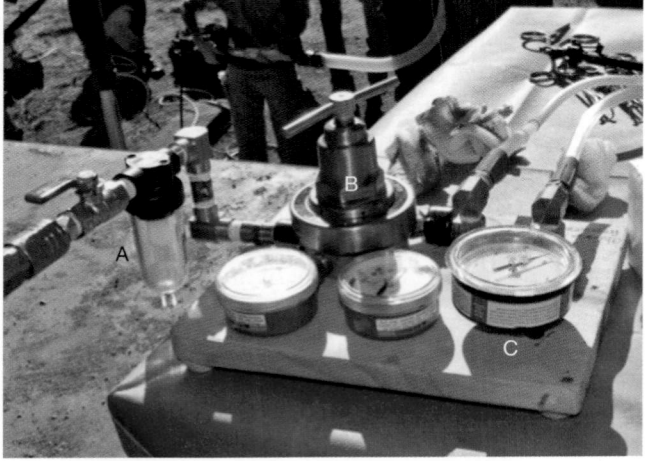

Figure 68-5

Photograph of a specially designed insufflator for megavertebrate laparoscopy. *A*, First filter. *B*, Acetylene welding regulator used to adjust air flow into the abdomen. *C*, Intra-abdominal pressure gauge.

Surgical Anatomy of the Elephant

Several different laparoscopic approaches have been evaluated and a flank approach, just rostral to the tuber coxae and ventral to the caudal ribs, has been deemed the best approach to the abdomen.[6,15-17,19] The ribs of the elephant extend into the traditional area of the paralumbar fossa and are very difficult to palpate under the thick skin. The tuber coxae is palpated and 5-inch, 18-gauge spinal needles are placed into the body wall and used to identify and avoid the ribs when the incision is made. The skin incision (approximately 15 cm) for the primary cannula is made approximately 10 cm rostral to the tuber coxae and immediately ventral to the ribs.[18] The skin is incised using a no. 60 BD scalpel blade on a no. 8 handle because the length of the blade is sufficient to penetrate the skin of even large bull elephants. A set of Finocetto rib spreaders is place into the skin incision and the skin edges are retracted to allow access to the external abdominal oblique fascia and muscle, which are transected using a similar scalpel handle and blade as for the skin. The Finocetto rib spreaders are removed and a specially designed, long-blade version of Finocetto rib spreaders (Scanlan Surgical Instruments, St. Paul, Minn) is inserted through the skin and muscle incision. A long-handled no. 4 scalpel handle with a no. 22 BD scalpel blade is used to divide the internal abdominal oblique muscle along the incision, and the rib spreaders are placed deeper into the incision. The transverse abdominus muscle is divided sharply along the same line as the skin and other muscles. Vulsellum forceps are introduced into the incision and the fibroelastic layer over the peritoneum is grasped at the center portion of the incision and pulled through the incision. An additional Vulsellum forceps is placed on the fibroelastic peritoneum at the dorsal and ventral portion of the incision. A long Mayo scissors is used to remove a portion of the fibroelastic peritoneum and fat. The Vulsellum forceps are released, a single Vulsellum forceps is again introduced into the central portion of the incision, and a portion of the peritoneum is exteriorized from the incision. Vulsellum forceps are again applied at the dorsal and ventral portions and a central portion is removed.

The actual peritoneum is relatively thin and difficult to differentiate from the fibrous portions until the glistening inner layer can be seen. Once the peritoneum has been penetrated, a purse-string suture is placed and the large diameter, primary cannula is placed into the peritoneal space. The purse-string suture is closed over the cannula and the abdominal space is insufflated to a

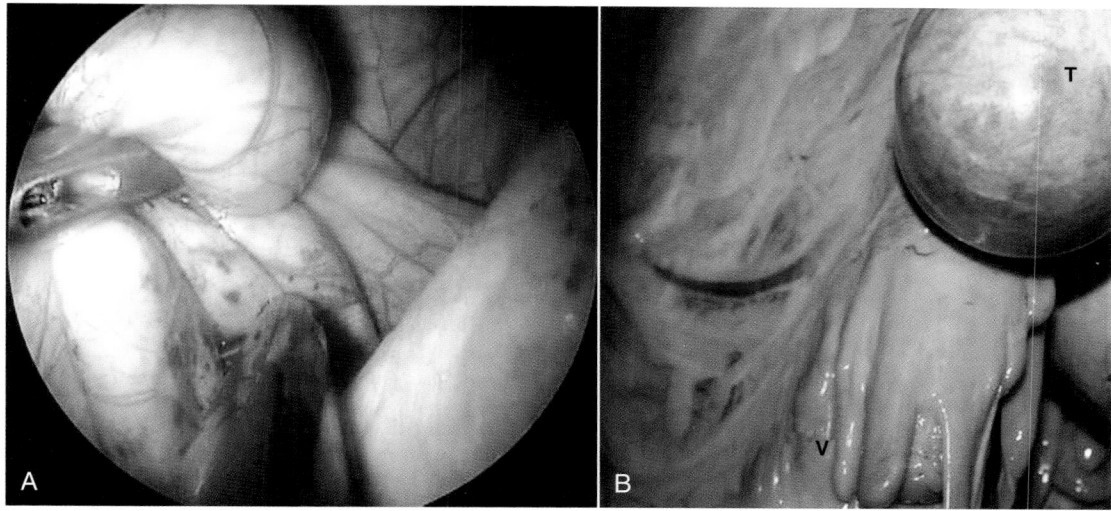

Figure 68-6

Intra-abdominal photographs of an elephant's right abdomen. **A,** Winter season, with 20-mm Hg pressure showing poor organ visibility because of gas-filled bowels. **B,** 75-mm Hg intra-abdominal pressure. *T,* Testes; *V,* vas deferens.

pressure of 0.5 to 1 psi (25 to 50 mm Hg). The rib spreaders are now removed, allowing the body wall and skin margins to come together and help seal the peritoneal space. One to two pairs of Vulsellum forceps are maintained on the peritoneum to stabilize the peritoneum during surgery. When performing the surgical incision on the second side, a similar approach is used. Once the billowing peritoneum is identified (the abdomen has been insufflated), a suture is placed for more rapid identification.

The telescope is introduced into the large cannula and an initial exploration is performed. After the telescope has been placed and insufflation is complete, an accessory portal is made. A 2-cm incision, located 10 cm rostral to the middle portion of the primary incision, is made through the skin, external abdominal oblique fascia and muscle, and internal abdominal oblique muscle.[6,17] The accessory cannula with a conical obturator, as described earlier, is introduced through the skin and muscle layers directed toward the testis. As soon as the cannula and obturator are noted to be tenting the peritoneum, the obturator is removed, a pair of small hooked scissors is introduced, and the peritoneum is sharply incised under direct visualization. The cannula is advanced through the hole created by the scissors and the small-hook scissors are removed and replaced with grasping forceps. Abdominal exploration, with visibility of the kidney, ureter, testes, ovary, uterus, testes, ductus deferens, colon, and portions of the small bowel, may be facilitated in this way.

Elephant Vasectomy Procedure

Unlike most mammals, elephants do not have a scrotum and external testes. The elephant's testes are intra-abdominal and located caudal and lateral to the kidneys[10,14] (Fig. 68-6). The vas deferens is more appropriately identified as the ductus deferens in elephants and is actually more similar to a long epididymis. It originates at the dorsal caudal pole of the testis and courses toward the bladder in a mesoductus.

A traumatic grasping forceps is advanced into the abdomen through the operating channel of the telescope and the ductus deferens is identified and grasped using the grasping forceps advanced through the telescope. As noted, if visualization is difficult, the intra-abdominal pressure may be increased as necessary up to 3 psi (150 mm Hg) for short periods of time.[6,17] Once identified and grasped, a scissors is introduced through the accessory portal, and a 4- to 8-cm segment of ductus deferens is resected and removed through the large-diameter primary cannula. After a segment of the ductus deferens has been removed on the first side, the abdomen is desufflated, the cannulas removed, and the peritoneum at the primary portal site is closed. It is important to create a gas-tight seal to be able to insufflate the abdomen on the second side. As soon as the ductus deferens is identified on the first side, a second group of surgeons begins a similar approach down to, but not including, the peritoneum on the second side. Either the elephant is rotated 180 degrees or the surgery teams switch sides, and the second ductus deferens is removed in similar fashion.

Closure

The peritoneum is closed with 0 polyglyconate suture in a simple continuous pattern. The external abdominal oblique fascia and muscle are also closed in this pattern. The skin is closed in multiple horizontal mattress sutures using no. 5 stainless steel and plastic stents in the large incision, and a single horizontal mattress suture using no. 5 stainless steel in each of the accessory portals. The two ends of the wire suture are tightly twisted together (i.e., like cerclage wire) rather than tied with a knot. Although the elephant is often laid back down on the side as soon as possible, it should be noted that it is often faster to suture the skin while the elephant is suspended from the crane truck. Once closure is complete, the patient's perisurgical area is scrubbed and the animal is lowered and placed in lateral recumbency for anesthesia reversal.

LAPAROSCOPY IN THE RHINOCEROS

Laparoscopy in the rhinoceros has similar challenges as in the elephant, although rhinoceros skin is also generally thicker than that of African elephants.[19] Surgery performed in the standing animal allows better visualization than in a laterally recumbent animal.[7,13] It is important to recognize that in the white rhinoceros, the skin over the ribs seems to be attached to the ribs, causing a depression in the skin. The fibroelastic tissue associated with the peritoneum is similar but much less extensive than in elephants and much more adherent to the body wall. At the time of this writing, we have performed laterally recumbent laparoscopy in two white and one black rhinoceros and standing sedated laparoscopy on one white rhinoceros. The uterus and ovaries are readily visible in the standing animal and are approachable in the laterally recumbent animal. Gas distension of the bowel occurs quickly, because it is often difficult to withhold feed prior to surgery. Consequently, surgery should be started as quickly as possible after anesthesia is induced in laterally recumbent animals. Surgical procedures have included uterine biopsy, liver biopsy, and ovariectomy. In general, the paralumbar fossa provides the best abdominal access for the urogenital tract. Access to the liver will require a more cranial approach, either between or just below the ribs. In some cases, a partial rib resection may be necessary to gain access to the dorsal abdomen.

REFERENCES

1. Byron HT, Olsen J, Schmidt MJ, et al: Abdominal surgery in three adult male Asian elephants. J Am Vet Med Assoc 187:1236–1237, 1985.
2. Foerner JJ, Houck RI, Copeland JF, et al: Surgical castration of the elephant (Elephas maximus and Loxodonta africana). J Zoo and Wildl Med 25:355–359, 1994.
3. Fowler ME, Hart R: Castration of an Asian elephant, using etorphine anesthesia. J Am Vet Med Assoc 163(6):539–543, 1973.
4. Gage, LJ, Schmitt D: Dystocia in an African elephant (Loxodonta africana). In Proceedings of the American Association of Zoo Veterinarians Annual Meeting, 2003, p 88.
5. Hendrickson DA: History and instrumentation of laparoscopic surgery. Vet Clin North Am Equine Pract 16:233–250, 2000.
6. Hendrickson DA, Stetter M, Zuba JR: Development of a laparoscopic approach for vasectomies in free-ranging African elephants. In Proceedings of the American College of Veterinary Surgeons Annual Symposium, 2008.
7. Hendrickson DA, Wilson DG: Laparoscopic cryptorchid castration in standing horses. Vet Surg 26:335–339, 1997.
8. Ikechebelu JI, Obi RA, Udigwe GO, et al: Comparison of carbon dioxide and room air pneumoperitoneum for day-case diagnostic laparoscopy. J Obstet Gynaecol 25:172–173, 2005.
9. Ishizaki Y, Bandai Y, Shimomura K, et al: Safe intra-abdominal pressure of carbon dioxide pneumoperitoneum during laparoscopic surgery. Surgery 114:549–554, 1993.
10. Jones RC, Brosnan MF: Studies of the deferent ducts from the testis of the African elephant, Loxodonta africana. I. Structural differentiation. J Anat 132:371–386, 1981.
11. Klein LV, Cook RA, Calle PP, et al: Etorphine-isoflurane-O₂ anesthesia for ovariohysterectomy in an Indian rhinoceros (Rhinoceros unicornis). In Proceedings of the American Association of Zoo Veterinarians Annual Meeting, 1997, pp 127–130.
12. Olsen J, Byron HT: Castration of the elephant. In Fowler ME, editor: Zoo and Wild Animal Medicine: Current Therapy 3. Philadelphia, 1993, WB Saunders, pp 441–444.
13. Radcliffe RM, Hendrickson DA, Richardson GL, et al: Standing laparoscopic-guided uterine biopsy in a southern white rhinoceros (ceratotherium simum simum). J Zoo Wildl Med 31:201–207, 2000.
14. Short RV, Mann T, Hay MF: Male reproductive organs of the African elephant, Loxodonta africana. J Reprod Fertil 13:517–536, 1967.
15. Stetter M, Grobler D, Zuba JR, et al: Laparoscopic reproductive sterilization as a method of population control in free-ranging African elephants (Loxodonta africana). In Proceedings of the AAZV, AAWV, AZA Nutrition Advisory Group, 2005, pp 199–200.
16. Stetter M, Hendrickson DA, Zuba JR, et al: Laparoscopic vasectomy as a potential population control method in free ranging African elephants (Loxodonta africana). In Proceedings of the International Elephant Conservation and Research Symposium, 2006, pp 177–.
17. Stetter M, Hendrickson D, Zuba JR, et al: Laparoscopic vasectomy in free ranging African elephants (Loxodonta africana). In Proceedings of the American Association of Zoo Veterinarians Annual Meeting, 2007, pp 185–188.
18. Trunzo JA, McGee MF, Cavazzola LT, et al: Peritoneal inflammatory response of natural orifice translumenal endoscopic surgery (NOTES) versus laparoscopy with carbon dioxide and air pneumoperitoneum. Surg Endosc 24:1727–1736, 2010.
19. Zuba JR, Stetter M, Dover S, Briggs M: Development of rigid laparoscopy techniques in elephants and rhinoceros, 2003 (http://elephantpmp.org/assets/files/news-scientific/Final AAZVZubaStetterLap14May03.PDF).

CHAPTER 69

Elephant Neonatal and Pediatric Medicine

Martha A. Weber and Michele A. Miller

Captive reproduction of elephants has had increasing success because of improved husbandry, medical and reproductive assessments, and assisted reproductive technology. Captive births have doubled worldwide during the last decade compared with the previous 10 years (1987 to 1996, 110 births; 1997 to 2006, 243 births).[9] Veterinarians are now more likely to see neonatal and pediatric elephant patients. Previously reported medical problems in elephant calves include umbilical infections or hernias, diarrhea (both infectious and dietary or nutritional), constipation, metabolic bone disease, elephant endotheliotropic herpesvirus (EEHV), trauma, septicemia, tooth eruption problems, and failure to gain weight. Treatment of EEHV is discussed further in Chapters 65 and 70.

NEONATES

Protocol for Neonatal Elephant Examinations

Captive elephant births are usually attended by elephant care staff, with veterinary staff available, allowing neonatal assessments to be performed shortly after birth (Box 69-1). Thorough examination of the calf should occur when the calf is first separated from the dam. This may be immediately after birth in the case of first-time dams, or during the first 24 to 48 hours with multiparous dams. Evaluation should include body weight and measurement of height, length, and girth, when possible, to develop correlates for growth. Average values, based primarily on data from Asian elephants, are as follows: birth weight, 105.5 kg (range, 53 to 150 kg); height, 88.9 cm (range, 66 to 107 cm). The initial evaluation should include a complete physical examination with special attention to periocular, oral, and anogenital regions, thoracic and abdominal auscultation,

assessment of limb conformation, and evaluation of the umbilical stalk. Initial treatment of the umbilicus with tincture of iodine may minimize the risk of umbilical infections as well as accelerate the closure and drying of the stalk.

Blood should be collected for a complete blood cell count (CBC), biochemical profile, and assessment of passive transfer of immunoglobulins (e.g., protein electrophoresis, glutaraldehyde coagulation, or zinc sulfate turbidity). If blood is collected prior to nursing, results of passive transfer tests are expected to be negative, because the elephant's placenta prevents the transfer of immunoglobulins in utero.[3] Whole blood in EDTA and frozen samples from the placenta should be submitted to the National Elephant Endotheliotropic Herpesvirus Laboratory to screen for EEHV (see the latest protocols at www.aazv.org or www.aza.org under the Elephant TAG page).

Regular monitoring of the neonate is crucial for the early detection of problems. In most cases (92%), passage of meconium occurs within 7 hours of birth. Failure to pass meconium by 2 days of age should alert the veterinarian to a potential problem, such as congenital defects (e.g., atresia ani or coli), constipation, dehydration, gastrointestinal stasis, or insufficient milk intake.

Ongoing Assessment of Calf Health

This includes the following:
- Umbilical stalk treatment. The umbilicus should be treated with diluted chlorhexidine solution four times daily for 1 day, then three times daily for 3 days. This may need to be accomplished while the calf is sleeping and/or the dam is restrained because it could cause discomfort or distress to the calf.

BOX 69-1	Neonate Examination and Emergency Supplies

KY Jelly
Endotracheal tubes (8-12 mm)
Flexible light source for intubation
Stylets for intubation
Laryngoscope with long blade
Oral speculum (e.g., baseball bat)
Large cotton swabs
Tie gauze
Nolvasan ointment
Umbilical tape
Large sterile hemostat to clamp umbilicus (if necessary)
Blood tubes (red, blue, EDTA, heparin)
Culturettes
Sharpie markers
Silver nitrate sticks
Pulse oximeter
Sharps container
50% dextrose
Ophthalmoscope
Stethoscope
Thermometer
Bandage scissors
Bulb syringe

- Body weight. Daily or when possible during the first 2 weeks. The calf should gain approximately 0.45 to 1.4 kg/day for the first year of life.
- Oral examination. Twice daily. Look for ulcers, swelling, and/or cyanosis of the tongue. These are relatively late signs of EEHV infection and may not occur in all cases.
- Respiratory rate. Twice daily (monitor trends). The normal rate in a 1-week-old calf is approximately 20 to 22 breaths/min.
- Heart rate. Ideally, twice daily (monitor trends). The normal heart rate in the first week is approximately 115 beats/min (range, 100 to 128 beats/min).
- Rectal body temperature. Ideally twice daily (monitor trends). The normal temperature range is 36.3° C to 37° C. Although not tested in elephant calves, the use of microchips that monitor body temperature passively (Bio-Therm chips, Riley Identification Systems, Carmel, Ind) may be a consideration for future use.
- CBC and chemistry panel, if indicated. Normal values have been published for elephant calves.[14]

- A first occurrence log should be kept to identify and monitor behavioral and other developmental signs that may assist in determining the health status of elephant calves.[7]

Nursing

Neonatal calves are often clumsy and may need assistance in learning to nurse. Prior to parturition a nulliparous dam should be trained to allow manipulation of the mammary glands. Approximately 74% of elephant calves attempt to nurse within 7 hours of delivery, but delays of up to 24 hours have been reported. If the calf has not nursed within the first 8 hours, elephant management and veterinary teams should review the calf's condition and behavior. If no nursing has occurred by 12 to 24 hours of age, a decision should be made whether to supplement the calf. This decision depends on many factors including: observations on the calf's vitality, strength of efforts to nurse, and assessment of the dam's receptivity to the calf.

Supplementary feedings may consist of colostrum collected from the dam, milk from the dam, milk replacer, or plasma. The supplements may be offered from a bottle (commercially available bovine bottles and nipples) or via stomach tube. Calves that have nursed from the dam may be reluctant to accept bottle feeding. One 2-month-old calf was sedated and given milk replacer by stomach tube once daily for 10 days because the dam's milk production had decreased as a result of low-grade metritis.

Failure of Passive Transfer

The zonary, endotheliochorial placenta of the elephant creates a barrier that prevents in utero transfer of immunoglobulins to the fetus.[3] The neonate must ingest colostrum prior to closure of the gap junctions of the intestinal mucosa to absorb colostral immunoglobulins. The time frame for immunoglobulin absorption is undocumented in elephants but probably ranges from 12 to 36 hours based on extrapolation from other species. Elephant calves have been reported to consume between 2 and 10 liters of colostrum during early nursing bouts.

Oral immunoglobulin supplementation may be provided by milking colostrum from the dam or feeding banked elephant plasma or commercial equine hyperimmune plasma. Even if given after an animal can no longer absorb antibodies systemically, orally administered immunoglobulins provide local immunity in the intestines. Elephant cows may be milked by hand or with a human breast pump. Oxytocin (30 to 60 IU IM) may be administered prior to milking attempts to facilitate milk let down. Milk yield may vary widely, from 300 to 1000 mL/milking.

Intravenous plasma may be administered to calves that have failure of passive transfer (FPT) and will tolerate the procedure or are deemed weak and particularly at risk for infection. Plasma transfusion was used successfully as part of the treatment of a 10-day-old Asian elephant calf that was failing to thrive.[13] Intravenous plasma should be administered at 40 to 80 mL/kg IV over 2 to 4 days. A single bolus of 10 to 20 mL/kg IV may be given in 30 to 60 minutes. Measurements of total protein and gamma globulin levels and tests for FPT should be repeated after the transfusion.

ELEPHANT CALVES

Training

Socialization of calves to humans should start shortly after birth so that the calf learns appropriate manners. Consistent interactions that do not allow undesirable behaviors toward humans to occur are crucial to prevent problems as the calf grows. Formal training is incorporated as the calf matures. It is not unreasonable to expect an elephant calf to present all parts of its body for examination, lie sternally and laterally on request, present its feet and limbs for radiographs, open its mouth for oral examinations, step on a platform scale for weighing, stand for urine collection, allow blood sample collection, and accept medications orally, rectally, and parenterally. Accounts of training and management of bull calves have been published.[3,19]

Preventive Health

Elephant calves should be trained for voluntary blood collection as soon as possible. Once the behavior is established, it is recommended that blood be collected monthly for a CBC and chemistry profile for the first 2 to 3 years to establish baseline values for the calf and assist in monitoring the health of the animal. At one institution, decreases in hematocrit levels were documented in the weeks prior to clinically evident signs of EEHV.

Elephant urine is typically a cloudy yellow color because of the presence of calcium crystals. Calves should be monitored for estimated urine volume, frequency, signs of stranguria, and discoloration as indicators of potential problems. Fecal consistency is usually a function of diet and feces may be lighter in color and less formed on a milk diet, with changes as the calf consumes more solid items. Excess mucus, blood, or sand should trigger further diagnostic testing. Salmonella culture and/or polymerase chain reaction (PCR) assay should be performed in any calf with diarrhea because infection in calves may be fatal.

Scale training to monitor normal weight gain should be initiated at an early age. Current growth charts for both African and Asian elephant calves have been presented by Olson.[14] Poor weight gain may be caused by either calf or cow illness. Adequate milk production by the dam and intake by the calf should be documented. Domperidone (500 to 5000 mg/day orally) has been used in elephants with agalactia.

Calves should be given tetanus toxoid at 3 and 4 months of age, followed by a vaccination at 1 year of age and then an adult vaccination schedule of vaccination every 5 years. Rabies vaccine should be given at 6 to 8 months of age, followed by annual vaccination if animals live in a rabies-endemic area and are considered to be at risk for exposure.

Hand Rearing

In 11 reported cases of elephant calves being completely hand-raised from birth, only 5 survived past infancy. In Asian working cows, agalactia was one of the leading causes of neonatal death.[12] Unfortunately there are times during which a calf may not be able to be reintroduced to the dam, such as when there is intractable aggression from the dam toward the calf or illness of the calf or dam.

The commercially available formulas recommended for elephant calves are Grober ElephantGro African and Asian elephant formulas (Grober Nutrition, Cambridge, Ontario, Canada) (Table 69-1). Elephant milk is significantly lower in lactose than cow's milk[15] and has a very different fatty acid profile.[10] The use of cow's milk–based formulas designed for human infants is not recommended because they may induce diarrhea. Some institutions have worked with nutritionists to create their own formulas based on reported elephant milk composition values.

Equipment needed for hand rearing include commercially available bovine bottles and nipples. Calves may aspirate or be frustrated by insufficient milk flow if the nipple hole size is inappropriate. Bottles should be washed with hot water and soap after every use. Sterilization of the bottles every 3 to 4 days is suggested.

TABLE 69-1	Comparison of Hand-Rearing Formulas Used in Elephant Calves					
Dry Matter Basis	African Elephant Milk[15]	Elephant-Gro (Grober)	Enfamil-Based Formula*	Pregestimil-Based Formula†	Lactogen (Nestlé, Vevey, Switzerland)[11]	Rice-Based Formula‡
Protein (%)	20.5	28	20.5	19.8	21.6	1-7
Fat (%)	38.7	41	36.8	23.9	18.9	1.5
Carbohydrate (%)	24.6	21.6	35.0	43.6	51.6	8.0
Solids (%)	11.5	11.8	11.7	12.6	—	12.4
kcal/g	5.29	6.0	5.54	4.63	—	—

*881 g water + 71 g Enfamil LIPIL with iron (Mead Johnson Nutrition, Glenview, Ill) + 20 g whey protein + 22 g coconut oil + 3 g dolomite powder + 3 g trace mineral salt.
†880 g water + 109 g Pregestimil LIPIL + 12 g whey protein + 6 g dicalcium phosphate + 4 g trace mineral salt.
‡0.5 kg milk powder + 0.5 kg red rice + 0.2 kg sucrose + 8.5 liters water.

TABLE 69-2	Reported Formula Volumes Bottle-Fed by Age[14]
Age	Liters/Day
Week 1	5.0-10.7
Week 2	8.75-11.6
Week 3	11.0-13.2
Week 4	11.8-12.0
Month 1	5.0-13.2
Month 2	12.0-18.0
Month 3	10.9-20.0
Month 4	12.1-24.0
Month 5	14.5-29.0
Month 6	13.7-31.0
Month 7	10.9-24.6
Month 8	12.7-25.8
Month 9	15.0-28.5
Month 10	10.6-28.3
Month 11	12.7-30.6

Newborn calves are initially fed on demand and may nurse up to 12 times in a 24-hour period. The intervals between feedings may gradually be increased so that by 1 year of age, a calf is offered bottles six or seven times a day. Volumes depend on caloric density and fluid requirements. Typically, calves will consume 10% to 15% of their body weight on a daily basis, although volumes fed depend on the formula (Table 69-2).[13] Caloric requirements have been estimated at 6000 to 8000 kcal/day for a 100-kg calf and 16000 to 20,000 kcal/day for a 200-kg calf.[11] Formulas should be analyzed for composition and energy.

Nutritional secondary hyperparathyroidism and bone fractures have occurred in formula-fed calves. These problems may be a result of improperly balanced formulas or malabsorption of nutrients from the intestinal tract. Monitoring ionized and total serum calcium levels is a relatively insensitive method for monitoring nutritional status because homeostatic mechanisms that will maintain these values within normal ranges until significant calcium depletion has occurred. Preliminary work has suggested that measuring urinary calcium and phosphorus excretion is a much more sensitive way to detect early deficiencies or imbalances in mineral status.[20] Treatment of fractures has generally not been successful.

Calves begin to experiment with solid foods at a relatively early age. Solid foods should be introduced at 1 to 2 months of age, even though significant intake may be minimal. Cows will usually gradually wean their calves by 3 to 5 years of age. Beginning at 12 to 14 months, there is a gradual decrease in milk intake and increased sampling of solid foods. Ideally, calves should not be weaned before 2 years because some nursing may occur until at least 3 years of age.

Management of Sick Calves

The size and strength of even very young elephants may prevent easy physical restraint, and manual restraint for diagnostic testing or treatment may be stressful for the calf and staff. Sedation allows medical intervention while a calf is still active and strong. Butorphanol (0.02 to 0.03 mg/kg IM) and detomidine (0.02 to 0.03 mg/kg IM) have been used to produce standing sedation in elephant calves as young as 2 months of age. Drug effects may be reversed with naltrexone (2.0 to 3.5 mg/kg IM) and atipamezole (0.1 to 0.16 mg/kg IM).

Fluids may be administered to elephant calves orally, rectally, intravenously, or even intraperitoneally. Subcutaneous administration of appropriate volumes of fluids is generally not feasible. Balanced electrolyte solutions may be administered via the auricular arteries, but no other substances should be administered intra-arterially because they may result in tissue necrosis. The auricular veins are the most easily accessed for catheter placement but maintenance of catheters is difficult because elephants may easily remove them by pulling at them or rubbing their ears on structures in their enclosures.

Trauma

Trauma is a potential cause of morbidity and mortality in young elephants. Causes of trauma to elephant calves may include herdmate aggression or physical encounters, accidental falls, and drowning. In one case, maternal trauma resulted in a fatal torsion of the root of the mesentery.[1] Preventive measures include assessment of postparturient cows for aggressive behavior toward offspring, provision of nonslip surfaces for the calf, limited access to pools and moats until the calf becomes familiar with these areas, and a proactive plan for introduction of the calf to other herd members.

Sepsis and Methicillin-Resistant
Staphylococcus aureus

Sepsis and septicemia have been reported[12a] in elephant calves following maternal rejection, FPT, transport, and trauma and through umbilical infection.[6] Salmonella infection may cause acute septicemia in juvenile elephants after a stressful event.[24] Antimicrobial drugs for elephant calves have been reported, although pharmacologic studies are lacking.[5]

Methicillin-resistant *Staphylococcus aureus* (MRSA) infection has been reported in one hand-reared African elephant calf.[6] This calf showed signs of discharge from skin wounds at 7 weeks of age. Despite resolution of the skin lesions following antibiotic therapy, the calf failed to thrive. Necropsy results showed evidence of enterococcal septicemia. Based on epidemiologic investigations, it appears that the calf acquired the staphylococcal infection from human caretakers.

Umbilical Hernias

Umbilical hernias have been reported in Asian elephant calves.[2,16,21] These may be detected during the neonatal examination, but some become apparent 2 to 4 weeks after birth. Large umbilical hernias typically are repaired surgically, but smaller hernias have successfully resolved with daily manual reduction, which stimulates second intention healing of the abdominal wall defect. Use of nonsurgical treatment is only recommended in cases in which the hernia is completely reducible, does not contain incarcerated viscera, and is not infected. Early detection and intervention are more likely to result in a good outcome. Repeated palpation and ultrasound examination of the umbilicus may allow detection of a developing umbilical hernia at an early stage.

Diarrhea and Other Gastrointestinal Problems

Fecal quality may vary widely depending on the calf's diet. Establishing normal parameters for color, consistency, and frequency of defecation for each individual will aid in monitoring changes that could indicate gastrointestinal disease. Diarrhea in elephant calves is a relatively common medical problem. Differential diagnoses include dietary intolerance, dietary indiscretion, imbalanced or abnormal bacterial flora, parasitism, and septicemia. Salmonellosis is a significant concern for elephant calves.[18] Workup of a calf with diarrhea should include a physical examination, blood collection for a CBC and chemistry panel, fecal culture, fecal cytology, and fecal examination for parasites. Treatments should include fluid therapy (intravenous, oral, or rectal) to maintain hydration and targeted antibiotic or antiparasitic treatment.

Some calves that begin ingesting substrates (sand or clay) at a young age seem to develop habitual intake and may develop intestinal impaction. Some institutions have had to change substrates completely to prevent calves from continuing to ingest foreign materials. Medical management of these animals may include maintaining hydration through the administration of intravenous or oral fluids, enemas, and psyllium or other oral fiber supplements. In one 3-year-old African elephant, the severity of the impaction required an enterotomy to remove the sand.[17]

Dental Problems

Tusk fracture may occur in young elephants. In calves, the risk of pulp exposure after a fracture is greater than in adults because of tusk length. Radiographs are useful in determining the length of the pulp canal if it is not apparent on physical examination. Necrotic or exposed pulp tissue should be removed surgically and the open canal sealed using dental synthetic bone graft material (Consil Bioglass, Nutramax Laboratories, Edgewood, Md) and chemical composite (Compcore, Premier Dental, Plymouth Meeting, Pa).[23] If a tusk is being excessively worn, a metal crown may be used to protect it from further damage (MM).[22]

Molar eruption varies among individuals, making it difficult to predict expected times for each molar to appear. Commonly reported problems affecting molars include malalignment, abnormal wear, and abscessation.

REFERENCES

1. Abou-Madi N: Personal communication, 2010.
2. Abou-Madi N, Kollias G, Hackett RP, et al: Umbilical herniorrhaphy in a juvenile Asian elephant *(Elephas maximus).* J Zoo Wildl Med 35:221–225, 2004.
3. Allen WR, Mathias S, Wooding FB, et al: Placentation in the African elephant *(Loxodonta africana):* II. Morphological changes in the uterus and placenta throughout gestation. Placenta 24:598–617, 2003.
4. Durham A: First year of growth and training of a bull calf at ZLS Whipsnade Zoo. J Elephant Managers Assoc 20:20–26, 2009.
5. Emanuelson K: Neonatal care and hand-rearing. In Fowler ME, Mikota SK, editors: Biology, medicine, and surgery of elephants. Ames, Iowa, 2006, Blackwell, pp 233–241.
6. Janssen DL, Lamberski N, Donovan T, et al: Methicillin-resistant *Staphylococcus aureus* infection in an African elephant *(Loxodonta africana)* calf and caretakers. In Proceedings of the American Association of Zoo Veterinarians Annual Meeting, 2009, pp 200–201.
7. Joseph S, Miller L: Documenting behavioral and physical development in African elephant *(Loxodonta africana)* calves. In Proceedings of the International Elephant Conservation and Research Symposium, 2004, pp 20.
8. Knauf S, Blad-Stahl J, Lawrenz A, et al: Plasma preparation and storage for African elephants *(Loxodonta africana).* J Zoo Wildl Med 40:71–75, 2009.
9. Koehl D: Elephant database, 2010 (http://www.elephant.se).
10. Mainka SA, Cooper RM, Black SR, et al: Asian elephant *(Elephas maximus)* milk composition during the first 280 days of lactation. Zoo Biol 13:389–393, 1994.
11. Manansang J, Prastiti S: Hand rearing Sumatran elephant *(Elephas maximus sumatrensis)* at Taman Safari Indonesia, 2004 (http://www.seaza.org/scientific_papers/hand_rearing_sumatran_elephant.htm).
12. Mar KU: The studbook of timber elephant of Myanmar with special reference to survivorship analysis, (http://www.fao.org/docrep/005/ad031e/ad031e0m.htm).
12a. Miller M: Personal communication, Feb 1, 2010.
13. Murray S, Bush M, Tell LA: Medical management of postpartum problems in an Asian elephant *(Elephas maximus)* cow and calf. J Zoo Wildl Med 27:255–258, 1996.
14. Olson D: The elephant husbandry resource guide. Silver Spring, Md, 2004, American Zoo and Aquarium Association.
15. Parrott JJ: Analysis of African elephant mature milk in early lactation and formulation of an elephant calf milk replacer. In Proceedings of the American Association of Zoo Veterinarians Annual Meeting, 1996, pp 102–111.
16. Pathak SC, Saikia J, Lahon DK, et al: Attempted ventral herniorrhaphy in an Asian elephant *(Elephas maximus)* using xylazine sedation. J Zoo Wildl Med 21:234–235, 1990.
17. Proudfoot JS, Ramer JC, Singleton CL, et al: Abdominal surgery and enterotomy in a juvenile African elephant *(Loxodonta africana).* In Proceedings of the International Elephant Conservation and Research Symposium, 2004, pp 6–7.
18. Ratanakorn P: Elephant health problems and management in Cambodia, Lao and Thailand. In Proceedings of the International Elephant Conservation and Research Symposium, 2001, pp 111–114.
19. Royals S: Raising Kandula: The first three years. Calf development update and behavioral management of a bull calf from birth to transition to protected contact. In Proceedings of the International Elephant Conservation and Research Symposium, 2004, pp 27.
20. Weber M, Junge R, Black P, et al: Management of critical juvenile Asian elephants *(Elephas maximus).* In Proceedings of the American Association of Zoo Veterinarians Annual Meeting, 2009, pp 61–63.
21. Wiedner EB, Gray C, Rich P, et al: Nonsurgical repair of an umbilical hernia in two Asian elephant calves *(Elephas maximus).* J Zoo Wildl Med 39:248–251, 2008.
22. Willis GP: Placement of protective metal crown on the tusk of a captive African elephant *(Loxodonta africana).* J Elephant Managers Assoc 17:36, 2006.
23. Willis GP, Proudfoot J, Ramer J: Pulpal treatment and restoration of a fractured tusk of an African elephant *(Loxodonta africana).* In Proceedings of the American Association of Zoo Veterinarians Annual Meeting, 2002, p 26.
24. Windsor RS, Ashford WA: Salmonella infection in the African elephant and black rhinoceros. Trop Anim Hlth Prod 4:214–219, 1972.

CHAPTER 70

Treatment of Elephant Endotheliotropic Herpesvirus

Ellen Wiedner, Lauren L. Howard, and Ramiro Isaza

Although the number of elephant endotheliotropic herpesvirus (EEHV) cases continues to increase, the survivor list has remained disappointingly small. This has confounded the identification of worthwhile treatment modalities. In addition, outcome is also likely affected by variables unrelated to treatment, such as viral load, strain virulence, and immune status. Nevertheless, growing evidence from antemortem blood work, case reports, and necropsies has suggested that shock and hypotension, along with possible disseminated intravascular coagulation (DIC), develop as EEHV progresses. In this way, EEHV infection, a peracute to acute hemorrhagic disease, clinically resembles some human hemorrhagic diseases, such Dengue fever and Ebola,[19] although the mechanisms underlying shock in elephants with EEHV are not known.

Human hemorrhagic diseases are mostly treated symptomatically by providing circulatory support, maintaining blood volume and tissue perfusion. Antiviral drugs are administered, if available. Presumably, a similar approach has value in elephants. Several recent EEHV survivors were treated with antiviral drugs, crystalloids, and colloids, lending credence to the idea that aggressive supportive care—in particular, fluid therapy—along with careful monitoring of vital signs, are likely to be as important to patient survival as antiviral medication.

Providing intensive care to these massive animals, however, is no easy task. Complicating factors include delays in confirming diagnosis, lack of physiologic data in elephants, progression and severity of the disease and, finally, the complexities involved in the hospitalization of a multiton patient who is often ambulatory, even in end-stage disease, including safety issues.

Strategic planning for the possibility of having an EEHV patient, including equipment, supplies, treatment protocols, and budget, should be done by all facilities with young elephants and reviewed regularly. Because EEHV cases often demand 24-hour care, staffing is another consideration, and a team approach is vital to avoid work force exhaustion. Some facilities should consider establishing liaisons with experienced outside individuals to create backup emergency teams of handlers and clinicians that may assist when called.

Many facilities now specifically train their juvenile elephants to accept various medical procedures to facilitate herd monitoring as well as crisis management. However, sedation is indicated for some animals, facilities, or procedures. A successful protocol that has been used in juvenile elephants is presented in Table 70-1. Risks of sedation may be decreased by having an accurate weight, choosing standing sedation over recumbent sedation, using reversible sedatives, having adequate padding to support the patient if recumbency occurs, and monitoring vital signs.

In general, standard equipment and basic physical examination tools are sufficient to manage elephants medically. A few specifics are described here. Because measurements of packed cell volume (PCV) and total protein (TP) are needed to guide fluid therapy, stall side results are highly desirable. Microhematocrit centrifuges offer the advantage of using capillary blood tubes that require minute quantities of blood; thus, buccal bleeds or similar methods may be used if venous access is not possible. In compromised elephants, veins may be severely vasoconstricted or even thrombosed, and filling standard vacuum tubes is not always possible.

Tools for medicating elephants are similarly straightforward. Soft tubing, attached to a large dosing syringe or an equine stomach pump, may be used for the administration of rectal medications and rectal fluids, respectively. In elephants willing to take oral medications, smaller dosing syringes and flavoring syrups may be helpful.

TABLE 70-1 Pharmacologic Treatment of Elephants With Elephant Endotheliotropic Herpesvirus

Drug	Dose	Route	Frequency	Type of Drug
Butorphanol	0.006-0.03 mg/kg	SC, IM, IV	tid	Opioid agonist, antagonist, analgesic
Ceftiofur	1.1-2.2 mg/kg	IM or IV	Once daily bid or tid	(IV) or, BID or TID (IM) Cephalosporin
Famciclovir	16 mg/kg, then 12 mg/kg	PO or per rectum antiviral	qid	Alphaherpes
Flunixin meglumine	0.2-0.5 mg/kg	IM, IV	bid	NSAID
Furosemide	0.25-1.0 mg/kg	IM, PO	bid	Loop diuretic
Ganciclovir	5 mg/kg	Slow IV	bid	β–herpes antiviral
Mannitol	0.25-2.0 g/kg	20% solution by slow IV	—	Osmotic diuretic
Sulfamethoxazole-trimethoprim	22 mg/kg	PO	Twice daily or bid	Antibiotic
Vitamin E	2.2 IU/kg	PO	Once daily	Antioxidant

EEHV, *Elephant endotheliotropic herpesvirus.*
Standing calf sedation[23]:
 Butorphanol, 0.02-0.03 mg/kg IM plus detomidine 0.02-0.03 mg/kg IM.
 Reversal: atipamezole, 0.1-0.16 mg/kg IM, and naltrexone, 2.0-3.5 mg/kg IM.

With the recent report of the death of an elephant caused by methicillin-resistant *Staphylococcus aureus* (MRSA) and the growing suspicion that some EEHV patients have compromised immune systems, attention to hygiene and biosecurity is paramount.[12] Frequent hand washing, removal of waste products from the environment, and excellent sanitization are strongly recommended. Additional equipment and supplies are described in the following sections.

PHYSICAL EXAMINATION AND MONITORING

Many facilities routinely monitor a variety of parameters in their herds, including complete blood counts (CBCs) and serum blood chemistries, to identify changes that may foreshadow clinical disease. Some institutions also ship blood regularly to the National Elephant Herpes Laboratory in Washington DC for polymerase chain reaction (PCR) testing of whole blood for EEHV. The recent finding that healthy elephants may shed virus in nasal secretions suggests that frequent trunk wash screening could be useful, although currently this is only available for research purposes.[22] Useful physical and blood monitoring parameters in elephants are listed in Box 70-1.

In fulminant disease, much more frequent evaluation is needed. Sometimes hourly, or even more

BOX 70-1 Parameters to be Monitored in Elephant Endotheliotropic Herpesvirus Patients

Heart rate and rhythm
Temperature
Respiratory rate and effort
Mentation
Edema check
Ophthalmic examination:
 • Scleral injection
 • Icterus
 • Retinal hemorrhage
Production of urine and feces
Eating, drinking, and nursing behavior
Urinalysis with dipstick and refractometer
Oral examination
Lameness
Presence or absence of edema (head, elsewhere)
Presence or absence of borborygmi
Abdominal pain
Feces: consistency and frequency
Blood pressure (tail cuff)
Ultrasound assessment of thorax, abdomen
Pulse oximetry
Weight
Blood work
 • PCV, TP
 • CBC, serum blood chemistry
 • Platelet count
 • Acid-base level
Coagulation

frequent, examinations are needed for the guidance of treatment, particularly fluid therapy. As the animal stabilizes, this may be decreased.

Physical Findings

In elephants less than 2000 kg, the heart may usually be clearly auscultated from both the left and right sides. This is aided by having the elephant lift its front leg and placing the stethoscope just cranial to the elbow. Tachycardia, arrhythmias, and murmurs have been reported in progressing EEHV cases, as have changes in respiratory rate. These findings may be related to cardiovascular deterioration, worsening anemia, or pericardial or pleural effusion. Transcutaneous ultrasound evaluation of the heart, thorax, and peritoneum is possible in most juveniles and may be used to identify and monitor effusions. Although no published reports exist of thoracocentesis or pericardiocentesis in elephants, both procedures are theoretically feasible in smaller animals and could be necessary if effusions become severe enough to impede respiration or cardiac output.

Mentation and behavior are subjective, and ideally should be observed by individuals familiar with the elephant. Some EEHV patients are described as lethargic or somnolent.[7] Others refuse to lie down to sleep. Brain imaging techniques are not currently possible in elephants, but procedures that might distinguish between general malaise and elevated intracranial pressure (ICP) caused by vasculitis include an ophthalmic examination to look for papilledema and retinal hemorrhage, as well as cranial nerve evaluation. In animals suspected to have increased ICP, oxygen therapy and mannitol in conjunction with fluid therapy to correct hypovolemia and maintain blood pressure should be considered. Oxygen may be administered at 10 to 20 liters/min from a portable tank through tubing placed into the trunk if the animal permits it, or in a flow-by manner.[9] Mannitol, an osmotic diuretic used to treat elevated ICP, has not been evaluated in elephants, but the equine dose might be an appropriate starting point.

Edema, especially of the head, neck, and tongue, may become severe enough to impede breathing, prevent swallowing, and cause skin fissures, although total protein and albumin levels may not immediately correlate with the severity of edema. Colloidal support, oxygen therapy, and diuretics may be helpful. Furosemide has been used in elephants at empirical doses extrapolated from equine data.[21] It must be used with caution in shocky patients and in patients receiving nonsteroidal anti-inflammatory drugs (NSAIDs).

The soft and hard palates, tongue, and buccal surfaces of the mouth should be examined for oral ulcers or vesicles. Discomfort from such lesions, or from others located in the larynx or esophagus, may contribute to anorexia. The conjunctiva and genital mucosa, as well as the sclera, should be assessed for lesions, injected vessels, and color changes. Cyanosis is a significant finding that ideally should be correlated with a pulse oximetry reading or measurement of PaO_2. Although pulse oximetry may be challenging in elephants, usable probe sites include the finger of the trunk, tongue, upper lip, pinna of the ear, and distal nasal septum. A caveat is that these devices are designed to read the oxygen saturation (SaO_2) of human hemoglobin (Hb), which has a lower oxygen affinity than elephant Hb. Thus, a high SaO_2 reading could, in fact, correlate with a lower PaO_2.[10] Supplemental oxygen should be provided to cyanotic patients and those with low SaO_2 and PaO_2.

Lameness associated with EEHV may be caused by leakage of blood into joints, muscle swelling, or other viral damage. Ruling out nonviral causes of lameness should be attempted. NSAIDs may relieve discomfort but, to avoid nephrotoxicity, they should be used at the lowest dose possible and only in hydrated animals. Flunixin meglumine appears to provide significant relief, but other NSAIDs can be used, as can other classes of analgesics. Stomach protectants or acid blockers might be warranted if NSAIDs are given. Their usage in elephants is empirical.

Abdominal pain, another nonspecific sign, is commonly reported.[7] Decreased borborygmi, inappetance, or scant manure may be caused by impaction from dehydration or viral damage to the gastrointestinal (GI) tract. Diarrhea may also be caused by viral injury. However, because elephants are prone to a variety of nonviral causes of colic, even in a confirmed EEHV case, other diagnoses should be considered. Treatment of colic signs is symptomatic.

Decreased urine output and/or the presence of blood or protein in the urine may indicate renal compromise caused by inadequate circulation. Except for very young calves, elephants do not concentrate their urine very well, and specific gravity does not indicate hydration status.[26] Standard signs of dehydration such as sunken eyes or decreased skin turgor are rarely observed in elephants. The patient's water and milk consumption should be assessed to correlate input with output. Sick elephants should be weighed daily, if possible.

EEHV patients often present with low-grade fever. Normal fecal ball temperatures are 35° C to 37° C

(96.8° F to 98.6° F).[1] A subcutaneous microchip that measures body temperature has been developed for horses and is currently being tested in elephants. Fever does not necessarily require treatment, but is a useful monitoring tool.

Blood Monitoring

Normal PCV and TP in adult elephants is 36 and 8.4 g/dL, respectively.[15] Concurrent decreases in both PCV and TP suggest peracute hemorrhage. Decreases in PCV with normal or slightly decreased TP occur with vasculitis in other species. This pattern is often seen in elephants with progressing EEHV infection. PCV and TP do not always immediately correlate with the severity of hemorrhage, and frequent repeat measurements are recommended. Serum should be clear and pale yellow; in EEHV, both hemolysis and opacity caused by increased blood lipids may occur. The presence and size of any buffy coat should be noted. Leukopenia, anemia, and thrombocytopenia are common on the CBC. Leukopenia often precedes clinical signs by days and possibly weeks, and a mild left shift has been observed in several cases at the onset of clinical signs. Changes in cell morphology have also been noted.

Blood smears may provide stall side information on platelet numbers. In other species, bleeding occurs if platelets decrease below 50×10^9/liter.[4] Profound thrombocytopenia has been reported in elephants just before death. Interestingly, in several cases, recovery from EEHV has been accompanied by a rebound hematopoiesis in all cell lines lasting days to weeks.

Electrolyte imbalances, hypoalbuminemia, and azotemia have been seen in serum blood chemistries. Correction requires fluid therapy. Hypertriglyceridemia, elevated liver enzyme levels, hypercholesterolemia, and elevated muscle enzyme levels have also been noted. Trending may be used to indicate disease progression.

Changes in acid-base status, particularly metabolic acidosis and elevated lactate level, are consequences of hypoperfusion in other species and should be assessed in elephants. Normalization of these values requires correction of the underlying problem, along with bicarbonate or oxygen therapy, as needed.[5]

In human hemorrhagic diseases, coagulation parameters may be dramatically altered. Hemostatic values have been published for normal Asian elephants,[8] but alterations during disease are unknown. Prolongation of clotting times might provide evidence of internal hemorrhage; decreases have been associated with DIC in other species.

Indirect blood pressure measurements may be done in elephants using a tail cuff.[23] Repeated measurements are needed to identify trends. Consistency in the position of both the elephant and cuff are necessary to interpret results. Persistent hypotension is indicative of hypovolemia or circulatory shock and requires appropriate fluid therapy. Neither vasopressor nor inotrope use has been reported in elephants.

TREATMENT

Antiviral Drugs and Other Medications

Treatment of EEHV infections with antiviral medications has been a cornerstone of therapy for the past decade. Most survivors, although not all, were started early on high doses of antiviral medications. Current recommendations are to start treatment in young animals immediately if nonspecific mild clinical signs such as depression or lethargy are present, and before diagnosis is confirmed.

Because antiviral medications are often costly and difficult to procure quickly in the large quantities necessary, proactive communication with a local hospital or pharmacy regarding drug availability is a critical part of any institution's overall EEHV treatment plan. Some institutions may choose to keep enough antiviral drugs on site to treat any elephant in their collection for at least 2 or 3 days, until new supplies are available.

To date, the three antiviral drugs that have been used to treat EEHV infection are aciclovir, famciclovir, and ganciclovir. All require phosphorylation by viral thymidine kinase into their active metabolites. It is unknown, however, whether all strains of EEHV have a functioning thymidine kinase gene. Aciclovir and famciclovir are effective against alphaherpesviruses in humans. Their efficacy against betaherpesviruses, such as EEHV, is unclear. Ganciclovir, however, is effective against human betaherpesviruses. All three are associated with risks during pregnancy.

Famciclovir is the most commonly used antiviral in EEHV treatment and was used to treat all known survivors, although many nonsurvivors received it as well.[7,21] Famciclovir is converted into its active compound penciclovir following oral or rectal administration. Pharmacokinetic data in elephants have shown that in healthy young Asian elephants, 8 to 15 mg/kg famciclovir given orally or rectally three times daily results in plasma concentrations of penciclovir considered therapeutic against herpes simplex virus in humans.[11] Famciclovir absorption in sick elephants in unknown. No adverse effects have been reported in elephants, although they occur in humans.

Many institutions use a loading dose of famciclovir of 16 mg/kg every 6 hours for the first day. The dose is decreased to 12 mg/kg every 6 hours on day 2, which is continued for at least 2 weeks. Total duration of treatment is usually a minimum of 2 weeks, until the animal is clinically normally and no longer viremic. Some institutions will treat any sick elephants for 2 weeks with famciclovir even in the face of a negative diagnosis because of concerns that current diagnostic methods cannot identify all strains of EEHV.

Ganciclovir has been used in two surviving elephant calves.[23,24] One of these elephants was started on oral famciclovir and switched to IV ganciclovir when her condition continued to deteriorate.[25] Measurable ganciclovir concentrations in serum were not documented although clinical improvement occurred. Ganciclovir is available as a lyophilized powder to be reconstituted, diluted, and administered via slow IV. In humans, ganciclovir may cause severe bone marrow suppression.

Broad-spectrum antibiotics such as sulfamethoxazole or ceftiofur are commonly administered prophylactically to elephants with EEHV. The use of analgesics, NSAIDs, ulcer treatments, and diuretics has already been discussed. Oral vitamin E has been given for its antioxidant properties. Suggested doses for various medications are listed in Table 70-1.

Fluid Therapy

Fluid therapy may be lifesaving in EEHV patients. Treatment of early shock, generally defined as a massive decrease in effective tissue perfusion, requires maintenance of blood pressure and tissue oxygenation and is accomplished by circulatory support. Determination of amount, route, and type of fluid must be based on trends noted during the ongoing monitoring of the patient, particularly clinical improvements in behavior and vital signs.[5] Data on fluid therapy in elephants are empirical.

The three routes of fluid administration possible in elephants are oral, rectal and IV. Oral fluids require a cooperative and willing elephant, and IV administration is associated with a high rate of complications. Rectal administration of plain warm water, however, is a simple and rapid method of providing circulatory support. A legitimate, albeit uncommonly used technique in human emergency medicine,[2] rectal fluid

administration may be effective in elephants who appear to absorb fluids quickly if they are needed and excrete all surplus.[20] Retention is aided by pausing if the elephant starts to strain and by holding the tail down firmly following administration. Rectal fluid administration, if started early, even in unconfirmed EEHV cases, may provide enough resuscitation in the early stages of shock to prevent further decompensation.

Although IV catheterization and catheter maintenance may be challenging in this species, IV administration of fluids is certainly possible in elephants,[14,16-18,20] and venous access is essential for plasma or blood transfusions and for the administration of certain medications. Both through the needle catheters (used in ear veins) and over the wire types (used in ear and saphenous veins) have been used in sizes ranging from 20 to 14 gauge and in lengths from 3 to 5 inches. Catheters manufactured from less thrombogenic materials are recommended. Aseptic technique should be used in placement, and numbing the area in advance with a topical lidocaine-based cream or intradermal lidocaine may be desirable. A bungee cord may serve a tourniquet to distend the saphenous vein. Either cyanoacrylate glue or suture are used to affix the catheter in place. Ear vein catheters may be protected with an adhesive sterile barrier such as an antimicrobial surgical incise (Ioban) drape, whereas saphenous catheters usually require bandaging. Anecdotal and reported problems include difficulty in placement, loss of patency, venous thrombosis, thrombophlebitis, hematoma formation, and removal or destruction of the catheter by the elephant or a herdmate.[23]

Any elephant with an IV catheter must be continuously observed by knowledgeable personnel.. Thus, clinicians might want to place a catheter, group together the administration of all IV medications and drugs, and then immediately remove the catheter. Extended compression of the puncture site is recommended to avoid hematoma formation.

With ambulatory elephants, fluids may be carried by a handler who walks along with the elephant or hung on an IV pole and pushed along. Large animal IV lines will deliver fluids at high flow rates. Fluid pumps or a pressure cuff may be helpful but are not required.

Whether rectal or IV, the fluid bolus technique of administration is useful in elephants and in domestic species. This method entails giving a bolus of crystalloids using a 20-mL/kg dose and then reassessing the patient. Usually, a maximum of three boluses are given, with evaluation of patient vital signs and attitude after each bolus.[3] In juvenile elephants, a dose of 10 mL/kg is often more practical, which means that boluses between 5 to 20 liters are used. Following this, IV fluids are continued at a maintenance rate or are discontinued. Equine maintenance rates of 40 mL/kg/day IV have been used in elephants.[14,20]

Fresh plasma, fresh-frozen plasma, and fresh whole blood are colloids that have all been administered to elephants.[13,14,18,20,23] Collection techniques have been described. Cross matching of donor and receipient should be performed prior to administration, as should donor screening for blood-borne diseases, including EEHV.[27] A very slow starting rate should be used initially and the patient assessed for transfusion reaction. If none is seen, the transfusion rate may be increased. Synthetic colloids such as hetastarch and dextrans, and hemoglobin-based oxygen carriers (e.g., Oxyglobin) have not been evaluated in elephants, but are generally a better source of oncotic pressure in hypoalbuminemic patients than natural colloids.

Almost all species benefit from blood transfusion at a hematocrit (Hct) less than 12%, and many clinicians elect to transfuse at a Hct less than 20%.[4] The ideal amount of blood and plasma to transfuse in elephants is unknown. In a report of a hemorrhaging adult elephant with a Hct of 13, a whole-blood transfusion of 8 liters produced tremendous clinical improvement, although the dose of blood was very low compared with transfusion recommendations for other species.[16] Similarly, small amounts of plasma (1 to 2 liters) have reportedly been of clinical benefit as well.[18,20] Donor guidelines do not exist for elephants but, in most species, 1% of body weight (in kilograms) is suggested as the maximum amount of blood to withdraw. Platelet products are not available for elephants. Thus, although fresh whole blood contains relatively small numbers of platelets, in a severely thrombocytopenic (platelets $<50 \times 10^9$/liter) elephant, it is currently the only choice.

Reports of parenteral nutrition are absent from the elephant literature, but in an animal with a damaged digestive tract or profound weakness, partial or even total parenteral nutrition should be considered. Equine guidelines might provide a useful starting point.[6]

In conclusion, although much remains unknown about EEHV pathophysiology, an intensive care unit approach combining circulatory support, antiviral medication, and careful monitoring has the potential to improve outcomes. Research on elephant physiology, pharmacokinetics, and new treatments will further extend the toolbox of the clinician treating this devastating disease.

Acknowledgments

We would like to acknowledge the elephant care staff at the Houston Zoo and the Ringling Bros. Center for Elephant Conservation as well as the many veterinarians and researchers worldwide dedicated to understanding and combating EEHV. We also offer thanks to those who shared their first-hand, and often heartbreaking experiences of this disease with us. And finally, we want to recognize Barack, who survived, and Mac, who didn't—who both continue to inspire us daily.

REFERENCES

1. Benedict FG, Fox EL, Baker ML: The surface temperature of the elephant, rhinoceros and hippopotamus. Am J Physio 56:454–459, 1921.
2. Bruera E, Pruvost M, Schoeller T, et al: Proctoclysis for hydration of terminally ill cancer patients. J Pain Symptom Manage 15:216–219, 1998.
3. Corley KTT, Axon JE: Resuscitation and emergency management for neonatal foals. Vet Clin North Am Equine Pract 21:431–455, 2005.
4. David JB: Blood-donor horses and whole blood transfusion in private practice. In Robinson NE, Sprayberry KA, editors: Current therapy in equine medicine, ed 6, Philadelphia, 2008, Elsevier Health Sciences, pp 224–226.
5. Day TK, Bateman S: Shock syndromes. In DiBartola SP, editor: Fluid, electrolyte, and acid-base disorders in small animal practice, ed 3, St. Louis, 2006, Saunders Elsevier, pp 540–566.
6. Dunkel BM, Wilkins PA: Nutrition and the critically ill horse. Vet Clin North Am Equine Pract 20:107–126, 2004.
7. Garner MM, Helmick K, Ochsenreiter J, et al: Clinico-pathologic features of fatal disease attributed to new variants of endotheliotropic herpesviruses in two Asian elephants (Elephas maximus). Vet Pathol 46:97–104, 2009.
8. Gentry PA, Ross ML, Yamada M: Blood coagulation profile of the Asian elephant (Elephas maximus). In Gentry PA, Ross ML, Yamada M: Zoo biology, vol 15, New York, 1996, Wiley-Liss, pp 413–423.
9. Heard DJ, Jacobson ER, Brock KA: Effects of oxygen supplementation on blood gas values in chemically restrained juvenile African elephants. J Am Vet Med Assoc 189:1071–1074, 1986.
10. Honeyman VL, Pettifer GR, Dyson DH: Arterial blood pressure and blood gas values in normal standing and laterally recumbent African (Loxodonta africana) and Asian (Elephas maximus) elephants. J Zoo Wildl Med 23:205–210, 1992.
11. Isaza R, Hunter RP, Richman LK, et al: Famciclovir pharmacokinetics in young Asian elephants (Elephas maximus). In Proceedings of the Annual Meeting of the American Association of Zoo Veterinarians, Minneapolis, 2003, American Association of Zoo Veterinarians, pp 82–83.
12. Janssen D, Lamberski N, Dunne G, et al: Methicillin-resistant Staphylococcus aureus skin infections from an elephant calf—San Diego, California, 2008. MMWR CDC Surveill Summ 58:194–198, 2009.
13. Knauf S, Blad-Stahl J, Lawrenz A, et al: Plasma preparation and storage for African elephants (Loxodonta africana). J Zoo Wildl Med 40:71–75, 2009.
14. Lawrenz A, Barhold D, Olbricht G, et al: [Infusiontherapie bei einem juvenilen Afrikanischen elefanten (Loxodonta africana) mit Salmonellenenteritis unter Berücksichtigung der Blutparameter.]

Intravenous fluid therapy in a juvenile African elephant *(Loxodonta africana)* with Salmonella diarrhoea with simultaneous control of the blood values. Verh ber Erkrg Zootiere 113–119, 1999.

15. Lewis JH: Comparative hematology on elephants, *Elephas maximus.* Comp Biochem Physiol A Comp Physiol 49:175–181, 1974.
16. Merkt H, Ahlers D, Bader H, et al: [Nachbehandlung und heilungsverlauf bei einer Elefantenkuh nach Geburtshilfe durch Dammschnitt.] Aftercare and recovery of a female Indian elephant after delivery of a dead fetus by episiotomy. Berl Münch Tieraerztl Wochen 99:329–333, 1986.
17. Miller RM: Use of commercially-bottled water in emergency intravenous fluid therapy for large animals. Vet Med Small Anim Clin 443–444, 1976.
18. Murray S, Bush M, Tell LA: Medical management of postpartum problems in an Asian elephant *(Elephas maximus)* cow and calf. J Zoo Wildl Med 27:255–258, 1996.
19. Rigau-Perez J, Clark GG, Gubler DJ, et al: Dengue and dengue haemorrhagic fever. Lancet 352:971–977, 1998.
20. Sanchez CR, Murray S, Montali RJ, et al: Diagnosis and treatment of presumptive pyelonephritis in an Asian elephant *(Elephas maximus).* J Zoo Wildl Med 35:397–399, 2004.
21. Schmitt DL, Hardy DA, Montali RJ, et al: Use of famciclovir for the treatment of endotheliotrophic herpesvirus infections in Asian elephants *(Elephas maximus).* J Zoo Wildl Med 31:518–522, 2000.
22. Stanton JJ, Zong J-C, Latimer E, et al: Detection of pathogenic elephant endotheliotropic herpesvirus in routine trunk washes from healthy adult Asian elephants *(Elephas maximus)* using a novel quantitative real-time polymerase chain reaction assay. Am J Vet Res 71:925–933, 2010.
23. Suedmeyer WK, Fine D: Indirect oscillometric blood pressure measurement in four African elephants *(Loxodonta africana)*. In Proceedings of the Annual Meeting of the American Association of Zoo Veterinarians, Minneapolis, 2006, American Association of Zoo Veterinarians, pp 170–172.
24. Weber M, Junge R, Black P, et al: Management of critical juvenile Asian elephants *(Elephas maximus)*. In Proceedings of the AAZV and AAWV Joint Conference, 2009, Tulsa, pp 61–63.
25. Wiedner E, Alleman RA, Isaza R: Urinalysis in Asian elephants *(Elephas maximus)*. J Zoo Wildl Med 40:659–666, 2009.
26. Wiedner E, Hale A: Evidence of specific blood types in Asian elephants *(Elephas maximus)* and significant incidence of positive crossmatch. In Proceedings of the AAZV and AAWV joint conference, 2010.

Perrissodactyla

CHAPTER 71

Rhinoceros Theriogenology

Robert Hermes and Thomas Bernd Hildebrandt

Over the last few decades, the six rhinoceros species have become important icons in the saga of wildlife conservation.[12] Recent surveys have estimated the wild black *(Diceros bicornis)*, southern white *(Ceratotherium simum)*, northern white *(Cerathoterium cottoni)*, Indian *(Rhinoceros unicornis)*, Javan *(Rhinoceros sondaicus)*, and Sumatran rhinoceros *(Dicerorhinus Sumatrensis)* populations to be, at most, 3610, 11,330, 7, 2500, 70, and 300, respectively. Protected against habitat loss, poaching, and left undisturbed, rhinoceroses reproduce well in the wild. However, small and decreasing populations make successful captive management increasingly important.

From the first descriptions of the reproductive anatomy and estrous cycle to the present use of advanced assisted reproduction technologies, researchers and veterinarians have attempted to understand the function and dysfunction of the reproductive biology of these charismatic species.[10,22] This chapter briefly reviews current knowledge on rhinoceros theriogenology.

MALE REPRODUCTIVE ANATOMY AND CLINICAL ASPECTS

The external and internal genitalia of the male rhinoceros include the prepuce, prepucial fold, penis, accessory sex glands, duct deferens, epididymis, and testes (Fig. 71-1).[44-47,59]

The relaxed musculocavernous penis is fully covered by the prepucial fold. During urination and territorial marking, the penis exits the sheath, pointing caudally between the hind legs. The fully erect penis points cranially; it has characteristic horizontal flaps and a mushroom-shaped process glandis, both being specific to each species. The horizontal flaps and process glandis suggest that the rhinoceros is a cervical inseminator. During up to a 45- to 60-minute intromission, the flaps unfold in the female's vagina while the process glandis locks into the portio and cervical folds.[44,59]

The paired set of accessory sex glands consists of cigar-shaped, multilobulated, seminal glands, the prostate with two triangular lobes and an isthmus across the urethra, and compact, round, or elongated bulbourethral glands. An ampulla at the end of the deferens ductus has not been described for the rhinoceros. In adult white rhinoceros, it has been shown that the volume of the accessory sex glands correlates with semen quality.[45,47,59]

The testes and tightly attached epididymides are located in the dorsal aspect of the prepucial fold. Their position in the prepucial fold shifts from vertical, clearly visible and palpable, caudal to the relaxed penis to more horizontal and nonpalpable, adjacent to the inguinal rings.[45,47,59] Thick skin, dense testicular capsule and changing positions limit possible conclusions from testicular palpation about functional status or pathologic lesions. Clinical examination of the testes and accessory sex glands relies on transcutaneous and transrectal ultrasound, respectively. Whereas transrectal examination of the accessory sex glands requires a chute-trained animal or sedation, transcutaneous ultrasound of the testes can be achieved through the bars of the enclosure with very little training.

Semen Collection, Evaluation, and Preservation

The evaluation of breeding soundness to determine a bull's reproductive potential consists of two components, clinical examination of the reproductive tract and semen collection. Semen collection and evaluation in rhinoceros are aimed at the determination of causes for reproductive failure or for semen donation and

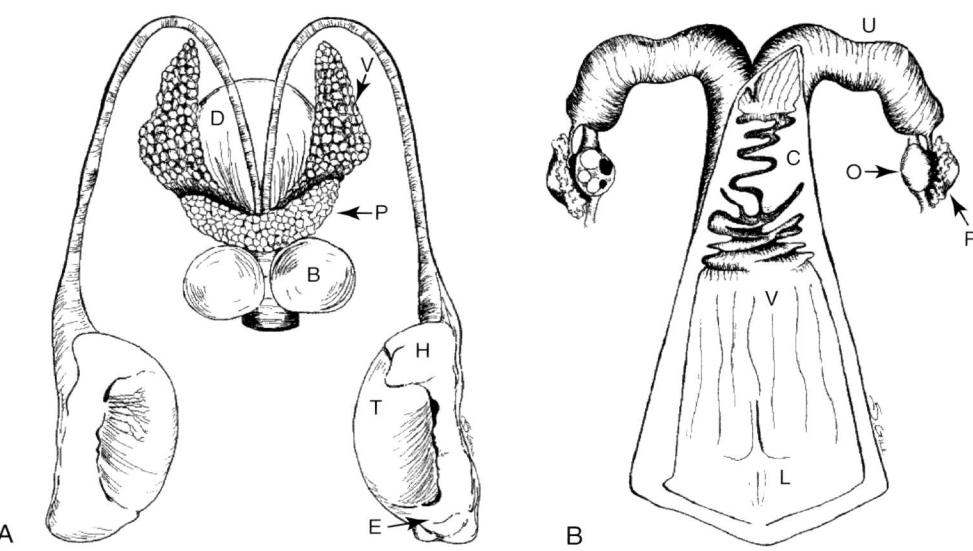

Figure 71-1

Male and female reproductive anatomy of the rhinoceros. **A,** Male reproductive organs from an Indian rhinoceros. **B,** Female reproductive organs from an African rhinoceros. *B,* Bulbourethral gland; *C,* cervix; *E,* tail of epididymis; *F,* fallopian tube; *H,* head of epididymis; *L,* vulva; *O,* ovary; *P,* prostate; *T,* testis; *D,* urinary bladder; *U,* uterine horn; *V,* vagina; *V,* vesicular gland. *(From Schaffer NE, Foley GL, Gill S, Pope CE: Clinical implications of rhinoceros reproductive tract anatomy and histology. J Zoo Wildl Med 32:31–46, 2001.)*

TABLE 71-1	Rhinoceros Semen Characteristics (Mean)					
Species	Collection Method	Volume (mL)	Concentration (Sperm × 10⁶/mL)	Motility (%)	Normal Morphology (%)	Post-Thaw Motility (%)
Black rhinoceros	Manual	62	15	—	—	—
	Electroejaculation	17-58	18-58	40-50	29	—
White rhinoceros	Manual	0.7	7	—	—	—
	Electroejaculation	30-80	165	71	69	20-78
Indian rhinoceros	Manual	4-17	1738	16	—	—
	Electroejaculation	92-160	124-377	48-72	34-39	50-55
Sumatran rhinoceros	Post coital	104	25	60	40	40-60
	Electroejaculation	21	1.5	55	8	—

preservation for assisted reproduction for males with known, good semen quality. Values generated might therefore differ greatly and their interpretation must be put carefully in context with the method of collection, the male's libido, presence or absence of mating or masturbation, territorial behavior, and diagnosed reproductive tract disease. Semen quality provides indications on the current breeding potential of a male. Poor semen quality does not exclude remaining chances of fertilization but is mostly associated with a lack of breeding activity.[17,36,41,44,53]

Semen Collection

Semen can be collected postcoitally, by manual stimulation, rectal massage, or electroejaculation, or postmortem (Table 71-1).[14,38] Postcoital collection, manual stimulation, and rectal massage give regular access to sperm for preservation and cryopreservation and later use in assisted reproduction without medical restraint. During postcoital semen collection, the ejaculatory fluid is captured draining from the vulva. Mating behavior, proper intromission, and ejaculation are prerequisites for this collection method, but are usually absent in males for which semen evaluation is warranted. Manual stimulation with or without light sedation has been successful in individual black, white, and Indian rhinoceroses. However, it is time-consuming, limited to well-trained individuals, and requires a restraint chute. It is characterized by inconsistent collection success and sometimes only a minute ejaculate volume 0.2 mL. Attempts to collect semen by the use of an artificial vagina have produced ejaculates but failed to produce sperm.

Electroejaculation under general anaesthesia is the method of choice for obtaining a semen sample in untrained, captive, or wild rhinoceroses. It has been adapted and applied in all captive rhinoceros species and provides reliable sampling for semen evaluation, assessment of current breeding potential, and sperm preservation for assisted reproduction purposes.* Prior to electrostimulation, ultrasound helps determine the position of the accessory sex glands, facilitating accurate placement of the electrostimulation probe and avoiding urine contamination from accidental stimulation of the bladder or bladder neck. The electrostimulation probe is placed onto the pelvic part of the urethra and prostate. Electric current induces ejaculatory contraction of the accessory sex glands and pelvic urethra. Manual massage of the pelvic and penile urethra between stimulation sets funnels the emitted ejaculatory fluids into the thermally and light-insulated collection tube. Sperm-rich fractions are emitted at the beginning of the induced ejaculatory process, followed by less concentrated fractions of sperm and aspermatic seminal plasma.

The core of semen evaluation is based on the sperm-rich fractions of the ejaculate. Semen evaluation involves assessment of ejaculate volume, color and odor, and sperm motility, morphology, viability and concentration (see Table 71-1). In general, ejaculates can be obtained from bulls as young as 6 and up to 42 years of age. Sperm quality is not affected by age and can remain high until advanced age, despite the presence of increasing testicular fibrosis. Sperm production and androgen concentration are consistent throughout the year and do not show seasonal influences.[17] Recorded ejaculate volumes range from 0.1 to 200 mL and seem to be greatly influenced by collection method, probe operator, probe design, or stimulation protocol applied. Ejaculates collected postcoitally or by electroejaculation show the most consistent mean volumes, from 17 to 160 mL, presumably representing the naturally ejaculated volume range.

*References 17, 36, 41, 44, 45, and 53.

The preparation of epidydimal sperm after castration or postmortem represents a unique opportunity for a final male gamete rescue. The extraction of spermatozoa from the epidymis or vas deferens rescues the remaining stock of mature gametes. Extraction is best performed on site shortly after the donor's death to avoid autolysis or heterolysis of the tissue and temperature changes affecting sperm quality. Cooled transport (4° C) of the testis and epidymis in saline solution is an alternative to on-site preparation if the death occurs unexpected Cryopreserved sperm conserves the male's ability to produce offspring posthumously. The authors used sperm extracted and cryopreserved postmortem for artificial inseminations, which have resulted in pregnancy.

Semen Assessment and Preservation
Rhinoceros spermatozoa are similar in size to those of the stallion.[2] Sperm characteristics show huge ranges (see Table 71-1). Good- and poor-quality semen has no significant differences in terms of ejaculate volume, pH (8.5 to 9.0), or osmolarity (290 to 300 mOsm/kg).[53] Sperm motility, viability, and morphology therefore represent the most relevant indicators to rate current semen quality. In domestic species, sperm motility and morphology are positively correlated with pregnancy rate. In the rhinoceros, analogous to domestic species, the percentages of motile and morphologically normal sperm in sperm-rich fractions are used to rate a bull's semen quality. Semen quality is considered as a prognostic indicator of the sperm's fertilizing potential and thus of the bull's breeding potential. Sperm with motility of 75% is considered to have excellent fertilizing potential. Fertilizing potential of sperm with motility of less than 75% or less than 50% is considered intermediate or poor.[17,36] However, samples with 60% motility have proven sufficient for assisted reproduction and semen preservation.[25] Variations in semen quality among collections may occur and repeated evaluations are suggested to confirm poor semen quality and limited breeding potential of a bull. In white rhinoceroses, social structure and subordinate behavior have been identified as a cause of the high incidence of reduced semen quality in males without or long past breeding history. The subordination of males in multimale institutions has corresponded with low sperm quality. Socially subordinated males display decreased reproductive fitness in the presence of a territorial male. Altering the captive social structure by separating nonbreeding but territorial males, exclusive access of subordinate males to breeding females, or introduction of new challenging males might improve libido and reproductive parameters.

Rhinoceros spermatozoa are not sensitive to slow chilling. The motility of white rhinoceros sperm chilled to 4° C after suspension in equine, bovine, or custom-made extenders remains almost constant for 24 hours.[17] In another study, we noted that high-quality sperm from Indian and black white rhinoceroses show reduced motility values after only 72 hours of chilling. This low sensitivity of rhinoceros sperm to chilling facilitates sperm transport to distant locations for use in regional AI breeding programs.[20]

Cryopreservation of sperm has been shown in white, Sumatran, and Indian rhinoceroses and was successfully used for artificial insemination in white and Indian rhinoceroses.* Cryopreservation of male gametes permits the use of sperm from unrepresented, wild, or deceased males, thus improving the genetic diversity of a population. In general, cryopreservation of sperm induces cell damage, resulting in cell death or loss of function. Motility, viability, morphology, and acrosome integrity of the sperm are the main characteristics used to assess semen quality after thawing. Single- or double-stranded sperm DNA fragmentation has recently been added as a critical parameter for assessing post-thaw sperm integrity.[32] Fast fragmentation of the rhinoceros sperm nucleus in comparison with other eutherian species, including the stallion, suggests that semen processing and current freezing methods used will need further substantial improvement to increase cell and DNA integrity and longevity of rhinoceros sperm after cryopreservation.

Cryopreservation of Sperm

A critical precondition to cryopreserving rhinoceros sperm is a high-quality semen sample. Even in one ejaculate, only few sperm-rich fractions with highly motile sperm qualify for preservation. Standard or modified equine extenders or a skim milk–egg yolk or TEST–egg yolk medium are used to cryopreserve the sperm, with good success. Glycerol and dimethylsulfoxide (Me_2SO) in concentrations of 5% or 6.25% are used as cryoprotectants.[17,24,25] In a Sumatran rhinoceros, Me_2SO was identified as the superior cryoprotectant compared with glycerol. In large-scale studies in white rhinoceroses, Me_2SO, as an exclusively tested cryoprotectant, produced reproducible good results.[36] However, in a recent comparative study in Indian rhinoceros, no significant difference in post-thaw results was found between glycerol and Me_2SO.[53] Sperm is generally frozen in 0.5-mL straws in liquid nitrogen vapor. This freezing method

provides good post-thaw results across species, and is relatively simple and easy to apply under field conditions. A new freezing technology, multithermal gradient directional freezing (Core Dynamics, Orangeburg, NY), facilitates freezing of large volumes (8 mL/vial).[16] Thanks to precise control over ice crystal formation, it is reported to result in less cell damage and higher gamete survival. In a comparative study, directional freezing has been superior to freezing over liquid nitrogen vapor in white rhinoceroses. However, high liquid nitrogen consumption and vulnerable electronics make this technology logistically more challenging.

Diseases of the Male Reproductive Tract

Penis

Mating or masturbation on foreign objects may cause trauma to the penis, resulting in superficial lesions, edema, or abrasion (Fig. 71-2). Superficial lesions are treated by and responsive to topical ointment. More severe abrasions might cause edema further, preventing retraction of the penis. With the penis permanently unprotected, edema increase and further secondary abrasions might occur to the free-hanging and swinging penis. Similar to the stallion, blood circulation of the glans is disturbed and aggressive therapy is necessary to prevent further abrasions, ulceration, and irreversible penile damage. Replacement of the penis into the sheath is the primary goal, best achieved by bandaging the penis to the abdominal wall. Blunt trauma of the erect penis can cause penile fracture, resulting in inability to obtain intromission thereafter.[21]

Accessory Sex Glands

Diseases of the accessory sex glands are rare. Prostate cysts have been documented in one white rhinoceros. Cystic formations in the prostate are presumably painful and could be interpreted as the reason for lack of libido.

Testis

Testicular fibrosis, atrophy, trauma, or neoplasia and epididymidal cysts are disorders described in the male rhinoceros (Fig. 71-3).[17,30,31,53] Testicular fibrosis is a common finding in older males. In white and Indian rhinoceroses, testicular fibrosis starts forming at the age of 15 years.[17,53] Fibrotic areas, located in the interstitium, appear in the ultrasound as bright dots (approximately 0.1-0.3 mm) within the testicular parenchyma. The size and number of fibrotic spots are positively correlated with age and are regarded as signs of testicular aging, but with no influence on semen characteristics.

*References 16, 17, 24, 25, 37, and 53.

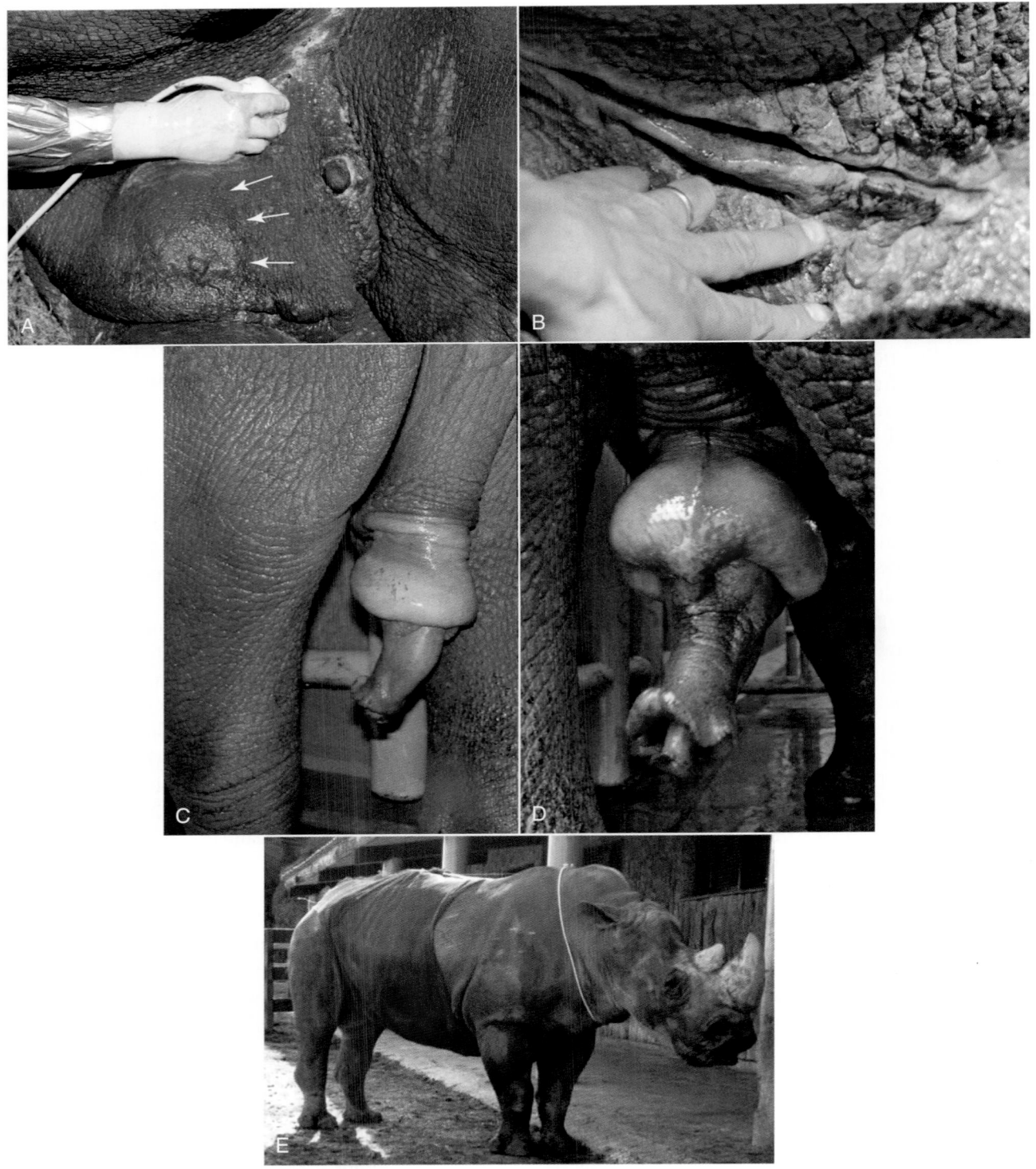

Figure 71-2

A, Swelling within the prepucial fold *(arrows)* diagnosed as a hematoma or seroma by ultrasound. **B,** Deep fissure and purulent infection in the upper inguinal area of a male after territorial fight. **C, D,** Increasing edema and prolapse of the penis. **E,** Complete body bandage to reposition the prolapsed penis into the sheath, reinitiating penile blood circulation.

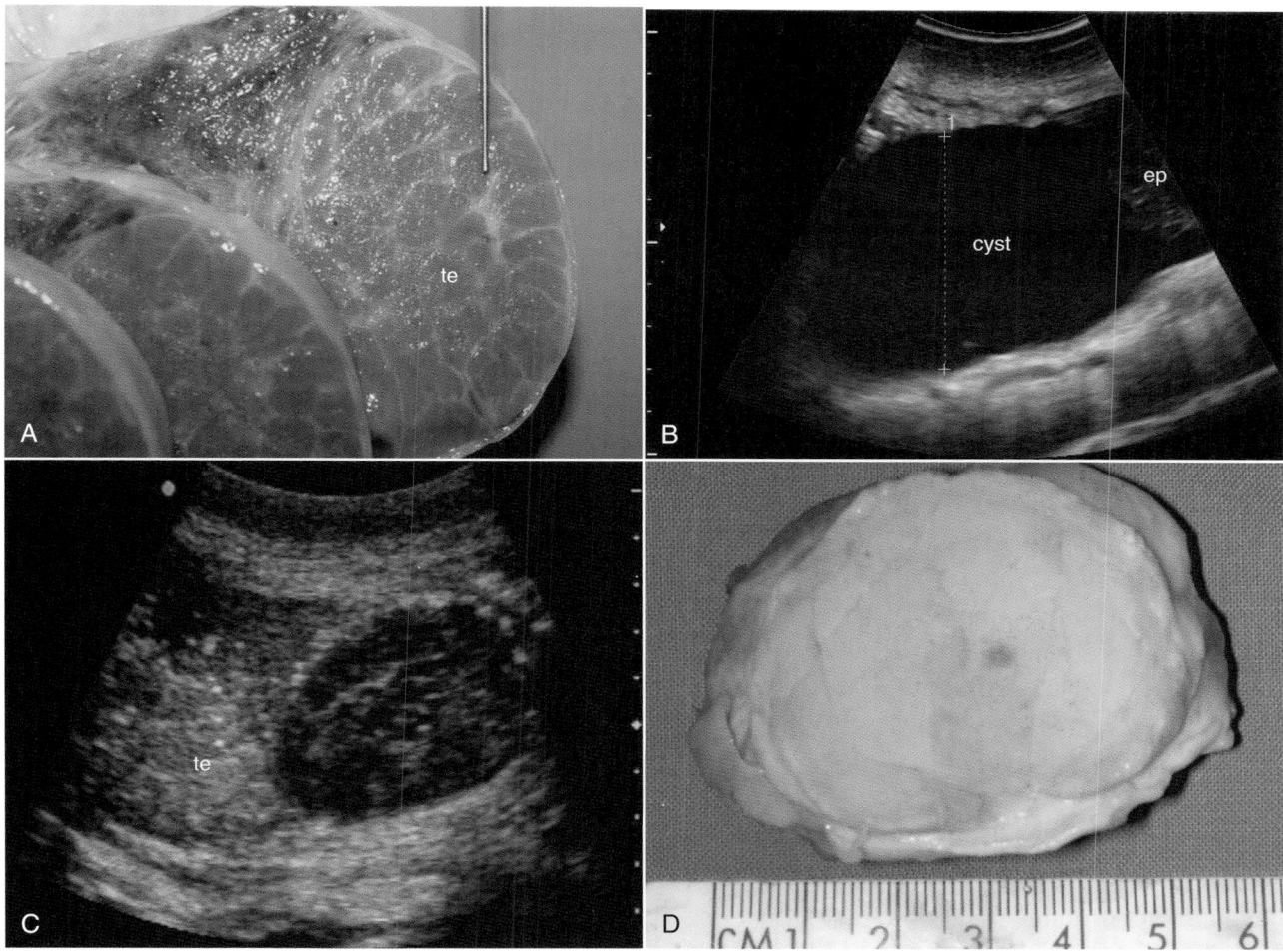

Figure 71-3

A, Interstitial fibrosis *(probe)* in the postmortem sliced testis *(te)* of an old Indian rhinoceros. **B,** Epidydimal cyst adjacent to the epidymis *(ep)* in a sterile white rhinoceros. **C, D,** Ultrasound image and postmortem preparation of a seminoma in the testis of a white rhinoceros.

Different from age related fibrosis, physical trauma, testicular neoplasia or epididydimal cysts may influence sperm production, causing subfertility or infertility.[30,31] During territorial fights or rough courtship, the opponent's horn forks into the inguinal area of the male, causing blunt trauma of the gonads (see Fig. 71-2). Hematoma or seroma of the testis may be visible as asymmetric swelling of the prepucial fold or by visualizing fluid cavities in and around the testis using ultrasound. Effects of hematoma or seroma on sperm production might be temporary. However, severe trauma might induce testicular necrosis and atrophy or permanent stenosis of the spermatic cord, resulting in infertility.

Testicular neoplasia is characterized as solid mass within the testicular parenchyma (see Fig. 71-3).[30,31] Diagnosed by ultrasound, it is further characterized by testicular biopsy. Seminoma has been described in black and white rhinoceroses. Hemicastration of the affected testis prevents further growth and possible metastasis and ensures the animal's breeding potential. A hemicastrated black rhinoceros resumed good-quality semen production after surgery, with proven fertility.

Epidydimal cysts as a defect of the gonaduct system have been detected in Sumatran and white rhinoceroses by the authors and Schaffer[43] (see Fig. 71-3). Filled with clear fluid, their dimensions can range from 1 to 10 cm. Ejaculates from effected males are consistently aspermatic or of low quality. The cause of these cysts is unclear. Previous trauma resulting in the formation of cysts might induce seroma and stenosis of the gonaduct system. Transcutaneous fine-needle aspiration of the cystic fluid can be attempted to resolve the cyst(s), resuming sperm passage and fertility.

TABLE 71-2   Female Reproductive Anatomy and Estrous Cycle

Rhinoceros Species	LENGTH OR DIAMETER							
	Vestibule (cm)	Vagina (cm)	Cervix (cm)	Uterine Body (cm)	Uterine Horns (cm)	Ovary (cm)	Ovulatory Follicle (cm)	Estrous Cycle (days)
Black rhinoceros	15	22-25	11-17	3-6	34-80	5-12	5.0	21-27
White rhinoceros	14-20	19-30	12-23	2-8	40-64	6-9	3.2-3.5	31-35 or 66-70
Indian rhinoceros	27	20	30	10	33	5	10-12	43-48
Sumatran rhinoceros	—	—	6-7	4	30-34	2-8	2-2.5	21-25

FEMALE REPRODUCTIVE ANATOMY AND CLINICAL ASPECTS

The female reproductive organs in the rhinoceros consist of the vulva, clitoris, vestibule, vagina, cervix, uterus bicornis, oviduct, and ovaries. The total length of the genital tract varies among species, from approximately 50 cm in the Sumatran to well over 100 cm in the white rhinoceros (Table 71-2). The hymenal membrane and cervix are uniquely shaped anatomic structures in the rhinoceros (see Fig. 71-1).[19,46,47,59]

The external genitalia are composed of vertical, symmetrical, outer and inner vulval labia and a prominent clitoris on the ventral commissure. The outer labia protrude caudoventrally and, in the white and greater one-horned rhinoceroses, are sometimes the only part of the external genitals visible from a distance. Changes of the external genitalia associated with estrous are small and subtle in all species. In most species, estrous is therefore noted only if the female vocalizes (Indian and Sumatran rhinoceroses) or if the male indicates estrous by his interest.

The vestibule and vagina in nulliparous females are separated by a hymenal membrane cranial to the urethral orifice. The patency of the hymen in young females is limited to small perforations of 0.1 to 0.5 cm. The hymen ruptures during first mating, with only vestiges of the membrane remaining thereafter. In females in which mating is rare or intromission is not observed, the hymenal status is often unknown. Reproductive failure in these females is generally associated with a persistent hymen. The presence or absence of the hymenal membrane in nulliparous females can be determined by vestibulovaginal palpation. In a study group of mature white rhinoceroses with reproductive failure, the incidence of a persistent hymen was 76%.[19] Specifically, in older females, the hymen becomes more fibrous and, despite dilated hymenal orifices (3 cm), is

more difficult to rupture. Blunt surgical rupture of the hymen is an option to resolve this mechanical breeding barrier for mating in older females.

The cervix consists of three to five very tight interdigitated folds of fibrous connective tissue. The cervical cannel is tortuous, with 90-degree turns and blind pockets. The length and tightness of the cervical folds allow catheter passage only during estrous. The cervix is well definable as a tight cylindrical structure during rectal palpation.

The uterus bicornis consists of a short body and long uterine horns. The horns first run alongside as a pseudo-uterine body before parting laterally at the bifurcatio uteri. In the white rhinoceros, the total length of the uterine horns can exceed 50 cm.

The size of the ovaries and their functional structures vary greatly among species (see Table 71-2). Unlike the horse, the closest related domestic species of the rhinoceros, follicles rupture on the surface of the ovary. Both the uterus and ovary are not accessible for conclusive palpation.

Because palpation is of limited value in the rhinoceros, clinical examination of the reproductive tract is commonly performed by transrectal ultrasound.[19,34,40,54] Ultrasound allows an efficient and accurate determination of the reproductive status, function, and diagnosis of reproductive pathology. Portable commercial systems equipped with 2- to 8-MHz ultrasound probes are sufficient for diagnostic imaging. In black, Indian, and Sumatran rhinoceroses, the genital tract is easily accessible for the examiner. In the white rhinoceros, the length of the genital tract might exceed the examiner's arm reach and custom-made extensions of the ultrasound probe might be necessary to access the cranial part of the reproductive tract.[19] In chute-trained animals, transrectal examinations can be performed on a daily basis. In animals not trained, standing sedation is adequate for reproductive assessment.

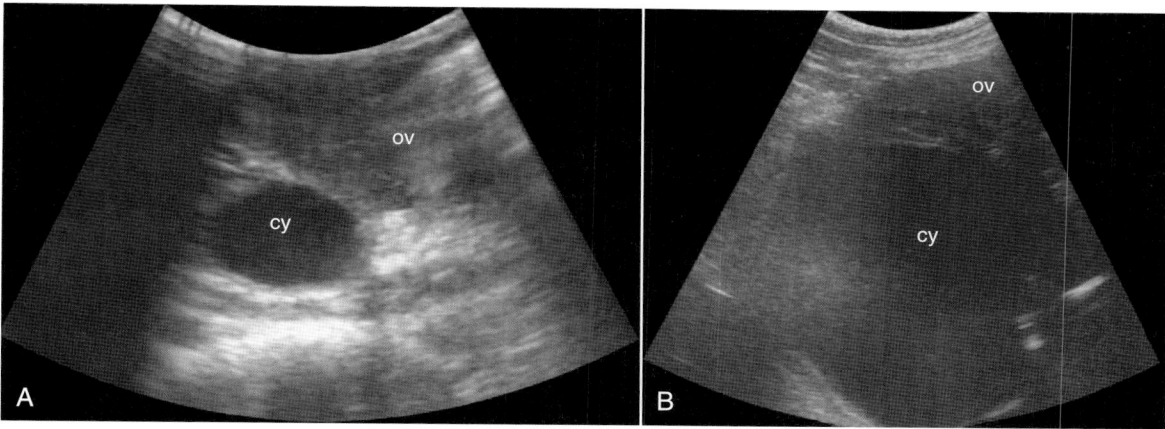

Figure 71-6

Ultrasonographic images of paraovarian cysts in white rhinoceroses. **A,** Small paraovarian cysts *(cy)* close to the ovary *(ov)* in a noncycling southern white rhinoceros. **B,** Paraovarian cyst. The small inactive ovary *(ov)* appears atrophic because of the mechanical pressure of the large cystic structure.

the most common uterine tumor across species, but endometrial adenoma and adenocarcinoma have also been documented to occur in white rhinoceroses.[58] The predominant location of neoplasia within the genital tract is species-specific. Although tumors occur mainly in the uterus in the white rhinoceros, the cervix and vagina are the most affected organs in the Indian rhinoceros. Excessive tumors may become necrotic or cause internal or external blood loss. In old females, regular bloody discharge from the vagina is a common clinical sign associated with genital tumours. Extensive chronic blood loss may even lead to anemia. In geriatric females, downregulation of ovarian activity using long-acting GnRH analogue formulations or GnRH vaccine might be an approach to stop further hormone-dependent tumor growth and blood loss. However, great care should be taken when managing old anestrous or artificially downregulated females in a herd together with a mature breeding bull. Old females with naturally ceased ovarian activity or artificially downregulated (GnRH vaccine) are disposed of any sexual signals and may be perceived as territorial rival to the breeding bull. Breeding bulls have repeatedly attacked or killed older females presumably in an attempt to eliminate a potential 'rival'.

Reproductive disorders, along with ovarian exhaustion, might render a female irreversibly infertile early during life. This phenomenon has been termed *asymmetrical reproductive aging*.[18] A reproducing female white rhinoceros in captivity may produce up to nine calves and, in between, exhibit approximately 90 estrous cycles during her reproductive life. Observations from the wild have confirmed that pregnancy and lactation represent the predominant endocrine status. With as few as 90 cycles, estrous is a relatively rare event during a female's reproductive life. These numbers are considerably lower than the up to 310 estrous cycles in captive, nonreproducing female rhinoceroses. By the age of 16 years, when first reproductive lesions are detected, nonreproducing females have already displayed the 90–estrous cycle allotment. The reproductive organs of nonreproducing female rhinoceros are exposed to prolonged periods of sex steroid fluctuations from continuous ovarian cycle activity. The central effects of this asymmetrical reproductive aging process include the progressive development of genital pathology, with subsequent subfertility or infertility and, presumably, the utilization of follicular stock at a higher rate. Because the incidence of reproductive disorders in parous females is significantly lower, achievement of pregnancy in young animals can be regarded as a prophylactic measure against reproductive disorders.[19]

Infectious diseases of the reproductive tract are rarely described. Endometritis caused by *Pseudomonas* or hemolytic streptococci has only been reported in several Indian rhinoceroses.[11,55] Vaginal purulent discharge was noted in these cases as the only clinical sign. Treatment consisted of vaginal lavage and systemic antibiotic treatment with penicillin and streptomycin.

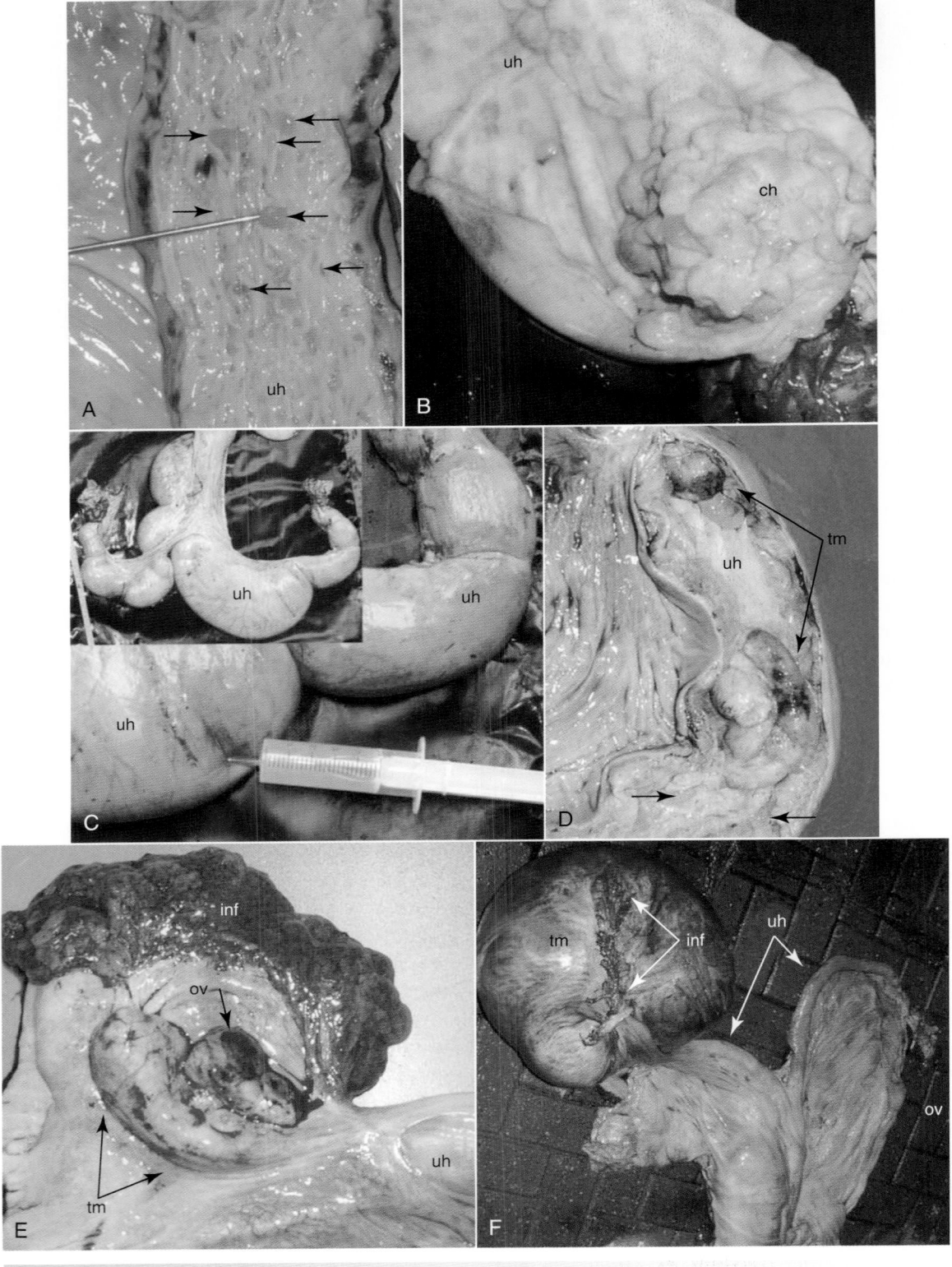

Figure 71-7

Postmortem preparations of genital pathology from white rhinoceroses. **A,** Multiple endometrial cysts (arrows) in the uterine horn. **B,** Multifocal cystic endometrial hyperplasia at the end of the uterine horn *(uh)* blocking the oviductal orifice. **C,** Hydromucometra. The uterine body and horns *(uh)* are filled with fluid. **D,** Cystic endometrial hyperplasia *(arrows)* and intraluminal adenoma *(tm)* in the uterine horn *(uh)*. **E,** Leiomyoma *(tm)* in the mesovarium close to the ovary *(ov)*, opposite the infundibulum *(inf)*. **F,** Paraovarian leiomyoma *(tm)*.

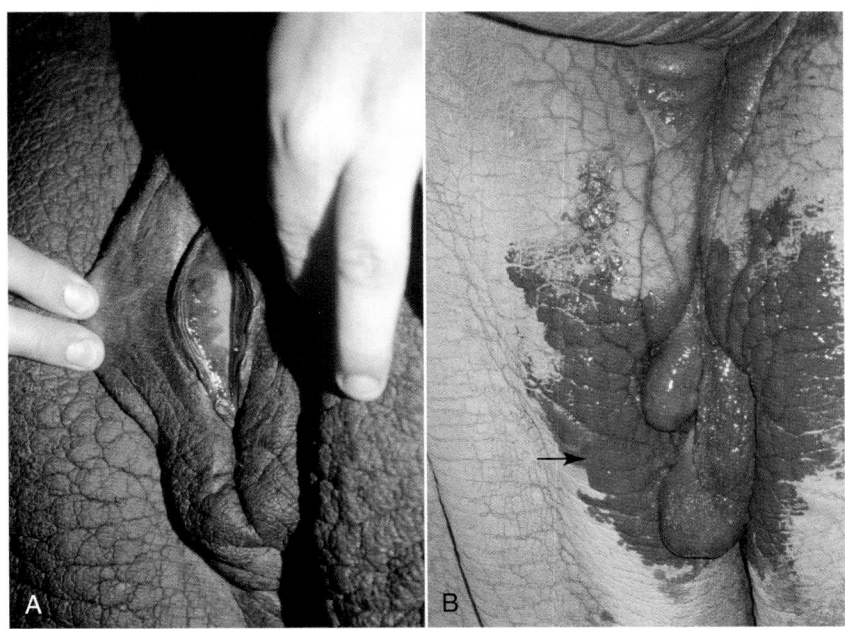

Figure 71-8

A, Symmetrical outer and inner vaginal labia in a white rhinoceros. B, Vaginal fissure of the outer labia *(arrow)* as the source for chronic vaginal discharge and reluctance to breed.

$PGF_{2\alpha}$ to enhance discharge should be used very carefully and in combination with a preceding cervical application of PGE to open the tightly closed cervix, facilitating passage prior to uterine contraction. Abortion and unnoticed fissures of the vulval labia, with purulent discharge from rough courtship or fights between rivals, should be considered as differential diagnosis to endometritis in animals with purulent vaginal discharge (Fig. 71-8).

ARTIFICIAL INSEMINATION

Artificial insemination (AI) has been successful using fresh and cryopreserved semen in white and Indian rhinoceroses.[16,20,37] So far, seven rhinoceroses have been conceived by AI worldwide. Yet only five of those were born alive. When considering the limited breeding success of both white rhinoceros species in captivity, skewed birth sex ratios in the Indian and black rhinoceros, and the disastrous situation of some rhinoceros species in the wild, AI might become a useful tool to overcome these crises.[1,60]

The estrous cycle in anestrous AI candidates has been induced using chlormadinone acetate plus GnRH analogue. The presence of a preovulatory follicle and accurate timing of ovulation were determined by preceding ultrasound examinations.[16,20] In cycling or postpartum females, GnRH analogue was used to hasten ovulation and to coincide with the insemination. The anatomic challenge for AI, the firm tortuous cervix, is overcome using a rhinoceros-specific AI catheter. Frequent use of AI in the future might help in establishing self-sustaining captive populations of threatened rhinoceros species and enhancing genetic diversity when using unrepresented captive or even wild semen donors.

ADVANCED ASSISTED REPRODUCTION TECHNOLOGIES

Sperm Sexing

In domestic species and a few wildlife species, using gender-biased sperm samples has been described as a tool to influence the gender of the offspring. AI in rhinoceros will facilitate the development and implementation of this technology in the future. The feasibility of sorting sperm by gender in black, white, and Indian rhinoceroses has been demonstrated by sorting the spermatozoa into X and Y chromosome–bearing populations based on their relative DNA differences.[2,3] A sorting purity of 94% for X chromosome–bearing spermatozoa was achieved. However, the slow sorting rate of 300 to 700 cells indicates that improvements could still be made before gender-sorted sperm can be used in future

AI programs. Using gender-sorted sperm might help in boosting critically small captive rhinoceros populations by producing more female offspring using X chromosome–bearing spermatozoa or adjusting skewed birth gender ratios, such as in the Indian or black rhinoceros.[1,60]

Gamete Rescue

In vitro fertilization (IVF), intracytoplasmic sperm injection (ICSI), and embryo transfer are well-established techniques for the production of embryos and as a solution to infertility in humans and domestic species. Although gamete rescue from male rhinoceroses is technically solved by different means of semen collection in vivo and postmortem epidydimal sperm extraction, the rescue of female gametes poses a bigger challenge. In the infertile rhinoceros, oocyte collection represents an option for female gamete preservation. Until recently, the collection of oocytes from deceased females has been the only source for these gametes. Successful ICSI of in vitro matured oocytes in a white rhinoceros collected postmortem was the first attempt at female gamete rescue and in vitro embryo production.[6] The repeated harvest of oocytes in live donors is a recent development. By transrectal, ultrasound-guided follicular aspiration, oocytes were collected from anesthetized live black and white rhinoceroses.[15,29] The ovaries of infertile females were superstimulated with a GnRH analogue to induce the development of a large number of follicles suitable for aspiration. Oocytes were collected by puncture of the follicles through the rectal wall under ultrasound guidance, using a long, flexible aspiration needle. The production of an embryo after IVF marked the first step toward banking and transfer of embryos produced in vitro from live oocyte donors.

Cell Lines

Skin sampling followed by in vitro culture of fibroblasts to establish and cryopreserve cell lines is another approach to preserving rhinoceros genetic diversity. The reprogramming of fibroblasts into omnipotent stem cells is one goal of cell line cryopreservation.[42]

REFERENCES

1. Association of Zoos and Aquariums (AZA): AZA Rhino Research Advisory Group: AZA species survival plan for rhinoceros, Silver Spring, Md, 2005, Association of Zoos and Aquariums.
2. Behr B, Rath D, Hildebrandt TB, et al: Germany/Australia index of sperm sex sortability in elephants and rhinoceros. Reprod Domest Anim 44:273–277, 2009.
3. Behr B, Rath D, Mueller P, et al: Feasibility of sex-sorting sperm from the white and the black rhinoceros (Ceratotherium simum, Diceros bicornis). Theriogen 72:353–364, 2009.
4. Berkeley EV, Kirkpatrick JF, Schaffer NE, et al: Serum and fecal steroid analysis of ovulation, pregnancy, and parturition in the black rhinoceros (Diceros bicornis). Zoo Biol 16:121–132, 1997.
5. Brown JL, Bellem AC, Fouraker M, et al: Comparative analysis of gonadal and adrenal activity in the black and white rhinoceros in North American by non-invasive endocrine monitoring. Zoo Biol 20:463–485, 2001.
6. Durant B: Personal communication.
7. Fouraker M, Wagener T: AZA rhinoceros husbandry resource manual, Forth Worth, Tex, 1996, Fort Worth Zoological Park.
8. Garnier JN, Holt WV, Watson PF: Non-invasive assessment of estrous cycles and evaluation of reproductive seasonality in the female wild black rhinoceros (Diceros bicornis minor). Reproduction 123:877–889, 2002.
9. Godfrey RRW, Pope CE, Dresser BL, et al: An attempt to superovulate a southern white rhinoceros (Ceratotherium simum simum) [abstract]. Theriogen 323:231, 1990.
10. Godfrey RW, Pope CE, Dresser BL, et al: Gross anatomy of the reproductive tract of female black (Diceros bicornis michaeli) and white rhinoceros (Ceratotherium simum simum). Zoo Biol 10:165–175, 1991.
11. Göltenboth R, Klös H-G: [Krankheiten der Zoo- und Wildtiere.] Berlin, 1995, Blackwell Wissenschaftsverlag.
12. Groves CP, Fernando P, Robovský J: The sixth rhino: A taxonomic re-assessment of the critically endangered northern white rhinoceros. PLoS One 5:e9703, 2010.
13. Guldenschuh G, von Houwald FF: Husbandry manual for the greater one-horned or Indian rhinoceros Rhinoceros unicornis Linne, 1758, Basel, Switzerland, 2002, Basel Zoo.
14. Hermes R Goeritz F, Streich WJ, et al: Assisted reproduction in female rhinoceros and elephants—Current status and future perspective. Reprod Domest Anim 42:33–44, 2007.
15. Hermes R, Göritz F, Portas TJ, et al: Ovarian superstimulation, transrectal ultrasound-guided oocyte recovery, and IVF in rhinoceros. Theriogen 72:959–968, 2009.
16. Hermes R, Göritz F, Saragusty J, et al: First successful artificial insemination with frozen-thawed semen in rhinoceros. Theriogen 71:393–399, 2009.
17. Hermes R, Hildebrandt TB, Blottner S, et al: Reproductive soundness of captive southern and northern white rhinoceroses (Ceratotherium simum simum, C.s. cottoni): Evaluation of male genital tract morphology and semen quality before and after cryopreservation. Theriogen 63:219–238, 2005.
18. Hermes R, Hildebrandt TB, Göritz F: Reproductive problems directly attributable to long-term captivity-asymmetric reproductive aging. Anim Reprod Sci 82-83:49–60, 2004.
19. Hermes R, Hildebrandt TB, Walzer C, et al: The effect of long non-reproductive periods on the genital health in captive female white rhinoceroses (Ceratotherium simum simum, C.s. cottoni). Theriogen 65:1492–1515, 2006.
20. Hildebrandt TB, Hermes R, Walzer C, et al: Artificial insemination in the anestrous and the post partum white rhinoceros using GnRH analogue to induce ovulation. Theriogen 67:1473–1484, 2007.
21. Horowitz I: Personal communication.
22. Kassam AH, Lasley BL: Estrogen excretory patterns in the Indian rhinoceros (Rhinoceros unicornis), determined by simplified urinary analysis. Am J Vet Res 42:251–255, 1981.
23. Kretzschmar P, Ganslosser U, Dehnhard M: Relationship between androgens, environmental factors and reproductive behavior in male white rhinoceros (Cerathoterium simum simum). Horm Behav 45:1–9, 2004.

24. Lubbe K, Bartels P, Kilian I, et al: Comparing motility and morphology of horse, zebra and rhinoceros epididymal spermatozoa when cryopreserved with two different cryodilutents or stored at 4 degrees Celsius. Theriogen 53:388, 2000.

25. O'Brien JK, Roth TL: Post-coital sperm recovery and cryopreservation in the Sumatran rhinoceros *(Dicerorhinus sumatrensis)* and application to gamete rescue in the African black rhinoceros *(Diceros bicornis)*. J Reprod Fertil 118:263–271, 2000.

26. Ochs A: Cyclopia—First description of a rare malformation in a greater one-horned rhinoceros *(Rhinoceros unicornis)* at the Berlin Zoo. [Zyklopie - Eine seltene Missbildung und erstmalige Beschreibung ihres Vorkommens beim Panzernashorn *(Rhinoceros unicornis)* im Zoo Berlin.] Bongo (Berlin) 39:17–26, 2009.

27. Patton ML: Personal communication.

28. Patton ML, Swaisgood RR, Czekala NM, et al: Reproductive cycle length and pregnancy in the southern white rhinoceros *(Ceratotherium simum simum)* as determined by fecal pregnane analysis and observations of mating behavior. Zoo Biol 18:111–127, 1999.

29. Portas TJ, Hermes R, Bryant BR: Anesthesia and use of a sling system to facilitate transvaginal laparoscopy in a black rhinoceros *(Diceros bicornis minor)*. J Zoo Wildl Med 37:202–205, 2006.

30. Portas TJ, Hermes R, Bryant BR: Seminoma in a southern white rhinoceros *(Ceratotherium simum simum)*. Vet Rec 157:556–558, 2005.

31. Portas TJ, Hildebrandt TB, Bryant BR: Seminoma in a southern black rhinoceros *(Diceros bicornis minor)*: Diagnosis, surgical management and effect on fertility. Aust Vet J 88:57–60, 2010.

32. Portas T, Johnston SD, Hermes R: Frozen-thawed rhinoceros sperm exhibit DNA damage shortly after thawing when assessed by the sperm chromatin dispersion assay. Theriogen 72:711–720, 2009.

33. Radcliffe RM, Hendrickson DA, Richardson GL, et al: Standing laparoscopic-guided uterine biopsy in a southern white rhinoceros *(Ceratotherium simum simum)*. J Zoo Wildl Med 31:201–207, 2000.

34. Radcliffe RW, Czekala NM, Osofsky SA: Combined serial ultrasonography and fecal progestin analysis for reproductive evaluation of the female white rhinoceros *(Ceratotherium simum simum)*: Preliminary results. Zoo Biol 16:445–456, 1997.

35. Radcliffe RW, Eyres AI, Patton ML, et al: Ultrasonographic characterization of ovarian events and fetal gestational parameters in two southern black rhinoceros *(Diceros bicornis minor)* and correlation to fecal progesterone. Theriogen 55:1033–1049, 2001.

36. Reid CE, Hermes R, Blottner S, et al: Split-sample comparison of directional and liquid nitrogen vapour freezing method on post-thaw semen quality in white rhinoceroses *(Ceratotherium simum simum* and *Ceratotherium simum cottoni)*. Theriogen 71:275–291, 2009.

37. Roth TL: Personal communication.

38. Roth TL: A review of the reproduction physiology of rhinoceros species in captivity. Int Zoo Yb 40:130–143, 2006.

39. Roth TL, Bateman HL, Kroll JL: Endocrine and ultrasonographic characterization of a successful pregnancy in a Sumatran rhinoceros *(Dicerorhinus sumatrensis)* supplemented with a synthetic progestin. Zoo Biol 23:219–238, 2004.

40. Roth TL, O'Brien JK, McRae MA: Ultrasound and endocrine evaluation of the ovarian cycle and early pregnancy in the Sumatran rhinoceros, *Dicerorhinus sumatrensis*. Reproduction 121:139–149, 2001.

41. Roth TL, Stoops MA, Atkinson MW: Semen collection in rhinoceroses *(Rhinoceros unicornis, Diceros bicornis, Ceratotherium simum)* by electroejaculation with a uniquely designed probe. J Zoo Wildl Med 36:617–627, 2005.

42. Ryder O, Lenk M: Personal communication. (Frozen Zoo, CRES Genome Resource Bank; Friedrich Löffler Institute, Greifswald, Germany.)

43. Schaffer NE: Personal communication.

44. Schaffer NE, Beehler B, Jeyendran RS, et al: Methods of semen collection in an ambulatory greater one-horned rhinoceros *(Rhinoceros unicornis)*. Zoo Biol 9:211–221, 1990.

45. Schaffer N, Bryant W, Agnew D, et al: Ultrasonographic monitoring of artificially stimulated ejaculation in three rhinoceros species *(Ceratotherium simum, Diceros bicornis, rhinoceros unicornis)*. J Zoo Wildl Med 29:386–393, 1998.

46. Schaffer NE, Foley GL, Gill S, Pope CE: Clinical implications of rhinoceros reproductive tract anatomy and histology. J Zoo Wildl Med 32:31–46, 2001.

47. Schaffer NE, Zainal-Zahari Z, Suri MSM, et al: Ultrasonography of the reproductive anatomy in the Sumatran rhinoceros *(Dicerorhinus sumatrensis)*. J Zoo Wildl Med 25:337–348, 1994.

48. Schaftenaar W, Fernandes T, Fritsch G, et al: Dystocia and fetotomy associated with cerebral aplasia in a greater one-horned rhinoceros *(Rhinoceros unicornis)*. Reprod Domest Anim 2010 (in press).

49. Schwarzenberger F: Personal communication.

50. Schwarzenberger F, Franke R, Goltenboth R: Concentrations of faecal immunoreactive progestagen metabolites during the estrous cycle and pregnancy in the black rhinoceros *(Diceros bicornis michaeli)*. J Reprod Ferti 98:285–291, 1993.

51. Schwarzenberger F, Walzer C, Tomasova K, et al: Faecal progesterone metabolite analysis for noninvasive monitoring of reproductive function in the white rhinoceros *(Ceratotherium simum)*. Anim Reprod Sci 53:173–190, 1998.

52. Sos E, Silinski S, Walzer C: Personal communication.

53. Stoops MA, Atkinson MW, Blumer ES, et al: Semen cryopreservation in the Indian rhinoceros *(Rhinoceros unicornis)*. Theriogen 73:1104–1115, 2010.

54. Stoops MA, Pairan RD, Roth TL: Follicular, endocrine and behavioral dynamics of the Indian rhinoceros *(Rhinoceros unicornis)* estrous cycle. Reproduction 128:843–856, 2004.

55. Von Maltzahn J: Personal communication.

56. Wagner DC, Edwards MS: Hand-rearing black and white rhinoceroses: A comparison, 2001 (http://www.rhinoresourcecenter.com/ref_files/1175857443.pdf).

57. Wallach JD: Hand-rearing and observations of a white rhinoceros Diceros s. simus. Int Zoo Yb 9:103–104, 1969.

58. Wilson M, Hermes R, Bainbridge J, Bassett H: A case of metastatic uterine adenocarcinoma in a southern white rhinoceros *(Ceratotherium simum simum)*. J Zoo Wildl Med 41:110–113, 2010.

59. Zainal-Zahari Z, Rosnina Y, Wahid H, et al: Gross anatomy and ultrasonographic images of the reproductive system of the Sumatran rhinoceros *(Dicerorhinus sumatrensis)*. Anat Histol Embryol 31:350–354, 2002.

60. Zschokke S, Studer P, Baur B: Past and future breeding of the Indian rhinoceros in captivity. Int Zoo News 45:5, 1998.

CHAPTER 72

Asian Wild Horse Reintroduction Program

Christian Walzer and Petra Kaczensky

The first documentation of Przewalski's-type wild horses dates from more than 20,000 years ago. Rock engravings, paintings, and decorated tools dating from 20,000 to 9,000 BC were discovered in European caves. Historically, wild horses *(Equus ferus)* ranged from Western Europe over the Russian Steppes east to Kazakhstan, Mongolia, and northern China.[1] The first written accounts of Przewalski's horse *(Equus ferus przewalskii)* were recorded by the Tibetan monk Bodowa around 900 AD. In the *Secret History of the Mongols,* there is a reference to wild horses that caused Chinggis Khaan's horse to rear up and throw him to the ground in 1226. Przewalski's horse is still absent from Linnaeus's *Systema Naturae* (1758) and remained essentially unknown in the West until John Bell, a Scottish doctor in the service of Tsar Peter the Great in 1719 to 1722, observed the species within the area of 85 to 97 degrees E and 43 to 50 degrees N (present-day Chinese-Mongolian border).[9] Subsequently, Colonel Nikolai Mikailovich Przewalski (1839-1888), a renowned explorer, obtained the skull and hide of a horse shot some 80 km north of Gutschen on the Chinese-Russian border. These were examined at the Zoological Museum of the Academy of Science in St. Petersburg by Poliakov, who concluded that they were from a wild horse, and he gave it the official name of *Equus przewalskii* (Poliakov, 1881). Present-day taxonomy places the Przewalski's horse as a subspecies of *Equus ferus.*[2]

The last wild population of Przewalski's Horses, called *takhi* in Mongolian, survived until recently in southwestern Mongolia and adjacent China in the provinces of Gansu, Xinjiang, and Inner Mongolia. The last recorded sightings of Przewalski's horse in the wild occurred in the late 1960s north of the Tachiin Shaar Nuruu in the Dzungarian Gobi in southwestern Mongolia.[12] Thereafter, no more wild horses were observed and the species was declared "extinct in the wild." The reasons for the extinction of Przewalski's horse were seen in the combined effects of pasture competition with livestock and overhunting. The species initially only survived because of captive breeding based on 13 founder animals.[17] Subsequent to the establishment of the International Przewalski's horse studbook at the Prague Zoo in the Czech Republic in 1959, the North American Breeders Group in the 1970s (which became the Species Survival Plan for the Przewalski's Horse), and the initiation of a European Endangered Species Programme (EEP) in 1986 under the auspices of the Cologne Zoo in Germany, the captive population grew to over 1000 individuals by the mid-1980s. In the early 1990s, reintroduction efforts started simultaneously in Mongolia, China, Kazakhstan, and Ukraine. However, Mongolia is currently the only country in which true wild populations exist within their historic range.[1] Reintroductions in Mongolia began in the Gobi Desert around Takhiin Tal in the Great Gobi B Strictly Protected Area (9000 km²) and in the mountain steppes of Hustai National Park (570 km²) in 1992. A third potential reintroduction site, Khomiin Tal (2500 km²), in the Great Lakes Depression, was established in 2004 as a buffer zone to the Khar Us Nuur National Park.

With the free-ranging population growing in Mongolia, the species was reassessed in 2008. According to the International Union for Conservation of Nature and Natural Resources (IUCN) criteria,[3] the population is currently estimated to consist of fewer than 50 mature individuals free-living in the wild for the past 5 years. Because the effective population size is still very small, Przewalski's horse is today listed as critically endangered.[1]

TAKHIIN TAL REINTRODUCTION PROJECT

In 1975, the Mongolian portion of the Dzungarian Gobi was established as part B of the Great Gobi Strictly Protected Area (SPA). The area was declared a United Nations Educational, Scientific, and Cultural Organization (UNESCO)–Man and the Biosphere Programme (MAB) Biosphere Reserve in 1990. The Great Gobi B SPA encompasses approximately 9000 km² of desert steppes and semideserts. Herder camps are allowed at preestablished locations in the surrounding zone. They are used by approximately 100 families with almost 60,000 livestock, predominantly during winter and spring and fall migration. In summer, human presence in the park is almost negligible and traffic is less than five vehicles/week. No paved roads exist and dirt tracks are not maintained. In winter, access and mobility within the park are often limited by snow cover. Poaching occurs but, based on the small number of wildlife carcasses encountered, seems to be of minor importance compared with that in other Gobi areas.[7,8]

The climate of the Great Gobi B SPA is continental, with long cold winters and short hot summers. In the northeastern section of the study area, average monthly temperatures were 11° C to 19° C during the summer months (May to September) and 5° C to −19° C during the winter months (October to April). Average annual rainfall is 96 mm, with a peak during the summer months. Average snow cover lasts 97 days. Rainfall and snowfall can be highly variable from year to year in space and time, and the annual coefficient of variance is 30% to 33%. The area is generally considered to follow a nonequilibrium dynamic. Biomass production and, as a consequence, ungulate population fluctuations, are driven by the amount and timing of rainfall events.

With Mongolia's independence, a private fund and the Mongolian Society for the Conservation of Rare Animals initiated the Takhiin Tal project with the support of various international sponsors.[8,20] In 1992, the first group of captive-born Przewalski's horses was airlifted to Takhiin Tal. In 1997, the first harem group was released into the wild from the adaptation enclosures and, in 1999, the first foals were successfully raised in the wild (Fig. 72-1).[11]

International criticism and recommendations resulted in the establishment of the International Takhi Group (ITG; www.savethewildhorse.org) in 1999 with the goal of continuing and extending the Takhiin Tal

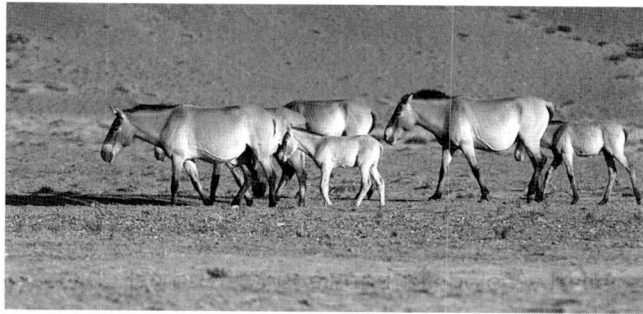

Figure 72-1

A group of Przewalski's horse mares with foals in the Greater Gobi B SPA near Takhiin Tal in southwestern Mongolia.

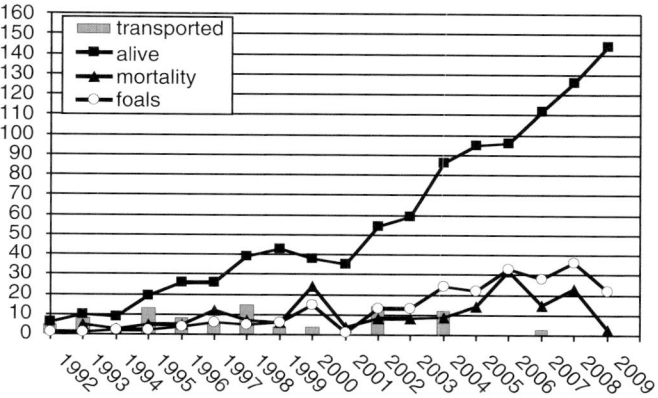

Figure 72-2

Population development of the Przewalski's horse population in the Great Gobi B SPA in southwestern Mongolia, as of December 2009. Years refer to horse years, from birth in May until the end of April, the following year.

project in accordance with the IUCN reintroduction guidelines.[14] Today, the Takhiin Tal project has received international recognition and, although it is still too early to judge whether the project is a success or failure, the positive trend of the free-ranging Przewalski's horse population is encouraging (Fig. 72-2). However, the population is still very small and is vulnerable to extinction subsequent to catastrophic environmental events, as witnessed in the winter of 2000 to 2001. At the time of this writing, southwestern Mongolia is experiencing a white *dzud*, a multifactorial natural disaster consisting of a summer drought with inadequate pasture followed by very heavy winter snowfall, winds, and lower than normal temperatures. Although continuing bad weather has not allowed for comprehensive evaluation, the losses to the Przewalski's horse population in the Great

Gobi B SPA appear to be massive. This situation clearly indicates the fragility of small populations to stochastic events in general, and specifically it emphasizes that the Gobi areas provide an edge, rather than an optimal habitat, for Przewalski's horses. Subsequently, only small and isolated pockets of suitable habitat remain as future habitat for Przewalski's horse.[7]

For the successful implementation of this reintroduction program, it needs to be embedded in a broader context of ecosystem conservation. We will describe how and why this project, which started as a single-species reintroduction, has significantly expanded in recent years.

Infrastructure

International transports from Europe to Mongolia were both a logistic and a financial challenge.[18] Initial efforts and research were focused on the survival of Przewalski's horses in and around the adaptation enclosures.[10,19] However, the establishment of a permanent field station with the necessary infrastructure (e.g., solar power, laboratory, office, vehicles, fuel) and communication capabilities (e.g., VHF communication, satellite-based email and telephone) proved equally important. In 2004, the Takhiin Tal camp hosted the Second International Workshop on the Re-introduction of the Przewalski's Horse. In 2005, facilities at the Takhiin Tal camp were further upgraded with the construction of the Great Gobi B SPA park headquarters, funded in part by the Austrian Ministry of Environment. Facilities at the Takhiin Tal camp now allow year-round living and workspace. Today, the camp is run by well-trained and motivated local staff, provides training opportunities for young Mongolian scientists, and has created local employment options (see www.savethewildhorse.org).

Monitoring

Monitoring is a key element in any reintroduction project. In the Great Gobi B SPA, monitoring has used standardized methods since 2002 with a focus on the following: (1) population dynamics and distribution of reintroduced Przewalski's horses; (2) distribution of wild and domestic ungulates; and (3) human impacts on the protected area. Park rangers are able to identify individual Przewalski's horses and check groups once or twice weekly. They determine the location of individual Przewalski's horses and groups based on a raster map, note group size and composition, and record any peculiarities in individual horses (e.g. injuries, poor body condition). The data are fed into a central database, and all data on population dynamics and group composition are passed on to the EEP coordinator for annual reporting. By the summer of 2009, the population in Great Gobi B SPA had increased to approximately 140 individuals (see Fig. 72-2).

Range use of the reintroduced Przewalski's horse population increased gradually and pasture use was largely confined to the northeastern corner of the protected area (Fig. 72-3). In 2005, one harem group was released at Takhiin Us water point, about 120 km west of the Takhiin Tal camp, to speed up the expansion of the distribution range. To facilitate monitoring and gain sound data on habitat and space use, 10 Przewalski's horses were monitored with satellite collars.[7] Range sizes based on telemetry differed only marginally from those determined by the ranger observational data. In Takhiin Tal, the individual horse groups cover non-exclusive home ranges of 152 to 826 km^2.[5] Additionally, the adaptation of newly released Przewalski's horses was also monitored through behavioral observations of selected groups.[13]

Wildlife surveys are conducted on a monthly basis, alternating between smaller surveys covering the northwestern part of the park (4000 km^2) with an entire park (9000 km^2) assessment in the following month. During these surveys, all wildlife and livestock seen from fixed transects are counted and mapped, thus providing qualitative data on ungulate distribution.[5] The surveys are also an excellent opportunity to meet local herders and patrol for illegal actions such as poaching or saxaul (*Haloxylon* spp.) collection. Additional monitoring data are obtained via interviews or questionnaires, mainly focusing on livestock numbers and herder camp positions, wolf (*Canis lupus*) predation on livestock, and wolf harvest data.[6]

Inventories

The Great Gobi B SPA connects the Aralo-Caspian with the central Asian region and thus shows a mixture of floral elements, which makes it rather unique within Mongolia.[16] To map plant biodiversity and vegetation types as a basis for habitat analysis studies, vegetation of the entire Great Gobi B SPA and its surroundings was mapped using a combination of ground surveys, multivariate statistics, and remote sensing tools (see Fig. 72-3).[15] Other inventories within the Great Gobi B SPA have focused on small mammals, birds, and an initial bat study.

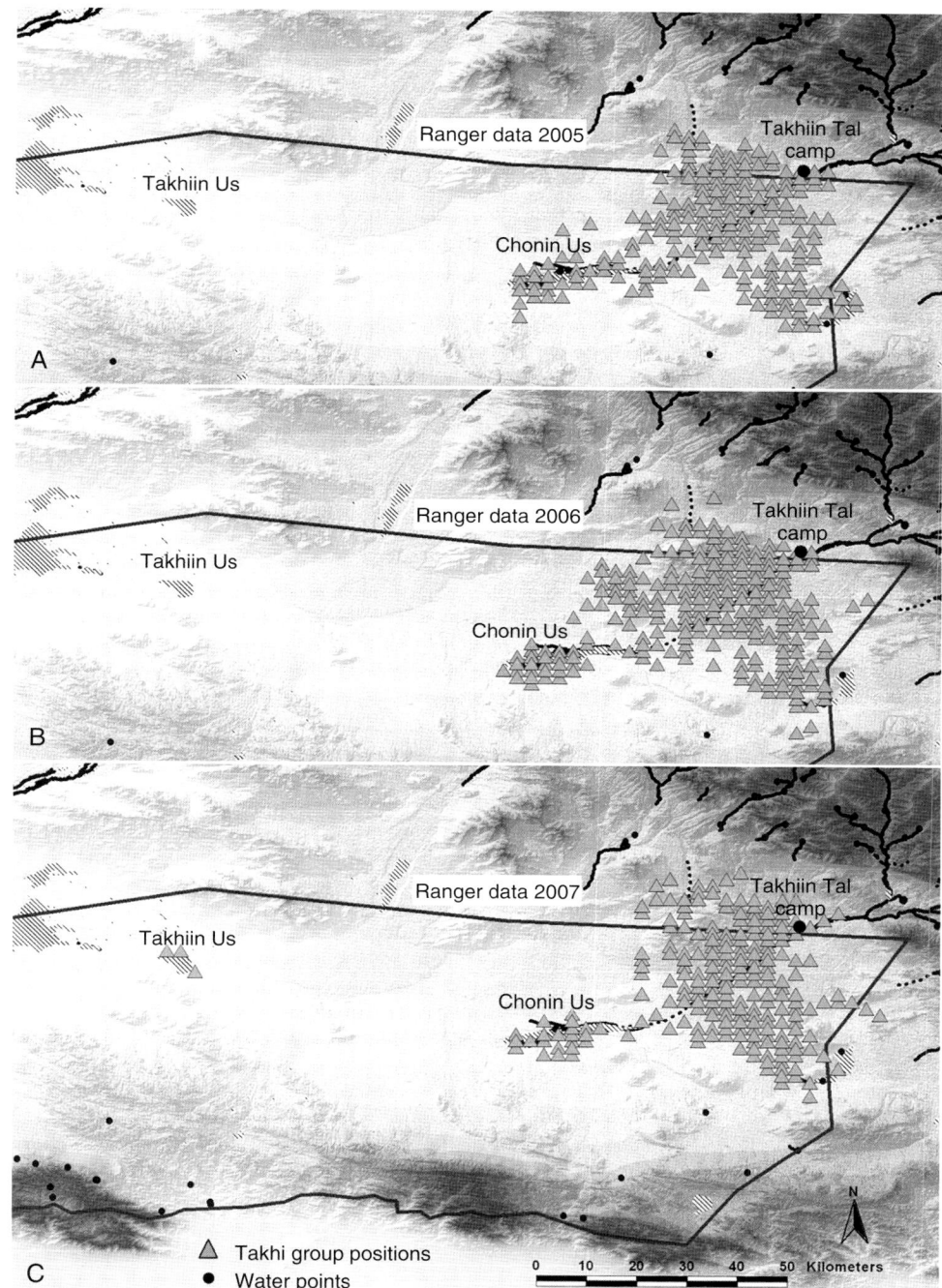

Figure 72-3

Range use by Przewalski's horses in Takhiin Tal as determined by ranger observations 2005 to 2007. Monitoring of the group released at Takhiin Us in 2005 was initially performed by satellite telemetry. Since 2007, this group is also included in ranger monitoring.

Specific Research Projects

In addition to the establishment of basic infrastructure, basic monitoring (designed to provide long-term data) and inventories (designed to derive baseline data),

several short- and mid-term research projects have been initiated. In respect to wildlife, one research focus is on the spatial organization and habitat use of the Asiatic wild ass *(Equus hemionus)* and another is on habitat use and feeding ecology of the grey wolf.[6,7]

Socioeconomic Projects

Another focus of the project involves socioeconomic aspects of local herders, their impact on the park and its surroundings, and their attitude toward wildlife and management issues.[4] In 2005, training workshops on the construction and application of fuel efficient stoves were conducted in Takhiin Tal to reduce the pressure on saxaul and juniper (*Juniperus* spp.) through illegal collection. In 2006, a concept for environmental education for children in Takhiin Tal was developed, but still needs to be implemented. In 2007, with support from the Italian Region of Lombardia and under the auspices of the Instituto Oikos (www.istituto-oikos.org), a transboundary project was initiated in collaboration with the Xinjiang Institute of Ecology and Geography of the Chinese Academy of Sciences. This project aims to support rural communities of nomadic pastoralists living in the transboundary area of the Dzungarian Gobi in China and Mongolia. Local livelihood will be improved through the strengthening of international collaboration on sustainable development issues and the integration of an environmental component in the development process. Recently, alternative income and sustainable tourism initiatives have been implemented in the Takhiin Tal area (see www.communitybasedtourism.info/en/our-destinations/mongolia-nature.asp). Strengthening local involvement and community development in the Great Gobi B area is of utmost importance for the future of the Przewalski's horse in this remote area.

CONCLUSION

Starting out initially as a single-species reintroduction project, the magnitude of conservation activities has greatly expanded in recent years. Seen from a species perspective, research projects dealing with the Mongolian wild ass, grey wolf, various rodent species, and vegetation have been implemented. Whereas the initial reintroduction efforts were driven mostly by veterinarians, the disciplinary scope has significantly broadened with zoologists, botanists, and remote sensing experts performing habitat mapping and assessment and community development experts establishing a socioeconomic framework for future project development. Away from the field, an important prerequisite for project advancement has proven to be lobbying activities both in Ulaanbaatar and the international community. Lobbying activities not only enhance information flow and political understanding for the project, but also create collaborative opportunities and necessary alliances. There is no consensus on when a reintroduction program is deemed successful. Clearly, viewing the self-sustainable reestablishment of a population as a successful end point is at best a short-term approach, constrained by time (today and now). Comprehensive interdisciplinary monitoring and research have been and are currently the foundation for management strategies and decisions regarding this project. However, a self-sustaining financial base, in conjunction with dedicated training and empowerment of local scientists and residents, constitute essential prerequisites for the project's future. Defining success and thereby inferring an end point can easily lead to complacency, compromising species persistence. The ultimate project objective must be a constantly reevaluated state of population persistence without intervention.

REFERENCES

1. Boyd L, Zimmermann W, King SRB: Equus ferus, 2010 (http://www.iucnredlist.org/apps/redlist/details/41763/0).
2. Groves CP: The taxonomy, distribution and adaptations of recent equids. In Meadow RH, Uerpermann HP, editors: Equids in the ancient world. Wiesbaden, Germany, 1986, Dr. Ludwig Reichert Verlag, pp 11–65.
3. International Union for Conservation of Nature and Natural Resources (IUCN): Categories & criteria (version 3.1), 2010 (http://www.iucnredlist.org/apps/redlist/static/categories_criteria_3_1).
4. Kaczensky P: Wildlife value orientations of rural Mongolians. Hum Dimensions Wildl 12:317–329, 2007.
5. Kaczensky P, Enkhsaikhan N, Ganbaatar O, et al: Identification of herder-wild equid conflicts in the Great Gobi B Strictly Protected Area in SW Mongolia. Explor Biol Resources Mongolia 10:99–116, 2007.
6. Kaczensky P, Enkhsaikhan N, Ganbaatar O, et al: The Great Gobi B Strictly Protected Area in Mongolia—refuge or sink for wolves Canis lupus in the Gobi? Wildl Biol 14:444–456, 2008.
7. Kaczensky P, Ganbaatar O, von Wehrden H, et al: Resource selection by sympatric wild equids in the Mongolian Gobi. J Appl Ecol 45:1762–1769, 2008.
8. Kaczensky P, Walzer C, Steinhauer-Burkart B: Great Gobi B Strictly Protected Area—A wild horse refuge, Oberaula, Germany, 2004, ECO Nature Edition, Steinhauer-Burkart OHG.
9. Mohr E: The asiatic wild horse, London, 1971, JA Allen.
10. Robert N, Walzer C, Rüegg SR, et al: Pathologic findings in reintroduced Przewalski's horses (Equus caballus przewalskii) in Southwestern Mongolia. J Zoo Wildl Medicine 36:273–285, 2005.
11. Slotta-Bachmayr L, Boegel R, Kaczensky P: Use of population viability analysis to identify management priorities and success in reintroducing Przewalski's horses to southwestern Mongolia. Jf WildlManage 68:790–798, 2004.
12. Sokolov VE, Orlov VN: Introduction of Przewalski horses into the wild. FAO Anim Prod Health Paper 61:77–88, 1986.
13. Souris AC, Kaczensky P, Julliard R, et al: Time budget, behavioral synchrony and body score development of a newly released Przewalski's horse group Equus ferus przewalskii, in the Great Gobi B strictly protected area in SW Mongolia. Appl Anim Behav Sci 107:307–321, 2007.

14. Van Dierendonck MC, Wallis de Vries MF: Ungulate reintroductions: Experiences with the takhi or Przewalski horse (*Equus ferus przewalskii*) in Mongolia. Conserv Biol 10:728–740, 1996.
15. Von Wehrden H, Wesche K, Miehe G, et al: Vegetation mapping in central Asian dry eco-systems using Landsat ETM+—A case study on the Gobi Gurvan Sayhan National Park. Erdkunde 60:261–272, 2006.
16. Von Wehrden H, Wesche K, Tungalag R: Plant communities of the Great Gobi B Strictly Protected Area, Mongolia. Mongol J Biol Sci 4:3–17, 2007.
17. Wakefield S, Knowles J, Zimmermann W, et al: Status and action plan for the Przewalski's horse (*Equus ferus przewalskii*). In Moehlman P, editor: Equids: Zebras, asses and horses: Status survey and conservation action plan. Cambridge, England, 2002, IUCN, pp 82–92.
18. Walzer C, Baumgartner R, Ganbataar O, et al: Boxing a wild horse for Mongolia—Tips, tricks and treats, 2004 (http://library.vetmed.fu-berlin.de/resources/global/contents/VET164623/EAZWV/Ebeltoft%20PDF/Microsoft%20Word%20-%20Walzer.pdf).
19. Walzer C, Baumgartner R, Robert N, et al: Medical aspects in Przewalski horse (*Equus przewalskii*) re-introduction to the Dzungjurian Gobi, Mongolia. In Baer CK, Patterson RA, editors: Proceedings of the American Association of Zoo Veterinarians and International Association of Aquatic Animal Medicine Joint Conference. New Orleans, 2000, pp 17–21.
20. Walzer C, Kaczensky P, Ganbataar O, et al: Coming home: The return of the Przewalski's horse to the Mongolian Gobi. In Dick G, Gusset M, editors: Building a future for wildlife—Zoos and aquariums committed to biodiversity conservation. Gland, Switzerland, 2010, World Association of Zoos and Aquariums (WAZA), pp 123–128.

Artiodactylids

Section 14

CHAPTER 73

Management of Cryptosporidiosis in a Hoofstock Contact Area

Edward C. Ramsay

Cryptosporidium spp. are protozoal enteric parasites of many vertebrate groups. Several but not all cryptosporidia species are zoonotic pathogens and outbreaks of human cryptosporidiosis have been linked to public contact with young ruminants. Although most of these outbreaks have occurred at open or educational farms, similar contact occurs in zoo hoofstock contact areas, and thus cryptosporidia are serious concerns for zoo managers and veterinarians.

The nomenclature of this group has undergone numerous revisions and may be confusing. *Cryptosporidium parvum* remains the most common cause of zoonotic infections and cattle are its principal host species.[5] Young calves, frequently animals younger than 8 weeks old, have been the source of almost all zoonotic cases of cryptosporidiosis involving direct animal contact. Numerous other species may be infected with *C. parvum*, including other domestic ruminants, pigs, and camels. Clinical cryptosporidiosis may occur in kids and lambs, and lambs have been linked to zoonotic cases as well. Adult cattle, sheep, and goats are infrequently identified as sources of zoonotic infections, and adult cattle may shed other nonzoonotic cryptosporidial species, such as *C. andersoni*.[6]

Clinical cryptosporidiosis occurs most commonly in neonatal and young animals. It has been estimated that more than 90% of dairies have infected stock.[5] Signs in calves vary from unformed stool to severe diarrhea. Mortality is considered moderate for uncomplicated infections, but coinfection with other enteric pathogens or accompanying stress (e.g., from cold weather or transport) may increase morbidity and mortality. There is no generally accepted, specific treatment for cryptosporidiosis in North America. Paromomycin has been used for the treatment of individual animals[4] and halofuginone is registered for the prevention and treatment of calf cryptosporidiosis in Europe.[2]

Cryptosporidiosis in immunocompetent people is typically a self-limiting gastroenteritis. It may occur in any older adult, but children younger than 2 years are most frequently and severely affected. Signs in humans include watery diarrhea that may contain mucus and be accompanied by abdominal pain and bloating. Signs typically are gone within 3 weeks, but shedding of oocysts may persist for a short time after signs abate. In immunocompromised individuals, cryptosporidiosis may be a severe and debilitating disease. Involvement of the pancreatic duct and gallbladder tree may occur, in addition to intractable diarrhea. Chronic diarrhea, cholera-like symptoms, and severe weight loss are predominant signs in the profoundly immunocompromised individual.[3]

Ingestion of oocysts is the major mode of transmission. *C. parvum* oocysts are sporulated and immediately infective when shed by the hosts, in contrast to other common ruminant coccidia *Eimeria* and *Isospora*. Clinical signs usually occur within 1 week of ingestion but longer incubation times may occur. Oocysts may persist in the environment for months and are resistant to many commonly used disinfectants.

DIAGNOSIS

Cryptosporidium spp. are tiny organisms (4.0 to 6.0 mm in diameter), and many laboratories use special techniques for their identification in fecal samples. There is disagreement on which test is the gold standard, but most agree that visualization of oocysts is confirmatory. Concentration techniques such as a centrifugal flotation technique using Sheather's sugar may be used (Fig. 73-1). Acid-fast staining of fecal smears or the use of auramine phenol fluorescent stains have been recommended. Many laboratories prefer immunofluorescent assays to sugar flotation; however, in one study there

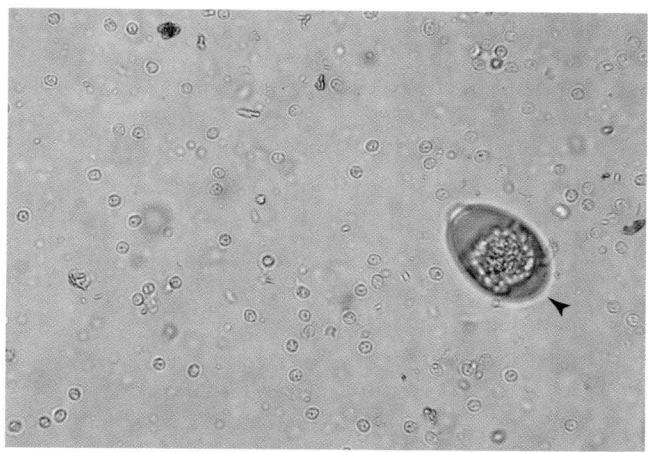

Figure 73-1

Photomicrograph of numerous cryptosporidial oocysts in feces of a goat with diarrhea. An *Eimeria* spp. oocyst is also present *(arrowhead)*. A sugar flotation with centrifugation methodology was used. *(Courtesy Aly Chapman.)*

was significant agreement between polymerase chain reaction (PCR) detection of *Cryptosporidium parvum* and the flotation technique.[7] Young animals with diarrhea shed millions of oocysts, but oocyst shedding may be infrequent in asymptomatic animals. Multiple fecal examinations are required to ensure that an asymptomatic individual is not infected.

PREVENTION AND CONTROL: ANIMALS

Because diagnosis, treatment, and disinfection are challenges with cryptosporidiosis, prevention is the most important strategy for control of its causative pathogen. Not importing or exhibiting very young dairy calves appears to be the single most important way to avoid having a clinical case of cryptosporidiosis on the grounds. All incoming ruminants, regardless of age, should undergo quarantine and be screened repeatedly for cryptosporidia. Routine fecal examinations for cryptosporidia species in all contact area ruminants are also prudent.

Any ruminant in a hoofstock contact area with diarrhea, particularly neonates and young animals, should be tested for cryptosporidiosis. If a case of cryptosporidiosis occurs in a contact area, a control plan should be immediately formulated and address the following points:

1. Preventing visitor and caretaker exposure to *Cryptosporidium* spp.
2. Preventing further contamination of grounds and infection of other animals
3. Determining whether infection has spread to other contact yard animals

Preventing Visitor and Keeper Exposure

The contact area should be immediately closed to the public and the number of keepers caring for animals in the area should be limited. These keepers should receive extensive training on the biology of cryptosporidia and how to protect themselves from infection. Those working in a contaminated enclosure should wear coveralls and boots that remain in that area. They should also wear disposable gloves while working there. Foot baths containing a germicidal detergent with activity against cryptosporidia may be placed at the entrances and exits of any contaminated area. The footbaths, if used, should be changed daily.

Keepers should not use leaf blowers to clean the contact area. All fecal material must be raked, bagged, and disposed of, instead of being composted. Tools used in contaminated areas should not be used in non-contaminated areas. Coveralls should be laundered on the zoo grounds. After laundering coveralls, an additional empty wash cycle should be run on the washing machine to remove any contaminants that might remain in the washing machine mechanically.

Contaminated facilities (e.g., fences, feed bowls, water tanks) should be thoroughly cleaned and disinfected. Soil yards cannot be adequately cleaned and disinfected so that complete destruction of all infective oocysts is accomplished. If the yard cannot be left empty of animals for a long period of time (more than 6 months), then the top 15 cm of the soil should be removed and replaced.

Prevention of Further Contamination

Any animal with diarrhea should be isolated and placed in an enclosure that can be thoroughly cleaned and disinfected, and where fecal material cannot reach other animals. If possible, contact area animals may be segregated into exposed and nonexposed populations. The nonexposed animals should be kept away from any contaminated sites.

Releasing an animal that has recovered from cryptosporidiosis back into a contact area is controversial. Although that animal may lead a healthy, normal life, there is no way to assure that it will not occasionally shed cryptosporidia. Most institutions will elect to permanently remove the animal from the contact population. Because responsible relocation of these animals to new owners may be difficult and considered by some to be ethically questionable, euthanasia of animals with cryptosporidiosis may be considered.

Determination of Infection in Other Contact Area Animals

All animals exposed to a clinical case should be closely observed for signs of diarrhea. Any exposed animal should be screened multiple times to determine whether it is shedding *Cryptosporidium* spp. I have used the following protocol successfully. One month after the last clinical case, small groups of animals (three or four animals/group) were moved to the zoo clinic (or off any contaminated yard), and three fecal flotation examinations were performed on each animal within a 7-day period. Moving the animals to the clinic was done to prevent identification of cryptosporidial organisms passing through each animal's system without causing infection.

If all the fecal flotations for each member of the group were negative for cryptosporidia oocysts, the group was considered to be clean and moved to a new, noncontaminated yard. All exposed animals had individual fecal examinations for cryptosporidia performed at 3 and 9 months after being moved to their new enclosure, and biannual herd fecal examinations were performed thereafter. All evidence to date indicates that none of the exposed contact yard animals became infected or, if they did become infected, their infections were completely resolved.

VISITOR SAFETY

Risk factors associated with cryptosporidiosis via animal contact include hand to mouth contact and failure to wash hands following animal contact.[1] A major strategy is to prohibit eating, drinking, smoking, and using pacifiers in contact areas, or immediately after leaving. A method of limiting the latter is to locate food sale stands or machines well away from contact yards. Education of the public about the importance of washing hands following animal contact is equally important. Providing adequate numbers of hand washing stations, located just outside all animal contact areas, is essential to limit potential infection. These precautions also help prevent the transmission of other fecal-oral zoonotic pathogens, such as *Escherichia coli* O157:H7 and *Salmonella* spp.

C. parvum is a serious zoonotic pathogen that may be controlled and prevented. Avoiding importation of nursing dairy calves, quarantining and screening for cryptosporidia all incoming contact area animals, and rapidly diagnosing any neonate with diarrhea will limit sources of the pathogen on grounds. Diligent visitor education to avoid hand to mouth contact within hoofstock contact areas, and to promote hand washing immediately after leaving contact areas, is also critical to protect zoo patrons and staff.

REFERENCES

1. Bender JB, Shulman SA: Reports of zoonotic disease outbreaks associated with animal exhibits and availability of recommendations for preventing zoonotic disease transmission from animals to people in such settings. J Am Vet Med Assoc 224:1105–1109, 2004.
2. Chako CZ, Tyler JW, Schultz LG, et al: Cryptosporidiosis in people: It's not just about cows. J Vet Intern Med 24:37–43, 2010.
3. Chalmers RM, Davies AP: Minireview: Clinical cryptosporidiosis. Exp Parasitol 124:138–146, 2010.
4. Johnson EH, Windsor JJ, Muirhead DE, et al: Confirmation of the prophylactic value of paromomycin in a natural outbreak of caprine cryptosporidiosis. Vet Res Comm 24:63–67, 2000.
5. Lejunne JT, Davis MA: Outbreaks of zoonotic enteric disease associated with animal exhibits. J Am Vet Med Assoc 224:1440–1445, 2004.
6. Robertson LJ: Giardia and *Cryptosporidium* infections in sheep and goats: A review of the potential for transmission to humans via environmental contamination. Epidemiol Infect 137:913–921, 2009.
7. Starkey SR, Kimber KR, Wade SE, et al: Factors associated with *Cryptosporidium* infection on dairy farms in a New York state watershed. J Dairy Sci 89:4229–4236, 2006.

CHAPTER 74

Bluetongue: Lessons from the European Outbreak 2006-2009

Stephanie Sanderson

Bluetongue is a ruminant disease of global importance causing significant economic losses due to the morbidity and mortality of susceptible species and also the impact of the legislative measures taken to control its spread. This chapter describes this disease and its management in captive, nondomestic ruminant species, drawing specifically from experience gained during the European outbreaks during 2006 to 2009.

CAUSE AND EPIDEMIOLOGY

Bluetongue (BT) is an insect-borne disease caused by the bluetongue virus (BTV), an *Orbivirus* in the family Reoviridae. BT viruses consist of 10 linear, double-stranded, RNA segments contained within three concentric structural protein shells. Variations in the proteins that make up the outermost shell, particularly the variable virus protein 2 (VP2), determine the virus serotype. 24 serotypes are currently recognized, with a 25th proposed.[1,13]

BT was first described in 1902 and was thought to be confined to Africa until reports of its spread to Israel in 1951, United States (1952), southern Europe (1956), Asia (1961), and Australia (1975).[20] It is now endemic to the tropics and subtropics but recent sustained outbreaks outside this geographic range, such as those in northwest Europe (2006 to 2009), indicate that this pattern may be changing.[9,11] Historically, incursions into Europe have been attributed either to movements of infected ruminants from the Maghreb to southern Europe or to infected vectors being blown to noninfected areas on the wind. Other sources include illegal importation of live attenuated BTV vaccines from the Republic of South Africa such as in the recent incursions of BTV6 and BTV11. The cause of the sudden appearance of BTV8 in Belgium in 2006 (a country in which BTV had never previously been recorded) remains unknown.

Phylogenetic studies have indicated the likely origin to be sub-Saharan Africa, and its introduction could have been by any one of the aforementioned routes.[6] A summary of the incursions of BTV serotypes into Europe since 1998 are shown in Figure 74-1.

BTV relies on hematophagous female midges for its primary route of transmission among ruminant hosts. Less than 50 of the known 1500 *Culicoides* species have been shown to be competent BTV vectors; hence viral distribution is largely dependent on the occurrence of suitable climatologic factors for these particular midge species. In addition, temperature variations may also have a marked effect on transmission rates, even within the geographic ranges of these competent midges. After ingestion of a blood meal, the virus must infect and replicate within the insect's midgut cells and again in their salivary gland cells prior to being inoculated into another ruminant. Only a small percentage of midges are susceptible to infection after viral ingestion via a blood meal; however, if reared at warmer temperatures, the infection rate and hence percentage of midges that may act as competent vectors increase. Warmer temperatures also lead to a reduction in the time required for the multiplication stage within the midge and increase the frequency of blood meals taken. At cool temperatures (<12° C), virus replication within the midge stops, and so does the midge's ability to transmit virus.[20]

Until the outbreak of BT in northwest Europe, it was thought that Palaearctic midge species such as *C. obsoletus* and *C. pulicaris*, although shown to be competent in laboratory conditions, would not be able to sustain transmission of BTV in the field because of wide fluctuations in seasonal temperature. Experience gained during this outbreak has shown that for this newly introduced strain of BTV serotype 8 (BTV8), low-grade secondary routes of transmission (such as transplacental and oral) in combination with suspected latent infection in

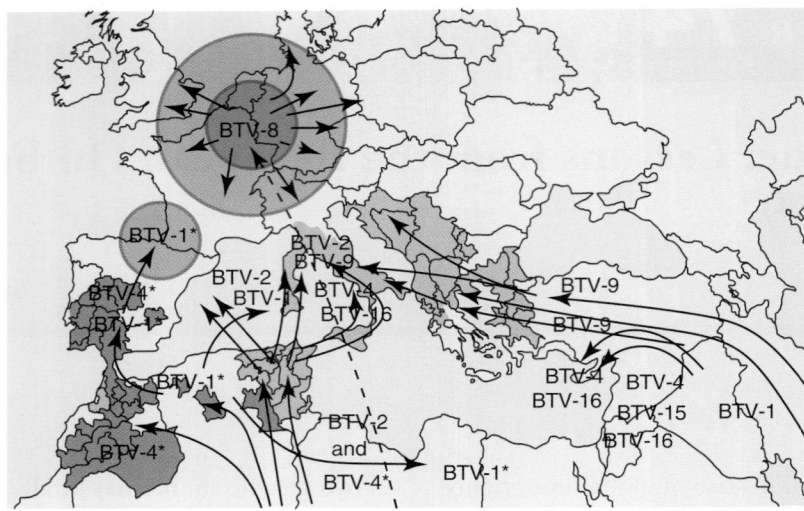

Figure 74-1

Spread of Bluetongue throughout Europe since 1998. (*Courtesy Institute of Animal Health, Pirbright Laboratory, Surrey, England.*)

ruminants and midges, may sustain infection over the cold winter months at levels sufficient for BTV to be maintained at these latitudes.[20] This newly apparent capability of BTV to maintain itself through temperate winters in conjunction with the highly temperature-dependent features of its epidemiology have led to a highly seasonal pattern of disease, with clinical cases in the northern European epizootics occurring almost exclusively between July and December each year.

CLINICAL PICTURE AND SPECIES SUSCEPTIBILITIES

It is generally accepted that all ruminant species and some camelids are likely to be capable of supporting BTV infection. Clinical expression of the disease is however highly variable and dependant on viral serotype, species, breed, immunologic status, environmental conditions and individual's health status. Animals indigenous to endemic areas appear to be clinically resistant—however the mechanism of their resistance is unknown and could be either attributed to natural or acquired immunity.[19]

The pathology and pathogenesis of the disease has been reviewed in detail by Maclachlan and colleagues[11] and the clinical picture seen in domestic species is well documented. The classic clinical signs of fever, nasal discharge, dyspnea, cyanosis of the tongue, oral lesions and ulcers, edema of the head and neck, lameness, and

hyperemia of the coronary band are caused by virus-mediated vascular injury. These signs are most frequently seen in sheep, in which mortality rates may be 30% or higher. Cattle rarely show clinical disease, with the exception of the European BTV8 strain.[20]

Little has been published about the clinical susceptibility of nondomestic species. In North America, white-tailed deer (*Odocoileus virginianus*), prong-horn antelope (*Antilocapra americana*), and desert bighorn sheep (*Ovis canadensis*) are known to develop severe disease similar to that described in domestic sheep.[19] Infection is not confined to ruminants and camelids but is also occasionally seen in carnivores. Abortion and death has been reported in dogs injected with a BT-contaminated vaccine and in a European lynx fed infected meat[6,10,11] and natural asymptomatic infection is known to occur in endemic African carnivores. The incursion of BTV8 into Europe has enabled European zoos to provide a unique contribution to our knowledge of species susceptibility as they hold immunologically naïve individuals representing a wide taxonomic and geographic spectrum.

A survey of all 313 European Association of Zoos and Aquariams (EAZA) zoos was undertaken in January 2008 to collate data on clinical disease seen during the 2007 BTV season. Of these, 49 zoos had confirmed BTV8 cases within 20 km and could be classified as at risk of infection. These 49 zoos held over 1000 susceptible individuals of 53 different species and seven ruminant families indigenous to Europe, North and South

America, Africa, and Asia. Clinical disease was seen in 62 individuals (6% of the at-risk population), spread among 13 zoos (27% of at-risk collections).[17]

Mortality and morbidity rates and the clinical picture seen in each affected species are summarized in Table 74-1. The subfamilies bovinae and caprinae are the most susceptible of the ruminants to clinical disease,

with four species showing morbidity rates higher than 20% and mortality rates higher than 10%. The average case-fatality rate for the affected bovinae and caprinae species was 69%. All the affected ruminant species in this study were indigenous to Europe, Asia, or South America. Clinical signs in these species are consistent with those recorded for BTV8 infection in

TABLE 74-1   Bluetongue in Ruminant Species in Zoos, August 2006-December 2007*

Affected Species	No. of At-Risk Individuals (BTV8 Within 20 km)	No. Clinically Affected	Morbidity Rate (%)[†]	Laboratory Confirmation (No.)	No. of Deaths	Mortality Rate (%)[‡]	Case-Fatality Rate (%)[§]	Clinical Signs Reported in Affected Animals
Bovidae	519	55	10.60	25	38	7.32	69.09	
American bison (*Bison bison*)	30	10	33.33	3	5	16.67	50.00	Lethargy, fever, mouth ulcers, drooling, difficulty eating, conjunctivitis, corneal edema, lameness, inflammation coronary band, sudden death
European wisent (*Bison bonasus*)	20	8	40.00	4	4	20.00	50.00	Lethargy, fever, mouth ulcers, drooling, difficulty eating, conjunctivitis, corneal edema, respiratory difficulty, lameness, inflammation coronary band, sudden death
Yak (*Bos grunniens*)	35	6	17.14	6	6	17.14	100.00	Nasal discharge, conjunctivitis, corneal edema, drooling, difficulty eating, respiratory difficulty, lameness, inflammation of coronary band, sudden death
Blackbuck (*Antilope cervicapra*)	17	2	11.76	2	2	11.76	100.00	Sudden death
Sheep, mouflon (*Ovis aries*)	101	6	5.94	5	2	1.98	33.33	Lethargy, fever, swelling head and neck, mouth ulcers, drooling, difficulty eating, conjunctivitis, respiratory difficulty, lameness, inflammation coronary band, sudden death

Continued

TABLE 74-1   Bluetongue in Ruminant Species in Zoos, August 2006-December 2007*—cont'd

Affected Species	No. of At-Risk Individuals (BTV8 Within 20 km)	No. Clinically Affected	Morbidity Rate (%)[†]	Laboratory Confirmation (No.)	No. of Deaths	Mortality Rate (%)[‡]	Case-Fatality Rate (%)[§]	Clinical Signs Reported in Affected Animals
Goat (Capra hircus)	208	2	0.96	2	2	0.96	100.00	Lameness
Alpine ibex, tur (Capra ibex)	34	2	5.88	2	2	5.88	100.00	Nasal discharge, sudden death
Siberian ibex (Capra sibirica)	4	1	25.00	0	0	0.00	0.00	Swelling of head and neck
Muskox (Ovibos moschatus)	5	1	20.00	1	0	0.00	0.00	Lethargy, fever, conjunctivitis, abortion
Cervidae	83	5	6.02	5	2	2.41	40.00	
Fallow deer (Dama dama)	43	2	4.65	2	2	4.65	100.00	Mouth ulcers, difficulty eating, drooling, lameness, sudden death
Camelidae	40	2	5.00	2	2	5.00	100.00	
Bactrian camel (Camelus bactrianus)	8	1	12.50	1	1	12.50	100.00	Sudden death
Alpaca (Lama pacos)	32	1	3.13	1	1	3.13	100.00	Sudden death

*Zoos situated within 20 km of confirmed BTV8 outbreaks during the period.[17]
[†]Morbidity rate = number clinically affected/number at risk.
[‡]Mortality rate = number that die/number at risk.
[§]Case-fatality rate = number that die/number clinically affected. Note that morbidity and mortality rates for the 2006 BTV8 epidemic in domestic livestock were 20% and 5% for domestic sheep and 7% and 3% in domestic cattle, respectively.[2]
From Sanderson S, Garn K, Kaandorp J: Species susceptibility to bluetongue in European zoos during the bluetongue virus subtype 8 (BTV8) epizootic Aug 2006-Dec 2007, 2008 (http://www.zoonosis.ac.uk/BTS2008/ext_abstract.pdf).

domestic livestock and with those reported in yak.[2,12] It is noteworthy that despite over 200 African ruminants of 20 species being held by zoos in at-risk areas, none of these were reported to have shown clinical signs of infection. This is consistent with observations in Africa that indigenous antelope do not develop clinical disease.[19]

Data were also gathered by European zoos on species' susceptibility to BTV1. The low number of submissions relating to animals known to be infected by BTV1 makes it difficult to draw any firm conclusions; however, anecdotal reports have suggested a similar clinical picture and species susceptibility as for BTV8.

DISEASE CONTROL

Bluetongue is recognized by the World Organization for Animal Health (Office International des Epizooties [OIE]) as a disease of global importance both due to its ability to cause death and debilitating disease across international borders—for example, the 2006 to 2009 European outbreak led to over 80,000 reported outbreaks and 100,000 cases across 14 countries—and due to the lack of effective treatments. The OIE consider BT of such significance that they have included it in their Terrestrial Animal Health Code: a document setting out international recommendations for disease control[13]

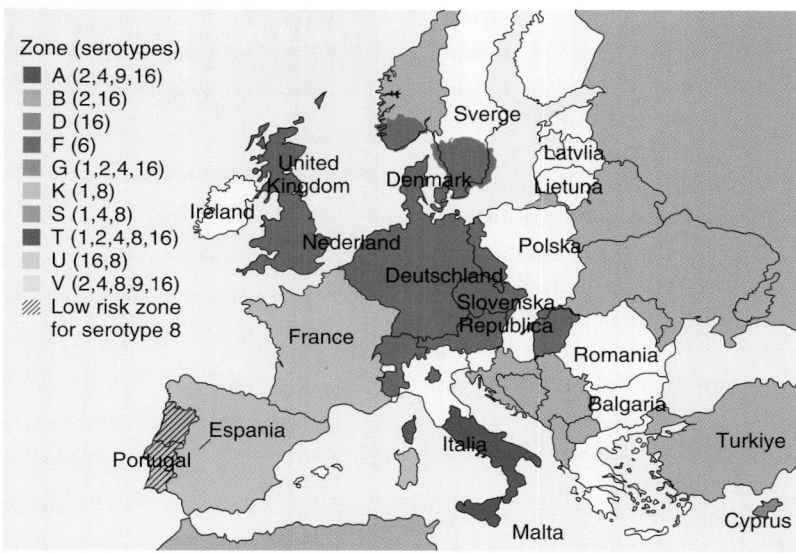

Zone (serotypes)
- A (2,4,9,16)
- B (2,16)
- D (16)
- F (6)
- G (1,2,4,16)
- K (1,8)
- S (1,4,8)
- T (1,2,4,8,16)
- U (16,8)
- V (2,4,8,9,16)
- Low risk zone for serotype 8

This map includes information on the bluetongue virus serotypes circulating in each restricted zone which permits, for the purposes of Articles 7 and 8 of Regulator No. 1266/2007, the indentification of the restriced zones demarcated in different Member States where the same bluetongue virus serotypes are circulating.

Figure 74-2

Restrictions during the 2006 to 2009 European outbreak covered most of the EU.

and also in their Manual of Diagnostic Tests and Vaccines that sets out standards for laboratory diagnosis and vaccine production.[14]

BTV's listing by the OIE also has implications for trade because it is recognized as a reference organization by the World Trade Organization (WTO). The trade implications in turn influence the types of control measures that different countries will put in place. Countries in which disease is endemic are likely to rely on rearing genetically resistant breeds of sheep and cattle in conjunction with protective vaccination and naturally acquired immunity. However, those countries in which disease incursions are rare will work hard to attempt to eradicate the disease to regain their disease-free status so that they may once again engage in free trade. Members of the European Union (EU) fall into this second category; their control and eradication provisions are laid out in Council Directive 2000/75/EC. These measures include vector control, restriction to movements of live ruminants and the controlled use of vaccines.

It should be noted that the economic impact of these control measures, particularly animal movement restrictions, may often be considerable. Because this is a vector-borne disease and midges have been shown to spread 100 km on the wind, restriction zones around outbreaks must be extensive to be effective. Restrictions

during the 2006 to 2009 European outbreak cover most of the EU (Fig. 74-2). In a study of the impact of BTV8 on the Dutch farming industry, the consequences of not being able to move animals were more costly to the industry than the value of the animals lost to the disease, even at the height of the epidemic.[20] In addition, movement restrictions have had a major impact on cooperative breeding programs among European zoos.

Other nonstatutory control measures have been suggested, such as housing animals at dawn and dusk when midges are most active, and removing standing water. Both these measures are likely to have little effect, because midges have been shown to enter buildings and their preferred breeding sites are moist soil and dung, rather than standing water.

VACCINATION

Vaccination is the mainstay of control in areas in which BTV has become established. Mass emergency vaccination campaigns may be used to achieve the following objectives[3,18]:

- Prevent clinical disease
- Limit regional spread of BT
- Allow regional and countrywide eradication
- Permit safe movement of animals between affected and disease-free zones

A variety of vaccines has been developed, of three different types: modified live vaccines (MLVs), inactivated vaccines (either prepared from whole killed virus or virus-like particles produced from recombinant baculovirus), and recombinant vaccinia, capripoxvirus, or canarypox virus-vectored vaccines.[6] The international standards for vaccine production have been published by the OIE in their *Manual of Diagnostic Tests and Vaccines for Terrestrial Animals.*[14] Only MLV and killed whole virus preparations will be discussed further here as they are the only vaccine types currently approved for national disease control programmes by the European Commission.

MLVs have been used for over 40 years in endemic bluetongue areas.[19] They can be produced quickly (8 to 10 weeks), are highly immunogenic, and may confer long-lasting protection after a single dose. Using live virus has significant disadvantages, however, because there is potential for under attenuation, causing symptomatic disease, milk drop, and fetal pathology, and for infection of the vector population, leading to local spread and potential for reassortment with field strains leading to new serotypes. For these reasons, inactivated vaccines are preferred, even though they take longer (6 to 8 months) to be developed, are more costly, and require regular boosters to maintain efficacy.[6,14]

There is little or no cross protection between different serotypes of BTV, so vaccines are produced specifically in response to circulating BTV serotypes and strains. All the vaccines currently available in the EU for the control of BTV1 and BTV8 are inactivated vaccines that use saponin and aluminum hydroxide as adjuvants (Table 74-2).

Safety

Trial and field experience has found these vaccines to be safe in domestic species.[3,4,8] An overview of field experience following the administration of over 60 million doses of BTV8 vaccine in 12 countries was undertaken by the European Medicines Agency.[2] Mass vaccination campaigns often necessitate deviations from normal procedure. Large groups of animals are brought together, less attention is paid to their individual health status, needle hygiene is worse, and government instructions may deviate from those of the manufacturers (e.g., minimum age of vaccination, target species, duration of immunity). In addition, compensation schemes in some countries may lead to overreporting of certain adverse reactions. Despite these factors, adverse reactions were seen in less than 1 in 10,000

TABLE 74-2	BTV1 and BTV8 Vaccines Licensed for Use in 2008	
	VACCINE TRADE NAMES	
Manufacturer	BTV8	BTV1
Intervet/Schering-Plough Animal Health	Bovilis BTV8	
CZ Veterinaria (Pontevedra, Spain)	Bluevac 8	Bluevac 1
Fort Dodge Animal Health (Fort Dodge, Iowa)	Zulvac 8 Bovis Zulvac 8 Ovis	Zulvac 1 Bovis Zulvac 1 Ovis
Merial (Essex, England)	BTVPUR AlSap 8	
Virbac		SYVAZUL 1

animals. Those recorded were typical for other inactivated vaccines; these include local reactions and non-severe general reactions, such as pyrexia (fever) and lethargy.

A survey of all 313 EAZA zoos was undertaken in February 2009 to collate data on vaccination in nondomestic species.[16] Over 2000 individuals of 57 species in 47 institutions in nine European countries were vaccinated for BTV8 using five of the products available in 2008. Adverse reactions occurred at a rate of 0.5% (equivalent to 50 in 10,000), with 50% of these being local reactions and 40% being abortions. The slightly higher rate could have been the result of the relatively small sample size and because the species studied were not used to handling and were likely to have been more stressed than their domesticated counterparts. Nonetheless, the abortion rate was still well below that considered acceptable for vaccines.[2]

Efficacy

Vaccine efficacy may be assessed by response to virus challenge (clinical and levels of viremia) and by the serologic response induced by immunization.[18] Although experimental virus challenge under laboratory conditions provides the most accurate measure of efficacy, is the mainstay of vaccine testing and is required for vaccine licensing, field experiences also provide useful data.[7] The licensed vaccines have been shown to be efficacious in domestic animals.[4,8] In addition, field data from the northern European outbreak would also seem to suggest that when vaccine uptake was high, virus transmission was effectively controlled and the numbers of clinical cases dropped dramatically.[20]

The February 2009 European Zoo Survey was used to gather data on nondomestic species. Results indicated that of the 37 Bovidae (cattle, sheep, goat, and antelope spp.) and Giraffidae tested postvaccination, 100% seroconverted postvaccination, as did 87% of the 40 South American camelids tested. Of the nine Cervidae (deer spp.) represented, only 50% seroconverted.[16] No vaccinated animals succumbed to clinical disease postvaccination, despite virus circulating in the area. These data suggest that the inactivated BTV8 vaccines are efficacious in bovids, giraffids and, to a lesser extent, camelids. The sample size in the cervids is too small to draw any firm conclusions and further work is needed to evaluate efficacy in these species.

CONCLUSIONS

The Northern European BT outbreaks (2006 to 2009) have demonstrated that BTV may now be sustained beyond its traditional tropical and subtropical distribution. Data gathered cooperatively by European zoos have demonstrated that as well as being a significant threat to the farming industry, BT also poses a significant risk of mortality and morbidity in a variety of naïve nondomestic ruminant species. The clinical picture seen was similar to that seen in domestic livestock. Species indigenous to temperate areas of Europe, Asia, and the Americas were most severely affected, whereas species indigenous to Africa, the putative source of BTV8, were clinically unaffected. This suggests that African species carry a degree of genetic resistance to BT.

Inactivated BTV8 and BTV1 vaccines have been used in many European zoos, both on a voluntary basis and as part of national control measures. Adverse reactions were rare and in line with those seen in the domestic species for which they were licensed. Vaccination produced a reliable immune response and no animals showed clinical evidence of infection postimmunization, despite the presence of circulating virus in the region. These vaccines would appear to be safe in nondomestic ruminants and efficacious in the Bovidae and Camelidae. Further work is needed to evaluate their efficacy in Cervidae.

Acknowledgments

The data on species susceptibilities and vaccine safety and efficacy in zoo ungulates were derived from two European Association of Zoo and Wildlife Veterinarians (EAZWV) and European Association of Zoos and Aquariums (EAZA) bluetongue Internet surveys of EAZA zoos covering the 2007 and 2008 outbreaks of BTV8 and BTV1. I would like to thank all the participants for their contributions to the surveys, particularly Katrin Garn and the EAZA office, Christine and Jacques Kaandorp, Christian Setzkorn of the National Zoonosis Centre, and Matthew Baylis and Sarah Jayne Edwards, Liverpool University, for their invaluable assistance with design and implementation of this project.

REFERENCES

1. Chaignat V, Worwa G, Scherrer N, et al: Toggenburg Orbivirus, a new bluetongue virus: Initial detection, first observations in field and experimental infection of goats and sheep. Vet Microbiol 138:11–19, 2009.
2. Committee for Medicinal Products for Veterinary Use (CVMP): An overview of field safety data from the EU for bluetongue virus vaccines serotype 8 emerging from the 2008 national vaccination campaigns, 2009 http://www.ema.europa.eu/docs/en_GB/document_library/Other/2009/12/WC500017480.pdf.
3. Commission of the European Communities: Commission Decision of 24 July 2008 approving the emergency vaccination plans against bluetongue of certain Member States and fixing the level of the Community's financial contribution for 2007 and 2008, 2008 http://ec.europa.eu/food/animal/diseases/controlmeasures/docs/decision_2008-288-bt-vaccination.pdf.
4. Eschbaumer M, Hoffmann B, Konig P, et al: Efficacy of three inactivated vaccines against bluetongue virus serotype 8 in sheep. Vaccine 27:4169–4175, 2009.
5. European Food Safety Authority: Epidemiological analysis of the 2006 bluetongue virus serotype 8 epidemic in northwestern Europe, 2007 (http://www.efsa.europa.eu/en/scdocs/doc/34br.pdf).
6. European Food Standards Agency (EFSA): Scientific Report of the Scientific Panel on Animal Health and Welfare on request from the Commission (EFSA-Q-2006-311) and EFSA Selfmandate (EFSA-Q-2007-063), 2007 (http://www.efsa.europa.eu/en/scdocs/doc/479rax1.pdf).
7. European Parliament and Council of the European Union: Directive 2001/82/EC of the European Parliament and of the Council of 6 November 2001 on the Community code relating to veterinary medicinal products, 2001 (http://www.biosafety.be/PDF/2001_82.pdf).
8. Gethmann J, Huttner K, Heyne H, et al: Comparative safety study of three inactivated BTV-8 vaccines in sheep and cattle under field conditions. Vaccine 27:4118–4126, 2009.
9. Hateley G: Bluetongue in northern Europe: The story so far. In Practice 31:202–209, 2009.
10. Jauniaux TP, De Clercq KE, Cassart DE, et al: Bluetongue in Eurasian lynx. Emerg Infect Dis 14:1496–1498, 2008.
11. Maclachlan NJ, Drew CP, Darpel KE, et al: The pathology and pathogenesis of bluetongue. J Comp Pathol 141:1–16, 2009.
12. Mauroy A, Guyot H, De Clercq K, et al: Bluetongue in captive yaks. Emerg Infect Dis 14:675–676, 2008.
13. Office International des Epizooties (OIE): Bluetongue. In Terrestrial animal health code, ed 18, OIE, 2010, Paris. http://www.oie.int/eng/normes/mcode/en_preface.htm#sous-chapitre-0.
14. Office International des Epizooties (OIE): Manual of Diagnostic Tests and Vaccines for Terrestrial Animals Bluetongue and

epizootic haemorrhagic disease, 2009 (http://www.oie.int/eng/normes/mmanual/2008/pdf/2.01.03_BLUETONGUE.pdf).

15. Sanderson S: Bluetongue in non-domestic ruminants: Experiences gained in EAZA zoos during the 2007 & 2008 BTV8 and BTV1 epizootics, In European Association of Zoo and Widlife Veterinarians, Infectious Diseases Working Group, Transmissible Diseases Handbook. 4th Edition. Ed Kaandorp J, Chai N & A Bayens 2010 (http://www.eaza.net/activities/TDH/09%20Blue%20tongue%20virus.pdf).

16. Sanderson S, Edwards SJ, Setzkorn C, et al: Survey of species susceptibility to bluetongue virus and bluetongue vaccine usage in European zoos during 2008. In Proceedings of the International Conference on Diseases of Zoo and Wild Animals, 2009, pp 1–2.

17. Sanderson S, Garn K, Kaandorp J: Species susceptibility to bluetongue in European zoos during the bluetongue virus subtype 8 (BTV 8) epizootic Aug 2006-Dec 2007. In Proceedings of the European Association of Zoo and Wildlife Veterinarians annual meeting, 2008, pp 225–227.

18. Savini G, MacLaclalan NJ, Sanchez-Vinaino JM, et al: Vaccines against bluetongue in Europe. Comp Immunol Microbiol Infect Dis 31:101–120, 2008.

19. Verwoerd DW, Erasmus BJ: Bluetongue. In Coetzer JAW, Tustin RC, editors: Infectious diseases of livestock. Oxford, 2004, Oxford University Press, pp 1201–1220.

20. Wilson AJ, Mellor PS: Bluetongue in Europe: Past, present and future. Philos Trans R Soc B 364:2699–2681, 2009. Council Directive 2000/75/EC of 20 November 2000 laying down specific provisions for the control and eradication of bluetongue OJ L 327, 22.12.2000, pp 74–83 http://eur-lex.europa.eu/LexUriServ/LexUriServ.do?uri=CELEX:32000L0075:EN:NOT.

CHAPTER 75

Alternatives for Gastrointestinal Parasite Control in Exotic Ruminants

Deidre K. Fontenot and James E. Miller

Internal nematode parasites are a significant health concern in ruminants, domestic and nondomestic, resulting in morbidity and mortality. In the southeastern United States, as well as in other warm humid climates, this is primarily caused by the abomasal worm, *Haemonchus* spp. Historically, parasite control programs in zoological institutions have relied heavily on an empirical, rotational drug program. Zoo veterinarians are being challenged with orally, parenterally, and topically medicating a variety of artiodactylid species in the face of estimated body weights, marginal compliance of oral medications, and unknown pharmacokinetic data. Consequently, subtherapeutic dosing and anthelmintic drug resistance are common. High development costs of new products are preventing new drugs from entering the market. In the domestic animal industry, anthelmintics alone may no longer be relied on to control parasites. Zoological institutions must take heed and look to the future for alternatives. Successful parasite control may be accomplished if holistic control programs are used with drug resistance prevention in mind, integrating diagnostic tools with strategic parasite control focusing on the animal and environment. Programs such as this are being used in the small ruminant industry and may serve as models.* Components of these programs include objective fecal parasite monitoring systems, fecal larval cultures and/or in vitro larval development assays to determine drug sensitivity and resistance patterns, fecal egg count reduction rate testing, pasture larval counts to identify hot zones for strategic environmental control, and nonchemical alternatives to reduce drug selection pressure and resistance issues.

*References 1, 11, 12, 15-18, 23, and 27.

PARASITE MONITORING STRATEGIES

Modified McMasters Fecal Egg Count

Accurate evaluation of nematode burdens cannot be made with subjective assessments of egg loads on fecal examinations. Fecal egg counts, such as the modified McMasters fecal egg count (MMFEC), are more objective for understanding patterns of infection and shedding, success of parasite management, when program changes are needed, and whether changes are helping. Annual and biannual fecal egg count monitoring may be suitable for some artiodactylid species; but higher risk species may need more frequent monitoring. The use of spreadsheet technologies may graph trends and establish in-house reference intervals by species or individual to aid in establishing strategic guidelines for monitoring and treatment. Many procedures exist for determining fecal egg counts, but it is important to use the same procedure each time. The MMFEC, with a sensitivity of 50 eggs/g (epg), is commonly used because of the quantitative data and simplicity of technique. Samples may be collected and refrigerated, not frozen, for up to 7 days to prevent larval hatch out in the fecal matter, typically within 12 to 24 hours at room temperature, rendering the sample nondiagnostic. Laboratory techniques for this procedure may be found at the website for the Southern Consortium for Small Ruminant Parasite Control (SCSRPC; http://www.scsrpc.org).[17] A McMasters slide (Chalex, Wallowa, Ore) is required for this procedure (Fig. 75-1). Trichostrongyle-type eggs (oval; ~80 to 90 μm) seen in the slide grid of the two chambers are counted on low-power (10×) objective. Notation of other parasites may be made but not counted because of poor correlation

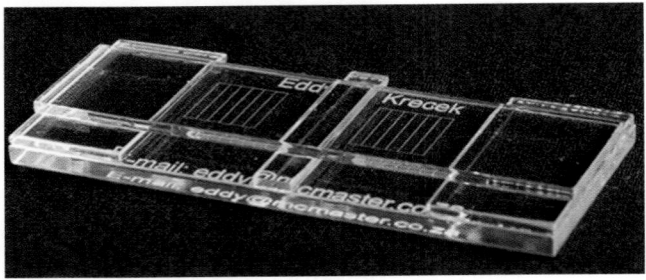

Figure 75-1

McMasters slide for FEC enumeration of nematode eggs, which are counted inside the slide grid areas of the two chambers using a low-power (10×) objective. The count (epg) is calculated by multiplying the total number of eggs counted in both chambers by 50.16. *(Courtesy Eddy Krecek.)*

with nematode infection. The count (epg) is calculated by multiplying the total number of eggs in both chambers by 50.

Fecal Larval Culture, Larval Development Assay, and Fecal Egg Count Reduction Test

Treatment strategies may be refined when trichostrongyle species and resistance status are identified in populations. Diagnostic options to consider include the in vitro larval development assay (LDA), which includes fecal larval culture (FLC), species identification, and/or FLC in combination with the fecal egg count reduction test (FECRT). A 2-year investigation of exotic artiodactylid nematode populations in four zoological facilities (three in Florida and one in California) using FLC showed individual, species, exhibit, and seasonal variability in nematode species.[20] Nematode species vary in their anatomic location of infection, potential for morbidity and mortality, and response to therapy. FLC testing may further characterize these factors to strategize treatment options better and may be done on individual or herd samples. The LDA and/or FECRT are also critical to your program. Similar to bacterial and fungal monitoring, the LDA may identify nematode populations and determine their resistance levels. Resistance, the ability of nematodes to survive anthelmintic drugs typically effective for the same species and dose, is the most critical problem facing our industry.

Nematodes have great genetic diversity, with a high rate of reproductive potential; *Haemonchus contortus* females may produce 5000 to 10,000 eggs/day. With this population growth, resistance will be an inevitable consequence of drug selection. Nematodes that survive because of evolved resistance transfer their alleles to the next generation.[12,15] Adding to this issue, animal transfers among conservation institutions permits the dispersal of resistant nematodes among multiple populations. Clinically, we see resistance when the normal therapeutic dose is no longer effective (<95% reduction in FECRT). Unfortunately, drug resistance occurs long before it is detected clinically. Because LDA and FECRT are not traditionally part of parasite monitoring programs, clinical resistance is often discovered too late. Zoo veterinarians should determine the resistance issues in their populations and implement testing during quarantine, preshipment, and routine monitoring program. When resistance is recognized in early stages through testing, anthelmintics may still be used but need to be managed appropriately. The LDA (DrenchRite, Microbial Screening Technologies, New South Wales, Australia) as well as the FLC are not suited for clinical use and may only realistically be performed in a parasitology diagnostic laboratory. A single DrenchRite test may detect resistance to three classes in one assay, including benzimidazoles, levamisole, and avermectin-milbemycin anthelmintics from a single herd sample.[18] The FECRT is an in-house means of determining whether resistance is present. For this test, FEC sampling is performed before and typically 10 to 14 days after treatment on individual animals. It is necessary to perform pretreatment FEC so that treatment efficacy may be balanced against the level of infection. An untreated control group should be included, if possible, to detect other factors that could influence FEC variations. The FECRT is calculated by the following:

$$FECRT(\%) = (\text{Pretreatment FEC} - \text{post-treatment FEC})/ \text{pretreatment FEC} \times 100$$

An FECRT of less than 95% indicates an incomplete therapy response and is likely a concern for resistance. Monitoring frequency is program-dependent. Consider performing FLC and LDA tests using monthly or bimonthly sampling for the first year to identify areas of concern and then an annual or biannual monitoring program may be adequate to monitor any significant change in population trends. FECRT should be completed after every treatment is performed. Feces should be submitted fresh or refrigerated but not frozen. Check with your laboratory partners to get specifics on sampling and shipping needs for FLC and LDA testing.

Pasture Larval Count

Exhibit populations, forage populations, seasonal changes, and rain accumulation may all influence which nematode populations are present in exhibits. A 2-year investigation of nematode populations in a Florida zoological facility using the pasture larval count (PLC) assay showed exhibit, exhibit region, species, and seasonal variability. This information has proven helpful for developing animal collection and exhibit management, fecal removal schedules, and savannah forage maintenance, including irrigation strategies. PLC is not an in-house test and also requires a partnership with a university parasite laboratory. Sampling and monitoring frequency are program-dependent and may not be critical to your strategic program. If testing is indicated, consider performing monthly or bimonthly sampling for the first year to identify areas of concern. Follow-up annual or biannual testing may be indicated to monitor any significant changes in population trends. Check with your laboratory partners to obtain specifics of sampling and shipping needs.

PARASITE CONTROL STRATEGIES

Drug Treatment

The current drug resistance crisis shows that total reliance on chemical control for parasites is no longer a viable strategy.[12,15] Intelligent use of anthelmintics is necessary because drugs are a valuable limited resource to be used conservatively, not on a rotational basis. Treatment decisions based on the biology and life stages of parasites, dynamics of resistance selection, biology of the host-parasite relationship, and needs of individual patients are critical. This approach, termed *smart drenching* in the domestic industry, uses the information about parasite, animal, and drugs to maximize effectiveness of treatments while decreasing the development of resistance.[27] Drug strategies should be based on current resistance patterns, with consideration of using only one drug class until resistance develops, synergistic use of classes (different modes of action) to enhance efficacy, and restricted use of one class of drugs only for crisis management. Studies in oral dosing in domestic ruminants have shown that the duration of drug availability is dependent on the flow rate of the rumen. With the benzimidazole and avermectin classes, fasting animals 24 hours prior to treatment decreases rumen motility and increases drug availability and efficacy through increased nematode contact.

Dosing accuracy to minimize resistance in exotic species may be a challenge with unknown pharmacokinetic data. Additionally, domestic ruminant studies have shown significant differences in dosing in cattle versus small ruminant species. For oral and parenteral anthelmintics, goats metabolize drugs more rapidly with rule of thumb dosages, resulting in dosages that are 1.5 to 2 times higher than those of sheep or cattle. Levamisole, however, has a narrow margin of therapeutic safety and should be used at no more than 1.5 times the dosage. Anthelmintic drugs are typically most effective orally, but moxidectin in goats has shown a superior pharmacokinetic profile with subcutaneous injection, resulting in slower resistance. The bioavailability of pour-ons in domestic nonbovid species is poor and the pharmacokinetics of absorption is highly variable because of differences in follicular density and skin lipid characteristic.[13] Studies have supported selective target treatment in domestics, with most parasite dispersal in only 20% to 30 % of animals, allowing treatment of animals only if clinically indicated. A standardized scoring system correlating conjunctival color with the level of anemia (FAMACHA; http://www.ars.usda.gov) was developed for the control of *H. contortus* and has resulted in a significant drop in individual and herd treatments, resulting in delayed resistance. This program requires anemia to be present before treatment is warranted. Animals are scored using the FAMACHA system histogram typically before parasite season and then every 2 to 3 weeks thereafter.[16] Developing a system such as this in our industry would require a large population data set, correlation of anemia with conjunctival color, and standardization among species, which presents challenges.

Animal Management

Mixed species exhibits that combine primary grazers with higher risk browsing species have shown to reduce nematode burdens on susceptible species by reducing grass length and larval exposure while increasing pass-through species and refugia. The term *refugia* refers to the population that is not under selection by drug treatment; it includes untreated animals as well as the eggs and larvae present in the pasture. This refuge of susceptible genes dilutes the frequency of resistant alleles. In the domestic animal industry, increasing refugia is recognized as the key animal management strategy to manage drug resistance, allowing nonclinical animals to harbor susceptible worms.[12,15,27]

Another novel concept that is currently in a trial phase in two exotic artiodactylid collections is the principle of selection against resistance. This method requires LDA testing in quarantine; susceptible nematodes are not being eliminated but rather introduced into current nematode populations in an effort to dilute resistant nematode strains and slow the rate of selection for resistance. Also, a critical part of this program is to use aggressive, synergistic, multidrug therapy against highly resistant nematodes to minimize introduction to the current nematode populations. It is hoped that the use of this strategy will preserve drug efficacy for as long as possible.

Environmental Control

Good environmental management may also play a role in minimizing disease and reducing drug use. Factors such as temperatures higher than 50° F, more than 2 inches of rain a month, exposure time to exhibit of more than 8 to 12 hours, grazing behaviors (<3 inches from the ground), immune or nutritionally challenged status, and stocking rates more than 5 animals/acre may negatively influence nematode burdens.[14] Environmental management of pastures and exhibits have been challenged in zoological exhibits by other factors, such as animal visibility for guest experience, staff time for fecal removal, and limited acreage for animal environment, but compromises may balance these issues. Limiting population densities and decreasing stocking rates on exhibit may be managed through proper collection planning and herd rotations to limit exhibit exposure time. Rotating species on exhibit, as well as multispecies populations, will increase the refugia population. Providing diet and enrichment items such as elevated browse and grass higher than 3 inches may minimize larval exposure and stereotypic grazing behaviors reported in browsing species such as giraffe. Parasite transmission is greatly reduced when animals are browsing or grazing high away from the larvae, which usually migrate 3 to 5 inches up the grass blade.

Tillage of exhibits prior to replanting between grazing seasons is another way to reduce larval contamination on exhibits, allowing most of the larvae to die buried under soil, resulting in a reduction of the PLC and concentration of infective larvae. Several chemicals have been investigated for use in killing larvae on pastures, but none have proven effective. Measures such as exhibit forage burning may be considered to kill larvae. Trees, although desirable for foraging and reduction of grazing behaviors, provide shade and humidity, causing animals to congregate, thus concentrating feces and allowing increased ingestion of infective larvae. Barns and watering areas may also contribute to animal concentration and exhibit plans should take this into account. Fecal removal strategies may be labor-intensive and exhibit geography-dependent, but may be cost-effective measures with vacuum systems and labor reinforcement. Water control by eliminating water leaks and pooling, controlling irrigation schedules, and removing animal exposure to moist areas may limit larval development and infection rates as well.

NONANTHELMINTIC CONTROL AND TREATMENT STRATEGIES

Alternatives to anthelmintics are needed to address resistance concerns as a result of no new products being developed. Copper oxide wire particles (COWPs), condensed tannin plants, and nematophagous fungi have shown promise for animal and environmental control in studies in domestic species.[1-7,10,11,19,21-26] Limited pilot studies and clinical trials in zoological collections have also shown promise for nonchemical methods.[9] Some alternative control measures have significant research data indicating that they work, some have limited data that merit further studies, but many lack data, especially in regard to exotic artiodactylids. As these methods are tested, animals should be closely monitored for morbidity through clinical examinations and FEC and potential toxicity issues should be addressed. Staying abreast of emerging technology in the domestic field and consideration of validating these methods in exotic species are critical.

Copper Oxide Wire Particle Therapy

The success of COWP therapy in domestic ruminants has been well documented and has shown good efficacy against *Haemonchus* spp. COWPs, as well as trace mineral boluses with copper, reduce FEC by 60% to 90% for 21 to 28 days.* COWPs are retained in the folds of the abomasa, with the low pH causing the release of high concentrations of soluble copper ions and creating an environment that causes death and/or expulsion of worms. The exact mechanism of action is unknown. Studies have shown that nematode cuticle damage likely disrupts the metabolic function of the

*References 4, 6, 7, 9, 11, and 22.

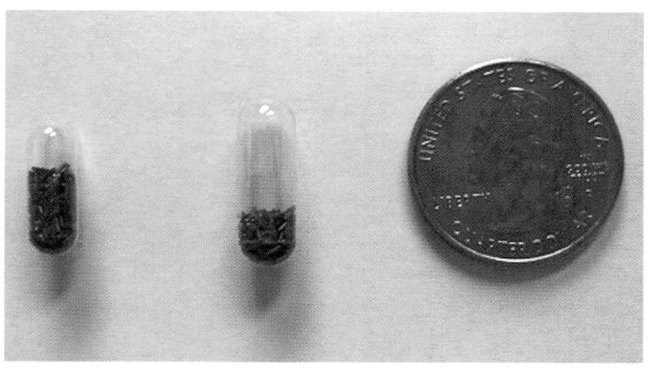

Figure 75-2

COWP boluses may be made and administered using commercially available copper boluses and repackaged into doses suitable for smaller species using gelatin capsules. *(Courtesy Joan Burke.)*

nematode through absorption of toxic levels of copper from the blood or abomasal fluids. Copper may also stimulate a local immune response. FEC reductions with COWPs are likely reflective of nematode kill versus decreased fecundity in the nematode population. A COWP study in four species of exotic artiodactylids has shown species variability, with an efficacy of FECRT more than 90% by 7 days post-treatment for three species and by 21 days for all species. Dosing was based on the manufacturer's recommendation of 12.5 g for cattle less than 227 kg, but lower dosages of 0.02 to 0.05 g/kg have been used with similar efficacy in domestic small ruminants.

Copper does not appear to affect intestinal nematodes, so FLC is critical before COWP therapy is used. Boluses may be administered using the commercially available product (Copasure, Butler Schein Animal Health, Dublin, Ohio), which may be repackaged into doses suitable for smaller species using gelatin capsules (Fig. 75-2). Copper tends to accumulate in the liver, and chronic elevations in copper levels could predispose to hepatic disease and anemia. In a study in lambs, copper dosages higher than the recommended supplemental dose (0.25 to 0.5 g/kg) were given without clinical side effects; however, liver copper levels were high. Until further studies may be completed, limit COWP administration to no more than once every 6 to 12 months to limit the risk of toxicity. Other factors contributing to toxicity include dietary sources, interactions of dietary minerals (e.g., molybdenum, sulfur, iron, zinc), and other environmental sources. There are complex mineral interactions that affect copper absorption and deficiencies in other minerals may increase the risk for copper

toxicity. COWPs should not be administered to animals with unknown copper status, those supplemented with other forms of copper, or animals with preexisting liver disease. Copper oxide is not as readily absorbed as copper sulfate, but COWPs may stay in the system for a few weeks, compared with a few days for copper sulfate and, in the long term, both may contribute to copper toxicity, depending on how often each is used. Concentrations higher than 1.5% copper sulfate may be caustic. One source has reported success with feeding a 3.3% mixture of copper sulfate in the salt for several months until sheep died from copper toxicity. When they reduced the concentration in the salt to 2%, it was ineffective at controlling worms.[3]

Condensed Tannins

Tannins are polyphenolic plant compounds that bind proteins and other molecules. There are two main types of tannins—hydrolyzable, which may have toxic effects on animals, and bioactive condensed tannins (CTs), found in legumes and other plants. Effects of CTs vary, depending on type of tannin, forage, CT concentration, and the animal. Domestic studies have shown efficacy with CT concentrations as low as 20 to 45 g CT/kg dry matter (DM; 2% to 4.5% DM), whereas high forage CT concentrations (>55 g CT/kg DM, 5.5%) may have negative effects such as reduced intake and digestibility (Table 75-1). Positive effects include an increase in bypass protein and a reduction in FEC, parasite numbers, and egg hatchability. Research has shown that CT-containing bioactive plants, such as sericea lespedeza *(Lespedeza*

TABLE 75-I	Condensed Tannin Content in Forage Used for Trichostrongyle Control		
Forage Species		g/kg DM CT	% DM
Birdsfoot trefoil *(Lotus corniculatus)*		48	4.8
Big trefoil *(Lotus uliginosus)*		77	7.7
Sanfoin *(Onobrychis viciifolia)*		29	2.9
Sulla *(Hedysarum coronarium)*		51-84	5.1-8.4
Sericea *(Lespedeza cuneata)*		46-152	4.6-15.2

From Coffey L, Hale M, Terrill T, et al: Tools for managing internal parasites in small ruminants: Sericea lespedeza, 2007 (http://attra. ncat.org/attra-pub/PDF/sericea_lespedeza.pdf).

cuneata), are useful in controlling internal parasite infection in sheep and goats. Sericea grows in marginally fertile and acid soils, is disease- and insect-resistant and heat- and drought-tolerant, and is widely planted to treat erosion and soil depletion. It grows throughout most of the southeastern and eastern United States but is listed as an invasive noxious weed in some states. Palatability of the coarse, heavy-stemmed plant is variable, but no issues have been reported with sericea hay or pellets.[1,19,21,24,26] Plant management and production information may be found at the SCSRPC website (http://scsrpc.org).

Studies have shown that a diet of 75% pelleted sericea lespedeza over a 2- to 4-week period and forage or hay products over a 7- to 8-week period result in FEC reductions of 50%. The FEC has shown increases after sericea feeding was stopped, indicating an effect on nematode fecundity. Pelleting of ground sericea hay increases ease of storage, transport, and feeding, with one study showing improved efficacy in goats compared with sericea hay. Pelleted sericea may facilitate its broader use, but further investigation is needed to determine the temperature at which heat inactivates the biologic activity of CT in the pelleting process. Investigations are currently underway in exotic artiodactylid collections with pelleted sericea and show promise. The mechanism of action is not yet known, but researchers believe that CTs may affect parasites directly through cuticle absorption, causing nematode dysfunction, and/or indirectly, by improving protein nutrition, amino acid absorption, and immune system stimulation. CTs also appear to reduce the hatching of eggs and larval development by binding to the larvae or feed nutrients, or by preventing bacterial growth in the feces (larvae feed on bacteria) and limiting the feed available for larval growth.

Nematophagous Fungus

Another treatment is a naturally occurring nematode-trapping fungus, *Duddingtonia flagrans*, which acts as a biologic control agent by parasitizing developing nematode larvae in feces. The fungus is ubiquitous, found worldwide, and normally present in the feces at low levels. Spores of this fungus may be incorporated into various diet items and, on ingestion, pass unchanged through the digestive tract and concentrate in the feces. After feces are deposited onto the pasture, the spores germinate, forming hyphae that are able to trap and kill the developing larval stages (Fig. 75-3). It is primarily used as a preventive, with no therapeutic benefits. It is

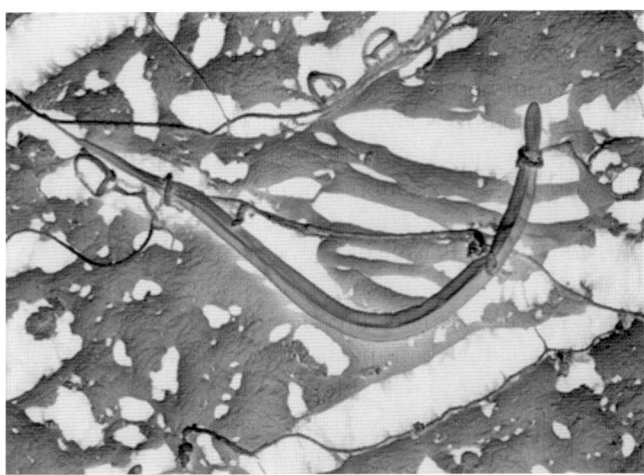

Figure 75-3

Electron microscopy photomicrograph of the nematode-trapping fungus, *Duddingtonia flagrans*. The spores germinate, forming hyphae that are able to trap and kill the developing parasite larval stages. *(Courtesy Jose Bresciani.)*

active against free-living larvae, with no effect on adult stages in vivo.[10,25] The eventual effect is reduction in pasture larval numbers and thus reduced reinfection. Studies in domestic ruminants have shown positive benefits and a study is currently underway in exotic ruminant species. The fungal spores must be fed daily for 2 weeks to achieve the full benefit, but alternate-day feeding has shown acceptable activity as well. Spores are fed at a dose of 250,000 to 500,000 spores/kg body weight, with larval reduction occurring 7 to 14 days after treatment starts.[5] Palatability does not appear to be a concern and spores should be fed with a dry diet to minimize moisture and prevent premature sporulation. No environmental impact studies have been performed to determine effects on soil health with increased concentration of fungus, but it is believed that the spores survive in the fecal environment for 3 to 4 days. A study in small ruminants has shown no effect of sporulation when used in combination with COWPs for parasite control, implying promise for using these two together in a control strategy program. Currently, there is a lack of a commercial source of spores in the United States. The spores are being produced in Australia (International Animal Health Products, Huntingtonwood, New South Wales), as well as in experimental settings in the United States.

Other Treatment Strategies

Other methods have been reported in the domestic small ruminant industry, with no clinical trials in exotic species. Parasite vaccines remain an elusive goal and it will likely be many more years before effective vaccines become commercially available.[15] Protein supplementation in small ruminants may be beneficial because increasing nutrition and amino acid availability could result in immune system stimulation.

Application in zoo species already receiving a high-quality diet with appropriate protein may limit efficacy and increasing amounts further may be a poor nutritional strategy long term. Historically, tobacco and nicotine sulfate have been recommended in for control of parasites. Dosing has not been well established with limited quantitative effects being reported. Nicotine sulfate is a nerve-paralyzing toxin with a narrow margin of safety to achieve nematode effect (worm release and excretion) without ill effects to host.[15] Diatomaceous earth is fossilized unicellular marine or fresh water algae and is used as a food ingredient and in swimming pool filters. Caution should be used in giving the nonfood-grade product to animals because of heavy metal contamination. Scientific studies in domestic goat and sheep species, combining it with mineral supplements, have shown minimal effects unless at a very high level in the diet (5% of the diet). It is postulated that this product may cause fecal pellets to dry out faster, which could reduce larval development; however, investigations have been inconclusive.[23] Commercially available herbal anthelmintics contain various mixtures of dried plants or plant products, such as *Artemisia absinthium* (wormwood), *Allium sativum* (garlic), *Juglans nigra* (black walnut), *Cucurbita pepo* (field pumpkin), *Artemisia vulgaris* (mugwort), *Foeniculum vulgare* (fennel), *Hyssopus officinalis* (hyssop), and *Thymus vulgaris* (thyme) and limited investigations have shown no measurable health benefits and failed to control nematode burdens in small ruminant species.[8] Use caution with commercial products, because some herbs may be toxic. Many producers swear by garlic and other herbs, but controlled studies have failed to see a positive response to these commercial herb preparations.[9] It is critical that these alternative chemical control products be objectively evaluated for zoological collections, monitoring for infectious (FEC, FECRT, and hematocrits), environmental (FLC and PLC), and adverse effects of these control methods.

REFERENCES

1. Coffey L, Hale M, Terrill T, et al: Tools for managing internal parasites in small ruminants: Sericea Lespedezas, 2007 (http://attra.ncat.org/attra-pub/PDF/sericea_lespedeza.pdf).
2. Burke J, Miller J: Control of Haemonchus contortus in goats with a sustained-release multi-trace element/vitamin rumen bolus containing copper. Vet Parasitol 141:132–137, 2006.
3. Burke J, Miller J: Dietary copper sulfate for control of gastrointestinal nematodes in goats. Vet Parasitol 154:289–293, 2008.
4. Burke J, Miller J, Brauer M: The effectiveness of copper oxide wire particles as an anthelmintic in pregnant ewes and safety to offspring, Vet Parasitol 131:291–297, 2005.
5. Burke J, Miller J, Larsen M, Terrill T: Copper oxide wire particles and Duddingtonia flagrans in lambs. Vet Parasitol 134:141–146, 2005.
6. Burke J, Miller J, Olcott D, et al: Effect of copper oxide wire particles dosage and feed supplement level on Haemonchus contortus infection in lambs. Vet Parasitol 123:235–243, 2004.
7. Burke J, Miller J, Terrill T: Use of copper oxide wire particles (COWP) to control barber poleworms in in lambs and kids, 2006 (http://www.scsrpc.org/SCSRPC/Files/Joan/COWP%20Use%203.pdf).
8. Burke J, Wells A, Casey P, Kaplan R: Herbal dewormer fails to control gastrointestinal nematodes in goats. Vet Parasitol 160:168–170, 2009.
9. Fontenot D, Kinney-Moscano A, Kaplan RM, Miller J: Effects of copper oxide wire particles bolus therapy on trichostrongyle fecal egg count in exotic artiodactylids. J ZooWildl Med 39:646–649, 2008.
10. Fontenot M, Miller M, Peña M, et al: Efficiency of feeding Duddingtonia flagrans chlamydospores to grazing ewes on reducing availability of parasitic nematode larvae on pasture. Vet Parasitol 118:203–213, 2003.
11. Hale M, Burke J, Miller J, Terrill T: Tools for managing internal parasites in small ruminants: Copper wire particles, 2007 (http://attra.ncat.org/attra-pub/PDF/copper_wire.pdf).
12. Kaplan R: Anthelmintic resistance and the changing landscape of parasite control, 2006 (http://scsrpc.org)
13. Kaplan R: Personal communication, 2009.
14. Kaplan R: Reduce the frequency of treatment through the use of sound pasture management, 2006 (http://www.scsrpc.com).
15. Kaplan R: Update on parasite control in small ruminants: addressing the challenges posed by multiple-drug resistant worms, 2006 (http://scsrpc.com/SCSRPC/Files/Files/Ray/AABP%202006%20SR%20proceedings.pdf).
16. Kaplan R, Miller J: FAMACHA information guide, 2007 (http://www.scsrpc.org/SCSRPC/FAMACHA/famachainfoguide.htm).
17. Kaplan R, Miller J: Modified McMaster egg counting for quantification of nematode eggs, 2006 (http://www.scsrpc.org/SCSRPC/Files/Files/RKJMMcMaster.pdf).
18. Kaplan R, Vidyashankar A, Howell S, et al: A novel approach for combining the use of in vitro and in vivo data to measure and detect emerging moxidectin resistance in gastrointestinal nematodes of goats, Int J Parasitol 37:795–804, 2007.
19. Lange K, Olcott D, Miller J, et al: Effect of sericea lespedeza (*Lespedeza cuneata*) fed as hay, on natural and experimental Haemonchus contortus infections in lambs. Vet Parasitol 141:273–278, 2006.
20. Muscona: Personal communication, 2009.
21. Shaik S, Terrill T, Miller J, et al: Effects of feeding sericea lespedeza hay to goats infected with Haemonchus contortus, S Afr J Anim Sci 34(suppl 1):248–258, 2004.
22. Soli F, Terrill T, Shaik S, et al: Efficacy of copper oxide wire particles against gastrointestinal nematodes in sheep and goats. Vet Parasitol 168:93–96, 2010.

23. Southern Consortium for Small Ruminant Parasite Control: Alternative dewormers, do they work? 2006 (http://www.scsrpc.org/SCSRPC/Publications/part5.htm).
24. Terrill T, Dykes G, Shaik S, et al: Efficacy of sericea lespedeza hay as a natural dewormer in goats: Dose titration study. Vet Parasitol 163:52–56, 2009.
25. Terrill T, Larsen M, Samples O, et al: Capability of the nematode-trapping fungus Duddingtonia flagrans to reduce infective larvae of gastrointestinal nematodes in goat feces in the southeastern United States: Dose titration and dose time interval studies. Vet Parasitol 120:285–296, 2004.
26. Terrill T, Mosjidis J, Moore D, et al: Effect of pelleting on efficacy of sericea lespedeza hay as a natural dewormer in goats. Vet Parasitol 146:117–122, 2007.
27. van Wyk J, Hoste H, Kaplan R, Besier R: Targeted selective treatment for worm management—How do we sell rational programs to farmers? Vet Parasitol 139:336–346, 2006.

CHAPTER 76

Thiafentanil Oxalate (A3080) in Nondomestic Ungulate Species

William R. Lance and David E. Kenny

Prior to the advent of potent opioids, the restraint and immobilization of nondomestic ungulates has been extremely problematic. There continues to be a need for pharmacologic agents that will quickly and safely immobilize nondomestic ungulates of all sizes. This group may range in weight from several hundred to several thousand kilograms. Opioids have been used for this purpose since the 1960s; opioids have been the primary immobilizing agents for this group of animals.

Thiafentanil oxalate is a potent opioid that is a synthetic fentanyl derivative, structurally similar to sufentanil. It has a molecular formula of $C_{24}H_{30}N_2O_2S$, a molecular mass of 506.57, and the molecular name 4-(methoxycarbonyl)-4-(N-phenylmethoxyacetamido)-1-[2-(thienyl)ethyl]piperidium oxalate. It represents the next generation of opioid immobilizing agents, following etorphine HCl and carfentanil citrate.

FEATURES OF THIAFENTANIL OXALATE

Structural Formula

Pharmacology

Thiafentanil oxalate has a morphine-like analgesic mode of action and produces rapid immobilization following intramuscular injection.

Clinical Considerations

The advantage of thiafentanil oxalate compared with the previously mentioned opioids (etorphine and carfentanil) is a shortened induction time, by as much as 50%, while still retaining equivalent agonist activity.[7] In an elk study, thiafentanil oxalate was found to have 63% the potency; in another study, it was found to have higher potency than carfentanil HCl and twice the potency of etorphine.[18,23,24] In cervids, the induction time was found to be shortened by 26% to 65% when compared with carfentanil. Thiafentanil appears to be not only more rapidly absorbed, but also more rapidly metabolized in those species in which it has been tested in. In ferrets, recovery from thiafentanil oxalate anesthesia was found to be two to four times more rapid when compared with carfentanil. Because of the shortened half-life, opioid renarcotization has not been a problem. This is a particularly important feature when working with free-ranging wildlife. Renarcotization is dangerous for free-ranging wildlife because prolonged struggling during recovery may lead to several life-threatening sequelae, such as hyperthermia, trauma, capture myopathy, and predation. There are multiple reports of complete thiafentanil oxalate reversal with the antagonist naltrexone, with no renarcotization.* Elk immobilized with thiafentanil oxalate and not reversed with an antagonist recovered spontaneously in 27 to 106 minutes, depending on the initial dose of thiafentanil oxalate. If the targeted free-ranging nondomestic ungulate escapes capture when darted, it may still successfully recover without the administration of an antagonist.

Thiafentanil oxalate is currently approved and registered for use in the Republic of South Africa. There is now a wealth of knowledge and experience with its use in African species. Published reports date back to a 1993 peer-reviewed study performed in Kruger National Park, South Africa.[12] Several current veterinary textbooks on

*References 2, 5, 12, 16, 20, 21, and 27.

exotic and wildlife capture recommend thiafentanil oxalate as a drug of choice.[8,26] A veterinary textbook on the subject of African wildlife anesthesia contains many protocols for the administration of thiafentanil oxalate to African ungulate species.[13] In North America, there have been several peer-reviewed articles on its use in North American ungulate species.* It has become the drug of choice for the American pronghorn antelope.[16] One of the authors (DK) has successful experienced using thiafentanil oxalate in several captive and free-ranging African, North American, and Asian nondomestic ungulate species.[3] Finally, perhaps the most popular veterinary textbook on wildlife and zoologic immobilization describes thiafentanil oxalate immobilization protocols for several North American ungulate species and many African species.[15] As is the case with carfentanil, thiafentanil oxalate does not seem to be effective in nondomestic ungulates in the family Equidae.[20] Specific mention was made of Burchell's zebra *(Equus burchellii)*. Thiafentanil oxalate plus a sedative was moderately effective with captive Grevy zebra *(Equus grevyi)* and Przewalski's horse *(Equus prezewalskii)* in a North American zoological institution but not equal to etorphine. If etorphine is available, it continues to be the drug of choice for Equidae.

As with other opioids, all species may show signs of excitement, tachycardia or tachypnea, bradycardia or bradypnea, hypertension or hypotension, depressed respiration, cyanosis, poikilothermia, and reaction to sudden noise when immobilized with thiafentanil oxalate. In elk, only high doses of thiafentanil oxalate (10 µg/kg body weight [BW]) have an effect on respiratory rate; very high doses (50 µg/kg BW) cause only modest decreases in respiratory rate and no significant decreases in heart rate.[25] Thiafentanil oxalate appears to produce less respiratory and cardiac depression when compared with other potent opioids such as fentanyl, carfentanil, and etorphine.

Thiafentanil oxalate is suitable for use by deep intramuscular injection using remote delivery systems (e.g., pistol, rifle, pole syringe) or by intramuscular or intravenous delivery by a handheld syringe with animals that are manually restrained. Opioid immobilizing agents should never be stored in aluminum darts because potency is lost in a matter of days.[14] On occasion, thiafentanil oxalate is used by itself as an immobilizing agent but is more typically combined with tranquilizers (e.g., azaperone), sedatives (e.g., xylazine, medetomidine), and dissociative agents (e.g., ketamine, telazol)

*References 10, 17, 18, 21, 25, and 27.

as a part of balanced anesthesia protocol. Balanced anesthesia lessens the dose of each agent maximizing their beneficial properties and minimizing the undesirable side effects.

The rapid immobilization provided by thiafentanil oxalate means that targeted animals may be handled and secured quicker than with carfentanil, mitigating problems with trauma, overheating, and escapes by free-ranging wildlife. Because the half-life is approximately 50% that of carfentanil, it is a safer drug because there is less potential for renarcotization. The concentration at 10 mg/mL also improves safety because it may be delivered in a dart, 3 mL, for most species. This improves dart ballistics and provides greater accuracy in delivery to the target.

Thiafentanil oxalate should only be used by zoologic, wildlife, or exotic animal veterinarians or field biologists who have received training and are supervised by the aforementioned veterinarians. Needles and syringes contaminated with thiafentanil oxalate should be secured and disposed of in a safe fashion. When dosed and delivered appropriately, thiafentanil oxalate has a wide margin of safety for target species.

Issues involving introduction of the drug into the human or animal food chain should be avoided. Users should refer to appropriate regulatory guidelines regarding use in animals that may be in the human food chain. This is not an issue with zoological animals.

Thiafentanil oxalate is commercially formulated as 10 mg/mL. Dosing for thiafentanil oxalate cannot be given on a strict millgram per kilogram basis because there is much species variability. Most species will require a total dose of 10 mg. At this formulation, the combination of thiafentanil oxalate and a sedative will fit in a dart of 3 mL or smaller. Darts of this size may typically be delivered safely and accurately (reliable ballistics) to most exotic ungulate species.

Doses will also vary depending on the situation: captive versus free-ranging animals, agitated versus quiet animals, healthy versus sick animals. In field conditions, it is often desirable to err on the side of overdosing so that the animal does not flee too long and too far, leading to trauma, overheating, and capture myopathy. Specific doses and recommendations are given in Table 76-1 for some nondomestic ungulate species.

HUMAN SAFETY

The same handling protocols currently in place for etorphine and carfentanil should be applied to handling thiafentanil oxalate. The handler should be

TABLE 76-1   Dosing Table Thianil

Species	Dose Thianil	Number	Recommended Dose	Additional Drugs
Personal Experience, David Kenny, V.M.D. & Scott Citino, D.V.M.				
Przewalskii horse	12.0-15.5 µg/kg[13]	2	4-6 mg[13]	10 mg med + 125 mg ket
Grevy zebra	20.0-26.0 µg/kg[13]	4	8-10 mg[13]	10-20 mg med + 300 mg ket
Bongo	53.0 µg/kg[13]	1	6 mg[13]	10 mg xylazine
Lesser kudu	94.0-140 µg/kg[13]	2	6-9 mg[13]	1-1.5 mg med + 100 mg ket
Rocky Mtn bighorn	10.0 µg/kg[13]	1	Male 10 mg[13]	4 mg med + 200 mg ket
Waterbuck	95.5 µg/kg[13]	1	10 mg[13]	2 mg med + 200 mg ket
White-lipped deer	54.5 µg/kg[13]	1	10 mg[13]	1.5 mg med
White-tailed deer	3 mg[13]	1	3 mg[13]	None
Brazilian tapir	2 mg[13]	1	2 mg[13]	30 mg xylazine
Mouflon	3 mg[13]	1	3 mg[13]	5 mg xylazine
Pronghorn	10 mg[13]	~5	10 mg[13]	35 mg xylazine
Gerenuk	40-45 µg/kg[3]	?	40-45 µg/kg[3]	40-60 µg/kg + ket 3.5 mg/kg
Nile Lechwe	20-22 µg/kg[3]	?	20-22 µg/kg[3]	16-22 µg/kg + ket 1.6-3.0 mg/kg
Clinical Expert Report , J. P. Raath, Bvsc.				
1st Study				
African buffalo	17.0-37.0 µg/kg[21]	9		Recommends adding a tranquilizer
Eland	37.0-110.0 µg/kg[21]	8		Recommends adding a tranquilizer
Greater kudu	37.0-120.0 µg/kg[21]	12		Recommends adding a tranquilizer
African elephant	15-40 mg total dose[21]	9	Male 15 mg[18] Female 12 mg	Recommends adding a tranquilizer
White rhino	4 mg total dose[21]	4		Recommends adding a tranquilizer
Warthog	40.0-123[21]	8	6 mg[18]	Recommends adding a tranquilizer
Waterbuck	34.0-43.0 µg/kg[21]	10	Male 7 mg[18] Female 5 mg	Recommends adding a tranquilizer
Clinical Expert Report, J. P. Raath, Bvsc.				
Lechwe	47.9 µg/kg[22]	5	4 mg[18]	Recommends adding a tranquilizer
Nyala	115.9 µg/kg[22]	8		Recommends adding a tranquilizer
Sable antelope	29.4 µg/kg[22]	14		Recommends adding a tranquilizer
Waterbuck	24.4 µg/kg[22]	9		Recommends adding a tranquilizer
White rhino	~2-3 µg/kg[22]	7	Male 5 mg[18] Female 4 mg	Recommends adding a tranquilizer
African buffalo	11-14 µg/kg[22]	16	Field 10 mg[18] Boma 5 mg	Recommends adding a tranquilizer
Roan antelope	26.3 µg/kg[22]	18		Recommends adding a tranquilizer
Summaries of Field Data, J. P. Raath, Bvsc.				
Common duiker	1-4 mg[23]	4	1 mg[18]	A. 0.1 ml domosedan + 50 mg ket B. 20 mg azaperone C. 10 mg xylazine
Bushbuck	2-4 mg[23]	14	3 mg[18]	A. 0.2 ml domosedan B. 80 mg azaperone C. 15 mg xylazine D. 80 mg azaperone
Blesbuck	1.5-3 mg[23]	3	3 mg[18]	20-40 mg azaperone
Impala	1.5-4 mg[23]	15	Male 2 mg[18] Female 1 mg	A. 0.2 ml domosedan B. 20-50 mg azaperone C. 20 mg xylazine D. 1.5 mg azap + 30 mg ket

Continued

TABLE 76-1 Dosing Table Thianil—cont'd

Species	Dose Thianil	Number	Recommended Dose	Additional Drugs
Summaries of Field Data, J. P. Raath, Bvsc.—cont'd				
Blue wildebeest	3-6 mg[23]	6	5 mg[18]	A. 30 mg azap + 10 mg ket
				B. 20 mg xylazine
				C. 7 mg domosedan
Eland	2-22 mg[23]	40	Male 15 mg[18] Female 10 mg	A. 25-60 mg azaperone
				B. 30-40 mg azap + 30 mg xylazine
				C. 100-200 mg xylazine
				D. 5 mg m99
				E. 17 mg domosedan
White rhino	1-4 mg[23]	9		A. 3-4 mg M99
				B. 2.5-3 mg M99 + 60-100 mg azap
Black rhino	1-2 mg[23]	4	4 mg[18]	A. 3 mg M99 + 100 mg azap
				B. 2-3 mg M99
Giraffe	2-16 mg[23]	38	12-15 mg[18]	A. 4 mg M99 + 30 mg azap
				B. 5-9 mg M99
				C. 20-50 mg azaperone
Sable antelope	1-10 mg[23]	36	5 mg[18]	A. 20-80 mg azaperone
				B. 4 mg M99 + 60 mg azap
				C. 3-5 mg M99
				D. 2.5 mg M99 + 60 mg azap + 100 mg ket
				E. 150 mg ketamine
				F. 40-100 mg azap + 10-20 mg xyl
				G. 40 mg azap + 30 mg fentanyl
				H. 100 mg xylazine
Roan antelope	0.6-14 mg[23]	20	6 mg[18]	A. 10-100 mg azaperone
				B. 2-4 mg M99 + 60 mg azap
				C. 50 mg azap + 50 mg xyl
				D. 1-2 mg M99
Waterbuck	3-10 mg[23]	23		A. 0.4 ml domosedan
				B. 24-100 mg azaperone
				C. 30 mg xylazine
				D. 4 mg M99
				E. 50 mg Azap + 50 mg xyl
Red hartebeest	2.5-8 mg[23]	6	4 mg[18]	A. 20-50 mg azaperone
				B. 2 mg M99 + 60 mg azap
				C. 3 mg M99
Reedbuck	2-8 mg[23]	14		A. 40 mg azaperone
				B. 10-15 mg xylazine
				C. 30 mg azap + 10 mg xyl
Tsessebe	1.5-7 mg[23]	25	3-4 mg[18]	A. 0.3 ml domosedan
				B. 10-60 mg azaperone
				C. 30-40 mg azap + 8-10 mg xyl
				D. 50 mg azap + 50 mg ket
				E. 150 mg ketamine
Steenbok	1 mg[23]	2	0.5 mg[18]	20 mg azaperone
Greater kudu	5-20 mg[23]	16	Male 15 mg[18] Female 8 mg	A. 30-100 mg xylazine
				B. 30-60 mg azaperone
				C. 30-50 mg azap + 15-60 mg xyl
				D. 5-20 mg domosedan
Gemsbok	3-8 mg[23]	7	7 mg[18]	A. 28 mg azaperone
				B. 40-120 mg azaperone
				C. 30-40 mg xylazine
Springbok	1 mg[23]	1	1 mg[18]	A. 3.5 mg M99
Klipspringer	0.5-1 mg[23]	2	0.5 mg[18]	A. 20 mg azaperone
Zebra	7 mg[23]	1	Not recommended	A. 150 mg azaperone

TABLE 76-1   Dosing Table Thianil—cont'd

Species	Dose Thianil	Number	Recommended Dose	Additional Drugs
Summaries of Field Data, J. P. Raath, Bvsc.—cont'd				
Black wildebeest	1.5-3 mg[23]	3	4 mg[18]	A. 40 mg azaperone
				B. 1.5 mg M99 + 40 mg azap
African buffalo	0.01-15 mg[23]	85		A. 10-120 mg azaperone
				B. 25-30 mg fentanyl +80 mg azap
				C. 4 mg M99
				D. 2.5-5 mg M99 + 50-60 mg azap
				E. 1 mg M99 + 150 mg ket + 20 mg xyl
				F. 40-70 mg azap + 20-60 mg xyl
				G. 3 mg M99 + 2 mg detom + 60 mg azap
Nyala	2-10 mg[23]	50	Male 10 mg[18]	A. domosedan? + 180-200 mg ket
			Female 6 mg	B. 20-60 mg azaperone
				C. 3-3.5 mg M99
				D. 20-200 mg xylazine
				E. 30-60 mg azap + 15-25 mg ket
				F. 40 mg stesnil + 20 mg xyl
				G. 3 mg M99 + 60 mg azap
				H. 45 mg stresnil
Oribi[4]			1 mg[18]	None provided
Reedbuck[4]			3 mg[18]	A. 2 mg detom + 30 mg xyl
Impala	30-80 µg/kg[12]	24	80.7 µg/kg[11]	None given
African buffalo[9]		10	0.025 µg/kg[11]	None given
Greater kudu[9]		10	0.077 µg/kg[11]	None given
Eland[9]		10	0.068 µg/kg[11]	None given
Waterbuck[9]		10	0.034 µg/kg[11]	None given
Attachment C Recommended Doses North American Species				
Elk	15 mg[19]	21	12 mg[18]	A. 50 mg xyl + 5 mg med
Pronghorn antelope	4-5 mg[15]		5 mg[18]	A. 25 mg xylazine
Moose	10 mg[30]	18	10 mg[18]	None provided
Mule deer			10-12 mg[18]	A. 100 mg xylazine
Literature Search Review				
Tibetan yak	Male 3.7-5.0 mg[2]	10	0.018 mg/kg[2]	0.15 mg/kg xylazine
	Female 4.0-7.5 mg			1 mg/kg propofol
Roan antelope	10-30 µg/kg[4]	20	10-13 µg/kg[4]	5-21 µg/kg med + 0.29-1.11 mg/kg ket
L. hartebeest	11-29 µg/kg[15]	13		5-10 µg/kg med + 0.7-1.4 mg/kg ket
Giraffe	Captive 5.8 µg/kg[6]	12		12.9 µg/kg med + 0.65 mg/kg ket
	FR ground 6.6 µg/kg[6]	29		15.9 µg/kg med + 0.5 mg/kg ket
	FR heli 10 µg/kg[6]	9		14.0 µg/kg med + 0.39 mg/kg ket
Nyala	45 µg/kg[7]	28	40-50 µg/kg[7]	60-80 µg/kg med + 200 mg ket
Gemsbok	22-45 µg/kg[18]	20		22-45 µg/kg med + 200 mg ket
Pronghorn antelope	0.1 mg/kg[-1 10]	5		None given
Impala	20-90 µg/kg[11]	50	51 µg/kg[11]	None given
Impala	80.7 µg/kg ED90	44	80.7 µg/kg ED90	None given
Giant eland	14.4 ug/kg[20]	5	Not recommended	8.6 ug/kg medetomidine + .86 mg/kg ketamine
Giant eland	12.5 ug/kg[20]	1	Not recommended	1.9 ug/kg medetomidine + .38 mg/kg azaperone + .91 mg/kg ketamine
Giant eland	15.7 ug/kg[20]	1	Not recommended	.52 mg/kg azaperone + .84 mg/kg ketamine
Axis deer	9 ug/kg[26]	9	Not recommended	3 ug/kg medetomidine + .33 mg/kg ketamine
Wapiti (elk)	.88 ug/kgED50[2]	69	2 ug/kg	None given
	2 ug/kg			
Mule deer	0.1 mg/kg[32]	6	0.15-0.2 mg/kg +	100 mg xylazine
	0.2 mg/kg	4	100 mg	Xylazine at various ratios from 3:1 to 30:1 to
	0.15-0.2 mg/kg	165	xylazine[32]	thiafentanil

paired with a second person who is also knowledgeable about the hazards of working with potent opioids and wear latex gloves and protective eyewear. All personnel involved in a capture should be informed that potent opioids are being used. Needles and syringes should be secured and safely disposed of following use.

Thiafentanil oxalate is a potent opioid and accidental human intoxication must be addressed immediately. Surface contamination sites should be treated aggressively with copious amounts of water to flush away any residual drug. If the intoxication is caused by an intramuscular injection, the patient needs to be treated expeditiously and aggressively. Individuals demonstrating opioid intoxication should be treated with the opioid antagonist naloxone hydrochloride intravenously or intramuscularly if a vein cannot be accessed quickly. The patient should be continuously monitored and supported while waiting for help from emergency medical services (EMS) personnel. Ideally, a person familiar with this opioid should accompany the patient, along with a copy of the package insert.

ANIMAL STUDIES

Table 76-1 illustrates immobilizations using thiafentanil oxalate in a variety of nondomestic ungulate species from South Africa and North America, and includes an extensive literature review. Raath has detailed the successful use of thiafentanil oxalate in 27 nondomestic African ungulates.[1,20] There are published reports for the use of thiafentanil oxalate in four North American free-ranging species.[17] Table 76-1 also details personal experience (of DK) with six African, three Asian, and three nondomestic ungulates in North and South American zoological parks.

Recommended Doses for Nondomestic Hoofstock

Doses used in nondomestic ungulate species to date have ranged from 0.5 mg (steenbok) to 15 mg (African elephant). Immobilization is usually achieved in 2 to 10 minutes following administration with a tranquilizer. The lower end of the dose range is suggested for those animals of quiet temperament, under confinement, that have not been hotly pursued prior to administration of the drug, or are in poor physical condition. The upper dose range is suggested for animals of excitable temperament following extensive pursuit or in situations in which an extremely short chase time is desirable. The upper end of the dose range may also be appropriate for animals being pursued by vehicle or aircraft when an extremely quick immobilization time is desired or when individuals are known to be highly excitable. In all cases, all factors, including nutritional, reproductive, and health status of an animal, as well as environmental conditions (e.g., temperature, cover, and terrain), must be evaluated and the best professional judgment used.

Administration

Inject the calculated dose deep into a large muscle mass of the neck, shoulder, back, or hindquarter. Intrathoracic, intra-abdominal, or subcutaneous injection is to be avoided. To ensure proper dosage for animals weighing less than 50 kg, remove the calculated dose of thiafentanil oxalate from the vial with a tuberculin syringe and dilute to an appropriate volume with sterile water for injection prior to administration. Always use safe technique by working in pairs, wearing disposable latex gloves, and wearing eye protection. Used syringes should be secured and disposed of in an appropriate biohazard container.

Antidote

Naltrexone (Trexonil) is the recommended antidote and rapidly reverses the effects of thiafentanil oxalate. The antagonist (naltrexone) should always be drawn up, labeled, and readily accessible prior to drawing up thiafentanil oxalate. Administer 10 mg of naltrexone for each milligram of thiafentanil oxalate. The total calculated dose of antagonist should be administered intramuscularly unless there is a medical or anesthetic emergency requiring immediate reversal; then, 25% of the calculated dose should be administered intravenously and 75% of the calculated dose should be administered intramuscularly. The entire dose may also be safely delivered intravenously but the operator should be prepared for occasional extrapyramidal activity and signs, and/or very rapid return to consciousness and mobility. Reversal of the effects of thiafentanil oxalate are usually observed in 2 to 10 minutes, with differences resulting from whether reversal is performed totally intramuscularly, split intravenous and intramuscular, or delivered completely intravenously, and according to the nature and reversal characteristics of the tranquilizer delivered with thiafentanil oxalate.

Warning

Thiafentanil oxalate must never be used unless an adequate amount of the reversal agent, naltrexone, is immediately available. Veterinarians using thiafentanil oxalate should be familiar with clinical procedures such as measurement of pulse and respiration, oxygen saturation, prevention of aspiration, relief of bloat, obstetric procedures, control of shock and hemorrhage, recognition of hyperventilation, heat exhaustion, capture myopathy, and immobilization of fractures. In cases of severe excitement during induction or delayed recovery, continued observation is necessary to correct any of these situations and to ensure that the animal does not injure itself.

Acknowledgments

We wish to recognize the valuable contributions to this chapter of Dr. Scott Citino of the White Oak Conservation Center, Yulee Florida; Dr. David Jessup of the California Department of Fish and Game; the Marine Wildlife Veterinary Care and Research Center, Santa Cruz, California; and Dr. J.PRaath of Wildlife Pharmaceuticals, Karino, South Africa. Their tireless fieldwork in wildlife anesthesia and academic excellence are greatly appreciated.

REFERENCES

1. Anonymous. 2009. Recommended A3080 dosages: South Africa and North America, pp 9–10.
2. Alcantar BE, McClean M, Chirife AD, et al: Immobilization of Tibetan yak (Bos gunnies) using A3080 (Thiafentanil) and xylazine in a wildlife park. In Proceedings of the American Association of Zoo Veterinarians Conference, 2007, pp. 47–48.
3. Citino SB: Personal communication. 2004.
4. Citino SB, Bush M, Grobler D, Lance W: Anaesthesia of roan antelope (Hippotragus equinus) with a combination of A3080, medetomidine and ketamine. J S Afr Vet Assoc 72:29–32, 2001.
5. Citino SB, Bush M, Grobler D, Lance W: Anesthesia of boma-captured Lichtenstein's hartebeest (Simoceros lichtensteinii) with a combination of thiafentanil, medetomidine, and ketamine. J Wildll Dis 38:457–462, 2002.
6. Citino SB, Bush M, Lance W, et al: Use of thiafentanil (A3080), medetomidine and ketamine for anesthesia of captive and free-ranging giraffe (Giraffa camelopardalis). In Proceedings of the American Association of Zoo Veterinarians Conference, 2006, pp 211–212.
7. Cooper DV, Grobler D, Bush M, et al: Anesthesia of nyala (Tragelaphus angasi) with a combination of thiafentanil (A3080), medetomidine and ketamine. J S Afr Vet Assoc 76:18–21, 2005.
8. Fowler ME, Miller RE: Zoo and wildlife animal medicine: Current therapy, ed 6, St. Louis, 2008, Saunders Elsevier.
9. Grobler D, Bush M, Jessup D, Lance W: Anaesthesia of gemsbok (Oryx gazella) with a combination of A3080, medetomidine and ketamine. J S Afr Vet Assoc 72:81–83, 2001.
10. Herbert J, Lust A, Fuller A, et al: Thermoregulation in pronghorn antelope (Antilocapra americana) in winter. J Exp Biol 211:749–756, 2008.
11. Janssen DL, Allen JL, Raath P, et al: Field studies with the narcotic immobilizing agent A3080. In Proceedings of the American Association of Zoo Veterinarians Conference, 1991, pp 340–342.
12. Janssen DL, Swan GE, Raath JP, et al: Immobilization and physiologic effects of the narcotic A-3080 in impala (Aepyceros melampus). J. Zoo Wildl Med 24:11–18, 1993.
13. Kock MD, Meltzer D, Burrows R, editors: Chemical and physical restraint of wild animals: A training and field manual for African species, Greyton, South Africa, 2006, International Wildlife Veterinary Services.
14. Kreeger TJ: Analyses of immobilizing dart characteristics. Wildl Soc Bull 30:968–970. 2002.
15. Kreeger TJ, Arnemo JM: Handbook of wildlife chemical immobilization, ed 3, Wheatland, WY, 2007, TJ Kreeger.
16. Kreeger TJ, Cook WE, Picho CA, Smith T: Anesthesia of pronghorns using thiafentanil or thiafentanil plus xylazine. J Wildl Mgmt 65:25–28, 2001.
17. Lance WR: Recommended dosages for adult animals, South Africa and North America, 2006, Attachment C. Fort Collins, Colo, Wildlife Pharmaceuticals, pp 9–10.
18. McJames SW, Smith IL, Stanley TH, Painter G: Elk immobilization with potent opioids: A3080 vs. carfentanil. In Proceedings of the American Association of Zoo Veterinarians Conference, 1993, pp 418–419.
19. Pye GW, Citino SB, Bush M, et al: Anesthesia of eastern giant eland (Taurotragus derbianus gigas) at White Oak Conservation Center. In Proceedings of the American Association of Zoo Veterinarians Conference, 2001, pp 226–231.
20. Raath JP: Clinical expert report: The use of thiafentanil oxalate (A3080) as an immobilizing agent in nondomestic species. pp 1–38, 2009.
21. Smith IL, McJames SW, Natte R, et al: A-3080 studies in elk: Effective immobilizing doses by syringe and dart injections. In Proceedings of the American Association of Zoo Veterinarians Conference, 1993, pp 420–421.
22. Smith KM, Powell DM, James SB, et al: Anesthesia of male axis deer (Axis axis): Evaluation of thiafentanil, medetomidine, and ketamine versus medetomidine and ketamine. J Zoo Wildl Med 37:513–517, 2006.
23. Stanley TH, McJames SW: Chemical immobilization using new high potency opioids and other drugs and drug combinations with high therapeutic indices, Washington DC, 1986, Final Report, U.S. Department of Defense, Contract DAAK11-84-K-0002.
24. Stanley TH, McJames SW, Kimball J: Chemical immobilization for the capture and transportation of big game. In Proceedings of the American Association of Zoo Veterinarians Conference, 1989, pp 13–14.
25. Stanley TH, McJames SW, Kimball J, et al: Immobilization of elk with A-3080. J Wildl Mgmt 52:577–581, 1988.
26. Tranquilli WJ, Thurmon JC, Grimm KA, editors: Lumb & Jones' Veterinary Anesthesia and Analgesia, ed 4, Ames, Iowa, 2007, Blackwell.
27. Wolfe LL, Lance WR, Miller MW: Immobilization of mule deer with thiafentanil (A-3080) or thiafentanil plus xylazine. J Wildl Dis 40:282–287, 2004.

CHAPTER 77

The Use of Butorphanol in Anesthesia Protocols for Zoo and Wild Mammals

Mitchell Bush, Scott B. Citino, and William R. Lance

Butorphanol tartrate is a synthetically derived opioid agonist-antagonist analgesic of the phenanthrene series, with a potency of about four to seven times that of morphine. In the United States, it is a U.S. Drug Enforcement Administration (DEA) class IV controlled substance. Butorphanol is a mixed agonist-antagonist with low intrinsic antagonist activity at receptors of the mu_1 (μ_1) and mu_2 (μ_2) opioid type (morphine-like), which are responsible for the significant opioid side effects and also an agonist with a high affinity for kappa (κ) opioid receptors. Butorphanol is also a sigma (σ) receptor agonist, which stimulates respiratory drive. Its interactions with these receptors in the central nervous system apparently mediate most of its pharmacologic effects, including analgesia. Generally, there is minimal cardiopulmonary depression with its use compared with other opioids and, at lower doses, there is a dose-dependent effect on respiratory depression but then a ceiling is reached and no further respiratory depression occurs. However, there is species variability, such as a fairly marked respiratory depression when used in primates.

In veterinary medicine, butorphanol tartrate is widely used as a sedative and analgesic in dogs, cats, and horses. It is administered either IM or IV, with its analgesic properties beginning to take effect about 15 minutes after IM injection and lasting about 4 hours. The elimination half-life is about 18 hours. For increased sedation or light anesthesia, it may be combined with sedatives such as α-adrenergic agonists (e.g., medetomidine, xylazine) or tranquilizers such as benzodiazepines (e.g., midazolam, diazepam) or phenothiazines (e.g., acepromazine) in dogs and cats. In horses, butorphanol is frequently combined with sedatives (e.g., xylazine, detomidine, romifidine) to make the horse easier to handle during veterinary procedures.

Butorphanol is relatively safe, with a high therapeutic index, and may be completely reversed rapidly with naloxone, nalmefene, or naltrexone, or partially reversed by diprenorphine, which antagonizes only the μ opioid receptors but not the κ opioid receptors. This partial reversal of the undesirable μ opioid receptor effects (muscle tremors, tachycardia-bradycardia, gastrointestinal stasis, euphoria-dysphoria, respiratory depression) while maintaining the sedative κ effect produces some useful and safer anesthetic protocols in nondomestic species.

As with other opioid analgesics, central nervous system effects (e.g., sedation, excitement) are considerations with the use of butorphanol. Nausea and vomiting are common. Less common are the gastrointestinal effects of other opioids, mostly constipation. Butorphanol is transported across the blood-brain and placental barriers and into milk. It is extensively metabolized in the liver with urinary excretion.

In zoo and wildlife species (mainly mammal), it is being used for one or more of the following: (1) pain control; (2) combined with sedatives to assist in minor manipulative procedures; (3) combined with α_2-adrenergic agonists and/or more potent opioids for anesthesia or neuroleptanalgesia. Butorphanol, when used alone, causes apathetic sedation that may allow arousal when the animal is stimulated, a potential danger when working with dangerous species.

Butorphanol combined with α_2-adrenergic agonists, potent opioids, dissociative anesthetics and/or tranquilizers may produce safer anesthesia procedures by minimizing many adverse effects. These combinations use lower doses of each agent and use the synergistic effects of the various drugs in the combination.

Butorphanol appears to be the opioid analgesic of choice for birds because analgesia is primarily regulated thorough κ receptors in birds; however, its analgesic efficacy is limited because of its short half-life in birds.[25] The development of a liposome-encapsulated formulation of butorphanol tartrate has extended its analgesic efficacy in birds to 3 to 5 days. Butorphanol has shown promise as a premedication for some avian species undergoing isoflurane inhalation anesthesia (see Chapter 41).

Butorphanol use in reptiles has shown limited analgesic effect and minor effects have also been seen when it is incorporated into various anesthetic protocols.[24,26] Because analgesia, in most reptiles studied to date, is μ opioid receptor–dependent, drugs such as morphine work best for analgesia.

The initial low commercial concentrations of butorphanol (10 mg/mL) made larger dart volumes necessary, which in turn adversely affected the performance and range of the dart. The various anesthetic protocols that use butorphanol are becoming more popular with the development of more concentrated formulations (30 and 50 mg/mL) that allow its use in remote delivery systems. One such formulation, containing butorphanol, azaperone, and medetomidine (BAM), has proved successful in a wide range of species.

Butorphanol combinations with tranquilizers and/or an α$_2$ agonist at low dosages are used together with restraint devices for standing restraint procedures in captive elephants, rhinoceros, giraffes, and tapirs.

USE IN VARIOUS SPECIES
Captive Elephant

As with other species, drug dosages for the sedation and anesthesia of elephants often vary among species and among individuals, so extrapolations should be used with caution. Butorphanol has been used mainly in combination with azaperone or α$_2$-adrenergic agonists (e.g., detomidine, xylazine) to manage excitable animals and/or for minor manipulative procedures.

In one report involving 14 standing clinical procedures in African elephants *(Loxodonta africana)*, a recommended starting dosage range of 14.7 to 16.2 μg/kg of both detomidine and butorphanol in a ratio of 1 : 1, on a microgram to microgram basis, were administered simultaneously IM. The initial effect was noted within 3.0 to 25 minutes (mean, 11.6 minutes; standard deviation [SD], ±5.9 minutes), with maximal effect occurring at 25 to 30 minutes for those procedures not requiring supplementation. This could subsequently be supplemented as needed using 4.0 to 7.3 μg/kg of each drug. Recovery after administration of reversal agents was rapid and complete, ranging from 2 to 20 minutes (mean, 9.0 minutes; SD, ±7.0 minutes).[18]

In Asian elephants *(Elephas maximus)*, a dose of 0.01 to 0.03 mg/kg administered IV, IM, or SC is suggested for minor manipulative procedures.[10] For aggressive adult African elephants, xylazine, 700 to 1000 mg/adult elephant (≈0.2 to 0. 3 mg/kg), followed by IV butorphanol, 50 to 180 mg/adult elephant (≈0.01 to 0.03 mg/kg), has proven effective.[22]

A xylazine-butorphanol combination was successfully used for standing restraint of Asian elephants at average doses of xylazine (70 μg/kg) and butorphanol (25 μg/kg) IV and reversal with naltrexone at approximately 50 μg/kg and yohimbine at 0.1 mg/kg. Atipamezole administered at 4 μg/kg IV provided better xylazine reversal than yohimbine.

Captive Rhinoceros

Butorphanol alone and in combinations with other tranquilizers and/or α$_2$-adrenergic agonists may facilitate many management and medical procedures, with or without restraint devices.

The use of a medetomidine-butorphanol combination for standing and recumbent chemical restraint of the white rhinoceros *(Ceratotherium simum)* has produced good results.[21] A mean dose of 63 ± 1.2 μg/kg butorphanol plus 2.64 ± 0.17 μg/kg medetomidine is given IM. Average doses for adult white rhinos are medetomidine, 5 to 7 mg, and butorphanol, 80 to 150 mg. Midazolam may be added to this cocktail at a total dose of 20 to 40 mg to improve relaxation. Animals become safe to work on in a standing position in about 8 to 20 minutes and then may be pulled down into recumbency, or supplemented with ketamine, 200 to 400 mg IV, to induce recumbency. Supplemental drugs used to maintain chemical restraint for long procedures include a constant rate IV infusion using guaifenesin 5% in dextrose, ketamine, butorphanol, medetomidine, propofol, or a combination of these. A wide range of procedures has been accomplished using these combinations, including electroejaculation, fiberoptic endoscopy, ophthalmic surgery, dental procedures, and daily repeated IV therapy. Reversal is accomplished with naltrexone, 233 ± 29 μg/kg (one to two times the butorphanol dose) and atipamezole, 14.7 ± 3.8 μg/kg (five times the medetomidine dose).[6]

Butorphanol is useful for modulating opioid receptor effects when etorphine is used in rhinoceroses. If etorphine combinations are used, partial reversal with butorphanol (titrate with 10 mg IV boluses) will reduce respiratory depression without getting arousal in the white rhinoceros.

For crate loading white rhinoceroses, a combination of etorphine-butorphanol-midazolam is useful. Doses are etorphine, 0.5 to 0.7 μg/kg, butorphanol, 15 to 25 μg/kg, and midazolam 15 to 25 μg/kg (average total doses for adults—etorphine 1.0 mg, butorphanol, 30 mg, midazolam, 30 mg). Etorphine causes the animal to continue to walk forward for loading. Once in the crate and loaded on the truck, the etorphine is reversed with diprenorphine at twice the etorphine dose; this only reverses the etorphine and leaves the butorphanol and midazolam on board for travel. Animals should be observed during travel for excessive pressing or getting into dangerous positions. If animals need to be fully reversed, they may be given naltrexone at one to two times the butorphanol dose. If various butorphanol combinations without etorphine are used for loading white rhinoceroses, the animals will tend to just stand and not move forward, so they may be difficult to load.

Two butorphanol combinations have been used in the captive black rhinoceros *(Diceros bicornis)*—butorphanol-azaperone and butorphanol-detomidine—but they are not recommend because restraint is not as good as with the white rhinoceros, which could be very dangerous for less experienced people. The black rhinoceros does not experience as much respiratory depression and other physiologic disturbances with etorphine as the white rhinoceros, so butorphanol combinations are generally not necessary.

Standing procedures on the Asian greater one-horned rhinoceros *(Rhinoceros unicornis)* using medetomidine-butorphanol-midazolam has been used successfully; average doses are medetomidine, 3 to 4 μg/kg, butorphanol, 50 to 60 μg/kg, and midazolam, 12 to 15 μg/kg. Most of these procedures have been for reproductive examinations on females (rectal ultrasound) and for IV therapy in sick rhinoceroses. Supplemental ketamine (200 to 400 mg IV) will produce recumbency. Reversal is with naltrexone at twice the butorphanol dose and atipamezole at five times the medetomidine dose. Standing sedation has also been produced in the Indian rhinoceros *(R. unicornis)* using a butorphanol-azaperone combination (adult, 100 mg of each).[20]

As with white rhinoceroses, butorphanol combinations are preferred in Sumatran rhinoceroses *(Dicerorhinus sumatrensis)* because better muscle relaxation and improved cardiopulmonary function are obtained when compared with the more potent opioids. A butorphanol (30 to 50 mg) and azaperone (50 to 60 mg) combination in adults may be used for standing sedation at the lower end of the dosage range or recumbency at the higher dosages.[20] A second combination using medetomidine (2.0 to 2.5 μg/kg) and butorphanol (70 to 72 μg/kg) produces a good standing chemical restraint in Sumatran rhinoceroses, after which they may be pulled into sternal recumbency. This combination also maintains acceptable physiology. Reversal is with naltrexone at twice the butorphanol dose and atipamezole at five times the medetomidine dose.

Captive Giraffe

The physical restraint of giraffe *(Giraffa camelopardalis)* in a confinement chute may be enhanced by the use of sedatives and tranquilizers. The combination of azaperone (250 to 350 μg/kg) plus detomidine (15 to 30 μg/kg) given IM produces good tranquilization and moderate analgesia. This combination facilitates blood sampling, reproductive examinations, tuberculin testing, joint taps, radiographs, suturing, and dystocia corrections. To increase sedation, 10 mg of butorphanol IV is used in adult animals. The detomidine is partially reversed with yohimbine (0.1 mg/kg) or atipamezole (0.2 mg/kg) and the butorphanol is reversed with naltrexone (2 mg naltrexone/1 mg butorphanol).

Captive Okapi

For standing chemical restraint in okapi *(Okapia johnstoni)*, combinations of either xylazine (0.4 to 0.8 mg/kg) and butorphanol (80 to 200 μg/kg) or detomidine (40 to 100 μg/kg) and butorphanol (80 to 200 μg/kg) provides good standing restraint for a variety of clinical procedures, including venipuncture, IV catheter placement, hoof trimming, endoscopy, bronchoalveolar lavage, insemination, rectal and transcutaneous ultrasound, thoracocentesis, and minor surgery. Animals will move around a bit, but otherwise the sedation is satisfactory. Reversal for the α_2-adrenergic agonist is with yohimbine, 0.1 to 0.2 mg/kg, or tolazoline, 0.5 mg/kg, and/or atipamezole, 30 to 50 μg/kg. The butorphanol is reversed with naltrexone at one to two times the butorphanol dose, if desired.

Other Ruminants

To improve analgesia and prolong down time in the gerenuk *(Litocranius walleri)* and other small ruminants anesthetized with medetomidine (60 to 70 μg/kg) and ketamine (2 to 3 mg/kg), butorphanol can be added to the anesthetic regimen. This has been very useful for electroejaculation in this species. Reversal is with atipamezole at five times the medetomidine dose and naltrexone at twice the butorphanol dose.

Medetomidine-butorphanol-ketamine has also been studied in Thomson's gazelles (Gazella thomsoni) with doses of medetomidine, 40.1 ± 3.6 μg/kg, butorphanol, 0.40 ± 0.04 mg/kg, and ketamine, 4.9 ± 0.6 mg/kg. This combination was successfully used for the castration of male Thompson's gazelles with the addition of local blocks at the surgical site. Mild hypoxemia and hypoventilation were seen in some animals not supplemented with intranasal oxygen. Animals stood within 12 minutes after reversal with atipamezole (0.20 ± 0.03 mg/kg) and naloxone (0.02 ± 0.001 mg/kg).[5]

The San Diego Zoo has reported excellent results using butorphanol (0.2 to 0.25 mg/kg) with medetomidine (0.03 mg/kg) for the chemical restraint of the takin (Budorcas taxicolor). Side effects included bradycardia and low oxygen saturation values. Nasal insufflation with oxygen helped maintain good oxygen saturation readings. Reversal with IM naltrexone (0.35 mg/kg) and atipamezole (five times the medetomidine dose) combination typically results in a smooth recovery in 7 to 8 minutes.[17]

A mixture of tiletamine-zolazepam (1.2 mg/kg) and butorphanol (0.1 mg/kg), and an equipotent sedative dose of α_2-adrenergic agonist (xylazine, detomidine, or medetomidine) was used in 18 different species of ungulates for routine medical procedures. To supplement the anesthesia, a 25-mg IV bolus of ketamine was given; this showed no after effect following reversal of the anesthesia with tolazoline (4 mg/kg) or atipamezole (1 mg/8 to 10 mg of xylazine) and naltrexone (1 mg/10 mg butorphanol). In some situations, the butorphanol was not reversed. Recovery times were not significantly affected by not reversing the butorphanol with naltrexone but the animals were not as alert following reversal. Rapid reversal with atipamezole was complete as expected in all combinations, with no recurrent sedation following antagonism. Despite being administered half IM and half SC, atipamezole reversed the effects more rapidly than tolazoline administered completely IV (1 to 8 minutes for atipamezole; 2 to 15 minutes for tolazoline). The zolazepam was not reversed.[19]

The San Diego Zoo uses a combination of medetomidine (70 to 100 μg/kg), butorphanol (300 μg/kg), and midazolam (300 μg/kg) for chemical restraint of its wild swine species and reversal with atipamezole (80 to 100 μg/kg) and naltrexone (350 to 700 μg/kg). If flumazenil is required to reverse midazolam; it is used at a ratio of 1 : 10 to 1 : 20 the dose of midazolam.[16]

A detomidine (59 to 79 μg/kg)-butorphanol (50 to 88 μg/kg) combination has been used for standing sedation in the banteng (Bos javanicus). For recumbent anesthesia, a combination of detomidine (69 to 104 μg/kg), butorphanol (71 to 83 μg/kg), and ketamine (0.60 to 2.78 mg/kg) has been used, with reversal with naltrexone and yohimbine.[7]

Tapir

In Baird's tapirs (Tapirus bairdii), a combination of medetomidine (6 to 8 μg/kg) and butorphanol (0.16 to 0.20 mg/kg) produces a good anesthesia. The combination can be reversed with atipamezole at five times the medetomidine dose and naltrexone at twice the butorphanol dose.[27]

Twenty immobilizations of 16 free-ranging Baird's tapirs in Corcovado National Park, Costa Rica, were successfully performed with a butorphanol-xylazine combination administered by remote injection. Tapirs were estimated to weigh between 200 and 300 kg. Butorphanol (48 ± 1.84 mg/animal) and xylazine (101 ± 2.72 mg/animal) were used. In some cases, ketamine was used IM or IV at 187 ± 40.86 mg/animal to prolong the anesthesia period. Naltrexone (257 ± 16.19 mg/animal) IM was used to reverse butorphanol. Yohimbine (34 ± 0.61 mg/animal) or tolazoline (12 ± 10.27 mg/animal) was used to reverse xylazine.[9]

A male Malayan tapir (Tapirus indicus; estimated weight of 340 kg) with oral squamous cell carcinoma was successfully treated under anesthesia using IM butorphanol (80 mg [0.24 mg/kg]) and either xylazine (120 mg [0.35 mg/kg]) or detomidine (12 mg [35 μg/kg]).[15]

Equids

Good standing restraint in Grevy's zebra (Equus grevyi) may be produced using a combination of detomidine (0.1 to 0.15 mg/kg) and butorphanol (0.2 to 0.25 mg/kg). Animals may then be induced to recumbency with an IV bolus of ketamine (200 to 500 mg total dose). Reversal can be accomplished with naltrexone at twice the butorphanol dose and yohimbine at 0.1 to 0.2 mg/kg plus tolazoline at 0.25 mg/kg.

The Somali wild ass (Equus asinus) may be anesthetized using a combination of etorphine (3 to 3.5 mg), detomidine (10 to 12 mg), and acepromazine (5 to 6 mg), but they developed significant respiratory depression ($SpO_2 = 70\%$ to 80%). Butorphanol (10 mg IV) can be used for partial reversal of the μ opioid effects of etorphine; within 5 minutes of administration, SpO_2 values rise to more than 90%.

For a more effective immobilization of the free-ranging Asiatic wild ass, butorphanol (10 mg) is added to the darting combination of etorphine (2.5 to 3.0 mg) and detomidine (10 mg), because butorphanol reduces respiratory depression and limits the etorphine-specific pacing, so that animals travel less distance after darting.[28]

Carnivores

For a completely reversible anesthesia in the cheetah (*Acinonyx jubatus*), a combination of medetomidine (35 ± 3.7 µg/kg), butorphanol (0.2 ± 0.02 mg/kg), and midazolam (0.15 ± 0.02 mg/kg) has proved successful. This combination has been used in more than 200 cheetahs, including very sick animals. Physiologic parameters remained good, except for bradycardia, accentuated sinus arrhythmia, and mild to moderate hypertension. This combination seems ideal for field procedures in which quick recovery and release are desirable. Reversal was complete with IM atipamezole at five times the medetomidine dose, naltrexone at 0.25 mg/kg, and flumazenil at 6 µg/kg.[13]

A reversible anesthetic combination using medetomidine (44.5 ± 9.1 µg/kg), butorphanol (0.24 ± 0.06 mg/kg), and midazolam (0.29 ± 0.1 mg/kg) was used successfully in a semi–free-ranging setting for the chemical restraint of African wild dogs (*Lycaon pictus*).[8] Mean induction times were 6 ± 5 minutes and acceptable physiology was monitored during a 38-minute working time (±6 minutes). The effects on the wild dogs were reversed with IM injections of atipamezole, 3 mg, naltrexone, 10 mg, and flumazenil, 0.2 mg. A similar successful study was done on free-ranging spotted hyena in Kruger National Park, with good results.[12]

A combination of IM medetomidine (0.4 mg/kg) and butorphanol (0.4 mg/kg) was evaluated in 16 red wolves (*Canis rufus*). Seven wolves received only medetomidine and butorphanol, and the other 9 wolves also received IV diazepam once the animal was down. Both these combinations produced a completely reversible anesthetic that also prevented the undesirable effects of hypertension and prolonged and rough recoveries; these were previously noted when an α_2-adrenergic agonist and ketamine were used for anesthesia. The reversal used IM atipamezole (0.2 mg/kg) for the medetomidine and naloxone (0.02 mg) for the butorphanol. The diazepam was reversed with IV flumazenil (0.04 mg/kg).[14]

Veterinary Wildlife Services, South African National Parks, have recently conducted a field trial (N = 30) in adult and subadult lions (*Panthera leo*) using a combination of butorphanol (0.3 mg/kg), medetomidine (0.05 mg/kg), and midazolam (0.2 mg/kg) and found it to be a very effective immobilizing drug combination.[2] Induction times were rapid, the animals were very stable while immobilized, and the combination could be reversed at any time. During the trial, the effects were reversed after 45 minutes, but subsequent use of the combination has shown it to be effective for at least 1.5 hours. In the initial stages of the study, all lions were blindfolded and had their front limbs hobbled in the event of a spontaneous recovery; at these dose rates, this still could happen. The antidotes are IV naltrexone (2.2 times the butorphanol dose), atipamezole, both IV and SC (2.5 times the medetomidine dose), and IV flumazenil (0.016 times the midazolam dose). We have subsequently found that it is not essential to administer the flumazenil, especially if the animals have been immobilized for longer than 1 hour. Reversal was smooth and rapid. This combination is proving to be very effective in immobilizing lions because the effects may be completely reversed; the main drawback is the costs of the drugs.

As a safety rule, it is a good idea to use caution and have some restraint of large dangerous carnivores when medetomidine and/or butorphanol are used without a dissociative anesthetic (ketamine or tiletamine-zolazepam) in the protocol, because sudden arousal may occur, especially at lower doses of medetomidine and/or butorphanol.

African Buffalo

The captive management of specific disease-free African buffalo (*Syncerus caffer*) is a major economic concern in Southern Africa. Presently, extensive testing is required to certify the disease status of those animals requiring repeated anesthesia and manipulation; also, there is extensive relocation of disease-free buffalo. The use of butorphanol has been shown to assist in and facilitate the management of these large, dangerous, and belligerent animals.[11] The buffalo are first anesthetized using etorphine-azaperone combinations at 8 and 12 mg total dosage, respectively, for bulls and 6 and 50 mg for cows. To move the animals to a transport vehicle or crate, the buffalo, which are blindfolded and have earplugs, are given IV butorphanol (25 mg for cows and 50 mg for bulls). After 45 seconds, the animals may be stimulated to stand and walk passively to the desired destination, which minimizes the physical effort of carrying them. The butorphanol also improves the respiration of the buffalo and thus the safety of the procedure.

BUTORPHANOL-CONTAINING ANESTHETIC COCKTAILS

The butorphanol combination that has rapidly come into use in hoofstock and large carnivores since 2008 is a mixture, BAM, in an approximate ratio of butorphanol (30 mg/mL), azaperone (18 mg/mL), and medetomidine (10 mg/mL). The combination concentrations and total dose volumes are adjusted slightly in some species. The total dose volumes range from 0.5 to 3 mL in most species. Table 77-1 lists various species and average doses.

This combination has been successfully used to anesthetize female white-tailed deer (65 to 75 kg) using 1.0 to 1.5 mL of the combination. Large, mature, white-tailed male deer may require up to 2.5 mL of this formulation. Over 1000 white-tailed deer have been anesthetized in Texas with this combination.[3] Large members of the family Felidae (lions, tigers, mountain lions) may be anesthetized with very small dart volumes of this combination (0.5 to 1.0 mL. In these large felids, the addition of ketamine to the protocol has resulted in a more effective anesthesia.[1] Induction to sternal recumbency usually requires 7 to 15 minutes and is extremely smooth and controlled.

Anesthesia with this combination is characterized by lack of postinduction hyperthermia, excellent respiration rates and patterns, and good muscle relaxation. The anesthesia may be reversed IM with atipamezole (3 mg/mg of medetomidine) or tolazoline (100 mg for every 10 mg of medetomidine) and naltrexone (50 mg for every 30 mg of butorphanol). The reversal is rapid and complete in less than 10 minutes in most species.

This BAM combination has not produced acceptable anesthesia in fallow deer. It has been tried for anesthesia for semen collection in white-tailed deer but the results have not been acceptable.

Rhinoceros Anesthesia

One study has compared a standard anesthesia protocol with the same protocol containing butorphanol in a capture cocktail for the capture of 31 white rhinoceroses. The control group contained 15 animals.[29] The standard anesthetic mixture used in both groups included etorphine, azaperone, and detomidine plus hyaluronidase, and dosages were adjusted for the age of the animal. In the study group, butorphanol (10 to 20 mg) was added to the anesthetic combination. No difference in induction time was noted, but the distance traveled following darting was shorter in the butorphanol group. They also reported no improvement in the measured physiologic parameters in the butorphanol group. Both groups showed metabolic acidosis, hypercapnia, and

TABLE 77-1	Butorphanol, Azaperone, and Medetomidine (BAM) Dosages in Hoofstock and Carnivores			
		BAM DOSAGES (MG/KG, AVERAGE)		
Study (Year)	Species	Butorphanol	Azaperone	Medetomidine
Seigal-Willot et al (2009)[23]; Wolfe (2010)*	White-tailed deer, *Odocolieus virginianus*	0.58	0.37	0.19
Wolfe (2010)*	Mule deer, *Odocoileus hemionus*	0.58	0.37	0.19
Wolfe (2010)*	Elk, *Cervus elaphus*	0.11	0.07	0.05
Wolfe (2010)*	Pronghorn, *Antilocapra americana*	0.74	0.68	0.28
Wolfe (2010)*	Bighorn sheep, *Ovis canadensis*	0.44	0.26	0.20
Shury (2010)†	Bison, *Bison bison*	0.29	0.14	0.07
Armstrong (2010)[1]; Wolfe et al (2008)[30]	Large felids	0.159	0.128	0.053
Wolfe (2010)*	Przewalski's horse, *Equus caballus przewalskii*	0.09	0.08	0.07
Citino (2010)‡	Nile hippopotamus, *Hippopotamus amphibibus*	0.10	0.10	60 µg/kg

*Wolfe L: Personal communication.
†Shury T: Personal communication.
‡Citino SB: Personal experience.

TABLE 77-2   Physiologic Data on Awake and Anesthetized White Rhinoceros

Time	pH	Po₂ (mm Hg)	Pco₂ (mm Hg)	O₂ Saturation (%)	Base Excess (mEq/liter)	Heart Rate (beats/min)	Respiratory Rate (breaths/min)	Systolic Blood Pressure (mm Hg)
Awake Rhinoceros (n = 12)								
—	7.391	98.2	49	97.2	3.5	39	19	160
Standard Protocol: Etorphine + Azaperone (n = 10) Ref 4								
0 time	7.175	35	62	49	−6.4	139	10	190
10 min	7.246	37	70	62	−0.3	122	11	151
20 min	7.244	41	64	69	−1.4	103	9	159
Protocol 1: Etorphine + Butorphanol + Midazolam (n = 48)								
0 time	7.270	56	48	89	−4.7	74	9	141
10 min	7.284	59	50	89	−3.0	65	9	143
20 min	7.305	59	51	90	−1.4	62	9	136
Protocol 2: Protocol 1 With a Partial Reverse Using Diprenorphine M50-50 (at 12 min; n = 16)								
0 time	7.289	46	52	82	−0.1	84	11	141
10 min	7.316	59	48	89	−2.1	65	10	140
20 min	7.350	67	48	92	−0.3	59	11	137

hypoxemia. Their conclusion was that the addition of butorphanol had little effect on the anesthetic procedure.

We have studied the anesthetic combination of etorphine, butorphanol, and midazolam in 64 free-ranging white rhinoceroses in South Africa and our results differ from the above report.[4] As in the study noted, we observed no mortality or morbidity in the study animals. We found that the following combination provides the best results: etorphine (1.5 ± 0.5 μg/kg), butorphanol (50 ± 15 μg/kg), plus midazolam (25 ± 5 μg/kg).

The data from captive awake white rhinoceroses has served as a baseline for evaluation of the effect of our anesthetic protocols (Table 77-2).[4] We compared these normal parameters with a previous standard protocol (etorphine-azaperone combination) used in white rhinoceroses. Note in this table the marked hypoxemia, elevated Pco₂, slight acidosis, and elevated heart rate observed when the standard protocol is used. We currently believe that the addition of butorphanol to the anesthetic combinations at the ratio of at least 20:1 butorphanol to etorphine for white rhinoceros anesthesia greatly improves the physiologic status and safety of the animal during the procedure compared with previous anesthetic protocols such as the etorphine-azaperone combination. This was indicated by improved hemoglobin oxygen saturation, decreased heart rate, and improved muscle relaxation, which in turn improves respiratory efficiency.

With this combination, an initial slightly higher dose of etorphine than usually used may be required to produce recumbency. It should be noted that although the down time is longer, the rhinoceroses tend to stop walking within 5 to 6 minutes. We also found it helpful to let the animals stand longer (5 minutes) before manipulation because this results in a smoother anesthesia. This combination offers another unique safety factor in the case of respiratory depression, The administration of a low IV dose of diprenorphine (M 50-50) (1 mg) will further antagonize the μ opioid effect of etorphine that caused the depressed respiration, muscle rigidity and tremors, and tachycardia, thus improving the physiologic parameters (see Table 77-1). Sedation and control of the animal are maintained by the κ opioid receptor sedation of the butorphanol and the tranquilizer midazolam. With this partial reversal of the anesthesia, the animal may be induced to stand and walked into a crate for transportation. Once loaded, the animal rides very well, with less head pressing because of the reversal of the μ opioid effect; sedation is maintained by the κ opioid effect of the butorphanol combined with midazolam. To reverse the etorphine and butorphanol, naltrexone is used because it reverses both μ and κ opioid effects, allowing the animal to regain its feet with only mild sedation remaining due to midazolam.

The differences reported in the results and conclusions from these two reports are probably the result of the use of both azaperone and detomidine with the etorphine, whereas we used only midazolam. Also, our ratio of butorphanol to etorphine was higher, at least 20:1 butorphanol to etorphine; they used a ratio of about 10:1 or lower.[29]

Drugs Mentioned in the Text

Atipamezole (Antisedan)—Farmos Pharmaceuticals; Turku, Finland

Azaperone (Stresnil)—Wildlife Pharmaceutical, Inc; Fort Collins, Colorado

Butorphanol (Butorphanol)—Wildlife Pharmaceutical, Inc; Fort Collins, Colorado

Etorphine (M99)—Wildlife Pharmaceutical, Inc; Fort Collins, Colorado

Flumazenil (Romazicon)—Roche Laboratories, Inc.; Nutley, New Jersey

Ketamine (Ketaset)—Fort Dodge Animal Health, Fort Dodge, Iowa

Naltrexone (Trexonil)—Wildlife Pharmaceutical, Inc; Fort Collins, Colorado

Medetomidine (Medetomidine)—Wildlife Pharmaceutical, Inc; Fort Collins, Colorado

Xylazine (Rompun)—Bayer Corporation; Shawnee, Kansas

Tiletamine–zolazepam (Telazol)—Fort Dodge Laboratories; Fort Dodge, Iowa

Tolozoline (Tolazine)—Lloyd Incorporated; Shenandoah, Iowa

Yohimbine (Antagonil)—Wildlife Pharmaceutical, Inc; Fort Collins, Colorado

REFERENCES

1. Armstrong D: Personal communication, 2010.
2. Bass P: Personal communication, 2010.
3. Bluntzer W: Personal communication, 2010.
4. Bush M, Citino SB, Grobler D: Improving cardio-pulmonary function for a safer anesthesia of white rhinoceros (*Ceratoherium simun*): use of opiate cocktails to influence receptor effects. In Proceedings of the AAZV, AZA/NAG Joint Conference, 2005, pp 259–260.
5. Chittick E, Horne W, Wolfe B, et al: Cardiopulmonary assessment of medetomidine, ketamine, and butorphanol anesthesia in captive Thomson's gazelles (*Gazella thomsoni*). J Zoo Wildl Med 32:168–175, 2001.
6. Citino SB: Use of medetomidine in chemical restraint protocols for captive African rhinoceroses. In Proceedings of the AAZV, ARAV Joint Conference, 2008, pp 108–109.
7. Curro TG: Non-domestic cattle. In West G, Heard D, Caulkett N, editors: Zoo animal and wildlife immobilization and anesthesia, Ames, Iowa, 2007, Blackwell, pp 635–642.
8. Fleming GJ, Citino SB, Bush M: Reversible anesthesia combination using medetomidine-butorphanol-midazolam in in-situ African wild dogs (*Lycaon pictus*). In Proceedings of the AAZV Conference, 2006, pp 214–215.
9. Foerster SH, Bailey JE, Aguilar R, et al: Butorphanol/xylazine/ketamine immobilization of free-ranging Baird's tapirs in Costa Rica. J Wildl Dis 36:335–341, 2000.
10. Fowler ME, Mikota SK: Chemical restraint and general anesthesia. In Fowler ME, Mikota SK, editors: Biology, medicine, and surgery of elephants, Ames, Iowa, 2006, Blackwell, pp 91–118.
11. Grobler D: Personal communication, 2010.
12. Hofmeyer M: Personal communication, 2010.
13. Lafortune L, Gunkel C, Valverde A, et al: Reversible anesthesia combination using medetomidine-butorphanol. midazolam (MBMZ) in cheetahs (*Acinonyx jubatus*). In Proceedings of the AAZV, AAWV, AZA/NAG Conference, 2005, pp 270.
14. Larsen RS, Loomis MR, Kelly BT, et al: Cardiorespiratory effects of medetomidine-butorphanol, medetomidine-butorphanol-diazepam, and medetomidine-butorphanol-ketamine in captive red wolves (*Canis rufus*). J Zoo Wildl Med 33:101–107, 2002.
15. Miller CL, Templeton RS, Karpinski L: Successful treatment of oral squamous cell carcinoma with intralesional fluorouracil in a Malayan tapir (*Tapirus indicus*). J Zoo Wildl Med 2:262–264, 2000.
16. Morris PJ, Bicknese B, Janssen DL, et al: Chemical immobilization of exotic swine at the San Diego Zoo. In Proceedings of the AAZV Conference, 1990, pp 150–153.
17. Morris PJ, Bicknese E, Janssen DL, et al: Chemical immobilization of takin (*Budorcas taxicolor*) at the San Diego Zoo. In Proceedings of the AAZV and IAAAM Joint Conference, 2000, pp 102–104.
18. Neiffer DL, Miller MA, Weber M, et al: Standing sedation in African elephants (*Loxodonta africana*) using detomidine-butorphanol combinations. J Zoo Wildl Med 36:250–256, 2005.
19. Parás A, Martínez O, Hernández A: Alpha-2-agonist in combination with butorphanol and tiletamie-zolazepam for immobilization of non-domestic hoofstock. In Proceedings of the AAZV Conference, 2002, pp 194–196.
20. Radcliffe RW, Morkel P: Rhinoceroses. In West G, Heard D, Caulkett N, editors: Zoo animal and wildlife immobilization and anesthesia, Ames, Iowa, 2007, Blackwell, pp 543–566.
21. Radcliffe RW, Shannon T, Ferrell ST, et al: Butorphanol and azaperone as a safe alternative for repeated chemical restraint in captive white rhinoceros (*Ceratotherium simum*). J Zoo Wildl Med 31:196–200, 2000.
22. Ramsay E: Standing sedation and tranquilization in captive African elephants (*Loxodonta africana*). In Proceedings of the AAZV Conference, 2000, pp 111–113.
23. Seigal-Willot J, Citino S, Wade S, et al: Butorphanol, azaperone, and medetomidine anesthesia in free ranging white-tailed deer (*Odocoileus virginianus*) using radio transmitters. J Wild Dis 45:468–480, 2009.
24. Sladky KK, Kinney ME, Johnson SM: Analgesic efficacy of butorphanol and morphine in bearded dragons and corn snakes. J Am Vet Med Assoc 233:267–273, 2008.
25. Sladky KK, Krugner-Higby L, Meek-Walker E, et al: Serum concentrations and analgesic effects of liposome-encapsulated and standard butorphanol tartrate in parrots. Am J Vet Res 67:775–781, 2006.
26. Sladky KK, Miletic V, Paul-Murphy J, et al: Analgesic efficacy and respiratory effects of butorphanol and morphine in turtles. J Am Vet Med Assoc 230:1356–1362, 2007.
27. Trim CM, Lamberski N, Kissel DI, et al: Anesthesia in a Baird's tapir (*Tapirus bairdii*). J Zoo Wildl Med 2:195–198, 1998.
28. Walzer C: Non-domestic equids. In West G, Heard D, Caulkett N, editors: Zoo animal and wildlife immobilization and anesthesia, Ames, Iowa, 2007, Blackwell, pp 523–531.
29. Wenger S, Boardman W, Buss P, et al: The cardiopulmonary effect of etorphine, azaperone, detomidine, and butorphanol in field-anesthetized white rhinoceroses (*Ceratotherium simum*). J Zoo Wildl Med 38:380–387, 2007.
30. Wolfe L, Goshorn CT, Baruch-Mordo S: Immobilization of black bears (*Ursus americanus*) with a combination of butorphanol, azaperone and medetomidine. J Wildl Dis 44:748–752, 2008.

CHAPTER 78

Importation of Nondomestic Ruminant Semen for Management of Zoological Populations Using Artificial Insemination

Linda M. Penfold and Justine O'Brien

Ruminants are in the order Artiodactyla and encompass a broad array of species, including the antelope (including pronghorn), cattle, sheep, goats, giraffe, okapi, bison, buffalo, deer, and yaks. The ruminant family contains some of the most endangered species, including the hirola, or Hunter's antelope *(Beatragus hunteri)*, dibatag *(Ammodorcas clarkei)*, Przewalski's gazelle *(Procapra przewalski)*, saiga *(Saiga tatarica)*, and the more recently discovered saola *(Pseudoryx nghetinhensis)*. Ruminants comprise a significant part of the collection in many zoo and wildlife institutions, and zoos have played a strong role in conserving species that are effectively extinct in the wild,[27] but that have sizable populations within the zoo community, such as the addax *(Addax nasomaculatus)*, scimitar-horned oryx *(Oryx dammah)*, and dama gazelle *(Gazella dama)*. Other species that were once abundant in their range countries, such as the Kenyan bongo *(Tragelaphus eurycerus eurycerus)*, are disappearing through overhunting and habitat loss, yet do well in captivity. Elsewhere, roan *(Hippotragus equinus)* numbers are similarly dwindling in southern African, purportedly because of their sensitivity to habitat disturbances.

Zoos and wildlife institutions have contributed significantly to ruminant conservation strategies, including reintroductions or repatriations, such as for the scimitar-horned oryx,[6] addax,[2] bongo (www.rarespecies.org/africa.html), and roan (http://www.backtoafrica.co.za/operations_roan.html). They continue to contribute through other projects, including surveillance to estimate populations accurately for updating their International Union for Conservation of Nature (IUCN) conservation status, such as for the okapi *(Okapi johnstonii)*.[9] Ongoing requirements for ruminant conservation include the following: clarification of taxonomy questions, such as whether the Jackson's hartebeest *(Acelaphus buselaphus jacksoni)* is a hybrid of the lelwel *(A.b lelwel)* and Coke's hartebeest *(A.b. cokei)*; nutrition studies on free-ranging counterparts to refine nutritional requirements in captivity, especially for browser antelope species; and basic research to elucidate species' biology. Zoos typically manage a limited number of individuals for every species, and problems associated with negative influences on populations become magnified in such small populations.[10] For a species to survive in the longer term, it is important that populations contain adequate genetic diversity to be evolutionarily flexible.[11,12] In recent years, the long-term sustainability of many ruminant populations in zoos and wildlife institutions has come under threat and new founders are needed to infuse new genes into the populations.[5] Because zoos actively support the concept of sustainable resources, the idea of moving frozen semen rather than translocating animals from the wild has become an attractive option. Not only would this approach create a permanent source of wild genetic material, but the ability to import new genes via frozen semen for use in artificial insemination (AI) confers the advantages of decreased disease risk (see later), decreased cost and, most importantly, enhanced animal welfare. The welfare improvements from this strategy occur because the animals would be temporarily captured for a quarantine period and for semen collection before release into the wild (or semiwild enclosures in the case of wildlife parks), rather than permanent translocation into captivity. Semen may thus be viewed as a sustainable resource.

For all these conservation strategies and research, biological samples such as feces, rumen contents, and frozen semen are imperative. However, importation of unfixed or untreated (effectively viable) ruminant samples into the United States is extremely difficult and, in the case of frozen semen, has yet to be achieved in nondomestic ruminants.

STATUS OF ARTIFICIAL INSEMINATION IN RUMINANT SPECIES

Because ruminants are in the Bovidae family, assisted reproductive techniques such as AI may be modified from techniques developed for domestic cattle. Because of the importance of the livestock industry in most countries, extensive research has been directed at developing techniques to maximize production, including the use of AI, which is widely used in the cattle and dairy industry. Such developments have proven advantageous to nondomestic ruminants because similar techniques may basically be applied and refined.

Ruminants represent the largest group of nondomestic animals to have been produced by AI, with offspring produced for seven antelope, seven cervid, two wild cattle, one caprid, and one ovid species[14] (Table 78-1). Artificial insemination of females with frozen-thawed rather than fresh sperm has resulted in pregnancies in most of these species. Although a significant amount of work is generally required to develop these techniques in each new species, the use of frozen-thawed sperm in conjunction with AI still represents a pragmatic option for infusing new genetic material into ex situ ruminant populations, both within and among countries. Importation of frozen semen for use in AI may enable animal managers to maintain or increase genetic diversity in captive populations of nondomestic ruminants. Organized sperm banks function as valuable repositories of genetic material that may be used long after the death of the semen donor, and therefore should be considered an important component of conservation efforts for nondomestic ruminants, particularly in view of dwindling numbers of many species in the wild. However, this approach is constrained by the very feature that facilitated the development of semen freezing and AI methods in the first place—the close relatedness of nondomestic bovidae to their domesticated counterparts means that nondomestic ruminants are susceptible to the same group of diseases that might threaten the livestock industry. Consequently, semen and other biologic samples from nondomestic ruminants present similar disease risks to agricultural industries and to zoological populations, and severe restrictions on sample transport and use exist. The full potential of AI as a means of managing the genetic diversity of captive populations will not be realized until regulatory processes for frozen semen importation are clarified and semen can be moved internationally.

FOREIGN ANIMAL DISEASE AND TRANSMISSION THROUGH SEMEN

The inadvertent importation of a foreign animal disease has serious implications for endangered species. Organisms that may be relatively harmless in their host and host country may wreak havoc in naïve species. For example, the relatively benign herpesvirus of the African elephant (Loxodonta Africana) is fatal in Asian elephants (Elephas maximus),[19] and the Great African rinderpest epizootic of the 1890s demonstrated the devastating effects that an introduced disease could have on wildlife species. Thought to have been introduced into Africa by domestic cattle imports from either India or Arabia, rinderpest decimated ruminant populations, reducing species such as roan and sable to small metapopulations.[1]

Rinderpest is a highly contagious disease, with spectacularly high mortality rates, rendering it a formidable disease for economic and social reasons. An extraordinary amount of historical information is available for this epizootic disease, with accounts throughout the centuries starting as early as 376 AD.[1] An African pandemic in 1895 decimated ruminant populations, with antelope being extremely susceptible. High numbers of waterbuck, kudu, giraffe, and wildebeest succumbed during this pandemic.

Many foreign animal diseases of concern to the agricultural industry in the United States and other nations may be carried in nondomestic ruminant biologic samples (Table 78-2).[7] These diseases may be virulent, with high morbidity, such as Rift valley fever, and/or economically devastating, such as foot-and-mouth disease (FMD) and bovine spongiform encephalopathy (BSE).

However, FMD is without question the most contagious animal virus disease[21] and has long been recognized as a disease transmissible by AI.[3] Endemic to all continents except Australia and North America, it is also one of the most economically important of the animal diseases because of its potential impact on international trade. There are seven serotypes of FMD—O, A, C, Asia 1, SAT1, SAT2, SAT3—and as few as 10 to 25 virus particles may be sufficient for disease transfer. Therefore, the emerging technique for semen washing may not be effective for FMD, although it is effective for HIV-1 and hepatitis C,[13] because the washing technique has the advantage of dramatically reducing the virus load but may not eliminate the virus completely from the semen.

Although an FMD vaccine is available, countries are reluctant to use it to avoid losing FMD-free status for

TABLE 78-1   Artificial Insemination (AI) in Nondomestic Bovidae

Species	Insemination Method	Semen	Pregnancies/AI (%)	Outcome
Bovinae				
Eland, *Taurotragus oryx*	TC	FT	1/4 (25)	1 live
		Epididymal		
Banteng, *Bos javanicus*	TC	FT	1/6 (17)	1 live
	TC	FT	7/15 (47)	2 live
Gaur, *Bos gaurus*	TC (presumed)	FT	2/6 (33)	2 live
	TC	FT	1/2 (50)	1 live
	TC	FT	0/4 (0)	0
Hippotraginae				
Addax, *Addax nasomaculatus*	TC	FT	1/1 (100)	1 live
	TC	FT	1/1 (100)	0
Scimitar horned oryx, *Oryx dammah*	TC	FT	2/4 (50)	2 live
	Vaginal	FT	0/1 (0)	0
	LIU	FT	1/4 (25)	0
	Not stated	2	0/2 (0)	0
	TC	FT	5/14 (36)	4 live
	TC	FT	0/14 (0)	0
	TC	FT	1/12 (8)	1 live
	TC	Chilled	0/12 (0)	0
	TC	FT	9/24 (38)	7 live
Fringe-eared oryx, *Oryx gazella callotis*	TC	FT	0/9 (0)	0
Antilopinae				
Suni, *Neotragus moschatus zuluensis*	LIU	Fresh	0/2 (0)	0
	LIU	FT	0/2 (0)	0
	TC	Fresh	1/2 (50)	Not reported
	TC	FT	2/2 (100)	Not reported
Blackbuck, *Antilope cervicapra*	TC	Fresh	3/4 (75)*	3 live
	TC	Fresh	2/4 (50)	2 live
	TC	FT	1/3 (33)	1 live
	LIU	FT	1/4 (25)	1 stillborn
	LIU	Fresh	0/3 (0)	0
Gerenuk, *Litocranius walleri walleri*	TC	FT	2/8 (25)	1 stillborn
	TC	Fresh	1/1 (100)	0
	TC	Fresh	4/6 (66%)	4 live
Speke's gazelle, *Gazella spekei*	Vaginal	FT	0/1 (0)	0
	Vaginal	Fresh	1/2 (50)	1 live
Mohor gazelle, *Gazella dama mhorr*	LIU	FT	3/7 (43)	1 stillborn
	LIU	FT	1/6 (17)	0
	LIU	FT		1 live
Springbok, *Antidorcas marsupialis*	Vaginal	FT	0/3 (0)	0
Caprinae				
Spanish ibex, *Capra pyrenaica hispanica*	LIU	FT, epididymal	1/6 (17)	1 live
	LIU	FT, epididymal	2/8 (25)	2 live
Barbary sheep, *Ammotragus lervia*	LIU	Fresh	2/4 (50)	2 live

Modified from Morrow CJ, Penfold LM, Wolfe BA: Artificial insemination in deer and non-domestic bovids. Theriogenology 2009;71:149-165.
FT, Frozen-thawed spermatozoa; LIU, laparoscopic intrauterine; TC, transcervical.
*SixAI attempts in 11 estrous blackbuck (i.e., over several cycles), overall pregnancy/insemination rate of 6/16 (37.5%).

TABLE 78-2	Viral and Bacterial Diseases Through Artificial Insemination in Ruminants*
Disease	**Ruminant Host Species**
Viral Infection	
Foot and mouth disease	Various artiodactylids
Rinderpest	Various artiodactylids
Peste de petite ruminants	Various artiodactylids
Bluetongue	Various artiodactylids
Malignant catarrhal fever	Various artiodactylids
Lumpy skin disease	Various artiodactylids
Rift Valley fever	Various artiodactylids
Sheep pox	Various artiodactylids
Enzootic bovine leucosis	Bovids
Infectious bovine rhinotracheitis	Bovids
Bovine viral diarrhea	Bovids
Epizootic hemorrhagic disease of deer	Cervids
Scrapie	Sheep
Rabies	Mammals
Bacterial Infection	
Tuberculosis	Mammals, birds
Brucellosis	Mammals
Paratuberculosis	Mammals
Salmonellosis	Various
Leptospirosis	Various
Haemophilus disease	Various
Campylobacter disease	Various
Chlamydiosis	Various
Mycoplasma disease	Various
Trichomoniasis	Various

Modified from Kirkwood JK, Colenbrander B: Disease control measures for genetic resource banking. In Watson P, Holt WV (eds): Cryobanking the genetic resource: Wildlife conservation for the future? London, 2001, Taylor and Francis, pp 69-84.
*Proven or probably transmitted.

which is noncontagious but transmitted by biting midges *(Culicoides imicola)*. Bluetongue is rarely clinically expressed in hoofstock but sheep are susceptible, with high fetal and neonatal mortality rates. For imports, polymerase chain reaction (PCR) testing, following positive serology testing, is sophisticated enough to identify individual strains, thus preventing importation of a strain not already present in the country.

Other diseases of importance that constrain ruminant sample importation include brucellosis, Rift Valley fever and, to a lesser degree, *peste des petite ruminants* (pest of small ruminants) and lumpy skin disease.

ADVANTAGES OF SEMEN IMPORTATION

The import of semen is considerably less expensive than the import of live animals, and animal welfare issues associated with relocation and quarantine procedures are avoided. As with semen, live animal imports run the risk of inadvertently importing foreign animal disease, but have the added risk of arthropod-transmitted diseases, such as trypanosomosis, theileriosis, African swine fever, and foreign arthropod species, such as the screwworm fly *(Cochliomyia hominivorax)*. Eradicated from the United States in the late 1950s,[28] the severe outbreak of screwworm in 1972 demonstrated the vulnerability of livestock to external parasites. Thus, there is inherently reduced disease risk when importing frozen semen versus a live animal because semen cannot inadvertently contain arthropod species.

RISK ASSESSMENT OF SEMEN VERSUS LIVE ANIMAL IMPORTATION

There are internationally agreed methods for the analysis of biosecurity risks associated with animal or animal product imports, developed by the World Organization for Animal Health (OIE).[16] Risk analysis basically assists the decision maker by answering the following questions[15]:
- What may go wrong?
- How likely is it to go wrong?
- What are the consequences of it going wrong?
- What may be done to reduce the likelihood and/or consequences if it goes wrong?

Theoretic modeling may allow identification of risk areas, also known as critical points. The likelihood of an adverse event and its consequences constitute the risk, and are measured mostly in economic, human health, and environmental terms. Sadly, animal welfare

trade. The main problem with the vaccine is not that vaccinated animals cannot be distinguished from infected animals, but that there is a risk that vaccinated animals that come into contact with live virus may become carriers.[8,22] Buffalo *(Syncerus caffer)* are notorious as carriers of FMD, although it is unclear whether antelope may act as carriers for the virus. Bluetongue was probably present on the African continent for centuries but, in 1943, the virus spread to Cyprus, followed by the United States, Europe, Asia, and Australia. Many hoofstock species have titers for bluetongue, especially those in warm climates in which biting flies are abundant. There are multiple strains of bluetongue, is seldom if ever a factor in disease risk modeling. Although the framework for risk assessment suggests that acceptable risk translates into acceptable economic losses, in reality the exercise of risk assessment is to introduce safeguards (to mitigate critical points) to avoid any economic losses. Because endangered species do not have an economic value per se, it is extremely difficult to balance the minimal or even negligible risk of inadvertently importing a foreign disease against the billion dollar U.S. agricultural industry, in which apparently even minor losses cannot be justified in the face of endangered species protection.

Although risk assessment may be a powerful tool, it is not without its own inherent limitations.[18] For example, consequences of an outbreak may not follow predicted patterns, changes in practices outside the model may weaken future predictions, or assumptions surrounding scenario prediction may carry unknown biases. Good examples of these include the incidence of BSE discovered in a cow of Canadian origin. In spite of the fact that BSE is not contagious and can be immediately controlled with the destruction of the individual, the border was closed for further imports for several months at a cost of millions of Canadian dollars. Ironically, another case of BSE, discovered in a cow of U.S. origin several months later, prompted a similar response by Japan which, in following the U.S. response, shut down all imports for months, resulting in a loss of millions of U.S. dollars. The consequential economic loss in this example seems completely disproportionate to the severity of the disease risk, which is in fact minimal and thus did not follow what would have been predicted in a risk analysis model.

An example of the impact of changed practices on disease outbreak patterns can be taken from the FMD outbreak in England in 2001. The rapid speed at which the disease spread was initially puzzling to governmental agencies. Later, it was found that in the time since England had joined the European Union (EU), farmers had become eligible for certain subsidies. The subsidies were calculated on a per head of sheep basis and subject to on-farm counts by EU inspectors. To take advantage of the subsidies, farmers were buying sheep in large numbers immediately before the count, and then selling them immediately after the count. These so-called bed and breakfast sheep moved the disease around with them, further aided by the practice of teeth checking used by vendees to determine the age of a sheep at sale, effectively spreading FMD from buccal lesions. Such changes in animal management practices may limit defined risk analysis protocols.

Similarly, disease testing to assess the health status of the animal adequately before importation of the animal or animal product should be the most robust factor of the modeling, but this is based on the knowledge that the tests are validated and sensitivity and specificity are known. For many endangered ruminant species, it is tacitly assumed that tests developed for domestic livestock will be adequate but, where possible, such tests should be validated for each species. Fortunately, PCR assay is most often a definitive test for virus detection and identification. Emerging molecular techniques based on PCR may also enhance risk assessment models and provide tools to promote greater confidence in disease testing.[17]

In contrast to live animals, disease risk associated with importing embryos has been determined as negligible, provided that the embryos are handled according to International Embryo Transfer Society guidelines.[22,24,26] Although it is important to note that in spite of the negligible disease risk, none have been imported into the United States from FMD countries, although embryos have been transported to Australia and Brazil from South Africa, where FMD-free status is occasionally open to debate.[4] The situation is less straightforward when dealing with semen because although embryos may be washed free of virus, semen most likely cannot, and there are several areas in which the animal or semen may become exposed to disease. When embarking on a project involving semen importation from a foreign country, a flow chart may be an important and useful exercise to map the project while identifying critical points. An abbreviated example of a flow chart is shown in Box 78-1. Once identified, measures may be taken to mitigate the critical points, reducing or eliminating the overall risk of foreign animal disease importation. At this point, a scenario or decision tree may be constructed, assigning probabilities at each node, where there are two probabilities of occurrence. Through this process, the likelihood of foreign animal disease importation may be quantified under different scenarios.

CURRENT STATUS OF SEMEN IMPORTATION

Import protocols for frozen semen from domestic ruminants in FMD-free countries have been established in the United States, although they do not exist for frozen semen importation from FMD countries for domestic or nondomestic ruminants. The import process is further complicated by differences in a country's regulatory

BOX 78-1	Ruminant Biologic Sample Treatment for Importation into the United States

For ruminant and swine material, the following is a list of APHIS-approved FMD inactivation treatments:
- Heat treatment at a minimum of 72° C for at least 30 min *or*
- pH ≤ 5.5 for at least 30 min *or*
- pH ≥ 10 for at least 2 hr *or*
- Immersion in 0.4% (or higher strength) beta-proprolactone for 12 hr at 4° C, pH 7 *or*
- Immersion in 0.2% (or higher strength) glutaraldehyde *or*
- Immersion in 10% (or higher strength) formalin *or*
- Treatment with proteinase K, followed by a heat treatment at 95° C for 15 min, followed by RNase (for DNA, RNA only)
- FTA card filter paper (for liquids only)
- Affinity chromatography
- Irradiation by United States Department of Agriculture 3 MRads (blood products)/6 MRads tissue, whole blood

policy for biologic sample import or export. The Regulatory Subcommittee of the International Embryo Transfer Society Parent Committee on Companion Animals, Non-domestic and Endangered Species (CANDES), was established to compile such information. Currently, import and export regulatory requirements for bio-materials have been compiled for 19 countries (www.omahazoo.com/iets/candeshomepage.htm). Whereas the information provided by the CANDES Regulatory Subcommittee may improve the accessibility of scientists and animal managers to pertinent information regarding permits and sample processing requirements, regulatory issues for semen transport when samples are destined for in vivo use become complex.

For the United States, ruminant biologic samples may be imported with the appropriate import and export permits, including Convention on International Trade in Endangered Species of Wild Fauna and Flora (CITES) permits, if necessary, provided that samples have undergone disinfection treatment (see Box 78-1). However, these treatments effectively render live cells nonviable and are thus unsuitable for use with frozen semen, or any biomaterial requiring intact DNA. Logically, if semen may be collected from males of known disease-free status, and samples are processed in a sterile environment, all using universally acceptable disinfection procedures, semen importation regulations should be less complicated. Unfortunately, this has not proven

to be the case, largely because of endemic disease in the export country and varying epidemiologic factors for each specific disease.

For the last decade, efforts have been focused on the gerenuk *(Litocranius walleri walleri)* as a nondomestic model for semen importation from a ruminant species into the United States. An initial application for a semen importation protocol from the U.S. Department of Agriculture (USDA)–Animal and Plant Health Inspection Service (APHIS) was requested in 2001, and a final protocol was received in 2004. An attempt at semen importation was made in 2004 but was unsuccessful after a positive serum antibody titer for FMD from one of the semen donors was found to be 1:20 (l:18 or lower is considered negative), even though PCR testing had determined that no virus was present. Suspicious lesions on two animals (that were not sampled for testing) were sufficient to prevent importation of any semen. At that time, a revision of the protocol was requested by the USDA-APHIS but, 6 years later, the resubmitted protocol is still under review.

In brief, the initial protocol requested a quarantine facility, approved by USDA inspection, surrounded by a perimeter fence of solid material, and situated 5 km from any outbreak of FMD or rinderpest. The gerenuk were to be captured from animals that were known not to have ranged within 50 km of any FMD outbreak for the last 5 years, and had to enter the facility over a 3-day period. Semen was to be collected in a room that could be cleaned and disinfected—a horse box was considered adequate—and processed in another room that could similarly be cleaned and disinfected. New supplies and equipment that could be disinfected should be used, together with virgin liquid nitrogen (contaminated liquid nitrogen) has been shown to transmit disease (Tedder et al., 1995) and extenders from known disease-free animals. Three sets of serum and esophageal-pharyngeal (O-P) samples would be collected at the time of entry into the quarantine facility, at the time of the last semen collection, and 30 days after the last semen collection. Semen samples (0.2 mL) would be frozen without extender for testing also. Negative results from disease testing would allow importation of the semen.

A disease risk assessment was performed for the importation of gerenuk semen and a projected flow chart constructed to identify critical points at which disease might inadvertently be introduced (Fig. 78-1). Steps were then taken to reduce or mitigate these perceived risks. For example, the use of virgin liquid nitrogen in the semen storage and transport tank

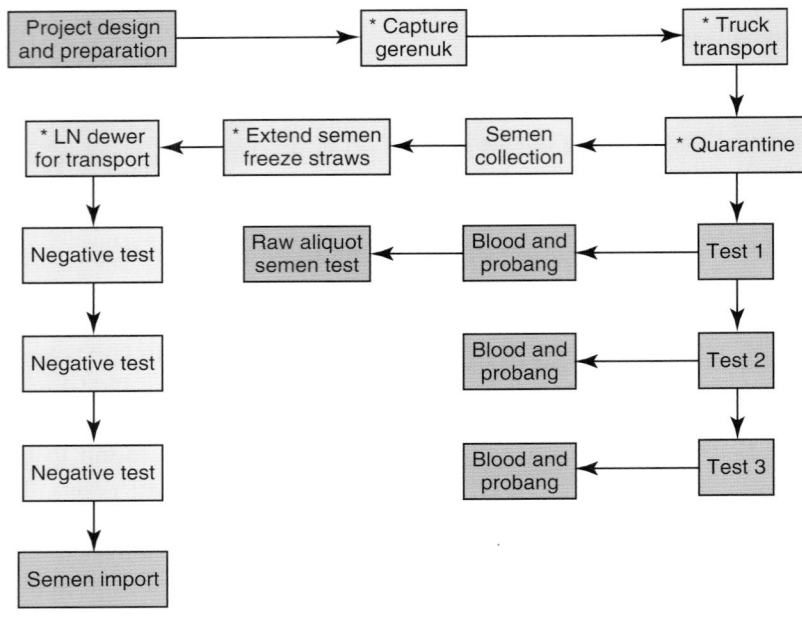

Figure 78-1

Simplified project flow chart for semen importation from an FMD country.

eliminates any risk associated with contamination of straws by pathogens present in the liquid nitrogen. Disinfection of the transport truck and quarantine area prior to use eliminates the probability of a gerenuk becoming infected through the use of a truck previously used for hauling infected animals or from a contaminated quarantine area. The use of semen extenders containing yolk from eggs of specific pathogen-free hens prevents the introduction of contagious disease to the poultry industry (e.g., Newcastle's disease). Furthermore, the use of semen extender containing egg yolk from hens that produce antiviral antibodies in their egg yolk after immunization may reduce the risk of contamination through the inactivation of semen-derived viruses. For example, bovine herpesvirus 1 (BHV-1) was inactivated in experimentally infected bovine semen through dilution of semen in an anti–BHV-1 hyperimmune egg yolk extender.[20]

Importantly, the gerenuk semen importation trial included collaborators from the Kenya government department responsible for wildlife (Kenya Wildlife Service; KSW) and participation from the Kenya Veterinary Services, the latter is the USDA counterpart in Kenya. A biomaterials transfer agreement signed by both the KWS and the U.S. importing institution (White Oak Conservation Center [WOCC], Yulee, Fla) confirmed that ownership of any samples was retained by Kenya. Also, WOCC established a training program for

veterinary technicians (previously identified as a high priority for KWS) and several technicians from KWS benefited from such training. Educational alliances such as this training program are crucial for maintaining effective collaborative efforts among range countries and importing nations; firm alliances among importing institutions, governmental agencies, and other stakeholders are imperative to ensure transparency and gain public trust.

Until endangered species are valued enough to gain sufficient economic importance, ruminant biomaterial importation, including semen, will continue to be viewed as a lower priority by regulatory agencies tasked with developing importation protocols, and ruminant conservation will continue to be hindered. Meanwhile, concerted efforts to work with government regulatory agencies and disease testing laboratories while investigating feasibilities of ruminant semen collection and importation are encouraged, because ultimately it is only through these partnerships that ruminant conservation goals will be realized.

REFERENCES

1. Blancou J: History of the surveillance and control of transmissible animal diseases, Paris, 2003, OIE (World Organization for Animal Health).
2. Convention on Migratory Species: Antelopes successfully reintroduced in Tunisia, 2007 (http://www.cms.int/news/Press/nwPR2007/12_Dec/Antelopes_Tunisiail_101207.htm).

3. Cottral GE, Gailiunas P, Cox BF: Foot-and-mouth disease virus in semen of bulls and its transmission by artificial insemination. Arch Virol 23:362–377, 1968.
4. De la Rey: Personal communication.
5. Fischer M: Personal communication.
6. Gilbert T, Woodfine T: The re-introduction of scimitar-horned oryx (*Oryx dammah*) to Dghoumes National Park, Tunisia, 2008 (http://www.marwell.org.uk/downloads/DghoumesEEPreport.pdf).
7. Kirkwood JK, Colenbrander B: Disease control measures for genetic resource banking. In Watson P, Holt WV, editors: Cryo-banking the genetic resource: Wildlife conservation for the future? London, 2001, Taylor and Francis, pp 69–84.
8. Kitching RP: Identification of foot and mouth disease virus carrier and sub-clinically infected animals and differentiation from vaccinated animals. Rev Sci Tech 21:531–538, 2002.
9. Kumpel N: Personal communication.
10. Lacy RC: Loss of genetic diversity from managed populations: Interacting effects of drift, mutation, immigration, selection and population subdivision. Conservation 1:153–158, 1987.
11. Lacy RC: Managing genetic diversity in captive populations of animals. In Bowles ML, Whelan CJ, editors: Restoration and recovery of endangered plants and animals, Cambridge, England, 1994, Cambridge University Press, pp 63–89.
12. Lacy RC: The importance of genetic variation to the viability of mammalian populations. J Mammalogy 78:320–335, 1997.
13. Loskutoff N, Huyser C, Singh R, et al: Use of a novel washing method combining multiple density gradients and combining trypsin for removing human immunodeficiency virus-1 and hepatitis C virus from semen. Fertil Steril 84:1001–1010, 2005.
14. Morrow CJ, Penfold LM, Wolfe BA: Artificial insemination in deer and non-domestic bovids. Theriogenology 71:149–165, 2009.
15. OIE (World Organization for Animal Health): Handbook on import risk analysis for animals and animal products: Volume 1. Introduction and qualitative risk analysis, Paris, 2004, OIE (World Organization for Animal Health).
16. OIE (World Organization for Animal Health): International animal health code: Special edition, Paris, 1997, Office International des Epizooties.
17. Paraguison RC, Flores EB, Cruz LC: Possible use of RNA isolate from inactivated vaccine for external positive control in reverse transcription-based detection of foot-and-mouth disease virus in bull semen. Biochem Biophys Res Commun 392:557–560, 2010.
18. Pharo, 2005.
19. Richman LK, Montali RJ, Garber RL, et al: Novel endotheliotropic herpesviruses fatal for Asian and African elephants. Science 283:1171–1176, 1999.
20. Silva N, Solana A, Castro JM: Inactivation of bovine herpesvirus 1 in semen using a hyperimmune egg yolk semen extender. J Vet Med 47:69–75, 2000.
21. Sutmoller P, Barteling SS, Olascoaga RC: Review: Control and eradication of foot and mouth disease. Virus Res 91:101–144, 2003.
22. Sutmoller P, Olascoaga RC: The risks posed by the importation of animals vaccinated against foot and mouth disease and products derived from vaccinated animals: A review. Rev Sci Tech 22:823–835, 2003.
23. Sutmoller P, Thomson GR, Hargreaves SK: The foot and mouth disease risk posed by African buffalo within wildlife conservancies to the cattle industry of Zimbabwe. Prev Vet Med 44:43–60, 2004.
24. Sutmoller P, Wrathall AE: The risks of disease transmission by embryo transfer in cattle. Rev Sci Tech 16:226–239, 1997.
25. Tedder RS, Zuckerman MA, Goldstone AH, et al: Hepatitis B transmission from contaminated cryopreservation tank. Lancet 346:137–140, 1995.
26. Thibier M, Stringfellow DA: Health and Safety Advisory Committee (HASAC) of the International Embryo Transfer Society (IETS) has managed critical challenges for two decades. Theriogenology 59:1067–1078, 2003.
27. Wiesner H, Müller P: On the reintroduction of the Mhorr gazelle in Tunisia and Morocco. Naturwissenschaften 85:553–555, 1998.
28. Wyss JH: Screwworm eradication in the Americas. Tropical veterinary diseases: Control and prevention in the context of the New World order. Ann N Y Acad Sci 916:186–193, 2000.

CHAPTER 79

Advances in Giraffe Nutrition

Eduardo V. Valdes and Michael Schlegel

In the last decade, numerous publications have been written with regard to the nutrition of giraffe and other ruminant browsers maintained in zoological institutions, inspired by several health problems suspected to have a nutritional origin. Thus, reports of rumen acidosis, chronic wasting, peracute mortality syndrome, energy malnutrition, hoof disease, inverse serum calcium and phosphorus levels, mortality caused by cold stress, overall poor body condition, urolithiasis, serous fat atrophy, chronic energy deficiency, dental disease, and pancreatic disease, among others, have been linked to nutritional imbalances in the giraffe diet.[4,7,11,26,29] Traditional giraffe zoo diets in North America consist mainly of low-fiber pellets (ADF-16) and alfalfa hay, with the original pellets designed based on the domestic ruminant.[20] Some zoos will occasionally add browse and some produce. This diet is high in soluble carbohydrates (sugars and starch) and low in total fiber. During the 1970s, and to cope with the peracute mortality syndrome reported in the giraffe, it was recommended to feed giraffes a diet containing low fiber and high protein (15% to 18% for adult nonlactating animals and 18% to 20% for calves and lactating cows). The idea of feeding zoo browsers, including giraffe, a low-fiber, high-protein pellet might be partly justified based on earlier studies that reported high levels of nitrogen in the rumen of free-ranging browsers when compared with grazers.

The claim that giraffes should have protein levels of 18% dry matter (DM) in their diet is not supported by any direct studies.[7] Traditional zoo commercial browser pelleted feeds such as ADF-16 are composed mainly of alfalfa meal, yellow corn grain, wheat middlings, and molasses. These pellets have the potential to supply high levels of readily fermentable carbohydrates (starch), increasing the availability of free glucose and stimulating the growth of certain ruminal bacteria,

thereby increasing the production of volatile fatty acids and decreasing ruminal pH and cellulitic bacteria. Studies with domestic sheep fed ADF-16 pellets, similar to the pellets used in giraffe diets, have shown sheep with a ruminal pH below 6 being maintained for more than 6 hours.[19] Starch is negligible in the natural diets of wild browsers. Research has shown that giraffe fed a diet of low- and high-fiber pellets, plus alfalfa hay, will selectively ingest the pellets and alfalfa hay with higher levels of neutral detergent fiber (NDF) and acid detergent fiber (ADF) and lower levels of gross energy, contrary to the idea that giraffe as browsers (concentrate selectors), will select a low-fiber easily digestible diet.[1] In 1973, for the first time, it was suggested that browsers such as the giraffe should be fed a diet higher in fiber and lower in protein.[11] It took over 30 years for the zoo community to develop similar recommendations.[26]

NATURAL DIET OF THE GIRAFFE

A thorough review of the giraffe natural diet has been given by Kearney.[14] The giraffe is classified as a concentrate selector (browser) that in the wild consumes mainly foliage, including leaves and twigs of trees and shrubs, herbs and forb, but these will vary with season and geographic location. The diet also includes wild fruits, flowers, bark, thorns, and seed pods.[13] Giraffe in their natural environment will strip leaves from terminal shoots with their tongues or bite off the new nonlignified shoot ends, but in the dry season they may consume a significant proportion of lignified material. In the Serengeti, giraffe consume 50% to 80% of the available shoots of favored *Acacia* species, exerting a major impact on *Acacia* regeneration. Reports have indicated that giraffe will spend 53% of the daylight hours searching for and consuming food, mainly woody plants. *Acacia* spp. seem to be consumed the most, but as many as 66 different plant species may be consumed by giraffe in a year.[16] Giraffe in their natural environment will consume little or no grass. Certainly, all the stimuli found in their natural habitat in the selection of browse and food are changed in zoo giraffe diets.

Despite the many in situ consumption and behavioral studies of giraffes, their nutrient requirements remain unknown.

GIRAFFE: SPECIALIZED BROWSER OR SPECIALIZED GRAZER?

The giraffe, being classified as a concentrate selector (browser),[3,13] will have different dietary and possibly nutritional requirements than wild grazers. The giraffe, like kudu, moose, gerenuk, and okapi, are considered tree and bush foliage selectors. Browsers, considered early evolved ruminants, had to deal with an inefficient fiber digestion in the rumen because of short retention times. Browsers, in general, focus on cell contents, whereas grazers focus on cell wall constituents.[1] As noted, giraffes in zoos have been offered diets high in soluble carbohydrates, low in fiber, and relatively high in protein. These diets originated from the time when wild herbivores were classified as grazers (grass and roughage eaters), concentrate selectors (browsers), and intermediate feeders. The latter might wrongly imply that browsers such as the giraffe are adapted to a diet high in soluble carbohydrates, with potential problems of producing rumen acidosis, as widely reported in domestic ruminants.[4] Although the giraffe had been classified as a concentrate selector (browser), there have been studies suggesting that giraffes are not truly concentrate selectors. Giraffes have more omasal laminae, whereas most browsers have few and thick omasal laminae, with the omasum serving as a filter between the reticulum and abomasum for coarse particulate matter, plus having an absorptive surface function. Giraffes, like grazers, have rumens well connected to the abdominal wall and an advanced compartmentalization of the rumen, in contrast with other browsers.[16] Furthermore, large ruminants require less energy per unit of volume of gastrointestinal tract, needing less energy-dense feeds than smaller ruminant-browsers. Thus, the giraffe as a large ruminant might not fit the classification of a true concentrate selector, but rather an intermediate feeder or a facultative concentrate selector.

RECENT RESEARCH
Serum Parameters

There are not many studies comparing zoo and free-ranging giraffe but, in one study, serum parameters were compared between zoo and free-ranging giraffes.[28] The results showed multiple differences in serum nutritional parameters between the two groups of giraffe. A total of 32 free-ranging giraffes and 20 zoo giraffes were used for the comparisons. Serum amino acid levels were higher in free-ranging animals, possible reflecting enhanced activity of the animals. Striking differences were found in the serum concentration of fatty acids. Free-ranging giraffes had higher concentrations of total omega-3 fatty acids because of elevations in α-linolenic, eicosatrienoic, eicosapentaenoic, and docosapentaenoic acids. Zoo animals, on the other hand, showed high levels of total omega-6 fatty acids, particularly linoleic and arachidonic acids due to their high levels in grains. The omega-3–to–omega-6 ratios were 0.48 ± 0.05 and 0.27 ± 0.07 for free-ranging and zoo giraffes, respectively, alerting the authors to recommend supplementation of omega-3 in the diet of zoo giraffes. In a more recent study, the addition of flax seed as a source of linolenic acid increased the serum omega-6 and omega-3 fatty acid levels, improving the omega-3–to–omega-6 ratios.[15] Serum cholesterol and saturated fatty acid levels have been seen to be higher in zoo giraffes, probably reflecting the composition of the dietary fatty acids. Serum retinol concentrations were significantly higher in zoo giraffes (89.3 µg/dL) when compared with free-ranging animals (24.1 µg/dL), although results reported in other studies showed less of a difference for retinol among these groups.[25] Serum α-tocopherol values in zoo giraffes were low (4.43 µg/dL) when compared with free-ranging animals (41.89 µg/dL),[28] although much higher levels of α-tocopherol (109 µg/dL)[23] have been reported in zoo giraffes.

Inverse serum calcium-phosphorus ratios were found in 62% of giraffes in a study that measured mineral values in 24 animals at two institutions from samples collected over 9 years.[23] Based on ISIS (International Species Information System) reports, captive adult giraffes in general show inverse calcium-phosphorus ratios. Mean serum calcium and phosphorus concentrations were 8.0 ± 0.8 mg/dL ($n = 142$) and 10.5 ± 2.9 mg/dL ($n = 135$), respectively.[31] In a more recent publication,[29] giraffes ($n = 10$) from five zoological institutions had higher serum calcium levels (8.6 to 10.6 mg/dL), lower serum phosphorus levels (3.1 to 6.2 mg/dL), and normal serum calcium-phosphorus (Ca:P) ratios, ranging from 1.4 to 2.9. The serum phosphorus concentrations were much lower than those reported by ISIS.[31] Two recent dietary studies of giraffes have shown positive effects on changing the serum calcium-phosphorus ratio after switching animals from a high-starch, low-fiber pellet (ADF-16) to a low-starch, high-fiber commercial pellet.[15,18] In both studies, the serum calcium level was not affected by diet, but the serum phosphorus level was reduced by diet. Calcium homeostasis in vertebrates is precisely regulated, unlike phosphorus and magnesium. The serum phosphorus level was significantly reduced in one of the studies[15] when changing from a high-starch, low-fiber to a low-starch, high-fiber diet that also reduced the level of phosphorus in the diet.

Physical Form of the Diet

A study[14] has been performed comparing giraffes fed a regular zoo diet (R) consisting of a mix of commercial pelleted feeds (Mazuri Browser Breeder and Purina Omolene 200, in a 75:25 mix), ad lib alfalfa hay and fresh browse, when available, with giraffes fed a coarse, nonpelleted, experimental browser feed similar in form to a TMR (total mix ration) fed to dairy cows. The coarse diet (C) was also developed with the intention to reduce the dietary starch (from 14.2% to 1.5%) and increase the total nonfiber carbohydrates (from 9.6% to 15%). Giraffes were fed the diets for 21 days. The study found that giraffes fed the C diet slightly increased the amount of time engaged in feeding behavior, closer to that observed in wild giraffes. Increased eating time may increase salivary rumen buffering. Giraffes fed the C diet showed lower blood glucose levels (82.3 mg/dl) compared with the blood glucose levels (99 mg/dl) of R-fed giraffes. However, no major statistical differences were found with regard to total feed intake as percentage of body weight, total dry matter intake, serum blood urea nitrogen (BUN) level (16.6 versus 20.6 mg/dL, for R versus C diets), serum parameters, or digestibility coefficients among dietary treatments. Giraffes in both groups showed inverse calcium-to-phosphorus ratios. Studies such as the one described are important, but probably require more time for the animals to be exposed to the positive effects of reducing dietary soluble carbohydrates, such as starch, to see any significant animal changes (e.g., in serum values).

Digestibility and Feed Intake

Early studies on diet digestibility have shown that nutrients in the giraffe diet are used efficiently. For example, in diets in which the main ingredients in the pellets were corn grain, soybean meal, dehydrated alfalfa meal, corn cob, wheat middlings, and molasses, digestibility coefficients measured using the acid-insoluble ash technique for DM, crude protein (CP), NDF, ADF, and gross energy (GE) were 85.2%, 79.5%, 74.8%, 72.5%, and 82.6%, respectively.[1] In other studies, different digestibility markers were tested in giraffe diets in which the main ingredients consisted of alfalfa hay, commercial pellets (Mazuri Browser Breeder) and beech (Fagus salvatica) browse.[6] In this study, the range of digestibility coefficients reported for DM, CP, NDF, and ADF were 63.5% to 74.3%, 73.4% to 82.4%, 49.9% to 62.2%, and 49.7% to 63.7%, respectively. In this study, the best digestibility markers were found to be acid-insoluble ash and alkanes (C36). Mean apparent digestibility of CP (59.7% to 82.4%), DM (52% to 85.2%), and NDF (32.5% to 74.8%) were reported for giraffes fed either a pelleted feed (Mazuri Browser Breeder and Purina Omolene 200, 75:25) and alfalfa hay or a coarse total mix diet plus alfalfa hay.[14] The average dry matter intake for a group of two giraffes was 13.06 kg/day, representing 1.22% of the body weight of a traditional alfalfa hay and pellet diet (87.4% DM, 16.2% CP, 29.6% NDF, 183% ADF, 3.8% acid detergent lignin [ADL]). In other studies, average feed intake (percentage of body weight) for a group of six adult female giraffes were 1.2% (7.6 kg DM/day) and 1.25% (7.91 kg DM/day) for a traditional pellet–alfalfa hay diet (ADF = 23%; starch = 14.2%) and a coarse TMR diet (ADF = 26%; starch = 1.47%), respectively. One report on the DM intake of free-ranging giraffes showed males consuming at 1.6% of their body weight (BW) whereas females consumed at 2.1% of their BW.[21]

Use of Woody Browse in Giraffe Feeding Programs

Browsers such as giraffes will benefit from the feeding of fresh woody browse that might provide nutrient supplementation or behavioral enrichment. Browse is particularly important for giraffes because giraffes are poor consumers of grass and alfalfa hay, even when offered ad lib,[10] something that might contribute to the chronic energy deficit reported in some animals.[3,4] The use of browse in giraffe and other antelope diets is considered important in their feeding and health and a recommendation has been given to feed giraffe in zoos between 10% and 25% of their diet as woody browse. Browse may include trees, shrubs, woody vines, and stems. However, although important in the diet of giraffe and other browsers, woody browse is difficult to produce for most zoological institutions. Recently, browse farms have originated to supply this demand in some locations in North America. Carolina willow (Coastal plain willow, *Salix caroliniana*) and Australian acacia has been extensively used in some institutions in the feeding program of giraffe and other browsers. Willow browse (including leaves, twigs, bark) has a nutrient profile for giraffe as follows (%): DM, 47.1; CP, 8.5; ADF, 52.2; lignin, 20.2; cellulose, 32; starch, 1.57; Ca, 1.39; P, 0.17; Mg, 0.14; Na, 0.19; K, 0.87. In addition, willow browse has a Ca:P ratio of 8.2 and contains the following: (ppm) Cu, 6.7; Fe, 44.4; Mn, 14.6; Mo, 9.6; and Zn, 114.4. Its GE (kcal/g) = 4.8.[24] The calculated digestibility of the willow browse for giraffe based on in vitro studies is 25.9%. Willow has been ensiled for the purpose of prolonging the browse season and research is underway to determine the acceptability of silage for giraffes and other browsers, as previously done for black rhinoceroses (willow, hazel, and maple silage). A practical way to estimate edible browse has been reported by equations based on branch weight and weight of the leaves, with the branch diameter, at the point of cutting.[5]

Water Intake

Giraffes may obtain all their water needs from the food they consume, given adequate moisture content, and will drink regularly if available.[8] In the Namib desert, giraffes were rarely seen drinking until the installation of artificial watering holes, at which giraffes have been observed drinking regularly, sometimes on consecutive days.[9] Water intake is dependent on the amount of water consumed in the diet, dry matter intake, ambient temperature, dietary salt, and precipitation. It is difficult to estimate the amount of water consumed by giraffes daily and therefore should be available at all times.

NUTRIENT RECOMMENDATIONS

Although the nutrient requirements of giraffe are unknown, new recommendations have been given based on the historical medical records of zoological institutions in North America and elsewhere.[2,26] The new recommendations have stimulated the feed

industry to start producing feeds that include new ingredients in their pellets, such as aspen, soybean hulls, oat hulls, and beet pulp, to reduce the starch content to less than 5% and to increase the ADF to more than 30% in giraffe and other browser feeds. The new nutrient recommendations[27] (Table 79-1) are different from those given in the *Giraffe Husbandry Resource Manual* of the Association of Zoos and Aquariums, Antelope and Giraffe Taxon Advisory Group,[30] and from the NAG (Nutrition Advisory Group, AZA),[17] but in general agree with the European recommendations.

Based on health conditions discussed earlier, nutrient recommendations have evolved to try to improve the nutritional health of giraffes without being based on nutrition research studies to establish nutrient requirements. Since initial recommendations were provided in 1997,[17] dietary CP concentrations have decreased because of the realization that high crude protein diets may exasperate rumen acidosis. Additionally, with the inverse Ca:P ratio observed in some giraffe populations,[24] recommended dietary calcium concentrations have narrowed, with a relative increase, and phosphorus concentrations have decreased.

PRACTICAL DIETS

Given the expected growth of giraffes (Fig. 79-1), three age-related diets may be developed for the juvenile (<12 months), the subadult (13 to 24 months) and adult (>24 months; Table 79-2). The maintenance energy requirements of giraffes have been calculated[2] using a range of 107.6 to 143 multiplied by the metabolic weight BW, $kg^{0.75}$. This is very similar to the estimate presented by Robbins[22] ($141.4 \times BW [kg]^{0.75}$), essentially twice the basal metabolic rate.

A typical diet may be prepared to include a low-starch complete feed (loose or pelleted) and hay (legume or legume-grass mixture), with the complete feed offered at 50% to 75% of the required calories and the hay offered at 25% to 50% of the daily caloric requirement. Woody browse should be offered daily to elicit appropriate behaviors and prevent stereotypies (see earlier). The quantity of browse offered should not exceed that which reduces the consumption of the complete feed. Produce may be offered for training and enrichment, but should include items that are low in starch and calories such as lettuce, green beans, and carrots.

In colder weather, energy requirements may increase by 24% ($175 \times BW [kg]^{0.75}$), with a subsequent need to increase dietary calories.[27] One of the concerns with giraffes is their inability to consume adequate amounts

TABLE 79-1 Evolution of Recommended Dietary Nutrient Requirements for Giraffe Diets				
	YEAR RECOMMENDATIONS PUBLISHED			
Nutrient, DM Basis	1997[18]	2005[27]	2006[8]	2009[28]
CP (%)	17.8-22.2	10-14	14	>14
ADF (%)	NR*	25-30	NR	NR
NDF (%)	NR	NR	35-50	>40
Fat (%)	NR	2-5	NR	4-8
Starch (%)	NR	<10	NR	7-10
Ca (%)	0.16-0.82	0.65-1.0	0.70-0.97	0.8
P (%)	0.11-0.49	0.35-0.5	0.36-0.40	0.3
Mg (%)	0.1-0.2	>0.3	0.18-0.24	0.3
Na (%)	0.06-0.18	NR	0.10-0.44	0.1
K (%)	0.5-0.89	NR	1.6-1.8	NR
Cu (ppm)	6.7-10.0	10-15	10-12	10-15
Fe (ppm)	30-50	NR	126-139	NR
I (ppm)	0.1-0.8	NR	0.3-0.4	NR
Mn (ppm)	20-40	NR	54-57	NR
Se (ppm)	0.08-0.20	NR	0.12-0.18	NR
Zn (ppm)	11-33	NR	54-68	NR
Vitamin A (IU/kg)	1111-3889	3900	1500-2200	5000-6000
Vitamin D3 (IU/kg)	556-1111	750	400-500	1200
Vitamin E (IU/kg)	133-389	60	120-178	100-150

NR, *No recommendation provided.*

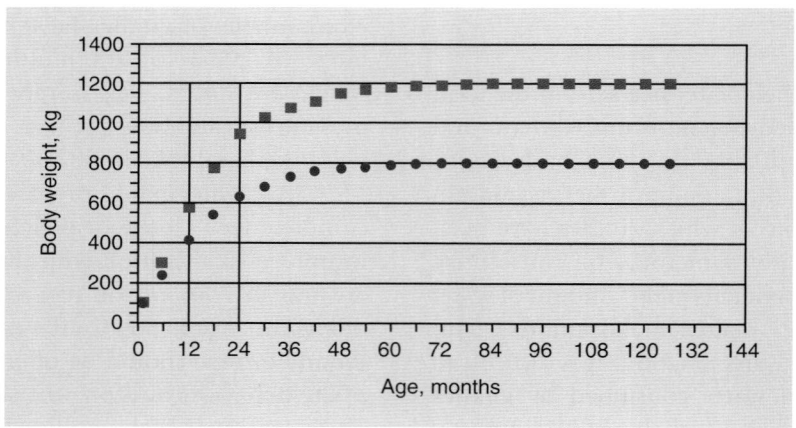

Figure 79-1

Average body weight of giraffe based on age for males (■) and females (●) based on equations developed by Hirst.[12]

TABLE 79-2 Diets Formulated for Three Age Classes of Male and Female Giraffe in Zoos

	MALES			FEMALES		
Item	Juvenile	Subadult	Adult	Juvenile	Subadult	Adult
Body weight (kg)	575	920	1200	425	630	800
ME required (Mcal/day)	16.6	23.6	28.8	13.2	17.8	21.3
Example Diet						
Complete feed (kg as fed/day)*	4.2-6.3[†]	6.0-9.0	7.3-10.9	3.4-5.1	4.5-6.8	5.4-8.1
Hay (kg as fed/day)	2.0-4.0[‡]	2.9-5.7	3.5-6.9	1.6-3.2	2.2-4.3	2.6-5.1
Browse[§]	At least one 2-m piece daily, when available including, leaves, bark and stems					
Produce (kg as fed/day)[‖]	0-1	0-1	0-1	0-1	0-1	0-1

ME, Metabolizable energy.
*Provides 1.98 Mcal ME/kg.
[†]Low-starch complete feed offered at 50% to 75% of the dietary calorie requirement.
[‡]Legume or legume-grass hay offered at 25% to 50% of the dietary calorie requirement.
[§]Browse may be offered in lieu of hay, but should not be fed to the extent that it decreases pellet consumption.
[‖]Low-starch produce items.

of food when their energy requirements increase. To compensate for the increased dietary requirements, dietary items that are more calorically dense need to be offered during periods of high energy needs to ensure adequate energy balance. In the example given in Table 79-2, if dietary energy increases 24%, the complete feed needs to have a 35% increase in caloric density to prevent the need for the animal to increase its daily dry matter intake.

Acknowledgment

Kathleen Sullivan is greatly acknowledged for her assistance with the manuscript.

REFERENCES

1. Baer DJ, Oftedal OT, Fahey GC: Feed selection and digestibility by captive giraffe. Zoo Biol 4:57–64, 1985.
2. Barta Z, Clauss M, Culik L, et al: EAZA Husbandry and Management Guidelines for Giraffa camelopardalis, Arnhem, The Netherlands, 2006, European Association of Zoo and Aquaria (EAZA).
3. Clauss M, Dierenfeld E: The Nutrition of Browsers. In Fowler ME, Miller RE, editors: Zoo and wild animal medicine: Current therapy 6, Philadelphia, 2007, Elsevier Saunders, pp 444–454.
4. Clauss M, Kienzle E, Hatt J-M: Feeding practice in captive wild ruminants: Peculiarities in the nutrition of browsers, concentrate selectors and intermediate feeders. A review. In Fidgett A, Clauss M, Ganslosser U, et al, editors: Zoo animal nutrition, vol II. Furth, Scotland, 2003, Filander Verlag, pp 27–52.
5. Clauss M, Kienzle E, Wiesner H: Feeding browse to large zoo herbivores: How much is "a lot," how much is "sufficient?" In Fidgett A, Clauss M, Ganslosser U, et al, editors: Zoo animal nutrition, vol II. Furth, Scotland, 2003, Filander Verlag, pp 17–25.
6. Clauss M, Lechner-Doll M, Flach EJ, et al: Comparative use of four different marker systems for the estimation of digestibility and low food intake in a group of captive giraffes (Giraffa camelopardalis). Zoo Biol 20:315–329, 2001.
7. Clauss M, Rose P, Hummel J, Hatt J-M: Serous fat atrophy and other nutrition-related health problems in captive giraffe (Giraffa camelopardalis). An evaluation of 83 necropsy reports. In 6th Congress of the European Association of Zoo and Wildlife Veterinarians, Budapest (Hungary), 24–28 May 2006. 2006, pp 233–235.
8. Dagg AI, Foster JB: The giraffe. Its biology, behavior and ecology, Malabar, India, 1976, Krieger.
9. Fennessy JT: Ecology of desert-dwelling giraffe Giraffa camelopardalis angolensis in northwestern Namibia, Ph.D. thesis, Sydney, Australia, 2004, University of Sydney.
10. Foose TJ: Trophic strategies of ruminants versus non-ruminant ungulates, Ph.D. thesis, Chicago, 1982, University of Chicago, 1982.
11. Fowler M: Peracute mortality in captive giraffe. J Am Vet Med Assoc 173:1088–1093, 1978.
12. Hirst SM: Ungulate-habitat relationships in a South African woodland/savanna ecosystem. Wildlife Monographs, No. 44, Lawrence, Kan, 1975, Allen Press.
13. Hoffman RR: The structure of digestive systems in the feeding of mammals: A comparative approach. In Nijboer J, Hatt H-M, Kaumanns W, et al, editors: Zoo animal nutrition, vol I. Furth, Scotland, 2000, Filander Verlag, pp 163–181.
14. Kearney CC: Effects of dietary physical form and carbohydrate profile in captive giraffe. Master's thesis, Gainesville, Fla, 2005, University of Florida (http://etd.fcla.edu/UF/UFE0009468/kearney_c.pdf).
15. Koutsos EA, Armstrong D, Ball R, et al: Influence of diet transition on serum calcium and phosphorus and fatty acids in zoo giraffe (Giraffa camelopardalis). Zoo Biol 2010 (in press).
16. Leuthold BM, Leuthold W: Daytime activity patterns of gerenuk and giraffe in Tsavo National Park, Kenya. E Afr Wildl J 16:231–243, 1978.
17. Lintzenich BA, Ward AM: Hay and pellet ratios: Considerations in feeding ungulates. AZA Nutrition Advisory Group Handbook, Fact Sheet 006, 1997 (http://www.nagonline.net/Technical%20Papers/NAGFS00697Hay_Pellets-JONIFEB24,2002MODIFIED.pdf).

18. Miller M, Weber M, Valdes EV, et al: Changes in serum calcium, phosphorus and magnesium levels in captive ruminants affected by diet manipulation. J Zoo Wildl Med 41:404–408, 2010.

19. Odongo NE, AlZahal O, Lindinger MI, et al: Effects of mild heat stress and grain challenge on acid-base balance and rumen tissue histology in lambs. J Anim Sci 84:447–455, 2006.

20. Oftedal O, Allen M: Specifications for feeds used in zoo animal diets. In Meehan TP, Allen ME, editors: Proceedings of the 6th and 7th Dr. Scholl Conferences on the Nutrition of Captive Wild Animals, Lincoln Park Zoo, Chicago, 1986, pp 13–27.

21. Pellew RA: Food consumption and energy budgets of the giraffe. J Appl Ecol 21:140–159, 1984.

22. Robbins CT: Wildlife feeding and nutrition, ed 2, San Diego, 1993, Academic Press.

23. Schlegel ML, Edwards MS, Miller M, Valdes EV: Mineral, vitamin A and vitamin E concentrations in serum, plasma and tissue of captive giraffe *(Giraffa camelopardalis)*. In Kirk-Baer C, editor: Proceedings of the 5th Biennial Symposium of the Comparative Nutrition Society, 2004, Hickory Corners, Michigan, pp 156–162.

24. Schlegel ML, Renjifo A, Valdes EV: Nutrient content of Carolina willow *(Salix caroliniana)* browse components fed to exotic herbivores. In Fidget A, Clauss M, Eulenberger K, et al, editors: Zoo animal nutrition, vol. III. Furth, Scotland, 2006, Filander Verlag, pp 213–224.

25. Schmidt DA, Ball RL, Grobler D, et al: Serum concentrations of amino acids, fatty acids, lipoproteins, vitamin A and E, and minerals in apparently healthy, free-ranging southern giraffe *(Giraffe camelopardalis giraffa)*. Zoo Biol 26:13–25, 2007.

26. Schmidt DA, Barbiers R: In The Giraffe Nutrition Workshop Proceedings, Chicago 2005, Lincoln Park Zoo, May 25–26.

27. Schmidt DA, Kendrick E: In Proceedings of the Browser Nutrition Workshop, Ed D. Schmidt and E.C. Kendrick; St. Louis, St. Louis Zoo, September 28–29, 2009.

28. Schmidt DA, Koutzos EA, Ellersieck R, et al: Serum concentration comparisons of amino acids, fatty acids, lipoproteins, vitamin A and E, and minerals between zoo and free-ranging giraffes *(Giraffa camelopardalis)*. J Zoo Wildl Med 40:29–38, 2009.

29. Sullivan K, van Heugten E, Ange-van Heughten K, et al: Analysis of nutrient concentrations in the diet, serum and urine of giraffe from surveyed North American zoological institutions. Zoo Biol 28:1–13, 2009.

30. The Antelope and Giraffe Taxon Advisory Group: The giraffe husbandry resource manual, Silver Spring, Md, 2004, Association of Zoo and Aquariums.

31. Teare JA, editor: Reference ranges for physiological values in captive wildlife, Apple Valley, Calif, 2002, International Species Information System.

CHAPTER 80

Hoof Disorders in Nondomestic Artiodactylids

Jeffery R. Zuba

Zoological institutions commonly exhibit nondomestic artiodactylids, or even-toed ungulates, because of their public appeal, educational value, and conservation message. These hoofed herbivorous mammals include the pigs, peccaries, hippopotami, camels, chevrotains, deer, giraffes, pronghorn, antelopes, sheep, goats, and cattle species.[15,20] Ungulates also include hoofed animals with an odd number of toes, or Perissodactyla (horse, tapir, rhinoceros), but are not discussed in this chapter.

Because of the variety in body size, coat color, and personality, nondomestic artiodactylids are charismatic and represent the diversity of the animal kingdom. Many adaptations are present in the hoof structure of these ungulates and reflect the contrasting natural environments in which they are found. Desert-dwelling species such as the addax *(Addax nasomaculatus)*, with hard, widely splayed hooves for travel in the sand, are readily differentiated from the elongate hooves and soft leathery heels adapted for traversing wetlands and bogs by species such as the sitatunga *(Tragelaphus spekeii)*.[20] Thus, the zoo veterinarian must recognize species differences and understand the range of normal structure and function of the nondomestic artiodactyl hoof. Anatomically, the foot of a two-toed artiodactyl is described as the limb distal to the fetlock joint but the focus of this chapter will be limited to the horn covered structure, interchangeably called the hoof or claw.

Just as in the domestic cow, sheep, goat, and pig, normal hoof structure may be compromised because of trauma, infection, or poor conformation, leading to clinical problems in nondomestic artiodactylids.* In my practice, hoof disease is a common cause of lameness and morbidity, which without proper medical attention may result in fatal consequences. Despite the clinical importance, specific epidemiologic information

on hoof health and diseases is lacking in the nondomestic animal literature.

An encyclopedic review of hoof disorders is beyond the scope of this chapter and the reader is directed to the many excellent veterinary references on the ungulate foot found on the domestic hoofstock library shelf. Extrapolation from a domestic prototype species is a familiar and clinically useful concept to the zoo and wildlife veterinarian. Because detailed information on hoof disorders does not exist on the approximately 220 species of nondomestic artiodactylids,[15,20] it is reasonable for their domestic cousins to serve as valid references for basic anatomy, physiology, biomechanics, diseases, and treatments of the hoof. The objective of this chapter is to provide the veterinarian with practical clinical review of the cause, diagnosis, and management of the common and unique hoof problems in nondomestic artiodactylids under their care.

FUNCTIONAL ANATOMY OF THE HOOF

It is important to understand the normal anatomy of the hoof to recognize, treat, and prevent common and uncommon diseases. The basic function of the hoof reflects an adaptation to minimize weight-bearing stress and protect it from injury and pathogens in the animal's natural environment. Most nondomestic two-toed ungulates have foot anatomy similar to that of cattle, sheep, goat, and swine.[4,20,22,23] Hippopotami, however, do not fit this classic description.[7,13] The hippopotamus has a widespread foot with four weight-bearing digits. Table 80-1 reviews the foot structure and number of weight-bearing digits in the nondomestic artiodactylid. The primary distinguishing feature of artiodactylids is the paraxonic limb structure, in which the symmetry of the foot passes between two well-developed middle digits. The first digit is absent in all

*References 2, 4, 6, 10, 14, and 18.

619

				No. of Weight-Bearing Digits	No. of Non–Weight-Bearing Digits (Dewclaws)	
TABLE 80-1	Number of Digits on Feet of Nondomestic Artiodactylids[7,13,15,20]					
Order	Family	Subfamily	Common Name	No. of Weight-Bearing Digits	No. of Non–Weight-Bearing Digits (Dewclaws)	Comment
Artiodactyla (even-toed ungulate, unguligrade locomotion)	Tayassuidae		Chacoan peccary	Two on front limb, two on rear limb, digits 3 and 4 are weight bearing, digitigrade locomotion	Two on front limb, none on rear limb	Has hoof and sole similar to domestic pig; digitigrade
			Collared peccary, white lipped peccary		Two on front limb, one on medial aspect of rear limb	
	Suidae		Warthog, babirusa, African pigs, Asian pigs		Two on front limb, two on rear limb	
	Bovidae	Bovinae	Bison, banteng, gaur, buffalo, eland, kudu, bongo			Has hoof and sole similar to domestic cattle, goat, sheep; digitigrade
		Antilopinae	Gazelle, gerenuk, klipspringer, saiga			
		Cephalophinae	Duikers			
		Reduncinae	Waterbuck, lechwe, kob, rhebok			
		Aepycerotinae	Impala			
		Caprinae	Sheep, goat, ibex, tar, takin, serow, musk ox			
		Alcelaphinae	Wildebeest, topi, hartebeest, bontebok			
		Hippotraginae	Oryx, addax, gemsbok, roan, sable antelope			
	Cervidae		Deer, elk moose, reindeer, muntjac, sika			
	Tragulidae		Chevrotain			
	Moschidae		Musk deer			
	Giraffidae		Giraffe, okapi			
	Antilocaprinae		Pronghorn		None on front and none on rear limb; no dewclaws present	
	Hippopotamidae		Hippopotamus	Four on front limb, four on rear limb	None on front and none on rear limb; no dewclaws; digitigrade, with fibrous pad	Rounded hooves/ toenails, walk on four toes on each foot

ungulates. The third and fourth digits are weight bearing, whereas the second and fifth are reduced, vestigial, or absent. Bovids are differentiated from other terrestrial animals by unguligrade locomotion, in which only a hoof or claw (the tip of one or two digits) touches the ground.

The bovine hoof is well described in the literature[22,24] and will be used as a prototype to describe its microscopic and macroscopic anatomy. The hoof, or claw, is descriptively composed of the coronary band, adjacent skin, horned wall, sole, lamina, heel, and encased bone of the distal or third phalanx (P3). Rear limbs are rigidly fixed to the body at the ball and socket of the hip joint, whereas the front limbs are more flexibly connected to the torso by soft tissue (muscle, ligaments, tendons). This biomechanical difference is proposed as a potential explanation for the more common lameness noted in the rear limbs of dairy cattle when compared with the front limbs. The hoof grows distally from the coronary band at a rate of approximately 5 to 7 mm/month in cattle but is dependent on genetics, weight distribution, environment, nutrition, and exercise. The outer claw of the rear foot grows more rapidly than the inside claw, whereas the inner grows more rapidly than the outer on the front foot. The heel, also called the bulb, functions as a shock absorber to normal compressive forces.

The lamina in bovid species is not as extensive as in the horse, but is a unique and important structure deserving special attention.[23] It is analogous to the dermis and consists of connective tissue and a rich supply of vasculature and nerves. The lamina provides a strong but flexible attachment between the weight-bearing bone of the third phalanx with the hard wall of the claw. Adjacent to the lamina, and moving outward to the claw surface, are the basement membrane, germinal epithelium, stratum spinosum and, finally, the outer horn layer, the stratum corneum. The interdigitating junction of dermal and epidermal laminae act as a suspensory apparatus between the bone and horny wall and is extremely sensitive to physical or vascular disturbances. The germinal epithelium is the active region of cell proliferation and differentiation. These cells differentiate into keratinocytes that produce and accumulate keratin proteins as they migrate away from the germinal epithelium, losing their supply of nutrients and oxygen. Keratinocytes then undergo a process of death and cornification, forming the cells of the tough outer horn of the claw that serves to protect inner structures and support the weight of the animal. Undoubtedly, any disorder that disrupts blood flow to the lamina will eventually have an effect on the integrity and health of the horny wall of the hoof or sole. Also of clinical significance, the rigid wall of the hoof precludes natural swelling of inflamed tissue, resulting in increased interstitial pressures, which may be greater than vascular pressures that cause obstruction to blood flow, with potential pathologic consequences.

EXAMINATION AND DIAGNOSIS

Just as with any clinical problem, obtaining a complete patient history and performing a thorough and systematic examination are standard when investigating hoof disorders. However, the generally noncompliant and potentially dangerous disposition of most of my nondomestic patients sometimes complicates early intervention and diagnosis. These animals are naturally skilled at concealing significant lameness; the risk associated with anesthesia or physical restraint simply to examine a medically suspicious nondomestic artiodactylid is sometimes met with justified caution and hesitancy. Despite these limitations, the veterinarian must remain clinically diligent to pursue hoof problems as they arise to ensure early management and favorable outcome. It is also good practice to perform opportunistic hoof evaluations during other hands-on procedures.

Prior to physical evaluation, the animal's legs and hooves should be observed at a distance, and from all views, for weight-bearing stance and conformation defects. The patient should be encouraged to walk or run for gait analysis and any initiation or change in reported lameness. The entire limb is inspected for symmetry, range of motion, and insightful defects. The hoof and associated structures are evaluated for normal appearance and structural integrity. Excessive wear marks or elongation on any area of the claw represent improper weight loading or abnormal biomechanics. Soft tissues are noted for indications of hair loss, ulcerations, cellulitis, swelling, erythema, and temperature. Horned areas of the claw are analyzed for evidence of infection, softened tissue, erosions, or ulcers and may need débridement or paring to evaluate fully. Suspect areas should be investigated with cultures and biopsies.

Further diagnostic techniques may be indicated if the hoof disorder is not found on initial examination. This includes blood tests, radiography, arthrocentesis, and ultrasound. More detailed assessment of a suspicious hoof is afforded by the use of computed tomography (CT), magnetic resonance imaging (MRI), and nuclear scintigraphy (bone scan).

CAUSES OF HOOF DISORDERS IN NONDOMESTIC ARTIODACTYLIDS

Lameness is defined as any condition that inhibits or modifies the gait of an animal and is typically the most obvious clinical sign of a hoof disorder. There are many causes of lameness that may originate in any anatomic structure of the limb, but the discussion here is limited to the hard and soft tissues of the hoof. Just as in domestic hoofed animals, lameness caused by disruption of hoof wall and sole integrity from physical trauma, laminitis, and infection is a common disorder in my nondomestic artiodactylid practice. Therefore, a lameness scoring system, adapted from the literature,[22] is used by the veterinary and animal care staff to provide consistency in description, documentation, and communication of lameness problems (Table 80-2). Although most lameness is caused by pain, nonpainful causes such as those that restrict normal biomechanics (e.g., fibrosis, arthrodesis, pregnancy) or neurologic dysfunction may mimic lameness and should be considered. Any persistent or significant lameness should not be neglected.

There are many predisposing factors that potentially contribute to hoof disorders in captive nondomestic artiodactylids. Enclosures with adequate space must be properly and carefully designed, with the natural history and welfare of the species in mind. Exercise promotes natural control of hoof growth while providing ideal circulation and nutrient delivery to the tissues of the hoof. Wire fences and other potentially harmful exhibit perimeters may cause traumatic wounds to the hoof and interdigitum of species known to jump and climb (e.g., nondomestic goat and sheep). Similar considerations must be made for hospital and temporary holding facilities. Poor nutrition and improper substrate (hard, soft, wet, dry) are recognized as contributing to hoof problems in domestic animals,[1,16,18,24,25] and similarly affects our collection artiodactylids. Excess moisture weakens the protective properties of the hoof and sole, which increases susceptibility to bruises, abscesses, and laminitis. Exhibition of certain species should be avoided if climatic and seasonal housing needs cannot be met. Poor living conditions and lack of hygiene predispose animals to many health problems, including those of the hoof. Hoof infections are commonly related to environmental conditions and increased abundance of causative organisms.[17] As noted, the inability to perform routine hoof evaluations and trims in noncompliant species may also jeopardize hoof health by allowing secondary hoof infections to occur. Healthy epithelium and horn tissue are naturally resistant to infections so any breach may increase susceptibility. Refer to Box 80-1 for review of potential hoof problems, by anatomic location, in the nondomestic artiodactylid.

TABLE 80-2	Lameness Scoring System for Nondomestic Artiodactylids			
Score (Grade)	Description	At Rest Analysis	Movement and Gait Analysis	Comment
0	Sound	Even distribution of weight on all limbs	Normal gait and movement	No lameness
1	Intermittent, mildly lame	Subtle, if any, redistribution of weight at rest	Subtle occasional lameness	Mostly normal posture at rest, intermittent limp when moving
2	Mildly lame	Occasional shifting of weight or lifting of leg	Slight head nod or quick gait but moves around freely with mild lameness	Occasional change in posture; may need to exercise to see lameness
3	Moderately lame	Consistent shifting weight, obvious toe touching	Grade 2 signs, with mild reluctance to move, consistent and obvious limp, short striding	Abnormal posture and gait at rest and when moving; may be trailing the herd
4	Very lame	Holds leg off ground at rest, obvious posture change	Grade 3 signs plus three-legged lameness at times, frequent stops, difficulty turning, moderately reluctant to move	Grade 3 signs plus taking deliberate steps one at a time; may be isolating from herd
5	Severely lame	Prefers to lie down	Grade 4 signs, depressed, inability or extremely reluctant to move	Severe pathology likely; behavior and well-being are affected, isolating from herd

BOX 80-1	Disorders of the Hoof in Nondomestic Artiodactylids by Anatomic Foot Location

1. Skin, interdigital space: Trauma, contusions, infection (foot rot, interdigital dermatitis, foot scald, digital dermatitis, MCF, FMD, dermatophilosis), foreign body, fibroma (corn), hyperplasia, heel erosion, impacted or infected sebaceous oil gland, extension of any hoof disease
2. Coronary band: Trauma, contusions, infection (foot rot, interdigital dermatitis, foot scald, digital dermatitis, MCF, FMD, Orf, VSV, BTV, dermatophilosis), extension of any hoof disease
3. Hoof wall: Trauma, foreign body, overgrowth, infection (foot rot, digital dermatitis), structural weakness (soft hooves, wet conditions, poor hygiene), laminitis, coronary band trauma, vertical wall fissures, horizontal wall fissures (laminitic or stress lines, hardship grooves), conformation defect, lack of exercise, nutrition, poor flooring or substrate (hard, rough surface), poor foot care, extension of any hoof disease
4. Sole or subsolar tissue: Trauma, contusions, foreign body, thinning (overuse, overtrimming), overgrowth, infection (foot rot, digital dermatitis, enteric pathogens), structural weakness (soft soles, wet conditions, poor hygiene), ulceration (toe, sole, heel), hemorrhage, abscess (sole, subsole), poor flooring or substrate (hard, rough surface), poor foot care, extension of any hoof disease
5. Heel or heel bulb: Trauma, contusions, foreign body, erosion caused by overgrowth, infection (foot rot, digital dermatitis, interdigital dermatitis), extension of any hoof disease
6. Lamina (corium): Trauma, contusions, foreign body, laminitis, white line disease (hemorrhage, inflammation, infection, horn separation), infection (foot rot, digital dermatitis, enteric pathogens, FMD, BTV), systemic disease (endotoxin release, rumen acidosis, metritis, mastitis, retained fetal membranes, fever), inappropriate nutrition (rumen acidosis, high-energy feed), poor foot care, extension of any hoof disease
7. Bone, joint: Trauma of third phalange (fracture, sprain, tendon or ligament rupture), infection (osteomyelitis, pedal osteitis, tenosynovitis); trauma, arthritis of distal interphalangeal joint (septic, aseptic), copper deficiency, extension of any hoof disease

BTV, Bluetongue virus; BVD, bovine viral diarrhea; FMD, foot-and-mouth disease; MCF, malignant catarrhal fever; Orf, contagious ecthyma, sheep poxvirus; VSV, vesicular stomatitis virus.

Noninfectious Disorders of the Hoof

Physical Injuries

Physical injuries of the hoof may be caused by primary trauma such as fracture of the distal phalanx, degenerative joint disease, or excessive wear of the hoof from pacing on an improper substrate. Secondary injuries caused by wet conditions, overgrown hooves, nutritional disorders, and metabolic disease will predispose the animal to hoof problems as well. Overgrown feet may cause gait abnormalities; places increased stress on joints, tendons, and ligaments; and are a source of pain.[12,16,22] Similarly, improper hoof trimming may lead to pain, thin soles, and abnormal weight bearing.

Laminitis

Laminitis (inflammation of the laminae) is caused by any disturbance of the microcirculation of blood in the lamina, which leads to a collapse of the dermal-epidermal junction between the wall and third phalanx.[1,11,21,23] Metabolic disturbances (e.g., rumen acidosis, lactic acidosis), endotoxemia (e.g., metritis, retained placenta, mastitis) and trauma may cause the release of vasoactive substances that initiate a cascade of events reducing blood flow to the sensitive lamina by vasoconstriction, thrombosis, ischemia, and hypoxia. This results in edema, hemorrhage, and necrosis, which compromise the integrity of laminar tissues. The suspensory function of the lamina fails, allowing for the rotation and sinking of the P3 bone within the claw, causing pain and predisposition to other disorders. A delayed clinical sequela to laminitis may be reduced or abnormal keratinization, which produces weak hoof horn that is less resistant to bacterial invasion and physical forces. Various degrees of laminitis are possible (e.g., subclinical, acute, or chronic) and play a major role in clinical hoof disorders such as sole hemorrhage, sole ulcers, and white line disease in domestic and predictably in nondomestic artiodactylids.

Nutritional Problems

Nutrition plays a vital role in hoof health in domestic animals[1,12,16,22,24] and it is reasonable to assume a similar importance in nondomestic species.[18] Micronutrients such as biotin, copper, and zinc are considered essential for the synthesis of keratin and general hoof health in domestic species. Diets too high in starch or low in fiber may cause rumen acidosis, which is a primary cause of laminitis in dairy cattle. The development of balanced and natural diets appropriate for the variety of nondomestic artiodactylid species is a challenge and continued research is needed to ensure optimum nutrition for hoof and general health.

Sole Lesions

Sole lesions are full-thickness breaks in the epidermis and are differentially named by location on the sole.[1,3,23] The common, or classic, sole abscess is located at the sole-heel junction, the toe abscess is near the apex of the toe, and the heel abscess is located on the heel. A sole hemorrhage is an indication of a contusion to deeper tissue, and may take weeks to become apparent, with clinical lameness and pain. Traumatic injuries, foreign bodies, and penetrating wounds have similar predispositions and clinical presentations. Treatment includes débridement of damaged horn and necrotic tissue to open the wound to air and decrease dirt and fecal entrapment. Application of a hoof block to the sole of the adjacent sound digit to relieve weight bearing on the affected digit will increase healing time and offer pain relief.[22]

Fissures and Cracks

Vertical fissures, or sand cracks, form on the hoof wall because of abnormal production of horn tissue, resulting in decreased toughness and quality.[1,3,21] Causes include improper diet, poor conditions, and trauma. Most cracks are not painful and do not require treatment unless they extend proximally into the coronary band. If cracks become wide and threaten deeper tissue, trimming and the use of wire stents across the vertical crack support the weakened hoof wall. Horizontal fissures and grooves, or stress lines, are sometimes noted on the hoof wall as a result of interrupted horn growth. If they extend into the sensitive lamina, lameness may occur. Causes and treatment options are similar to those of laminitis.

White Line Disease

White line disease is the separation or avulsion of the fibrous junction between the sole and wall on the abaxial border of the sole at the heel-sole junction.[1,3,12,21] The lamina becomes infected secondarily through this opening and tracks of infection may cause abscessation of superficial and deep tissues. Early signs may include black marks in the area of the white line; these must be trimmed and investigated for potential deeper sites of infection. Causes are comparable to those of laminitis and treatment options are similar to those for sole ulcers.

Worn Soles

Thin soles may cause lameness because of aggressive trimming or increased wear from pacing on hard substrates. Worn soles are then susceptible to trauma, bruising or hemorrhage, and laminitis because of inadequate protection from external forces. Thin soles from pacing are problematic especially in noncompliant anxious artiodactylids when moved to new exhibits or to hospital, quarantine, or shipping pens. Quiet enclosures with soft substrate, visual barriers for hiding, and the use of neuroleptic agents should be considered as the animal adapts to novel surroundings.

Interdigital Hyperplasia

Interdigital hyperplasia is a proliferative reaction caused by chronic irritation of the interdigital skin.[1,3] A focal area of dermatitis may form, progressing to a hyperkeratotic protuberance of skin in the interdigital space. Chronic foot rot lesions may also contribute to this condition. Traumatic injuries to the interdigital space may have the same causes as those of the sole. Because of similar clinical presentation, infectious diseases of the hoof (see later) must also be considered, especially if lameness develops concurrently in several animals.

Infectious Disorders of the Hoof

Infectious Pododermatitis

Foot rot, or infectious pododermatitis, is a highly contagious disease of artiodactylids and is the term used to describe an acute to chronic infection and inflammation of the skin and adjacent soft tissue of the hoof.[1,8,9,16,17] It is characterized by diffuse swelling, fetid odor, necrosis of interdigital skin, laminitis with progressive separation of the horny tissues, and varying degrees of lameness. Historically, it was believed to be caused by a dual infection of various strains of the anaerobic bacteria *Fusobacterium necrophorum* and *Dichelobacter nodosus* but advances in diagnostic capabilities have also implicated other bacteria.[5] This disease may be a problem for any hoofed animal persistently exposed to wet, poorly drained, muddy, and fecal-contaminated lots, enclosures, or pastures. Foot rot caused by *D. nodosus* has been described in wild ibex and mouflon[2] and has been diagnosed in my practice in several species of artiodactylids during the winter rainy season. Infection is facilitated by the maceration of the interdigital skin caused by constant exposure to moisture and mechanical trauma. Because susceptibility and severity of foot rot are dependent on several risk factors, a multifaceted approach to its management is necessary. Treatment depends on the severity of the clinical signs and includes therapeutic trimming and foot baths, antibiotics, analgesics, and recuperating affected animals in a dry pen or pasture. Eradication of foot rot is difficult because of the numerous implicated strains of *F. necrophorum* and *D. nodosus*. Current vaccines are not effective against all strains but may be helpful in reducing transmission.

Interdigital Dermatitis

The term *foot scald*, or *interdigital dermatitis*, is used in domestic hoofed species to describe a mild form of infectious pododermatitis caused by a primary infection by *F. necrophorum* and may be a precursor to foot rot.[1,12,17] Interdigital dermatitis in cattle has been a source of controversy because clinical and histopathologic findings are sometimes similar to those of digital dermatitis (see later) but will be considered distinct disorders in this chapter. Any outbreak in lameness within the herd should be investigated thoroughly for potential infectious causes, especially those reportable to public health officials. Dermatophilosis (strawberry foot rot) affects the hairy skin of the coronet and pastern and may be mistaken for foot scald. Certain important viral diseases (see later) may produce lesions that might be confused with foot scald or foot rot because of similar initial clinical signs involving the coronary band, interdigitum, and adjacent skin. *F. necrophorum* may also secondarily infect viral hoof lesions and may distract from an early diagnosis of the primary cause. Most foot scald lesions heal rapidly following the wet season or removal to dry and clean pastures. Treatment options are similar to those for foot rot. Although *F. necrophorum* vaccines are available, they are not clinically effective in all situations.

Papillomatous Digital Dermatitis

Digital dermatitis (DD), also known as papillomatous digital dermatitis, is a highly contagious, proliferative skin disease of the foot in cattle, sheep, and goats caused by primary or secondary spirochete infection.[1,17] Lesions are characteristically found on the plantar aspect of the rear foot, near the interdigital space or heel bulbs, but may invade the horny structure of the claw. It may be a major cause of pain, lameness, and financial loss in infected herds. The advent of improved molecular diagnostics has increased the incidence of DD and its importance was likely underestimated in the past. It has become widespread in the United States dairy industry in the past 10 years. The causative agent most commonly identified histologically is an anaerobic spirochete of the genus *Treponema*. Its occurrence and transmission

seem to be dependent on numerous factors such as environment, host, microbe, and husbandry. Because of variability in initial clinical signs, DD may be misdiagnosed as foot rot or foot scald. Treatment choices are similar to those for foot rot but there are no *Treponema* vaccines commercially available for control of DD at this time.

Viral Diseases

As noted, there are several viral diseases that may cause important hoof disorders in the domestic artiodactylid and are presumed or documented to occur in nondomestic species. The severity of the disease depends on infectious dose, viral serotype, age, species, and health status. Clinically, these viral diseases may resemble each other or hoof infections of bacterial origin, such as foot rot. Possibly the most important is foot-and-mouth disease because of the devastating consequences of misdiagnosis.

Foot-and-Mouth Disease

Foot-and-mouth disease (FMD) is a highly contagious and sometimes fatal disease that affects swine, sheep, goats, deer, water buffalo, bison, antelope, and likely other wild artiodactylids.[19] Clinical lesions may include vesicles and erosions between the hooves and may be confused with several similar but less harmful viral diseases, including bluetongue, bovine viral diarrhea, vesicular stomatitis, contagious ecthyma, malignant catarrhal fever, and swine vesicular disease. The ability of FMD virus to remain viable in the environment for up to 1 month and its persistence in wildlife reservoirs contribute to the difficulty in regard to eradication and control. This disease was last diagnosed in North America in 1929 and is considered endemic in regions of Africa, Asia, South America, and Europe. If unusual or suspicious signs of disease are noted, immediate reporting to animal health officials is indicated. Because zoological collections contain a variety of artiodactylids from around the world, it behooves the zoo and wildlife clinician to provide careful opportunistic inspection of the hooves of nondomestic artiodactylids, especially of imports during quarantine, to identify potentially infected animals.

PREVENTION AND TREATMENT

As with other medical disorders, it is ethically and economically important to prevent rather than treat. Despite the difficulty in handling nondomestic artiodactylids, early intervention and treatment of hoof problems are vital for overall health. Zoos must make thoughtful efforts to create healthy, hygienic, and natural enclosures for all artiodactylids to meet their mental and physical requirements for longevity and health. Stress management, enclosure comfort, regular removal of waste, and disease control are general principles that should not be overlooked. For ungulates, enclosures need to be designed to promote hoof health by providing sufficient space for exercise, with a variety of natural substrates under foot. Facilities used for seasonal housing should be creatively designed with hoof health in mind. In my practice, temperamental species are known to pace excessively when separated from the herd or transferred to novel locations (e.g., hospital, quarantine, shipping, new exhibit); therefore, the prophylactic use of neuroleptic or tranquilizing agents should be anticipated and strongly considered. Climate may play a role in hoof health and should always be considered when acquiring and exhibiting artiodactylids in weather conditions inconsistent with those found in their natural environment. As noted, proper nutrition is extremely important in the maintenance of hoof fitness. The role of observant animal caretakers trained in the early detection of lameness and hoof disorders cannot be overemphasized.

While in quarantine, new acquisitions must have thorough hoof health evaluations, assessment for infectious hoof disease, and therapeutic hoof trims prior to entry into an established herd. Routine and opportunistic corrective hoof trims are an integral component of preventive health programs for captive nondomestic hoofstock. To reduce spontaneous lameness, hoof trimming is necessary to ensure proper balance and weight loading on all limbs and to avoid any disparity in natural growth and adequate wear. Despite the variety in foot structure of our collection artiodactylids, the principles of therapeutic hoof trimming and care are similar to those for domestic species and excellent references are available for specific techniques.[22] The zoo veterinarian is often required to be the collection's farrier, so becoming skilled in this specialty is highly advised. It is important to clean trimming equipment in between animals to decrease the possibility of disease transmission.

The general treatment, control, and management of common hoof disorders in nondomestic artiodactylids is supportive and, because of similarities, the literature for domestic species is a valid reference. Aggressive and competent but considerate intervention is warranted to avoid the development of secondary problems. Débridement of affected hoof to expose healthy tissue with appropriate follow-up treatment greatly enhance healing. The use of systemic antibiotics, tetanus vaccination, protective bandaging, hydrotherapy, rest on dry substrate, and foot baths may not be appropriate in all situations but should be considered. More invasive treatments such as cast or splint application, regional perfusion, bone débridement, intra-articular medication, and the use of hoof repair material (with or without antibiotics) are useful in suitable cases. Combination of treatments may be the best for resolution and control of hoof problems. The ethical use of analgesics is recommended to comfort the patient.

REFERENCES

1. Aiello SE, Mays A: Musculoskeletal system. In Aiello SE, Mays A, editors: The Merck veterinary manual, ed 8, Whitehouse Station, NJ, 1998, Merck, pp 755–882.
2. Belloy L, Giacometti M, Boujon P, Waldvogel A: Detection of *Dichelobacter nodosus* in wild ungulates (*Capra ibex ibex* and *Ovis aries musimon*) and domestic sheep suffering from foot rot using a two-step polymerase chain reaction. J Wildl Dis 43:82–88, 2007.
3. Collick DW, Weaver AS, Greenough PR: Interdigital space and claw. In Greenough PR, Weaver AD, editors: Lameness in cattle, ed 3, Philadelphia, 1997, WB Saunders, pp 101–122.
4. deMaar TW, Ng'ang'a MM: Normal hoof angles and other parameters of selected African ungulates. In Proceedings of the Annual Meeting of the American Association of Zoo Veterinarians, 2000, pp 488–491.
5. Dubreuil P: Small ruminant infectious disease of the foot. In Anderson DE, Rings AM, editors: Current veterinary therapy: Food animal practice, ed 5, St. Louis, 2009, WB Saunders, pp 251–258.
6. Fowler ME: Hoof, nail and claw problems in mammals. In Fowler ME, editor: Zoo and wild animal medicine, ed 2, Philadelphia, 1986, WB Saunders, pp 550–556.
7. Fowler ME: Integumentary system. In Fowler ME, editor: Medicine and surgery of South American camelids: llama, alpaca, vicuna, guanaco, ed 2, Ames, Iowa, 1998, Iowa State University Press, pp 250–269.
8. Jahnke JJ: Interdigital necrobacillosis (foot rot) in cattle. In Smith BP, editor: Large animal internal medicine, ed 4, St. Louis, 2009, Mosby, pp 1234–1236.
9. Jahnke JJ: Infectious foot rot in sheep and goats. In Smith BP, editor: Large animal internal medicine, ed 4, St. Louis, 2009, Mosby, pp 1236–1239.
10. Lavin S, Ruiz-Bascaran M, Marco I, et al: Foot infections associated with *Arcanobacterium pyogenes* in free-living Fallow deer (*Dama dama*). J Wildl Dis 4(3):607–611, 2004.
11. Linford RL: Laminitis (founder). In Smith BP, editor: Large animal internal medicine, ed 4, St. Louis, 2009, Mosby, pp 1224–1231.
12. Matthews JG: Lameness in adult goats. In Matthews J, editor: Diseases of the goat, ed 3, Ames, Iowa, 2009, Blackwell, pp 87–111.
13. Miller MA: Hippopotamidae (hippopotamus). In Fowler ME, Miller RE, editors: Zoo and wild animal medicine, ed 5, Philadelphia, WB Saunders, 2003, pp 602–612.
14. Morris PJ, Shima AL: Suidae and Tayassuidae. In Fowler ME, Miller RE, editors: Zoo and wild animal medicine, ed 5, Philadelphia, WB Saunders, 2003, pp 586–602.
15. Nowak RM: Artiodactyla. In Nowak RM, editor: Mammals of the world, ed 5, Baltimore, 1991, John Hopkins University Press, pp 1334–1499.

16. Reilly LK, Baird AN, Pugh DG: Diseases of the musculoskeletal system. In Pugh DG, editor: Sheep and goat medicine, Philadelphia, 2001, Elsevier, pp 223–254.

17. Shearer JK: Infectious disorders of the foot skin. In Anderson DE, Rings AM, editors: Current veterinary therapy: Food animal practice, ed 5, St. Louis, 2009, WB Saunders, pp 224–242.

18. Sikarskie JG, Brockway CR, Ullrey DE, et al: Dietary protein and hoof growth in juvenile female white-tailed deer *(Odocoileus virginianus)*. J Zoo Wildl Med 19:18–23, 1988.

19. Thomson GR, Bengis RG, Brown CC: Picornavirus infections. Foot and mouth disease. In Williams ES, Barker IK, editors: Infectious diseases of wild mammals, ed 3, Ames, Iowa, 2001, Iowa State University Press, pp 119–130.

20. Ultimate Ungulate: Ungulates of the world, 2010 (http://www.ultimateungulate.com/ungulates.html).

21. van Amstel SR: Noninfectious disorders of the foot. In Anderson DE, Rings AM, editors: Current veterinary therapy: Food animal practice, ed 5, St. Louis, 2009, WB Saunders, pp 222–234.

22. van Amstel SR, Shearer J. Biomechanics of weight (load) bearing and claw trimming. In van Amstel SR, Shearer J, editors: Manual for treatment and control of lameness in cattle, Ames, Iowa, 2006, Blackwell, pp 42–126.

23. van Amstel SR, Shearer J: Horn formation and growth. In van Amstel SR, Shearer J, editors: Manual for treatment and control of lameness in cattle, Ames, Iowa, 2006, Blackwell, pp 16–30.

24. van Amstel SR, Shearer J: Introduction to lameness in cattle. In van Amstel SR, Shearer J, editors: Manual for treatment and control of lameness in cattle, Ames, Iowa, 2006, Blackwell, pp 1–15.

25. van Amstel SR, Shearer J: Nutrition and claw health. In van Amstel SR, Shearer J, editors: Manual for treatment and control of lameness in cattle, Ames, Iowa, 2006, Blackwell, pp 31–41.

CHAPTER 81

Johne's Disease and Free-Ranging Wildlife

Elizabeth J.B. Manning and Jonathan Mark Sleeman

This chapter addresses the current status of *Mycobacterium avium* subsp. *paratuberculosis* (MAP) infection in free-ranging wildlife, taking care to distinguish between the simple presence of the organism and true infection, the significant differences seen for MAP infection in ruminant versus nonruminant hosts, and the important distinctions between indicators of the organism in a host and actual disease. Attentiveness to these distinctions is needed to assess the risk of Johne's disease for wildlife population health accurately.

CAUSE

The mycobacterial organism causing Johne's disease in ruminants belongs to the *Mycobacterium avium* complex (MAC), and is now broadly referred to as a subspecies of *M. avium*, itself a ubiquitous opportunistic pathogen for humans and animals alike. The members of this mycobacterial complex, previously classified phenotypically but now under reclassification via molecular typing methods, are acid-fast, slow- to very slow-growing, nonpigmented, rod-shaped bacteria with complex, lipid-rich cell walls.[27] The elaboration of MAP strain K-10's genome in 2005 sparked a proliferation of molecular typing analyses in concert with the elucidation of the complementary genome of its cousin, *M. avium* subsp. *hominissuis*.[13,19] These studies have parsed MAP isolates into numerous strain groups beyond the S (sheep) and C (cattle) categories previously used. These strain discriminations are not diagnostically critical for wildlife managers, although analyses of the genetic polymorphisms and potential virulence variations across strains that have been revealed are valuable from a research standpoint, because MAP strain types are not restricted to host species—for example, so-called sheep strains have been

isolated from cattle, and cattle strains from bison, sheep, and deer. Each strain is capable of infecting and eventually causing disease in ruminants and each strain may be isolated through culture by an experienced laboratory. In the United States, the organism's genome is highly conserved, with most (78%) isolates from cattle belonging to the same genetic node (e.g., the cattle strain now referred to as type I).[17] For wildlife managers, a reasonable working hypotheses is that any strain of MAP may infect any ruminant host, the organism may be subsequently shed by an infected animal in milk and feces, and any such infection will eventually kill the ruminant host.

MAP is resistant to heat, cold, drying, and acidic conditions, but does not replicate in the environment. An obligate pathogen, MAP in the environment does eventually die off completely, but not quickly. When a premise is contaminated by MAP-containing manure, approximately 90% of the organisms are believed to die off within a few months, but MAP in low numbers may be recovered for more than 1 year. The relevance of this persistence at low levels to new cases of infection is unknown. In Australia, MAP could be isolated (albeit from fewer and fewer samples over time) from shaded soil (including soil shaded by crops) for up to 55 weeks, and in shaded trough water at 48 weeks. Even greater longevity was noted in trough sediment. MAP was isolated from grasses germinating through manure-laden soil, again in the pattern observed for MAP isolation from soil; greater MAP longevity was seen in grasses grown from completely shaded versus 70% shaded soil boxes (24 versus 9 weeks).[28] This study's comparison of shaded versus partially shaded sites led the authors to conclude that diurnal temperature fluctuation was more relevant in hastening complete MAP die-off than was ultraviolet (UV) radiation, and removal of vegetation to maximize temperature changes at soil level may be beneficial. Based on these data, contaminated drinking water may remain a reservoir for new infections longer than contaminated ground.

EPIDEMIOLOGY

The primary route whereby wildlife may encounter MAP is by sharing range with infected domestic agricultural ruminant species. Because of long-standing patterns of husbandry (e.g., high animal density, bottle-feeding pooled milk and colostrum, fecal contamination of calf water, premises, and feed), in addition to a history of low biosecurity trade across states and countries, the global dairy industry reports the highest prevalence of Johne's disease. The U.S. Department of Agriculture recently stated that the organism was detected on 68% of U.S. dairy premises (based on pooled environmental sample culture data; http://www.aphis.usda.gov/vs/ceah/ncahs/nahms/dairy/dairy07/Dairy07_is_Johnes.pdf). Given that a cow produces 100 pounds of manure daily and that manure spreading on fields is a common agricultural practice, the environmental (soil and water) burden of MAP is highest in intensively farmed areas. Browsing ruminants are likely primarily at risk through shallow sources of contaminated water and grazing ruminants through both contaminated water and grasses in these areas.

The fecal-oral route is the primary means of transmission. Most new cases of infection occur when MAP is ingested by a susceptible animal (<6 months old) and sufficient organisms are successfully taken up by M cells in the distal ileal Peyer's patches to reside (and replicate) in the phagosomes of subepithelial macrophages. For months to years, the animal's immune system appears to ignore the intracellular pathogen. During this long silent infection phase, the animal appears healthy but is still capable of contaminating pastures and transmitting the infection through intermittent shedding of MAP in feces. Calves, fawns, lambs, or kids may be born infected because in utero transmission is possible, even in subclinical cases. At some point during adulthood, for reasons not yet understood, the infection spreads to regional lymph nodes and then disseminates throughout the body.

Most young animals acquire the organism by suckling from manure-soiled teats, drinking water contaminated by feces from infected animals, drinking colostrum or milk carrying MAP from an infected dam, or in utero. The transmission risks increase as dams move into later stages of the infection; thus, clinically affected hoofstock are more likely to infect offspring than dams still in good condition.

As noted, MAP is an obligate pathogen believed capable of replicating only within a host; therefore, it eventually disappears from an environment and its recovery in low numbers from the environment does not guarantee that spillover into ruminant wildlife will occur. Interrelated conditions must exist before a new case of infection is achieved, much less before a wild ruminant reservoir of infection is established—that is, a ruminant must be susceptible, 6 months of age or younger, and ingest a sufficient dose frequently enough to ensure MAP's residence in the ileal epithelial macrophages. Experimental infection studies have indicated that an infective oral dose for young cattle, deer, and goats is 4×10^6 colony-forming units (CFUs; total of 200 mg wet weight pelleted MAP). Therefore, the risk of infection for a susceptible animal due to remote contact—for example, by crossing barn corridors in the path of a contaminated keeper's boot or traversing a road driven on by a veterinary truck that had crossed a pasture containing infected cattle—is low. However, given that infected cattle may shed 10^6 CFUs/g of manure, this environmental contamination presents a risk to wildlife via contaminated feed and water in some circumstances.

RUMINANT INFECTIONS

Johne's disease is primarily a concern for ruminant species. Disease and death caused by MAP infection has been reported for captive and free-ranging ungulates of all taxonomic groups. All ruminant species are thought to be susceptible to infection and clearing the infection is unlikely, although anecdotal cases of test-positive animals maintaining good health until killed by another fatal illness have been reported. Broadly, similar patterns of transmission, subclinical incubation, immunologic responses, and clinical illness prevail across the Artiodactyla order, although differences do exist among species that may affect diagnosis and control.

Clinical Signs

After infection, the clinical disease known as paratuberculosis is slow to develop; affected wild ruminants are generally 1 year of age and usually much older. The vague and nonspecific primary clinical signs are loss of body condition, poor hair coat, and diarrhea in the later stages of the disease, which may be intermittent and may not appear at all in some species (Fig. 81-1).

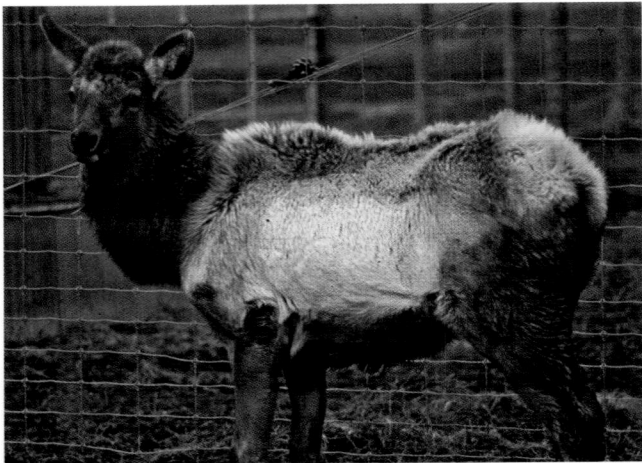

Figure 81-1

Elk *(Cervus elaphus)* showing the typical nonspecific clinical signs of Johne's disease, including loss of body condition and poor hair coat.

Pathology

Lesions may range from inapparent to florid, depending on the stage of infection at the time of necropsy and the species being examined. For example, in some cases of infection in sheep, bison, and perhaps other nondomestic species, the gastrointestinal tract may appear completely normal, even when the animal is clinically affected. At the other extreme, the ileum may be thickened, corrugated, and reddened, with dilated lymphatic vessels coursing over its serosal surface as well as the serosa of enlarged mesenteric lymph nodes. Clinically ill animals are often emaciated, with a total absence or necrosis of abdominal fat stores. Microscopically, acid-fast rod-shaped organisms (scarce to numerous) may be noted within macrophages as part of a granulomatous infiltrate (Fig. 81-2). This inflammation may be slight or may completely efface ileal villi.

Bison

Several articles in the literature have addressed Johne's disease in bison in the United States.[2] Each article relied on the same samples, herd history, and isolates obtained from a single population in Montana. Unfortunately, extrapolations from this population to general conclusions about MAP in bison (e.g., that MAP in bison is unusually difficult to detect via culture or that serology is ineffective) have turned out to be inaccurate, at least for bison in other parts of the country. Several but not all the commercial enzyme-linked immunosorbent assays (ELISA) detect antibody in bison and, in

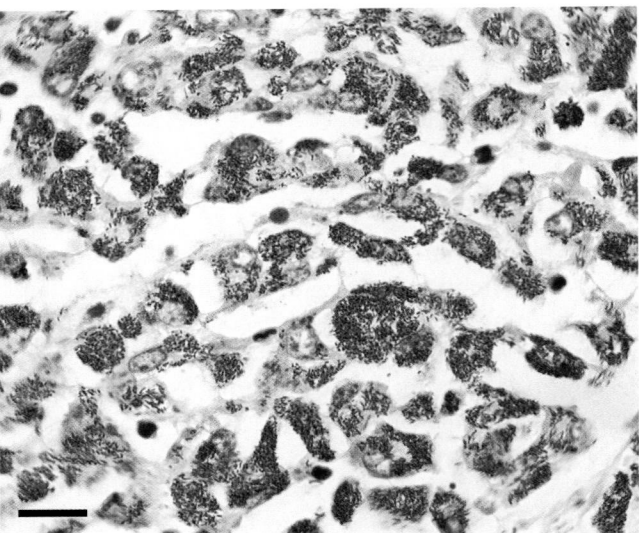

Figure 81-2

Photomicrograph of colon from a white-tailed deer with Johne's disease demonstrating accumulations of epithelioid macrophages in the lamina propria, with myriad intracytoplasmic bacilli consistent with *M. avium* subsp. *paratuberculosis* (acid-fast stain). Bar = 30 μm. *(From Sleeman JM, Manning EJB, Rohm JH, et al: Johne's disease in a free-ranging white-tailed deer from Virginia and subsequent surveillance for* Mycobacterium avium *subspecies* paratuberculosis, *J Wildl Dis 45:201-206, 2009.)*

numerous cases, the MAP strain has been easily isolated and characterized as the same that is detected in other U.S. species.[17] Clinical signs and pathologic lesions mirror those seen in cattle and transmission of the organism is the same. In Canada, surveillance of bison with the polymerase chain reaction (PCR) assay produced positive results in several herds, but the organism was not recovered. A serologic survey of banked sera collected over multiple years from free-ranging bison managed in four western national parks was completed under the auspices of the National Park Service. ELISA results for more than 1200 serum samples did not indicate the presence of MAP infection in these populations.[15]

Deer and Elk

Infected tule elk *(Cervus elaphus nannodes)* were first detected in 1979 at the Point Reyes National Seashore (PRNS; Marin County, Calif). The infection has been confirmed in adult animals since that time.[16] Reserve managers have reported no obvious effect on herd health or reproduction in the approximately 450-member herd because of Johne's disease; diagnostic testing is no longer part of the management plan.[8] No evidence of MAP infection has been found in native black-tailed deer *(Odocoileus hemionus columbianus)* also located at PRNS. Although an infection prevalence in two non-native cervid species—axis deer *(Axis axis)* and fallow deer *(Dama dama)*—sharing the range with tule elk was estimated at 8% to 9% 20 years ago, the infection appears also to have had minimal impact on population-based health parameters. Surveys in Arkansas[4] and Montana, and in Wyoming elk,[22] did not reveal indicators of MAP infection in these free-ranging populations.

The causative organism has also been isolated from tissues of clinically normal free-ranging white-tailed deer *(Odocoileus virginianus)*.[5] However, clinical disease as a result of infection with MAP in free-ranging white-tailed deer is rarely reported as opposed to several reports of clinical cases in captive white-tailed deer.[10,14] Paratuberculosis was first diagnosed in an endangered Florida Key deer (a subspecies of white-tailed deer; *O. virginianus clavium*) in 1996 and later in six additional Florida Key deer from 1998 to 2004. Subsequent surveys have indicated that the organism persists in the Florida Key deer population and environment at a low prevalence, but its distribution is limited to a relatively small geographic area within their range.[20] A single clinical case in a 2-year-old male white-tailed deer from Virginia has also been reported.[26] Subsequent surveillance failed to reveal additional cases or infected animals. The authors concluded that infection with MAP is an infrequent occurrence in these deer, and speculated that a local cattle farm was the likely source of infection. A study that performed multistate surveys of wild white-tailed deer in the southeastern United States also revealed a very low prevalence of infection (0.3%).[5] It thus appears that white-tailed deer do not currently constitute a broad regional reservoir for this organism.

Clinical Johne's disease has also been reported on occasion in other free-ranging ungulate species, including Rocky Mountain bighorn sheep *(Ovis canadensis canadensis)*, Rocky Mountain goats *(Oreamnos americanus)*, and free-ranging red *(Cervus elaphus hippelaphus)* and fallow deer in Europe.[9]

A quicker progression from infection to clinical signs has been reported in farmed cervids (red deer or elk) than bovids, with animals younger than 2 years of age rapidly losing weight, developing severe pathology, and dying of the infection.[6,14] Whether this is a function of stress, dose, or other factors caused by high animal density under intensive husbandry as opposed to a factor innate to cervids' response to MAP is not known.

NONRUMINANT INFECTIONS

Although evidence of MAP infection has been reported on occasion over the last decade in nonruminant wildlife species, disease caused by this infection has not.[3,6,7] Few studies have noted any pathologic changes or visible acid-fast organisms in sampled tissues and fewer still have confirmed shedding of the organism in these nonruminants. Conclusions on interspecies MAP transmission based on the presence of the organism in nonruminant tissue, especially if the presence is indicated solely by PCR results as opposed to isolation of the living organism, in the absence of lesions, disease, or shedding, should be made cautiously. It may be that these surveys captured non-ruminant animals in early subclinical phases of infection, but the prevailing opinion of experts is that MAP does not cause clinical cases of paratuberculosis in nonruminant species and histopathologic changes are mild to nonexistent. (See later for the sole exception, lagomorphs.) In reviewing these reports, the species range suggests a greater likelihood for the presence of MAP in carnivorous predators or scavengers such as stoat, crows, opossum, starling, fox, coyote, and raccoon (implying ingestion of infected prey) or in species found in close proximity to infected domestic agricultural animals and structures (barn cats and rodents). Molecular analysis has confirmed in numerous cases that the MAP strains obtained from wildlife are the same as those recovered from domestic ruminants on the same property.

The most extensive research addressing MAP in a nonruminant species has focused on rabbits *(Oryctolagus cuniculus)* sharing pastures with a herd of cattle with Johne's disease in Tayside, Scotland.[11] At necropsy, these rabbits displayed intestinal granulomatous inflammatory lesions, ranging from minimal to extensive, with intracellular acid-fast bacilli detectable in numerous cases. The rabbits shed the organism in fecal pellets and one study[11a] has described both horizontal and vertical transmission in this population. Because this species apparently may maintain the infection within its population and excrete the organism in a form ingestible by other species (cattle, at least, do not avoid rabbit pellets while grazing), this population must be considered a reservoir of MAP infection for domestic animals and other wildlife species. The reason why rabbits are apparently the sole nonruminant species to develop disease caused by MAP infection is unknown; perhaps the caecotrophic and denning habits of rabbits create an exposure to the organism once introduced that is not experienced by other nonruminant species.

Isolation of MAP has been noted in other lagomorph species (*Sylvilagus floridanus* in the United States, *Lepus europaeus* in Chile), but neither lesions nor acid-fast organisms were noted in tissue samples and clinical disease was not seen.[3,23] To date, the circumstances that created a rabbit MAP reservoir appear to be unique to the Tayside population.

Camelids

Free-ranging guanacos (*Lama guanicoe*) on Tierra del Fuego Island, Chile, were found to be shedding MAP in a recent report.[24] The prevalence was low (4.2%, 21/501 fecal samples); in all cases, the isolate was characterized as the cattle-type strain. The economic basis of this region is livestock production. Johne's disease has not been reported in sheep or cattle in the area but surveillance for the infection is not performed. The authors made no comments about the clinical condition of these guanacos. Paratuberculosis in camelids under domestic husbandry has also been reported, including alpacas (*Lama pacos*) in Australia and camels (*Camelus dromedarius*) from Egypt and Saudi Arabia. From these few reports, it appears that the epidemiology, diagnostic findings, and pathology of the disease are similar to those seen in ruminant species.

DIAGNOSIS

Effective and affordable diagnostic assays are available to determine the infection status of a herd or confirm a Johne's disease diagnosis in an individual animal of any species. Because of various factors, such as inherent sample contamination (particularly for fecal samples), potential for isolation of mixed mycobacterial species, prolonged incubation, isolation variations caused by MAP strain type, it is recommended that wildlife managers use laboratories experienced in MAP diagnostics specifically. In the United States, laboratories may elect to demonstrate their competency in serologic, culture, and PCR detection of MAP infection with samples collected from cattle. Laboratories successfully passing these annual assay-specific check tests provided by the U.S. Department of Agriculture (USDA)–Animal and Plant Health Inspection Service (APHIS) can be found online (http://www.aphis.usda.gov/animal_health/lab_info_services/approved_labs.shtml).

There are two approaches for MAP diagnostics; the first is to look for evidence of the organism itself (culture or direct PCR) and the second is to screen for animals' response to infection (antibody, cytokine pro-

duction). Assays useful for the former are available for any species, whereas validated assays targeting the latter are limited to cattle, sheep, and goats. However, an ELISA for deer has been evaluated and is currently in use in Australia.[14]

Culture

The capacities of bacterial culture for MAP isolation have been expanded to include such diverse samples as blood, milk, water, soil, and forage, as well as the commonly collected fecal and tissue samples. Pooling of fecal or environmental samples permits culture to be done at a fraction of the cost of individual animal testing. Many laboratories have adopted liquid media systems with automated growth detection and have found them to be more sensitive than solid media for this slow-growing organism—generation time of 1 to 4 days, depending on initial inoculum.[25] Liquid cultures are automatically monitored daily, whereas solid media slants are usually inspected weekly, or perhaps only monthly. Samples are incubated for at least 7 weeks before the sample is considered to be free of MAP; samples with a heavy burden of MAP may signal positive within a single week, however. The identity of the organism triggering a positive signal in these liquid media systems must be determined, usually via acid-fast staining to confirm a mycobacterial species followed by PCR targeting the MAP genetic insertion sequence IS*900*.[18] Identification of the organism from samples tested with solid media slants is accomplished by assessing growth rate, colony morphology, and mycobactin (an iron chelator required by MAP) dependency status. Quantification of the number of MAP in the sample, useful for assessing level of environmental contamination, may be accomplished if requested of the laboratory at sample submission by standard plate counting or through an algorithm developed for one of the liquid culture systems. It should be noted that in heavily contaminated premises, an isolation of MAP from a fecal sample may simply be the organism passing through the gastrointestinal tract as opposed to its being shed by a truly infected animal.

Not only is there now a broader range of sample types that may be tested and more sensitive media in use, but experienced laboratories may now establish the infection status of a herd or enclosure at a significantly lower cost by pooling individual samples (usually five/pool) with minimal loss of assay sensitivity. Because of the recognized challenges of this technique, wildlife managers are recommended to submit samples for pooling to check-test approved laboratories listed on the USDA-APHIS website, as noted earlier.

Polymerase Chain Reaction

Assays based on PCR testing are used in two ways in MAP diagnostics. One is to confirm the identity of an acid-fast organism isolated from a cultured sample and the other is applied directly to a fecal sample without culture. The PCR's target is usually the MAP gene insertion sequence IS900, a sequence believed to be unique to this organism. Other targets are also used; in fact multiplex (multiple target) PCR assays are helpful when dealing with members of the *M. avium* complex, especially when a sample may contain more than one subspecies.

PCR assays are notoriously finicky, requiring multiple precisely calibrated steps with reagents that are prone to molecular contamination. Most commercially available direct PCR kits for MAP have been validated for bovine feces only. Interpretation of the assay for samples from other species should be done cautiously because biologic inhibitors in other types of samples may be present, leading to false-negative results. The assay may also be confounded by suboptimal sample processing protocols—for example, processing protocols describe the amount of sample needed by weight but because the moisture content of fecal samples varies considerably by factors such as species' diet or environmental exposure, the actual amount of sample matrix processed also varies considerably. Protocols to manage samples, ranging from desiccated to dripping, are now being optimized.

Tests for MAP by PCR assay are not infallible. For some laboratories and for some MAP strains, its sensitivity is less than what is seen with culture, and there have been a few reports of IS900-like elements producing false-positive results.[21] For this reason, it is critical that culling decisions not be made on the basis of direct PCR fecal results only. Reliance on PCR confirmation in the absence of proof of the living organism is not recommended. Isolation of the living organism through culture and/or presence of other indicators of infection (e.g., clinical disease, test-positive serologic test, PCR-positive on subsequent sample) are needed to avoid erroneous euthanasia.

Wildlife research has another epidemiologic tool thanks to PCR technology; the assay may be used to assess paraffin-embedded tissues for MAP. Paraffin block repositories kept for populations of interest may now be screened retrospectively for this infection, adding

more specificity to the histopathologic identification of acid-fast organisms. This assay may also be an adjunct at necropsy for the diagnosis of individual animals. The sensitivity of this diagnostic approach is greater for tissues with visible intracellular MAP.[15]

Serologic Testing

Antibodies, produced as an infected animal moves into the late and clinical stages of MAP infection, neither clear the infection nor slow the progress of Johne's disease, because intracellular pathogens are unaffected by this facet of the immune system. Antibodies do serve as useful surveillance analytes detectable via ELISA or the agar-gel immunodiffusion (AGID) test to determine herd prevalence. Serologic assays are a quick and inexpensive way to raise the index of suspicion for MAP infection; sensitivity is highest for clinically ill animals. The numerical result provided by the ELISA (versus the AGID test's bimodal positive-negative interpretation) is correlated with the level of shedding—that is, the higher the value above the ELISA cutoff, the more likely an animal is contaminating the premises with MAP in feces and, if female, shedding into milk and producing offspring infected in utero. The assays are validated for domestic (primarily bovine) species; however, an assay has also been approved by the USDA for use in small ruminants. False-negative results will occur if the infected animal is tested when not yet producing antibody. False-positive results may occur if the animal is infected with or vaccinated for a different organism eliciting antibodies that cross-react on a Johne's disease ELISA (e.g., another mycobacterial species such as *M. bovis* or *Corynebacterium pseudotuberculosis*). Neither AGID nor ELISA have been validated for use with nondomestic hoofstock and cannot be relied on to establish a definitive diagnosis of Johne's disease for an individual animal.[1] On a herd basis, however, the pattern of ELISA results provides an index of suspicion concerning the likelihood of MAP infection in the tested population. This information is useful for deciding whether further, more specific, testing is warranted, and permits managers to compare populations or monitor the infection status of the same population over time.

Postmortem Testing

The best tissues for assessment are the ileum and mesenteric lymph nodes, even if no gross lesions are seen. Two sets of these tissues should be collected, one set for culture, and one for staining by both hematoxylin and eosin and an acid-fast stain, such as Ziehl-Neelsen. Typical paratuberculosis lesions are noncaseating granulomatous inflammation (caseation has been noted in red deer), composed predominantly of epithelioid macrophages within the intestinal lamina propria and submucosa. The cortex and paracortex of the mesenteric lymph nodes are good sites to scrutinize for the multinucleated inflammatory giant cells that may be the sole indication of infection. The acid-fast stain may highlight the intracellular rod-shaped organism; macrophages may be packed with them, or only a single bacillus may be seen after examining multiple fields. As noted, PCR analysis of paraffin blocks for MAP may be rewarding.

TREATMENT AND VACCINES

Few treatment trials have been attempted for infected ruminants because of high cost and infeasibility; multiple drugs must be given daily orally or injected over many months. The drugs tested have mirrored those used to treat other mycobacterioses, such as rifampin, clarithromycin, and isoniazid. In one small study with infected adult cattle, signs abated during treatment but returned when therapy was discontinued. Recent studies have attempted to detail MAP's specific susceptibility to antibiotics.[12]

Killed vaccines are approved in numerous countries for use under veterinary supervision in cattle (Mycopar in the United States) or small ruminants (Gudair in other countries, such as Australia, New Zealand, and Spain). Other vaccines are under development for domestic agriculture species. Currently available vaccines reduce the amount of clinical disease in a herd and the level of shedding of infected vaccinates, but transmission continues and new cases will arise in a vaccinated herd or flock. Vaccinated animals will test positive to any serologic assay; therefore, only organism detection methods may be used for Johne's disease surveillance in vaccinated herds or flocks.

MANAGEMENT AND CONTROL

Preventing transmission in free-ranging species is difficult because intervention to address a contaminated range or to limit transmission in free-ranging animals is usually not feasible. Management should be directed at preventing introduction into new populations. This may include measures such as minimizing contact between wildlife and domestic species (farm biosecurity) and moving individuals only from MAP test-negative herds; surveillance for MAP as part of herd health monitoring is recommended. Infected wild animals should not be used for reintroduction or translocation programs. Capture and release programs should ensure that animals to be moved are unlikely to have been infected and are moved to an uncontaminated location some months before the birthing season begins. If it is possible that the new location was contaminated with MAP, shallow pools or ponds should be fenced off for as long as possible and the grassy vegetation cut close to the ground and removed to increase heating and cooling cycles at soil level. Feeders and water troughs should be placed in sunny areas and the sediment from troughs removed and not dumped on the nearby ground.

Although MAP infection does not yet appear to be a significant threat to free-ranging wildlife health, with the greater infection pressure seen by the rising prevalence in domestic livestock and the shrinking wildlife habitat, the risk of infection may increase.

Acknowledgments

The authors thank Kathy Wesenberg for assistance in preparing this chapter and Drs. Joe Corn and Mike Collins for their helpful comments. Mention of trade, product, or firm names does not imply endorsement by the U.S. Government.

REFERENCES

1. Buddle BM, Wilson T, Denis M, et al: Sensitivity, specificity, and confounding factors of novel serological tests used for the rapid diagnosis of bovine tuberculosis in farmed red deer (Cervus elaphus). Clin Vaccine Immunol 17:626–630, 2010.
2. Buergelt CD, Layton AW, Ginn PE, et al: The pathology of spontaneous paratuberculosis in the North American bison (Bison bison). Vet Pathol 37:428–438, 2000.
3. Corn JL, Manning EJ, Sreevatsan S, et al: Isolation of Mycobacterium avium subsp. paratuberculosis from free-ranging birds and mammals on livestock premises. Appl Environ Microbiol 71:6963–6967, 2005.
4. Corn JL, Cartwright ME, Alexy KJ, et al: Surveys for disease agents in introduced elk in Arkansas and Kentucky. J Wildl Dis 46:186–194, 2010.
5. Davidson WR, Manning EJB, Nettles VF: Culture and serologic survey for Mycobacterium avium subsp paratuberculosis infection among Southeastern white-tailed deer (Odocoileus virginianus). J Wildl Dis 40:301–306, 2004.
6. de Lisle GW, Yates GF, Montgomery H: The emergence of Mycobacterium paratuberculosis in farmed deer in New Zealand—A review of 619 cases. N Z Vet J 51:58–62, 2003.
7. Florou M, Leontides L, Kostoulas P, et al: Isolation of Mycobacterium avium subspecies paratuberculosis from non-ruminant wildlife living in the sheds and on the pastures of Greek sheep and goats. Epidemiol Infect 136:644–652, 2008.
8. Gates N: Personal communication, 2010.
9. Glawischnig W, Steineck T, Spergser J: Infections caused by Mycobacterium avium subspecies avium, hominissuis, and paratuberculosis

in free-ranging red deer *(Cervus elaphus hippelaphus)* in Austria, 2001-2004. J Wildl Dis 42:724–731, 2006.

10. Hattel AL, Shaw DP, Love BC, et al: A retrospective study of mortality in Pennsylvania captive white-tailed deer *(Odocoileus virginianus)*: 2000-2003. J Vet Diagn Invest 16:515–521, 2004.

11. Hutchings, MR, Stevenson K, Greig A, et al: Infection of nonruminant wildlife by *Mycobacterium avium* subsp. *paratuberculosis*. In Behr MA, Collins DM, editors: Paratuberculosis: organism, disease, control, Cambridge, Mass, 2010, CAB International, pp 188–200.

11a. Judge J, Kyriazakis I, Greig A, et al: Clustering of *Mycobacterium avium* subsp. *paratuberculosis* in rabbits and the environment: How hot is a hot spot? Journal of Applied Environmental Microbiology 71:6033–6038, 2005.

12. Krishnan MY, Manning EJ, Collins MT: Effects of interactions of antibacterial drugs with each other and with 6-mercaptopurine on in vitro growth of *Mycobacterium avium* subspecies *paratuberculosis*. J Antimicrob Chemother 64:1018–1023, 2009.

13. Li L, Bannantine JP, Zhang Q, et al: The complete genome sequence of *Mycobacterium avium* subspecies *paratuberculosis*. Proc Natl Acad Sci U S A 102:12344–12349, 2005.

14. Mackintosh CG, Griffin JF: Paratuberculosis in deer, camelids and other ruminants. In Behr MA, Collins DM, editors: Paratuberculosis: Organism, disease, control, Cambridge, Mass, 2010, CAB International, pp 179–187.

15. Manning EJB: Unpublished data, 2009.

16. Manning EJB, Kucera TE, Gates NB, et al: Testing for *Mycobacterium avium* subsp. *paratuberculosis* infection in asymptomatic free-ranging tule elk from an infected herd. J Wildl Dis 39:323–328, 2003.

17. Motiwala AS, Amonsin A, Strother M, et al: Molecular epidemiology of *Mycobacterium avium* subsp. *paratuberculosis* isolates recovered from wild animal species. J Clin Microbiol 42:1703–1712, 2004.

18. Okwumabua O, Shull E, O'Connor M, et al: Comparison of three methods for extraction of *Mycobacterium avium* subspecies *paratuberculosis* DNA for polymerase chain reaction from broth-based culture systems. J Vet Diagn Invest 22:67–69, 2010.

19. Paustian ML, Zhu X, Sreevatsan S, et al: Comparative genomic analysis of *Mycobacterium avium* subspecies obtained from multiple host species. BMC Genomics 9:135, 2008.

20. Pedersen K, Manning EJ, Corn JL: Distribution of *Mycobacterium avium* subspecies *paratuberculosis* in the lower Florida Keys. J Wildl Dis 44:578–584, 2008.

21. Pithua P, Wells SJ, Godden SM, et al: Experimental validation of a nested polymerase chain reaction targeting the genetic element ISMAP02 for detection of *Mycobacterium avium* subspecies *paratuberculosis* in bovine colostrum. J Vet Diagn Invest 22:253–256, 2010.

22. Rhyan JC, Aune K, Ewalt DR, et al: Survey of free-ranging elk from Wyoming and Montana for selected pathogens. J Wildl Dis 33:290–298, 1997.

23. Salgado M: Personal communication, 2010.

24. Salgado M, Herthnek D, Bolske G, et al: First isolation of *Mycobacterium avium* subsp. *paratuberculosis* from wild guanacos *(Lama guanicoe)* on Tierra del Fuego Island. J Wildl Dis 45:295–301, 2009.

25. Shin SJ, Han JH, Manning EJ, et al: Rapid and reliable method for quantification of *Mycobacterium paratuberculosis* by use of the BACTEC MGIT960 system. J Clin Microbiol 45:1941–1948, 2007.

26. Sleeman JM, Manning EJB, Rohm JH, et al: Johne's disease in a free-ranging white-tailed deer from Virginia and subsequent surveillance for *Mycobacterium avium* subspecies *paratuberculosis*. J Wildl Dis 45:201–206, 2009.

27. Turenne CY, Collins DM, Alexander DC, et al: *Mycobacterium avium* subsp *paratuberculosis* and *M. avium* subsp *avium* are independently evolved pathogenic clones of a much broader group of *M. avium* organisms. J Bacteriol 190:2479–2487, 2008.

28. Whittington RJ, Marsh IB, Reddacliff LA: Survival of *Mycobacterium avium* subsp. *paratuberculosis* in dam water and sediment. Appl Environ Microbiol 71:5304–5308, 2005.

CHAPTER 82

Practical Aspects of Ruminant Intensive Care

Nadine Lamberski and Jeanette Fuller

Ruminant intensive care often requires intervention, even before a diagnosis is made. The patient's condition may be from an acute illness or injury, a chronic illness that has decompensated, or from an unexpected complication of another illness or condition. When managing complex cases, it is helpful to remember to treat the most life-threatening problems first.[4]

Anticipation, not reaction, has been cited as the key to successful management of severely ill animals. The Rule of Twenty was designed to assist the clinician in anticipating what might happen next with an intensive care patient. This rule is a list of 20 critical parameters that should be evaluated regularly in such cases.[4,7] Using it as a guide to assess the status and therapeutic strategy, the Rule of Twenty is adapted and applied to the intensive care needs of nondomestic ruminants. Despite the usefulness of the Rule of Twenty, good intensive care must include careful consideration of the patients' problems along with compassionate nursing care and attention to detail. The most important monitoring tools available are our own eyes, ears, hands, and stethoscope. Although advances in technology have greatly improved the ability to assess a patient's status objectively, there is no substitute for a carefully repeated physical examination.[2]

Many nondomestic ruminant species exhibit aggressive, fractious, or flighty behavior and, therefore, cannot tolerate frequent handling. The use of neuroleptics may improve patient compliance as well as decrease stress.[1,10] Successful case management also hinges on the ability to deliver the appropriate therapeutic and supportive care. Placing an indwelling intravenous catheter (IVC) facilitates the remote delivery of fluids and adjunct therapies. Materials and procedures used at the Harter Veterinary Medical Center at the San Diego Zoo Safari Park are listed in Table 82-1 and Boxes 82-1 and 82-2.

RULE OF TWENTY FOR RUMINANTS

1. Fluid Balance

One of the most important decisions will be based on the animal's hydration and perfusion status. The type of fluid should be chosen carefully so that it maintains adequate intravascular volume and hydration without overloading the interstitial space. Shock results when there is inadequate tissue oxygenation, most often caused by decreased perfusion. The systemic inflammatory response syndrome (SIRS) involves the release of vasoactive and inflammatory mediators that accompany shock; it may be initiated by bacteremia, endotoxemia, traumatic shock, localized infections, hyperthermia, hypothermia, dehydration, and hypotension. Any organ injury that causes hypoxia and the release of vasoactive or inflammatory mediators may result in SIRS. SIRS may reduce circulation to the digits and therefore laminitis is a potential sequela. Animals with SIRS diseases may require much more fluid than expected because of massive losses into the third body fluid space or into the interstitium because of the loss of endothelial integrity.[7]

Dehydration and poor perfusion are different problems requiring different therapeutic strategies. Perfusion deficits result from deficits in the intravascular fluid compartment, whereas hydration deficits result from deficits in the extravascular (interstitial and intracellular) compartments. Perfusion deficits are detected by changes in the heart rate, pulse intensity, capillary refill time, mucous membrane color, limb temperature, and rectal temperature. Blood pressure and central venous pressure are other ways to detect intravascular volume deficits but are used less often in conscious nondomestic ruminants. Most animals with an intravascular deficit (poor perfusion) also have concurrent extravascular deficits (dehydration). Hydration deficits are detected

636

acutely anemic or suffering from SIRS diseases, the packed cell volume (PCV) should be maintained at more than 20%. The PCV may be allowed to become much lower before transfusion in cases of hemolytic or chronic anemia. Conversely, the PCV should be kept lower than 55% with IV fluid therapy. In cases of absolute polycythemia, phlebotomy should be performed to prevent microvascular sludging and hypertension that could develop as a result of the increased blood viscosity.[4,7]

12. Renal Function

Urine output should be assessed on an ongoing basis as a reflection of renal function, perfusion, and fluid balance. Urine output should be at least 1 mL/kg/hr. For a 100-kg ruminant, urine output is minimally 2.4 liters/day. Urine sediment examination and urea and creatinine levels should be regularly checked. Serial urinalyses to detect glucosuria, proteinuria, or cylindruria are useful for evaluating acute tubular injury before the damage progresses to overt renal failure and azotemia. This is especially important when administering potentially nephrotoxic drugs such as aminoglycosides or nonsteroidal antiinflammatory drugs (NSAIDs). Inadequate urine production should be managed by ensuring adequate fluid therapy and blood pressure. If that does not improve urine production, then mannitol, 50% dextrose, or furosemide should be considered.[4,7]

13. Immune Status, Antibiotic Selection, and White Blood Cell Count

Antibiotics are selected based on the site of infection and the most likely types of bacterial infection. Ultimately, antibiotic selection should be based on the results of culture and sensitivity, including blood culture if multisystemic disease is present or suspected. However, empirical treatment is often necessary pending these results. Broad-spectrum antibiotics (including anaerobic coverage) are indicated for a critical patient with a compromised immune system. The numbers of antibiotics administered empirically on a routine basis should be minimized to reduce the development of resistant organisms in the hospital environment, such as *Salmonella*, methicillin-resistant *Staphylococcus aureus*, *Clostridium perfringens*, and *C. difficile*. Wash hands and wear gloves before and after handling or treating an ill animal.[4,7]

14. Gastrointestinal Motility and Mucosal Integrity

Critically ill ruminants, even those without a primary GI disease, are prone to ileus and stress-induced gastric ulceration. Auscultation for rumen contractions and visual inspection for signs of bloat, which is often difficult if the animal is recumbent, may help confirm abnormal motility. Metoclopramide may be useful because of its ability to increase progressive gastric and intestinal motility but should be used cautiously, because it may cause central nervous system (CNS) stimulation. Sedation and extrapyramidal effects may also be seen. Erythromycin is used as a prokinetic agent in monogastrics and may be of some benefit in ruminants. Cimetidine or ranitidine should be considered to treat or prevent GI ulcerations. Oral omeprazole may be useful in neonatal ruminants but the benefits for an adult ruminant are not known.

Placement of a nasogastric tube to allow removal of accumulated gas and fluid reduces the possibility of aspiration of refluxed rumen contents and allows continuous decompression. The nasogastric tube also may be used to introduce small amounts of a liquid diet to provide nutrition to the enterocytes, which will help prevent gastric ulceration and intestinal mucosal compromise with secondary bacterial translocation.[4,7]

Just as important as these conditions, rumen dysbiosis may occur in the ill patient as a direct result of the primary disease or secondary to chronic debilitation and/or the use of antibiotics. Rumen fluid analysis may help identify the cause of the indigestion or abnormal fermentation. Rumen transfaunation is often indicated but may be problematic from a practical perspective if a rumen donor is not immediately available.

15. Drug Dosages and Metabolism

If renal or hepatic function is compromised, some drug dosages should be decreased to account for decreased elimination. Also, drug treatments should be reviewed daily to ensure that the dose has been calculated correctly and that it is appropriate for the animal's current weight and interactions with concurrent medications.[4,7]

16. Nutrition

Patients that refuse to eat, or are unable or too weak to eat, rapidly become protein-energy deficient. Enteral feeding is always preferred if the GI tract may tolerate it, but this is often problematic in the anorectic non-domestic ruminant. Because most patients are handled infrequently, parenteral nutrition is a good option. Partial parenteral nutrition, using amino acid solutions, may be given in a peripheral vein and provide part of the animal's caloric requirements in a form that may be readily metabolized. The acutely ill animal, unlike the chronically malnourished animal, uses protein preferentially as a fuel source. Total parenteral nutrition should be initiated early in the course of treatment in the anorectic patient.[4,7] Regardless of the level of enteral or parenteral support, food should be available at all times for voluntary consumption. Offering browse may help stimulate the animal's appetite.

17. Pain Control

Pain may be assumed in many diseases and postoperatively. Pain activates the stress hormone systems of the body and contributes to morbidity and mortality. Pain may be manifested as tachycardia, pale mucous membranes, restlessness, reluctance to move or stand, anorexia, and/or severe mental depression and poor attitude. These signs mimic those of shock. The control of pain is vital to normal cardiovascular function and quality of life. Analgesics should be administered pre-emptively for maximum benefit.[4]

Morphine is a potent inexpensive analgesic that may be given IV as a slow bolus, followed by a constant rate infusion (CRI) or intermittent IM injections. A very small dose of ketamine does not cause an increase in sympathetic tone and is frequently used with opioids for analgesia given as a CRI. A CRI provides constant analgesia and is often more convenient and less painful and stressful than intermittent IM or SC injections. When using a CRI, the drugs may be titrated to effect. This reduces the total amount of drug used, causes fewer side effects, and improves cost-effectiveness. A disadvantage to CRI is the slow rise in drug plasma concentration to therapeutic levels, necessitating a loading dose. A syringe pump or IV infusion pump is also needed. Transdermal fentanyl patches are another option but require up to 12 hours to reach therapeutic blood levels.[7]

Antagonists may be used to reverse the unwanted side effects of opioid administration. Naloxone is a μ and κ antagonist. Naloxone may reverse the sedation, respiratory depression, and bradycardia, but this may cause pain, excitement, delirium, and hyperalgesia. Low-dose naloxone (0.004 mg/kg titrated slowly IV) may be used to reverse CNS depression without

affecting analgesia but the duration is short. Butorphanol may also be used to reverse μ CNS depression without antagonizing κ analgesia effects. Butorphanol should be administered at 0.4 mg/kg IV to reverse only the sedative and respiratory side effects.[6]

NSAIDs are another option for the alleviation of acute postoperative and traumatic pain. These drugs inhibit prostaglandin synthesis, which may lead to gastrointestinal erosion, impaired renal function, and bleeding. In critical patients, an advantage to the use of NSAIDs is for the control of inflammation in endotoxemia.[7]

18. Nursing Care

Providing nursing care to critically ill animals requires a skilled, knowledgeable, attentive, and highly trained support staff. The patient's physical and psychologic needs should be considered. Recumbent animals should be repositioned on well-padded bedding and encouraged to stand to prevent decubital ulcers. Attempts should be aborted if this results in increased morbidity or trauma to the patient or poses a danger to staff. Placing the animal in a sling or whirlpool bath has some advantages in certain situations. Similarly, physical therapy is important for maintaining range of motion, muscle tone, and blood flow, but this should be evaluated for feasibility on a case by case basis. Recumbent patients may not urinate or defecate normally so special attention should be paid to estimating urine and fecal volume. The stall and patient must be kept clean and dry. The catheter sites should be inspected frequently for signs of infection or displacement. Catheters should be labeled and marked with the date of placement. When catheters are removed, the tips should be saved for possible culture if there is evidence of inflammation at the catheter site. Patients also need to be kept warm with hot water bottles, blankets, portable heaters, heat lamps, or ambient heat.[4,7]

19. Wound Care and Bandage Changes

Wet, soiled, or contaminated bandages should be changed as needed. Good wound hygiene, drainage, and débridement are essential. Bandages should be changed whenever they become soiled or wet.[4,7]

20. Tender Loving Care

If the patient is tractable, keeper visits should be encouraged. Animals should be handled and spoken to gently to minimize stress and anxiety. Consolidating several treatments at one time and turning down the lights at night allow the animal some time to rest and sleep undisturbed.[4,7]

Acknowledgments

We gratefully acknowledge the staff of the San Diego Zoo Safari Park Veterinary Services Department for their daily contributions, dedication, and teamwork that continuously improve the quality of care for our patients.

REFERENCES

1. Blumer ES: A review of selected neuroleptic drugs in the management of nondomestic hoofstock. In Proceedings of the American Association of Zoo Veterinarians Annual Conference, 1991, pp 326–332.
2. Boag AK: What constitutes intensive care? British Small Animal Veterinary Congress, 2007 (http://www.vin.com/Members/Proceedings/Proceedings.plx?CID=BSAVA2007&Category=&PID=16371&O=VIN).
3. Jandrey KE: Current overview of intensive care. Western Veterinary Conference, 2007 (http://www.vin.com/Members/Proceedings/Proceedings.plx?CID=WVC2007&Category=&PID=15423&O=VIN).
4. Kirby R: Golden rule of emergency medicine—And more! International Veterinary Emergency and Critical Care Symposium, 2009 (http://www.vin.com/Members/Proceedings/Proceedings.plx?CID=IVECCS2009&Category=&PID=52956&O=VIN).
5. Kirby R: The physiology of fluid therapy. International Veterinary Emergency and Critical Care Symposium, 2009 (http://www.vin.com/Members/Proceedings/Proceedings.plx?CID=IVECCS2009&Category=&PID=52950&O=VIN).
6. Lamont L, Tranquilli W: Alpha2 agonists. In Gaynor JS, Muir WW, editors: Handbook of veterinary pain management, St. Louis, 2002, Mosby, pp 199–220.
7. Merck Veterinary Manual: The rule of twenty, 2008 (http://www.merckvetmanual.com/mvm/index.jsp?cfile=htm/bc/160501.htm&word=Rule%2cof%2c20).
8. Miller M, Weber M, Neiffer D, et al: Use of commercially available plasma for transfusion in exotic ungulates. In Proceedings of the American Association of Zoo Veterinarians Annual Conference, 2002, pp 175–178.
9. Rivera AM: Concepts of critical illness, 2003 (http://www.vin.com/Members/Proceedings/Proceedings.plx?CID=ACVIM2003&Category=&PID=3978&O=VIN).
10. Zuba JR, Oosterhuis JE: Treatment options for adverse reactions to haloperidol and other neuroleptic drugs in non-domestic ruminants. In Proceedings of the American Association of Zoo Veterinarians Annual Conference, 2007, pp 53–57.

83 *Mycoplasma haemolamae* in New
World Camelids
Susan J. Tornquist

CHAPTER 83

Mycoplasma haemolamae in New World Camelids

Susan J. Tornquist

In 1990, the first descriptions of a newly identified organism found on red blood cells of llamas were published in two reports from Colorado and Kentucky.[6,10] The organism was called an *Eperythrozoon*-like organism, based on light and scanning electronic microscopic morphology.

In the initial reports of infections with this organism, some affected llamas had mild to severe anemia that was associated with the variable presence of anisocytosis, reticulocytes, and nucleated red blood cells. Some of the more severely anemic llamas also had low serum iron levels, hypoalbuminemia, and hypoglycemia. These severely affected llamas also tended to have poor body condition and evidence of other concurrent disease. Other infected llamas did not have significant clinical signs nor hematologic or biochemical abnormalities.[6,10]

Sera from some of these infected llamas reacted positively with antigen from *Eperythrozoon suis*–infected swine red blood cells (RBCs), leading to speculation that this organism could be a previously named *Eperythrozoon* or *Hemobartonella* that had found a new host species.[6,7] Attempted transmission to cats, sheep, and swine was unsuccessful, even when the cats and pigs were splenectomized. This suggested that the camelid organism was, in fact, a new species.

Johnson and colleagues[5] attempted to reproduce the infection in llamas experimentally by intravenous or subcutaneous injection of infected blood into six healthy adult and yearling llamas. Only one of these llamas became more than transiently infected, as detected by examination of blood smears. However, later dexamethasone suppression showed that some of these llamas did appear to be infected. This early experiment suggested both that infectivity of the organism might be relatively low in healthy animals and that a chronic carrier state might exist.

Reports in 1992 and 1997 of eperythrozoonosis in immunodeficient llamas provided support for the idea that the organism caused clinical disease, primarily in camelids that were not immunocompetent.[2,4]

POLYMERASE CHAIN REACTION ASSAY DEVELOPMENT

In 2001, a polymerase chain reaction (PCR)–based assay was developed to provide a more sensitive and specific diagnostic technique for diagnosis of the infection and to study the kinetics of infection, response to treatment, and prevalence of infection.[11,12] The assay was developed using blood from a naturally infected alpaca from Oregon. The primers for the assay were chosen to amplify a 318–base pair (bp) sequence that was unique to the hypervariable region of the organism's 16S rRNA region, as identified in GenBank accession AF306346.[8] Specificity of the assay was demonstrated by failure of the primers to amplify several related organisms. The lower detection limit was shown to be approximately 28 gene copies, or one organism in 3.8 to 7.7×10^9 erythrocytes. The assay was able to detect the organism in samples from llamas and alpacas from almost every state in the United States, as well as a variety of locations in Canada, Australia, and the United Kingdom, thus demonstrating that the assay was not geographically limited.

CLASSIFICATION AND CHARACTERISTICS

In 2002, Messick and associates[9] reported that the 16S rRNA sequence of an *Eperythrozoon*-like organism amplified from a heavily infected alpaca was closely related

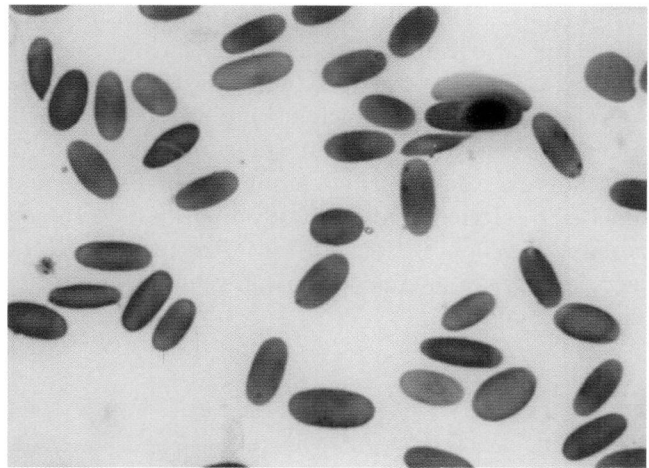

Figure 83-1

Photomicrograph of a blood smear from an infected alpaca showing ring form and coccoid-shaped organisms.

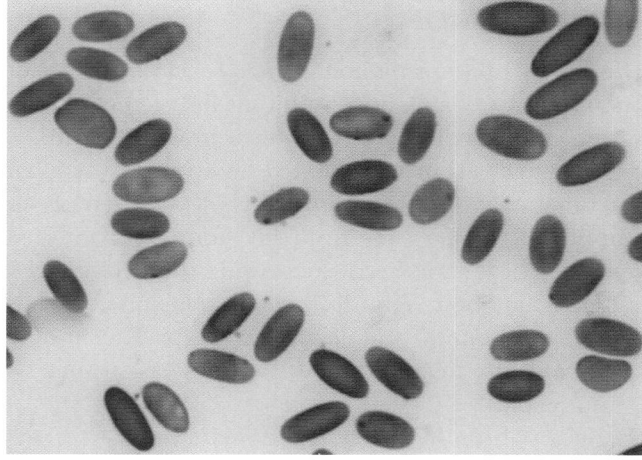

Figure 83-2

Photomicrograph of a blood smear from an alpaca showing some heavily infected erythrocytes.

to the hemotropic mycoplasmas present in cattle, pigs, cats, and opossums. The new name, *Candidatus Mycoplasma haemolamae* was proposed for this organism based on morphologic, genomic, and structural characteristics. Although this organism has not yet been cultured, precluding an official species designation, it is often referred to as *Mycoplasma haemolamae*.

M. haemolamae, along with the other related hemotropic mycoplasmas, are small (0.4 to 0.6 μm) bacteria that lack a cell wall. They may appear as coccoid, linear, or ring-shaped and most often appear to be on the edge of the erythrocyte or free in the background, especially if there is a delay between blood collection and making blood smears (Figs. 83-1 and 83-2). Scanning electron micrographs have shown that there is often a slight depression in the red blood cell membrane where the organisms are located, but the bacteria do not actually enter the cell.[10]

EXPERIMENTAL INFECTIONS AND TREATMENT STUDIES

Following the development of the PCR assay, a number of experimental infections in llamas and alpacas were undertaken to study the efficacy of treatment regimens on infection. With very rare exceptions, healthy adult llamas and alpacas became infected when transfused with blood from a chronically infected alpaca. Infection is most often detectable by PCR assay within 4 days of infection. Organisms are usually seen on blood smears approximately 2 to 4 days later, but they are never seen

in some experimentally infected camelids that have positive PCR results.[11,12]

Clinical signs such as fever and depression are almost never seen in healthy, experimentally infected camelids. Laboratory abnormalities are variable and do not inevitably include anemia. When anemia develops, it is often mild (packed cell volume [PCV] = 23% to 27%), with evidence of regeneration such as reticulocytosis, anisocytosis, polychromasia, and increased numbers of nucleated red blood cells being inconsistently present. Although anemia is often transient, some infected camelids remain mildly anemic for many months, although there is no evidence of organisms on blood smears and PCR positivity is intermittent. Hypoglycemia has not been observed in these experimentally infected animals.

Treatment of experimentally infected llamas and alpacas with oxytetracycline, florfenicol, and oral and injectable enrofloxacin did not effectively clear infection. This was shown when infected animals that appeared to be negative following antibiotic treatment were still positive when they were immunosuppressed with dexamethasone 2 to 6 months later.

Overall, the experimental infection studies have shown that many, perhaps most, infected camelids that are otherwise healthy do not show clinical signs of infection and may have no associated laboratory abnormalities. In addition, these studies have shown that most infected camelids appear to remain chronic carriers with organisms suppressed to very low levels unless the animals are immunosuppressed.

TRANSMISSION

The mode of transmission of M. haemolamae is not known, but transmission by biting insect vectors and vertical transmission are considered most likely. Insect vector transmission is suspected, as it is in several of the other hemotropic mycoplasmas.[9] My attempts to amplify M. haemolamae from lice found on infected camelids have not been successful; they have been sporadic at best. Transplacental transmission has been hypothesized and is supported by the finding of organisms in the blood of crias as young as 24 hours old.[1,3]

An opportunity to test the hypothesis that the organism could be transmitted transplacentally or via colostrum was created when five pregnant alpacas were found to be positive by PCR assay at the time of parturition. Whole blood samples were taken from the crias prior to and shortly after nursing on the dams. Three of the crias were negative by PCR both prior to and following the ingestion of colostrum. Both of these crias continued to test negative for 3 months thereafter. Two other crias born to positive dams tested positive prior to and after nursing on the positive dams.[13] A conclusion that may be drawn from this very small sample is that transplacental transmission may occur, but that it is not inevitable and that transmission via colostrum is unlikely.

PREVALENCE

Using the PCR assay to test over 6000 llama and alpaca blood samples from the United States, as well as Canada, Australia, and the United Kingdom, the prevalence rate appears to be approximately 30%, with the prevalence being somewhat higher in older animals. Gender and species (llama versus alpaca) do not appear to be risk factors. Within groups of camelids kept together, the percentage of positive animals is similar, around 30%. In herds of five or more camelids tested, it is uncommon to find a 0% positive rate, although a few such groups have been identified. This is consistent with an organism that is not spread directly from one animal to another. Also, although animals in groups are likely to be exposed to similar potential insect vectors, it is clear that not all will develop infections. This may be the result of the relatively low infectivity of the organisms, prompt and effective immune responses in some animals, or other factors.

Anecdotally, the percentage of positive animals in the United States appears to be greater in the late summer and early fall than in other times of the year. There are also numerous cases in which previously healthy camelids developed clinical signs and were found to be positive following shipping, animal movement, or other potentially stressful situations.

Samples from smaller numbers of llamas and alpacas in selected herds in South America have shown a lower prevalence, from 10% to 20% positive.[14] No association with anemia or clinical signs was found in these animals.

REFERENCES

1. Almy FS, Ladd SM, Sponenberg P, et al: Mycoplasma haemolamae infection in a 4-day-old cria: Support for in utero transmission by use of a polymerase chain reaction assay. Can Vet J 47:229–233, 2006.
2. Barrington GM, Parish SM, Tyler JW: Chronic weight loss in an immunodeficient adult llama. J Am Vet Med Assoc 211:294–298, 1997.
3. Fisher DJ, Zinkl JG: Eperythrozoonosis in a one-day-old llama. Vet Clin Pathol 25:93–94, 1996.
4. Hutchison JM, Garry FB, Belknap EB, et al: Prospective characterization of the clinicopathologic and immunologic features of an immunodeficiency affecting juvenile llamas. Vet Immunol Immunopathol 49:209–227, 1995.
5. Johnson LW, Garry FM, Weiser GM, et al: In Proceedings of the Symposium on Health and Disease of Small Ruminants, 1990.
6. McLaughlin BG, Evans CN, McLaughlin PS, et al: An Eperythrozoon-like parasite in llamas. J Am Vet Med Assoc 197:1170–1175, 1990.
7. McLaughlin BG, McLaughlin PS, Evans CN: An Eperythrozoon-like parasite of llamas: Attempted transmission to swine, sheep, and cats. J Vet Diagn Invest 3:352–353, 1991.
8. Messick JB: Hemotrophic mycoplasma (hemoplasmas): A review and new insights into pathogenic potential. Vet Clin Pathol 33:2–13, 2004.
9. Messick JB, Walker PG, Raphael W: 'Candidatus Mycoplasma haemodidelphidis' sp. nov., 'Candidatus Mycoplasma haemolamae' sp. nov. and Mycoplasma haemocanis comb. nov., haemotrophic parasites from a naturally infected opossum (Didelphis virginiana), alpaca (Lama pacos) and dog (Canis familiaris): Phylogenetic and secondary structural relatedness of their 16S rRNA genes to other mycoplasmas. Intl J Syst Evol Microbiol 52:693–698, 2002.
10. Reagan WJ, Garry F, Thrall MA, et al: The clinicopathologic, light, and scanning electron microscopic features of eperythrozoonosis in four naturally infected llamas. Vet Pathol 27:426–431, 1990.
11. Tornquist SJ, Boeder, LJ, Cebra CK, Messick J: Use of a polymerase chain reaction assay to study response to oxytetracycline treatment in experimental 'Candidatus Mycoplasma haemolamae' infection in alpacas. Am J Vet Res 70:1102–1107, 2009.
12. Tornquist SJ, Boeder LJ, Parker JE, et al: Use of a polymerase chain reaction assay to study the carrier state in infection with camelid Mycoplasma haemolama, formerly Eperythrozoon spp. infection camelids. Vet Pathol 39:616, 2002.
13. Tornquist SJ, Boeder LJ, Lubbers S, Cebra CK: Investigation of Mycoplasma haemolamae infection in crias born to infected dams. Accepted for publication, Vet Record, 2010.
14. Tornquist SJ, Boeder L, Alarcon V, Rios-Phillips C: Prevalence of Mycoplasma haemolamae infection in Peruvian and Chilean llamas and alpacas. J Vet Diagn Invest 22:766–769, 2010.

Index

Note: Page numbers followed by "f" refer to illustrations; page numbers followed by "t" refer to tables; page numbers followed by "b" refer to boxes.

Greater kudu, 101
Green iguanas, 248t, 250
Green technology, 89-90
Grevy's zebra, 599
Guanacos, 632
Gyps vultures, 350-352
Gyrodactylids, 203

H

Haemobartonellosis, 461
Haemonchus contortus, 582
Haemosporidian parasites
  in captive populations, 357
  definition of, 356
  eradication of, 361-362
  in Hawaii, 357-358
  hosts of, 356, 358
  impact of, 359t-360t
  life cycle of, 356, 357f
  pathogenicity of, 356-357
  Plasmodium spp. *See Plasmodium* spp.
  summary of, 362
  in zoo populations, 357
Hair samples, 60-62, 61t
Halogen oxidizers, 193
Hamadryas baboons, 25f
Hantavirus, 142-143
Hatchers, 325
Hazard identification, 3
Hazardous materials
  disaster preparation considerations, 41
  identification of, 41
Health for Animals and Livestock Improvement Project, 158-159
Heart rate monitoring
  in elephant endotheliotropic herpesvirus, 539
  in ruminants, 640
Heat exchanger devices, 194
Heavy metals
  description of, 197
  toxicosis, in kakapo, 309-310
Hedgehogs, 120
Hellbenders
  anesthesia of, 262
  Batrachochytrium dendrobatidis in, 261, 263
  biologic data regarding, 260
  captive husbandry of, 260
  congenital abnormalities in, 262
  diagnostic techniques in, 262-263, 263f
  diet of, 260
  habitat of, 260
  hyperthermia treatment in, 263-264
  infectious diseases in, 261
  limb amputations in, 262
  noninfectious conditions in, 261-262
  parasites in, 261
  phlebotomy in, 262-263
  radiography of, 262, 263f
  restraint of, 262
  surgery in, 262
  treatment of, 263-264
  ultrasonography of, 262, 263f
Hemagglutination inhibition, 258
Hemoglobin concentration, 640-641
Hemolymph sampling, 206

Hemoparasites, 308
Hepatic mycobacterial granuloma, 267f
Hepatozoonosis, 463
Hermann's tortoise, 149-150, 150f
Herpesvirus simiae, 27
Herpesviruses
  in amphibians, 236-237
  avian, 27-28
  caprine, 26
  characteristics of, 256-257
  diagnosis of, 257
  elephant endotheliotropic. *See* Elephant endotheliotropic herpesvirus
  equine, 27
  gammaherpesvirus, 26
  human, 255, 257
  Ranid herpesvirus 1, 236-237
  Ranid herpesvirus 2, 236-237
  in reptiles, 256-257
  in sea turtles, 257
  in tortoises, 28, 257
  virulent strains of, 446
Heterakis gallinarum, 166
Heterophilia, 339
Highly pathogenic avian influenza viruses
  definition of, 343-344
  description of, 140
  ecology of, 344
  H5N1. *See* H5N1
  outbreaks of, 343-345, 346t
High-performance liquid chromatography, 66
High-terminal bacteremia, 103-104, 104f
High-throughput experiments, 69-70
Hippopotamus, 619-621, 620t
Histoplasma capsulatum, 122
Histoplasmosis, 122
H1N1, 123, 141
H5N1, 343-344
  description of, 140
  outbreak of, 343
  source of, 344-345
  vaccinations against, 345-348
  zoo outbreaks of, 345, 346t
Hoof disorders
  anatomic location of, 623b
  anatomy, 619-621, 620t
  causes of, 622-625
  cracks, 624
  description of, 619
  diagnosis of, 621
  examination for, 621
  facility design to prevent, 625-626
  fissures, 624
  foot rot, 624-625
  foot-and-mouth disease, 625
  infectious, 624-625
  infectious pododermatitis, 624-625
  interdigital dermatitis, 625
  interdigital hyperplasia, 624
  laminitis, 623
  noninfectious, 623-624
  nutritional causes of, 623-624
  papillomatous digital dermatitis, 625
  predisposing factors, 622
  prevention of, 625-626
  quarantine for, 626
  sole lesions, 624

Hoof disorders *(Continued)*
  treatment of, 625-626
  viral diseases, 625
  white line disease, 624
  worn soles, 624
Hoofstock, cryptosporidiosis in, 570-572
Hormones, 66
Hornbills
  casque squamous cell carcinoma in
    antiangiogenic topical treatment for, 283
    clinical presentation of, 281-282, 282f
    description of, 281
    diagnosis of, 282
    ongoing investigations of, 284
    pathology of, 282-283, 283f
    prognosis for, 284
    radical resection for, 283, 283f
    treatment of, 283-284, 283f
  characteristics of, 281
  Rhinoceros, 284
Horn-induced trauma, 24
Hospital buildings
  case studies of, 95-97, 96f
  construction of, 92-95
  design of, 92-95
  energy efficiency considerations, 93
  environmental considerations, 90
  green technology applications, 92-93, 93b, 95
  indoor environmental quality, 94
  inventory analysis for, 91t
  location of, 90-92
  low-impact, 90-97
  maintenance of, 92-95
  materials management, 94-95
  site development, 92-93
  waste management, 95
  water efficiency considerations, 93-94
Hot spots, 16-17, 157
Hounsfield units, 425
Howler monkey, 138f
Human choriogonadotropin, 508
Human herpesvirus 1, 255, 257
Human immunodeficiency virus, 136
Human population
  agricultural practices affected by, 139-141
  growth of, 139
Humane Farm Animal Care group, 72
Hunting, 137-139
Hydrogen sulfide, 178t-180t, 196-197
Hydrometer, 183-184
Hydromucometra, 558f
Hygrometer, 324
Hymenolepiasis, 120
Hyperkalemia, 639
Hyperprolactinemia, 512-513
Hyperthermia, 263-264
Hypoalbuminemia, 640
Hypobromite, 199
Hypobromous acid, 199
Hypochlorous acid, 193
Hypokalemia, 639
Hypothermia
  analgesic uses of, 252
  in sea turtles, 243
Hypovitaminosis A, 472-473, 475
Hypoxia, 639